2017.

PARKES'

Occupational Lung Disorders

Fourth Edition

Sir Anthony Newman Taylor, CBE, FRCP, FFOM, FMedSci
Professor of Occupational and Environmental Medicine
Faculty of Medicine, National Heart & Lung Institute, Imperial College, London, UK

Paul Cullinan, MD, FRCP
Professor of Occupational and Environmental Respiratory Disease
Faculty of Medicine, National Heart & Lung Institute, Imperial College, London, UK

Paul Blanc, MD, MSPH
Professor of Occupational and Environmental Medicine
University of California, San Francisco, USA

Anthony Pickering, FRCP, FFOM, DIH
Professor of Occupational Medicine
University Hospital of South Manchester, Manchester, UK

CRC Press
Taylor & Francis Group
Boca Raton London New York

CRC Press is an imprint of the
Taylor & Francis Group, an **informa** business

CRC Press
Taylor & Francis Group
6000 Broken Sound Parkway NW, Suite 300
Boca Raton, FL 33487-2742

Printed and bound in India by Replika Press Pvt. Ltd.

Printed on acid-free paper
Version Date: 20160208

International Standard Book Number-13: 978-1-4822-4070-2 (Pack - Book and Ebook)

Visit the Taylor & Francis Web site at
http://www.taylorandfrancis.com

and the CRC Press Web site at
http://www.crcpress.com

Contents

Preface

It is now 20 years since the last edition, the third, of this now classic text book. Raymond Parkes wrote the first edition, published in 1974, himself. By the time of the third, published in 1995, he had collaborated with experts in 18 of the 25 chapters. This was a reflection, he wrote, of the pace of change in the field and of the difficulty of any one individual having sufficient expertise across the expanding field of occupational lung disease. While several other books have been written about this subject, ever since the first edition, Parkes' has remained an authoritative and comprehensive text. In editing a new edition we have been very aware of this legacy. We have invited contributors with international reputation in their field, who have closely considered the new issues and emerging knowledge that continues to inform the field.

At the time of the first edition the dominant occupational lung diseases remained the pneumoconioses caused primarily by coal, silica and asbestos; of these, Parkes had an unrivalled experience. While these conditions remain important globally, other conditions, particularly cancers (including both lung cancer, attributable to a variety of exposures, and mesothelioma due to asbestos), asthma and COPD caused by occupation are now recognised to be of increasing importance.

It is our intention in this new edition to reflect these changes, while retaining the authority and comprehensiveness of the earlier editions. We have included new chapters, such as 'Investigating Outbreaks' and 'Compensation and Attribution' as well as chapters on coal, silica and asbestos by contemporary experts familiar with current, international developments in these areas. With one exception, all of the chapters in this new edition have been rewritten. This exception is Parkes' chapter on 'Elements of Geology and Geochemistry', which we carried forward unchanged as an excellent introduction to a complex but relevant topic; we recognise the irony that, in his preface to the last edition, Parkes noted that he had considered deleting this section.

Other innovations include a new chapter on interstitial lung diseases, which considers recently recognised causes of interstitial lung disease, including organising pneumonia and fibrosis in textile spray workers ('Ardistyl' disease), nylon flock worker's lung in textile manufacturers, and obliterative bronchiolitis in popcorn workers, diseases first identified in outbreaks in Spain and the United States. In keeping with this international perspective, the authors of this new edition come from Europe, United States, Asia and Australia.

The contribution to respiratory disease of exposures in the workplace is considerable, both as specific causes of pathognomonic disease, such as in the pneumoconioses, and as causes of diseases with multiple aetiologies such as asthma, COPD and lung cancer. The American Thoracic Society has estimated that approximately 15% of asthma and 15% of COPD are attributable to occupation, and a recent investigation of the occupational burden of cancer in the United Kingdom estimated some 20% of lung cancer to be attributable to occupation. Recognizing and understanding the occupational causes of respiratory disease is essential for all whose work encompasses the prevention, diagnosis and management of respiratory disease. It is our intention that this new edition will not only inform but also stimulate those engaged in these fields.

Anthony Newman Taylor
Paul Cullinan
Paul Blanc
Anthony Pickering

Contributors

Jerrold L. Abraham
State University of New York Upstate Medical University
Syracuse, New York

Raymond Agius
Centre for Occupational and Environmental Health
The University of Manchester
Manchester, United Kingdom

Eduardo Algranti
Division of Medicine
Coordination of Health and Work
FUNDACENTRO
São Paulo, Brazil

Christopher M. Barber
Northern General Hospital
Sheffield, United Kingdom

Paul Blanc
Department of Medicine
University of California
San Francisco, California

Fraser J. H. Brims
Curtin Medical School
Curtin University
and
Department of Respiratory Medicine
Sir Charles Gairdner Hospital
Perth, Australia

Sherwood Burge
Heart of England NHS Foundation Trust
Birmingham, United Kingdom

Melanie Carder
Centre for Occupational and Environmental Health
The University of Manchester
Manchester, United Kingdom

David C. Christiani
Department of Environmental Health
Harvard School of Public Health
and
Department of Medicine
Massachusetts General Hospital
Boston, Massachusetts

Anne Cockcroft
CIET/PRAM, Department of Family Medicine
McGill University
Montreal, Canada

David Coggon
MRC Lifecourse Epidemiology Unit
University of Southampton
Southampton, United Kingdom

Robert A. Cohen
Division of Environmental and Occupational Health Sciences
University of Illinois at Chicago School of Public Health
and
Division of Pulmonary and Critical Care Medicine
Feinberg School of Medicine, Northwestern University
Chicago, Illinois

William Osmond Charles Cookson
Asmarley Centre for Genomic Medicine
National Heart and Lung Institute
Imperial College London
London, United Kingdom

Paul Cullinan
National Heart and Lung Institute
Imperial College London
London, United Kingdom

Nick H. de Klerk
Telethon Kids Institute and School of Population Health
University of Western Australia
Crawley, Australia

Rafael E. de la Hoz
Department of Preventive Medicine
Icahn School of Medicine at Mount Sinai
New York, New York

Ken Donaldson
Queens Medical Research Institute
University of Edinburgh
Edinburgh, United Kingdom

Shona C. Fang
Department of Environmental Health
Harvard School of Public Health
Boston, Massachusetts

Johanna Feary
Royal Brompton and Harefield NHS Foundation Trust
London, United Kingdom

R. William Field
Department of Occupational and Environmental Health
and
Department of Epidemiology
College of Public Health
University of Iowa
Iowa City, Iowa

David Fishwick
Health and Safety Executive
Buxton, United Kingdom

Matthew C. Frise
Department of Physiology, Anatomy and Genetics
University of Oxford
Oxford, United Kingdom

John Gibson
Respiratory Medicine
Newcastle University
Newcastle upon Tyne, United Kingdom

Mark Glover
Medical Director, Hyperbaric Medicine Unit
St. Richard's Hospital
Chichester, United Kingdom

Leonard H. T. Go
Division of Environmental and Occupational Health Sciences
University of Illinois at Chicago School of Public Health
and
Division of Pulmonary and Critical Care Medicine
John H. Stroger Hospital of Cook County
Chicago, Illinois

Francis H. Y. Green
Pathology and Laboratory Medicine
University of Calgary
Calgary, Canada

David M. Hansell
Royal Brompton and Harefield NHS Foundation Trust
London, United Kingdom

Dick Heederik
Institute for Risk Assessment Sciences
Utrecht University
Utrecht, the Netherlands

David J. Hendrick
University of Newcastle upon Tyne
and
Consultant Physician, Royal Victoria Infirmary
Newcastle upon Tyne, United Kingdom

Julia Heptonstall
London, United Kingdom

Remko Houba
Netherlands Centre for Occupational Respiratory Disorders
Utrecht, the Netherlands

Sarah E. Howie
Queens Medical Research Institute
University of Edinburgh
Edinburgh, United Kingdom

Ryan F. Hoy
Department of Allergy, Immunology and Respiratory Medicine
Alfred Hospital
and
Department of Epidemiology and Preventive Medicine
Monash University
Melbourne, Australia

Jennifer Hoyle
North Manchester Hospital
Manchester, United Kingdom

Kathleen Kreiss
Division of Respiratory Disease Studies
National Institute for Occupational Safety and Health
Morgantown, West Virginia

Mona Lärstad
Occupational and Environmental Medicine
Gothenburg University
Gothenburg, Sweden

Lisa A. Maier
National Jewish Health
Denver, Colorado

and

Colorado School of Public Health
and
School of Medicine
University of Colorado
Aurora, Colorado

and

State University of New York Upstate
Medical University
Syracuse, New York

Steven Markowitz
Queens College
City University of New York
Queens, New York

Annyce S. Mayer
National Jewish Health
Denver, Colorado

and

Colorado School of Public Health
Aurora, Colorado

Charles P. McSharry
Greater Glasgow and Clyde NHS
Research & Development
University of Glasgow
Glasgow, United Kingdom

Margaret Mroz
National Jewish Health
Denver, Colorado

Nicola Murgia
Department of Occupational and
Environmental Medicine
University of Gothenburg
Gothenburg, Sweden

and

Section of Occupational Medicine
Respiratory Diseases and Toxicology
University of Perugia
Perugia, Italy

Jill Murray
School of Public Health
University of the Witwatersrand and Pathology Division
National Institute for Occupational Health
National Health Laboratory Service
Johannesburg, South Africa

Bill Musk
The University of Western Australia
Crawley, Australia

Anthony J. Newman Taylor
National Heart and Lung Institute
Imperial College London
London, United Kingdom

Anna-Carin Olin
Occupational and Environmental Medicine
Gothenburg University
Gothenburg, Sweden

Neil Pearce
Department of Medical Statistics
London School of Hygiene and Tropical Medicine
London, United Kingdom

and

Centre for Public Health Research
Massey University Wellington Campus
Wellington, New Zealand

Nayia Petousi
Nuffield Department of Medicine
University of Oxford
Oxford, United Kingdom

C. A. C. Pickering
Wythenshawe Hospital
North West Lung Centre
Manchester, United Kingdom

Craig A. Poland
Institute of Occupational Medicine
Edinburgh, United Kingdom

David Rees
Occupational Medicine Division
National Institute for Occupational Health
and
Occupational Health School of Public Health
University of the Witwatersrand
Johannesburg, South Africa

Carl J. Reynolds
Department of Occupational and Environmental Medicine
National Heart and Lung Institute
Imperial College London
London, United Kingdom

Peter A. Robbins
Department of Physiology, Anatomy and Genetics
University of Oxford
Oxford, United Kingdom

Alastair Robertson
Heart of England NHS Foundation Trust
Birmingham, United Kingdom

Cecile Rose
National Jewish Health
Denver, Colorado

Paul-André Rosental
Sciences Po
and
Institute National d'Etudes Démographiques
Paris, France

Anita K. Simonds
NIHR Respiratory Biomedical Research Unit
Royal Brompton and Harefield NHS Foundation Trust
London, United Kingdom

Chris Stenton
The Newcastle upon Tyne NHS Hospitals
Newcastle, United Kingdom

Hille Suojalehto
Occupational Medicine Team
Finnish Institute of Occupational Health
Helsinki, Finland

Joanna Szram
Royal Brompton and Harefield NHS Foundation Trust
London, United Kingdom

Kjell Torén
Department of Occupational and Environmental Medicine
University of Gothenburg
Gothenburg, Sweden

and

Section of Occupational Medicine
Respiratory Diseases and Toxicology
University of Perugia
Perugia, Italy

Olivier Vandenplas
Department of Chest Medicine
Centre Hospitalier Universitaire de Mont-Godinne
Université Catholique de Louvain
Yvoir, Belgium

1 The History of Occupational Lung Diseases

A Long View

Paul-André Rosental

CONTENTS

Occupational lung diseases have been a scourge whose history is as old as that of human labour, to the point that in 1915 the great industrial hygienist Edgar Collis wondered—no doubt wrongly—whether even cavemen had suffered from the most infamous of such diseases, namely silicosis. In the mid-twentieth century, eminent physicians such as Luigi Carozzi (1880–1963), the director of the International Labour Office's industrial hygiene section, and George Rosen (1910–1977), a Yale University medical historian, undertook projects to identify references to these diseases in old medical texts (Carozzi, 1941–1942; Rosen, 1943; Meiklejohn, 1951–1952). Such references date back to antiquity, abounded in the seventeenth century and morphed into a dense scientific debate beginning in the nineteenth century, which was also the era of the Industrial Revolution.

The history of knowledge about these diseases is not one of cumulative and steady progress, however (Fleck, 1979). Over time, a number of theories that had been raised, such as the blood origin of the 'black pigmentation' of underground miners' lungs or the pathogenic role of 'miasma', were later discarded, while the roles of dust, and later of radiation, were eventually aetiologically recognized. But clinicians ran into recurring problems; thus, while 'nanoparticles' have only been cited since the 1980s, the existence of pathogens too small to be observed had been suspected since the nineteenth century, and toxicological concepts pertaining to them were developed throughout the twentieth century (Oberdörster et al., 2007; Donaldson and Seaton, 2012).

Another obstacle, which was greater here than in other areas of medicine, was the major role that political, economic and social history played in the lifecycle of the diseases and the perceptions of doctors and workers themselves. Technological change constantly altered the hazards to which lungs were exposed. 'Corporate' medical systems run by employers (historically beginning with the mines) and, after the Industrial Revolution, public regulations, insurance and the struggle between labour movements and industry regarding the recognition of workplace hazards, all shaped the knowledge of occupational lung diseases, including their definitions and classifications. The importance of the non-medical context explains the endurance, particularly in the International Commission on Occupational Health's (ICOH) Committee on the History of Prevention of Occupational and Environmental Diseases, of the tradition of 'clinician–historians', who delve into history as a means of contributing to current medical research (Blanc and Dolan, 2012).

THE SLOW EMERGENCE AND CONTESTED ROLE OF THE 'WORK ENVIRONMENT'

Let us begin with medicine's difficulty in recognizing lung diseases arising from dust, which continues to be an ongoing problem in the twenty-first century, in particular in emerging economies. For example, consider a Limoges porcelain workshop in central France in 1855, right before these diseases became prominent in industrial hygiene. Dr. Déperet-Muret described 'this fine and smooth dust covering the walls, the partitions, the boards, the machines and the work instruments with a thick coat that the slightest movement causes to spread through the air, enter the airways, and deposit on nasal, pharyngeal, laryngeal, and bronchial mucous membranes [...];

to permeate clothes, deposit on the skin in a barely adherent layer, or become embedded in some areas like some kind of tattoo; finally, even to enter the digestive track with food, which is too often consumed in the workshops without taking proper measures of cleanliness beforehand; colic, dyspepsia, and diarrhoea ensue, creating yet another cause of nutritional deficiency and economic impoverishment' (Dépéret-Muret, 1860, pp. 211–213). Dépéret-Muret, along with the porcelain workers themselves, saw dust as the cause of 'coughing, dyspnoea and frequent recurrences of bronchitis, laryngitis, and pneumonia that more or less quickly but almost inevitably lead to tubercular phthisis', especially in cases where 'due to work requirements this inhalation is common, continual, and persistent'.

Yet, this doctor lamented at the time, 'the impact of mineral dusts is still debated today'. Why has the medical field taken so long to agree on their importance? Rather than attacking the irrationality of past scientists, answering this question involves understanding the history of their observational methods, their reasoning and their own working conditions. This historical analysis will reconcile a number of considerations that, at first glance, might seem contradictory.

Risks linked to professional activity have long and variously been commented on. In antiquity, such commentaries came from doctors such as Hippocrates, Celsus and Dioscorides, as well as polymath non-clinician observers such as Teophrastus and Pliny the Elder, and even anonymous texts such as the *Satire of Trades* from the Egyptian papyrus Sallier II. Several points of convergence can be detected in this body of work. From antiquity through to the early modern period, both in Europe and elsewhere (Thomann, 2009), while authors made myriad comments on craft trades (Figure 1.1), they also focused on mining activity, particularly gold, sulphur and mercury. Mining was also the domain *par excellence* of reports that associated it with despised slave labour or even with the world of demons, as was the case made by Agricola during the Renaissance and, still at the dawn of the eighteenth century, by Bernardino Ramazzini. These documents show the long history of certain symptoms such as asthma (Bueß and Lerner, 1956; Pepys and Bernstein, 1999), and of the effects of certain toxins such as mercury (Kobal and Grum, 2010; Menéndez-Navarro, 2011, pp. 47–59). Finally, they reveal, as in the case of Pliny the Elder's *Historia Naturalis*, the attempts of affected workers to protect themselves from risk, in particular by wearing makeshift masks.

However, this retrospective coherence is partly misleading. It masks the great diversity of scientific frameworks in which these observations were made. In Greek and Roman medicine, and particularly in the Galenic tradition that predominated through the Renaissance, breathing did not have the vital function ascribed to it today: it was seen as an activity regulating the temperature of the *pneuma*, the vital breath animating the body that was sometimes identified with the soul (Worthen, 1970; Furley and Wilkie, 1984; Hirai, 2005). From this perspective, lung history underwent a revolution in the seventeenth century, with William Harvey's (1578–1657) new theories on blood circulation (Frank, 1980; Gregory, 2001), and another one several decades later, when the medical field embraced new principles of mechanical physics exemplified by Robert Boyle's air pump (Merton, 1952; Schaffer, 1989; Bertoloni Meli, 2008).

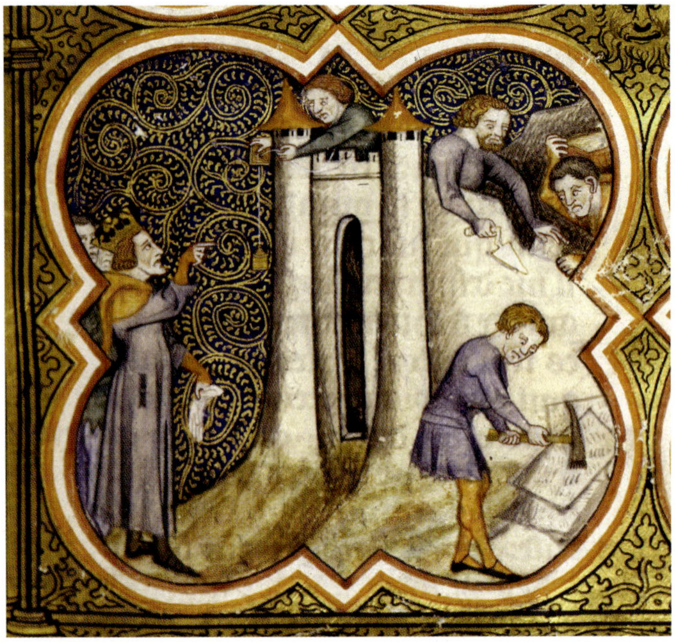

FIGURE 1.1 Architect, stoneworkers and masons building a castle in the fifteenth century. (Courtesy of Municipal Library, Bordeaux, Coll, Jean Vigne/Kharbine Tapabor.)

While it had been a subject of university studies beginning in the Middle Ages, medicine was not a self-contained discipline. In the sixteenth century, it was often inseparable from chemistry, which itself heterogeneously gathered data, 'through accumulation of data by miners, alchemists, craftsmen, and by pharmaceutical application of drugs' (Hellman 1955, p. 196). By today's standards, the Saxon Georgius Agricola (1494–1555) was primarily a mineralogist, a geologist and a philologist: he aimed to reshape the ancient Greco–Roman terms that were used in the science of his day by integrating German terms handed down by oral tradition in mining communities across Central Europe where he practiced medicine (Halleux and Yans, 1990; Hannaway, 1992).* At the same time, Paracelsus (1493–1541), an itinerant physician also with mining town experience, placed his observations in a framework combining alchemical and magical concepts with a form of Catholic enlightenment in response to the Protestant Reformation (Weeks, 1996; Webster, 2002). Paracelsus focused on the relationships between human beings and their mineral environment (Sigerist, 1996). The role he attributed to sulphur, mercury and saltpetre in place of the 'four elements' left little room for the issue of dust in his treatise on mountain diseases, *Von der Bergsucht und anderen Bergkrankheiten*, which is often cited as the first book-length work dedicated to occupational diseases.

A century and a half later, the same need to reposition medical knowledge in the context of its broader development was expressed by Bernardino Ramazzini, whose 1700 treatise (further expanded in 1713) on occupational diseases (as well as observations that have elements of ethnography) resonates with contemporary medical issues (Ramazzini, 1705; Sakula, 1983; Bisetti, 1988; Carnevale and Baldasseroni, 2000; Carnevale et al., 2009). His work is often considered, in retrospect, to be the modern foundation of occupational health as a distinct discipline. But to the contrary, Ramazzini's work, which focused on workplaces as one of the 'environments' to which human health is subject, also could be used today to break down the division between occupational and environmental diseases (Camuffo et al., 2000; Riva and Cesana, 2010; Vincent, 2012). The discussion on the relative position of bodily and environmental explanations was not simply a matter of doctrine; it evolved in step with the observational techniques that became available at that time. With the increased use of autopsies in the early modern period, and later the anatomo-pathological observations in the nineteenth century (Foucault, 1973), the discovery of a 'black pigment' in lung tissues led some doctors to favour a completely endogenous pathogenesis for certain occupational diseases.† From the end of the seventeenth century, when Richard Morton (1637–1698) proposed this interpretation, up until the 1860s, when it was abandoned, several pathways were proposed in order to explain the genesis of these melanotic diseases: tracheobronchial, intestinal, haematic and, finally, cellular. As many of these observations related to coalminers, the interpretation was that of a failure in the decarbonisation of the blood, which at the time was often seen as a key function of breathing. In the middle of the nineteenth century, the 'internal' thesis was reformulated in Germany by Rudolf Virchow (1821–1902), who adopted what we would call today a cytopathic approach.

Many doctors, especially in England, countered this with an 'external' explanation of such disease. While they were convinced of dust's pathogenic role, they did not see it as the sole explanatory factor. From the seventeenth through to the nineteenth centuries, practitioners who had been closely observing various work-related environments (no longer only underground miners, but increasingly discrete trades such as stone-cutters, granite cutters, potters, slate-quarry workers, knappers, needle manufacturers and workers who sharpen knives, forks or sickles on abrasive rocks) considered more general environments, including, but not limited to, the workplace. These observers alternately or concomitantly blamed: poor postures constraining breathing; deplorable living conditions (housing, food and drink); exceedingly low or high temperatures; multiple toxic gases, vapours or smoke; excessive working hours; and night work. 'Dust' itself was hard to grasp as an entity, since it included, as it does today, a mix of very different components.

Many observations accumulated without referencing each other, or remained compartmentalized by country or sector of activity. The various respiratory diseases affecting the miners of deposits located in the hills of Central Europe were lumped together under a specific category: *Bergsucht*, or 'mountain disease'. It was not until the end of the nineteenth century that the category was broken down in order to differentiate between pneumoconioses and, in the Schneeberg mines to the south of Dresden, occupational lung cancer. The cause of the latter—radiation from uranium—was not identified until well into the twentieth century (Greenberg and Selikoff, 1993; Piekarski and Morfeld, 1997; Proctor, 2012a). The various approaches were fragmented as well. In the absence of sufficient empirical knowledge, experiments by Claude Bernard and his students in the nineteenth century overestimated the ability of the lungs to expel dusts by simply making animals inhale dusts for very short periods of time (several days), a time period that did not bear any relationship to human working conditions. Despite all of these obstacles, Dépéret-Muret's analysis of the mid-nineteenth century marked the dawn of a scholarly revolution: entry into the 'dust century'.

* A translation into English of *De Re Metallica* was edited in 1912 by the future president of the United States, Herbert Clark Hoover, who graduated in geology, and his wife Lou Henry Hoover (London, *The Mining Magazine*, 1912).

† The references cited in the next four paragraphs are taken from Carozzi (1941–1942) and Rosen (1943). I am placing them in a general analytical framework here.

THE DUST CENTURY (MID-NINETEENTH TO MID-TWENTIETH CENTURY)

In the nineteenth century, anatomical–pathological and experimental observations were able to explain the path and effect of dusts in the respiratory tract in increasingly precise detail. In 1838, the Englishman Thomas Stratton (1816–1886) used the term 'anthracosis' to refer to the disease he believed was caused by coal dust (Meiklejohn, 1959). The decade of the 1860s was particularly decisive. In 1867, Friedrich Albert von Zenker (1825–1898) noticed the red pigmentation of lungs exposed to iron particles; he named the disease 'siderosis' in a nod to the processes it shared with anthracosis, and placed these two afflictions in a broader category, which he called pneumonokoniosis that later became 'pneumoconiosis' (von Zenker, 1867, p. 171). Five years later, in Milan, Achile Visconti (1836–1911) was the first to use the term 'silicosis' (Rovida, 1871).

But identifying the specific pathogenic effects of a given type of dust and 'creating' new diseases was challenging, as the case of byssinosis exemplifies. Long after Ramazzini, who had noticed respiratory illnesses among flax, hemp and silk workers, medical observation of symptoms affecting the workers employed in the cotton and linen industries multiplied. This had especially been the case in England since the 1830s, in particular with the Manchester physician James Phillips Kay and the brilliant but prematurely deceased Charles Thackrah (Bowden and Tweedale, 2002, p. 562; Blanc, 2007, p. 178 et seq.). But the challenge was to demonstrate the specificity of the disease to the medical body. It was often noted to be a 'Monday' syndrome, because its symptoms were particularly strong at the start of the week. It was also known as strippers' asthma, by reference to the syndromes affecting the workers employed in the cardroom. The Frenchman Villermé had failed to successfully promote the term 'cotton phthisis', which he suggested in 1839. His fellow-countryman Adrien Proust—Marcel's father—finally coined the term 'byssinosis' (after the Greek *byssos* for 'fine fibre') in 1877. It took repeated statistical observations and a thorough epidemiologic study to which Collis was associated in 1908 for 'byssinosis' to finally establish itself at a distinct entity (Beck and Schachter, 1983, pp. 404–412; Levenstein et al., 1987; Bowden and Tweedale, 2003).

Medicine favoured deterministic explanatory factors (Campaner, 2012) at the time and adopted a new aetiological framework that lasted a century. It sought to *causally* link a given type of dust to a specific disease. Socioeconomic and political factors contributed to this transition. With the mechanization and intensification of industrial activity that began in England and then extended abroad in the second half of the nineteenth century, occupational diseases grew in number and kind and attracted the concern of public, sanitary and economic authorities. Throughout Western Europe, these diseases were the subject of dedicated commissions, including medical experts, engineers, administrators and employers. Public authorities were committed to the new cause of 'public health' and to the search for common causes of mortality, but also acted out of a utilitarian concern for looking after a valuable workforce, especially in skilled trades. High-profile investigations (such as a succession of surveys concerning the Sheffield grinders in England throughout the nineteenth century) explored the pathogenic role of dust. Doctors using different approaches (pathological, clinical, experimental, toxicological and, increasingly, statistical) in different professional settings were encouraged to bring together their views, and in doing so they transformed medical knowledge more and more markedly in the second half of the nineteenth century.

Around 1900, this dynamic grew as the working class gained union and electoral strength. Social conflicts denouncing the hazards of certain industrial products (phosphorus and white lead) were relayed via the booming popular press. To guard against the threat of revolution, the reformist bourgeoisie called for social legislation. Occupational diseases became medico-legal and were compensated by social insurance (beginning in the 1880s in Europe) and private insurance (particularly in the United States), thereby giving statistics a greater role in the area of health. The process of defining these diseases thus played out in the intense struggles between workers, employers and the state.

The diffusion of the terms 'pneumoconiosis' and 'silicosis' was inextricably linked to the emergence of labour issues, labour law and insurance frameworks, as epitomized in England in the Milroy Lecture given by Edgar Leigh Collis in 1915, which can be considered as the outcome of a review of dust hazards undertaken by the Royal Commission on Metalliferous Mines and Quarries (Collis, 1915; Melling and Sellers, 2011). Four years later, the United Kingdom decided to recognize silicosis as an occupational disease, except, that is, in the mining sector. Collis, the Home Office's medical inspector of factories since 1908, was the leading authority in industrial medicine, a speciality in which England was a pioneer. He combined fields of knowledge from several industries, the use of professional morbidity and mortality statistics on an experimental basis (Schweber, 2006), as well as a familiarity with radiological data—a new science that revolutionized the understanding of lung diseases (Figures 1.2 and 1.3).

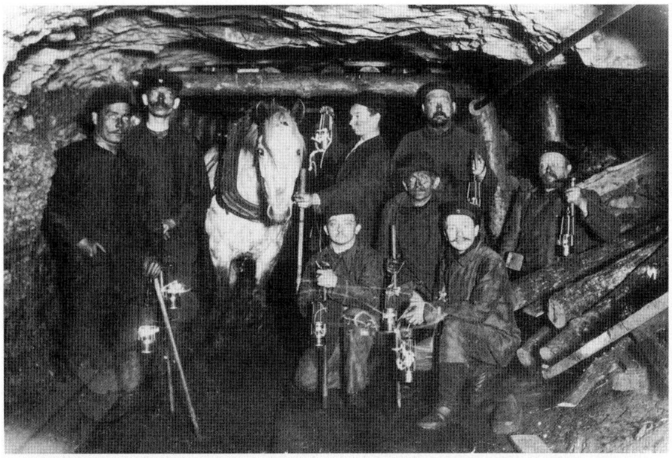

FIGURE 1.2 Coal mine gallery in the Ruhr Basin (Germany), c. 1880. (Copyright: Imagno.)

This institutional framework was key to countering the microbial interpretation of pneumoconioses. Since Robert Koch (1843–1910) had identified the tuberculosis bacillus in 1882, industry experts had proffered a microbial and therefore 'private' explanation for occupational lung diseases, allowing them to refuse to provide compensation (Markowitz and Rosner, 1991; Menéndez-Navarro, 2008; Rosental, 2009; Gallo and Valderrama, 2011). The issue had to move to the transnational level in order to overcome this resistance. In conjunction with international labour unions, Luigi Carozzi, director of the 1919-established International Labour Office's (ILO) Industrial Hygiene Section (IHS) (Carnevale and Baldasseroni, 1999; Cayet et al., 2009), made it a priority to medico-legally recognize silicosis as the 'king of occupational diseases' (Selikoff, quoted by Markowitz and Rosner, 1991, p. 4). In 1930, Carozzi dedicated a decisive conference to it in Johannesburg, which led to the adoption four years later of an international convention on silicosis (Rosental et al., 2015).

As was typical in what could be called the political economy of occupational diseases, this conference was co-funded by the South African gold mining industry, which had been working over the previous 20 years to optimize the use of its skilled workforce (Katz, 1994; McCulloch, 2012). Its conclusions took the form of adopted resolutions that defined the disease as a three-stage process (*Silicosis*, 1930). At a time when the notion of chronic disease was growing (Weisz, 2014), silicosis was conceived as a slow-onset disease, an outgrowth of the long-term employment of (often white) skilled workers in South African mines. But if fitted badly with the extreme forms of exposure to silica dust that unskilled black workers experienced (Packard, 1989), nor with the prevailing conditions in then-emerging industries such as the production of abrasive powders or sandblasting (Middleton, 1929; Blanc, 2015) (Figure 1.4).

More broadly, out of a desire to jettison the microbial explanation and to reach consensus (Weindling, 1995), the ILO focused the debate on a manageable disease; that is, silicosis, rather than on the pneumoconioses in general. This scaling back to a disease that was highly publicized at the time (Markowitz and Rosner, 1991) capped the era that had begun in the 1860s. But the framework thus forged was too restrictive to withstand the evolution of medical thought and the expansion of the chemical and nuclear industry after the Second World War.

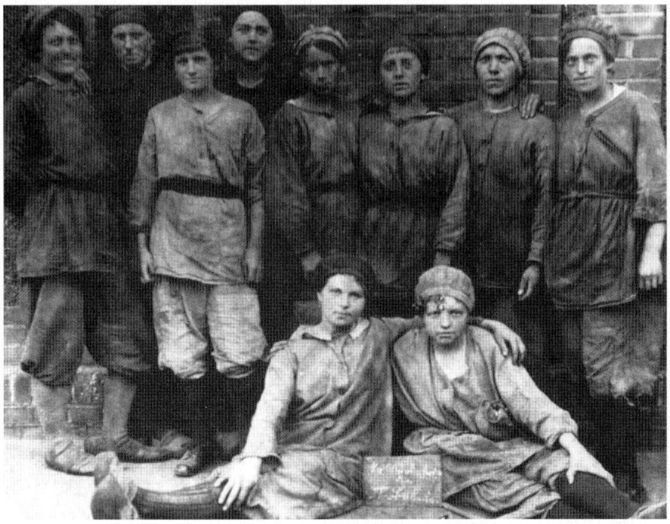

FIGURE 1.3 Women working in the Ruhr coal mines in Buer, near Gelsenkirchen, during the First World War. (Copyright: Imagno.)

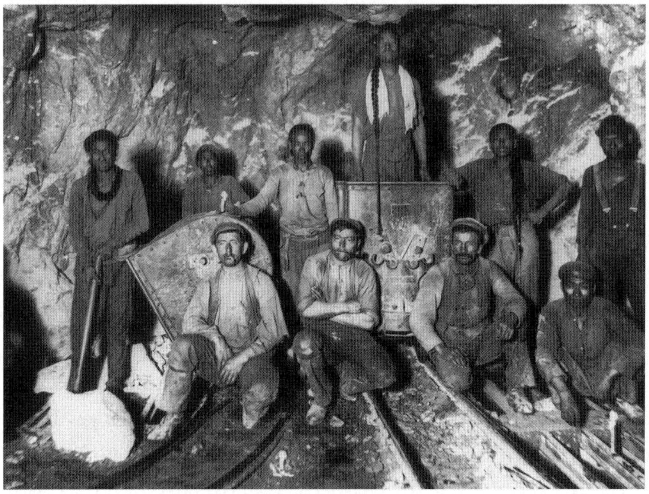

FIGURE 1.4 Black, Chinese and white workers in a South African gold mine, c. 1900. (Copyright: The Granger Collection NYC.)

CHALLENGING INVISIBILITY (MID-TWENTIETH CENTURY ONWARDS)

Within the family of the pneumoconioses itself, important studies by the Medical Research Council's Industrial Pulmonary Diseases Committee in Wales at the end of the 1930s had already led to the 'rediscovery of coal dust disease' (Heppleston, 1992; McIvor and Johnston, 2007, p. 82) under the name of coal workers' pneumoconiosis (CWP). But the two processes (the accumulation of silica and of coal dust) could be difficult to distinguish using clinical, radiological and lung function tests. This was all the more so the case because the technical conditions of production were rapidly changing, and also because, in most work situations, miners inhaled a mixture of minerals present in dusts. A comparison between the medico-legal treatment of these two diseases (silicosis and CWP) in the United Kingdom, France and the United States illustrates the importance of political arrangements in the history of pneumoconiosis (Rosental, 2017).

In the United Kingdom, the 1919 law on silicosis had been extended to the mining sector in 1928, but it only granted the right to compensation to miners who had worked with ores containing at least 50% silica, placing the burden of proof on the miners at risk. Labour shortages during the Second World War strengthened the hand of miners, who requested the full enforcement of silicosis legislation. The 1943 Pneumoconiosis Compensation Scheme, which extended the previous legislation to 'other dusts', was a compromise of sorts that recognized coal dust hazards without loosening the strict conditions imposed on miners for receiving compensation for silicosis (McIvor and Johnston, 2007, p. 86).

By contrast, France only recognized silicosis in 1945 due to fierce resistance from employers. But the government, which then included the Communist Party, promoted the recognition so heavily that 'silicosis' became the established diagnostic umbrella covering all miners' ailments (Figure 1.5). The 1945 arrangement provided the legal framework to compensate coal miners until 1980, when CWP was finally recognized, too. In the United States, the mining industry refused to recognize CWP, leading miners and social rights activists in the 1960s to largely mobilize around 'black lung'. Coined by cardiologist and independent activist Isidore Buff (1908–1974), the term was 'the descendant of miners' asthma in the vernacular tradition' (Derickson, 1998, p. 147) and relied on workers' experiences rather than conventional scientific knowledge. In 1969, a US federal (as opposed to state-based) compensation plan on 'Black Lung Benefits' was established for occupational pneumoconiosis. However, as in the two other countries,

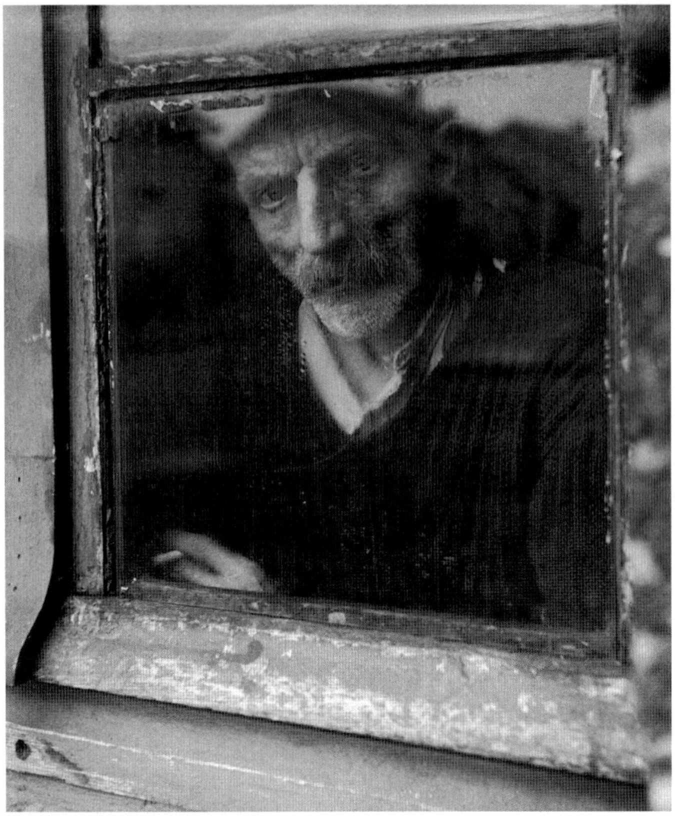

FIGURE 1.5 Willy Ronis, silicotic miner in Lens (Northern France), 1951 (the worker died shortly afterwards at the age of 47). (Copyright: Succession Willy Ronis/Diffusion Agence Rapho.)

the successive recognition of silicosis and CWP left out chronic obstructive pulmonary disease and emphysema. As noted elsewhere in this volume, the occupational origins of the latter two are amply discussed in the biomedical literature today. The key point, though, is that the reductionist interpretation of occupational lung diseases as equating with pneumoconioses was shattered after 1945. The recognition of the carcinogenic effects of asbestos symbolized the dawn of this new era.

The dangers of asbestos had initially only been considered in the nosological framework of pneumoconioses, with the creation of the term 'asbestosis' and its identification in several European countries in the 1900s (Auribault, 1906; Kotelchuck, 1987; Carnevale, 1997). Since it was recognized as an occupational disease when silicosis reigned supreme (in 1931 in the United Kingdom and in 1945 in France), asbestosis was initially seen as an extension of the former, and was even included in the same medico-legal category (Wikeley, 1992; Tweedale and Hansen, 1998). This hierarchy was reversed in the 1950s. With the drop in infectious diseases after the antibiotic revolution, research on cancer exploded. This shift was particularly evident in the field of lung cancers, an almost exclusively man-made disease. While the occupational origin of some cancers had started to be identified at the end of the nineteenth century, it was the publication in 1942 of *Occupational Tumors and Allied Diseases* by W. C. Hueper that marked the beginning of this new era. Asbestos became an established carcinogen for bronchogenic carcinoma and mesothelioma; mesothelioma went on to become a symbol of occupational disease in the second half of the twentieth century.

The transition was marked by the Johannesburg conference of 1959, during which the South African pathologist John Christopher Wagner (1923–2000) exposed the relationships between asbestos and mesothelioma (Wagner, 1960; McCulloch, 2003). This shift in medical opinion took place at the same time as change regarding cigarettes, and the two shared many common features. The role of these two products in causing lung cancer had been suspected since the 1930s, but was only established in the 1950s through epidemiologic research. The British epidemiologist Richard Doll (1912–2005) made a major contribution in both cases. The risks of asbestos and tobacco faced the same 'agnotologic' processes, or in other words, according to the historian Robert Proctor, active strategies by the industry to weaken this emerging knowledge and produce ignorance and doubts (Proctor, 2012b). After hiding their hazardousness (McCulloch and Tweedale, 2008), industry sought to take apart the accumulating medical evidence; intense legal and media mobilization was needed in both cases to establish recognition (Henry, 2011).

This chronology has applied *mutatis mutandis* to other products such as radon (George, 2008; McLaughlin, 2013), but it is not universal. On the one hand, the geological ubiquity of a mineral such as silica, which is the primary component of the Earth's crust, paradoxically made it difficult to recognize its carcinogenicity, despite the International Agency for Research on Cancer's (IARC's) unambiguous reiteration of its conclusions on that topic (Tse et al., 2011; Carnevale et al., 2012). On the other hand, the proliferation of new chemical materials with poorly monitored medical effects put toxicology in a race to catch up. Examples include the epidemiology of beryllium in the 1940s (Zwerling, 1987), of chloromethylether and lung cancer in the 1970s (DeFonso and Kelton, 1976; Weiss et al., 1979) and of the numerous products that this volume addresses for the current time period; in 2001, of the 100,000 chemical substances in circulation in Europe, only 3% had been properly risk assessed (Jouzel and Lascoumes, 2011). Occupational asthma, although long recognized as a clinical phenomenon, is another pathological syndrome that has only emerged as a distinct occupational challenge in the later part of the twentieth century (Pepys and Bernstein, 1999). More generally, the second half of the twentieth century saw the disruption of the delicate balances that had developed around industrial hygiene (mid-nineteenth century), medico-legal occupational diseases (1900), occupational medicine and the *pax toxicologica* (1920s) (Sellers, 1997). With long historical hindsight, it appears that the current era is characterized by several features.

The first one is a challenge to the notion of diseases being limited to the workplace, which resulted from the political and scholarly compromise that had created the notion of 'occupational diseases' around 1900. A growing number of cases of chemical materials affecting the health of both workers producing or using them, as well as local residents living close by, initiated this challenge (Tweedale and McCulloch, 2004). Later came evidence that the 'contamination' of the working environment could spread to the domestic sphere, particularly through the handling of work clothes at home, the victims of which were wives, children and even unborn babies. Asbestos was probably the most recognized symbol of spill-over from the narrow context of the workplace: 'ironically, what was to become one of the great occupational health discoveries of the 20th century was based principally on cases drawn from outside the workplace' (McCulloch, 2006, p. 610). More recently, the case of radon offers another example. It was first recognized as an occupational pollutant and only later as an element that could be widespread in the home (Mazur, 1987).

The second challenge to the old paradigm of occupational lung disease comes from the erosion of the managerial model that had held sway since the 1920s in occupational medicine, which was designed to reconcile utilitarian concerns with the health of workers. For example, the spirometer, which was invented in its current form, and its name coined, in England in the 1840s, measured both workers' respiratory capacities and productive capacities (Hutchinson, 1846; Yernault, 1997). Acceptable thresholds for harmful substances or exposures (dusts and then radiation and chemical products) were determined on the basis of the technological capabilities of the time, rather than strictly epidemiological criteria (Markowitz and Rosner, 1995). By showing the limitations of this approach, the asbestos tragedy challenged the notion of 'controlled' risk. Another challenge today is to balance the utility and the danger of products such as nanoparticles or radon, which are both hazardous and medically useful.

The third is the challenge to the tripartite forum (employees, unions and public and judicial authorities) that had determined the recognition of occupational lung and other work-related diseases for over a century. As trade unionism weakened in the old industrial countries and faltered in emerging countries, and as the importance of traditional media and information dissemination has grown in the 'information age', struggles around occupational diseases have unfolded in various configurations geared towards broadening the problems affecting isolated communities to the national and even international levels (Brugge et al., 2006). In the coal mines of the Jaintia Hills district in north-eastern India, for instance, where an estimated 70,000 Nepalese and Bangladeshi children are forced to work, the mobilization of the Impulse NGO Network against silicosis does not exclusively target the workers, who are mostly males working in other exposed industries, but rather joins forces with other types of movements focused on the fight against child labour, the advancement of women and, more generally, the defence of human rights (Carnevale et al., 2012).

Finally, with the emergence of diseases linked to irradiation and, more recently, nanoparticles, the issue of disease invisibility has become central to today's occupational and environmental medicine (Nash, 2004; Hecht, 2012a,b; Boudia and Jas, 2013). Despite the impression of control created by progress in electron microscopy, this struggle between the visible and invisible is not new: it is part and parcel of medical thought on diseases, especially those created as a result of human labour (Wilson, 1988). This also means that the old model of inhaled dusts as being relevant to respiratory deposition and, for the most part, local effects, cannot be applied to nanoparticles that can be displaced and enter the circulation (thus being more analogous to an inhaled gas). The upending of a cognitive framework limited to the workplace makes it more important than ever to move beyond set perspectives on past medical theories and observations. Because it enables understanding of the genesis of diseases that have been caused by human activities, and more broadly because it provides models of relationships between work and the environment, history has become a valuable research tool for contemporary medicine.

REFERENCES

Auribault, E. 1906. Note sur l'hygiène et la sécurité des ouvriers dans les filatures et tissages d'amiante [Note on the hygiene and security of workers milling and weaving asbestos]. *Bulletin de l'Inspection du Travail [Work Inspectorate Bulletin]* 14:120–32.

Beck, G. J. and Schachter, E. N. 1983. The evidence for chronic lung disease in cotton textile workers. *Am Stat* 37:404–12.

Bertoloni Meli, D. 2008. The collaboration between anatomists and mathematicians in the mid-seventeenth century with a study of images as experiments and Galileo's role in Steno's myology. *Early Sci Med* 13:665–709.

Bisetti, A. 1988. Bernardino Ramazzini and occupational lung medicine. *Ann N Y Acad Sci* 534:1029–37.

Blanc, P. D. 2007. *How Everyday Products Make People Sick: Toxins at Home and in the Workplace*. Berkeley, CA: University of California Press.

Blanc, P. D. 2015. 'Acute' silicosis in the 1930 Johannesburg conference and its aftermath. *Am J Ind Med* 58(Suppl. 1):539–47.

Blanc, P. D. and Dolan, B. (eds). 2012. *At Work in the World*. San Francisco, CA: University of California Medical Humanities Press: 68–83.

Boudia, S. and Jas, N. (eds). 2013. *Toxicants, Health and Regulation since 1945*. London: Pickering & Chatto.

Bowden, S. and Tweedale, G. 2002. Poisoned by the fluff: Compensation and litigation for byssinosis in the Lancashire cotton industry. *J Law Soc* 29:560–79.

Bowden, S. and Tweedale, G. 2003. Mondays without dread: The trade union response to byssinosis in the Lancashire cotton industry in the twentieth century. *Soc Hist Med* 16:79–95.

Brugge, D., Benally, T. and Yazzie-Lewis, E. (eds). 2006. *The Navajo People and Uranium Mining*. Albuquerque, NM: University of New Mexico Press.

Bueß, H. and Lerner, R. 1956. Über Asthma bronchiale und Asthmoide Bronchitis in der chemischen Industrie [On bronchial asthma and asthmatic bronchitis in the chemical industry]. *Zeitschrift für Präventivmedizin [Journal of Preventive Medicine]* 1:59–74.

Campaner, R. 2012. *Philosophy of Medicine: Causality, Evidence and Explanation*. Bologna: Archetipolibri.

Camuffo, D., Daffara, C. and Sghedoni, M. 2000. Archaeometry of air pollution: Urban emission in Italy during the 17th century. *J Archaeol Sci* 27:685–90.

Carnevale, F. 1997. Sentenza del Tribunale Civile e Penale di Torino, Sezione II, nella causa The British Asbestos Company Ltd contro Il progresso del Canavese e delle Valli di Stura (31.8.1906) [Ruling by the civil and criminal court of Turin, section II, in the suit of the British Asbestos Company versus Il Progresso del Canavese e delle Valli di Stura]. *Epidemiologia e Prevenzione [Epidemiology and Prevention]* 21:65–73.

Carnevale, F. and Baldasseroni, A. 1999. *Mal da lavoro. Storia della salute dei lavoratori [Sick from Work: A History of Worker Health]*. Rome, Laterza.

Carnevale, F. and Baldasseroni, A. 2000. The *De morbis artificum diatriba* editions since 1700 and their legacy. *Epidemiologia and Prevenzione [Epidemiology and Prevention]* 24:270–5.

Carnevale, F., Mendini, M. and Moriani, G. (eds). 2009. *Bernardino Ramazzini Works*. Caselle di Sommacampagna: Cierre Edizione.

Carnevale, F., Rosental, P.-A. and Thomann, B. 2012. Silice, silicose et santé au travail dans le monde globalisé du 21e siècle [Silica, silicosis and occupational health in the globalized world of the 21st century]. In C. Courtet and M. Gollac (eds), *Risques du travail. La Santé Négociée [Occupational Risk. Negotiated Health]*. Paris: La Découverte: 83–101.

Carozzi, L. 1941–1942. Contributo bibliografico alla storia della pneumoconiosi 'silicosi' (dal 17 sec. A.C. al 1871) [Bibliographical contribution to the history of silica-related pneumoconiosis (from the 17th century AD to 1871)]. *Rassegna di Medicina industriale [Industrial medicine review]* Seven articles from 12, 10 to 13, 5.

Cayet, T., Rosental, P.-A. and Thébaud-Sorger, M. 2009. How international organisations compete: Occupational safety and health at the ILO, a diplomacy of expertise. *J Mod Eur Hist* 2:173–94.

Collis, E. L. 1915. Industrial pneumonoconioses, with special reference to dust-phthisis. Public Health, Milroy Lecture 1915 [four articles from 29, 8 to 29, 11].

DeFonso, L. R. and Kelton, S. C. Jr. 1976. Lung cancer following exposure to chloromethyl ether: An epidemiological study. *Arch Environ Health* 31:125–30.

Dépéret-Muret. 1860. Hygiène et maladies spéciales des porcelainiers et des tisserands [Hygiene and diseases particular to porcelain makers and weavers]. *Congrès Scientifique de France [French Scientific Congress], 26th Session, Limoges*, Session of 22 September 1859, Paris: Libr. Derache and Limoges, Chapoulaud Frères: 209–16.

Derickson, A. 1998. *Black Lung: Anatomy of a Public Health Disaster.* Ithaca, NY: Cornell University Press.

Donaldson, K. and Seaton, A. 2012. A short history of the toxicology of inhaled particles. *Part Fibre Toxicol* 9:13.

Fleck, L. 1979 [or. ed. 1935]. *The Genesis and Development of a Scientific Fact.* Chicago, IL: University of Chicago Press.

Foucault, M. 1973 [or. ed. 1963]. *The Birth of the Clinic: An Archaeology of Medical Perception.* New York: Pantheon Books.

Frank, R. J. 1980. *Harvey and the Oxford Physiologists.* Berkeley, CA: University of California Press.

Furley, D. J. and Wilkie, J. S. (eds). 1984. *Galen on Respiration and the Arteries.* Princeton, NJ: Princeton University Press.

Gallo, Ó. and Valderrama, J. M. 2011. La silicosis o tisis de los mineros en Colombia, 1910–60 [Miner silicosis or phthisis in Colombia, 1910–1960]. *Salud Colectiva [Collective Health]* 7:35–51.

George, A. C. 2008. World history of radon research and measurement from the early 1900s to today. *AIP Conf Proc* 1034:20–33.

Greenberg, M. and Selikoff, I. J. 1993. Lung cancer in the Schneeberg mines: A reappraisal of the data reported by Harting and Hesse in 1879. *Ann Occup Hyg* 37:5–14.

Gregory, A. 2001. *Harvey's Heart: The Discovery of Blood Circulation.* Cambridge: Icon Books.

Halleux, R. and Yans, A. (eds). 1990. *Bermannus (Le Mineur): Un dialogue sur les mines [Bermannus (The Miner): A Dialogue on Mines].* Paris: Les Belles Lettres.

Hannaway, O. 1992. Georgius Agricola as humanist. *J Hist Ideas* 53:553–60.

Hecht, G. 2012a. *Being Nuclear: Africans and the Global Uranium Trade.* Cambridge, MA: MIT Press.

Hecht, G. 2012b. The work of invisibility: Radiation hazards and occupational health in South African uranium production. *Int Labor Working-Class Hist* 81:94–113.

Hellman, C. D. 1955. Science in the renaissance: A survey. *Renaissance News* 8:186–200.

Henry, E. 2011. A new environmental turn. How the environment has come to the rescue of occupational health: Asbestos in France c. 1970–1995. In C. Sellers and J. Melling (eds), *Dangerous Trades: Histories of Industrial Hazard across a Globalizing World.* Philadelphia, PA: Temple University Press: 140–52.

Heppleston, A. G. 1992. Coal workers' pneumoconiosis: A historical perspective on its pathogenesis. *Am J Ind Med* 22:905–23.

Hirai, H. 2005. Alter Galenus: Jean Fernel et son interprétation platonico-chrétienne de Galien [Alter Galenus: Jean Fernel and his Platonic-Christian interpretation of Galen]. *Early Sci Med* 10:1–35.

Hutchinson, J. 1846. On the capacity of the lungs, and on the respiratory functions, with a view of establishing a precise and easy method of detecting disease by the spirometer. *Medico-Chirurgical Trans* 29:137–252.

Jouzel, J. N. and Lascoumes, P. 2011. L'inversion de la charge de la preuve dans la gestion des risques. L'exemple du règlement européen REACH de 2006 sur le contrôle des substances chimiques [The reversal of the burden of proof in risk management. The example of the European REACH regulation of 2006 on controlling chemical substances]. *Politique Européenne [European Policy]* 33:185–214.

Katz, E. 1994. *The White Death: Silicosis on the Witwatersrand Gold Mines, 1886–1910.* Johannesburg: Witwatersrand University Press.

Kobal, A. B. and Grum, D. K. 2010. Scopoli's work in the field of mercurialism in light of today's knowledge: Past and present perspectives. *Am J Ind Med* 53:535–47.

Kotelchuck, D. 1987. Asbestos: 'The funeral dress of kings' – and others. In D. Rosner and G. Markowitz (eds), *Dying for Work. Workers' Safety and Health in Twentieth Century America.* Bloomington, IN: Indiana University Press: 192–207.

Levenstein, C., Plantamura, D. and Mass, W. 1987. Labor and bissynosis, 1941–1969. In D. Rosner and G. Markowitz (eds), *Dying for Work. Workers' Safety and Health in Twentieth Century America.* Bloomington, IN: Indiana University Press: 208–23.

Markowitz, G. and Rosner, D. 1991. *Deadly Dust: Silicosis and the Politics of Occupational Disease in Twentieth Century America.* Princeton, NJ: Princeton University Press.

Markowitz, G. and Rosner, D. 1995. The limits of thresholds: Silica and the politics of science, 1935–1990. *Am J Public Health* 85:253–62.

Mazur, A. 1987. Putting radon on the public's risk agenda. *Sci Technol Human Values* 12:86–93.

McCulloch, J. 2003. The discovery of mesothelioma on South Africa's asbestos fields. *Soc Hist Med* 16:419–36.

McCulloch, J. 2006. Saving the asbestos industry, 1960–2006. *Public Health Rep* 121:609–14.

McCulloch, J. 2012. *South Africa's Gold Mines and the Politics of Silicosis*. Woodbridge: James Currey.

McCulloch, J. and Tweedale G. 2008. *Defending the Indefensible: The Global Asbestos Industry and Its Fight for Survival*. Oxford: Oxford University Press.

McIvor, A. and Johnston, R. 2007. *Miners' Lung: A History of Dust Disease in British Coal Mining*. Aldershot: Ashgate.

Mc Laughlin, J. 2013. Radon: Past, present and future. *Rom Rep Phys* 58:S5–13.

Meiklejohn, A. 1951–1952. History of lung diseases of coal miners in Great Britain, 1800–1952. *Br J Ind Med* Three articles from 8, 127 to 9, 208.

Meiklejohn, A. 1959. The origin of the term anthracosis. *Br J Ind Med* 16:324–5.

Melling, J. and Sellers, C. 2011. Objective collectives? Transnationalism and 'invisible colleges' in occupational and environmental health from Collis to Selikoff. In J. Melling and C. Sellers (eds), *Dangerous Trades: Histories of Industrial Hazard across a Globalizing World*. Philadelphia, PA: Temple University Press: 113–25.

Menéndez-Navarro, A. 2008. The politics of silicosis in interwar Spain: Republican and Francoist approaches to occupational health. *Dynamis* 28:77–102.

Menéndez-Navarro, A. 2011. Global markets and local conflicts in mercury mining: Industrial restructuring and workplace hazards at Almaden mines in the early twentieth century. In J. Melling and C. Sellers (eds), *Dangerous Trades: Histories of Industrial Hazard across a Globalizing World*. Philadelphia, PA: Temple University Press: 47–59.

Merton, E. S. 1952. Sir Thomas Browne's theories of respiration and combustion. *Osiris* 10:206–23.

Middleton, E. L. 1929. The present position of silicosis in industry in Britain. *Br Med J* 2:485–92.

Nash, L. 2004. The fruits of ill-health: Pesticides and workers' bodies in post-World War II California. *Osiris* 19:203–19.

Oberdörster, G., Stone, V. and Donaldson, K. 2007. Toxicology of nanoparticles: A historical perspective. *Nanotoxicology* 1:2–25.

Packard, R. M. 1989. *White Plague, Black Labor: Tuberculosis and the Political Economy of Health and Disease in South Africa*. Berkeley and Los Angeles, CA: University of California Press.

Pepys, J. and Bernstein, I. L. 1999. Historical aspects of occupational asthma. In: I. L. Bernstein, M. Chan-Yeung, J. L. Malo, and D. I. Bernstein (eds), *Asthma in the Workplace*, second edition, New York, NY: Marcel Dekker: 5–26.

Piekarski, C. and Morfeld, P. 1997. Occupational health aspects of uranium mining in Thuringia and Saxony: An historical view. *Applied Occup Environ Hyg* 12:915–8.

Proctor, R. N. 2012a. Occupational disease and labor health and safety under the Nazis. In P. D. Blanc and B. Dolan (eds), *At Work in the World*. San Francisco, CA: University of California Medical Humanities Press: 68–83.

Proctor, R. N. 2012b. *Golden Holocaust: Origins of the Cigarette Catastrophe and the Case for Abolition*. Berkeley, CA: University of California Press.

Ramazzini, B. 1705 [or. ed. 1700]. *A Treatise of the Diseases of Tradesmen*. London: Andrew Bell.

Riva, M. A. and Cesana, G. C. 2010. La 'salubrità' dell'aria: Analisi storica degli studi della correlazione tra salute ed inquinamento dell'aria negli ambienti di vita e di lavoro [The 'healthiness' of air: Historical analysis of studies of the correlation between health and air pollution in living and working environments]. *Giornale Italiano di Medicina del Lavoro ed Ergonomia [Italian Journal of Occupational and Ergonomics]* 32:37–40.

Rosen, G. 1943. *The History of Miners' Diseases: A Medical and Social Interpretation*. New York, NY: Schuman's.

Rosental, P.-A. (ed.). 2009. La silicose, un cas exemplaire [Silicosis, an exemplary case]. *Revue d'Histoire Moderne et Contemporaine [Modern and Contemporary History Review]* 56:83–176.

Rosental, P.-A. (ed). 2017. *Silicosis: A World History*. Baltimore, MD: Johns Hopkins University Press.

Rosental, P.-A., Rosner, D. and Blanc, P. D. (eds). 2015. From silicosis to silica hazards: An experiment in medicine, history, and the social sciences. *Am J Ind Med* 58:S1,S3–5.

Rovida, C. 1871. Un caso di silicosi del polmone, con analisi chimica [A case of silicotic lungs, with chemical analyses]. *Annali di Chimica Applicata alla Medicina [Annals of Chemistry Applied to Medicine]* 53:102–6.

Sakula, A. 1983. Ramazzini's '*De Morbis Artificum*' and occupational lung disease. *Br J Dis Chest* 77:349–61.

Schaffer, S. 1989. The glorious revolution and medicine in Britain and the Netherlands. *Notes Records R Soc London* 43:167–90.

Schweber, L. 2006. *Disciplining Statistics: Demography and Vital Statistics in France and England, 1830–1885*. Durham, NC: Duke University Press.

Sellers, C. C. 1997. *Hazards of the Job: From Industrial Disease to Environmental Health Science*. Chapel Hill, NC: University of North Carolina Press.

Sigerist, H. E. (ed.). 1996. *Paracelsus: Four Treatises*. Baltimore, MD: Johns Hopkins University Press.

Silicosis. 1930. Records of the International Conference held at Johannesburg, 13–27 August 1930. Geneva, ILO [Available at http://www.ugr.es/~amenende/investigacion/ILO-Silicosis-Conference-1930.pdf].

Thomann, B. 2009. L'hygiène nationale, la société civile et la reconnaissance de la silicose comme maladie professionnelle au Japon (1868–1960) [National hygiene, civil society and the recognition of silicosis as an occupational disease in Japan (1868–1960)]. *Revue d'Histoire Moderne et Contemporaine [Modern and Contemporary History Review]* 56:142–76.

Tse, L. A., Yu, T. S. I., Au, J. S. K., Qiu, H. and Wang, X. 2011. Silica dust, diesel exhaust, and painting work are the significant occupational risk factors for lung cancer in nonsmoking Chinese men. *Br J Cancer* 104:208–13.

Tweedale, G. and Hansen P. 1998. Protecting the workers: The medical board and the asbestos industry, 1930s–1960s. *Med Hist* 42:439–57.

Tweedale, G. and McCulloch, J. 2004. Chrysophiles versus chrysophobes: The white asbestos controversy, 1950s–2004. *Isis* 95:239–59.

Vincent, J. 2012. Ramazzini n'est pas le précurseur de la médecine du travail: Médecine, travail et politique avant l'hygiénisme [Ramazzini is not the forerunner of occupational medicine. Medicine, work and politics before the hygiene era]. *Genèses [Geneses]* 89:84–107.

von Zenker, F. A. 1867. Über Staubinhalationskrankheiten der Lungen [On lung diseases from dust inhalation]. *Deutsches Archiv für Klinische Medizin [German Clinical Medicine Archives]* 2:116–72.

Wagner, J. C. 1960. Pathological aspects of asbestosis in South Africa. In A. J. Orenstein (ed.), *Proceedings of the Pneumoconiosis Conference held at the University of Witwatersrand, Johannesburg, 9th–24th February 1959.* London: Churchill: 373–81.

Webster, C. 2002. Paracelsus, paracelsianism, and the secularization of the worldview. *Sci Context* 15:9–27.

Weeks, A. 1996. *Paracelsus: Speculative Theory and the Crisis of the Early Reformation.* Albany, NY: State University of New York Press.

Weindling, P. (ed.). 1995. *International Health Organisations and Movements, 1918–1939.* Cambridge: Cambridge University Press.

Weiss, W., Moser, R. L. and Auerbach, A. 1979. Lung cancer in chloromethyl ether workers. *Am Rev Respir Dis* 120:1031–7.

Weisz, G. 2014. *Chronic Disease in the Twentieth Century: A History.* Baltimore, MD: Johns Hopkins University Press.

Wikeley, N. 1992. The asbestos regulations 1931: A licence to kill? *J Law Soc* 19:365–78.

Wilson, C. 1988. Visual surface and visual symbol: The microscope and the occult in early modern science. *J Hist Ideas* 49:85–108.

Worthen, T. D. 1970. Pneumatic action in the Klepsydra and Empedocles' account of breathing. *Isis* 61:520–30.

Yernault, J. Y. 1997. The birth and development of the forced expiratory manoeuvre: A tribute to Robert Tiffeneau (1910–1961). *Eur Respir J* 10:2704–10.

Zwerling, C. 1987. Salem sarcoid: The origins of beryllium disease. In D. Rosner and G. Markowitz (eds.), *Dying for Work. Workers' Safety and Health in Twentieth Century America.* Bloomington, IN: Indiana University Press: 103–18.

2 Global Patterns

Neil Pearce and Paul Cullinan

CONTENTS

INTRODUCTION

It is indisputable that occupational lung diseases are a global health issue and that, through worldwide increases in production and consumption, the extent of the problem is greater now than ever. Curiously, the routine exposure of many millions of workers to serious occupational hazards is a matter that is omitted from virtually every generic discussion of 'global public health'; the few notable exceptions are discussed below.

The changes in the global economy over the last half century, whereby manufacturing and its attendant hazards have shifted out of Europe and North America to rapidly developing economies, are well recognized (Pearce and Matos, 1994a). The process has a long history, as discussed in Chapter 1, and is graphically—if a little speciously—highlighted by a plot of the global 'economic centre of gravity' over the last two millennia (Figure 2.1).

Two sectors, each with well-known occupational risks, are especially illustrative. At the turn of the twentieth century, shipbuilding was very largely a European and North American enterprise, a position maintained until after the Second World War. It is a labour-intensive industry, and with rising costs of labour in these economies, activity moved to low-wage Asia—first to Japan and, more recently, to South Korea and China (Figure 2.2), Indonesia and the Philippines (Stopford, 2009).

The story of textile manufacturing is very similar (Figure 2.3); half of the world's textiles are now manufactured in China, and a high proportion of the remainder in other parts of east and south-east Asia.

These patterns are accelerating with an inexorable, worldwide rise in both population and consumption.

Arguably, the shifts in location have not been matched by a shift in knowledge of occupational disease prevention and good occupational health practice. This is not to claim that the only examples of good practice are to be found in the post-industrial western economies, whose histories in this respect are far from laudable (Pearce and Matos, 1994b), but it is very likely that, globally, there are now far more workers exposed to significant and unregulated risks of occupational lung disease than ever previously, an example of 'risk transition'. The International Labour Organisation (ILO), for example, estimates that 2 million of the world's 2.5 billion workers die each year from occupational accidents or diseases, a third of the latter comprising respiratory cancers and interstitial lung disease; these figures are almost certainly a significant underestimate. Significantly, many of these workers are confronted with exposures whose hazards are well known and for which there are effective means of control (Kjellstrom and Rosenstock, 1990). An egregious example is the aggressive marketing of both tobacco and asbestos, with their synergistically high contribution to lung cancer, in parts of the world where the regulation of both remains lax (Jamison et al., 2006).

MODES OF EMPLOYMENT

Definitions of a 'worker' are blurred in many parts of the world. In advanced economies, the standard model, whereby employees are paid wages in a dependent

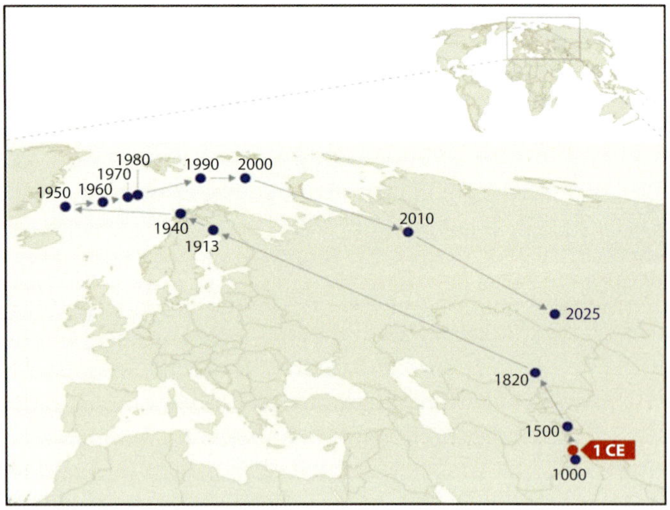

FIGURE 2.1 The shift in the global 'economic centre of gravity' from the year 1 CE to 2010 with projection to 2025. (Reproduced with permission from Dobbs, R. et al. 2012. *Urban World: Cities and the Rise of the Consuming Class*, London, UK: McKinsey Global Institute.)

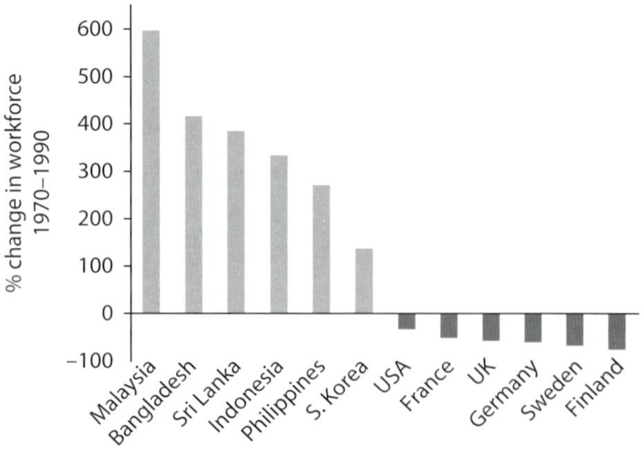

FIGURE 2.3 Proportional changes in the textile manufacturing workforces of 12 countries, 1970–1990.

relationship with an employer, is increasingly in decline. In emergent economies, informal employment, with short-term contracts and irregular hours of work, remains widespread, as do jobs in the 'informal' economy and unpaid family work (Figure 2.4).

These patterns are strong determinants of occupational risks, and tend to blur the boundary between 'general' and 'occupational' health, particularly for respiratory diseases such as tuberculosis, chronic obstructive pulmonary disease (COPD) and lung cancer, where risks are present both at and outside work.

Two patterns pose peculiar problems. The first is the increasing use of migrant workforces, both intra- and trans-national, a pattern now found in most parts of the world, and accounting for at least 150 million workers. Dislocated from home and often on short-term contracts in working conditions deemed unacceptable by local resident workers, migrant labourers have rates of occupational disease and risk behaviours that tend to be higher than average. Second is the still widespread use of children in some sectors, particularly in agriculture, but also in the services and industrial sectors (Figure 2.5). While numbers have declined (ILO, 2013), an estimated 168 million children aged between 5 and 17 years are labourers, more than half of them (85 million) involved in work deemed to be hazardous. The risks incurred through exposure to occupational respiratory hazards at a young age are unknown, but the developing lung is considered especially vulnerable to airborne pollutants. At the very least, childhood exposures will incur a younger age of onset for occupational lung diseases of both short and long latency.

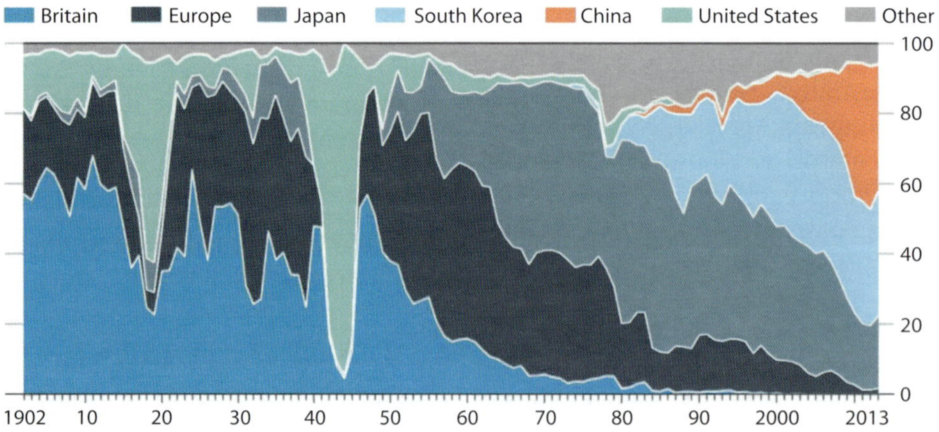

FIGURE 2.2 World shipbuilding between 1902 and 2013 in terms of percentage of total in gross tonnage. (From The Economist Newspaper Limited, London. 8 August 2014.)

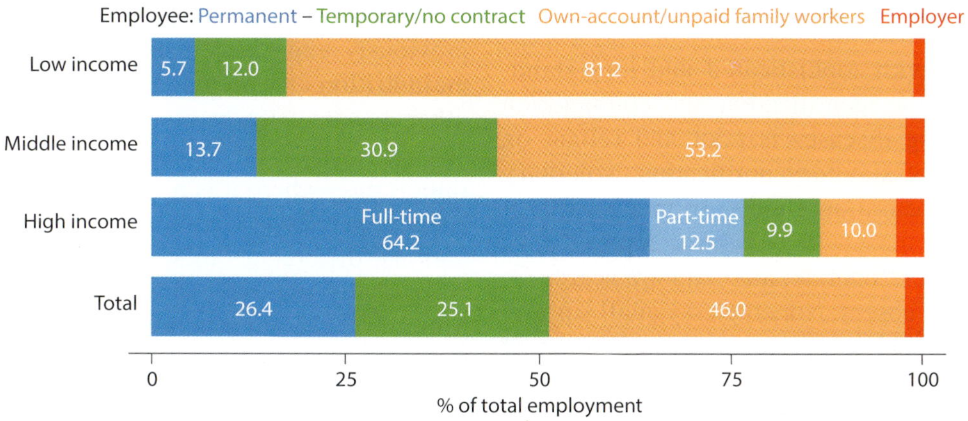

FIGURE 2.4 Distribution of employment status by income group for 90 countries, representing 84% of global employment. (Adapted from ILO Research Department. 2015. World Employment and Social Outlook—Trends 2015. Available at: http://www.ilo.org/global/research/global-reports/weso/2015/lang—en/index.htm.)

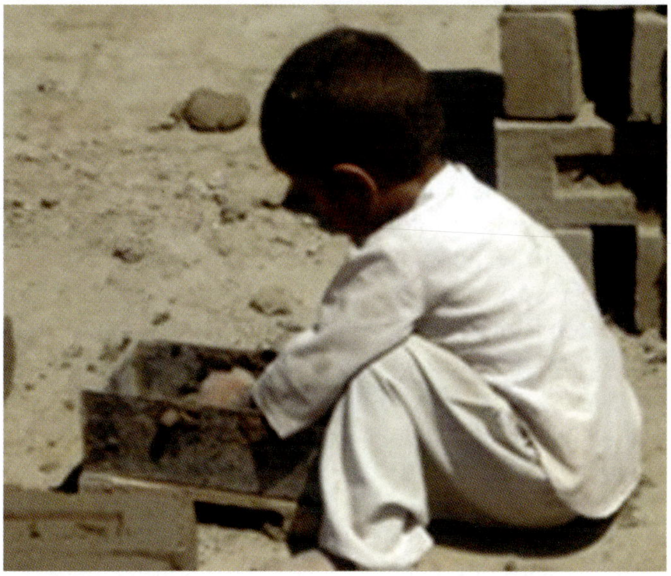

FIGURE 2.5 Young child working in a brickfield in Afghanistan. (Adapted from ILO. 2015. Breaking the mould. Occupational safety hazards faced by children working in brick kilns in Afghanistan. Available at: http://www.ilo.org/ipec/Informationresources/WCMS_IPEC_PUB_25295/lang—en/index.htm.)

EXPOSURES

For the most part, it seems that workers around the world face the same, familiar respiratory hazards, even if the scale of exposure is unprecedented. In India, for example, an estimated 11.5 million workers are exposed to silica dust with, in some reports, extraordinarily high rates of silicosis and attendant tuberculosis (Jindal, 2013). In China, over half a million cases of silicosis were recorded between 1991 and 1995, with more than 24,000 deaths annually (WHO, 2000). A particularly depressing example of a novel exposure to a recognised hazard is the high incidence of silicosis in Turkish men employed in the sandblasting of denim jeans in order to allow wealthy consumers to parade an ‘industrial’ chic (Akgun et al., 2006).

An important exception to this general rule is asbestos, by a wide margin the most important occupational cause of lung cancer. In many ways, asbestos is the ideal construction material: tough, durable, light in weight, inflammable and very cheap; but total bans are in place in over 50 countries, including those of the European Union, Australia, South Africa and Japan (International Ban Asbestos Secretariat, 2011), and its use is tightly restricted in the USA, New Zealand and Canada—the last, ironically, historically among the world’s largest exporters of the material. In many other parts of the world, its production and use continue to flourish, largely in the manufacture of roofing material and pipes for sanitation and irrigation, in contrast to the uses once common in Europe and North America. In India, for example, the use of asbestos has doubled in the last decade, to approximately 300,000 tonnes a year, by an industry that now employs an estimated 100,000 workers (Burki, 2011). Other major users/producers include China, Brazil, Russia, the Ukraine, Kazakhstan and Indonesia. Almost all of the estimated 2 million tonnes mined each year is now chrysotile asbestos with very little deliberate extraction of amphibole types; the attendant risks of malignant mesothelioma are thus lower, but this is unlikely to be the case for lung cancer and asbestosis.

ESTIMATING THE GLOBAL BURDEN

Even in countries with sophisticated and long-standing bureaucracies, the identification and enumeration of occupational lung diseases is poor and reliant on an imperfect mix of statutory notification, voluntary reporting and compensation claims. In many parts of the world, including those with very large exposed populations, none of these operate, and data are scarce or, more often, entirely absent. Nonetheless, small surveys of specific occupational groups suggest that in many of these settings the prevalence of occupational respiratory disease is high. The problems are compounded by important variations in diagnosis, disease labelling and attribution. In a description of malignant mesothelioma in the Ukraine, for example, just two of almost 5000 cases identified between 1992 and 2011 were deemed to have an occupational aetiology (Varivonchik, 2014); it is virtually impossible to interpret or contextualise information such as this. Further difficulties arise from the fact that when information is available, it is not widely so. Almost all of the (scanty) literature on the epidemiology of asbestos-related disease in Russia—a major producer and consumer of the mineral—is unavailable to non-Russian speakers (Kogan, 1998). An analysis of the scientific literature on asbestos-related diseases published since 1970 reported that, of the 28 most prolific countries, the bottom four, after adjustment for population and economic parameters, were (in descending order) Brazil, Russia, India and China—each major producers and/or users of asbestos (Ugolini et al., 2015).

Despite these difficulties, several useful estimates of global burden have been produced through extrapolation of the available data. This process carries several important caveats (Driscoll et al., 2005b). Most estimates are expressed as a population-attributable risk (PAR), which is calculated using the relative risk of developing a disease due to an exposure and the proportion of the population that has that exposure. Risk information is usually available from a small number of epidemiological studies undertaken in a limited number of (usually) developed countries. To make global estimates, these relative risks must be assumed to be universal, although they are in fact specific to the levels of exposure in the studies from which the risk estimates are derived. As described above, there are important variations in employment patterns between countries, and even if the rates within a given industry are similar in different countries, extrapolation can lead to considerably biased estimates of the overall rates of injury or disease. For example, the hazards of occupational exposures may be much greater in populations that have previously experienced or currently are experiencing malnutrition or who may have greater susceptibility for other reasons (Pearce et al., 1994). This makes extrapolating rates on an industry-specific basis particularly important—where it is possible—but even then there is a risk of serious inaccuracy if there are significant international differences in specific exposure intensities, as is generally the case, or in susceptibility to exposure. Moreover, the distributions of relevant co-exposures (such as smoking) often differ.

A particular difficulty arises in the consideration of long-latency diseases where there have been important temporal reductions in exposure. In these instances, exposure prevalences ought to be based on workers who have *ever* been exposed, rather than only those who are currently being exposed, and current exposure levels will underestimate historical exposures that continue to increase cancer risk in former asbestos workers. Otherwise significant underestimates of the true burden—current and future—are inevitable. In practice, because the required information is seldom available, most estimates include an arbitrary 'fix'. Estimations of global burden using the WHO's comparative risk assessment methodology, for example, applied a factor of four to the population of current workers exposed to asbestos in order to estimate an ever-exposed population (Nelson et al., 2005); others (Lim et al., 2012) have used mesothelioma mortality in order to estimate asbestos exposure, with the assumption of a fixed ratio of attributable lung cancers to mesothelioma, but this approach cannot readily be used for other causes of occupational cancer.

Despite these concerns, it seems reasonable to assume that in many circumstances risks are similar between populations that have similar exposures, and if information on exposure prevalence is available, then a PAR for any country or region can be calculated. Estimates of the worldwide burden of occupational lung disease have been published as part of the Global Burden of Disease (GBD) project, the most comprehensive effort to date aimed at measuring epidemiological levels and trends worldwide, with estimates for 1990 (Murray and Lopez, 1996) and 2010 (Lim et al., 2012). The GBD project involves not only estimation of total global mortality for specific causes or attributable to specific risk factors such as occupation, but also the estimation of disability-adjusted life-years (DALYs) lost, a measure that combines both years of life lost due to premature mortality and years lived with a disability (taking into account the severity of the disability).

LUNG CANCER

The 2010 GBD study involved five steps in estimating the disease burden attributable to a risk factor: (i) selection of risk–outcome pairs based on criteria regarding causal association; (ii) estimations of distributions of exposure to each risk factor; (iii) estimation of aetiological effect sizes (using the relative risk); (iv) choice of 'counterfactual' alternative exposure distributions (e.g. no occupational exposure); and (v) computation of burden attributable to each risk factor. The estimates for lung cancer included only ten known occupational causes, whereas many others have been established or are suspected. For example, a recent assessment of the burden of occupational cancer in the United Kingdom (Rushton et al., 2008) included all of the occupational lung carcinogens included in the GBD reports, but also considered cobalt, dioxins, lead, mineral oils, radon, steel foundry work and welding. Overall, these accounted for 19% of the estimates of occupational lung cancer in males and 39% of the estimates in females. Furthermore, some workers may be exposed to these ten carcinogens in other industries apart from those included in the GBD estimates; for example, diesel exhaust exposure is widespread. A third limitation is that there are undoubtedly a number of occupational lung carcinogens yet to be discovered. This particularly applies to female workers, where the relevant industries (in which women predominate) have not yet been studied as extensively.

All of these factors imply that the GBD figures are likely to be underestimates, particularly for women. On the other hand, the GBD estimates apply to the broad grouping of 'trachea, bronchus and lung' cancer, so are likely to be overestimates of the burden of lung cancer alone. Many of these considerations also apply to the estimates for asthma and COPD, which are once again likely to be underestimates. More generally, the estimated number of deaths due to occupational causes in the GBD study (852,107 deaths in 2010) is substantially less than those produced from other sources such as the ILO, as above. Nevertheless, and bearing these limitations in mind, the GBD findings are of considerable interest. In particular, they provide approximate estimates of the overall numbers of deaths and DALYs, but more importantly can be used to assess the relative importance of the various types of lung disease, and the associated trends over time.

Table 2.1 summarises the GBD findings for cancer of the trachea, bronchus and lung with regards to occupational carcinogen exposure (Lim et al., 2012). Occupational lung carcinogens accounted for an estimated 117,696 deaths in 2010, a small (but non-trivial) proportion of overall deaths, but 32% of all occupational

TABLE 2.1
Estimates of the Global Burden of Cancers of the Trachea, Bronchus and Lung due to Occupational Exposures in 2010

	Deaths			Disability-Adjusted Life-Years		
	Men	**Women**	**Total**	**Men**	**Women**	**Total**
Asbestos	25,563	7,047	33,610	521,000	132,000	653,000
Arsenic	1,915	747	2,662	45,000	18,000	63,000
Beryllium	114	49	163	3,000	1,000	4,000
Cadmium	410	145	555	10,000	3,000	13,000
Chromium	1,361	570	1,931	32,000	13,000	45,000
Diesel engine exhaust	18,773	3,431	22,187	442,000	81,000	523,000
Second-hand smoke	17,189	7,046	24,235	405,000	167,000	572,000
Nickel	6,443	2,702	9,145	151,000	64,000	215,000
Polycyclic aromatic hydrocarbons	3,092	993	4,086	73,000	23,000	96,000
Silica	14,205	2,072	16,277	333,000	49,000	382,000
Sulphuric acid	2,606	239	2,845	66,000	6,000	71,000
Total occupational lung cancer	91,671	25,041	117,696	2,081,000	557,000	2,637,000
All occupational lung diseases	288,588	80,704	370,276	10,122,000	3,678,000	13,799,000

Source: Adapted from Lim, S. S. et al. 2012. *Lancet* 380: 2224–60.

Note: Population exposures were derived from the distributions across nine industries, except in the case of asbestos, where mesothelioma rates were used in a smoking impact ratio analogue.

TABLE 2.2
Estimates from Four Countries of The Proportions of Lung Diseases Attributable to Occupational Exposures

		Attributable Fraction			
Disease	**Country**	**Men**	**Women**	**Total**	**Reference**
Lung cancer	New Zealand	12.3%	2.6%		't Mannetje and Pearce (2005)
	United States			6.3%–13.0%	Steenland et al. (2003)
	United Kingdom	16.5%	4.5%	11.6%	Rushton et al. (2008)
	Finland			24.0%	Nurminen and Karjalainen (2001)
Pneumonia	New Zealand	1.4%	0.3%		't Mannetje and Pearce (2005)
	Finland			<0.1%	Nurminen and Karjalainen (2001)
Chronic obstructive pulmonary disease	New Zealand	14.0%	3.8%		't Mannetje and Pearce (2005)
	Finland			11.7%	Nurminen and Karjalainen (2001)
	United States			5%–24%	Steenland et al. (2003)
Asthma	New Zealand	17.8%	18.4%		't Mannetje and Pearce (2005)
	Finland			18.6%	Nurminen and Karjalainen (2001)
	United States			11%–21%	Steenland et al. (2003)
Pulmonary tuberculosis	United States			5%–6%	Steenland et al. (2003)

lung disease deaths. A more valid comparison is obtained by calculating work-related lung cancer deaths as a proportion of all lung cancer deaths. Estimates for four industrialised countries are provided in Table 2.2 and indicate that between 6% and 24% of all lung cancer deaths are attributable to occupational causes. These estimates are likely to (approximately) apply globally, since the GBD study found that occupational cancer was of relatively similar importance in each region of the world—occupational carcinogens were the 37th most important risk factor globally, with a range of 26th–42nd across the 21 regions considered.

NON-MALIGNANT OCCUPATIONAL RESPIRATORY DISEASES

Table 2.2 also includes attributable fractions for non-malignant occupational respiratory diseases: asthma, COPD, pneumonia and pulmonary tuberculosis. Global numbers of deaths for the first two of these, estimated from the GBD studies, are shown in Table 2.3. Occupational COPD accounted for 370,276 deaths, or 59% of all occupational lung disease deaths, a proportion that is approximately twice as high as that for occupational lung cancer.

In addition, the table summarises global estimates of DALYs lost to occupational asthma or COPD, again with a particularly high estimate for the latter. These were examined in more detail by the WHO, with analyses by geographical region, sex (Table 2.4) and age (Driscoll et al., 2005a). The estimates are considerably lower than those produced for the GBD project, a reflection of the many assumptions and approximations that have to be made in producing them. Rates within regions vary significantly depending on their levels of economic development, with much higher estimates for nations with less developed economies. Half of the burden of occupational COPD (deaths and DALYs) is borne by the population of the 'western Pacific B' region, which comprises China, Vietnam (and neighbouring countries) and Indonesia. Rates are consistently higher in men. For asthma, DALYs were evenly distributed across all ages between 30 and 59 years; as expected, the age distribution for COPD was a little higher (30–79 years).

A similar method—but reliant on absolute rather than relative risks because of their clearer relationships with occupational exposure—was used to estimate the global burden of deaths and DALYs from pneumoconioses (Table 2.5), diseases that are almost exclusive to men. The authors note (Driscoll et al., 2005a) that their figures almost certainly underestimate the true burden, particularly for asbestosis, where it is very difficult—even in developed countries—to judge accurately the prevalences and levels of exposure. Coal workers' pneumoconiosis remains an important cause of death globally, with approximately half of the burden falling, as with occupational COPD, on the population of the 'western Pacific B' nations. This same region and that of 'western Pacific A' (Australia and New Zealand) together contributed approximately half of the deaths and DALYs attributed to asbestosis or silicosis.

TABLE 2.3
Estimates of the Global Burden of Asthma and Chronic Obstructive Pulmonary Disease due to Occupational Exposures in 2010

	Deaths			Disability-Adjusted Life-Years		
	Men	Women	Total	Men	Women	Total
Asthma	25,364	8,352	33,716	1,359,000	661,000	2,020,000
Chronic obstructive pulmonary disease	171,553	47,311	218,864	6,682,000	2,460,000	9,142,000
All occupational lung diseases	288,588	80,704	370,276	10,122,000	3,678,000	13,799,000

Source: Adapted from Lim, S. S. et al. 2012. *Lancet* 380: 2224–60.
Note: Population exposures were derived from the distributions across eight (asthma) or nine (chronic obstructive pulmonary disease) occupational groups.

TABLE 2.4
Disability-Adjusted Life-Years (Thousands) from Asthma and Chronic Obstructive Pulmonary Disease Caused by Workplace Exposures, by Global Region in 2000

	Asthma			Chronic Obstructive Pulmonary Disease		
	Men	Women	Total	Men	Women	Total
Africa	63–84	27–56	90–141	43–57	10–12	53–69
Americas	16–98	4–27	19–125	6–147	0–21	6–168
Eastern Mediterranean	18–74	3–27	21–100	20–75	1–13	20–87
Europe	30–41	9–14	41–55	75–176	19–34	94–205
South-east Asia	44–310	26–166	70–476	90–552	21–149	111–701
Western Pacific	23–241	9–115	33–356	44–1485	9–378	53–1862
Global	1110	511	1621	3020	713	3733

Source: Adapted from Driscoll, T. et al. 2005a. *Am J Ind Med* 48: 432–45.
Note: The ranges reflect variations in the relative wealth of different countries in the regions—see text.

TIME TRENDS

GBD estimates are available for both 1990 (Murray and Lopez, 1996) and 2010 (Lim et al., 2012), permitting consideration of temporal changes, albeit over a very short period. Overall, the estimated number of lung disease deaths due to occupational causes fell a little (from 389,462 to 370,276) between 1990 and 2010. COPD was the largest contributor in both time periods, but the proportion of occupationally related lung disease deaths due to lung cancer increased substantially (from 18% to 32%). In contrast, there was a small increase in the estimated DALYs related to occupational lung disease between 1990 and 2010 (from 13,400,000 to 13,799,000). Once again, COPD was the major contributor, but the proportion due to lung cancer increased substantially (from 13% to 19%).

CONCLUSIONS

Although beset by uncertainties and replete with assumptions, the best available evidence confirms that occupational exposures are of major importance in the global burden of lung disease; regional analyses indicate that the burden falls most heavily on the populations of western Asian countries undergoing industrial

TABLE 2.5
Deaths and Disability-Adjusted Life-Years (Thousands) from Pneumoconiosis, by Global Region in 2000

	Deaths			Disability-Adjusted Life-Years		
	Silicosis	Asbestosis	CWP	Silicosis	Asbestosis	CWP
Africa	0.2	0.2	0	8	9	0
Americas	0.1–0.5	0–0.2	0–0.5	3–20	1–11	0–12
Eastern Mediterranean	0.2–0.3	0.1–0.2	0	11–18	5–14	0
Europe	0.2–0.7	0.1–0.3	0.9–2.4	11–47	5–22	24–75
South-East Asia	0.3–1.1	0.2–1.0	0.1–0.8	10–78	8–78	1–27
Western Pacific	2.3–2.4	1.6–2.3	0.1–6.7	97–149	95–104	3–172
Global	8.8	6.7	13.8	486	376	366

Source: Adapted from Driscoll, T. et al., *Am J Ind Med* 48, 432–45, 2005a.
Note: The ranges reflect variations in the relative wealth of different countries in the regions—see text. CWP: coal workers' pneumoconiosis.

(and 'risk') transitions. This is entirely to be expected, given the history of European and North American nations that underwent very similar experiences; history, after all, teaches that people and governments have never learned anything from history. It is doubly unfortunate that discussions of non-communicable diseases in developing countries often make no mention of occupational exposures; instead, the emphasis is on personal risks such as tobacco, salt and alcohol overuse and obesity. The tragedy of this focus on lifestyle factors is that they are difficult to change, while occupational risk factors—which are of major global importance—are relatively easier to ameliorate (Pearce et al., 1994).

REFERENCES

Akgun, M., Mirici, A., Ucar, E. Y., Kantarci, M., Araz, O. and Gorguner, M. 2006. Silicosis in Turkish denim sandblasters. *Occup Med (Lond)* 56:554–8.

Burki, T. 2011. Health experts concerned over India's asbestos industry. *Lancet* 375:626–7.

Dobbs, R., Remes, J., Manyika, J., Roxburgh, C., Smit, S. and Schaer, F. 2012. *Urban World: Cities and the Rise of the Consuming Class.* London, UK: McKinsey Global Institute.

Driscoll, T., Nelson, D. I., Steenland, K., Leigh, J., Concha-Barrientos, M., Fingerhut, M. and Pruss-Ustun, A. 2005a. The global burden of non-malignant respiratory disease due to occupational airborne exposures. *Am J Ind Med* 48:432–45.

Driscoll, T., Takala, J., Steenland, K., Corvalan, C. and Fingerhut, M. 2005b. Review of estimates of the global burden of injury and illness due to occupational exposures. *Am J Ind Med* 48:491–502.

ILO. 2013. Marking progress against child labour. Global estimates and trends 2000–2012. Available at: http://www.ilo.org/wcmsp5/groups/public/—ed_norm/—ipec/documents/publication/wcms_221513.pdf.

ILO. 2015. Breaking the mould. Occupational safety hazards faced by children working in brick kilns in Afghanistan. Available at: http://www.ilo.org/ipec/Informationresources/WCMS_IPEC_PUB_25295/lang—en/index.htm.

ILO Research Department. 2015. World Employment and Social Outlook—Trends 2015. Available at: http://www.ilo.org/global/research/global-reports/weso/2015/lang—en/index.htm.

International Ban Asbestos Secretariat. 2011. Available at: http://ibasecretariat.org/index.htm.

Jamison, D., Breman, J., Measham, A., Alleyne, G., Claeson, M., Evans, D., Jha, P., Mills, A. and Musgrove, P. (eds) 2006. *Disease Control Priorities in Developing Countries.* Washington: Oxford University Press and the World Bank (co-publication).

Jindal, S. K. 2013. Silicosis in India: Past and present. *Curr Opin Pulm Med* 19:163–8.

Kjellstrom, T. and Rosenstock, L. 1990. The role of environmental and occupational hazards in the adult health transition. *World Health Stat Q* 43:188–96.

Kogan, F. 1998. Asbestos-related diseases in Russia. In D. Banks, and J. Parker, (eds), *Occupational Lung Disease; An International Perspective.* Philadelphia, PA: Chapman and Hall, pp. 247–254.

Lim, S. S., Vos, T., Flaxman, A. D., Danaei, G., Shibuya, K., Adair-Rohani, H., Amann, M. et al. 2012. A comparative risk assessment of burden of disease and injury attributable to 67 risk factors and risk factor clusters in 21 regions, 1990–2010: A systematic analysis for the Global Burden of Disease Study 2010. *Lancet* 380:2224–60.

Murray, C. and Lopez, A. D. 1996. *The Global Burden of Disease: A Comprehensive Assessment of Mortality and Disability from Diseases, Injuries, and Risk Factors in 1990 and Projected to 2020.* Geneva and Boston, MA: World Health Organization and Harvard School of Public Health. Distributed by Harvard University Press.

Nelson, D. I., Concha-Barrientos, M., Driscoll, T., Steenland, K., Fingerhut, M., Punnett, L., Pruss-Ustun, A., Leigh, J. and Corvalan, C. 2005. The global burden of selected occupational diseases and injury risks: Methodology and summary. *Am J Ind Med* 48:400–18.

Nurminen, M. and Karjalainen, A. 2001. Epidemiologic estimate of the proportion of fatalities related to occupational factors in Finland. *Scand J Work Environ Health* 27:161–213.

Pearce, N. and Matos, E. 1994a. Occupational cancer in developing countries. Introduction. In N. Pearce, E. Matos, H. Vainio, P. Boffeta and M. Kogevinas (eds), *Occupational Cancer in Developing Countries.* IARC Scientific Publications No 129. Lyon: IARC, pp. 1–3.

Pearce, N. and Matos, E. 1994b. Strategies for prevention of occupational cancer in developing countries. In N. Pearce, E. Matos, H. Vainio, P. Boffeta and M. Kogevinas (eds), *Occupational Cancer in Developing Countries.* IARC Scientific Publications No 129. Lyon: IARC, pp. 173–183.

Pearce, N., Matos, E., Vainio, H., Boffeta, P. and Kogevinas, M. 1994. *Occupational Cancer in Developing Countries.* IARC Scientific Publications No 129. Lyon: IARC.

Rushton, L., Hutchings, S. and Brown, T. 2008. The burden of cancer at work: Estimation as the first step to prevention. *Occup Environ Med* 65:789–800.

Steenland, K., Burnett, C., Lalich, N., Ward, E. and Hurrell, J. 2003. Dying for work: The magnitude of US mortality from selected causes of death associated with occupation. *Am J Ind Med* 43:461–82.

Stopford, M. 2009. *Maritime Economics 3e.* Oxford, UK: Routledge.

't Mannetje, A. and Pearce, N. 2005. Quantitative estimates of work-related death, disease and injury in New Zealand. *Scand J Work Environ Health* 31:266–76.

Ugolini, D., Bonassi, S., Cristaudo, A., Leoncini, G., Ratto, G. B. and Neri, M. 2015. Temporal trend, geographic distribution, and publication quality in asbestos research. *Environ Sci Pollut Res Int* 22:6957–67.

Varivonchik, D. V. 2014. [Epidemiologic situation in Ukraine, concerning malignant mesothelioma prevalence]. *Med Tr Prom Ekol* (1):18–22.

WHO. 2000. Silicosis. Available at http://web.archive.org/web/20070510005843/http://www.who.int/mediacentre/factsheets/fs238/en/.

3 Taking an Occupational History

Alastair Robertson, Sherwood Burge and Paul Cullinan

CONTENTS

INTRODUCTION

Few textbooks on occupational disease do not include Bernardo Ramazzini's famous exhortation from the first years of the eighteenth century:

> When a doctor arrives to attend some patient of the working class, let him condescend to sit down, if not on a gilded chair then on a three-legged stool. He should question the patient carefully … so says Hippocrates in his work '*Affections*'. I may venture to add one more question: What occupation does he follow?
>
> **Ramazzini**
> *1964*

Unhappily, it appears that Ramazzini's counsel frequently goes unheeded. Family doctors in the United Kingdom, for example, recorded an occupation in only one in seven of their patients with asthma who were of working age (Walters et al., 2012), and in Canada, 40% of patients with occupational asthma reported that a failure to enquire into their work was a major cause of the delay in their diagnosis (Poonai et al., 2005). Doctors in specialist centres seem to do no better: in the United States, an 'occupational history' was recorded in just 28% of adult inpatient case records at a tertiary centre (Politi et al., 2004), with physicians (32%) scoring little better than surgeons (23%). Notably, single-word records such as 'unemployed' or 'receiving benefits' qualified as an 'occupational history' in this survey. This uninspiring experience is repeated in many other surveys, with the result that a substantial proportion of occupational disease is unrecognised, or is diagnosed late, with important consequences for patients, employers and regulatory authorities. Quite why doctors find the matter so difficult is unclear, but it may reflect the insularity—mistaken as privacy—of the conventional doctor–patient relationship, and perhaps the socioeconomic demography of most doctors, relatively few of whom have had any experience—direct or indirect—of traditional labour. This in turn is reflected in the low priority given to occupational health in most medical school curricula, despite evidence that such training is effective (Storey et al., 2001).

Arguably, a detailed occupational history is not always necessary, although some enquiry—if only to establish context and display good manners—would seem appropriate in every first medical encounter. In the investigation of (adult) respiratory disease, the issue needs to be taken more seriously, since a substantial proportion of the caseload is directly attributable to workplace exposures, and patients with non-occupational respiratory disease frequently find that their symptoms are provoked by exposures or activities in their work, which may threaten their employment.

AN OCCUPATIONAL HISTORY: FOCUSED OR FULL?

A full occupational history requires considerable time and expertise, both of which are in short supply. It is for this reason—and to counter the difficulties described above—that some authorities advocate simple screening questions to be used by every physician caring, for example, for an adult of working age with asthma, and referral onwards for more specialist enquiry and investigation if appropriate (Fishwick et al., 2012). This approach has the virtue of pragmatism, but it does not seem unreasonable that every respiratory specialist should be confident in taking a more detailed history themselves.

With experience and a little forethought, a focused approach can be used. For many putative occupational respiratory diseases, the question is not so much 'what is this disease?' but 'what, if any, is or was its occupational aetiology?' Some diseases, such as coal workers' pneumoconiosis (CWP), are specific to occupational exposures and have a clinical (radiological) picture that is not seen otherwise. In contrast, others (lung cancer, asbestosis and chronic obstructive pulmonary disease [COPD]) are clinically indistinguishable from cases with a non-occupational cause and require a detailed consideration of work histories, while yet others fall somewhere in between these extremes. In each case, an understanding of the types and levels of exposure required to induce disease will help to focus the occupational history.

There are two broad categories of occupational causation: those that reflect cumulative exposure and those reflective of hypersensitive or toxic mechanisms. Table 3.1 separates diseases that have, in general, a cumulative exposure–response relationship from those in which the intensity of exposure is probably more important than cumulative exposure. These in turn are reflected in the usual latent periods between (first) exposure and the clinical onset of disease, thus providing a focus for enquiry into the probably relevant occupational exposures in an individual case.

By way of example, with knowledge that the usual latency for mesothelioma is approximately 40 years (and very rarely under 20 years), an occupational history would efficiently be focused on exposures incurred 30–50 years prior to diagnosis, an approach that is well supported by the epidemiology of the disease. In a study of over 600 cases of mesothelioma in the UK, the occupational risks were essentially confined to jobs held before the age of 30 years (Rake et al., 2009). The initiation of occupational lung cancer requires time for the tumour to increase in size sufficiently for detection. Tumour doubling times vary from approximately 35 days for small-cell cancers to 160 days for adenocarcinomas, meaning that exposures in the previous 3 years (small-cell cancers) to 10 years (adenocarcinomas) before detection are unlikely to be causes (Usuda et al., 1994). In contrast, for diseases in which the known latency is short—exemplified by acute hypersensitivity pneumonitis or, most obviously, by inhalation accidents—a focus can be applied to exposures that are far closer in time to their onset. Diseases with the same clinical presentation, such as asthma and alveolitis, may occur with or without a latent interval. If the disease follows the first ever exposure to an agent, the asthma is likely to be due to an irritant mechanism (acute irritant-induced asthma) or the alveolitis to one of the fume fevers (such as organic dust toxic syndrome), in which cases sensitisation should not have occurred and subsequent low-level exposures should be tolerated.

Diseases such as CWP, occupational COPD, asbestosis and asbestos-related lung cancer generally require high levels of exposure, which can only be assessed

TABLE 3.1
Categorisation of Occupational Lung Diseases Based on Their Probable Exposure Requirement and the Usual Interval between First Exposure and Disease Onset

Cumulative Exposure		Hypersensitive or Toxic	
Onset Usually During Exposure	**Onset Possible or Usual After Exposure Ceases**	**Onset Possible with First Exposure**	**Latent Interval Required**
Silicosis	Asbestosis	Acute irritant-induced asthma	Occupational asthma due to sensitisation
Coal workers' pneumoconiosis	Occupational chronic obstructive pulmonary disease	Inhalation fever	Hypersensitivity pneumonitis
Byssinosis	Occupational lung cancer	Pneumonia (*Legionella*, Q fever, etc.)	Chronic beryllium disease
	Mesothelioma	Toxic pneumonitis	Occupational rhinitis
	Benign asbestos pleural disease	Asphyxiation	

from more complete exposure histories. There have been very substantial reductions of exposures in most western countries, generally dating from around 1975, so shorter periods of exposure in earlier years relate to higher levels of cumulative exposure.

Collecting and Recording an Occupational History

The occupational history aims to identify causative exposures, but patients are on the whole better at recollecting jobs than exposures; indeed, there is good evidence that some exposures are poorly or inaccurately recollected. Patients with asthma, for example, are more likely to report, erroneously, 'dusty' occupations than those without asthma (Bakke et al., 1991). Thus, an occupational history starts with the collection of a job history, focused or otherwise as above. Understanding the jobs that patients have done can be difficult and the likely exposures they incur may not be immediately obvious. Jobs such as 'machine operator' or 'civil servant', for example, give no clues as to actual exposures. Industries and the workers in them often have their own jargon that at first can seem impenetrable, but most patients are perfectly happy to educate their doctors. Having some background knowledge of the social and industrial history of the area helps, and as consecutive patients contribute their occupational histories, it soon becomes possible to build a better understanding of the details of the industrial processes and exposures that have taken place in a particular geographical area over time. The more occupational histories that one takes, the greater becomes the appreciation of the likely exposures involved.

Case History

A 49 year old man presented with 2 years of breathlessness and a chest X-ray showing widespread nodules without mediastinal adenopathy. He had been a coal miner from 1975 to 1985 in a low-rank coal mine, and again from 1992 to 1998 without any coal face work. He had also spent 2 years fettling welded steel.

CWP would be very unlikely with just 10 years of face work exposure in a low-rank coal mine. Fettling steel could result in iron deposits in the lung (siderosis), but these can usually be distinguished radiologically because of their higher density. Further detail is needed in order to determine what he was actually doing as a miner.

From 1975 to 1977, he was a hard header. This is somebody who cuts the access tunnels to the coal seam, which involves mining through whatever strata are present, often through silica-containing rock. From 1997 to 1998, he became a mine deputy in charge of blasting the access tunnels. From 1992 to 1998, he was in charge of the maintenance of the underground roadways (tunnels), including 1 year roof bolting, where long bolts are drilled into the rock above the tunnels in order to fix roof supports. Again, this may have involved drilling into siliceous rock.

From this history, it is much more likely that his significant exposures have been to silica rather than coal dust, and that silicosis explains his radiological findings. Silicosis results from much lower cumulative exposures than coal pneumoconiosis.

Patients may need time to remember and recount their jobs, and there may be gaps where they cannot remember; friends or relatives may be helpful in this respect. Some patients, particularly those who have been self-employed, may be reluctant to declare certain jobs with high-risk exposures. Exposures can also be generated from adjacent processes, and therefore enquiry should be made about all other processes within the same work area. Understanding the details of processes is important in assessing how the exposures are being generated; for instance, in the form of a vapour, gas, dust or fume. Patients may, of course, hold more than one job at a time. Some specialists send their patients an occupational history template and request them to complete their employment history prior to their first consultation; while this practice has merits in a specialist referral clinic, it is probably not efficient in routine practice.

In some cases it is useful to enquire into control measures. These would include factors such as whether the process was enclosed or extracted or other local measures were implemented to control exposure. Enquiry should be made about respiratory protection and its nature. The type of respiratory protection needs to be appropriate for the agent and the nature of the exposure; for instance, a simple dust mask will not prevent isocyanate exposure during two-pack paint spraying. Periods where respiratory protection was worn, and more importantly periods where protection was not worn or was inappropriate, may need to be noted.

If respiratory surveillance has been carried out, then an individual's results can be requested from the employer (or their occupational health service) with appropriate consent. In some countries, including the

United Kingdom, the patient has a right of access to this information and should have been given the results after each screening. The information that is released may include the results from both a respiratory questionnaire and spirometry and, more occasionally, chest radiography. Surveillance should have been carried out at regular intervals and many years of data may be available. Using historical spirometry data can be helpful; for instance, when looking for a patient's 'normal' lung function prior to exposure or for evidence of an accelerated decline in lung function during exposure.

Identifying Exposures

With experience, the physician becomes familiar with the types, levels and natures of exposure associated with particular jobs. No physician, however, can expect to understand all types of work, and further enquiry is often necessary, as outlined below.

- With permission from the patient – not always granted – safety or occupational health personnel at the place of work may be consulted; they should be able to provide a full list of the chemicals and other agents in use and to provide details on the processes and controls in place. In many countries, this information should also be available to the employee. Discussions such as these require considerable delicacy; employees may not wish to risk being identified and employers and their representatives may take defensive positions or cite commercial confidentiality.
- Patients can be asked to bring in whatever information they have with regards to their workplace exposures. This may simply be a list of agents or a picture of whatever information can be gained from the packaging or labelling of the products. A great deal of information is now available online and, in some cases, visiting the company website can be helpful for understanding the products that are being produced and the processes used in their production. When the cause, for instance, of occupational asthma remains unclear, a written request, with suitable reassurance over confidentiality, can be made to the manufacturer or distributor of a product, requesting that all agents contained within it be identified, as this may be more than that which is routinely disclosed in the Material Safety Data Sheet (MSDS).
- Most developed countries require that employees are informed about chemicals that they are exposed to and the associated risks to their health. The information should include access to MSDSs, as well as relevant risk assessments. SDSs should list all of the chemical hazards contained within the product, as well as the likely route of absorption, the specific nature of the health hazards and the country-specific occupational exposure standards. The system of chemical hazard classification is currently in transition for compliance with the United Nations Globally Harmonised System on the classification and labelling of chemicals; this will principally affect the ways in which hazard classification and labelling are expressed (Regulation [EC] No. 1272/2008).
- Most MSDSs are readily available from the web, but while they are useful starting points for identifying potentially hazardous agents, they are not necessarily comprehensive or even accurate.

Case History

A 29 year old man was referred by an occupational physician after 'failing' respiratory surveillance. He had had deteriorating asthma over the past 9 years, with improvement on days away from work. Since leaving school at the age of 17, he had worked at a metal finishing company. For the first 2 years, he had worked on 'jigging up', which involved placing metal components onto a wire frame prior to being plated in an adjacent series of plating baths. He was then moved into the paint spraying area. He described using a number of different paints including epoxy- and polyurethane-based paints. Extraction was poor and his respiratory protection had been variable, but mostly inappropriate for working with isocyanates. Serial peak flow recordings were consistent with occupational asthma. MSDSs identified that the epoxy-containing paints and the polyurethane paints contained isocyanates. He was relocated onto the plating baths in order to be away from these exposures, but his asthma persisted. A visit to the paint manufacturer's website showed that the paints contained significant quantities of hexavalent chrome that were not mentioned within the MSDS. Subsequent inhalational challenge tests showed no reaction to the epoxy or isocyanate paints, but there was a 28% fall when exposed to potassium dichromate. Several of the plating baths contained hexavalent chrome, hence his continuing occupational asthma when relocated to this job. Two further workers with occupational asthma were identified at the same factory.

Speciation

Speciation refers to the specific physical form of a substance that influences disease causation; some examples are shown in Table 3.2. For chrome, for example, increased risks of lung cancer follow exposures to hexavalent and not trivalent forms (IARC, 1990). The increased risks of lung and nasal sinus cancers in nickel refiners were initially unexplained, and appeared to resolve spontaneously after the transfer of primary refining close to the site of mining. Many years later, increased lung cancer was found in the primary refiners of sulphide ores; sulphide ores, perhaps nickel subsulphide, are the likely carcinogens in humans, rather than metallic nickel (IARC, 1990). CWP is related to the carbon content of coal; anthracite, with the highest carbon percentage, has the highest risk, which reduces progressively as the carbon content reduces (Bennett et al., 1979). Platinum refiners have historically had one of the highest incidences of occupational asthma, which has been reduced significantly by replacing hexachloroplatinates with tetramine dihydrochlorides in catalyst manufacture (Linnett and Hughes, 1999).

Workplace Visits

Ramazzini was a proponent of physicians making visits to the workplaces of their patients:

> I have not thought it beneath me to step into workshops of the meaner sort now and again and study the obscure operations of the mechanical arts.

TABLE 3.2
Examples of Speciation Where Different Forms of a Substance Have Large Effects on the Risks of Exposure

	High Risk	Lower/No Risk
Chrome and lung cancer	Hexavalent	Trivalent
Nickel and lung cancer	Sulphide ores	Carbonate ores
Coal and pneumoconiosis	Anthracite	Brown coal
Asbestos and mesothelioma	Amphibole fibres	Serpentine fibres
Platinum and asthma	Hexachloroplatinates	Tetraamineplatinum dichloride

A visit to the workplace is often helpful for identifying the precise cause of a putative occupational respiratory disease, especially those of a short latency, such as occupational asthma or hypersensitivity pneumonitis. This particularly applies when the patient is the first from a particular workplace. In many countries, including the UK, the physician will need to make the visit, while in other countries there are occupational hygienists attached to departments of occupational medicine who are better equipped to make these visits. The consent of the patient is required before any contact is made with their employer; if there is an occupational health service, it is best to arrange the visit through them. 'Clean-ups' before visits are common, and problem processes may not be working on the day of such a visit. The main aim of a workplace visit is to identify exposures to possible causes of occupational disease; it is not the physician's job to identify negligent exposures or practices or to provide advice about remedies. Nearly all relevant exposures are by inhalation; particular attention should be paid to the area in and near to which the patient works, identifying material that can form aerosols (such as metal-working fluid, paints and electroplating baths) and vapours from volatile or heated agents (especially isocyanates, solder fluxes, welding fumes, etc.). The exposures may come from a neighbouring process, or occasionally from the ventilation system (for instance, from humidifiers in the air supply).

Workplace Visit

A 55 year old man had wheeze, chest tightness and breathlessness, which was better on holidays, since 2005. He had worked in a school as a technician in the woodwork and metalwork department since 1995. He had to saw medium-density fibreboard (MDF) regularly, did some sanding, less commonly helped set up metalwork lathes and did occasional soldering. Serial peak flow records were consistent with work-related asthma. He was admitted for specific inhalation challenges with MDF, solder fume and a cleaning solution containing benzalkonium chloride used at work; all tests were negative. A visit to his workplace showed visible mould in his office. A section of the drain pipe from the gutter one floor above was missing, resulting in penetrating water. This had been there for so long that he took no notice of it. Relocation of his office while continuing the same job resulted in resolution of his asthma.

TABLE 3.3
Studies Showing Increased Asbestos-Related Pleural Disease from Environmental Sources

Country	Fibre	Plaques (%)	Mesothelioma/ Million/Year	Source
Turkey	Erionite	65	–	Farming
	Tremolite	1–25	High	White wash
Greece: Metsovo	Tremolite	47	280	White wash
Macedonia	Tremolite	24	High	
Corsica	Tremolite	41	High	Population
Finland	Anthophyllite	6.5–9	Not increased	–
Bulgaria	Anthophyllite	Female 2.8	Not increased	Tobacco growers
	Tremolite	Male 5.6		
Austria	Tremolite	5.3	Not increased	Vineyards
South Africa	Amosite crocidolite	2.5–6.6	High	Around mine

Source: Adapted from Hillerdal, G. 1999. *Occup Environ Med* 56:505–13.

Domestic and Environmental Exposures

New cases of asthma or extrinsic allergic alveolitis in adulthood may arise from exposures in the home, commonly to new pets, hobbies or water-damaged rooms. An appropriate history should identify these as potential aetiologies.

In some cases, the jobs of any working adults sharing the childhood home should be sought, paying special attention to those working with asbestos and returning home in their working clothes. When an occupational source of asbestos has not been found in patients with asbestos pleural disease (including mesothelioma), a full list of residences and schools should be included. 'Neighbourhood' exposures to asbestos arising from industrial contamination have been responsible for pleural disease—sometimes in large numbers—in cities across the world, including in the UK (Newhouse and Thompson, 1965), Egypt (Madkour et al., 2009), Spain (Lopez-Abente et al., 2005), Japan (Kurumatani and Kumagai, 2008) and Italy (Marinaccio et al., 2015). Asbestiform exposures may also come from local soil, with exposures being sufficient to cause benign and malignant pleural disease (Table 3.3).

Case History

A man of 48 years of age has multiple pleural plaques identified on chest computed tomography undertaken during the investigation of his ischaemic heart disease. He left Cairo at the age of 28 and moved to Malta and then the UK, where he worked in the hotel trade and as a chef. He recalls no occupational exposure to asbestos. In Egypt, he spent 3 years working for a firm that bought second-hand car parts from Europe. These included brake pads and clutches, but they were always packaged and his work was confined to an office. None of those in his childhood home worked with asbestos. Detailed questioning, followed by some online enquiries, revealed that he had spent the first 23 years of his life in the Helwan district of Cairo, close to the Sigwart asbestos factory; this was the most probable explanation for his plaques.

NOTES ON SOME DISEASES

Inhalation Accidents

In cases of inhalation accident, it is not uncommon for the specialist to be taking a detailed occupational history sometime after the event. Two areas require particular attention: first is the nature of the exposure; in some cases, this will be straightforward, but in others further enquiry is necessary, in which case communication with the patient's occupational health provider or workplace safety representative may be useful. Some exposures—particularly those that arise through fire smoke—may never be characterised in any detail. Second, it is helpful to enquire into the likely intensity of the exposure. This is rarely known with any certainty, but may be inferred from: knowledge of the quantity (and its physical properties) of the material involved; the ventilation of the area in which the incident took place (including whether it was inside or outside); the duration of exposure; the nature and intensity of the initial symptoms; the nature and extent of any first aid and immediate care of the victim; and whether others were similarly affected and, if so, what their fate was.

Occupational Asthma

Most cases of occupational asthma arise from agents that are recognised to be respiratory sensitisers; exceptions occur, of course (new agents are constantly being identified), and the question of occupational asthma should occur to any physician whose patient describes symptoms that have a close temporal relationship with work. Workers may attribute their disease to an incident that took place at the time of disease onset, such as a chemical spill, whereas their asthma is more likely to be due to something to which they have been exposed without symptoms for some time. Latent intervals vary for occupational asthma arising from sensitisation; some are as short as a few weeks, but most are measured in a few months or years, and exposures within this interval prior to the onset of symptoms are likely to be the most informative. Work relatedness may be identified by asking whether symptoms are (or were initially) the same, better or worse on rest days or holidays; in long-standing cases, improvement away from work may be less obvious. In addition, patients should be asked if their symptoms are worse during or after any particular work tasks or exposures. Frequently, they are concerned over materials that are readily volatile and have a pungent odour (solvents, chlorine and industrial perfumes), but many of these are not sensitising agents. 'Work with a sensitiser' does not necessarily imply 'exposure to a sensitiser'; several diisocyanates, for example, do not vaporise at room temperature and are therefore not inhaled unless heated. Occupational asthma rarely occurs in isolation, and patients should be asked whether they have regular surveillance and whether any colleagues have (had) similar symptoms.

Inhalation Fevers

In most cases of inhalation fevers, polymer fume, metal fume and organic dusts, an occupational exposure can be readily identified as the cause, usually by the individual(s) affected. However, aerosol exposures from humidification systems may be more difficult in terms of identifying an exposure. While localised humidification (spinning disc humidifiers) or wall air-conditioning units are visible to the employees and their maintenance can be checked, central humidification is 'invisible' and, in most outbreaks of humidifier fever, poorly maintained. In cases presenting with symptom patterns consistent with humidifier fever who work in an air-conditioned building, the building manager or the firm's occupational physician should be approached by the employee or preferably by the specialist consultant and asked to provide details of the ventilation system and request an opportunity to view the system.

Asbestos Diseases

Asbestosis and lung cancer arising from asbestos exposure require heavy exposures over long periods of time. In Europe and parts of the world with similar industrial histories, exposures to asbestos declined markedly over the second half of the twentieth century (Table 3.4), resulting in incident disease becoming increasingly less common in these locations.

Pleural diseases (benign and malignant) arising from asbestos exposure can be caused by far lower levels of exposure, which may be more difficult to detect without a careful occupational history. Increasingly, these

TABLE 3.4
Typical Asbestos Exposures in German Industry 1950–1990—Estimates are of Airborne Fibre Concentrations (Fibres/cm^3) in Former 'West' and 'East' Germany

	1952		1972		1980		1990	
Manufacture of Asbestos	**'West'**	**'East'**	**'West'**	**'East'**	**'West'**	**'East'**	**'West'**	**'East'**
Textiles	100	100	10	12	4	6	0.9	2.2
Gaskets	60	60	7	8	5	8	0.7	1.6
Cement	200	200	11	13	1	2	0.3	0.7
Brake pads	150	150	9	11	1	2	0.7	1.6
Insulation	15	18	15	18	9	14	0.2	0.5

Source: Adapted from Hagemeyer, O., Otten, H. and Kraus, T. 2006. *Int Arch Occup Environ Health* 79:613–20.

diseases reflect exposure to 'secondary' sources of encountering asbestos; for example, in the refurbishment of commercial or domestic buildings by building labourers, carpenters, electricians and plumbers, who may not be aware of the extent (or even existence) of their exposure. Asbestos-related pleural diseases (with the possible exception of benign effusion) generally require at least 15 years between first exposure and identifiable disease.

Extrinsic Allergic Alveolitis

A diagnosis of extrinsic allergic alveolitis (EAA) may be suspected from a typical history of symptoms in an individual with a recognised exposure, commonly a farmer, bird breeder or metal turner. In many other cases, EAA is only suspected after a computed tomography scan, and a detailed occupational and environmental history is then taken. EAA requires allergic sensitisation, which commonly takes several years of regular exposure to develop. A detailed smoking history is also relevant here, as EAA is uncommon in smokers. Cases of EAA have, however, been reported to have developed within a year of quitting smoking and in individuals who have kept birds for many years without symptoms.

Identifying the causative exposure in EAA is crucial, as prognosis is significantly better where further contact can be prevented. In some cases, this may be very obvious (e.g. during an outbreak of EAA from a single factory), whereas in other cases, the cause remains obscure even after a visit to the home and workplace. The relationship between symptoms and particular exposures varies widely and is easier to recognise in acute EAA a few hours after a heavy exposure to an organic dust than with chronic decline over several years of low-level exposure. A history of improvement away from work or away from home on a 2–3-week holiday should be sought.

In terms of identifying potential causes, the majority relate to avian proteins or microbial contamination of either an organic dust or a water-containing material. Any process in the home or workplace that involves these should be enquired into in detail, followed by any other identifiable exposures to dusts, fumes, vapours or mists. A screening checklist of common causative exposures is used by some centres and covers rarer causes, such as contact with domestic moulds or damp; use of hot-tubs, saunas or humidifiers; exposure to feathers from pillows and duvets; and the use of waterproofing sprays.

Outbreaks of EAA have been reported in a number of work environments, usually due to microbial contamination of metalworking fluids, humidifiers, air conditioners or swimming pools. A good occupational history will include whether there are similarly exposed co-workers with known alveolitis or undiagnosed symptoms, and whether the employer is aware of the problem.

REFERENCES

Bakke, P., Eide, G. E., Hanoa, R. and Gulsvik, A. 1991. Occupational dust or gas exposure and prevalences of respiratory symptoms and asthma in a general population. *Eur Respir J* 4:273–8.

Bennett, J. G., Dick, J. A., Kaplan, Y. S., Shand, P. A., Shennan, D. H., Thomas, D. J. and Washington, J. S. 1979. The relationship between coal rank and the prevalence of pneumoconiosis. *Br J Ind Med* 36:206–10.

Fishwick, D., Barber, C. M., Bradshaw, L. M., Ayres, J. G., Barraclough, R., Burge, S., Corne, J. M. et al. 2012. Standards of care for occupational asthma: An update. *Thorax* 67:278–80.

Hagemeyer, O., Otten, H. and Kraus, T. 2006. Asbestos consumption, asbestos exposure and asbestos-related occupational diseases in Germany. *Int Arch Occup Environ Health* 79:613–20.

Hillerdal, G. 1999. Mesothelioma: Cases associated with non-occupational and low dose exposures. *Occup Environ Med* 56:505–13.

IARC. 1990. *Chromium, Nickel and Welding, IARC Monographs on the Evaluation of Carcinogenic Risks to Humans*, vol. 49. Lyon: IARC.

Kurumatani, N. and Kumagai, S. 2008. Mapping the risk of mesothelioma due to neighborhood asbestos exposure. *Am J Respir Crit Care Med* 178:624–9.

Linnett, P. J. and Hughes, E. G. 1999. 20 years of medical surveillance on exposure to allergenic and non-allergenic platinum compounds: The importance of chemical speciation. *Occup Environ Med* 56:191–6.

Lopez-Abente, G., Hernandez-Barrera, V., Pollan, M., Aragones, N. and Perez-Gomez, B. 2005. Municipal pleural cancer mortality in Spain. *Occup Environ Med* 62:195–9.

Madkour, M. T., El Bokhary, M. S., Awad Allah, H. I., Awad, A. A. and Mahmoud, H. F. 2009. Environmental exposure to asbestos and the exposure–response relationship with mesothelioma. *East Mediterr Health J* 15:25–38.

Marinaccio, A., Binazzi, A., Bonafede, M., Corfiati, M., Di Marzio, D., Scarselli, A., Verardo, M. et al. 2015. Malignant mesothelioma due to non-occupational asbestos exposure from the Italian national surveillance system (ReNaM): Epidemiology and public health issues. *Occup Environ Med* 72:648–55.

Newhouse, M. L. and Thompson, H. 1965. Mesothelioma of pleura and peritoneum following exposure to asbestos in the London area. *Br J Ind Med* 22:261–9.

Politi, B. J., Arena, V. C., Schwerha, J. and Sussman, N. 2004. Occupational medical history taking: How are today's physicians doing? A cross-sectional investigation of the frequency of occupational history taking by physicians in a major US teaching center. *J Occup Environ Med* 46:550–5.

Poonai, N., Van Diepen, S., Bharatha, A., Manduch, M., Deklaj, T. and Tarlo, S. M. 2005. Barriers to diagnosis of occupational asthma in Ontario. *Can J Public Health* 96:230–3.

Rake, C., Gilham, C., Hatch, J., Darnton, A., Hodgson, J. and Peto, J. 2009. Occupational, domestic and environmental mesothelioma risks in the British population: A case–control study. *Br J Cancer* 100:1175–83.

Ramazzini, B. 1964. *Diseases of the Workers (De Morbis Artificum Diatriba, 1713)*. W. C. Wright (Translator). New York, NY: Hafner.

Regulation (EC) No. 1272/2008 of the European Parliament and of the Council of 16 December 2008 on classification, labelling and packaging of substances and mixtures, amending and repealing Directives 67/548/EEC and 1999/45/EC, and amending Regulation (EC) No. 1907/2006 *Official Journal of the European Union* L 353/1, 31.12.2008.

Storey, E., Thal, S., Johnson, C., Grey, M., Madray, H., Hodgson, M. and Pfeiffer, C. 2001. Reinforcement of occupational history taking: A success story. *Teach Learn Med* 13:176–82.

Usuda, K., Saito, Y., Sagawa, M., Sato, M., Kanma, K., Takahashi, S., Endo, C. et al. 1994. Tumor doubling time and prognostic assessment of patients with primary lung cancer. *Cancer* 74:2239–44.

Walters, G. I., McGrath, E. E. and Ayres, J. G. 2012. Audit of the recording of occupational asthma in primary care. *Occup Med (Lond)* 62:570–3.

4 Respiratory Function Tests in Occupational Lung Disorders

John Gibson

CONTENTS

SCOPE AND ROLES OF RESPIRATORY FUNCTION TESTS

Tests of respiratory function are commonly used in the diagnosis, assessment and monitoring of respiratory symptoms and disease. Their role in specific diagnosis usually depends on pattern recognition, with the results supporting or excluding a particular condition or group of conditions. One exception to this generalisation is asthma, for which demonstration of the characteristic variability of airway function may be diagnostic in itself. Breathing tests are also used to detect impaired function, to quantify its severity and to aid location of the likely anatomical site(s) of disease (e.g. airway, lung parenchyma, pulmonary vasculature, etc.). Sequential spirometric measurements are frequently employed in order to monitor the progress of disease and the response to treatment, and in many conditions they give useful information on the prognosis.

In the occupational context, respiratory function tests are of particular value in recognising occupational asthma, in assessing the severity of pneumoconioses and, using longitudinal measurements, in identifying an abnormal rate of decline (i.e. greater than would be expected from the normal effects of ageing) due to potentially hazardous exposures.

The commonly used tests are conveniently grouped into those of respiratory mechanics, pulmonary gas exchange and exercise. In the workplace, tests of forced expiration using a portable spirometer are by far the most commonly used, because of their simplicity of performance and equipment, reproducibility and high information content. Other tests will be described only briefly. For detailed accounts of individual tests, their performance and interpretation, the reader is referred to guidelines produced by the American Thoracic Society and European Respiratory Society (MacIntyre et al., 2005; Miller et al., 2005a,b; Pellegrino et al., 2005; Wanger et al., 2005).

TESTS OF RESPIRATORY MECHANICS

The volume of air in the lungs at the end of a tidal expiration at rest (functional residual capacity [FRC]) represents the 'neutral' volume of the thorax (i.e. the volume pertaining when the respiratory muscles are inactive). Expansion of the lungs above FRC is achieved by contraction of the inspiratory muscles (predominantly the diaphragm), while, in health, resting tidal expiration is essentially passive, with the driving force provided by elastic recoil of the lungs. The main expiratory muscles are those of the abdominal wall; their contraction increases abdominal pressure, which is transmitted to the thorax. The expiratory muscles become active when ventilation is increased markedly, as upon exercise or during coughing, when high intrathoracic pressure aids the clearance of airway secretions.

Measurements of Static Lung Volumes

A spirometer records only the air that can be displaced from the lungs, with the unmeasured residual volume (RV) remaining in the lungs after full expiration (Wanger et al., 2005). The maximum volume that can be expired after a full inspiration (or inspired after a full expiration) is known as the vital capacity (VC) or, if measured during forceful expiration, the forced VC (FVC); in health, these are effectively the same, but in subjects with more severe airway disease, VC often exceeds FVC. The total lung capacity (TLC) represents the volume of air in the lungs after full inspiration—the sum of VC and RV (Figure 4.1). Two main clinical methods are used for the measurement of absolute lung volume: inert gas dilution and whole-body plethysmography. Because of the nature of the equipment, the latter is essentially laboratory based, but transportable versions of the former are occasionally used.

Inert Gas Dilution

From a closed circuit, the subject rebreathes a gas mixture containing an inert marker gas such as helium. This gradually equilibrates with the air in the lungs so that its concentration falls progressively and stabilises once mixing is complete. In a healthy individual, this occurs in less than 10 minutes, but in patients with diffuse airway disease such as asthma or chronic obstructive pulmonary disease (COPD), equilibration is much slower due to uneven ventilation, and the end point may be much less definite. The volume measured is that in the lungs upon connecting the subject to the circuit (usually the

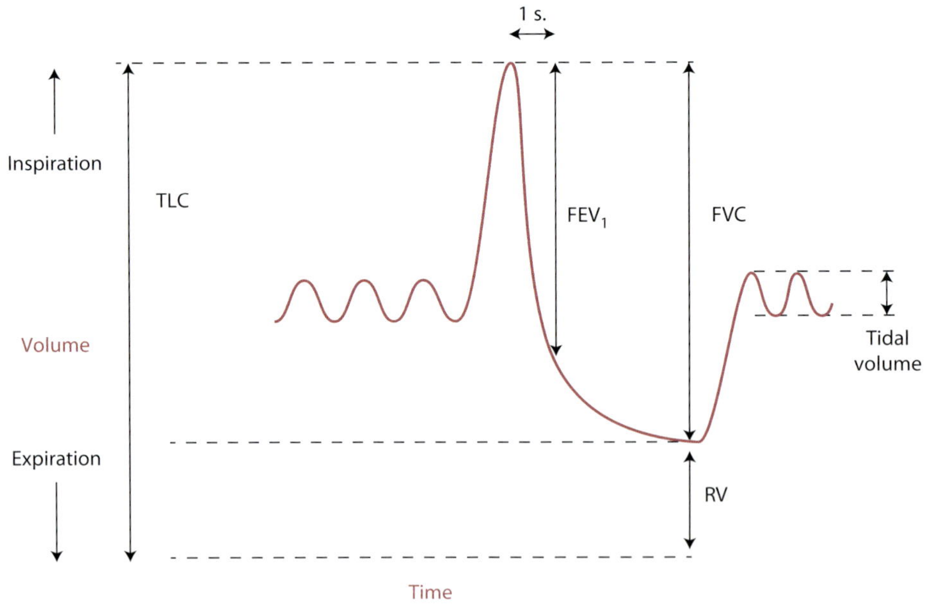

FIGURE 4.1 Schematic static and dynamic lung volumes with volume inspired and expired plotted against time. The subject has taken three tidal breaths, followed by an inspiration to total lung capacity (TLC) and then a forceful maximal expiration. The volume expired in the first second of the forced expiration is the FEV_1 and the maximum expired is the forced vital capacity (FVC). In healthy subjects, FVC is effectively the same as the vital capacity (VC); in patients with more severe airway obstruction, VC often exceeds FVC). At the end of the maximal expiration, the lungs contain the residual volume (RV).

FRC). After disconnection, the subject inspires fully and the volume inspired when added to the FRC gives the TLC, from which subtraction of VC gives RV (Figure 4.1). With moderate or severe airway disease, the uneven distribution of the inspired gas and poor mixing in the lungs cause underestimation of lung volumes.

Whole-Body Plethysmography

The subject, seated within an air-tight rigid chamber, makes gentle breathing efforts against a shutter that closes the airway at the mouth. According to Boyle's law, as intrathoracic pressure falls during an inspiratory effort, the air in the lungs is rarefied and lung volume increases by a small amount. This causes the pressure in the rigid plethysmograph to increase, with the converse occurring during expiratory efforts; the thoracic gas volume is derived from the pressure changes after calibrating the instrument by measuring the rise in pressure accompanying the introduction of a measured volume of air. Immediately upon opening the shutter, the TLC and RV are derived by having the subject take a full inspiration and expiration. This method measures the volume of any air spaces within (or without) the lung that share the pressure changes occurring during breathing efforts; consequently, poorly ventilated areas of lung (or even those that are totally unventilated, such as a bulla) are included.

Measurements During Forced Expiration

The strengths of forced expiratory tests include the simplicity of both the manoeuvre and equipment required, as well as the relative independence of the measurements of the effort applied by the patient (Miller et al., 2005b). Inevitably, forced expiratory tests are effort dependent to the extent that a preceding full inspiration is required. However, during forced expiration, the larger intrathoracic airways are subject to dynamic compression by the surrounding pleural pressure and, provided a modest effort is applied, increasing the effort merely compresses the airway further and produces no increase in flow. This relative effort independence is more marked as forced expiration proceeds, and is also more marked in patients with airway obstruction than in healthy subjects. Maximum expiratory flow is, however, more dependent on effort at higher lung volumes (i.e. closer to full inflation). Since peak expiratory flow (PEF) is attained very rapidly at the start of forced expiration, it is more effort dependent than the forced expiratory volume in 1 second (FEV_1), which effectively integrates flow over a large proportion of the expired volume. PEF is measured with a simple peak flow meter and is often used in the workplace in order to investigate suspected occupational asthma.

Spirometry: Volume Expired Versus Time

Although originally the term 'spirometry' referred to the measurement of any volume breathed in or out, it is now effectively synonymous with measurements made during forced expiration, of which the FEV_1—the volume expired forcefully in 1 second after full inspiration (Figure 4.1)—is the most commonly used. It is usually obtained together with the FVC, which is the maximum volume expired during a forced expiration.

The characteristic feature of diffuse airway obstruction is slowing of the rate of expiration, so that the ratio of FEV_1 to FVC (the forced expiratory ratio) is reduced. In symptomatic airway disease, FVC is usually reduced, but the reduction is proportionally less than that in FEV_1.

In patients with airway obstruction, the measurements are often repeated a few minutes after inhalation of a short-acting bronchodilator (usually two puffs from a pressurised aerosol). The bronchodilator response is expressed as the increase in FEV_1, either as an absolute value or a percentage increase. A large increase (e.g. 0.4 L or more) suggests probable asthma, but smaller increases are non-diagnostic, as patients with airway narrowing of other causes (e.g. COPD) usually show some response (as do healthy subjects as well). Equally, a 'negative' result does not exclude asthma.

Maximum Flow–Volume Curves

Maximum expiratory flow–volume (MEFV) curves (Figure 4.2) are obtained during the same manoeuvre as FEV_1 and, indeed, contain the same information, albeit displayed in a different fashion. Forceful expiration of the FVC may be followed by maximal inspiration in order to give the maximum inspiratory flow–volume (MIFV) curve. Older spirometers responded too slowly to allow accurate measurement of instantaneous flow, but modern portable devices readily allow accurate display of flow against volume expired and inspired. Unlike the MIFV curve, which typically has a symmetrical semi-circular appearance, the MEFV curve has a characteristic flow peak early in expiration (equivalent to the PEF recorded by a peak flow meter), followed by a progressive decline in maximum flow as volume is expired (Figure 4.2). In young healthy subjects (Figure 4.2a), the descending limb of the curve approximates a straight line, whilst in older normal subjects (Figure 4.2b), maximum flow is lower, particularly in the latter part of forced expiration, and the curve becomes concave to the volume axis. Notably, in patients with diffuse airway obstruction (such as COPD or asthma),

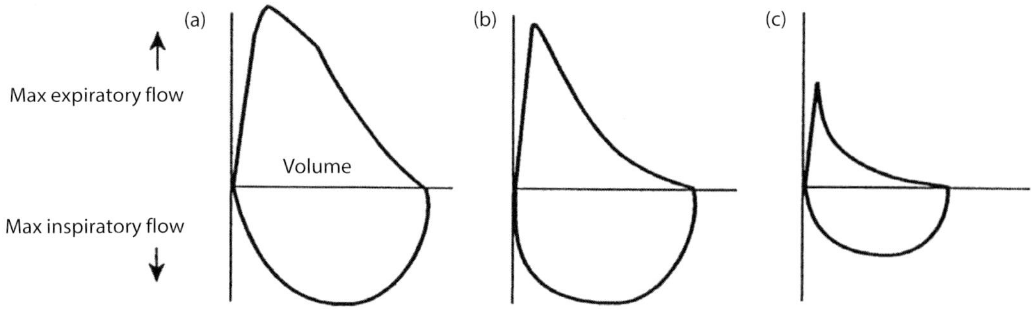

FIGURE 4.2 Schematic maximum expiratory and inspiratory flow–volume curves in (a) a normal young adult, (b) a normal middle-aged or elderly adult and (c) a patient with severe chronic obstructive pulmonary disease. The expiratory curve shows a characteristic early peak, equivalent to the peak expiratory flow (PEF) recorded by a peak flow meter. In (a), the down-stroke of the expiratory curve is almost a straight line, while in the older individual (b), it shows concavity towards the volume axis, with slightly lower PEF and forced vital capacity (the displacement on the volume axis). The inspiratory curve has a more symmetrical appearance. The abnormalities seen in (c) are an exaggeration of the normal age-related change (i.e. greatly diminished maximum expiratory flow, more marked concavity of the curve and much smaller forced vital capacity); maximum inspiratory flow is also reduced, but less markedly.

the appearance is qualitatively similar to that of healthy ageing, although greatly exaggerated, with expiratory flow reduced more markedly as lung volume declines (Figure 4.2c).

The shape of the flow–volume curve does not distinguish between different causes of diffuse airway narrowing and so does not enable the distinction of asthma from COPD or emphysema. In theory, measurements of maximum expiratory flow in the latter part of forced expiration should be more sensitive to milder degrees of airway narrowing. In practice, however, use of indices such as maximum flow after 75% of the FVC has been expired (FEF_{75}) has proved disappointing because the very wide normal range seriously reduces its discriminating power. Another widely used measurement is the average maximum flow over the central 50% of expiration (FEF_{25-75}; formerly known as maximum mid-expiratory flow). Again, however, the value of this index is seriously compromised by its wide variation in the healthy population and also by its dependence on VC, such that subnormal values are not specific for airway disease.

Restrictive and Obstructive Ventilatory Defects

Classically, two patterns of abnormality of mechanical function of the lungs are described in disease: restrictive and obstructive. The hallmark of a *restrictive* ventilatory defect is an abnormally low TLC; this may be due either to shrinkage of the lungs themselves (intrapulmonary restriction) or to limitation of full inflation of the lungs by factor(s) outside the lungs (extrapulmonary restriction). A restrictive defect is seen in numerous conditions, in particular, in the context of occupational lung disease, diffuse pulmonary fibrosis or extensive pleural disease (effusion or diffuse pleural thickening). Characteristically, a restrictive defect is accompanied by approximately proportional reductions in FEV_1 and FVC, such that the ratio of FEV_1 to FVC remains normal (or may be a little above normal). However, this pattern is not necessarily specific for a restrictive defect, as it can occur in some individuals with mild airway disease, causing an increase in RV such that TLC is normal.

An *obstructive* ventilatory defect is characteristic of diffuse airway narrowing, as in COPD, asthma and widespread bronchiectasis; it is recognised by a reduction below normal in the forced expiratory ratio, although a normal ratio can accompany significant disease of the smaller airways. Patients with diffuse airway disease also typically develop marked increases in RV and TLC and in the ratio of RV to TLC. A large increase in TLC is characteristic of emphysema, but is not specific for this condition; an increase is also common in asthma, even in relative remission.

While a low ratio of FEV_1 to FVC indicates the *presence* of airway obstruction, it is usually a poor guide to its *severity*, which is better assessed by comparing the FEV_1 alone with relevant normal reference values (see below).

Combined obstructive (low FEV_1/FVC) and restrictive (low TLC) defects are not uncommon, either because of dual pathology or because some diseases can affect both airways and lung parenchyma. Sometimes TLC may be within the normal range due to opposing influences with, for example, lung fibrosis tending to reduce it and airway obstruction tending to increase it.

Airway and Respiratory Resistance

Although forced expiratory tests assess airway calibre only indirectly, they are adequate for most purposes. Direct measurement of airway or respiratory resistance demands more sophisticated equipment and, in general, the results have poorer reproducibility than forced expiratory measurements.

Direct measurement of airway resistance (R_{AW}) requires estimation of both airflow (easy) and the pressure difference along the airway between the alveoli and mouth (technically demanding). The most commonly used technique for estimating alveolar pressure is body plethysmography, as used for measuring lung volumes (see above), with which measurement of R_{AW} can be combined. Resistance measurements require the subject to make gentle panting efforts with the airway unobstructed, as well as against a shutter at the mouth.

R_{AW} falls as lung volume increases due to an expanding effect of more negative pleural pressure and the increased tension in the lung tissue surrounding the intrapulmonary airways. R_{AW} is often expressed as its reciprocal, airway conductance (G_{AW}), which, in turn, can be divided by the lung volume at which it is measured to give the specific G_{AW}, which largely allows for the variation of G_{AW} with volume.

The resistance of the airway is dominated by its narrowest part, which in the healthy individual is the upper airway (larynx and trachea). Although individual airways become progressively smaller towards the periphery of the lung, the effect of this on total R_{AW} is greatly outweighed by the considerable increase in their number with sequential branching; consequently, the overall cross-sectional area of the airways increases towards the alveoli. Since COPD has its greatest impact on peripheral airways, plethysmographic measurements of R_{AW} are not sensitive to the earlier stages of the disease. As with measurement of lung volumes, plethysmographic measurement of R_{AW} is impracticable for fieldwork, although it is sometimes used in laboratory-based challenge tests, especially in subjects with initially normal function.

An alternative and increasingly popular method for evaluating airway function is the use of forced oscillation (Oostveen et al., 2003; Goldman and Saadeh, 2005). This technique involves superimposition of small oscillating pressures at the mouth during tidal breathing, with the pressure produced by a sinusoidal generator oscillating at different frequencies (e.g. a loudspeaker) or by an impulse generator. The resulting varying pressure and flow measured at the mouth are used to compute the total respiratory resistance; in this context, the measurement includes the mechanical behaviour not only of the airways, but also of the lung tissue and chest wall. Oscillation at different frequencies has been shown to generate characteristic patterns depending on the site(s) and severity of airway narrowing. The technique uses portable equipment and requires little cooperation from the subject, as measurements are made during resting quiet breathing. It can show abnormal function with disease of the peripheral airways even when spirometric volumes are normal. It may also be particularly helpful in subjects who are unable to cooperate sufficiently for reproducible forced expiratory measurements.

TESTS OF PULMONARY GAS EXCHANGE

Arterial Blood Gases and Oxygen Saturation

The main roles of the lungs are to maintain normal blood oxygenation and to remove carbon dioxide (CO_2), with the latter also maintaining normal acid–base balance. Classically, the efficacy of pulmonary gas exchange is assessed by the arterial pH and the partial pressures of oxygen (PaO_2) and CO_2 ($PaCO_2$). Alternatively, oxygenation can be measured simply and non-invasively using a pulse oximeter clipped over a finger. This gives a valid estimate of arterial oxygen saturation (designated SpO_2 when measured by pulse oximetry), which represents the proportion of oxygen binding sites on haemoglobin occupied by oxygen (normally 96%–98%). The relationship between the partial pressure and percentage saturation of oxygen in the blood is described by the classical sigmoid-shaped haemoglobin–oxygen dissociation curve (Figure 4.3). In health, blood gases and oxygen saturation are maintained within narrow limits, with the only common cause of normal variation being altitude, which reduces the PO_2 of inspired air and, therefore, also reduces PaO_2 and SaO_2.

The chemical combination of oxygen with haemoglobin creates a considerable functional 'reserve' of oxygen in the blood; this comes into play, for example, during exercise, when the increased metabolic demands are met by the exercising muscles extracting a greater proportion of the oxygen supplied by the arterial blood. This reduces the oxygen in the venous blood returning to the heart, but in health has no effect on the arterial PO_2 or saturation. In general, resting arterial blood gas measurements are relatively insensitive to mild–moderate lung disease, but a fall in oxygenation with exercise is sometimes used to detect early functional impairment or assess its severity. Elevation of $PaCO_2$ (hypercapnia) is seen only in advanced disease (usually very severe airway obstruction).

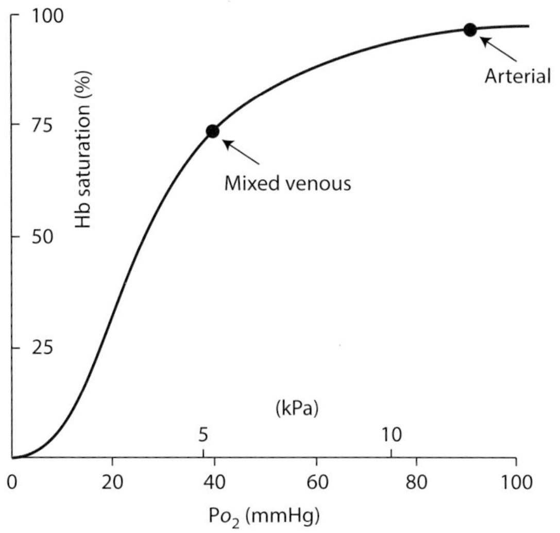

FIGURE 4.3 The sigmoid-shaped haemoglobin (Hb)–oxygen dissociation curve showing the relationship between the partial pressure of oxygen in blood and the percentage saturation of Hb. Arrows indicate typical arterial and mixed venous (pulmonary arterial) values in a healthy subject at rest. Normal arterial saturation is 96%–98%; the curve shows how even small reductions below this range are accompanied by relatively greater falls in arterial PO_2. At rest, the blood returning to the heart still has a relatively high oxygen saturation of approximately 75%; this important 'reserve' of oxygen in the blood is utilised during exercise when the metabolising muscles extract more oxygen and venous saturation falls.

Carbon Monoxide Uptake

Carbon monoxide (CO) diffusing capacity (D_LCO) (also known as the transfer factor [T_LCO]) is widely used as a simple test of the integrity of the alveolar–capillary membrane and the overall gas exchanging capacity of the lungs (MacIntyre et al., 2005). The sensitivity of D_LCO to disease is relatively good but its specificity is poor, as impairment can result from several pathological mechanisms, including uneven distribution of inspired air or pulmonary blood flow and reduction in surface area or thickening of the alveolar walls.

The rate of uptake of CO is measured during a single breath hold for 10 seconds following full inspiration of a gas mixture containing a very low concentration of CO. In most situations, the most important factor determining CO uptake is the 'effective' surface area of alveoli available for gas exchange. Thus, D_LCO is reduced, for example, after surgical removal of lung tissue, but it is also reduced with widespread emphysema, as the terminal air spaces are much larger than normal, with a consequently greatly diminished area. D_LCO is also reduced when there is loss of the 'effective' alveolar volume (V_A) in which the test gas is distributed (e.g. in diffuse airway obstruction of any cause when the distribution of inspired gas is inevitably more uneven than normal). The inspired test gas also includes an inert gas (usually helium); since CO and helium are distributed similarly, comparison of inspired and expired helium concentrations enables the calculation of the 'effective' V_A that has been exposed to the CO. The transfer coefficient (KCO) represents the uptake of CO per litre of 'effective' V_A:

$$\text{i.e.}\quad KCO = \frac{D_LCO}{V_A}$$

Assessing both D_LCO and KCO improves the specificity of the former. For example, following surgical resection of the lung, both D_LCO and V_A are reduced, but KCO is typically normal or increased.*

In asthma, KCO is usually normal (or sometimes mildly increased), as any reduction in D_LCO is due only to an uneven distribution of ventilation secondary to airway narrowing. By contrast, in widespread emphysema, D_LCO is reduced due not only to maldistribution of inspired gas, but also because, even in the better-ventilated parts of the lung, the total surface area of the alveoli is diminished. Consequently, in emphysema, KCO is also reduced. Reductions in both D_LCO and KCO are also characteristically seen in pulmonary fibrosis and pulmonary vascular disease.

Notably, both indices are dependent on the blood haemoglobin concentration; this should be checked if D_LCO is measured and a simple arithmetic correction is made if the subject is anaemic. If the subject fails to take a full inspiration prior to the measurement, or if full inflation of the lungs is impeded due to disease outside of the lungs (e.g. very extensive pleural thickening), D_LCO may be somewhat reduced, but KCO is typically greater than the predicted value because, although the alveolar surface area at full inflation is less than normal, the density of pulmonary capillaries per litre of V_A is greater than it would be at a normal TLC.

EXERCISE TESTS

The respiratory (as opposed to cardiological) indications for exercise testing include evaluation of breathlessness, assessment of disability and assessing the likely factors limiting performance.

* The higher-than-normal value of KCO is due to a disproportion between alveolar and pulmonary capillary blood volumes resulting from unchanged overall blood flow through a reduced capillary bed; the resulting greater density of red blood cells in the remaining pulmonary capillaries results in higher CO uptake per litre of functioning lung.

In health, the maximum oxygen consumption (maximum aerobic capacity) is determined by the ability of the circulation to supply oxygen to exercising muscle, rather than by the maximum ventilation that can be achieved. In patients with significant lung disease, however, the maximum attainable ventilation is reduced approximately in proportion to the mechanical abnormality. The maximum attainable ventilation may then come to determine exercise capacity, although circulatory factors and deconditioning often also contribute.

Exercise tests vary considerably in complexity, ranging from detailed laboratory-based measurements of respiratory and cardiovascular performance to simple walking tests that are suitable for field use (Holland et al., 2014). The latter include the 6-minute walk test, a self-paced test in which the subject is asked to walk as far as possible in 6 minutes along a measured level route such as an internal corridor; this has the disadvantages of relative insensitivity to mild disease and, inevitably, is dependent on motivation. An alternative is the incremental shuttle walk test, an externally paced progressive exercise test in which the subject increases his or her walking speed in response to a series of pre-recorded signals until he or she is no longer able to continue; this gives more reproducible results than the 6-minute walk test. In the endurance shuttle walk test, which is a derivative of the incremental test, the subject walks for as long as possible at a predetermined percentage of his or her maximum performance as determined in a preceding incremental shuttle walk.

A simple exercise test can also be used for the identification of exercise-induced asthma. During exercise, most individuals with asthma show bronchodilatation, while with exercise-induced asthma, bronchoconstriction typically develops *after* a brief period of exercise (this should be distinguished from the breathlessness *during* exercise, which affects many asthmatic individuals with impaired respiratory function). In susceptible individuals, the intensity of exercise necessary to provoke asthma is relatively high and, for this reason, exercise-induced asthma is relevant mainly to children and young adults. Optimally, it is demonstrated after exercising for at least 5 minutes at a constant rate that has been chosen to increase ventilation to approximately 50% of maximal or to increase heart rate to approximately 80% of maximal. FEV_1 or peak flow should be measured beforehand and for up to 30 minutes afterwards.

NORMAL AND ABNORMAL

To determine whether a breathing test result is 'normal' or 'abnormal' requires comparison with an appropriate reference range from a healthy population. The main contributors to variation within the healthy population are sex, age, height and ethnicity. For the most commonly used indices, FEV_1 and FVC, larger values are seen in males and in taller individuals, while results decline with age from the mid-20s, and most non-white ethnic groups have values of between 5% and 20% lower than whites. Moderate or severe obesity, which is seen increasingly in Western societies, also reduces spirometric volumes. Posture (seated or sitting) has a very small effect, but this may be relevant for longitudinal monitoring, when a consistent recording posture should be used.

Modern automated spirometers usually incorporate a choice of reference equations based on sex, age, height and sometimes ethnicity, from which mean predicted values and standard deviations (SDs) are calculated. Those responsible for interpreting results need to be aware of the default settings of the equipment and the limitations of the equations being used. Globally, more than 300 reference equations for spirometric volumes have been published, but none is universally applicable. The most commonly used in Europe have been the summary equations originally derived for the European Coal and Steel Community (Quanjer et al., 1993). As these take no account of ethnicity, it has been conventional with results from non-Caucasian individuals to apply a proportional reduction to predicted values of spirometric and static lung volumes, most commonly multiplying by 0.88. Variation due to ethnicity is gradually being incorporated into reference equations such as the National Health and Nutrition Examination Survey (NHANES) III equations now recommended for use in North America (Hankinson et al., 1999) and those derived by the ongoing Global Lung Function Initiative of the European Respiratory Society (ERS) (Quanjer et al., 2012).

Inevitably, the level at which an individual result is considered 'abnormal' is somewhat arbitrary. The historical method of expressing individual results as a percentage of the mean predicted value and considering values between 80% and 120% predicted as 'normal' is not valid. Rather, the deviation of a given result from the mean predicted value should be viewed in light of the SD of results for that test in the reference population. The number of SDs by which the result deviates from the mean predicted is the 'standardised residual' or 'z score' (e.g. a measured value of 1 SD less than the mean predicted has a z score of −1). Defining the limits of normality represents a balance between the sensitivity and specificity of the test: if narrow limits are set, the test becomes more sensitive but less specific, while wider limits have the converse effect. For respiratory function tests, the limits of normality are usually set

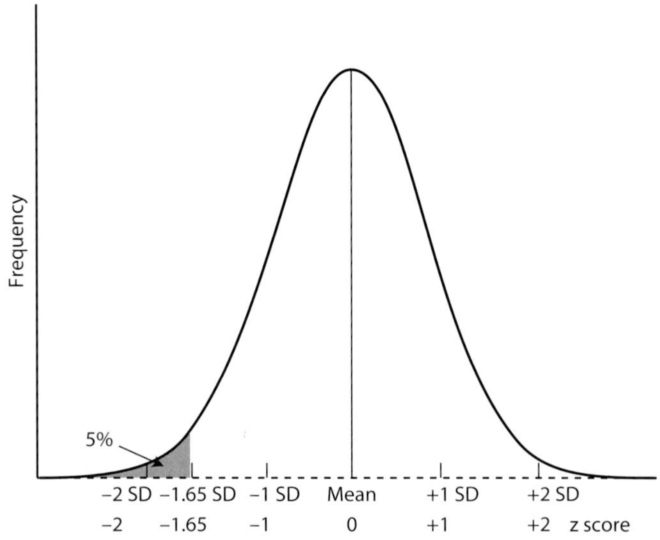

FIGURE 4.4 Schematic normal distribution in the population of, for example, forced expiratory volume in 1 second. The range from approximately +1.65 to −1.65 standard deviations (SDs) encompasses 90% of the results, leaving 5% with values above and 5% below. The lower limit of normal is usually taken as more than 1.65 SD below the mean predicted, but 1 in 20 of the healthy population would be expected to have results in this 'abnormal' range (false positives). The standardised residual (z score) is the number of SDs by which a given result deviates from the mean predicted value.

by z scores of between −1.65 and +1.65 (sometimes abbreviated to +/−1.65) which, with a normal distribution, encompasses 90% of the healthy population (Figure 4.4). For spirometric indices, the 5% of values above 'normal' are unlikely to be of interest, but it is important to appreciate that using this compromise implies that 5% of the healthy population have results that would be classified as abnormally low.

One contentious area of interpretation relates to defining a normal ratio of FEV_1 to FVC, a point of considerable importance as abnormal airway narrowing (airway obstruction) is defined by this ratio. Many authorities use a ratio of <0.7 as a blanket cut-off indicating airway obstruction. While this has the apparent advantage of simplicity (and is incorporated in some diagnostic criteria for identifying COPD), it ignores the normal age-related decline in the ratio. Many healthy elderly individuals have values of <0.7, so its use as a cut-off between 'normality' and 'abnormality' results in significant overdiagnosis of COPD in subjects older than 60 years of age. On the other hand, a value of FEV_1/FVC of 0.7 in a 25 year old would be very abnormal, so its use also risks failure to recognise significant airway obstruction in young adults. The alternative—and preferred—approach is to use appropriate reference data for the FEV_1/FVC ratio in order to define the limits of normality with which to compare the z score in the same manner as for other measurements.

PRACTICAL APPLICATIONS IN OCCUPATIONAL MEDICINE

Longitudinal Monitoring of Spirometry

Sequential monitoring of respiratory function in the workplace is usually based on measurements of FEV_1 repeated at intervals in order to detect an abnormally rapid rate of decline from initial baseline measurements (Hnizdo et al., 2010; Redlich et al., 2014). If monitoring for slowly developing conditions such as COPD or pneumoconiosis, testing every 2–3 years may suffice, whereas with exposure to potential occupational causes of asthma, shorter intervals of 6–12 months are recommended. With long-term monitoring, it is important to take account of the normal age-related decline of FEV_1. In middle-aged non-smokers, the average rate of decline is approximately 30 mL per year, but it is appreciably greater in smokers. Self-evidently, the greater the intrinsic variability ('noise') of the measurement, the more difficult it is to detect a true decline ('signal'). Since relatively small changes are being sought in surveillance spirometry, it is particularly important to minimise background noise by careful attention to detail; this implies adequate training of personnel, accurate calibration and consistency of equipment and subject posture (either seated or standing). Even with optimal procedures and conditions of testing, variation of FEV_1 over the short to medium term is approximately 4%. Various methods have been proposed in order to define abnormal decline, the most common being a reduction of >15% from the baseline, after taking account of the expected average age-related decline. Alternatively, the within-subject SD can be calculated from the earlier measurements of FEV_1 as a reference against which to judge subsequent decline. In order to establish an accurate baseline variability, it may therefore be helpful to record FEV_1 more frequently over the first couple of years of surveillance. In practice, accurate determination of the rate of decline of FEV_1 is likely to take 5–8 years. Consequently, only relatively large declines are identifiable in the early years, but the sensitivity of the method improves with the duration of surveillance. Computer software to aid analysis of longitudinal measurements is available (National Institute for Occupational Safety and Health); this also helps with the recognition of unexpected excess variability and thus improves quality control.

Workplace Peak Flow Monitoring

Self-monitoring of PEF is widely employed for the diagnosis or exclusion of occupational asthma, offering ease of use, portability and sequential measurements during and after realistic exposure to potential sensitisers (Fishwick et al., 2008; Tarlo et al., 2008; Moore et al., 2010). As mentioned above, PEF is intrinsically more dependent on effort than other forced expiratory tests, so a learning effect is to be expected and careful instruction is necessary. At least three recordings of PEF should be made on each occasion, and the highest two should differ by <20 L/minute. Some devices incorporate a data logger, which reduces the risk of fabrication of results. Measurements should be made frequently (e.g. every 2 hours) throughout the working day, and continued at home in order to detect a late asthmatic reaction. The recommended minimum period of recording for detecting a work-related change is 4 weeks, with at least 1 week away from work. Care needs to be taken in order to ensure that the same meter is used throughout the monitoring period, that asthma treatment remains as constant as possible during work and non-work days and that any respiratory infections are noted.

Several patterns of peak flow variation are recognised as suggestive of, or compatible with, occupational asthma (Moore et al., 2010). These include: (i) a rapid fall in PEF shortly after arriving at work; (ii) a delayed decrease occurring later in the working day or after leaving work; (iii) a progressive decrease over the working week; and, rarely, (iv) a pattern of tolerance with a marked fall in PEF on the first working day which becomes less as the working week progresses. Subsequent recovery may be either rapid (within a few hours of leaving work) or delayed (taking several days to return to baseline values).

There is no consensus on how best to evaluate the results but, most commonly, a typical pattern is identified by visual inspection by an expert in occupational asthma. The recordings can be analysed statistically (e.g. by comparing mean PEF or diurnal variation of PEF on work and non-work days). Analysis can be aided by computer software such as Oasys (Occupational Asthma SYStem). When independent methods such as workplace challenge or specific inhalation challenge are used as the reference for diagnosis, computer-aided diagnosis has a slightly lower sensitivity but higher specificity than expert visual analysis. Using computer software has the additional advantage of minimising observer variation, and it can be used by non-experts (Moore et al., 2010).

Inhalation Challenge Tests

Bronchial challenge testing includes: testing with nonspecific agents (most commonly methacholine) in order to detect nonspecific airway reactivity; monitoring the airway response to exposure under normal working conditions; and laboratory testing with specific work-related agents that are suspected of causing occupational asthma. Inhalation challenge should not be performed in individuals with more severe airway obstruction; a pre-challenge FEV_1 of >70% predicted is usually taken as a precondition for safe challenge. Prior to challenge, bronchodilators, etc., should be withheld according to the duration of action of the individual agents. FEV_1 is by far the most common measurement that is used to assess responses; occasionally, resistance/conductance measurements by either plethysmography or forced oscillation may give complementary information.

Nonspecific Inhalation Challenge

Bronchoconstriction following inhalation of various directly or indirectly acting agents is a characteristic feature of asthma in general, and challenge testing is routinely used in some centres in order to measure airway responsiveness in diagnosis and monitoring (American Thoracic Society, 2000; Cockcroft, 2003). Previously, histamine was used as the challenge agent, but most laboratories now favour methacholine due to its fewer side effects. Two main inhalation techniques are used: in the tidal breathing method, the subject inhales a solution of methacholine via a jet nebuliser and facemask or mouthpiece for 2 minutes at each increasing concentration; while with the dosimeter method, the subject takes a sequence of five slow, full inspirations, each followed by a breath hold for 5–10 seconds. Inhalation of the active agent is preceded by inhalation of saline or the diluent alone in order to give baseline measurements of FEV_1. Methacholine is inhaled in increasing (usually doubling) concentrations with a constant time interval (usually 5 minutes) between doses. At 30 and 90 seconds after each dose, FEV_1 is re-measured; in order to avoid fatigue from repeated measurements, it is acceptable to curtail the forced expiration after 1 second. The procedure continues until either a fall of FEV_1 of 20% from baseline is reached or the highest concentration has been inhaled. Bronchial responsiveness is measured in terms of either the provocative concentration (PC_{20}) or provocative dose (PD_{20}) that produces a 20% fall in FEV_1, with graphical interpolation between measurements if necessary. PD_{20} is increasingly preferred to PC_{20} as it allows for more valid comparison between methods (Cockcroft, 2015).

In occupational practice, demonstration of greater nonspecific bronchial responsiveness following a period of exposure compared to a period of absence from the workplace is suggestive of occupational asthma.

Specific Inhalation Challenge

Specific inhalation challenge is generally regarded as the most definitive ('gold standard') diagnostic test for occupational asthma; it is usually preceded by workplace monitoring that has shown a suspected response (Vandenplas et al., 2014). The individual is then exposed in a controlled fashion under laboratory conditions to the agent under suspicion. The aim is gradually to increase exposure to the relevant chemical, with conditions and the degree of exposure being as close as possible to those encountered in the workplace. In order to allow for the effect of nonspecific bronchial responsiveness and spontaneous variation of airway function, the test day should be preceded by a control day during which the subject is exposed to an appropriate inert control substance. Where feasible, on both the control and challenge days, asthma treatment should be withheld according to the duration of action of the individual agent. If the control day results in a reduction in FEV_1 exceeding 10%, the active challenge should be deferred until the asthma has stabilised. The dose of the suspected agent is increased by increasing either the duration of exposure or the concentration of the agent with monitoring of FEV_1. The test is usually considered positive if there is a sustained fall in FEV_1 of at least 15% from the pre-challenge value and provided that fluctuations of FEV_1 were <10% on the control day. If FEV_1 falls by >10% but <15%, it should be re-measured in order to confirm resolution before further exposure. Patients should be monitored with periodic measurement of FEV_1 in the laboratory for 6–8 hours post-challenge, after which self-monitoring of FEV_1 or PEF should continue for a total of 24 hours. False-negative results can occur if the potential cause of occupational asthma is chosen incorrectly or if the amount or form of the agent is not comparable with the workplace exposure.

If the suspected pulmonary reaction is alveolar as well as—or rather than—in the airways, additional monitoring of D_LCO and SaO_2 may be helpful.

Measurement of nonspecific airway responsiveness pre- and post-challenge is a useful adjunct, as increased responsiveness despite no change in baseline function is suggestive of a response.

Patterns of Abnormality in Disease

Some individuals with symptoms that are potentially related to occupational exposure are likely to undergo detailed evaluation in a respiratory function laboratory. As mentioned in the introduction, the interpretation of pulmonary function tests and their use in differential diagnosis often depend on pattern recognition. Table 4.1 shows some typical patterns that are relevant to occupational disease, but the examples shown should not be regarded rigidly, as test results in many individuals are less clear cut. Furthermore, mixed patterns are quite common, especially in a smoking population. Optimal interpretation requires consideration of many other factors in addition to the results themselves, with the most relevant including the type and duration of exposure, the subject's smoking status and radiographic and computed tomography scan appearances.

TABLE 4.1
Typical Patterns of Respiratory Function Tests Relevant to Occupational Medicine

Disease	FEV_1	FVC	FEV_1/FVC	TLC	RV	D_LCO	KCO
COPD[a]	Reduced	Mildly reduced	Reduced	Increased	Increased	Reduced	Reduced
Asthma[a]	Reduced/normal	Mildly reduced/normal	Reduced/normal	Increased	Increased	Normal/mildly reduced	Normal/increased
Pulmonary fibrosis (e.g. asbestosis)	Reduced	Reduced	Normal	Reduced	Normal	Reduced	Reduced/normal
Diffuse pleural thickening	Reduced	Reduced	Normal	Reduced	Normal	Mildly reduced	Increased/normal

Abbreviations: FEV_1: forced expiratory volume in 1 second; FVC: forced vital capacity; TLC: total lung capacity; RV: residual volume; D_LCO: carbon monoxide diffusing capacity; KCO: carbon monoxide transfer coefficient.

[a] Depending on severity of airway narrowing.

REFERENCES

American Thoracic Society. 2000. Guidelines for methacholine and exercise challenge testing—1999. *Am J Respir Crit Care Med* 161:309–29.

Cockcroft, D. W. 2003. Bronchoprovocation methods. *Clin Rev Allergy Immunol* 24:19–27.

Cockcroft, D. W. 2015. Methacholine challenge: PD_{20} versus PC_{20}. *Ann Am Thorac Soc* 12:291–2.

Fishwick, D., Barber, C. M., Bradshaw, L. M., Harris-Roberts, J., Francis, M., Naylor, S., Ayres, J. et al. 2008. Standards of care for occupational asthma. *Thorax* 63(3):240–50.

Goldman, M. D., Saadeh, C. and Ross, D. 2005. Clinical applications of forced oscillations to assess peripheral airway function. *Respir Physiol Neurobiol* 148:179–94.

Hankinson, J. L., Odencrantz, J. R. and Fedan, K. B. 1999. Spirometric reference values from a sample of the general U.S. population. *Am J Respir Crit Care Med* 159:179–87.

Hnizdo, E., Glindmeyer, H. W. and Petsonk, E. L. 2010. Workplace spirometry monitoring for respiratory disease prevention: A methods review. *Int J Tuberc Lung Dis* 14:796–805.

Holland, A. E., Spruit, M. A., Troosters, T., Puhan, M. A., Pepin, V., Saey, D., McCormack, M. C. et al. 2014. An official European Respiratory Society/American Thoracic Society technical standard: Field walking tests in chronic respiratory disease. *Eur Respir J* 44(6):1428–46.

MacIntyre, N., Crapo, R. O., Viegi, G., Johnson, D. C., van der Grinten, C. P. M., Brusasco, V., Burgos, F. et al. 2005. Standardisation of the single-breath determination of carbon monoxide uptake in the lung. *Eur Respir J* 26(4):720–35.

Miller, M. R., Crapo, R., Hankinson, J., Brusasco, V., Burgos, F., Casaburi, R., Coates, A. et al. 2005a. General considerations for lung function testing. *Eur Respir J* 26(1):153–61.

Miller, M. R., Hankinson, J., Brusasco, V., Burgos, F., Casaburi, R., Coates, A., Crapo, R. et al. 2005b. Standardisation of spirometry. *Eur Respir J* 26(2):319–38.

Moore, V. C., Jaakkola, M. S. and Burge, P. S. 2010. A systematic review of serial peak flow measurements in the diagnosis of occupational asthma. *Ann Respir Med* 1:31–44.

National Institute for Occupational Safety and Health. Spirometry long term data analysis (SPIROLA) software v3.0.2. Available at: http://www.cdc.gov/niosh/topics/spirometry/spirola-software.html (accessed 28 March 2014).

Oostveen, E., MacLeod, D., Lorino, H., Farre, R., Hantos, Z., Desager, K., Marchal, F. and ERS Task Force on Respiratory Impedance Measurements. 2003. The forced oscillation technique in clinical practice: Methodology, recommendations and future developments. *Eur Respir J* 22(6):1026–41.

Pellegrino, R., Viegi, G., Brusasco, V., Crapo, R. O., Burgos, F., Casaburi, R., Coates, A. et al. 2005. Interpretative strategies for lung function tests. *Eur Respir J* 26(5):948–68.

Quanjer, P. H., Stanejovic, S., Cole, T. J., Baur, X., Hall, G. L., Culver, B. H., Enright, P. L. et al. 2012. Multi-ethnic reference values for spirometry for the 3–95-yr age range: The global lung function 2012 equations. *Eur Respir J* 40(6):1324–43.

Quanjer, P. H., Tammeling, G. J., Cotes, J. E., Pedersen, O. F., Peslin, R. and Yernault, J. C. 1993. Lung volumes and forced expiratory flows. *Eur Respir J* 6(Suppl. 16):5–40.

Redlich, C. A., Tarlo, S. M., Hankinson, J. L., Townsend, M. C., Eschenbacher, W. L., Von Essen, S. G., Sigsgaard, T. et al. 2014. Official American Thoracic Society technical standards: Spirometry in the occupational setting. *Am J Respir Crit Care Med* 189(8):983–93.

Tarlo, S. M., Balmes, J., Balkissoon, R., Beach, J., Beckett, W., Bernstein, D., Blanc, P. D. et al. 2008. Diagnosis and management of work-related asthma. *Chest* 134(3 Suppl.):1S–41S.

Vandenplas, O., Suojalehto, H., Aasen, T. B., Baur, X., Burge, P. S., de Blay, F., Fishwick, D. et al. 2014. Specific inhalation challenge in the diagnosis of occupational asthma: Consensus statement. *Eur Respir J* 43(6):1573–87.

Wanger, J., Clausen, J. L., Coates, A., Pedersen, O. F., Brusasco, V., Burgos, F., Casaburi, R. et al. 2005. Standardisation of the measurement of lung volumes. *Eur Respir J* 26(3):511–22.

5 Non-Invasive Methods for Assessing the Respiratory Tract in Occupational Lung Disease

Bronchoalveolar Lavage and Induced Sputum

Mona Lärstad and Anna-Carin Olin

CONTENTS

BRONCHOALVEOLAR LAVAGE

Bronchoalveolar lavage (BAL), performed via flexible bronchoscopy, is a useful and commonly implemented tool in clinical diagnosis and in research. The technique uses a flexible fibrescope and was introduced in the late 1960s and gained widespread acceptance as a minimally invasive method that provides important information about immunologic, inflammatory and infectious processes taking place at the alveolar level (Meyer et al., 2012). As early as 1974, a seminal article reporting the application of BAL in the study of secretions obtained from the human lung was published by Reynolds and Newball, introducing BAL as a research tool (Reynolds and Newball, 1974). The use of BAL involves a fibre optic bronchoscope for washing sub-segments of the lung with sterile physiological saline in order to sample components from the peripheral air spaces (Haslam and Baughman, 1999). The lung epithelium is lined with the epithelial lining fluid (ELF) which can be sampled by a saline wash (BAL) of the area of interest. BAL is a valuable tool for assessing complex pathogenic mechanisms involving the lower respiratory tract, as well as characterizing the effects of specific exposures, both occupational and environmental. Furthermore, BAL provides information that may be helpful for characterizing the prognosis and response to therapy in a variety of lung diseases. Beyond microbiological sampling, the mediators or agents that can be measured include: immune and inflammatory cells; pathological cells or features; cytokines, enzymes, lipids, nucleic acids or other secreted products; and inhaled environmental or occupational agents (if they are retained). For both research and routine applications, a standardized BAL procedure should be followed in order to minimize differences due to the dilution factor from the lavage, as well as many other potential sources of variability (Haslam and Baughman, 1999). The BAL technique requires trained personnel who can perform the procedure correctly. Minor clinical complications can include cough, chest pain and shortness of breath or fever, with major—albeit uncommon—complications including bronchospasm, laryngospasm and, with concomitant biopsy, pneumothorax and haemoptysis. Furthermore, repeated or serial BAL is a cause of airway inflammation in itself, not limited to the site of first lavage and characterized by increased proportions of inflammatory cells in BAL (mainly neutrophils) (von Essen et al., 1998).

Despite its degree of invasiveness, BAL has been used in occupational medicine for quite some time, particularly as an assessment tool in mineral dust-associated diseases such as asbestos and talc pneumoconiosis (Karjalainen et al., 1994; Scancarello et al., 1996; Vathesatogkit et al., 2004; Kokkinis et al., 2011). Characteristic cytological features of the above-mentioned patient groups are asbestos bodies and talc bodies, respectively, in the cells (Haslam and Baughman, 1999). Other BAL findings in asbestos-exposed individuals have shown moderate increases in neutrophils with or without increased eosinophils or lymphocytes. In a study of coal workers' pneumoconiosis, BAL cytokine and antioxidant enzyme level increases were related to disease status (Ulker et al., 2008). In silica, the amount of alveolar silica particles in different forms of silicosis has been studied by BAL (Moreira et al., 2005). Patients manifested an increase in BAL silica particles compared to controls; when comparing simple to complicated silicosis, however, no significant difference was observed. In acute silicosis, with massive silica dust exposure, more than 70% of BAL alveolar macrophages contained silica particles. When duration of exposure and retirement from work were evaluated, an inverse correlation between duration of exposure and the amount of alveolar dust was found, and there was a trend of less involvement of macrophages with a greater period since retirement from work. These results suggest that particle analysis in BAL may be important in order to establish the nature and intensity of exposure. In a report by Schuyler et al. (1980), patients with complicated silicosis who had been working as sandblasters were investigated by BAL. The patients had last been exposed to silica 1–12 years prior to lavage. Compared to controls, no differences were detected in cell number, viability, adherence or ability to phagocytize and kill *Listeria monocytogenes*, but significantly increased numbers of type II pneumocytes were present in lavage samples from the patients with silicosis.

Another occupational lung disease that has been investigated using BAL is chronic beryllium disease (CBD). Beryllium exposure leads to cell-mediated immunological sensitization in a small percentage of workers exposed to beryllium aerosols, dusts or fumes, and of the sensitized workers, many develop a granulomatous disease (Kreiss et al., 1997). There is a blood test referred to as the beryllium lymphocyte proliferation test that measures beryllium-specific T-cell-proliferative responses in the blood of beryllium-exposed workers (Tinkle et al., 1999; Newman et al., 2005). This test can be used to detect both beryllium sensitization and CBD. Among workers identified as having beryllium sensitization, clinical evaluation with BAL is used to confirm the diagnosis of CBD (Newman et al., 2005). This subject is covered at greater length elsewhere in this text.

BAL has also been used to in the diagnosis of parenchymal immuno-inflammatory conditions such as hypersensitivity pneumonitis (HP). This condition can arise from a wide variety of occupational as well as environmental exposures. Bird fancier's lung, which is typically avocational rather than from salaried employment, is one of the most common types of HP, for which BAL classically shows greater than 25% lymphocytosis with a CD4:CD8 ratio of less than 1.0 and greater than 1% mast cells in the acute phase (Chan et al., 2012). In a study by Tsushima et al. (2001) of HP in the mushroom industry, employees exposed to buna-shimeji spores underwent BAL. The percentages of lymphocytes, macrophages and neutrophils in BAL fluid were significantly different between the exposed group and controls. In four of the exposed subjects with HP, the CD4:CD8 ratio was less than 1.0 in BAL fluid. Another common type of HP occurs in farmers. In a study by Behr et al. (2000), the number of neutrophils in BAL fluid was increased in farmer's lung (FL) patients as compared to asymptotic farmers. The concentrations of total and reduced glutathione (GSHT and GSH, respectively) in ELF were decreased in FL patients and increased in asymptotic farmers. Pig farmers working in large swine-confinement buildings are exposed to high concentrations of respirable dust particles containing feed and faecal particles, dander from pigs, bacteria, fungi, endotoxins and gases, such as hydrogen sulphide and ammonia (Pedersen et al., 1996). Larsson et al. (1992) reported that the concentrations of total cells and granulocytes were increased, as well as the concentrations of albumin, fibronectin and hyaluronan, in BAL samples from pig farmers. Pedersen et al. (1996) showed that young, large-scale pig farmers had a significantly increased percentage of lymphocytes and neutrophils, and that their alveolar macrophages showed biological signs of activation, compared to controls.

BAL has also been used in experimental air-pollution models in which, for example, exposure to diesel particles was investigated (Ghio et al., 2012). Exposure to air pollution in road tunnels has been studied, and BAL results showed increased levels of inflammatory cells (Larsson et al., 2007). This is also likely to be relevant to those exposed occupationally to diesel combustion by-products. Exposure to water-damaged buildings has been shown to cause an increase of lymphocytes in BAL from patients who are referred to an indoor air health clinic (Wolff et al., 2009), findings that could be relevant to indoor air occupational exposure scenarios. In a study in which BAL samples from food-grain workers were analysed, aflatoxins (metabolites from *Aspergillus* moulds) were detected in 33% of the samples compared to in 9% of non-food-grain workers, and a significant difference was also found in BAL fluid that was cultured for *Aspergillus* growth (Malik et al., 2014).

To conclude, BAL provides cells and solutes from alveolar lung regions and, in selected protocols, selectively from the airways, as well as yielding information that is relevant to the assessment of the health status of the lung in different occupational and environmental settings. BAL can facilitate the diagnosis of lung disease, but is also useful as a research tool. More scientific observations using BAL from individuals with diseased and/or affected small airways will likely continue to be forthcoming. Nonetheless, even though BAL is an important method in assessing the respiratory tract, it is too invasive to be used routinely in occupational monitoring. To address this, techniques that are less invasive have been developed. These can be complementary to BAL findings or, in some cases, can substitute for BAL altogether.

INDUCED SPUTUM

Analysis of induced sputum (IS) has emerged as a very valuable tool for characterizing the inflammatory pattern in the respiratory tract after exposure to high- and low-molecular-weight agents (Malo et al., 2011), but also for recognizing different endotypes of responses (inflammatory and otherwise) in occupational respiratory diseases (Quirce et al., 2010). IS likely reflects predominantly, but not exclusively, the larger airways.

The European Respiratory Society's task force on sputum induction in 2002 agreed upon general principles for a standard protocol for sputum induction (Paggiaro et al., 2002). These include safety and performance considerations, with a goal of consistency and reduced variability similar to BAL standardized protocols. There is also a specific IS protocol for persons at higher risk from the procedure, which is predominantly excessive cough and bronchospasm.

It is recommended that sputum be processed as soon as possible or within 2 hours in order to ensure optimum cell counting and staining. The volume of the IS sample is determined and then mixed with an equal volume of 0.1% dithiothreitol for homogenization in order to enable correct identification of cells. Filtration through a nylon mesh is commonly used to remove mucus and debris. The sample is spun in a centrifuge to separate sputum cells from the fluid phase. Centrifugal forces used in studies to date have ranged from 300 to 1500 × g and the duration of centrifugation from 5–10 minutes. After centrifugation, the cell-free supernatant is aliquoted and can be stored at −80°C until analysis. The cell pellets are re-suspended and the distribution of the different cell types can be analysed.

There are a number of potential endpoints that can be studied using IS. The differential count is the most common way to analyse the IS sample. It provides information on whether there is an increase in eosinophils or neutrophils in the sample, and can be presented both as absolute (i.e. the number of cells present) and relative (%) amounts of cell types.

Sputum induction has also been used to study soluble mediators of inflammatory pathways after various exposures. Concentrations of a number of biomarkers can be analysed in the supernatant of the IS; for example, those associated with eosinophilic inflammation, such as eosinophil cationic protein, and neutrophilic inflammation (elastase), as well as lipid mediators (leukotrienes), proteinases (tryptase and matrix metallopeptidases), nitrite/nitrate and cytokines (IL-1β, IL-5, IL-6, IL-8, TNF and VEGF). Data on the within-individual reproducibility of these measures are scarce, partly due to the difficulties in reliably repeating IS, as the method in itself can induce airway inflammation.

Interestingly, recent data suggest that IS also can be used to quantify the burden of particle exposure, as described by Fireman et al. She and her co-workers have developed a method for analysing shape, size and burden of particles in IS. This is achieved by using a laser technique to assess particle size and shape (Fireman et al., 2015). The results suggest that particles in the size of 2–3 μm in IS are related to the inhaled cumulative dose.

There is also a potential role for IS in assessing occupational asthma (OA). In the diagnosis of OA, specific inhalation challenge (SIC) is the reference test in many countries and has contributed to an increased knowledge of the disease. The SIC technique can induce an immediate, late or dual asthmatic reaction, defined by the pattern of forced ejection volume in 1 second (FEV_1) after challenge, where a 20% drop in FEV_1 is defined as a positive test. It is generally believed that low molecular weight (LMW) agents induce a late reaction (but this is not always the case), whereas high molecular weight (HMW) substances may induce any of the asthmatic reaction types, likely depending on individual host factors and perhaps previous exposure. SIC has been used in combination with IS to potentially yield new insights into the inflammatory response following exposure. In parallel with spirometric changes, the influx of inflammatory cells into the airways may have certain time kinetics, but these are difficult to elucidate with sequential testing, given that if IS is repeated within 6 hours, it itself induces inflammatory changes, as already noted.

In combination with SIC, IS has been used to classify the effects of exposure to a large variety of substances that have the potential to induce asthma, in terms of both LMW and HMW agents. In a retrospective study by Malo et al. (2011), data from 519 subjects who underwent SIC testing for the suspected diagnosis of OA were analysed. When including all examined subjects, the positive predictive value (PPV) and negative predictive value (NPV) for identifying subjects with OA were similar for change in sputum eosinophils as for change in the provocative concentration, causing a 20% fall in FEV_1 (PC_{20}) after SIC. In order to discriminate OA from other forms of asthma, the measure of increased levels of eosinophils in IS performed better than PC_{20} (PPV 44% vs. 35%, NPV 58% vs. 30%). Interestingly, on a control non-exposure day, increased levels of sputum eosinophils were only found in half of the patients diagnosed with OA, and as many as 27% had normal bronchial hyper-responsiveness, pointing to the lack of sensitivity of these methods for diagnosing OA when ongoing exposure may have ceased.

Vandenplas et al. (2009) have investigated whether adding IS after SIC improves the predictive value of the test as compared to post-SIC lung function testing alone. Sixty-eight consecutive patients with respiratory symptoms suggestive of OA were examined with SIC. They were first challenged with a sham agent and then challenged up to three or more times with the suspected agent, and both HMW and LMW agents were included. IS and histamine challenge tests were performed 6–8 hours after the end of each challenge each day. Thirty-nine out of 68 subjects had a positive SIC. Receiver–operator curve analysis indicated that an increase in sputum eosinophils after the first challenge had the highest discriminating power for predicting a positive response to SIC. An increase of at least 3% in IS eosinophils achieved the best combination of specificity (97%) and sensitivity (67%) for the diagnosis of OA. This suggests that a specific endotype (i.e. eosinophilic airway inflammation) is associated with bronchoconstriction independently of type of exposure.

Sputum induction has been used to study inflammatory pathways more specifically after various exposures. Hur et al. (2008) studied IS after challenge with methylene diphenyl diisocyanate (MDI) in 13 MDI-exposed workers with respiratory symptoms and two controls. Exposure was associated with mast cell activation, as indicated by an increase in tryptase, IL-8 and VEGF in IS, as well as eosinophilic activation.

In a study by Lemiere et al. (2010), 19 subjects with diagnoses of OA after a SIC test were followed at 2 weeks, 6 months and 1, 2, 3 and 4 years after diagnosis and examined with IS, spirometry and metacholine challenge test at each time point. Thirteen subjects had OA due to HMW agents and 11 subjects had OA due to LMW agents. In this study, there was no significant improvement in clinical parameters, but inhaled steroids were stopped in nine subjects, and among the rest, the dose was decreased. Subjects with a neutrophilic predominance in sputum after SIC at diagnosis had a worse prognosis and there was an inverse correlation between eosinophil counts at diagnosis and PC_{20} at 3 years after removal from exposure. Subjects having less than 2% increases in eosinophils by IS, but reacting with an increase in neutrophils after SIC challenge, also had significantly lower lung function (FEV_1 predicted 81.3% vs. 89.2%) after 4 years.

Occupational eosinophilic bronchitis is believed to be a diagnostic entity that is distinct from OA, in which IS plays a particular diagnostic role. Eosinophilic bronchitis is defined as chronic cough in patients with no symptoms or objective evidence of variable airflow obstruction or non-specific airway hyper-responsiveness, and yet manifesting sputum eosinophilia (Brightling, 2010). Data on the prevalence of occupational eosinophilic bronchitis are limited (Pala et al., 2012) and the diagnosis may be missed when IS is not performed.

Despite its usefulness, IS has its pitfalls as well. One major limitation with the IS method is that it is rather cumbersome and time consuming to perform and hence not suitable in many screening situations (e.g. as a surveillance tool). When analysing differential cell counts, the samples have to be prepared within 2 hours after sampling, and the handling is not straightforward. This has meant that IS can be used only rarely in the natural exposed environment (i.e. at the worksite), but rather is used in exposure challenge studies. It may also be difficult to achieve a representative sample (i.e. reflecting the lining fluid of the airways and not merely saliva).

Another major limitation with the method of IS is that approximately 20% of subjects cannot produce an adequate sputum sample. The method in itself also irritates the airways and gives rise to neutrophilic influx, reducing the possibility of performing repeated sampling within the same subject, as noted above (Holz et al., 1998), even though it seems safe to repeat the test within 24 hours (Quirce et al., 2010). Hence, methodological aspects make it difficult to repeat the test in order to identify when maximal inflammatory response of exposure occurs. This also limits the possibilities of examining the reproducibility of the results. Short-term variability (2 days) in cell counts in subjects with stable asthma have been shown to be moderate to good (in 't Veen et al., 1996; Rossall et al., 2014).

In summary, IS has been used in occupational medicine mainly to assess airway inflammation after SIC, and in that context, it does provide insight into inflammatory patterns and mechanisms, as well as improving diagnostic accuracy. An interesting new approach of IS is to use it to quantify the cumulative exposure burden of inhaled particles, which is also crucial for the diagnosis of eosinophilic bronchitis, a diagnosis that has been associated with occupational exposures. Major limitations remain, most notably that IS is cumbersome to perform and that it is not possible to elicit sputum samples in approximately one in five persons tested.

REFERENCES

Behr, J., Degenkolb, B., Beinert, T., Krombach, F. and Vogelmeier, C. 2000. Pulmonary glutathione levels in acute episodes of Farmer's lung. *Am J Respir Crit Care Med* 161:1968–71.

Brightling, C. E. 2010. Cough due to asthma and nonasthmatic eosinophilic bronchitis. *Lung* 188(Suppl. 1):S13–7.

Chan, A. L., Juarez, M. M., Leslie, K. O., Ismail, H. A. and Albertson, T. E. 2012. Bird fancier's lung: A state-of-the-art review. *Clin Rev Allergy Immunol* 43:69–83.

Fireman, E., Bliznuk, D., Schwarz, Y., Soferman, R. and Kivity, S. 2015. Biological monitoring of particulate matter accumulated in the lungs of urban asthmatic children in the Tel-Aviv area. *Int Arch Occup Environ Health* 88:443–53.

Ghio, A. J., Smith, C. B. and Madden, M. C. 2012. Diesel exhaust particles and airway inflammation. *Curr Opin Pulm Med* 18:144–50.

Haslam, P. L. and Baughman, R. P. 1999. Report of ERS task force: Guidelines for measurement of acellular components and standardization of BAL. *Eur Respir J* 14:245–8.

Holz, O., Richter, K., Jorres, R. A., Speckin, P., Mucke, M. and Magnussen, H. 1998. Changes in sputum composition between two inductions performed on consecutive days. *Thorax* 53:83–6.

Hur, G. Y., Sheen, S. S., Kang, Y. M., Koh, D. H., Park, H. J., Ye, Y. M., Yim, H. E. et al. 2008. Histamine release and inflammatory cell infiltration in airway Mucosa in methylene diphenyl diisocyanate (MDI)-induced occupational asthma. *J Clin Immunol* 28:571–80.

in 't Veen, J. C., De Gouw, H. W., Smits, H. H., Sont, J. K., Hiemstra, P. S., Sterk, P. J. and Bel, E. H. 1996. Repeatability of cellular and soluble markers of inflammation in induced sputum from patients with asthma. *Eur Respir J* 9:2441–7.

Karjalainen, A., Anttila, S., Mantyla, T., Taskinen, E., Kyyronen, P. and Tukiainen, P. 1994. Asbestos bodies in bronchoalveolar lavage fluid in relation to occupational history. *Am J Ind Med* 26:645–54.

Kokkinis, F. P., Bouros, D., Hadjistavrou, K., Ulmeanu, R., Serbescu, A. and Alexopoulos, E. C. 2011. Bronchoalveolar lavage fluid cellular profile in workers exposed to chrysotile asbestos. *Toxicol Ind Health* 27:849–56.

Kreiss, K., Mroz, M. M., Zhen, B., Wiedemann, H. and Barna, B. 1997. Risks of beryllium disease related to work processes at a metal, alloy, and oxide production plant. *Occup Environ Med* 54:605–12.

Larsson, B. M., Sehlstedt, M., Grunewald, J., Skold, C. M., Lundin, A., Blomberg, A., Sandstrom, T. et al. 2007. Road tunnel air pollution induces bronchoalveolar inflammation in healthy subjects. *Eur Respir J* 29:699–705.

Larsson, K., Eklund, A., Malmberg, P. and Belin, L. 1992. Alterations in bronchoalveolar lavage fluid but not in lung function and bronchial responsiveness in swine confinement workers. *Chest* 101:767–74.

Lemiere, C., Chaboillez, S., Welman, M. and Maghni, K. 2010. Outcome of occupational asthma after removal from exposure: A follow-up study. *Can Respir J* 17:61–6.

Malik, A., Ali, S., Shahid, M. and Bhargava, R. 2014. Occupational exposure to *Aspergillus* and aflatoxins among food-grain workers in India. *Int J Occup Environ Health* 20:189–93.

Malo, J. L., Cardinal, S., Ghezzo, H., L'Archeveque, J., Castellanos, L. and Maghni, K. 2011. Association of bronchial reactivity to occupational agents with methacholine reactivity, sputum cells and immunoglobulin E-mediated reactivity. *Clin Exp Allergy* 41:497–504.

Meyer, K. C., Raghu, G., Baughman, R. P., Brown, K. K., Costabel, U., Du Bois, R. M., Drent, M. et al. 2012. *American Thoracic Society Committee On BAL in Interstitial Lung Diseases.* An official American Thoracic Society clinical practice guideline: The clinical utility of bronchoalveolar lavage cellular analysis in interstitial lung disease. *Am J Respir Crit Care Med* 185:1004–14.

Moreira, V.B., Ferreira, A.S., Soares, P.J., Gabetto, J.M. and Rodrigues, C.C. 2005. The role of bronchoalveolar lavage in quantifying inhaled particles in silicosis. *Rev Port Pneumol* 11(5):457–75.

Newman, L. S., Maier, L. A., Martyny, J. W., Mroz, M. M., Vandyke, M. and Sackett, H. M. 2005. Beryllium workers' health risks. *J Occup Environ Hyg* 2:D48–50.

Paggiaro, P. L., Chanez, P., Holz, O., Ind, P. W., Djukanovic, R., Maestrelli, P. and Sterk, P. J. 2002. Sputum induction. *Eur Respir J Suppl* 37:3s–8s.

Pala, G., Pignatti, P. and Moscato, G. 2012. Occupational nonasthmatic eosinophilic bronchitis: Current concepts. *Med Lav* 103:17–25.

Pedersen, B., Iversen, M., Bundgaard Larsen, B. and Dahl, R. 1996. Pig farmers have signs of bronchial inflammation and increased numbers of lymphocytes and neutrophils in BAL fluid. *Eur Respir J* 9:524–30.

Quirce, S., Lemiere, C., De Blay, F., Del Pozo, V., Gerth Van Wijk, R., Maestrelli, P., Pauli, G. et al. 2010. Noninvasive methods for assessment of airway inflammation in occupational settings. *Allergy* 65:445–58.

Reynolds, H. Y. and Newball, H. H. 1974. Analysis of proteins and respiratory cells obtained from human lungs by bronchial lavage. *J Lab Clin Med* 84:559–73.

Rossall, M. R., Cadden, P. A., Molphy, S. D., Plumb, J. and Singh, D. 2014. Repeatability of induced sputum measurements in moderate to severe asthma. *Respir Med* 108:1566–8.

Scancarello, G., Romeo, R. and Sartorelli, E. 1996. Respiratory disease as a result of talc inhalation. *J Occup Environ Med* 38:610–4.

Schuyler, M. R., Gaumer, H. R., Stankus, R. P., Kaimal, J., Hoffmann, E. and Salvaggio, J. E. 1980. Bronchoalveolar lavage in silicosis. Evidence of type II cell hyperplasia. *Lung* 157:95–102.

Tinkle, S. S., Kittle, L. A. and Newman, L. S. 1999. Partial IL-10 inhibition of the cell-mediated immune response in chronic beryllium disease. *J Immunol* 163:2747–53.

Tsushima, K., Fujimoto, K., Yamazaki, Y., Takamizawa, A., Amari, T., Koizumi, T. and Kubo, K. 2001. Hypersensitivity pneumonitis induced by spores of *Lyophyllum aggregatum*. *Chest* 120:1085–93.

Ulker, O., Yucesoy, B., Demir, O., Tekin, I. and Karakaya, A. 2008. Serum and BAL cytokine and antioxidant enzyme levels at different stages of pneumoconiosis in coal workers. *Hum Exp Toxicol* 27(12):871–7.

Vandenplas, O., D'alpaos, V., Heymans, J., Jamart, J., Thimpont, J., Huaux, F., Lison, D. and Renauld, J. C. 2009. Sputum eosinophilia: An early marker of bronchial response to occupational agents. *Allergy* 64:754–61.

Vathesatogkit, P., Harkin, T. J., Addrizzo-Harris, D. J., Bodkin, M., Crane, M. and Rom, W. N. 2004. Clinical correlation of asbestos bodies in BAL fluid. *Chest* 126:966–71.

Von Essen, S. G., Scheppers, L. A., Robbins, R. A. and Donham, K. J. 1998. Respiratory tract inflammation in swine confinement workers studied using induced sputum and exhaled nitric oxide. *J Toxicol Clin Toxicol* 36(6):557–65.

Wolff, H., Mussalo-Rauhamaa, H., Raitio, H., Elg, P., Orpana, A., Piilonen, A. and Haahtela, T. 2009. Patients referred to an indoor air health clinic: Exposure to water-damaged buildings causes an increase of lymphocytes in bronchoalveolar lavage and a decrease of CD19 leucocytes in peripheral blood. *Scand J Clin Lab Invest* 69:537–44.

6 Non-Invasive Methods for Assessing the Respiratory Tract in Occupational Lung Disease

Exhaled Breath and Particles

Anna-Carin Olin and Mona Lärstad

CONTENTS

EXHALED NITRIC OXIDE

Fraction of exhaled nitric oxide (FENO) has gained a lot of interest as a biomarker for inflammation since it was discovered in exhaled air at the beginning of the 1990s. Nonetheless, its utility in occupational lung disease is not fully established. The current concept underlying the relevance of FENO is that it is linked to Th2-driven inflammation (Bjermer et al., 2014) and thereby to eosinophilic airway inflammation. Numerous studies have shown that FENO is associated with eosinophils in sputum and in bronchoalveolar lavage (BAL), even if this association is only modest (Berry et al., 2005), whereas the association of FENO with the blood eosinophil concentration is poor. In the occupational lung disease field, FENO has mainly been used in cross-sectional studies and in combination with specific inhalation challenge (SIC) testing. The results of these studies are summarized below.

There is a standard protocol for the measurement of FENO as set up by the American Thoracic Society (ATS) and European Respiratory Society (ERS) (2005). In this protocol, it is recommended that FENO be measured during a slow single exhalation at a fixed flow rate of 50 mL/second against an oral pressure of at least 5 cm H_2O. In order to avoid ambient NO influencing the measured levels, inhalation of NO-free air is also recommended. This initial protocol was based on large, fixed-place, laboratory-based equipment.

So-called 'off-line' methods using portable devices are far more attractive to occupational investigations. Although early attempts were associated with methodological difficulties, today considerable technology improvements, including constant and well-defined exhalation flow, inhalation of NO-free air prior to measurements and an increased mouth pressure to ensure closure of the velum, are incorporated into the off-line methods in order to ensure correct measurements.

There has also been substantial research aimed at discriminating the proportion of FENO produced in the small/terminal airways (a surrogate of the alveolar concentration) as opposed to large airways, based on modelling of measured NO concentrations using different exhalation flow rates. When exhaling with high flow rates, the measured concentrations in the exhaled air will have higher contributions of nitric oxide from small airways, and when using a low exhalation flow, the concentration is more representative for NO produced in central airways. The basic principle is simple: multiplying the NO concentration by the flow rate achieved will create a value of the NO output (i.e. the amount of excreted NO) at that specific flow rate. The NO outputs can then be plotted against the different flows, and the slope will represents the 'alveolar' NO concentration (Tsoukias and George, 1998). Several mathematical models have, however, been created, but so far none is perfect (Verbanck et al., 2012), and obstruction in small airways seems to be an important factor to consider when interpreting such results (Verbanck et al., 2012).

Smoking is known to down-regulate the NO synthases, resulting in substantially lower FENO values.

For this reason, whether or not FENO is a useful marker for airway inflammation associated with occupational exposures in smokers remains unclear. Conflicting results have been reported in this regard: in some studies, NO production is increased among those with occupational exposures that induce airway inflammation (Malinovschi et al., 2012), while in other studies, this does not seem to be the case (Smit et al., 2009). At a minimum, analyses of FENO in occupational cohorts should be stratified for current smoking (Rouhos et al., 2011; Malinovschi et al., 2012).

The measurement of FENO also seems to be systematically affected by narrowing in obstructive airway disease, decreasing the observed levels (de Gouw et al., 1998; Ho et al., 2000; Ferrazzoni et al., 2009). If possible, FENO should preferably be measured after bronchodilatation in those with airflow obstruction. The implication of this association is that some of the data related to FENO measurement after specific airway challenge testing may be difficult to interpret, given that such challenges often induce airway constriction that, in turn, reduces FENO, systematically impacting the observed results. Repeated spirometric manoeuvres may, however, also lower FENO (Deykin et al., 2000), which implies that study design when using FENO in occupational settings is also important.

A summary of the findings on FENO and exposure to high-molecular-weight asthma-causing agents is found in Table 6.1. Adisesh et al. (1998) performed the first study in an occupational setting in 1998, showing an increase in FENO levels with a higher degree of symptoms in laboratory animal allergy: those sensitized to animal dander with rhino-conjunctivitis had higher levels of FENO than non-sensitized workers, but lower levels than those with frank asthma. More recently, Hewitt et al. (2008) followed 50 laboratory animal workers and measured FENO at the end of a working week (Friday) and every morning and at the end of the workday during the following weekend. Eleven subjects had work-related symptoms and two were seropositive for laboratory animal antigens. In one of the seropositive individuals, but not the other, there was a progressive increase in FENO during the working week. Two other subjects also had an increase of FENO of more than 25 ppb during the working week, but no symptoms nor changes in peak expiratory flow rate measurements. In all other subjects, no significant changes in FENO occurred during the working week.

Chan-Yeung et al. (1999) found no relationship between FENO and respiratory impairment (lung function, bronchial hyperresponsiveness [BHR] or response to bronchodilator and medication) among 71 workers with western red-cedar asthma. Sputum eosinophilia, on the other hand, was correlated significantly with FENO (r = 0.42). Seventeen subjects with suspected western red-cedar asthma were challenged with plicatic acid in

TABLE 6.1
Fraction of Exhaled Nitric Oxide and Exposure to High-Molecular-Weight Agents

Reference	Exposure	n	Design	Outcome	FENO
Adisesh et al. (1998)	Laboratory animals	39	Cross-sectional	Asthma	↑ FENO in those with symptoms
				Rhinitis	↑
Hewitt et al. (2008)	Laboratory animals	50	Before and after working week	Symptoms (n = 11)	→
				Sensitized (n = 2)	↑
Chan-Yeung et al. (1999)	Red-cedar	71	Cross-sectional	BHR, sensitization	→ No correlation
Shiryaeva et al. (2014)	Fish industry	139	Cross-sectional	Effect of exposure	→
		249			↑ FENO in controls
				Dry cough at work	↑ FENO
Tossa et al. (2010)	Bakers, pasta makers, hairdressers	351	Apprentices Before and three times during a 2-year period	Increased BHR	↑ FENO 20% (non-atopics) ↑FENO 16% (atopics)
Obata et al. (1999)	Red-cedar	17	Challenge	Responders	→
				Non-responders	↑ (24 hours)
Tan et al. (2001)	Latex	12	Challenge	Responders	↑ FENO: 1 out of 6
Allmers et al. (2000)	Methylene diphenyl diisocyanate	12	Challenge	3 responders	↑ FENO:1 out of 3

Abbreviation: FENO: fraction of exhaled nitric oxide.

a study from Obata et al. (1999). Nine of the subjects were defined as 'responders' on the basis of a bronchoconstriction after the challenge. Levels of exhaled NO increased at 24 hours after the exposure, although only significantly among the non-responders, and the changes were not related to changes in lung function. Note that the phenomenon described above of airflow constriction reducing FENO could have come into play in this study.

Tan et al. have challenged eight subjects with self-reported latex sensitivity (3/8 radioallergosorbent test [RAST] positive for latex and 6/8 skin-prick test positive) and eye or nasal symptoms with latex (Tan et al., 2001). No change in FENO was found after the challenge. Allmers et al. (2000) challenged 12 subjects with natural rubber latex allergy (positive skin-prick test) and six controls. Three of the subjects reacted with bronchoconstriction, of whom one also reacted with increased FENO. Shiryaeva et al. (2010) examined 139 salmon workers from fish-processing facilities who were exposed to both fish proteins as well as endotoxins, comparing these to 214 control subjects (administrative workers). The control subjects had higher FENO levels than the exposed group. In a multivariable regression analysis, however, FENO was associated with work-related dry cough.

van der Walt et al. (2010) examined FENO in three spice-mill workers reporting symptoms of asthma and allergy. They were examined four times daily for 2 working weeks, 2 weeks away from work and 2 weeks back at work. In one out of three workers, FENO was elevated both before (84 ppb) and after the work shift (76 ppb), while the other two subjects had normal-range FENO (generally less than 40 ppb) without any changes during the work shifts. The subject with increased FENO had very high levels of specific IgE against garlic (208 kU/L); the other subjects had lower levels (2.37 and 0.63 kU/L, respectively). In another example of exposure to high-molecular-weight antigens, Tossa et al. (2010) followed 351 apprentices for 2 years; before being exposed and then three times during the following 2-year period of apprenticeship. The apprentices were working as bakers, pasta makers or hairdressers. In those with increased BHR, the level of FENO increased by 20% in non-atopic and 16% in atopic subjects, respectively. In a multiple regression model, the odds ratio for developing BHR was 2 for each log-ppb increase of FENO. The sensitization rate was 11.8% among bakers, 8.1% among pasta makers and 4.1% among hairdressers.

A summary of the findings on FENO and exposure to low-molecular-weight sensitizing agents and non-specific irritants is shown in Table 6.2. Non-smoking aluminium pot-room workers (n = 99) exposed to fluorides and dust had 63% higher FENO as compared to 40 non-smoking controls (Lund et al., 2000). The increased FENO, however, was not related to respiratory symptoms. Ulvestad et al. (2001) compared 29 non-smoking underground tunnel workers who had been exposed to a variety of substances, including dust and nitrogen dioxide, with 26 controls working in the open air. The tunnel workers had 50% higher FENO compared with non-smoking controls. Those workers reporting wheeze also had the highest levels of FENO Olin et al. have investigated bleachery workers in three pulp-mills, who were repeatedly exposed to high levels of ozone in Swedish pulp-mills, and dust-alone exposure referent workers (Olin et al., 1999, 2004). In the first small study, the 29 highest-exposed workers had 63% higher FENO.

In addition to antigens and irritants, there has also been interest in FENO in relation to occupational exposure to endotoxin. Von Essen et al. have showed slightly elevated FENO and an increased prevalence of respiratory symptoms among workers who had been exposed to swine dust (Von Essen et al., 1998), which is likely to contain endotoxin. A large cohort (n = 425) of farmers and agriculture workers in Holland has also been examined with FENO, along with a thorough assessment of exposure to endotoxin (Smit et al., 2009). FENO was associated with endotoxin exposure but only in non-atopic, non-smoking exposed persons. Subjects with wheezing and asthma symptoms had increased FENO, irrespective of atopy. Further, the association between exposure and symptoms was marginally affected by FENO.

Sundblad and Kölbeck et al. have performed many studies in endotoxin-exposed swine workers and in healthy volunteers exposed to endotoxin. The evolving picture is that endotoxin exposure in swine husbandry induces a predominantly neutrophilic inflammation, as well as an increase in exhaled nitric oxide. In contrast, Kölbeck et al. (2000) exposed 17 healthy subjects to swine dust and found no significant changes of FENO, although the measurement was made after repeated spirometry, which is known to decrease FENO, as noted previously. In a more recent study, 33 healthy non-atopic subjects were exposed to a swine confinement environment (Sundblad et al., 2002). Among the 22 subjects who were not wearing respiratory protection, FENO increased from 7.5 to 13.4 ppb. Among those using such protection, the FENO was unaltered, going from 8.3 ppb at baseline to 8.6 ppb after exposure. The same research group also compared the effect of real-life exposure in a swine barn, experimental lipopolysaccharide (LPS) exposure and the effect of previous/chronic exposure (Sundblad et al., 2009). Swine farmers (n = 11), current smokers (n = 12) and controls (n = 11) spent 3 hours

TABLE 6.2
Fraction of Exhaled Nitric Oxide and Exposure to Low-Molecular-Weight Agents and Irritants

Reference	Exposure	n Exp. Contr	Design	FENO
Lund et al. (2000)	Aluminium pot-room workers	99 40	Cross-sectional	↑ FENO Exposed had 63% higher FENO No association with symptoms
Ulvestad et al. (2001)	Tunnel workers	29 26	Cross-sectional	↑ FENO Exposed had 50% higher FENO
Olin et al. (1999)	Ozone, pulp industry	65 39	Cross-sectional	↑ FENO Most exposed had 69% higher FENO
Olin et al. (2004)	Ozone, pulp industry	228 63	Cross-sectional	↑ FENO 23% higher FENO
Allmers et al. (2000)	Diisocyanate (MDI)	9	Challenge	FENO increased in 2/3 positive challenges
Pronk et al. (2009)	Isocyanate (mainly HDI)	229	Cross-sectional	→ in exposed ↑ FENO among non-atopic subjects with respiratory symptoms
Sue-Chu et al. (1999)	Professional skiers with asthma	9	Cross-sectional	→ FENO
Fell et al. (2011)	Cement workers	85	Change-over shift	↓ FENO over shift
Carlsten et al. (2007)	Cement workers/electricians (control)	11 21	Cross-sectional	→ FENO
Sastre et al. (2011)	Cleaners	13	Chlorine challenge	→ FENO In all, 3 out of 13 challenges positive
Demange et al. (2009)	Lifeguards in swimming halls	39	Cross-sectional	↑ FENO in those with BHR
Mauer et al. (2011)	Firemen in World Trade Center	92 141	6 years after 9/11	→ FENO 10 highly exposed non-smokers had ↑ FENO
Järvelä et al. (2013)	Welders	20	Change-over shift	No change of FENO on group level, 3 subjects had ↑ FENO
Ndlovu et al. (2014)	Female workers exposed to pesticides	211	Cross-sectional	→ FENO Those with low cholinesterase levels had high FENO (>50 ppb) OR 4.80 (95 CI: 0.80–28.00)

Abbreviations: FENO: fraction of expired nitric oxide; HDI: hexamethylene diisocyanate; MDI: methylene diphenyl diisocyanate; OR: odds ratio; CI: confidence interval.

in the barn, and FENO increased both in smokers and controls, but not in farmers, possibly explained by their higher pre-exposure FENO levels; post-exposure FENO levels were similar in all groups. Experimental LPS challenge, on the other hand, did not change FENO in any of the groups. This group of authors has carried out an intervention study in order to examine the effects of introducing robot cleaning of the piggery stables on reducing exposure to endotoxins. In comparison with no robot cleaning, FENO levels increased significantly less ($p = 0.0047$) in healthy volunteer cleaners (Hiel et al., 2009).

In addition to swine husbandry, other occupational sources of endotoxin have also been studied. Heldal et al. (2010) examined 44 sewage workers exposed to endotoxin and 36 controls (office workers). They did not find any significant changes of FENO, despite high levels of endotoxin exposure (220 EU [endotoxin units]/m^2, SD [standard deviation]: 570). Mirmohammadi et al. examined 89 male cotton workers before and after work shifts who were exposed both to cotton dust and endotoxins (Mirmohammadi et al., 2014). FENO increased significantly after work shifts (mean FENO before 7.69 ppb vs. 10.65 ppb after shift, $p < 0.001$). Those with respiratory complaints associated with workplace exposure showed significantly increased FENO compared with those without symptoms (post-shift FENO: 14.88 vs. 9.65 ppb, $p = 0.011$).

Moore et al. (2010), having examined 60 workers currently exposed to both high- and low-molecular-weight agents, suggest that, based on FENO data, there are two variants of occupational asthma: one with increased FENO and lower provocative concentration causing a 20% fall in forced expiratory volume in 1 second (FEV_1) and one with normal FENO without BHR, even though both groups may have similar peak expiratory flow rate (PEFR) changes in relation to work.

In light of this, the results of FENO following SIC are of interest. Five studies have compared the results of sputum induction and FENO after SIC (Piirila et al., 2001; Swierczynska-Machura et al., 2008, Ferrazzoni et al., 2009; Lemiere et al., 2010) with somewhat contradicting results. The methodological aspect of FENO measurement noted previously, in which a decrease in FEV_1 is regarded as a positive test outcome for SIC but may also decrease the levels of exhaled FENO, may explain the heterogeneity of this literature.

This possible bronchoconstrictive effect on FENO is apparent in the study by Ferrazzoni et al. (2009), in which 15 subjects with isocyanate asthma, three subjects with isocyanate-induced rhinitis and 24 control subjects were exposed to a SIC with isocyanate. They were examined on 5 consecutive days and then 7 and 30 days after SIC. There was a strong correlation observed in that study between the fall in FEV_1 and the decrease in FENO at the corresponding time point among the early responders ($r = 0.76$, $p < 0.001$). Further, the results showed that the FENO levels were only significantly increased 24 hours after exposure, a time point when FEV_1 was on its way back to normal. The maximum FENO levels were reached at between 24 and 48 hours after exposure, a time point that is not normally examined. In comparison, among those with a positive SIC, the sputum eosinophil count only returned to normal after 7 days. Changes in sputum eosinophil count and changes in FENO levels were correlated at 24 hours ($\mathcal{P} = 0.66$, $p = 0.001$) and 48 hours ($\mathcal{P} = 0.66$, $p = 0.002$).

Lemiere et al. compared FENO and sputum eosinophils following SIC tests performed in Belgium and Canada (Lemiere et al., 2010). On a control day (day 1), subjects were exposed to a sham substance, and on a second and a third day (if there was a negative response on day 2), they were exposed to the offending agent. Sputum cell counts, FENO and metacholine challenge tests were performed at the end of the control day, 7 hours after the end of an exposure (giving rise to an asthmatic reaction) and then repeated 24 hours after that. In the event of a negative SIC, the measurements were performed on the last day of exposure. Twenty subjects with a positive SIC test and 16 subjects with a negative SIC test were finally included in the comparison. In subjects with a positive SIC test, there was a significant increase in both sputum eosinophil count and FENO, whereas no significant changes were found in those with a negative SIC. In addition, there was a moderate correlation between change in percentage of sputum eosinophils and change in FENO ($\mathcal{P} = 0.4$, $p = 0.007$). Using receiver–operator characteristic curves in order to identify those with a positive SIC (i.e. a fall in FEV_1 of 20%), a 2.2% change in sputum eosinophil counts provided the best sensitivity and specificity. No relevant cut-off value for FENO could be identified, and using a 10% increase in FENO as an arbitrary cut-off value achieved much lower sensitivity and specificity than sputum eosinophil counts.

Swierczynska-Machura et al. (2008) also measured FENO and performed induced sputum testing after SIC in 42 persons, including bakers, farmers and healthcare workers with suspected occupational asthma. Nineteen subjects had a positive SIC test and were diagnosed with occupational asthma. They all had increased FENO. Along the same lines, in a study from Finland, SIC tests were performed in 40 persons with suspected occupational asthma (Piirila et al., 2001). In those challenges in which a bronchoconstriction occurred, a significant increase in FENO was also noted, but only in those with normal or only slightly elevated basal NO levels. There was no increase among the subjects with high basal FENO levels. Finally, Walters et al. retrospectively examined data from 16 subjects that used SIC challenges and found positive test results (Walters et al., 2014). Most had increased FENO at baseline, but only one was increased following SIC.

As noted previously, efforts have been made to discriminate the peripheral and central origin of the exhaled NO by using different exhalation flows during the measurement and mathematical modelling. Indeed, subjects with allergic alveolitis have increased FENO at an exhalation flow of 300 mL/second, but almost normal FENO values at 50 mL/second (Lehtimaki et al., 2001). The same group has also reported interesting results showing increased alveolar NO in persons exposed to silica dust (Sauni et al., 2012) and in asbestosis (Lehtimaki et al., 2010).

In summary, the usefulness of FENO for monitoring occupational respiratory disease remains unclear. FENO seems to give a clear signal of eosinophilic inflammation after exposure to high-molecular-weight compounds in non-smokers, but the signal may be blurred by other concomitant (non-occupational) exposures. FENO also seems to increase after low-molecular-weight exposures (including irritants), but the increase is much less pronounced and may be absent despite inflammation. The results of FENO used in challenge studies may be confounded by a decrease in FENO related to airway obstruction counterbalancing an increase from the SIC itself. It does seem clear that there is large intra-individual variation in the FENO response to the same exposure in symptomatic persons, and that the different subtypes of inflammation (i.e. eosinophilic vs. neutrophilic) may be induced in different individuals, thus manifesting in differing FENO effects. Nevertheless, despite these limitations, there is a place for FENO in occupational respiratory disease, especially for monitoring the effects of exposure to high-molecular-weight agents, and particularly in the early identification of asthma. Thus, repeated measurement of FENO in the same individual may be an effective strategy for identifying workers in whom exposure induces airway inflammation, thereby identifying those with eosinophilic inflammation after exposure to high-molecular-weight agents. Finally, measurement of alveolar NO may have a role in the assessment of the occupational disease processes affecting the small airways, but more research is needed in order to evaluate this question.

EXHALED BREATH CONDENSATE

Collection of exhaled breath condensate (EBC) is a technique that is based on the cooling of exhaled breath that then condenses; that is, the water vapour turns to water and simultaneously captures the non-volatile and semi-volatile substances in the exhaled breath. Different cooling devices are used, and tidal breathing using a nose-clip is typically performed during the manoeuvre. It is likely that the non-volatile matter contained in the condensate is transported from the respiratory tract lining fluid in the form of small particles (droplets) in an aerosol. Condensation is affected by temperature and the surface of the condenser, which can have different adhesive properties. For example, proteins can be trapped (Rosias et al., 2006), explaining some of the contradictory results that have been observed with EBC. The anatomical site of origin of non-volatiles in EBC has been explored by Bondesson et al. by using an aqueous aerosol containing technetium-99m in healthy, non-smoking subjects (Bondesson et al., 2009). Their findings indicate that EBC mainly derives from the central airways, but oral contamination also seems to take place. This is supported by Trischler et al. (2012) who performed fractionated sampling of EBC. The fractions mainly represented the airway and alveolar fractions, respectively, and hydrogen peroxide (H_2O_2; a semi-volatile compound) was quantified. The latter study does not determine, however, the origin of the non-volatiles in EBC.

EBC potentially contains a wide range of mediators of inflammation and oxidative stress. These are potential biomarkers of effect that reflect the biochemical reactions of the epithelial lining fluid and are exhaled in bio-aerosol form. Important compounds in EBC that can be used for diagnosis, assessment of severity or follow-up in airway diseases include leukotrienes, prostaglandins, cytokines, hydrogen ions (pH/acidity), H_2O_2, 8-isoprostane, malondialdehyde, nitrite/nitrate, nitrotyrosine and nitrosothiols (Hoffmeyer et al., 2009). Additionally, biomarkers of exposure have been measured in EBC; for example, metals such as manganese and chromium (Corradi et al., 2010; Felix et al., 2013).

In EBC, pH—reflecting the presence of hydrogen ions (H^+)—is perhaps the biomarker that has been most commonly used to date in a variety of studies, including in asthma, chronic obstructive pulmonary disease (COPD) and occupational exposures. It has been reported that the pH in EBC decreases during an asthma exacerbation; that is, the respiratory tract lining fluid becomes more acidic, possibly due to an increase in the concentration of acetic acid (Caffarelli et al., 2014). Water-soluble acids are exhaled and then trapped in EBC and lower its pH. In studies of COPD, conflicting results have been reported, with some finding that the pH drops (Koczulla et al., 2010) and others finding that it is unchanged (Koczulla et al., 2009). One of the worries regarding the measurement of pH in the condensate is that the presence of ammonium ions in the oral cavity may affect the pH (Effros, 2003), although Wells et al. reported that EBC pH assays are not influenced by oral ammonia (Wells et al., 2005). To achieve stable pH of the collected condensate, the sample needs 'de-aeration' (bubbling of an inert gas into the sample) so that carbon dioxide (CO_2) that is absorbed from the ambient air disappears (Vaughan et al., 2003). Another approach is to saturate the sample with CO_2, which takes approximately 40 minutes (Kullmann et al., 2007). Although the full interpretation of pH measurement in EBC is not yet clear, the pH of the airways may be important in respiratory disease.

EBC has been used as a non-invasive tool in occupational settings, with most of these studies focusing on pulmonary biomarkers of effect. For example, EBC has been collected in grain workers who were exposed to dust and endotoxin (Do et al., 2008). In this study, airway acidity reflected in the EBC was evaluated in relation to the duration and intensity of exposure. The authors found that chronic exposure is more associated with airway acidity, whereas acute exposure is more closely associated with oxidative stress, specifically increased 8-isoprostane. Respiratory inflammatory responses among occupants of water-damaged office buildings were studied by Akpinar-Elci et al. (2008) using EBC. They showed that IL-8 was a relevant biomarker of effect as it reflects airway inflammation after indoor exposure. The pH in EBC as a biomarker of air pollution-related inflammation in street traffic controllers and office workers was studied by Lima et al. (2013). The mean pH values were 8.12 in EBC in office workers compared to a pH of 7.80 in traffic controllers. Both groups presented similar cytokines concentrations in EBC. A study by Chow et al. described increases in the EBC biomarkers of inflammation and oxidative stress in persons with asbestos-induced diseases, an observation further indicating that 8-isoprostane as well as H_2O_2 and total protein in EBC may be useful in assessing persons with asbestosis (Chow et al., 2009). Another study supported the hypothesis that oxidative stress due to asbestos exposure is the main cause of increased 8-isoprostane levels (Pelclova et al., 2008). In this study, the mean level of 8-isoprostane was increased in the whole group of asbestos-exposed subjects as compared to the controls.

EBC has also been used as a medium for biomarkers of exposure, mainly in the case of occupational exposure to toxic metals (Corradi et al., 2010), as noted previously. Goldoni et al. also demonstrated that metals can be detected in the EBC of exposed workers (Goldoni et al., 2004). These authors studied workers exposed to cobalt and tungsten and found that the EBC levels were higher in samples collected at the end of the working shift and also paralleled the measurements in urine samples. In a study by Fireman et al., measurements of pH and H_2O_2 in EBC demonstrated the presence of airway inflammation in asymptomatic welders, which was modulated by the different metal fumes and gases generated according to the material and method used for the welding process (Fireman et al., 2008; Hoffmeyer et al., 2009). Hulo et al. determined concentrations of manganese, nickel, iron and chromium in EBC as potential indicators of exposure to fumes from metal inert gas welding processes (Hulo et al., 2014). Concentrations of manganese and nickel in EBC were significantly higher among welders than controls, but were not correlated with their respective levels in urine.

The EBC method also has some limitations. During condensation, the exhaled air is cooled and the water vapour is released in aqueous form, in which particles/droplets contained in the breath also are trapped, but only to a limited extent. Hence, EBC essentially consists of water, and the substances in EBC are diluted and only present at extremely low concentrations that are difficult to measure with existing enzyme-linked immunosorbent assay (ELISA). Condensation of the particles is random, and many of the exhaled particles may pass the condenser without being collected. This was clearly indicated by a study in which two condensers were connected in series and similar levels of analytes were identified in both condensers (Corradi et al., 2008). The extent to which the degree of dilution with water vapour varies between and within subjects remains uncertain. Attempts to overcome this have been made by measuring conductivity in samples, but this has not been shown to yield more reproducible results (Effros et al., 2003). Rosias et al. have developed a new capacitor that partially overcomes this problem: the exhaled air passes through the capacitor twice, resulting in a greater exchange of material (Rosias et al., 2010). Another potential problem is contamination of the EBC with substances present in the saliva. For example, Marteus et al. compared nitrate in EBC from intubated persons from whom samples were collected from the mouth and from the tracheal tube before and after intake of nitrate (Marteus et al., 2005). They showed that nitrate concentrations were much higher in the samples collected during normal tidal breathing through the mouth compared to EBC collected from the tracheal tube.

The above concerns with the EBC method are particularly disturbing when the method is used to study non-volatile substances. For semi-volatile substances, the problem is somewhat different, but contamination from the oral cavity is probably an even bigger problem. The first ATS/ERS recommendations on EBC were published in 2005 (Horvath et al., 2005). Important areas for future research involve ascertaining mechanisms, the determination of dilution markers, improving reproducibility, the employment of EBC in longitudinal studies and determining the utility of EBC measures for the management of individual patients.

In summary, EBC is a non-invasive method that reflects changes in the epithelial lining fluid within the airways. The method has been used in a number of studies regarding respiratory diseases and occupational exposures, and at a group level, the use of EBC presents interesting results. Yet there are limitations, as described above, which have to be overcome.

OTHER EXHALED VOLATILES

The major components in exhaled air are water vapour, nitrogen, oxygen, CO_2 and inert gases (Miekisch et al., 2004). The remaining fraction consists of a great number of components in the parts per billion to trillion (ppb–ppt) ranges. These components may be endogenous (i.e. generated by the body) or exogenous (i.e. contaminants from the environment that are inhaled). Endogenous compounds include volatile organic compounds (VOCs) such as acetone, methane, isoprene, ethane, pentane, small aldehydes and various inorganic compounds, such as NO and carbon monoxide.

Hundreds of VOCs have been identified in exhaled air. The composition of VOCs in breath varies widely from person to person, both qualitatively and quantitatively.

To date, there have not been many studies on exhaled volatiles in occupational exposure settings. In a study by Svedahl et al., short-term exposure to moderate concentrations of cooking fumes was studied (Svedahl et al., 2013). There was a trend of an increase of ethane in exhaled air and, in a sub-analysis of 12 subjects, there was also an increase in the levels of ethane, from 2.83 ppb on the morning before exposure to cooking fumes to 3.53 ppb on the morning after exposure.

In a study of three groups (patients with histology-established diagnoses of malignant pleural mesothelioma, persons with long-term certified professional exposure to asbestos and healthy control subjects without exposure to asbestos), exhaled breath samples were analysed using gas chromatography/mass spectrometry (de Gennaro et al., 2010). Cyclopentane was the dominant compound in the discrimination between asbestos-exposed subjects and the other groups (both mesothelioma and controls). Benzene was measured in the blood and alveolar air of 168 men subdivided into four groups: blood donors, hospital staff, chemical workers occupationally exposed to benzene and chemical workers not occupationally exposed to benzene (Brugnone et al., 1989). The group of exposed workers was found to be significantly different from the other three groups in terms of both blood and alveolar benzene concentrations. The alveolar benzene concentration was significantly higher in smokers than in non-smokers in the groups of the hospital staff and non-exposed workers, but not in the blood donors and exposed workers. In the three groups without occupational exposure considered altogether, the alveolar benzene concentration correlated significantly with environmental benzene concentration measured at the time of the individual examinations, both in the smokers and non-smokers in the same three groups, and in the exposed workers alveolar benzene concentration showed a significant correlation with the blood benzene concentration.

A study of firefighters exposed to wildland fire smoke included the measurement of exhaled volatiles (Miranda et al., 2012). Firefighter levels of carbon monoxide, nitrogen dioxide and VOCs were measured in wildfires during three fire seasons in Portugal. There was a significant increase in carbon monoxide and a decrease in nitrogen dioxide in the exhaled air of the majority of the firefighters. In a study by Chen et al., the relationship between environmental exposure to toluene, xylene and ethyl benzene and the exhaled breath concentrations for these among gasoline service workers was investigated (Chen et al., 2002). The breath concentrations of toluene and xylene were significantly correlated with personal monitoring concentrations. Furthermore, multiple regression analysis showed that exhaled toluene levels were highly influenced by personal toluene concentrations and the amount of personal gasoline sold, whereas exhaled xylene levels depended on wind speed and personal xylene exposure concentrations. Regarding exposure to organic solvents specifically, breath analysis is an attractive, non-invasive procedure for screening workers (Wilson and Monster, 1999). It has been used in numerous laboratory-based studies and also for field research, but has not yet become widely accepted as a tool in occupational hygiene. It is, however, likely to become more widely used in the future.

Breath analysis research is being successfully pursued using a variety of analytical methods, prominent amongst which are gas chromatography with mass spectrometry, ion mobility spectrometry, the fast-flow and flow-drift tube techniques called selected ion flow tube mass spectrometry and proton transfer reaction mass spectrometry (Smith et al., 2014). Apart from gas chromatography with mass spectrometry, these methods have seldom been reported as being used in occupational field studies to date. Different 'omics' techniques can assess the patterns of VOCs. One such technique that is suitable for breath analysis is represented by electronic noses (e-noses), which provide fingerprints of the exhaled VOCs, called 'breath prints'. An e-nose is an artificial sensor system that generally consists of an array of chemical sensors for the detection of the VOC profiles and an algorithm for pattern recognition (Montuschi et al., 2013). E-noses are handheld, portable devices that provide immediate results. They are able to discriminate between patients with respiratory diseases, including asthma, COPD and lung cancer, and healthy control subjects, as well as differentiating among different respiratory diseases. The potential use of an e-nose for monitoring the headspace volatiles in biological samples from benzene-exposed workers and non-exposed controls has been investigated (Mohamed et al., 2014). The e-nose technology successfully classified and distinguished benzene-exposed workers from non-exposed controls for all measured samples of blood, urine and the exhaled air with a very high degree of precision.

EXHALED NON-VOLATILES (PARTICLES IN EXHALED AIR)

In recent years, a novel technique for sampling non-volatiles in exhaled breath has been introduced based on impaction: the sampling of particles in exhaled air

(PExA) (Almstrand et al., 2009). By applying a breathing manoeuvre that allows for airway closure followed by re-opening, a substantial increase in particle (or droplet) formation takes place. This indicates that the exhaled particles sampled derive from the small airways, a region of the respiratory tract that is very difficult to reach by other non-invasive methods. This region of sample derivation is further supported by the absence of mucins in PExA samples from healthy individuals (there are no goblet cells present in non-cartilaginous airways in healthy subjects). The increase in particle formation also implies that the sampled amount of material is increased, which facilitates chemical analyses of the samples. In fact, the PExA method has been shown to be highly reproducible within the same subject, and to be much more efficient than EBC when sampling non-volatiles (Larsson et al., 2012). Comparing levels of surfactant protein A, which is the most abundant surfactant protein, the PExA method samples 10–50-times higher concentrations than the EBC method when using the same volume of exhaled air (Larsson et al., 2012). The method also overcomes the problem of contamination from the oral cavity: no amylase (a saliva marker) is found in the PExA samples (Bredberg et al., 2012).

A total of 124 proteins have been identified in the PExA samples (approximately three-times more than previously detected in EBC), and the protein profile resembles that of BAL (Bredberg et al., 2012). The most abundant lung-specific protein in PExA, surfactant protein A, has been shown in small exploratory studies to be decreased in COPD (Larstad et al., 2015) and chronic rejection (broncho-obliterans) (Eriksson et al., 2015).

More than 80% of the exhaled particles in PExA consist of lipids, mainly phospholipids, from the surfactant. In a pilot study of asthma, the phospholipid composition was also shown to be altered as compared to healthy controls (Almstrand et al., 2012). In parallel, the phospholipid composition has also been shown to be altered in smokers as compared to non-smokers (Bredberg et al., 2013). There has also been an attempt to use this method in order to assess exposure to inhaled materials (i.e. metals in welding fumes, even though the clinical utility of this purpose still needs to be shown) (Bredberg et al., 2014).

The PExA method is easy to perform and possible to repeat several times within the same subject over a short time period, as it does not interfere with airways, in contrast to both BAL and induced sputum. It therefore has great potential for use in assessing the inflammatory effects of various exposures. However, the sample does not contain any cells, and the sample amount is still a limiting factor for analyses. In summary, data on the PExA method in the occupational setting are so far lacking, but the method seems highly reproducible and specifically to reflect pathological changes in small airways, making it interesting to explore further in the monitoring of occupational respiratory disease.

REFERENCES

Adisesh, L. A., Kharitonov, S. A., Yates, D. H., Snashell, D. C., Newman-Taylor, A. J. and Barnes, P. J. 1998. Exhaled and nasal nitric oxide is increased in laboratory animal allergy. *Clin Exp Allergy* 28:876–80.

Akpinar-Elci, M., Siegel, P. D., Cox-Ganser, J. M., Stemple, K. J., White, S. K., Hilsbos, K. and Weissman, D. N. 2008. Respiratory inflammatory responses among occupants of a water-damaged office building. *Indoor Air* 18:125–30.

Allmers, H., Chen, Z., Barbinova, L., Marczynski, B., Kirschmann, V. and Baur, X. 2000. Challenge from methacholine, natural rubber latex, or 4,4-diphenylmethane diisocyanate in workers with suspected sensitization affects exhaled nitric oxide [change in exhaled NO levels after allergen challenges]. *Int Arch Occup Environ Health* 73:181–6.

Almstrand, A. C., Josefson, M., Bredberg, A., Lausmaa, J., Sjovall, P., Larsson, P. and Olin, A. C. 2012. TOF-SIMS analysis of exhaled particles from patients with asthma and healthy controls. *Eur Respir J* 39:59–66.

Almstrand, A. C., Ljungstrom, E., Lausmaa, J., Bake, B., Sjovall, P. and Olin, A. C. 2009. Airway monitoring by collection and mass spectrometric analysis of exhaled particles. *Anal Chem* 81:662–8.

American Thoracis Society, European Respiratory Society. 2005. ATS/ERS recommendations for standardized procedures for the online and offline measurement of exhaled lower respiratory nitric oxide and nasal nitric oxide. *Am J Respir Crit Care Med* 171:912–30.

Berry, M. A., Shaw, D. E., Green, R. H., Brightling, C. E., Wardlaw, A. J. and Pavord, I. D. 2005. The use of exhaled nitric oxide concentration to identify eosinophilic airway inflammation: An observational study in adults with asthma. *Clin Exp Allergy* 35:1175–9.

Bjermer, L., Alving, K., Diamant, Z., Magnussen, H., Pavord, I., Piacentini, G., Price, D. et al. 2014. Current evidence and future research needs for FeNO measurement in respiratory diseases. *Respir Med* 108:830–41.

Bondesson, E., Jansson, L. T., Bengtsson, T. and Wollmer, P. 2009. Exhaled breath condensate-site and mechanisms of formation. *J Breath Res* 3:016005.

Bredberg, A., Gobom, J., Almstrand, A. C., Larsson, P., Blennow, K., Olin, A. C. and Mirgorodskaya, E. 2012. Exhaled endogenous particles contain lung proteins. *Clin Chem* 58:431–40.

Bredberg, A., Josefson, M., Almstrand, A. C., Lausmaa, J., Sjovall, P., Levinsson, A., Larsson, P. et al. 2013. Comparison of exhaled endogenous particles from smokers and non-smokers using multivariate analysis. *Respiration* 86:135–42.

Bredberg, A., Ljungkvist, G., Taube, F., Ljungstrom, E., Larsson, P., Mirgorodskaya, E., Isaxon, C. et al. 2014. Analysis of manganese and iron in exhaled endogenous particles. *J Anal Atom Spectrom* 29:730–5.

Brightling, C. E. 2010. Cough due to asthma and nonasthmatic eosinophilic bronchitis. *Lung* 188(Suppl. 1): S13–7.

Brugnone, F., Perbellini, L., Faccini, G. B., Pasini, F., Danzi, B., Maranelli, G., Romeo, L., Gobbi, M. and Zedde, A. 1989. Benzene in the blood and breath of normal people and occupationally exposed workers. *Am J Ind Med* 16:385–99.

Caffarelli, C., Dascola, C. P., Peroni, D., Rico, S., Stringari, G., Varini, M., Folesani, G. et al. 2014. Airway acidification in childhood asthma exacerbations. *Allergy Asthma Proc* 35:51–6.

Carlsten, C., De Roos, A. J., Kaufman, J. D., Checkoway, H., Wener, M. and Seixas, N. 2007. Cell markers, cytokines, and immune parameters in cement mason apprentices. *Arthritis Rheum* 57:147–53.

Chan-Yeung, M., Obata, H., Dittrick, M., Chan, H. and Abboud, R. 1999. Airway inflammation, exhaled nitric oxide, and severity of asthma in patients with western red cedar asthma. *Am J Respir Crit Care Med* 159:1434–8.

Chen, M. L., Chen, S. H., Guo, B. R. and Mao, I. F. 2002. Relationship between environmental exposure to toluene, xylene and ethylbenzene and the expired breath concentrations for gasoline service workers. *J Environ Monit* 4:562–6.

Chow, S., Campbell, C., Sandrini, A., Thomas, P. S., Johnson, A. R. and Yates, D. H. 2009. Exhaled breath condensate biomarkers in asbestos-related lung disorders. *Respir Med* 103:1091–7.

Corradi, M., Gergelova, P. and Mutti, A. 2010. Use of exhaled breath condensate to investigate occupational lung diseases. *Curr Opin Allergy Clin Immunol* 10:93–8.

Corradi, M., Goldoni, M., Caglieri, A., Folesani, G., Poli, D., Corti, M. and Mutti, A. 2008. Collecting exhaled breath condensate (EBC) with two condensers in series: A promising technique for studying the mechanisms of EBC formation, and the volatility of selected biomarkers. *J Aerosol Med.* 21:34–44.

De Gennaro, G., Dragonieri, S., Longobardi, F., Musti, M., Stallone, G., Trizio, L. and Tutino, M. 2010. Chemical characterization of exhaled breath to differentiate between patients with malignant pleural mesothelioma from subjects with similar professional asbestos exposure. *Anal Bioanal Chem* 398:3043–50.

De Gouw, H. W., Hendriks, J., Woltman, A. M., Twiss, I. M. and Sterk, P. J. 1998. Exhaled nitric oxide (NO) is reduced shortly after bronchoconstriction to direct and indirect stimuli in asthma. *Am J Respir Crit Care Med* 158:315–9.

Demange, V., Bohadana, A., Massin, N. and Wild, P. 2009. Exhaled nitric oxide and airway hyperresponsiveness in workers: A preliminary study in lifeguards. *BMC Pulm Med* 9:53.

Deykin, A., Massaro, A. F., Coulston, E., Drazen, J. M. and Israel, E. 2000. Exhaled nitric oxide following repeated spirometry or repeated plethysmography in healthy individuals. *Am J Respir Crit Care Med* 161:1237–40.

Do, R., Bartlett, K. H., Dimich-Ward, H., Chu, W. and Kennedy, S. M. 2008. Biomarkers of airway acidity and oxidative stress in exhaled breath condensate from grain workers. *Am J Respir Crit Care Med* 178:1048–54.

Effros, R. M. 2003. Do low exhaled condensate NH4+ concentrations in asthma reflect reduced pulmonary production? *Am J Respir Crit Care Med* 167:91; author reply 91–2.

Effros, R. M., Biller, J., Foss, B., Hoagland, K., Dunning, M. B., Bosbous, M., Castillo, D. et al. 2003. A simple method for estimating respiratory solute dilution in exhaled breath condensates. *Am J Respir Crit Care Med.* 168:1500–5.

Eriksson, P., Almstrand, A.-C., Mirgorodskaya, E., Lärstad, M., Viklund, E., Riise, G. C. and Olin, A.-C. 2015. Surfactant protein A in exhaled particles is decreased in lung transplant patients with chronic rejection. *Am J Respir Crit Care Med* 187:A6138.

Felix, P. M., Franco, C., Barreiros, M. A., Batista, B., Bernardes, S., Garcia, S. M., Almeida, A. B., Almeida, S. M., Wolterbeek, H. T. and Pinheiro, T. 2013. Biomarkers of exposure to metal dust in exhaled breath condensate: Methodology optimization. *Arch Environ Occup Health* 68:72–9.

Fell, A. K., Noto, H., Skogstad, M., Nordby, K. C., Eduard, W., Svendsen, M. V., Ovstebo, R., Troseid, A. M. and Kongerud, J. 2011. A cross-shift study of lung function, exhaled nitric oxide and inflammatory markers in blood in Norwegian cement production workers. *Occup Environ Med* 68:799–805.

Ferrazzoni, S., Scarpa, M. C., Guarnieri, G., Corradi, M., Mutti, A. and Maestrelli, P. 2009. Exhaled nitric oxide and breath condensate pH in asthmatic reactions induced by isocyanates. *Chest* 136:155–62.

Fireman, E., Lerman, Y., Stark, M., Schwartz, Y., Ganor, E., Grinberg, N., Frimer, R. et al. 2008. Detection of occult lung impairment in welders by induced sputum particles and breath oxidation. *Am J Ind Med* 51:503–11.

Goldoni, M., Catalani, S., De Palma, G., Manini, P., Acampa, O., Corradi, M., Bergonzi, R., Apostoli, P. and Mutti, A. 2004. Exhaled breath condensate as a suitable matrix to assess lung dose and effects in workers exposed to cobalt and tungsten. *Environ Health Perspect* 112:1293–8.

Haslam, P. L. and Baughman, R. P. 1999. Report of ERS Task Force: Guidelines for measurement of acellular components and standardization of BAL. *Eur Respir J* 14:245–8.

Heldal, K. K., Madso, L., Huser, P. O. and Eduard, W. 2010. Exposure, symptoms and airway inflammation among sewage workers. *Ann Agric Environ Med* 17:263–8.

Hewitt, R. S., Smith, A. D., Cowan, J. O., Schofield, J. C., Herbison, G. P. and Taylor, D. R. 2008. Serial exhaled nitric oxide measurements in the assessment of laboratory animal allergy. *J Asthma* 45:101–7.

Hiel, D., Von Scheele, I., Sundblad, B. M., Larsson, K. and Palmberg, L. 2009. Evaluation of respiratory effects related to high-pressure cleaning in a piggery with and without robot pre-cleaning. *Scand J Work Environ Health* 35:376–83.

Ho, L. P., Wood, F. T., Robson, A., Innes, J. A. and Greening, A. P. 2000. Atopy influences exhaled nitric oxide levels in adult asthmatics. *Chest* 118:1327–31.

Hoffmeyer, F., Raulf-Heimsoth, M. and Bruning, T. 2009. Exhaled breath condensate and airway inflammation. *Curr Opin Allergy Clin Immunol* 9:16–22.

Horvath, I., Hunt, J. and Barnes, P. J. 2005. Exhaled breath condensate: Methodological recommendations and unresolved questions. *Eur Respir J* 26:523–48.

Hulo, S., Cherot-Kornobis, N., Howsam, M., Crucq, S., De Broucker, V., Sobaszek, A. and Edme, J. L. 2014. Manganese in exhaled breath condensate: A new marker of exposure to welding fumes. *Toxicol Lett* 226:63–9.

Karjalainen, A., Anttila, S., Mantyla, T., Taskinen, E., Kyyronen, P. and Tukiainen, P. 1994. Asbestos bodies in bronchoalveolar lavage fluid in relation to occupational history. *Am J Ind Med* 26:645–54.

Koczulla, A. R., Noeske, S., Herr, C., Jorres, R. A., Rommelt, H., Vogelmeier, C. and Bals, R. 2010. Acute and chronic effects of smoking on inflammation markers in exhaled breath condensate in current smokers. *Respiration* 79:61–7.

Koczulla, R., Dragonieri, S., Schot, R., Bals, R., Gauw, S. A., Vogelmeier, C., Rabe, K. F., Sterk, P. J. and Hiemstra, P. S. 2009. Comparison of exhaled breath condensate pH using two commercially available devices in healthy controls, asthma and COPD patients. *Respir Res* 10:78.

Kolbeck, K. G., Ehnhage, A., Juto, J. E., Forsberg, S., Gyllenhammar, H., Palmberg, L. and Larsson, K. 2000. Airway reactivity and exhaled NO following swine dust exposure in healthy volunteers. *Respir Med* 94:1065–72.

Kullmann, T., Barta, I., Lazar, Z., Szili, B., Barat, E., Valyon, M., Kollai, M. and Horvath, I. 2007. Exhaled breath condensate pH standardised for CO_2 partial pressure. *Eur Respir J* 29:496–501.

Larsson, P., Mirgorodskaya, E., Samuelsson, L., Bake, B., Almstrand, A. C., Bredberg, A. and Olin, A. C. 2012. Surfactant protein A and albumin in particles in exhaled air. *Respir Med* 106:197–204.

Larstad, M., Almstrand, A. C., Larsson, P., Bake, B., Larsson, S., Ljungstrom, E., Mirgorodskaya, E. and Olin, A. C. 2015. Surfactant protein A in exhaled endogenous particles is decreased in chronic obstructive pulmonary disease (COPD) patients: A pilot study. *PLoS One* 10(12):e0144463.

Lehtimaki, L., Kankaanranta, H., Saarelainen, S., Hahtola, P., Jarvenpaa, R., Koivula, T., Turjanmaa, V. and Moilanen, E. 2001. Extended exhaled NO measurement differentiates between alveolar and bronchial inflammation. *Am J Respir Crit Care Med* 163:1557–61.

Lehtimaki, L., Oksa, P., Jarvenpaa, R., Vierikko, T., Nieminen, R., Kankaanranta, H., Uitti, J. and Moilanen, E. 2010. Pulmonary inflammation in asbestos-exposed subjects with borderline parenchymal changes on HRCT. *Respir Med* 104:1042–9.

Lemiere, C., D'Alpaos, V., Chaboillez, S., Cesar, M., Wattiez, M., Chiry, S. and Vandenplas, O. 2010. Investigation of occupational asthma: Sputum cell counts or exhaled nitric oxide? *Chest* 137:617–22.

Lima, T. M., Kazama, C. M., Koczulla, A. R., Hiemstra, P. S., Macchione, M., Fernandes, A. L., Santos Ude, P. et al. 2013. pH in exhaled breath condensate and nasal lavage as a biomarker of air pollution-related inflammation in street traffic-controllers and office-workers. *Clinics (Sao Paulo)* 68:1488–94.

Lund, M. B., Oksne, P. I., Hamre, R. and Kongerud, J. 2000. Increased nitric oxide in exhaled air: An early marker of asthma in non-smoking aluminium potroom workers? *Occup Environ Med* 57:274–8.

Malinovschi, A., Backer, V., Harving, H. and Porsbjerg, C. 2012. The value of exhaled nitric oxide to identify asthma in smoking patients with asthma-like symptoms. *Respir Med* 106:794–801.

Marteus, H., Tornberg, D. C., Weitzberg, E., Schedin, U. and Alving, K. 2005. Origin of nitrite and nitrate in nasal and exhaled breath condensate and relation to nitric oxide formation. *Thorax* 60:219–25.

Mauer, M. P., Hoen, R. and Jourd'heuil, D. 2011. FE NO concentrations in World Trade Center responders and controls, 6 years post-9/11. *Lung* 189:295–303.

Miekisch, W., Schubert, J. K. and Noeldge-Schomburg, G. F. 2004. Diagnostic potential of breath analysis—Focus on volatile organic compounds. *Clin Chim Acta* 347:25–39.

Miranda, A. I., Martins, V., Cascao, P., Amorim, J. H., Valente, J., Borrego, C., Ferreira, A. J., Cordeiro, C. R., Viegas, D. X. and Ottmar, R. 2012. Wildland smoke exposure values and exhaled breath indicators in firefighters. *J Toxicol Environ Health A* 75:831–43.

Mirmohammadi, S. J., Mehrparvar, A. H., Safaei, S., Nodoushan, M. S. and Jahromi, M. T. 2014. Across-shift changes of exhaled nitric oxide and spirometric indices among cotton textile workers. *Int J Occup Med Environ Health* 27:707–15.

Mohamed, E. I., Mahmoud, G. N., El-Sharkawy, R. M., Moro, A. M., Abdel-Mageed, S. M. and Kotb, M. A. 2014. Electronic nose for tracking different types of leukaemia: Future prospects in diagnosis. *Hematol Oncol* 32:165–7.

Montuschi, P., Mores, N., Trove, A., Mondino, C. and Barnes, P. J. 2013. The electronic nose in respiratory medicine. *Respiration* 85:72–84.

Moore, V. C., Anees, W., Jaakkola, M. S., Burge, C. B., Robertson, A. S. and Burge, P. S. 2010. Two variants of occupational asthma separable by exhaled breath nitric oxide level. *Respir Med* 104:873–9.

Ndlovu, V., Dalvie, M. A. and Jeebhay, M. F. 2014. Asthma associated with pesticide exposure among women in rural Western Cape of South Africa. *Am J Ind Med* 57:1331–43.

Obata, H., Dittrick, M., Chan, H. and Chan-Yeung, M. 1999. Sputum eosinophils and exhaled nitric oxide during late asthmatic reaction in patients with western red cedar asthma. *Eur Respir J* 13:489–95.

Olin, A. C., Andersson, E., Andersson, M., Granung, G., Hagberg, S. and Toren, K. 2004. Prevalence of asthma and exhaled nitric oxide are increased in bleachery workers exposed to ozone. *Eur Respir J* 23:87–92.

Olin, A. C., Ljungkvist, G., Bake, B., Hagberg, S., Henriksson, L. and Toren, K. 1999. Exhaled nitric oxide among pulpmill workers reporting gassing incidents involving ozone and chlorine dioxide. *Eur Respir J* 14:828–31.

Pelclova, D., Fenclova, Z., Kacer, P., Kuzma, M., Navratil, T. and Lebedova, J. 2008. Increased 8-isoprostane, a marker of oxidative stress in exhaled breath condensate in subjects with asbestos exposure. *Ind Health* 46:484–9.

Piirila, P., Wikman, H., Luukkonen, R., Kaaria, K., Rosenberg, C., Nordman, H., Norppa, H., Vainio, H. and Hirvonen, A. 2001. Glutathione S-transferase genotypes and allergic responses to diisocyanate exposure. *Pharmacogenetics* 11:437–45.

Pronk, A., Preller, L., Doekes, G., Wouters, I. M., Rooijackers, J., Lammers, J. W. and Heederik, D. 2009. Different respiratory phenotypes are associated with isocyanate exposure in spray painters. *Eur Respir J* 33:494–501.

Rosias, P. P., Robroeks, C. M., Niemarkt, H. J., Kester, A. D., Vernooy, J. H., Suykerbuyk, J., Teunissen, J. et al. 2006. Breath condenser coatings affect measurement of biomarkers in exhaled breath condensate. *Eur Respir J* 28:1036–41.

Rosias, P. P., Robroeks, C. M., Van De Kant, K. D., Rijkers, G. T., Zimmermann, L. J., Van Schayck, C. P., Heynens, J. W. Jobsis, Q. and Dompeling, E. 2010. Feasibility of a new method to collect exhaled breath condensate in preschool children. *Pediatr Allergy Immunol* 21:e235–44.

Rouhos, A., Kainu, A., Piirila, P., Sarna, S., Lindqvist, A., Karjalainen, J. and Sovijarvi, A. R. 2011. Repeatability of exhaled nitric oxide measurements in patients with COPD. *Clin Physiol Funct Imaging* 31:26–31.

Sastre, J., Madero, M. F., Fernandez-Nieto, M., Sastre, B., Del Pozo, V., Potro, M. G. and Quirce, S. 2011. Airway response to chlorine inhalation (bleach) among cleaning workers with and without bronchial hyperresponsiveness. *Am J Ind Med* 54:293–9.

Sauni, R., Oksa, P., Lehtimaki, L., Toivio, P., Palmroos, P., Nieminen, R., Moilanen, E. and Uitti, J. 2012. Increased alveolar nitric oxide and systemic inflammation markers in silica-exposed workers. *Occup Environ Med* 69:256–60.

Shiryaeva, O., Aasmoe, L., Straume, B. and Bang, B. E. 2015. Respiratory symptoms, lung functions, and exhaled nitric oxide (FE) in two types of fish processing workers: Russian trawler fishermen and Norwegian salmon industry workers. *Int J Occup Environ Health* 21:53–60.

Smit, L. A., Heederik, D., Doekes, G. and Wouters, I. M. 2009. Exhaled nitric oxide in endotoxin-exposed adults: Effect modification by smoking and atopy. *Occup Environ Med* 66:251–5.

Smith, D., Spanel, P., Herbig, J. and Beauchamp, J. 2014. Mass spectrometry for real-time quantitative breath analysis. *J Breath Res* 8:027101.

Sue-Chu, M., Henriksen, A. H. and Bjermer, L. 1999. Non-invasive evaluation of lower airway inflammation in hyper-responsive elite cross-country skiers and asthmatics. *Respir Med* 93:719–25.

Sundblad, B. M., Larsson, B. M., Palmberg, L. and Larsson, K. 2002. Exhaled nitric oxide and bronchial responsiveness in healthy subjects exposed to organic dust. *Eur Respir J* 20:426–31.

Sundblad, B. M., Von Scheele, I., Palmberg, L., Olsson, M. and Larsson, K. 2009. Repeated exposure to organic material alters inflammatory and physiological airway responses. *Eur Respir J* 34:80–8.

Svedahl, S. R., Svendsen, K., Tufvesson, E., Romundstad, P. R., Sjaastad, A. K., Qvenild, T. and Hilt, B. 2013. Inflammatory markers in blood and exhaled air after short-term exposure to cooking fumes. *Ann Occup Hyg* 57:230–9.

Swierczynska-Machura, D., Krakowiak, A., Wiszniewska, M., Dudek, W., Walusiak, J. and Palczynski, C. 2008. Exhaled nitric oxide levels after specific inhalatory challenge test in subjects with diagnosed occupational asthma. *Int J Occup Med Environ Health* 21:219–25.

Tan, K., Bruce, C., Birkhead, A. and Thomas, P. S. 2001. Nasal and exhaled nitric oxide in response to occupational latex exposure. *Allergy* 56:627–32.

Tossa, P., Paris, C., Zmirou-Navier, D., Demange, V., Acouetey, D. S., Michaely, J. P. and Bohadana, A. 2010. Increase in exhaled nitric oxide is associated with bronchial hyperresponsiveness among apprentices. *Am J Respir Crit Care Med* 182:738–44.

Trischler, J., Merkel, N., Konitzer, S., Muller, C. M., Unverzagt, S. and Lex, C. 2012. Fractionated breath condensate sampling: H_2O_2 concentrations of the alveolar fraction may be related to asthma control in children. *Respir Res* 13:14.

Tsoukias, N. M. and George, S. C. 1998. A two-compartment model of pulmonary nitric oxide exchange dynamics. *J Appl Physiol* 85:653–66.

Ulvestad, B., Lund, M. B., Bakke, B., Djupesland, P. G., Kongerud, J. and Boe, J. 2001. Gas and dust exposure in underground construction is associated with signs of airway inflammation. *Eur Respir J* 17:416–21.

van der Walt, A., Lopata, A. L., Nieuwenhuizen, N. E. and Jeebhay, M. F. 2010. Work-related allergy and asthma in spice mill workers—The impact of processing dried spices on IgE reactivity patterns. *Int Arch Allergy Immunol* 152:271–8.

Vaughan, D. J., Brogan, T. V., Kerr, M. E., Deem, S., Luchtel, D. L. and Swenson, E. R. 2003. Contributions of nitric oxide synthase isozymes to exhaled nitric oxide and hypoxic pulmonary vasoconstriction in rabbit lungs. *Am J Physiol Lung Cell Mol Physiol* 284:L834–43.

Verbanck, S., Malinovschi, A., George, S., Gelb, A. F., Vincken, W. and Van Muylem, A. 2012. Bronchial and alveolar components of exhaled nitric oxide and their relationship. *Eur Respir J* 39:1258–61.

Von Essen, S. G., Scheppers, L. A., Robbins, R. A. and Donham, K. J. 1998. Respiratory tract inflammation in swine confinement workers studied using induced sputum and exhaled nitric oxide. *J Toxicol Clin Toxicol* 36:557–65.

Von Essen S. G., Robbins R. A., Spurzem J. R., Thompson A. B., McGranaghan S. S. and Rennard S.I. 1991. Bronchoscopy with bronchoalveolar lavage causes neutrophil recruitment to the lower respiratory tract. *Am Rev Respir Dis* 144:848–54.

Walters, G. I., Moore, V. C., McGrath, E. E. and Burge, S. 2014. Fractional exhaled nitric oxide in the interpretation of specific inhalational challenge tests for occupational asthma. *Lung* 192(1):119–24.

Wells, K., Vaughan, J., Pajewski, T. N., Hom, S., Ngamtrakulpanit, L., Smith, A., Nguyen, A., Turner, R. and Hunt, J. 2005. Exhaled breath condensate pH assays are not influenced by oral ammonia. *Thorax* 60:27–31.

Wilson, H. K. and Monster, A. C. 1999. New technologies in the use of exhaled breath analysis for biological monitoring. *Occup Environ Med* 56:753–7.

7 The Consequences of Chronic Respiratory Disease for Employment and Employability

Kjell Torén and Nicola Murgia

CONTENTS

INTRODUCTION

Respiratory diseases, whether or not they are caused by occupational exposures, are common in the working population (Balmes et al., 2003). Respiratory diseases are important predictors of work-life participation, especially diseases such as asthma, which are common among younger populations. Chronic obstructive pulmonary disease (COPD), which peaks later in life, is more of a problem for older segments of the workforce. This has different implications for how to approach a patient whose work is affected by respiratory disease. A young person with asthma may be encouraged to change jobs. A 60 year old smoking welder with COPD may be advised to continue his or her work, stop smoking and, in cooperation with an occupational health service, reduce his or her exposure on the job. Until the 1980s, much of the literature on occupational respiratory disease and work ability concerned the assessment of impairment and disability among patients with pneumoconiosis, mainly silicosis (Morgan and Seaton, 1975). In the last few decades, however, disability assessments and research in relation to asthma and COPD have gained increased attention. More recently, patients with cystic fibrosis (CF) and transplanted lungs have gained attention as new groups joining the workforce, with implications for how to improve their work-life participation.

DEFINITIONS AND GENERAL BACKGROUND

There are many confusing definitions in this field. At the beginning of the 2000s, the International Classification of Functioning, Disability and Health (ICF) was proposed and has gained increased use (ICF, 2001). The ICF classification focuses on the capabilities of the subjects. The areas of the ICF are body functions, activities and participation and environmental factors. In the field of occupational medicine, the shift from using the term 'work disability' to 'work ability' is probably influenced by the ICF concept. Nonetheless, beyond that, the ICF concept has not been applied extensively in the field of respiratory diseases.

The older concept comprising impairment, disability and handicap is still in frequent use. These terms are easier to conceptualize. 'Impairment' refers to impairment in a function. In the respiratory field, impairment is often quantified using physiologic measures. The most common measure is lung function as measured by spirometry (forced expiratory volume in 1 second [FEV_1] and forced vital capacity [FVC]), and the use of these measures is based on the existence of normal (reference) values.

Disability is a reflection of the affected individual's capacity given the existing impairment and the demands from the workplace (environment). Work disability represents a specific subset of disability; for instance, a violinist lacking a little finger may have a minor impairment but a major work disability. A blind person, with an obvious impairment, can manage a form of work if the workplace is arranged in a certain way. This reflects the notion that the demands from the workplace are important parts of the nature of work disability. Another important feature of work disability, as compared to impairment, is that work disability is based on self-report from the affected person (patient) and is not based on assessments from a physician. Impairment can often be measured using different physiological parameters, but work disability is more complex to measure. One frequently used measure in respiratory research is a composite of disease-related complete cessation of work, change of workplace or occupation or change of work tasks. Another common measure is lost workdays or decreased productivity at work. 'Handicap' is defined along the lines of the person as a social being (i.e. the interaction at a personal level between impairment and disability and the demands from the society). However, in current classifications, the term 'handicap' has been dropped mainly because of its pejorative connotations.

Another method that has emerged is the assessment of work ability and the use of the Work Ability Index (WAI). The WAI originated from Finnish researchers who constructed an instrument (questionnaire) based on a multidimensional model comprising seven domains of importance for work-life participation (Tuomi et al., 1991). These domains include: the subject's global assessment of current work ability; self-assessment of work ability in relation to the physical and mental demands of the work; subjective estimation of the work impairment due to disease; sickness absence; self-estimation of future work ability; and self-assessment of psychological resources. These items have been used to construct a summary index (the WAI), which has been shown to be a good predictor of work-life participation (van den Berg et al., 2009).

Work disability is related mainly to two different factors that are often inter-related. The first one is disease severity, which could influence directly work ability. The other important factor is work-related exposure to agents that are capable of affecting work ability, often through symptoms or disease worsening (Murgia et al., 2011).

ASTHMA

Work Disability and Work Ability

Work disability is an important component for evaluating the consequences of occupational exposures among persons with asthma. Asthma-related work disability occurs both among persons with work-related asthma and among those who have asthma in whom the onset is totally unrelated to occupational exposures. Asthma is quite common in the working population. Hence, asthma-related work disability may carry large consequences for work-life participation in the form of absenteeism or restrictions in possible job duties or tasks.

In a longitudinal study on random population samples from many European countries, it was found that during 9 years of follow-up, 5% of the subjects with asthma reported changes of work due to respiratory problems (Torén et al., 2009). Further, it was found that exposure to biological dust or gases and fumes markedly increased the risk of changing work because of respiratory complaints compared to randomly selected population controls. Exposure to mineral dust (stone, quartz, sand, etc.) was not associated with any increased risk for asthma-related work disability. Atopy was not a modifying factor in this study. Nevertheless, these findings indicated that these work-related exposures induce asthma exacerbations, causing the subject to change job, although the magnitude of the effect was lower than one might have expected. An explanation for this may be that this was a study of a broad group of persons with asthma. A much more severe impact of occupational exposures was found in a US study of subjects with severe asthma (Eisner et al., 2006). Among 465 ever-employed adults with clinically ascertained asthma, 14% reported asthma-related complete work disability, and among those without current employment, 25% attributed their unemployment to previous occupational exposures.

Regarding sickness absence, the number of workdays lost by workers with asthma has been found to be related both to severity of asthma (Gozalez Barcala et al., 2011) and to current exposure to vapour, gas, dust and fumes, where such exposures seem to double the risk for respiratory sickness absence among subjects with asthma or respiratory symptoms (wheeze or breathlessness) (Kim et al., 2013a). A similar observation was made among healthcare workers, where cleaners had an increased prevalence of respiratory symptoms and significantly higher sickness absence than other working groups (Kim et al., 2013b). There are a number of studies indicating that employed asthmatics have reduced productivity because of their disease (Balder et al., 1998, Blanc et al., 2001).

Among workers with occupational asthma, longitudinal studies have consistently shown that occupational asthma is associated with a high risk of work disability, defined either as complete work cessation or reduced income levels (Vandenplas et al., 2003). The magnitude differs between countries, with the lowest unemployment rate in Finnish populations (Piirilä et al., 2005).

In conclusion, longitudinal studies and a number of cross-sectional studies have clearly shown that subjects with asthma have an increased risk for unemployment and job change due to the disease. Workplace exposure and disease severity interact with each other in causing the disability.

Exacerbations of Asthma

Exacerbation of asthma is a condition that is relevant to respiratory work disability. There are relatively few studies of this topic, but the existing literature indicates that occupational exposure to vapour, gas, dust and fumes increases the prevalence of symptoms among asthmatics, increasing the risk for respiratory disability. Table 7.1 summarizes the findings from relevant studies of asthmatics from random population samples.

Vocational Advice

In Scandinavia, there is an opinion among vocational counsellors that allergic adolescents should be advised to avoid occupations with exposure to irritants and allergens, including jobs such as painters, bakers, hairdressers or veterinarians. However, the evidence in favour of advising adolescents to avoid certain occupations is quite weak. There are longitudinal studies of apprentices showing that subjects with bronchial hyper-reactivity or positive skin-prick tests experience an increased risk of developing asthma or asthma symptoms (Kennedy et al., 1999; Gautrin et al., 2008). When apprentices in animal health technology were followed, those with sensitization to laboratory animals at the start of the study had a high risk of developing asthma, but there was also a high risk among those without sensitization (Gautrin, 2008). The non-sensitized at baseline was the largest group, consisting of 75% of the population. This indicates that vocational advice based on sensitization has low accuracy (poor predictive power). In a Dutch study, it was found that asthmatics were slightly more often vocationally advised compared to non-asthmatics, and they also more often sought white collar occupations (Orbon et al., 2006). This of course could be a consequence of the vocational advice. Despite this, this group more frequently reports work disability and has a slightly higher absence rate from work compared to non-asthmatics (Orbon et al., 2006). In addition, there is also an element of self-selection: it seems that subjects with rhinitis or severe asthma tend to select low-risk jobs, whereas as those with mild or moderate asthma have similar occupational careers as others.

TABLE 7.1
Description of Epidemiologic Studies Analyzing Association between Occupational Exposures and Asthma Exacerbations

Reference	Source Population (n = Number with Asthma)	Definition of Asthma Exacerbation	Exposure/Occupation	Exposures or Occupations that Increase the Risk for Exacerbations
Henneberger et al. (2003)	US population from an health maintenance organisation (n = 1461)	Is your current work impairing your asthma?	Current branch	Sales, administration, transports and public services
Saarinen et al. (2003)	Population-based case–control study (n = 969)	Occurrence of asthma symptoms during work over the last 12 months	1. Job exposure matrix (JEM); dust, gas and fumes in current occupation 2. Self-reported exposure	JEM for gas, dust and fumes Self-reported exposure: dust, chemicals, non-normal temperature, bad indoor quality or physical demanding work
Henneberger et al. (2006)	US population from an health maintenance organisation (n = 557)	Self-reported symptoms	Expert assessment 0, 1 och 2	Exposure to allergens and irritants
Henneberger et al. (2010)	European Community Respiratory Health Survey (n = 966)	Self-reported unplanned care for asthma in the past 12 months	Job exposure matrix (biological dust, mineral dust, gas and fumes)	High exposure to biological dust and gas/fumes was associated with at least doubled risk for severe exacerbations

Note: 0: no exposure; 1: low exposure; 2: high exposure.

A key issue relates to whether persons with atopy should be advised to avoid high-risk occupations, such as work with laboratory animals. There is increasing evidence that this is a futile strategy. As already described, the fractional numbers of prevented cases of asthma is quite low compared to the disadvantages of excluding atopics from certain workplaces. One example using bakers is illustrative: among bakers, 20% of atopics become sensitized to flour dust and 4% of non-atopics become sensitized to flour dust (Brisman et al., 1999). Hence, there is a fivefold increased risk for the atopics becoming sensitized. Is this a reason for advising atopics to avoid baking work? Assume that 500 bakers are employed and 15% of them (n = 75) are atopics. Among them, 15 workers (20%) will become flour dust sensitized. Among the non-atopics, 4% will develop a flour dust allergy, (i.e. 17 workers [425 × 0.04]). Thus, had the atopics been excluded from employment, only half of the sensitized cases would have been prevented. Hence, persons should be informed about the risks involved, but the individuals should make their own choice. It is also important to realize that one gets asthma from certain exposures, but not from occupation per se. This means that more emphasis has to be placed on exposure levels and exposure interventions, rather that avoiding certain occupations (Consensus Report, 2001).

CHRONIC OBSTRUCTIVE PULMONARY DISEASE

COPD is a disease that occurs late in working life with a long 'silent' period with deteriorating lung function but without symptoms. COPD has previously been regarded as a solely tobacco-induced disease, but in recent years there has been growing recognition that occupational exposures are important factors in the aetiology of COPD (Torén and Balmes, 2007). Whether occupational factors play a role in established disease has been less investigated. One of the first studies of work disability showed that males with COPD who have stopped working have had more dusty and heavy work and lower FEV_1 values compared to those still working (Diener and Burrows, 1967). Following this study, a number of publications have essentially confirmed this observation. Occupational exposure to fumes, but not to dust, increased the decline in lung function among male subjects with COPD (Harber et al., 2007). Occupational exposure to gas, dust and fumes was associated with increased severity of COPD and an increased risk of permanent work disability (Rodriguez et al., 2008). In a prospective study of 386 subjects with COPD, 23% had left work due to their lung disease (Blanc et al., 2004). Exposure to vapour, gas, dust and fumes resulted in a doubled risk for respiratory work disability. In a cross-sectional study from the USA, the subjects with COPD with occupational exposure to gas, dust or fumes reported decreased quality of life (both generic and specific), more symptoms, more exacerbations and shorter walking distance (6 minutes) as compared to COPD subjects without occupational exposure (Paulin et al., 2015). An editorial accompanying this publication stated that the study confirmed that occupational exposure is associated with worse clinical markers of disease effect (Martinez and Declos, 2015). Further, it underscored the importance of taking an occupational history of patients with COPD, especially if they have an exacerbation.

There are also a number of studies describing absence from work and sickness absence among subjects with COPD (Patel et al., 2014). The conclusion is that approximately 15% of gainfully employed persons report limitations regarding their work, with a higher prevalence among subjects with emphysema, indicating a more severe COPD. There are also studies showing that individuals with COPD who are still in the workforce are absent from 1 to almost 20 days a year. The conclusion is that COPD is probably associated with significant work disability, but the importance of occupational exposures in such disability has not been studied.

CYSTIC FIBROSIS

The survival of patients with CF has increased dramatically since 1936, the year in which the disease was first formally recognized (Fanconi et al., 1936). This increased survival means that today most patients reach adulthood and the majority of individuals with CF are working. There are a number of descriptive, uncontrolled studies of patients with CF with regards to work disability. In all studies, approximately 50% of the patients are currently employed, and a substantial proportion reports that their disease has hampered their career. However, in some studies, CF patients seems to have higher educational levels than the population in general. An early study from the UK investigated 866 subjects with CF with a questionnaire (Walters et al., 1993). Of the responders, 54% were in paid employment compared with 69% in the general population, and there was a higher proportion of non-manual occupations in the CF group. A similar but smaller study from the USA found that 27% were currently employed, and almost 50% attributed job change or work cessation to the disease (Gillen et al., 1995). The majority (84%) had non-manual occupations, but nearly 100% reaching adulthood had some labour force participation. In a multiple regression model, work disability was associated with adult onset of CF, female gender and living alone. A later study from Australia demonstrated that 72% of those with CF were currently employed and 40% worked more than 30 hours/week (Hogg et al., 2007). Nevertheless, over 50% attributed job changes or ceased work to CF. In a regression model, disease severity was associated with work disability, but there were no factors reflecting the workplace.

Further studies give the impression that the employability of subjects with CF is increasing. In a more recent French study from 2012, 70% of those with CF were employed and 94% reported having a job in the past (Laborde et al., 2012). The majority had non-manual employment, while only 4% were classified as blue-collar workers. Half of those studied had been counselled to avoid certain jobs such as healthcare work, physical work or dusty work. In a multiple regression model, disease severity and education were significantly associated with employment status. The most recent study from the UK reported that 65% were in employment or in education and 80% had worked at some time (Targett et al., 2014). Forty percent reported that CF had negatively affected their work (approximately 20% had blue-collar occupations). In a regression model, disease severity, male gender, quality of life and education were associated with employment status.

The survival of CF patients has increased, and now working-life participation is a reality for most persons with CF. Despite this increasing labour force participation, there is a lack of knowledge regarding the importance of workplace exposures, including psychosocial factors, even if it seems plausible that dusty and heavy work is not beneficial for the CF group.

ALLERGIC ALVEOLITIS (HYPERSENSITIVITY PNEUMONITIS)

This is a disease that occurs in certain occupations such as farming and other sectors in which organic material is handled. A Finnish study of the clinical course of 86 farmers with allergic alveolitis with 5 years of follow-up found that 57 (66%) continued as farmers, two farmers changed occupation and the rest gave up their work (Mönkäre et al., 1987). Those who gave up their work had more severe disease. In a metalworking shop series, 35 workers were diagnosed as having allergic alveolitis (Bracker et al., 2003). After 2 years, 51% had returned to work without any information about the predictors for returning to work.

LUNG TRANSPLANTATION

Several of the patients in the CF group described above had undergone lung transplantation. This intervention is increasing, leading to larger numbers of persons who are participating in the labour force after transplantation. Indeed, return to work has become increasingly important as part of the rehabilitation process among such patients. The first study in this field described 99 lung transplant patients from Canada and the USA, and of these, 60% were considered to have work ability (Paris et al., 1998). Of these, 37% were indeed working. Positive factors for work-life participation were pre-transplantation employment, self-report of work ability, good lung function and physical capacity after the transplantation. In a study from Belgium of 281 different organ transplantations, those who had undergone lung transplantation had a significantly lower rate of return to work compared to kidney transplantation (De Baere et al., 2010). Positive factors for return to work were employment before the transplantation, high self-assessed work ability, being married and male gender. It has been argued that heart–lung-transplanted patients have an inferior return to work compared to other transplanted patient (Paris et al., 2005). However, this is a field that is marked by a scarcity of data, and probably, as in the field of CF, we can anticipate that there are improvements to be made.

One exposure-specific topic that has been considered in lung transplantation is whether a patient with a suspected occupational lung disease, such as a pneumoconiosis or emphysema caused by α_1-antitrypsine deficiency with concomitant occupational exposure, could return back to dusty work. Based on clinical experience, the advice would be to avoid dusty workplaces. This clinical impression is supported by a review of 31 transplanted subjects with hypersensitivity pneumonitis, of whom two developed recurrent hypersensitivity pneumonitis (Kern et al., 2015). Both of these individuals returned to exposure conditions after the transplantation.

RHINITIS

Without concomitant asthma, rhinitis was regarded as a trivial medical condition until many studies highlighted its importance in causing sleep disturbance, daytime fatigue and psychomotor and cognitive impairment (Nathan, 2007). The burden of rhinitis, which is a common disease, would also be anticipated to affect work ability. In practice, many studies on this subject are characterized by the common coexistence of asthma and rhinitis, making it more difficult to estimate the real occupational impact of rhinitis alone. In a French study, almost 80% of patient with rhinitis reported some work disability due to their disease (Demoly et al., 2002). In an American study, subjects with rhinitis had a higher risk of ceasing work compared to those without disease, but the risk estimate was lower compared to asthma and COPD (Yelin et al., 2006). The number of work days lost to rhinitis in a year can vary greatly, ranging from 0.03 to 8/year per capita, accounting for the majority of rhinitis-related indirect costs (Vandenplas et al., 2008). In another study, it was shown that asthma and rhinitis have similar adverse effects on absenteeism, while rhinitis seems to have a more prominent impact on job effectiveness (Blanc, 2001).

There are several aspects of rhinitis that could have an impact on work functioning. First of all, symptom severity is a factor, given that subjects with more severe rhinitis symptoms have been found to be likely to have their work impacted (Bousquet et al., 2006). Moreover, allergen exposure could play a role in work ability, as higher concentrations of airborne allergens, when measured objectively, were associated with a greater impact on work impairment (Kessler et al., 2001). This can be specific to an occupational allergen, such as bell-pepper exposure among greenhouse workers (Groenewoud et al., 2006). Finally, patients who are treated for rhinitis have better outcomes in terms of work impairment than those who are not treated (Hanrahan et al., 2003).

CONCLUSIONS

Respiratory tract diseases are often work related, but can also exert a significant impact on occupational status, regardless of their aetiology, by leading to work disability. There is still no agreement in the scientific community as to whether it is more useful to assess work ability, which is often by self-report, or impairment at work, which is evaluated by more objective measurement. By whatever measure, asthma, COPD, rhinitis and more uncommon conditions, such as CF and allergic alveolitis, are able to affect work productivity, work absence and work cessation. Moreover, job choice, as in the case of apprentices, can also be impacted, either on a self-selection basis or due to formal vocational counselling.

Several studies have pointed toward occupational exposures as important determinants of work disability, regardless of whether the disease is asthma, COPD or another respiratory condition. This underscores the critical importance of taking an occupational history in patients with chronic respiratory tract disease presenting with exacerbations on the job or work disability. In a wider aspect, it is also important for physicians to act in order to prevent or decrease occupational exposures to vapours, gas, dust and fumes.

REFERENCES

Balder, B., Lindholm, N. B., Löwhagen, O., Palmqvist, M., Plascke, P., Tunsäter, A. and Torén, K. 1998. Predictors of self-assessed work ability among subjects with recent onset asthma. *Respir Med* 92:729–34.

Balmes, J., Becklake, M., Blanc, P., Henneberger, P., Kreiss, K., Mapp, C., Milton, D. et al. 2003. ATS statement on occupational contribution to the burden of airway disease. *Am J Crit Care Respir Med* 167:787–97.

Blanc, P. D., Trupin, L., Eisner, M., Earnest, G., Katz, P. P. and Israel, L. 2001. The work impact of asthma and rhinitis: Findings from a population-based survey. *J Clin Epidemiol* 54:610–8.

Blanc, P. D., Eisner, M. D., Trupin, L., Yelin, E. H., Katz, P. P. and Balmes, J. R. 2004. The association between occupational factors and adverse health outcome in chronic obstructive pulmonary disease. *Occup Environ Med* 61:661–7.

Bousquet, J., Neukirch, F., Bousquet, P. J., Gehano, P., Klossek, J. M., Le Gal, M. and Allaf, B.. 2006. Severity and impairment of allergic rhinitis in patients consulting in primary care. *J Allergy Clin Immunol* 117:158–62.

Bracker, A., Storey, E., Yang, C. and Hodgson, M. J. 2003. An outbreak of hypersensitivity pneumonitis at a metalworking plant: A longitudinal assessment of intervention effectiveness. *Appl Occup Environ Hyg* 18:96–108.

Brisman, J. and Järvholm, B. 1999. Bakery work, atopy and the incidence of self-reported rhinitis and hay-fever. *Eur Respir J* 13:502–7.

Consensus Report. 2001. Airway allergy and worklife. *Scand J Work Environ Health* 27:422–5.

De Baere, C., Delva, D., Kloeck, A., Remans, K., Vanrenterghem, Y., Verleden, G., Vanhaecke, J. et al. 2010. Return to work and social participation: Does type of organ transplantation matter? *Transplantation* 89:1009–15.

Demoly, P., Allaert, F. A. and Lecasble, M. 2002. ERASM, a pharmacoepidemiologic survey on management of intermittent allergic rhinitis in every day general medical practice in France. *Allergy* 57:546–54.

Diener, C. F. and Burrows, B. 1967. Occupational disability in patients with chronic airway obstruction. *Am Rev Respir Dis* 96:35–42.

Eisner, M. D., Yelin, E. H., Katz, P. P., Lactao, G., Iribarren, C. and Blanc, P. D. 2006. Risk factors for work disability in severe adult asthma. *Am J Med* 119:884–91.

Fanconi, G., Uelinger, E. and Knauser, C. 1936. The coeliac syndrome with congenital cystic pancreatic fibromatposis and bronchiectasis. *Wien Med Woschenschrift* 86:753–6.

Gautrin, D., Ghezzo, H., Infante-Rivard, C., Magnan, M., L'Archveque, J., Suarthana, E. and Malo, J.-L. 2008. Long term outcomes in a prospective cohort of apprentices exposed to high-molecular-weight agents. *Am J Respir Crit Care Med* 177:871–9.

Gillen, M., Lallas, D., Brown, C., Yelin, E. and Blanc, P. D. 1995. Work disability in adults with cystic fibrosis. *Am J Respir Crit Care Med* 152:153–6.

Gonzalez Barcala, F. J., La Fuente-Cid, R. D., Alvaraez-Gil, R., Tafalla, M., Nuevo, J. and Caamaño-Isorna, F. 2011. Factors associated with a higher prevalence of work disability among asthmatic patients. *J Asthma* 48:194–9.

Groenewoud, G. C., de Groot, H. and van Wijk, R. G. 2006. Impact of occupational and inhalant allergy on rhinitis-specific quality of life in employees of bell pepper greenhouses in the Netherlands. *Ann Allergy Asthma Immunol* 96:92–7.

Hanrahan, L.P. and Paramore, L.C. 2003. Aeroallergens, allergic rhinitis, and sedating antihistamines: Risk factors for traumatic occupational injury and economic impact. *Am J Ind Med* 44:438–46.

Harber, P., Tashkin, D. P., Simmons, M., Crawford, L., Hnizdo, E. and Connett, J. 2007. Effect of occupational exposures on decline of lung function in early chronic obstructive pulmonary disease. *Am J Respir Crit Care Med* 176:994–1000.

Henneberger, P. K., Deprez, R. D., Asdigan, N., Oliver, L. C., Derk, S. and Goe, S. K. 2003. Work-place exacerbation of asthma-symptoms: Findings from a population-based study in Maine. *Arch Env Health* 58:781–8.

Henneberger, P. K., Derk, S. J., Sama, S. R., Boylstein, R. J., Hoffman, C. D., Preusse, P. A. and Milton, D. K. 2006. The frequency of workplace exacerbation among health maintenance organisation members with asthma. *Occup Environ Med* 63:551–7.

Henneberger, P. K., Mirabelli, M. C., Kogevinas, M., Plana, E., Dahlman-Höglund, A., Jarvis, D. L., Olivieri, M. et al. 2010. The occupational contribution to severe exacerbation of asthma. *Eur Respir J* 36:743–50.

Hogg, M., Barithwaite, M., Baiuley, M., Kotsimbos, T. and Wilson, J. W. 2007. Work disability in adults with cystic fibrosis and its relation to quality of life. *J Cyst Fibr* 6:223–7.

International Classification of Functioning, Disability and Health (ICF). 2001. Geneva: WHO Press.

Kennedy, S. M., Chan-Yeung, M., Teschke, K. and Karlen, B. 1999. Changes in airway responsiveness among apprentices exposed to metalworking fluids. *Am J Respir Crit Care Med* 157:87–93.

Kern, R. M., Singer, J. P., Koth, L., Mooney, J., Golden, J., Hays, S., Greenland, J. et al. 2015. Lung transplantation for hypersensitivity pneumonitis. *Chest* 147:1558–65.

Kessler, R. C., Almeida, D. M., Berglund, P. and Stang, P. 2001. Pollen and mold exposure impairs the work performance of employees with allergic rhinitis. *Ann Allergy Asthma Immunol* 87:289–95.

Kim, J. L., Blanc, P. D., Zock, J. P., Kogevinas, M., Radon, K., Kromhout, H., Antó, J. M. et al. 2013a. Predictors for respiratory-related sickness absence in subjects with asthma, wheeze, breathlessness or chronic bronchitis. *Am J Ind Med* 56:541–9.

Kim, J. L., Torén, K., Lohman, S., Lötvall, J., Lundbäck, B. and Andersson, E. 2013b. Respiratory symptoms and respiratory-related absence from work among health care workers in Sweden. *J Asthma* 50:174–9.

Laborde-Castérot, H., Donnay, C., Chapron, J., Burgel, P.R., Kanaan, R., Honoré, I., Dusser, D. et al. 2012. Employment and work disability in adults with cystsic fibrosis. *J Cyst Fibr* 11:137–43.

Martinez, C. H. and Declos, G. L. 2015. Occupational exposure and chronic obstructive pulmonary disease. Causality established, time to focus on effect and phenotypes. *Am J Crit Care Med* 191:499–500.

Mönkäre, S. and Haahtela, T. 1987. Farmer's lung—A 5-year follow-up of eighty-six patients. *Clin Allergy* 17:143–51.

Morgan, W. M. K. C. and Seaton A. 1975. *Occupational Lung Diseases*. Philadelphia, PA: WB Saunders.

Murgia, N., Torén, K., Kim, J. L. and Andersson, E. 2011. Risk factors for respiratory work disability in a cohort of pulp mill workers exposed to irritant gases. *BMC Public Health* 11:689.

Nathan, R. A. 2007. The burden of allergic rhinitis. *Allergy Asthma Proc* 28:3–9.

Orbon, K. H., van der Gulden, J. W., Schermer, T. R. and Folgering, H. T. 2006. Vocational and working career of asthmatic adolescents is only slightly affected. *Respir Med* 100:1163–73.

Paris, W., Diercks, M., Bright, J., Zamora, M., Kesten, S., Scavuzzo, M. and Paradis, I. 1998. Return to work after lung transplantation. *J Heart Lung Transplant* 17:430–6.

Paris, W. and White-Williams, C. 2005. Social adaptation after cardiothoracic transplantation. *J Cardiovasc Nurs* 20:567–73.

Patel, J. G., Nagar, S. P. and Dalal, A. A. 2014. Indirect costs in chronic obstructive pulmonary disease: A review of the economic burden on employers and individuals in the Unites States. *Int J COPD* 9:289–300.

Paulin, L. M., Diette, G. B., Blanc, P. D., Putcha, N., Eisner, M. D., Kanner, R. E., Belli, A. J. et al. 2015. Occupational exposures are associated with worse morbidity in patients with chronic obstructive pulmonary disease. *Am J Crit Care Med* 191:557–65.

Piirilä, P. L., Keskinen, H. M., Luukkonen, R., Salo, S. P., Tuppurainen, M. and Nordman, H. 2005. Work, unemployment and life satisfaction among patients with diisocyanate induced asthma—A prospective study. *J Occup Health* 47:112–8.

Rodriguez, E., Ferrer, J., Marti, D. S., Zock, J. P., Plana, E. and Morell, F. 2008. The impact of occupational exposures on severity of COPD. *Chest* 134:1237–43.

Saarinen, K., Karjalainen, A., Martikainen, R., Uitti, J., Tammilehto, L., Klaukka, T. and Kurppa, K. 2003. Prevalence of work-aggravated symptoms in clinically established asthma. *Eur Respir J* 22:305–9.

Targett, K., Bourke, S., Nash, E., Murphy, E., Ayres, J. and Devereux, G. 2014. Employment in adults with cystic fibrosis. *Occup Med* 64:87–94.

Torén, K. and Balmes, J. 2007. Chronic obstructive pulmonary disease: Does occupation matter? *Am J Respir Crit Care Med* 176:951–2.

Torén, K., Kogevinas, M., Zock, J.-P., Sunyer, J., Kromhout, H., Jarvis, D., Payo, F. et al. 2009. A prospective longitudinal general population study of respiratory work-disability among adults. *Thorax* 64:339–44.

Tuomi, K., Ilmarinen, J., Eskelinen, L., Järvinen, E., Toikkanen, J. and Klockars, M. 1991. Prevalence and incidence rates of diseases and work ability in different work categories of municipal occupations. *Scan J Work Environ Health* 17(Suppl. 1):40–7.

van den Berg, T. I., Elders, L. A., de Zwart, B. C. and Burdorf, A. 2009. The effects of work-related and individual factors on the Work Ability Index: A systematic review. *Occup Environ Med* 66:211–20.

Vandenplas, O., D'Alpaos, V. and Van Brussel, P. 2008. Rhinitis and its impact on work. *Curr Opin Allergy Clin Immunol* 8:145–9.

Vandenplas, O., Torén, K. and Blanc, P. D. 2003. Health and socio-economic impacts of work-related asthma. *Eur Respir J* 22:689–97.

Walters, S., Britton, J. and Hodson, M.E. 1993. Demographic and social characteristics of adults with cystic fibrosis in the United Kingdom. *Br Med J* 306:549–52.

Yelin, E., Katz, P., Balmes, J., Trupin, L., Earnest, G., Eisner, M. and Blanc, P. 2006. Work life of persons with asthma, rhinitis, and COPD: A study using a national population-based sample. *J Occup Med Toxicol* 1:2.

8 Surveillance at a Population Level

Raymond Agius and Melanie Carder

CONTENTS

INTRODUCTION

Public policy for preventing occupational disease needs to be informed by good-quality data regarding the population burden and the risks of ill health associated with specific exposures, occupations and industries, so as to target appropriate action. Investigation of trends helps to monitor growing risks as well as to evaluate their mitigation following intervention. Therefore, in many industrialised countries, systems exist to monitor the occurrence of occupational lung disorders. These include statutory reporting systems (often linked to compensation), voluntary physician-based reporting networks, mortality records, cancer registries and other routine data sources such as labour market surveys. With careful interpretation, most of these data can be used to determine the burden of occupational lung disorders including secular (temporal) changes and the determinants of risk. However, each has its own strengths and weaknesses, which must be considered when interpreting and comparing data from different sources. Matters such as diagnostic criteria, case ascertainment, data quality and representativeness all need to be taken into account. This chapter provides an illustrated overview of these issues.

DATA SOURCES

Statutory Reporting

Many countries have statutory reporting systems in place for the reporting of work-related and/or occupational diseases. These are usually (but not always) linked to compensation, and are typically coordinated by government bodies and/or insurance companies. The person responsible for notifying the system varies between countries, and may be the individual themselves, if they believe that their condition has been caused by their work, or their employer, but frequently it is the (often legal) responsibility of the physician seeing the patient with a suspected occupational disease to notify the system. The type of diseases that can be reported (and/or compensated) also varies between countries. For some, the disease must be on a prescribed list and it must be linked to a prescribed occupation or occupational conditions, whilst others may allow other diseases (i.e. not on a prescribed list) to be reported and, if proven to be occupational in nature, compensated. In the USA, the health departments of each state are largely responsible for occupational disease monitoring, and the degree to which this has been implemented and the availability of compensation varies from state to state (Wolfe and Fairchild, 2010).

The main strength of statutory reporting systems as a data source is that they should have a good case ascertainment, with a high degree of accuracy both in the diagnosis and in the attribution of work relatedness. For example, most compensation-based systems require proof that the disease has been caused by workplace exposure, although the degree of proof required may vary between systems (and between diseases). Thus, for systems in some countries, a medical diagnosis and proof of employment in a relevant job might be sufficient, whilst others might require additional information, such as a description of the types of tasks undertaken (and for how long), the types of agents exposed to or even airborne measurements. Similarly, a lower level of proof might be required for those diseases that are almost exclusively occupational, such as mesothelioma, compared to others, such as asthma, that are not. Statutory reporting systems also tend to be well established and long running, with any changes to the data collection process well documented. However, cases are often significantly under-reported. For example, a worker may be unaware of the link between their condition and their work or of the availability of compensation, or they may be discouraged or excluded by the eligibility criteria for compensation. The extent to which factors such as these result in under-reporting will vary between systems (and between diseases). For example, the degree of under-reporting is likely to be less for those countries where the requested compensation is expected to cover all or most of the healthcare costs associated with the disease (which is the situation in many European countries) compared to countries such as the UK, where general healthcare costs are covered by the National Health Service and statutory compensation values may be low. Moreover, in the UK. Industrial Injuries Disablement Benefit (IIDB) scheme, some occupational lung disorders, such as asbestos plaques, per se, are not compensatable, nor is any compensation paid if the disorder arose from self-employment.

Physician-Based Reporting Systems

Besides statutory reporting systems, many countries have national systems set up that are based on the voluntary participation of physicians who report cases of occupational and work-related illnesses seen during their usual clinical practice, either continuously or during a specified sampling period (e.g. 1 month per year) (Table 8.1). These systems have tended to be established in response to perceived limitations of statutory systems, such as compensation-based systems, regarding fulfilling epidemiological purposes. Typically, physicians are asked to assign a diagnosis and also to report, in addition to basic demographic information such as age and gender, associated information such as the type of job undertaken by the individual, including any workplace agent(s) that they are exposed to.

In addition to national schemes, some countries may have smaller, more localised schemes, such as 'SHIELD' in the UK, a surveillance scheme for occupational asthma primarily covering the West Midlands (Gannon and Burge, 1993). The main strength of these voluntary physician-based systems is that they typically capture cases at a much broader level than compensation-based systems and therefore may represent a 'truer' picture of the burden of disease. This is particularly the case for those systems that are designed to capture data at the primary care level (Hussey et al., 2008). The main limitation of a primary care-based approach is that there is bound to be greater uncertainty in the accuracy of the diagnosis and the ascertainment of work relatedness. However, even amongst specialists, the degree of uncertainty in the accuracy of both the diagnosis and the work relatedness may vary depending on the type of disease and the competence and expertise of the physician reporting the case, or for other reasons (Turner et al., 2010). Systems based on voluntary physician participation may also be less sustainable than those based on statutory reporting because of difficulties in recruiting, rewarding and retaining the interest of participating physicians.

Sentinel Event Reporting Systems

Besides measuring disease incidence and trend, occupational disease surveillance should be able to identify new and emerging risks. These signal or sentinel cases can act as early warning signs, highlighting areas that require further investigation and informing the implementation of control measures in similar workplaces. Whilst physician-based systems that are not linked to compensation tend to be more suitable for this purpose, identifying sentinel cases from 'routine' surveillance is often difficult and, additionally, resources may not be in place to provide the necessary follow-up/translation into actions. Approaches that have been applied to 'routine' surveillance data in order to improve their capacity to identify new hazards include the use of methods derived from pharmaco-vigilance for identifying new disease–occupation–agent combinations (Bonneterre et al., 2012) and quantitative structure–activity relationships for predicting sensitisation risks to asthma (Jarvis et al., 2005). However, whilst approaches such as these can aid in the

TABLE 8.1
Physician-Based Reporting Systems for Occupational and Work-Related Lung Disorders

Country	System	Reporters	Linked to Compensation?	Type of Diseases Reported[a]
Australia	Surveillance of Australian Workplace Based Respiratory Events (SABRE) (Elder et al., 2004)	Chest physicians, occupational physicians, general practitioners	No	Any respiratory
Belgium	Belgium Compensation Fund for Occupational Diseases (FBZ, 2012)	All physicians	Yes	Any respiratory
Czech Republic	Czech Registry of Occupational Disease (Urban et al., 2000)	All physicians	Yes	Prescribed list
Finland	Finnish Register of Occupational diseases (Riihimäki et al., 2004)	All physicians	Yes	Prescribed list
France	Observatoire National des Asthmes Professionnels (ONAP2) (Ameille et al., 2003)	Chest physicians, occupational physicians, pathologists, allergists	No	Asthma
	The French National Program for Mesothelioma Surveillance (PNSM) (Goldberg et al., 2006)	Occupational physicians, pathologists, pneumologists, oncologists		Mesothelioma
	Maladies à Caractère Professionnel (MCP) (Valenty et al., 2012)	Occupational physicians		Any
	Réseau National de Vigilance et de Prévention des Pathologies Professionnelles (RNV3P) (Bonneterre et al., 2010)	Occupational physicians	No	Any
Germany	German Statutory Accident Insurance (DGUV, 2015)	All physicians	Yes	Any
Hungary	National Registry of Occupational Diseases and Excessive Exposure Cases (HIOH, 2015)	All physicians	Yes	Any
Italy	MALattie PROFessionali (MALPROF) Surveillance System of Occupational Diseases (INAIL, 2015)	All physicians	No	Any
Macedonia	Register of Occupational Diseases (Institute for Occupational Health, 2015)	All physicians	No	Prescribed list
The Netherlands	National Notification and Registration System (Molen et al., 2012)	Occupational physicians, dermatologists, chest physicians	No	Any, any skin, any respiratory
Norway	Registry of Work-Related Diseases, Illnesses, and Disorders at the Labour Inspectorate (Samant et al., 2008)	All physicians	No	Any
	National Institute of Occupational Health (NIOH) registry (NIOH, 2015)	All physicians	No	Any
South Africa	Surveillance of Work-Related and Occupational Respiratory Diseases Programme in South Africa (SORDSA) (Hnizdo et al., 2001)	Occupational physicians, occupational health nurses, pneumologists	No	Any
Spain	Occupational Diseases Registry of the Social Security System (Seguridad Social, 2015)	All physicians	Yes	Any

(*Continued*)

TABLE 8.1 (*Continued*)
Physician-Based Reporting Systems for Occupational and Work-Related Lung Disorders

Country	System	Reporters	Linked to Compensation?	Type of Diseases Reported[a]
United Kingdom	Surveillance of Work-Related and Occupational Respiratory Disease (SWORD) (Meredith et al., 1991)	Chest physicians	No	Any respiratory
	Occupational Physicians Reporting Activity (OPRA) (Cherry et al., 2000)	Occupational physicians	No	Any
	THOR in General Practice (THOR-GP) (Hussey et al., 2008)	General practitioners	No	Any
	Surveillance Scheme for Occupational Asthma (SHIELD) (Gannon and Burge, 1993)	Chest physicians	No	Asthma
United States	Work-Related Lung Disease Surveillance System (eWoRLD) (NIOSH, 2015)	The National Institute for Occupational Safety and Health (NIOSH) supports a number of work-related respiratory disease surveillance programmes across selected US states. Each state employs a variety of data sources, some of which include reports from physicians		

[a] Work-related and/or occupational.

initial identification of a new risk, for disease vigilance to have an impact in protecting workers, these findings then need to be followed by preventative actions.

Such a 'closed-loop' approach is exemplified by the Sentinel Event Notification System for Occupational Risks (SENSOR) in the USA, which was initiated by the National Institute for Occupational Safety and Health (NIOSH) in the late 1980s and implemented across ten states (Baker, 1989). The concept of SENSOR is that (within each state) a network of sentinel healthcare providers reports cases of selected occupational diseases to a surveillance centre, where they are analysed and form the basis of intervention activities aimed at workers and workplaces.

Mortality Records and Cancer Registries

Death registries can be useful sources of information on occupational and work-related ill health, as most countries have them and the cause of death is standardised by the use of the International Classification of Diseases. In many countries, the death certificate will also contain information about the (last known) occupation of the deceased. Advantages of mortality records as data sources include the generically consistent format of 'numerator' data collection based on a population denominator over time. The main limitation is that it is not necessarily possible to link the cause of death to occupational exposures. These data sources are therefore of most use for those diseases that are almost exclusively occupational, such as mesothelioma or asbestosis (Leigh and Driscoll, 2003). However, even for these diseases, under-reporting may occur because the physicians certifying the deaths may not recognise and record mesothelioma or asbestosis as the cause of death. Conversely, there may be over-reporting, for example, if the term 'asbestosis' is used incorrectly on the death record (i.e. to indicate that asbestos exposure took place rather than the presence of the disease itself).

Many countries also have registries recording the incidence rates of different cancers. Although these might not be collecting information specifically on cancers due to occupational exposures, it may be possible to estimate the attributable fraction (i.e. the proportion of cases that would not have occurred in the absence of exposure) from these data (Rushton, 2012).

Surveys of the Labour Force

Information on occupational and work-related illness may also be collected via surveys of the labour market. A labour force survey (LFS) is a standard household-based survey of work-related statistics. All European Union (EU) member states are required to conduct a LFS annually, with similar surveys also carried out in many non-EU countries, including Australia, New Zealand and the USA (International Labour Organisation, 2015). As part of the survey, respondents are often asked about any recent illness(es) that they have had that they believe to have been caused/aggravated by their work. The advantage of LFSs and similar surveys as data sources is that they capture cases at the very bottom of the 'disease

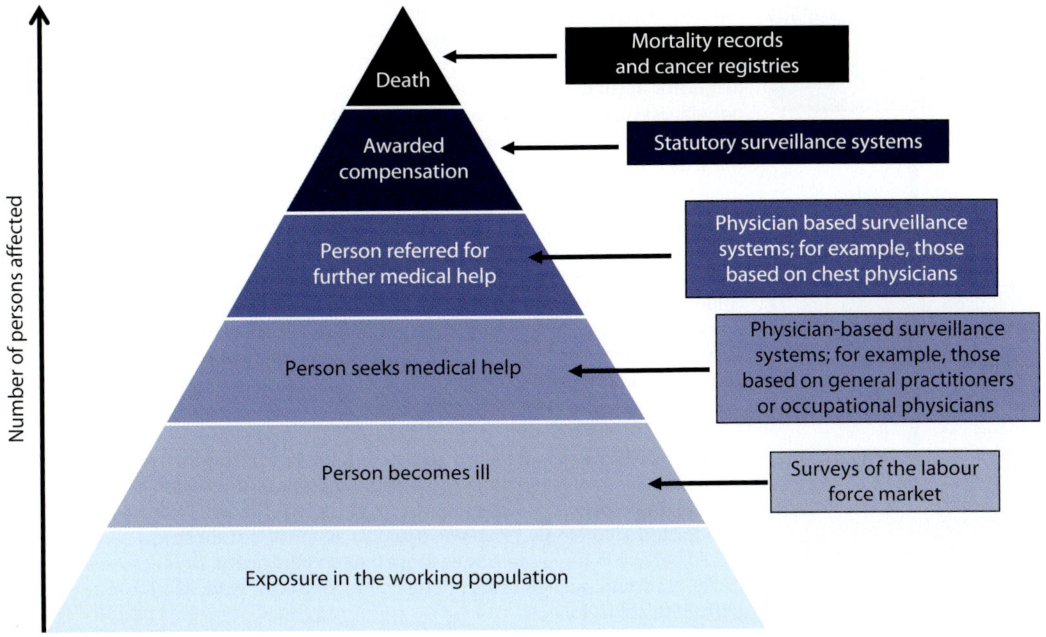

FIGURE 8.1 Disease severity and surveillance pyramid.

severity pyramid' (Figure 8.1). However, since they are generally based on the individuals' own perceptions of disease (rather than a physician's medical opinion), there is likely to be less diagnostic accuracy. In addition, because lung diseases are often not disaggregated beyond 'breathing and lung problems', it may not be possible to use such data in order to investigate the incidence of specific diseases.

METHODOLOGICAL ISSUES

Two of the principal objectives of disease surveillance are to be able to measure incidence (the number of new cases seen during a defined period) and to measure any change in incidence over time (with an additional aim being one of disease vigilance; i.e. detecting new and emerging risks). In describing the suitability of the data sources for meeting these objectives, there are a number of issues that need to be considered, especially when interpreting and comparing data from multiple sources (Figure 8.2). Broadly speaking, these can be divided into those that affect the reported cases themselves (i.e. the numerator) and those that affect the underlying population from which the cases are drawn (i.e. the denominator).

INCIDENCE

When comparing disease incidence from multiple sources, it is important to ensure that the populations from which the cases are drawn (and any differences between them) are taken into account. This can be illustrated by comparing reports of occupational lung disorders captured by different sources (voluntary physician reporting by primary care and secondary care physicians, compensation claims and workforce surveys) within (as an example) Great Britain (GB). During 2010–2012, there was an annual average of 4253 compensation awards from IIDB for occupational lung disorders (IIDB, 2014), compared to 1858 case reports of work-related respiratory disease from chest physicians to surveillance of work-related and occupational respiratory disease (SWORD), 120 from occupational physicians to occupational physicians reporting activity (OPRA) and 62 from general practitioners to the health and occupation research network in general practice (THOR-GP), and approximately 13,000 self-reports of breathing or lung problems to the Labour Force Survey (LFS) (2014). These counts of case reports, however, do not take into account differences in the underlying populations covered by the data sources and, if considered in isolation, could misinform about disease incidence. It is therefore more informative to apply a denominator to each of these figures in order to obtain incidence rates. Most statutory, national compensation-based systems (such as IIDB) should (in theory) cover and capture cases from the whole of the working population (perhaps with the exception of the self-employed). As such, national estimates of the working population (e.g. from the LFS) are usually applied as the denominator, preferably taking latency into account. However, in reality, because of under-reporting, such systems do not capture cases from the whole of the working population, and

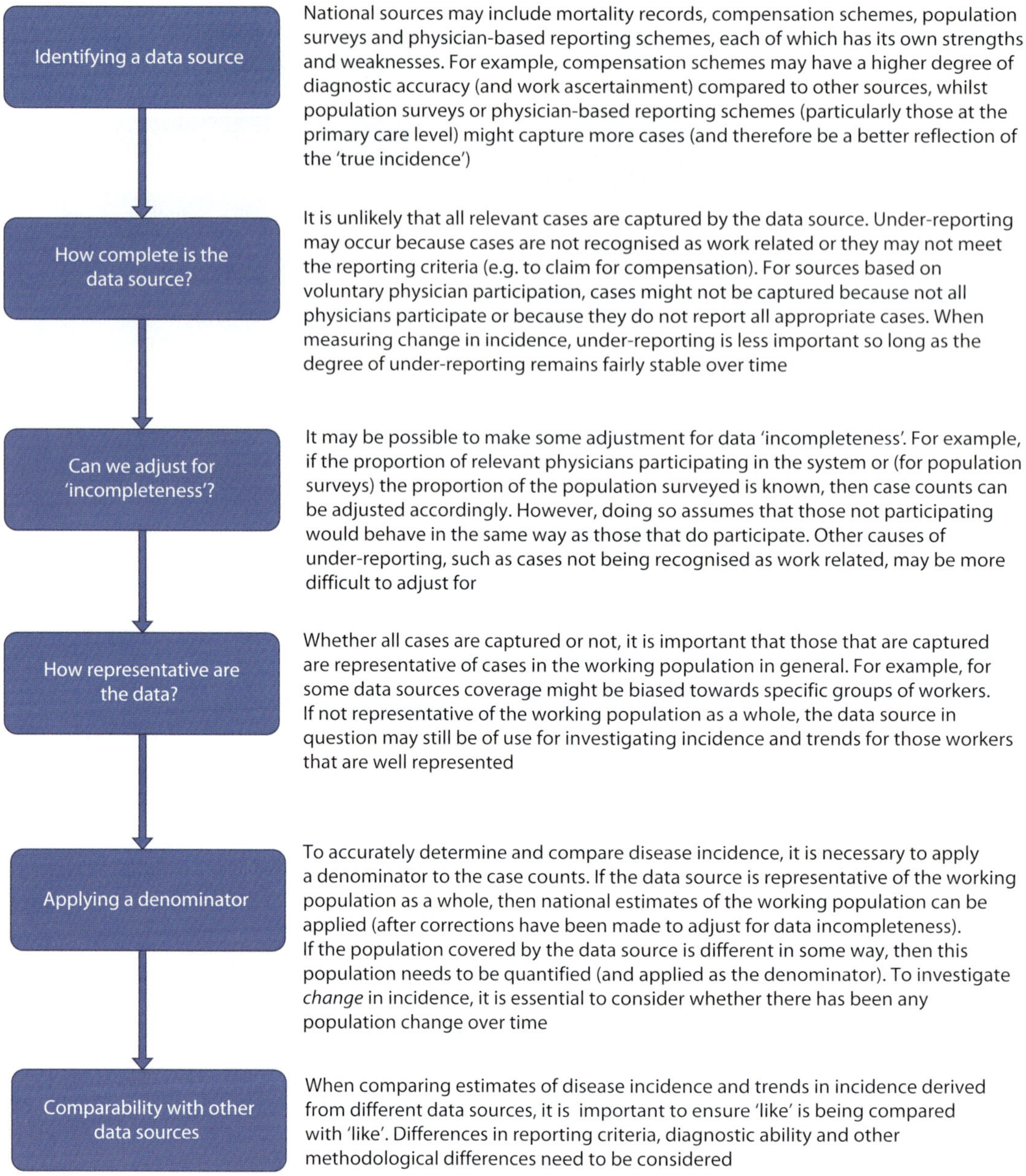

FIGURE 8.2 Methodological issues for determining incidence and trends in incidence of occupational diseases and work-related illnesses.

therefore incidence rates calculated this way are likely to be underestimated (although, as discussed, this is likely to vary between diseases and between countries).

Many voluntary physician-based surveillance systems (such as SWORD, OPRA and THOR-GP) are also established to cover and capture relevant cases from the whole of the working population. However, especially since physician participation is voluntary, it is unlikely that every relevant case will be captured. In some systems, the participating physicians (or a representative sample thereof) have been surveyed in order to specifically ask them about the workforce that they cover (Spreeuwers et al., 2008; Carder et al., 2014). This is of particular importance for those systems for which coverage might be biased towards certain industries (Carder et al., 2014). If this is the approach taken, a further issue to consider is how often participants need to be surveyed. This may be less frequently for systems in which the workforce that is covered by the physicians remains fairly stable compared to systems in which coverage is more changeable. Alternatively, if the proportion of relevant physicians participating in the system is known and there is no reason to believe that the population they covered is different to the population covered in general, then the

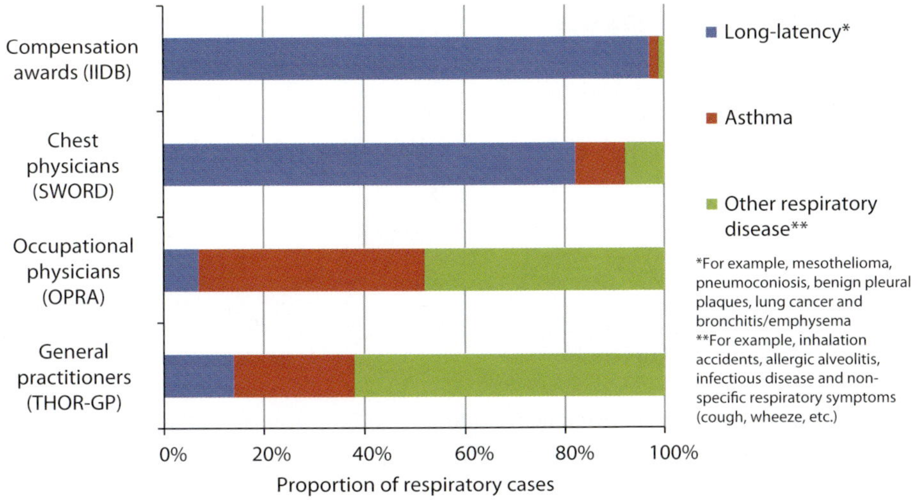

FIGURE 8.3 Proportionate distribution of occupational lung disorders in Great Britain (2010–2012). A comparison of awards for compensation from Industrial Injuries Disablement Benefit (IIDB) and reports from chest physicians (SWORD), occupational physicians (OPRA) and general practitioners (THOR-GP).

numerator (or denominator) can be adjusted accordingly (Carder et al., 2011). Other factors that might unduly influence incidence estimations include the opposing biases of 'harvesting' (reporting prevalent cases as though they were incident) and of 'reporter fatigue'. Both of these phenomena are the subject of continuing study (McNamee et al., 2010). Making comprehensive adjustments for under-reporting (such as under-recognition or non-response) would require assumptions or methods that have not yet been fully developed.

Continuing with the example above, if the (appropriate) denominators were to be applied to the numerator data, incidence rates for occupational and work-related lung disease of 15 per 100,000 employed (IIDB), 14 (SWORD), 15 (OPRA), 29 (THOR-GP) and 42 (LFS) would be obtained. Although these estimates are generally internally consistent, it might be expected that the incidence rate based on IIDB data would be the lowest, because of more stringent criteria for compensation awards. A further consideration, as illustrated in Figure 8.3, is that the 'case mix' of these different data sources varies widely, showing that some are better than others at identifying and measuring the frequency of specific diseases. Thus, in many countries, compensation claims for occupational lung disorders are primarily for pneumoconiosis and asbestos-related diseases such as mesothelioma. Similarly, physician-based reporting systems based on lung specialists are also likely to capture a higher proportion of long-latency diseases such as mesothelioma and pneumoconiosis, whereas occupational physicians tend to identify proportionately more asthma cases (since long-latency diseases often manifest after working age). The 'true' value of the overall incidence of occupational lung disorders is therefore likely to be derived from the integration of best estimates from different sources. The all-encompassing incidence might therefore be appreciably higher than that determined from any single source. Restricting the illustration to asthma, incidence rates per 100,000 employed of approximately <1 (IIDB), 1 (SWORD), 7 (OPRA) and 7 (THOR-GP) are observed (the LFS data in GB are not disaggregated beyond 'breathing and lung problems'). These rates follow the 'expected' pattern of the surveillance pyramid, with higher rates in primary care and lower rates associated with specialist reports and compensated cases.

Amongst the various considerations in determining the denominator for the purposes of calculating the incidence rate, an important factor is disease latency. Thus, for mesothelioma, a typical latency period may range from 20 to 50 years, and hence it can be difficult to identify which denominators would be most appropriate. This is particularly an issue if comparing incidence rates for specific industries or occupations, as the numbers working in these areas might have changed substantially over time, such as shipyard workers.

Incidence by Occupation, Industry, Causal Agent, etc.

Although it is useful to know the extent of occupational and work-related lung disorders in the population overall, it is probably of more practical use to be able to identify particular groups of workers who are at an increased risk, thereby enabling policies and resources

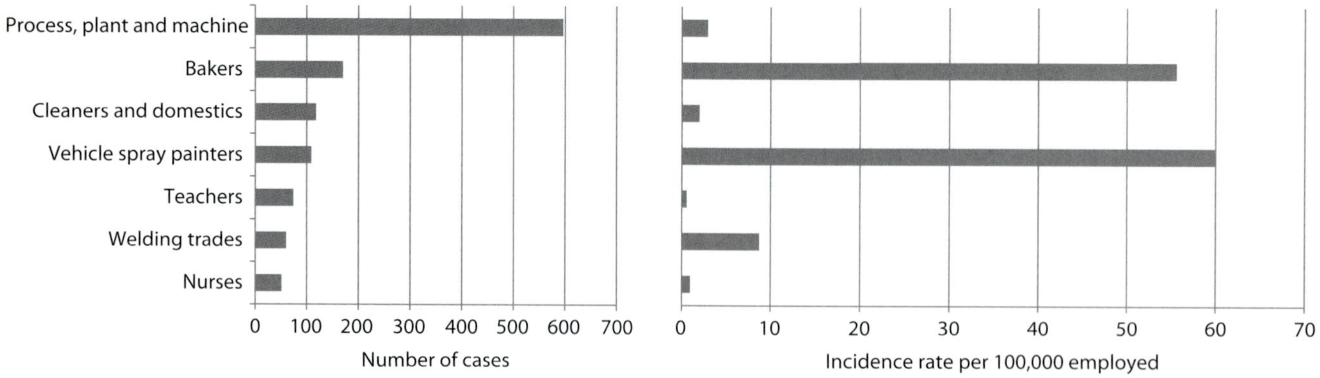

FIGURE 8.4 Number of cases and annual average incidence rates (per 100,000 employed) for work-related asthma by frequently reported occupations (as reported by chest physicians to SWORD, 2005–2014): the importance of applying a denominator.

aimed at reducing the incidence of these diseases to be targeted more efficiently. However, comparing disease incidence at the level of specific occupations, industries or causal agents introduces further methodological challenges. The number of people employed in different industries and occupations will vary considerably. It is therefore of even greater importance to adjust the case counts for the appropriate denominators (Figure 8.4). One potential limiting factor here is the availability of appropriate denominators. In many countries, the LFS provides counts of workers who are classified to specific occupational and industrial groups. However, these classification systems often vary both between countries and over time, making comparability difficult. Another issue to consider is whether the data source in question is representative of the occupation/industry of interest. For example, in GB (and elsewhere), employees in larger, public industries tend to have better access to occupational health services compared to those in smaller, private industries. If this 'bias' is not taken into account, it could lead to misinterpretation of apparent differences in disease incidence between industries/occupations (Carder et al., 2014). Furthermore, whilst it might be reasonable to make an adjustment for under-reporting when calculating overall disease incidence, it might be less appropriate to make this adjustment at the level of specific industries/occupations.

The proportion of asthma cases by most frequently reported agents is shown in Figure 8.5. In this instance, the numerator data have not been adjusted for a

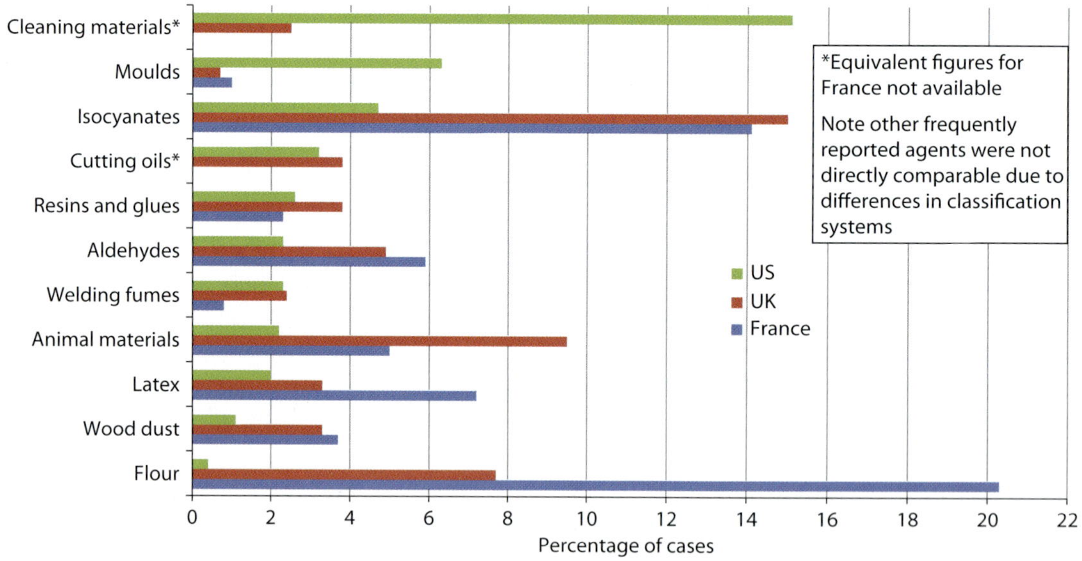

FIGURE 8.5 Distribution of frequently reported suspected agents for work-related asthma as reported in the USA. (to SENSOR, 1993–2008), the UK (to SWORD, 1993–2008) and France (to ONAP, 1996–1999). (From National Institute for Occupational Safety and Health [NIOSH]. 2015. Centers for Disease Control and Prevention [CDC]. Work Related Lung Disease Surveillance System [eWoRLD]. Available at: http://wwwn.cdc.gov/eworld/. Accessed 31 July 2015; Ameille, J. et al. 2003. *Occup Environ Med* 60(2):136–41.)

denominator. This is because the denominator here—the number of people exposed to each agent—is typically much more difficult to quantify. Therefore, when interpreting data such as these, it is beneficial to cross-reference with other data, such as incidence rates for occupations and/or industries. For example, two of the most frequently reported causal agents for asthma are isocyanates and flour. Rather than indicating a higher risk for workers exposed to these agents, this could simply reflect the fact that relatively high numbers of workers are exposed to these agents. However, data have also suggested higher (than the workforce as a whole) incidence rates for bakers (for whom the main exposure is flour) and vehicle spray painters (for whom the main exposure is isocyanates). Taken in conjunction, these data would therefore suggest a higher (than average) risk of asthma associated with these two agents.

Trends in Incidence

An equally important aim of disease surveillance is to know whether there has been any change in disease incidence over time, both in order to identify whether there are new/emerging risks that need to be addressed and to evaluate whether there has been any change in response to the implementation of policies aimed at reducing disease. Methodological issues that are important when measuring disease incidence are not necessarily the same as those that are important when measuring change in incidence. For example, when measuring change, it is less important that the system captures all of the relevant cases, so long as those that it does capture are representative of what is being measured and the degree of under-reporting does not vary significantly over time. In general, the best systems for measuring trends are those for which the data collection process and the population being sampled remain fairly stable over time, or if they do not, then any changes are well documented. At the simplest level, it is possible to investigate trends in incidence by plotting the number of new cases over time. However, these 'trends' do not take into account other factors that might vary over time, which, if not taken into account, might unduly influence the 'true' trend. These include changes in the population from which the cases are drawn, the number of physicians reporting to the system or seasonal patterns in reporting or a harvesting effect. In order to investigate how factors such as these impact on the trends that are derived from surveillance data, a method was developed by McNamee et al. (2008) using a multi-level model (MLM). The MLM enables the relationship between annual incidence rate and time to be investigated, after adjusting for potential confounders. This methodology was initially applied

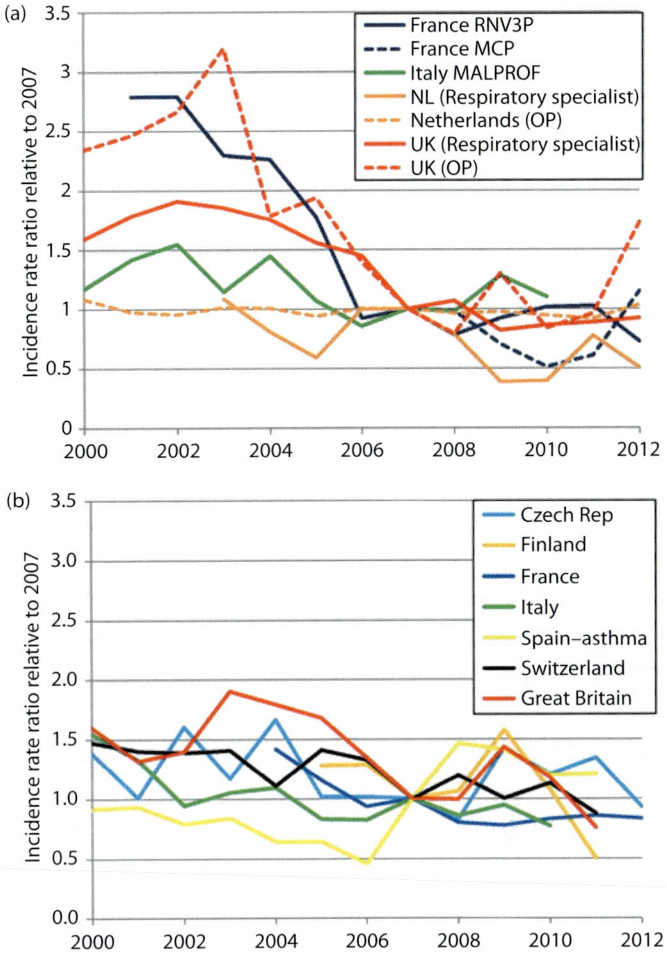

FIGURE 8.6 Estimated annual changes in the incidence of occupational asthma; physician reported (a) and recognised compensation claims (b). Abbreviations: NL: the Netherlands; OP: occupational physician. (From Stocks, S. J. et al. 2015. *Occup Environ Med* 72:294–303.)

to THOR data and has subsequently been adopted by researchers elsewhere in order to investigate asthma trends in France (Paris et al., 2012), Belgium (Vandenplas et al., 2011) and across ten European countries (Stocks et al., 2015) (Figure 8.6). As previously stated, the potential bias of reporter 'fatigue' on the observed trends remains a matter of concern.

In addition to investigating 'overall' trends, it is also of use to be able to investigate trends in incidence for specific industries or occupations, or those that can be attributed to specific agents. This can be achieved using the MLM methods in order to investigate, for example, trends in asthma attributed to flour (which, compared to the general decrease in incidence seen for asthma overall, has been shown to be increasing) (Stocks et al., 2013a). It is also possible to adapt these methods in order to investigate the impact of interventions aiming to decrease the incidence of occupational and work-related asthma. Examples include regulatory activity by the UK. Health and safety executive (HSE) in order to reduce asthma due to exposure to isocyanates or metal working fluids (Stocks et al., 2013a), or the impact of the introduction of workplace exposure limits/market forces in order to reduce exposure to specific agents (Stocks et al., 2013b). A critical methodological challenge here is to (a priori) clearly define the periods of interest to be compared (before, during and after the intervention) and to include a valid control group.

CONCLUSION

The measurement of frequency and trends in occupational lung disease is beset by many methodological challenges. Nevertheless, as shown here, it is possible to iterate the methodology such that occupational circumstances associated with high risk are identified and trends following intervention can be demonstrated.

REFERENCES

Ameille, J., Pauli, G., Calastreng-Crinquand, A., Vervloët, D., Iwatsubo, Y., Popin, E., Bayeux-Dunglas, M. C. and Kopferschmitt-Kubler, M. C. 2003. Reported incidence of occupational asthma in France, 1996–99: The ONAP programme. *Occup Environ Med* 60(2):136–41.

Baker, E. L. 1989. Sentinel event notification system for occupational risks (SENSOR): The concept. *Am J Public Health* 79(Suppl.):18–20.

Bonneterre, V., Bicout, D. J. and de Gaudemaris, R. 2012. Application of pharmacovigilance methods in occupational health surveillance: Comparison of seven disproportionality metrics. *Saf Health Work* 3(2):92–100.

Bonneterre, V., Faisandier, L., Bicout, D., Bernardet, C., Piollat, J., Ameille, J., de Clavière, C. et al. 2010. Programmed health surveillance and detection of emerging diseases in occupational health: Contribution of the French National Occupational Disease Surveillance and Prevention Network (RNV3P). *Occup Environ Med* 67(3):178–86.

Carder, M., McNamee, R., Turner, S., Hussey, L., Money, A. and Agius, R. 2011. Improving estimates of specialist-diagnosed, work-related respiratory and skin disease. *Occup Med* 61(1):33–9.

Carder, M., Money, A., Turner, S. and Agius, R. 2014. Workforce coverage by GB occupational physicians and disease incidence rates. *Occup Med* 64:271–8.

Cherry, N. M., Meyer, J. D., Holt, D. L., Chen, Y. and McDonald, J. C. 2000. Surveillance of work-related diseases by occupational physicians in the UK: OPRA 1996–1999. *Occupational Med* 50(7):496–503.

Deutsche Gesetzliche Unfallversicherung (DGUV). 2015. German statutory accident insurance. Available at: http://www.dguv.de/de/index.jsp (accessed 31 July 2015).

Elder, D., Abramson, M., Fish, D., Johnson, A., McKenzie, D. and Sim, M. 2004. Surveillance of Australian workplace based respiratory events (SABRE): Notifications for the first 3.5 years and validation of occupational asthma cases. *Occup Med* 54(6):395–9.

Fonds Voor de Beroepszieketen (FBZ). 2012. Belgium Compensation Fund for Occupational Diseases. 2012. Available at: http://www.fmp-fbz.fgov.be (accessed 31 July 2015).

Gannon, P. F. G. and Burge, P. S. 1993. The SHIELD scheme in the West Midlands Region, United Kingdom. *Br J Ind Med* 50:791–6.

Goldberg, M., Imbernon, E., Rolland, P., Gilg Soit Ilg, A., Savès, M., de Quillacq, A., Frenay, C. et al. 2006. The French national mesothelioma surveillance program. *Occup Environ Med* 63(6):390–5.

Hnizdo, E., Esterhuizen, T. M., Rees, D. and Lalloo, U. G. 2001. Occupational asthma as identified by the surveillance of work-related and occupational respiratory diseases programme in South Africa. *Clin Exp Allergy* 31(1):32–9.

Hungarian Institute of Occupational Health (HIOH). 2015. National registry of occupational diseases and excessive exposure cases. Available at: http://www.omfi.hu/index.php (accessed 31 July 2015).

Hussey, L. J., Turner, S., Thorley, K. J., McNamee, R. and Agius R. 2008. Work-related ill health in general practice, as reported to a UK-wide surveillance scheme. *Br J Gen Pract* 58(554):637–40.

Industrial Injuries Disablement Benefit Scheme. 2014. Table IIDB01: Prescribed industrial diseases: New cases of lung diseases in England, Wales and Scotland by disease (2003 to latest available year). Available at: http://www.hse.gov.uk/Statistics/tables/index.htm#iidb (accessed 31 July 2015).

Institute for Occupational Health. 2015. Macedonia. Available at: http://www.iph.mk/en/ (accessed 31 July 2015).

Instituto Nazionale per L'assicurazione Contro Gli Infortuni Sul Lavoro (INAIL). 2015. The Malattie Professionali surveillance system (MalProf). Available at: https://appsricercascientifica.inail.it/statistiche/index_mp.asp?p=dati (accessed 31 July 2015).

International Labour Organisation. 2015. Labour force surveys. Available at: https://www.ilo.org/dyn/lfsurvey/lfsurvey.home (accessed 31 July 2015).

Jarvis, J., Seed, M. J., Elton, R., Sawyer, L. and Agius, R. 2005. Relationship between chemical structure and the occupational asthma hazard of low molecular weight organic compounds. *Occup Environ Med* 62(4):243–50.

Labour Force Survey—Self-reported work-related ill-health and workplace injuries. 2014. Table SWIT6W12: Estimated incidence and rates of self-reported illness caused or made worse by work, by type of illness, for people working in the last 12 months. Office for National Statistics (ONS). Available at: http://www.hse.gov.uk/Statistics/lfs/index.htm (accessed 31 July 2015).

Leigh, J. and Driscoll, T. 2003. Malignant mesothelioma in Australia, 1945–2002. *Int J Occup Environ Health* 9(3):206–17.

McNamee, R., Carder, M., Chen, Y. and Agius R. 2008. Measurement of trends in incidence of work-related skin and respiratory diseases, UK 1996–2005. *Occup Environ Med* 65(12):808–14.

McNamee, R., Chen, Y., Hussey, L. and Agius R. 2010. Randomised controlled trial comparing time-sampled versus continuous time reporting for measuring incidence. *Epidemiology* 21(3):376–8.

Meredith, S. K., Taylor, V. M. and McDonald, J. C. 1991. Occupational respiratory disease in the United Kingdom 1989: A report to the British Thoracic Society and the Society of Occupational Medicine by the SWORD project group. *Br J Ind Med* 48(5):292–8.

National Institute for Occupational Safety and Health (NIOSH). 2015. Centres for Disease Control and Prevention (CDC). Work Realted Lung Disease Surveillance System (eWoRLD). Available at: http://wwwn.cdc.gov/eworld/ (accessed 31 July 2015).

National Institute of Occupational Health (NIOH). 2015. Norway. Available at: http://www.nifu.no/en/institutes/statens-arbeidsmiljoinstitutt/ (accessed 31 July 2015).

Paris, C., Ngatchou-Wandji, J., Luc, A., McNamee, R., Bensefa-Colas, L., Larabi, L., Telle-Lamberton, M. et al. 2012. Work-related asthma in France: Recent trends for the period 2001–2009. *Occup Environ Med* 69:391–7.

Riihimäki, H., Kurppa, K., Karjalainen, A., Palo, L., Jolanki, R., Keskinen, H., Mäkinen, I. et al. 2004. Finnish Register of Occupational Diseases (FROD). Occupational diseases in Finland in 2002: New cases of occupational diseases reported to the Finnish Register of Occupational Diseases. Available at: http://www.ttl.fi/en/publications/Electronic_publications/Documents/Occupational_diseases_2002.pdf (accessed 31 July 2015).

Rushton, L. 2012. The burden of occupational cancer in Great Britain. Health and Safety Executive research report RR931. Available at: http://www.hse.gov.uk/research/rrpdf/rr931.pdf (accessed 31 July 2015).

Samant, Y., Parker, D., Wergeland, E. and Wannag, A. 2008. The Norwegian Labour Inspectorate's registry for work-related diseases: Data from 2006. *Int J Occup Environ Health* 14:272–9.

Seguridad Social. 2015. Occupational Diseases Registry of the Social Security System. Spain. Available at: http://www.seg-social.es/Internet_1/index.htm (accessed 31 July 2015).

Spreeuwers, D., de Boer, A. G., Verbeek, J. H., de Wilde, N. S., Braam, I., Willemse, Y., Pal, T. M. et al. 2008. Sentinel surveillance of occupational diseases: A quality improvement project. *Am J Ind Med* 51(11):834–42.

Stocks, S. J., McNamee, R., Turner, S., Carder, M. and Agius, R. 2013a. Assessing the impact of national level interventions on workplace respiratory disease in the UK: Part 2—Regulatory activity by the Health and Safety Executive. *Occup Environ Med* 70(7):483–90.

Stocks, S. J., McNamee, R., Turner, S., Carder, M. and Agius, R. 2013b. Assessing the impact of national level interventions on workplace respiratory disease in the UK: Part 1—Changes in workplace exposure legislation and market forces. *Occup Environ Med* 70(7):476–82.

Stocks, S. J., McNamee, R., van der Molen, H. F., Paris, C., Urban, P., Campo, G., Sauni R. et al. 2015. Trends in incidence of occupational asthma, contact dermatitis, noise-induced hearing loss, carpal tunnel syndrome and upper limb musculoskeletal disorders in European countries from 2000 to 2012. *Occup Environ Med* 72:294–303.

Turner, S., McNamee, R., Roberts, C., Bradshaw, L., Curran, A., Francis, M., Fishwick, D. et al. 2010. Investigation of occupational asthma diagnoses using respiratory case studies: SWORD and OPRA. *Occup Environ Med* 67:471–8.

Urban, P., Cikrt, M., Hejlek, A., Lukáš, E. and Pelclová, D. 2000. The Czech national registry of occupational diseases. Ten years of existence. *Cent Eur J Public Health* 8(4):210–2.

Valenty, M., Homère, J., Mevel, M. et al. 2012. Surveillance programme of work-related diseases (WRD) in France. *Saf Health Work* 3:67–70.

van der Molen, H. F., Kuijer, P. P. F. M., Smits, P. B. A., Schop, A., Moeijes, F., Spreeuwers, D. and Frings-Dresen, M. H. W. 2012. Annual incidence of occupational diseases in economic sectors in the Netherlands. *Occup Environ Med* 69:519–21.

Vandenplas, O., Lantin, A. C., Alpaos, V. D., Larbanois, A., Hoet, P., Vandeweerdt, M., Thimpont, J. 2011. Time trends in occupational asthma in Belgium. *Respir Med* 105:1364–72.

Wolfe, D. and Fairchild, A. L. 2010. The need for improved surveillance of occupational disease and injury. *JAMA* 303(10):981–2.

9 Epidemiological Methods

David Coggon

CONTENTS

Epidemiology is concerned with the distribution and determinants of health and disease in populations. It has diverse applications in the prevention and management of illness, injury and disability and has contributed importantly to our understanding of occupational lung disorders. This chapter gives a brief overview of epidemiological methods and illustrates the ways in which they have been exploited in order to identify, characterise and control occupational causes of lung disease. At the end of the chapter, a list of references is provided for readers who wish to explore the topic in greater depth.

MEASURES OF DISEASE

Fundamental to epidemiology is the ascertainment and quantification of disease. Some measures, such as forced expiratory volume in 1 second (FEV_1) and forced vital capacity (FVC), occur in a continuum, while others, such as severity of pneumoconiosis on chest X-ray, are graded to ordinal categories. Most often, however, disease is classified simply as present or absent. For example, a person might be deemed to have, or be 'a case' of, asthma if they showed a 12% increase in FEV_1 or FVC after inhalation of a short-acting bronchodilator or a 20% decrease in FEV_1 after exercise challenge. Such definitions are often to some extent arbitrary—in the example given, the required reduction in FEV_1 after exercise challenge could reasonably be 25% rather than 20%. However, it is important that diagnostic criteria be explicit and unambiguous. Otherwise, comparisons between populations cannot be interpreted reliably.

QUANTIFYING THE OCCURRENCE OF DISEASE IN POPULATIONS

Meaningful comparison between populations requires that counts of cases be related to the numbers of people 'at risk' (i.e. those who would be counted as cases if they experienced the disease outcome at the time of, or during the period of, measurement). This is done by expressing the occurrence of disease in the form of rates, among which the most widely used are incidence, mortality and prevalence.

Incidence is the rate at which new cases occur in a specified population over a specified period of time. It is calculated as the ratio of the number of new cases to the sum of the times for which each member of the study population is at risk of becoming a case during the measurement period. If the outcome is rare and the population under study is fairly constant, this approximates closely to $N/(P \times T)$, where N is the number of new cases, P is the number of people in the population and T is the duration of the study period. Incidence is expressed in units such as cases per 100,000 per year or cases per million per year, and is the measure of disease occurrence that is most relevant in studies of causation.

A *mortality rate* (also known as a *death rate*) is the incidence of death from a specified cause. It has the advantage that, in many countries, the outcome can readily be ascertained from death certificates, and for diseases with high fatality (e.g. pleural mesothelioma and lung cancer), it provides a good proxy for incidence. However, where only a small proportion of cases are fatal and/or death occurs at a prolonged and variable interval after disease onset (e.g. chronic obstructive pulmonary disease [COPD]), differences in mortality may reflect differences not only in incidence, but also in survival once disease has developed.

Prevalence is the proportion of a population who are cases at a specified point in time (point prevalence) or during a specified period (period prevalence), and may be expressed, for example, as cases per 100,000 or cases per cent. The prevalence of a disease depends not only on its incidence, but also on how long people remain cases once they have developed the disorder (i.e. before they recover or die). Thus, associations with higher prevalence may reflect effects on the duration of a disorder, as well as on its development.

CRUDE AND SPECIFIC RATES

Rates that apply to a population as a whole are described as 'crude'. However, because the occurrence of many health outcomes varies importantly by sex and age, it may be more informative to derive sex- and age-specific rates. This is particularly important when comparing populations that differ in their demographic structures. For example, one occupational group might have a higher rate of disease than another simply because, on average, its members were older. Comparison of rates for each band or 'stratum' of sex and age would eliminate this 'confounding' effect.

Sex- and age-specific rates are derived in the same way as crude rates, but the enumeration of cases and of persons at risk is limited to the stratum of sex and age that is under consideration.

STANDARDISED RATES

Comparing sex- and age-specific rates can be rather unwieldy, especially if there are many strata to consider. Moreover, if based on only small numbers of cases, stratum-specific rates may be statistically unstable, some being unrepresentatively high or low simply by chance.

These problems may be overcome by the use of 'standardised' rates (Box 9.1).

Easiest to understand are *directly standardised rates*, which are simply weighted averages of the sex- and age-specific rates for a population. The weighting factors are defined by the sex and age distribution of a specified standard population. For example, the World Health Organisation has proposed a standard population with an age and sex structure that is typical of developed countries. Essentially, a directly standardised rate is that which would occur in the standard population if it experienced the sex- and age-specific rates of the population under study.

Indirect standardisation compares rates of a health outcomes in a study population with those in a specified standard population, which is often the national or regional population of which the study population is a subset. The total number of cases that is observed in the study population during the period of measurement is compared with the number that would have been expected had the study population experienced the same sex- and age-specific rates as the standard population. The comparison is expressed either as a simple ratio or as a percentage, these being termed a standardised incidence ratio, standardised mortality ratio (SMR) or standardised prevalence ratio, according to the type of rate that is being compared. A standardised ratio with a value of 1 or a percentage of 100% implies that after allowance for any differences in demographic structure, the study population has the same rate of the health outcome, on average, as the standard population. A higher ratio would indicate that after allowance for sex and age, the outcome tended to be more frequent in the study population.

Standardisation, whether direct or indirect, is most often applied to account for differences in the age and sex structure of populations, but it can be extended to cover other demographic determinants of health, such as social class. This would be done by defining strata according to combinations not only of sex and age, but also of social class.

Rates and Risks

The rates that have been described quantify the occurrence of health outcomes in populations, but they are numerically equivalent to the risks of those outcomes in individual members of the populations concerned. For example, if the annual incidence of coal workers' pneumoconiosis in a group of miners is 3%, then an individual member of the group has a 3% probability or risk of developing the disease over the course of a year.

BOX 9.1 DIRECT AND INDIRECT STANDARDISATION OF DISEASE RATES

The rate of disease in a study population is compared with that in a specified standard population. Assume that when broken down into combinations of sex and age, the populations and occurrences of disease are as set out in the table below.

Stratum of	Study Population			Standard Population	
Sex and Age	Number of People	Number of Cases in Unit Time	Disease Rate	Number of People	Disease Rate
1	p_1	c_1	$d_1 = c_1/p_1$	P_1	D_1
2	p_2	c_2	$d_2 = c_2/p_2$	P_2	D_2
.	.	.	.	.	.
.	.	.	.	.	.
.	.	.	.	.	.
n	p_n	c_n	$d_n = c_n/p_n$	P_n	D_n

The directly standardised rate of disease in the study population is calculated as $(P_1d_1 + P_2d_2 + \cdots + P_nd_n)/(P_1 + P_2 + \cdots + P_n)$.

The indirectly standardised rate ratio of disease in the study population is calculated as

$$\frac{(c_1 + c_2 + \cdots + c_n)}{(p_1D_1 + p_2D_2 + \cdots + p_nD_n)}$$

Note that the numerator of the standardised rate ratio represents the total number of cases in the study population in unit time across all strata. Provided this total is known, it is not necessary to know the number of cases in each individual stratum.

Proportional Mortality

Sometimes, information is available about the numbers of deaths from a disease in different groups, but the populations at risk cannot be enumerated. In these circumstances, proportional mortality may be used as a proxy for true mortality rates. For example, by using data from death certificates, it is possible to calculate the proportions of deaths in different occupations in England and Wales during 2001–2010 that were ascribed to COPD, and to compare them with the corresponding proportion in all occupations combined. Here, the number of deaths from all causes is used as a proxy measure of the population at risk. As with true mortality rates, such proportions can be indirectly standardised for sex and age, giving a standardised proportional mortality ratio (PMR).* The results of such an analysis are shown in Table 9.1. It is important to recognise that proportional mortality depends not only on the death rate from the cause of interest, but also on total mortality. Thus, for example, nurses might have a high PMR for COPD not because their mortality from the disease was higher than in other occupations, but because they had lower than average total mortality from all causes combined.

TABLE 9.1
Occupations with High Proportional Mortality from Chronic Obstructive Pulmonary Disease, Men Aged 20–74 Years, England and Wales, 2001–2010

Occupation	Number of Deaths	PMR	(95%CI)[a]
Armed forces	343	148	(131–163)
Publicans and bar staff	490	139	(127–152)
Nurses	103	153	(125–186)
Mine (excluding coal) and quarry workers	88	153	(123–189)
Painters and decorators	1109	131	(123–138)
Coal miners combined	1245	128	(121–136)
Ambulance staff	73	147	(115–184)

Source: Data provided by Office for National Statistics.
Abbreviations: PMR: proportional mortality ratio; CI: confidence interval.
[a] Proportional mortality ratio (%) and 95% confidence interval.

* In this case, the expected number of deaths is that which would be expected if the sex- and age-specific proportions of deaths from the cause of interest in the standard population applied to the observed numbers of deaths by sex and age in the study population.

MEASURES OF ASSOCIATION

Epidemiology often entails comparison of rates or risks between populations. For example, the incidence of lung cancer in welders might be compared with that in the general population. Such comparisons can be summarised by various measures of association, each with its own particular applications (Box 9.2). This section describes the measures of association that are used most often when comparing the incidence or prevalence of disease in populations or groups of people who differ in their exposure to a 'risk factor'. For example, the risk factor might be current employment as a baker or cumulative occupational exposure to respirable crystalline silica in excess of a specified value.

Attributable Risk

Attributable risk (AR) is the difference in risk between people who are exposed to a risk factor and a referent group that is unexposed or exposed at a different specified level. It is the measure that is most relevant when managing risks to individuals. For example, when deciding whether it is acceptable for a coal miner to continue working underground despite early changes of pneumoconiosis on chest X-ray, what matters is the AR of serious disease and disability (i.e. the absolute increase in risk) from remaining in such employment as compared with moving to a job entailing lower exposure to coal mine dust. AR is measured in the same units as the risks that are being compared; for example, a difference in incidence of 20 cases per 100,000 per year, or a 2% difference in prevalence.

BOX 9.2 MEASURES OF ASSOCIATION AND THEIR APPLICATION

Measure of Association	Application
Attributable risk	Managing risks to individuals
Relative risk, odds ratio	Identifying causes and predictors of health outcomes
Attributable fraction in exposed	Determining eligibility for compensation
Population attributable risk, population attributable fraction	Managing risks at population level

Relative Risk

Relative risk (RR) is the ratio of risk between people who are exposed to a risk factor and a referent group that is unexposed or exposed at a different specified level. Of all the measures of association, RR provides the best index of contrast between groups. Moreover, for a given risk factor, RR tends to be more constant than AR across strata of sex and age, making it easier to characterise.

Odds Ratio

Closely related to RR is the odds ratio, defined as the ratio of the odds of the disease in people who are exposed to a risk factor to the odds in a referent group that is unexposed or exposed at a different specified level. If R is the risk of an outcome, then the odds of that outcome are $R/(1 - R)$. Thus, the odds ratio corresponding to a RR of R_1/R_2 is $(R_1/[1 - R_1])/(R_2/[1 - R_2]) = R_1/R_2 \times ([1 - R_2]/[1 - R_1])$. If R_1 and R_2 are both <0.1 (i.e. the outcome is rare in both the exposed and referent groups), $(1 - R_2)/(1 - R_1)$ is close to 1, and the odds ratio is close to the RR. In practice, diseases of interest are usually rare. Thus, in most circumstances, the odds ratio is a good proxy for RR. Odds ratios have convenient mathematical properties, making it easier to model the combined effects of multiple risk factors.

SMRs and PMRs are also indicators of RR.

If a disease occurs with frequency F in the referent group, AR can be calculated from RR by the formula: $AR = F(RR - 1)$. From this, it should be noted that even with a large RR, AR will be small if the frequency of the health outcome is low. In other words, high RRs do not necessarily translate into high ARs.

Attributable Fraction in Exposed

The attributable fraction in exposed (AF_{exp}) is the proportion of cases among people exposed to a risk factor that would be eliminated if the risk in exposed persons were the same as that in those who are unexposed (or exposed at some other specified level). It is related to RR by the formula $AF_{exp} = (R - 1)/R$. Its main use is in quantifying the probability of attribution to a cause in claims for compensation because of diseases such as cancer that occur stochastically.* For example, when the AF_{exp} for a cause of disease exceeds 0.5, it is more likely than not that an exposed case would not have developed the disorder had he/she not been exposed.

* Diseases occur stochastically when their development behaves as a chance event. Causes of diseases that occur stochastically increase the probability of their occurrence.

Population Attributable Risk

Another measure of association is the population AR (PAR). Defined as the reduction that would occur in the rate of disease in a population if the risk in exposed persons were the same as that in those who are unexposed (or exposed at some other specified level), it is related to the AR by the formula $PAR = AR \times P$, where P is the prevalence of the risk factor in the population. It indicates the extent to which a disease might be eliminated from a population by control of a risk factor, and its main use is in the management of risk at a population level. For example, when deciding whether the costs of tighter regulatory controls on a hazardous exposure would be justified, one consideration might be the resulting reduction in incidence that could be expected in the national population (i.e. the PAR for exposure at current levels as compared with the situation in which no exposures exceeded the new control limit).

Population Attributable Fraction

Also relevant to decisions at a population level is the population attributable fraction (PAF), defined as the proportion of cases in a population that would be eliminated if the risk in exposed persons were the same as that in those who are unexposed or exposed at some other specified level. It depends on the prevalence of exposure to the risk factor in the population, P, and the RR associated with such exposure, R, according to the formula $PAF = P \times (R - 1)/([P \times R] + 1 - P)$. It should be noted that where a disease has multiple known causes, their PAFs can sum to more than 1. This is because the disease might be prevented in an individual by eliminating any of several causes to which he/she was exposed.

Associations with Continuous and Ordinal Health Outcomes

The measures that have been described in the preceding sections quantify associations between risk factors and dichotomous health outcomes. They can also be applied to continuous or ordinal health outcomes if a cut-point is defined in their distribution in order to distinguish cases from non-cases. For example, one might estimate the RR of having an FEV_1 of <80% expected, or of pneumoconiosis with profusion of opacities on chest X-rays graded 2 or higher, in coal miners employed at a pit for longer than 20 years. However, potentially important information about disease severity is lost when continuous or ordinal measures are dichotomised in this way. Alternative approaches are to estimate the average difference in the continuous outcome between exposed subjects and unexposed referents (e.g. the mean reduction in FEV_1), or the RR for several different grades of the ordinal outcome (e.g. different severities of pneumoconiosis).

SOURCES OF ERROR IN EPIDEMIOLOGICAL RESEARCH

The aim of epidemiological research is usually to estimate one or more parameters in a target population about which conclusions are to be drawn. Examples of such parameters might be the RR of occupational asthma from exposure to isocyanates in atopic as compared with non-atopic workers or the average decrement in FEV1 caused by a specified cumulative exposure to coke oven emissions. Such estimates are liable to error from bias, chance and confounding.

Bias

Bias is a systematic tendency to overestimate or underestimate a parameter of interest because of a deficiency in the design or execution of a study. It can arise in many ways, but broadly biases fall into two main categories: selection bias and information bias.

Selection bias occurs when the sample of people studied (study sample) is systematically unrepresentative of the target population with regard to the parameter of interest. For example, if a cross-sectional survey were carried out in a sample of laboratory workers in order to assess the relationship of asthma to contact with experimental animals, risk would tend to be underestimated if development of the disease caused affected workers to move to other jobs so that they were no longer employed at the time of the survey and therefore were excluded from the study sample.

Information bias arises from inaccuracies in the information that is collected about subjects. For example, in a study comparing mortality from lung cancer in coal miners and other occupations, risk estimates might be inflated if a higher rate of autopsies in miners meant that early lung tumours were less likely to be missed than in other workers.

Chance

Even where the methods by which subjects are recruited would not be expected to cause any systematic bias, it remains possible that a study sample could be unrepresentative simply by chance. The likelihood of resultant error tends to be greater when the study sample is relatively small. Two approaches are used to gauge the potential contribution of chance to results.

The first, known as hypothesis testing, starts with an assumption (*null hypothesis*) about a theoretically infinite population of which the study sample is intended to be representative. For example, suppose that a study is conducted in order to explore whether silicosis predisposes to tuberculosis, and an association between the two diseases is observed in the study sample. As a null hypothesis, it might be assumed that overall among workers with silicosis, there is no increased risk of contracting tuberculosis. With this assumption, the probability is then calculated that a random sample of the size studied would show an association as strong as that observed, simply by chance. Other things being equal, the smaller this probability (known as a *p-value*), the less plausible the null hypothesis becomes and the more inclined one would be to accept the alternative hypothesis that there is a true association between silicosis and tuberculosis. P-values are a measure of *statistical significance*, and smaller p-values are said to imply greater statistical significance.

It should be noted that statistical significance depends on the size of the study sample as well as the extent to which it deviates from the null hypothesis. A finding may be highly significant statistically, not because the deviation from the null hypothesis is large or important, but simply because it is observed in a large sample. Conversely, even a large and potentially important deviation from the null hypothesis may have little statistical significance if it is observed in only a small sample.

Because of this ambiguity in the interpretation of p-values, a preferable method of quantifying the possible contribution of chance is through *confidence intervals*. Here, the parameter of interest in the target population (e.g. the RR of tuberculosis in the general population of workers with silicosis) is estimated by the corresponding sample statistic (the RR in the study sample) with an associated confidence interval. In the absence of other information, and assuming there is no bias, a confidence interval is a range within which the population parameter might be expected to lie. Most often, 95% confidence intervals are derived. A 95% confidence interval is calculated in such a way that in the absence of bias, 95% of such intervals would be expected to include the population parameter that is being estimated.

Hypothesis testing and confidence intervals both indicate the potential contribution of chance to observed results. However, assessment of the role of chance should also take into account the consistency of findings with other relevant knowledge. For example, a positive association between occupational exposure to styrene and lung cancer, even if highly significant statistically, might nevertheless be attributed to chance if it was inconsistent with a strong body of evidence from other sources that there is no such association.

Confounding

One of the main applications of epidemiology is in the investigation of known or suspected causes of disease. However, estimates of causal impact may be misleading if the risk factor of interest is associated with a 'confounding factor' or 'confounder' that independently determines the risk of the disease. For example, a study to assess the effect of diesel fumes on risk of lung cancer in a sample of bus drivers might be misleading if it failed to account for the confounding effects of differences in smoking habits between the bus drivers and a control group with which they were being compared.

DESIGNS OF EPIDEMIOLOGICAL STUDY

This section provides a brief overview of the types of study that are used most often in epidemiological research.

Descriptive Studies

Descriptive studies aim simply to characterise the occurrence of health outcomes or their determinants in defined populations. Thus, in the UK, a reporting scheme involving chest physicians has been used to monitor trends in the incidence of occupational asthma overall and by occupation (McNamee et al., 2008). In another example, analyses of mortality from mesothelioma showed differences in risk by year of birth (Figure 9.1). Descriptive exercises of this type contrast with *analytical studies*, which investigate relationships between risk factors and health outcomes.

Ecological Studies

Ecological studies are analytical investigations in which the units of comparison are populations or groups of people. For example, the mortality of coal miners from COPD and coal workers' pneumoconiosis has been compared by county of residence (Figure 9.2). It may be possible to conduct such studies fairly cheaply and quickly using published data that have already been collected for other purposes. However, they are often limited by a potential for confounding, which may be difficult to take into account in comparisons at a population level. For this reason, ecological studies are used mainly to generate hypotheses and to determine priorities for more detailed research in which information is collected at the level of individuals.

Experimental Studies

In an experimental study, individuals (or groups of individuals) are allocated to receive differing exposures (e.g. to a possible treatment or preventive measure) and their subsequent health outcomes are compared. The method has

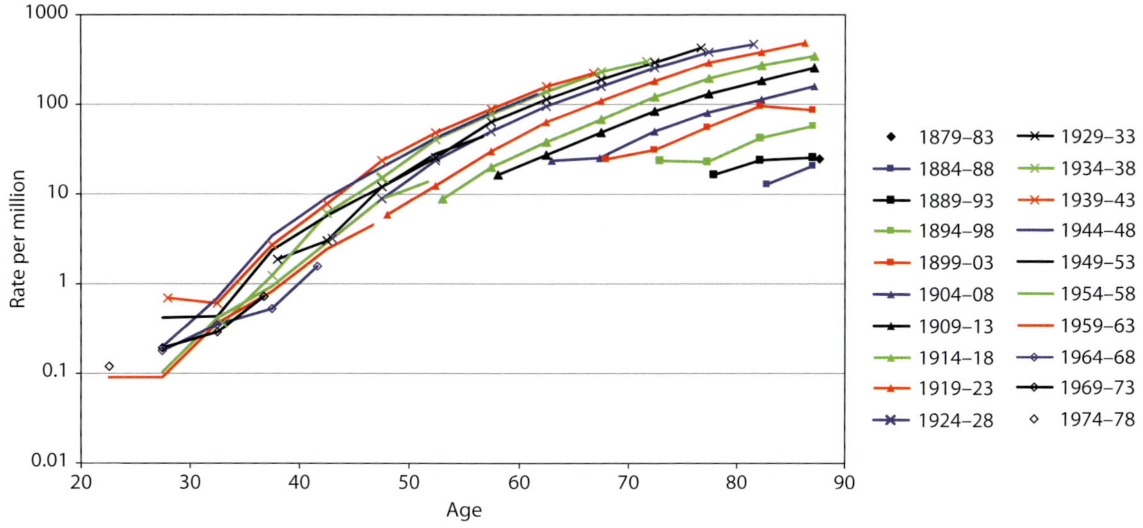

FIGURE 9.1 Death rates for mesothelioma in Great Britain by birth cohort and age group, men aged 20–89 years, 1968–2008. Rates are presented by age according to period of birth. Note that at almost all ages, the highest mortality occurred among men born during 1929-43. This is an example of a 'cohort effect' and suggests that relevant exposures to asbestos were higher in that generation of men than in those born earlier or later. (Data from Darnton, A. et al. 2012. *Occup Med* 62:549–52.)

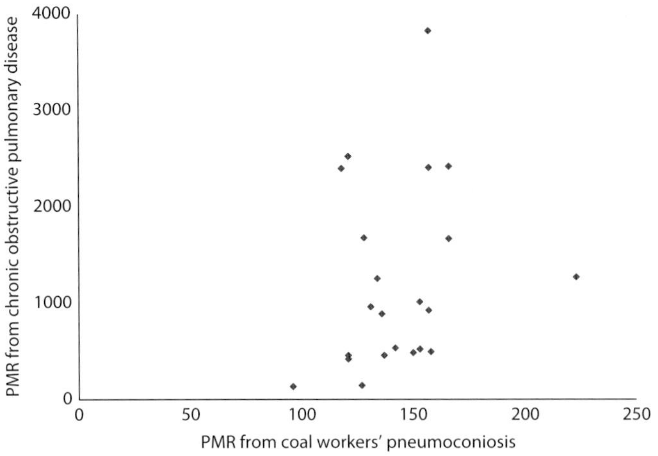

FIGURE 9.2 Mortality from chronic obstructive pulmonary disease and coal workers' pneumoconiosis in coal miners by county of residence in men aged 20–74 years in England and Wales for 1979–1980 and 1982–1990. Each point represents a county. The lack of correlation between mortality from the two diseases suggests that exposure–response relationships for the two diseases differ importantly, or that risk depends on different features of coal mine dust. PMR: proportional mortality ratio. (Based on data from Coggon, D. et al. 1995. *Occup Environ Med* 52:554–5.)

the advantage that the experimental exposure is controlled by the researcher and therefore generally well characterised, and it is particularly strong where the allocation to exposures is random (*randomised controlled trials*). This is because if sufficient numbers of individuals or groups are randomised, potential confounding factors (even if unrecognised) will tend to balance out between the exposure arms, and their effects will thus be minimised.

Cohort Studies

While it may be acceptable to allocate human subjects experimentally to exposures that could be beneficial, experimental exposure to possible hazards can rarely be justified ethically. To assess the impact of such exposures, it is instead necessary to conduct *observational* research in which subjects are studied according to differences in exposure that happen to occur for other reasons.

A cohort study is similar in design to an experimental study in individuals, except that it does not modify participants' exposures as part of the investigation. Subjects who differ in exposures of interest are identified and followed up to establish subsequent health outcomes, and the occurrence of those outcomes is compared according to exposures. If suitable sources of information are available, it may be possible to identify and follow up subjects retrospectively, which is particularly useful for outcomes such as cancer that are rare, or for which risk does not increase until some years after exposure.

Case–Control Studies

In a case–control study, patients with a disease (cases) are identified and their past exposures to risk factors of interest are ascertained and compared with those of *controls* or *referents* who do not have the disease. The method is relatively efficient for the study of rare diseases, but may be liable to bias from inaccurate assessment of exposures, especially if ascertained from subjects' recall. Another challenge is in the choice of appropriate controls, who should be representative (in their exposure to risk factors) of the population at risk of becoming cases (i.e. people who would have been included in the study as cases had they developed the disease).

Cross-Sectional Studies

Cross-sectional studies collect information about exposures and/or health outcomes in a defined study sample at a single point in time or over a short period. They may enable assessment of associations between exposure and disease, and for this purpose have the advantage of being relatively quick and cheap. However, care is needed in their interpretation because associations may be biased by factors that influence eligibility for inclusion in the study (for an example, see the section above on bias). In addition, when associations are observed, the direction of cause and effect may not always be clear.

INTERPRETATION OF EPIDEMIOLOGICAL FINDINGS

Not infrequently, epidemiological studies produce apparently conflicting answers to the same question. For example, two studies assessing the relationship of fibrosing alveolitis to metal machining might generate different estimates of risk. It could be that one found a positive association, while the other indicated no relationship, or even an inverse association. Such discrepancies can result from the interplay of up to six factors, all of which should be considered when interpreting epidemiological findings.

Nature of Exposure

Studies may ostensibly examine the same exposure when in fact the exposures experienced by subjects are importantly different. For example, in a community-based case–control study, participants might be classed as 'exposed' to asbestos on the basis of what, in many cases, were relatively low exposures, whereas in a cohort study of shipyard workers, the average exposure of 'exposed' workers was much higher.

Nature of Disease

Even where two studies focus on the same disease category, the mix of cases that they include may differ importantly. For example, one case–control study of lung cancer might predominantly include patients with squamous cell carcinomas, while in another, the case group might mainly comprise people with small-cell tumours. These histological subtypes could differ in their associations with the risk factors under investigation.

Bias

Studies may produce discordant results because they are subject to different biases.

Confounding

Similarly, discrepancies could arise because of differences between studies in terms of the nature and extent of confounding effects.

Chance

There is always a possibility that two studies of the same question could produce different results simply by chance. The likely potential for such chance variation can be assessed statistically.

Effect Modification

Effect modification occurs when the effect of a risk factor varies according to the presence or level of a second factor, known as an effect modifier. For example, the risk of occupational asthma from work with laboratory animals varies according to whether or not individuals are atopic. Two studies could produce different estimates of risk because their study populations differed in the prevalence or level of an effect modifier.

Other Considerations

When interpreting the results of an epidemiological study, it is important to consider their consistency not only with other epidemiological research, but also with relevant information from other scientific disciplines. For example, the causality of an epidemiological association between a chemical and cancer is more plausible if the substance has demonstrable genotoxicity and has been shown to cause cancer in laboratory animals.

APPLICATIONS OF EPIDEMIOLOGY TO OCCUPATIONAL LUNG DISORDERS

Epidemiology contributes to the recognition and management of occupational lung disorders in various ways.

Hazard Identification

The first step in controlling occupational diseases is identification of the hazard posed by work. A good example of an occupational disease that was first discovered through epidemiology is the increased susceptibility to infectious pneumonia that occurs following recent exposure to metal fume. The existence of this hazard emerged from national analyses of occupational mortality in England and Wales, which showed consistently high death rates from pneumococcal and unspecified lobar pneumonia in welders and several other metal-working occupations (Coggon et al., 1994).

Hazard Characterisation

Once an occupational hazard is identified, optimal planning of preventive measures requires information about the exact cause of the adverse health effect and the quantitative relationship of risk to exposure. Thus, for example, cohort studies of workers exposed to asbestos have provided information about the risk of lung cancer according to cumulative exposure to different forms of the mineral, and the results of those investigations have informed regulatory control limits on exposure.

Risk Characterisation

Related to this, epidemiology may sometimes provide direct information on the effects of a hazardous agent in a particular occupational setting. For example, demonstration of a major risk of occupational asthma in a factory making biological detergents (Flindt, 1969) led to encapsulation of the sensitising enzyme and improved engineering processes (Brant et al., 2004).

Effectiveness of Controls

Once measures have been put in place to control an occupational hazard, it is important to check that they are effective. In 1995, analysis of trends in mortality from mesothelioma in Britain indicated that rates were still increasing in men born up to 1948 (Peto et al., 1995), suggesting either that the regulatory control limits introduced in 1969 had not been sufficiently robust or that they had not been adequately enforced.

Effectiveness of Treatment

Epidemiological methods have also been used to evaluate clinical treatment for occupational lung disorders, particularly through randomised controlled trials.

Compensation

Another application of epidemiology is in determining eligibility to compensation for occupational lung diseases, both through social security and in the courts. This has been particularly useful when cases of a disease that are caused by work are clinically indistinguishable from the same disease occurring in the absence of relevant occupational exposures (e.g. lung cancer in coke oven workers and COPD in coal miners). In these circumstances, attribution has been probabilistic and has depended on the demonstration that the AF_{exp} is ≥ 0.5 (i.e. the disease is attributable to occupation in at least 50% of exposed cases) or that, on average, the occupational exposure makes a material contribution to the severity of the disease.

FURTHER READING

The following books may be helpful to readers seeking a more detailed description of epidemiological methods.

Coggon, D., Rose, G. and Barker, D. J. P. 2003. *Epidemiology for the Uninitiated*, Fifth edition. Chichester: Wiley (a brief introduction to epidemiology).

Coggon, D. 2002. *Statistics in Clinical Practice*, Second edition. Chichester: Wiley (an introduction to statistical methods for non-mathematicians).

Checkoway, H., Pearce, N. and Kriebel, D. 2004. *Research Methods in Occupational Epidemiology*, Second edition. Oxford: Oxford University Press (the most comprehensive textbook of occupational epidemiology).

Rothman, K. J., Greenland, S. and Lash, T. L. 2008. *Modern Epidemiology*, Third edition. Philadelphia, PA: Lippincott, Williams and Wilkins (a rigorous and detailed account of epidemiological methods).

REFERENCES

Brant, A., Hole, A., Cannon, J., Helm, J., Swales, C., Welch, J. et al. 2004. Occupational asthma caused by cellulose and lipase in the detergent industry. *Occup Environ Med* 61:793–5.

Coggon, D., Inskip, H., Winter, P. and Pannett, B. 1994. Lobar pneumonia—An occupational disease in welders. *Lancet* 344:41–3.

Coggon, D., Inskip, H., Winter, P. and Pannett, B. 1995. Contrasting geographical distribution of mortality from pneumoconiosis and chronic bronchitis and emphysema in British coal miners. *Occup Environ Med* 52:554–5.

Darnton, A., Hodgson, J., Benson, P. and Coggon, D. 2012. Mortality from asbestosis and mesothelioma in Britain by birth cohort. *Occup Med* 62:549–52.

Flindt, M. L. H. 1969. Pulmonary disease due to inhalation of derivatives of *Bacillus subtilis* containing proteolytic enzyme. *Lancet* 1:1177–81.

McNamee, R., Carder, M., Chen, Y. and Agius, R. 2008. Measurement of trends in incidence of work-related skin and respiratory diseases, UK 1996–2005. *Occup Environ Med* 65:808–14.

Peto, J., Hodgson, J. T., Matthews, F. and Jones, J. R. 1995. Continuing increase in mesothelioma mortality in Britain. *Lancet* 345:535–9.

10 Investigating an Outbreak

Kathleen Kreiss

CONTENTS

INTRODUCTION

Much of what we know about occupational lung disease is derived from outbreak investigation, triggered by a suspicion of increased cases in a defined population. The population and setting in which suspected cases are recognized often dictate whether an investigation is feasible and whether it can yield actionable information for clinicians, patients, employers or government.

This chapter provides examples of diverse investigations of suspected occupational or environmental lung disease (Table 10.1) in order to illustrate the triggers for investigation, settings of investigation, epidemiologic tools, challenges and outcomes. Some investigations attempt to establish new aetiologies of disease, such as fibrosis and alveolar proteinosis in indium workers, obliterative bronchiolitis in microwave popcorn workers and springtime deaths from interstitial disease in Korea. Other investigations explore new diseases such as pathologically unique lymphocytic bronchiolitis in nylon flock workers. In investigation of well-established occupational lung disease, the purpose is often to better understand risk factors and exposure–response relations; examples are hypersensitivity pneumonitis and damp-building-associated asthma. As in all science, each investigation builds on what is known before and contributes an advance that motivates further work in many disciplines pertinent to controlling occupational health risks. Any single outbreak investigation rarely contributes sufficient information to prevent a specific occupational lung disease across an industry. Nevertheless, the broad context of information needed to prevent occupational lung disease is useful to keep in mind when planning an investigation in order to maximize impact.

SUSPECTING EXCESSES OF LUNG DISEASE REQUIRING INVESTIGATION

For clinicians, suspecting excesses of disease is usually based on clinical cases, supplemented by published case reports and conferring with colleagues as to whether they have seen cases in similar settings. For example, an initial case report of interstitial pneumonia in an indium–tin oxide worker in Japan stimulated the reporting of another case with pulmonary fibrosis and eventual workforce investigation of employees in nine indium plants. These case reports alerted US investigators to pursue two cases of alveolar proteinosis in an indium–tin oxide facility; an international workshop reviewing ten cases of indium lung disease established that the disease starts with alveolar proteinosis and progresses to interstitial fibrosis and emphysema (Figure 10.1). A second example is the suspicion of occupational interstitial lung disease by a physician providing occupational health services to a company manufacturing flocked velvet-like upholstery who had seen two ill young men within 15 months. For occupational lung diseases that are known to be caused by occupational exposures, such as hypersensitivity pneumonitis, an isolated case with a temporal pattern of work-related exacerbation is sufficient to trigger investigation for the identification of an antigen, associated work process and co-worker risk, as in lifeguard lung. For common diseases such as asthma, suspecting a novel occupational cause warranting investigation is more difficult because the disease occurs so often in the general

TABLE 10.1
Illustrative Outbreak Investigations by Disease, Cause, Investigation Setting and References for Sentinel Cases and Outbreak Investigation

Disease	Cause	Setting	References
Fibrosis/emphysema	Indium–tin oxide	Nine indium workplaces	Homma et al. (2003, 2005); Nakano et al. (2009)
Alveolar proteinosis	Indium–tin oxide	Indium–tin oxide target manufacture	Cummings et al. (2010, 2013)
Lymphocytic bronchiolitis	Nylon flock	Flock upholstery manufacture	Kern et al. (1997); Washko et al. (2000)
Hypersensitivity pneumonitis	Contaminated water features	Leisure swimming pool	Rose et al. (1998)
Asthma	Dampness	Damp office building	Cox-Ganser et al. (2005)
Asthma	3-amino-5-mercapto-1,2,4-triazole	Pesticide manufacturing plant	Hnizdo et al. (2004)
Acute silicosis	Silica sandblasting of denim	Community cases	Akgun et al. (2005, 2008, 2015)
Interstitial lung disease	Humidifier disinfectant	81 hospitals nationwide	Kim et al. (2014)

(a)

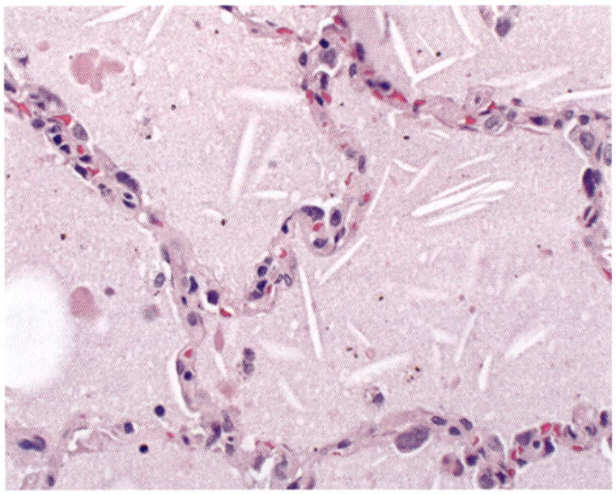

(b)

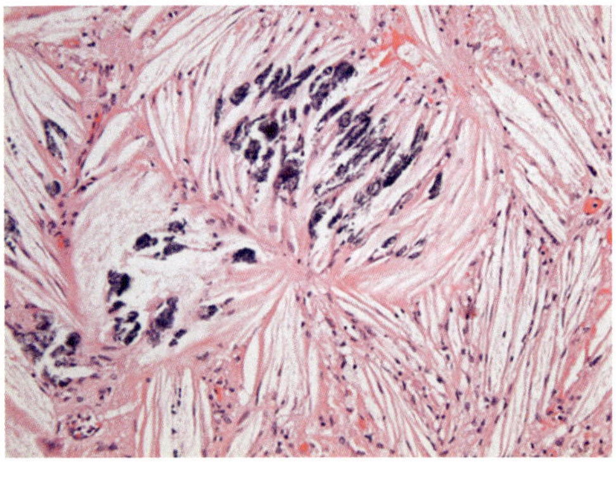

FIGURE 10.1 Photomicrographs demonstrating the common characteristics of indium lung diseases seen in Japan and the United States. (a) Alveolar proteinosis with filling of alveolar spaces with proteinaceous material and some cholesterol clefts. (b) Fibrosis with disruption of alveolar architecture by cholesterol clefts and cholesterol granulomas from a fatal Japanese case. Review of radiology and pathology of ten cases showed progression of disease from early alveolar proteinosis to fibrosis often accompanied by emphysema. (Reproduced from Cummings, K. J. et al. 2012. *Chest* 141:1512–21. With permission from the American College of Chest Physicians.)

population. In such diseases, workers often suspect an occupational cluster before their clinicians do, both because of temporal relationships of symptoms with work and because other incident asthma may be known by co-workers but rarely by physicians. Many instances of occupational asthma clusters coming to investigative attention exist in the setting of damp buildings.

In public health agencies, surveillance of physician reports of occupational asthma enables the identification of case clusters from a workplace that might otherwise go unrecognized; an example is reports by different physicians of eight cases of occupational asthma in a chemical plant making a herbicide. Two cases of end-stage lung disease among teenage workers in a small textile company in Turkey resulted in the identification of acute and accelerated silicosis caused by sandblasting of denim jeans, with hundreds of other cases subsequently being identified. Mortality data can even be a source of outbreak investigation; an example is the investigation of childhood deaths from interstitial lung disease in the springtime, often accompanied by similar illnesses in adult family members, which was found to be associated with humidifier disinfectant use in Korea. This outbreak was solved with a case–control study involving patients in 81 hospitals, and disappeared with the banning of the disinfectants.

GOALS OF OUTBREAK INVESTIGATION

The first goal of outbreak investigation is to develop actionable knowledge that will lead to the prevention of disease. In the setting of a sentinel cluster of clinically recognized illness, co-workers often have evidence of adverse health effects that have not resulted in clinical consultation. A workforce population-based approach allows epidemiological study of potential aetiology by examining risk factors, exposure–response relations and intervention effectiveness. Causality needs to be inferred for epidemiological associations to be actionable for prevention, and Sir Austin Bradford Hill's guidelines for assessing the likelihood of causation are useful, involving: strength of association; exclusion of other causes; demonstration that the cause precedes the effect (temporality); exposure–response relationship; replicability among investigators and in different populations; biological plausibility; and experiment (reduction in incidence following an intervention to reduce or avoid exposure) (Hill, 1965). The latter three often require efforts by others following an outbreak investigation. Together, the outbreak investigation and accumulation of evidence from other investigators can support societal action for prevention across industries.

A cluster of eight cases of obliterative bronchiolitis in former workers of a microwave popcorn manufacturing facility illustrates common outbreak investigation goals. These eight former workers, four of whom were listed for lung transplants, lacked work-related exacerbation of their symptoms (Centers for Disease Control and Prevention, 2002). They had developed their severe respiratory impairment, often within months of employment, between 1992 and 2000. None of them suspected that they had work-related disease, although the two pulmonologists who had provided clinical care were concerned that so many young non-smokers from the same workplace had developed spirometric obstruction that did not respond to bronchodilators or corticosteroid treatment. When brought to the attention of public health authorities, this eight-case cluster triggered a cross-sectional workplace investigation of current workers with a goal of identifying other possible cases by the occurrence of increased abnormalities consistent with obliterative bronchiolitis (Kreiss et al., 2002). Of 117 current employees, 25% had abnormal spirometry, some with forced expiratory volume in 1 second abnormalities in the range of the former worker cases listed for lung transplant. The current worker population had a 3.3-fold excess of spirometric obstruction, which was constituted by nearly equal numbers of those with pure obstruction and those with mixed obstructive and restrictive abnormalities. Of 21 workers with any obstructive abnormalities, 19 lacked substantial improvement with bronchodilators, consistent with the investigators' conception of fixed obstruction as characteristic of obliterative bronchiolitis. Thus, the cluster of former worker cases was a sentinel of current worker risk of abnormalities, which was probably largely related to the same exposure, a finding that fulfilled one goal of the investigation to describe the extent and range of disease and establish the existence of an ongoing outbreak.

However, the outbreak had no known cause at the time of the investigation. Textbook descriptions of obliterative bronchiolitis were based largely on cases from workplace accidents resulting in pulmonary oedema preceding the evolution of fixed obstructive lung disease. Indolent onset of obliterative bronchiolitis in individual patients had not been attributed to the workplace. Thus, a second goal was hypothesis generation in order to establish the aetiology of this disease by evaluating risk factors. To this end, the investigators collected job history and work location information in order to obtain hints about possible causes from uneven distributions of abnormalities in the plant workforce. The workers with flavourings exposure had symptom prevalences and spirometric abnormalities in excess of the 20 remaining workers without flavourings exposure. Half of the eight sentinel cases occurred in mixers of flavourings in oil, which suggested that flavourings were involved (Figure 10.2). The predominant chemical in butter flavouring and plant air was diacetyl (2,3-butanedione).

A third goal of the investigation was to evaluate exposure–response relations. Knowing the exposure levels associated with risk can lead to guidance regarding health-protective levels of exposure. The investigative

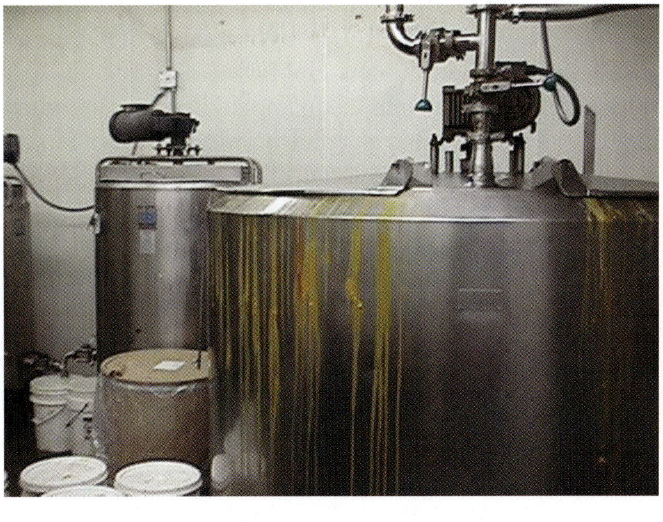

FIGURE 10.2 The mixers in the microwave popcorn plant had the highest exposure to diacetyl in this room, shown before preventative interventions. The large lidded tank on the right contains heated soybean oil, to which heated flavourings were added from 5-gallon buckets in the left foreground, with evident spillage. The two smaller tanks on the left contain heated flavourings that were transferred to the 5-gallon buckets.

team measured concentrations of diacetyl by job and area. This exposure information, linked with job histories of individual current workers in the workforce, enabled the estimation of cumulative exposure to diacetyl in months–mg/m^3. The investigators then demonstrated that average pulmonary function measurements, as well as the prevalence of pulmonary function abnormalities, decreased with increasing cumulative diacetyl exposure. This fulfilled the goal of defining exposure–response relations, substantiating that diacetyl was the likely cause of the respiratory abnormalities in the current workforce.

Sometimes measurements of causes of occupational lung disease do not correlate with disease risk, and process is a more holistic exposure index. When measurements do not predict risk, those responsible for worker health must consider several possible explanations: the measurement might not be biologically relevant; air concentration may not be a risk factor for disease; forms of the material may not have biological equivalency (e.g. in solubility or persistence in tissue); and historical exposure reconstruction may have led to misclassification.

Finally, once occupational disease is recognized, outbreak investigation may evolve to the goal of establishing the effectiveness of preventative interventions. This goal is especially important in settings in which environmental measurement techniques for monitoring occupational lung health risk are absent, as is largely the case for damp-building-related lung diseases such as asthma and hypersensitivity pneumonitis. In the microwave popcorn manufacturing facility, repeated cross-sectional evaluations of the workforce while lowering flavouring exposures documented that new employees maintained their pulmonary function, and mean annual declines in forced expiratory volume in 1 second normalized over nearly 3 years of follow up (Kreiss, 2007; Kanwal et al., 2011). The effectiveness of these interventions in terms of protecting most workers helped fulfil the Hill guidelines for experiment (i.e. cessation of exposure eliminated the respiratory hazard for new employees).

EPIDEMIOLOGIC TOOLS OF OUTBREAK INVESTIGATIONS

To maximize the potential impact of an outbreak investigation, an epidemiological approach to a worker population with a suspected range of exposures and high response rate is necessary (Table 10.2). An outbreak investigation in a workplace should not be limited to screening for additional cases beyond the cluster that may have triggered an investigation. Population-based information on job titles, work location, tenure, processes and exposures enables the identification of risk factors that can be used to set priorities for intervention and guidance about unsafe processes or exposure levels. In occupational asthma, workers may have changed jobs or even left work in order to avoid exacerbation of symptoms in particular areas. This healthy worker survival effect may preclude the identification of work-related aetiologies unless symptom onset can be associated with prior job titles in the work history. For diseases arising after employment, such as pneumoconiosis, consideration of community-based surveys is a possibility, such as were performed in Turkish denim sandblasters (Akgun et al., 2008, 2015).

Using standardized questionnaires is critical to making external comparisons between observed prevalence and expected rates derived from population-based surveys, such as to the National Health and Nutrition Examination Surveys and Behavioral Risk Factor Surveillance Surveys in the United States and the European Community Respiratory Health Survey. External comparisons are valuable when a range of exposures in the workplace is narrow, precluding exposure–response analyses. An approach that addresses temporality used in damp building investigations is the

TABLE 10.2
Tools for Outbreak Investigations by Advantages

Tool	Advantage
Population-based epidemiological approach	Range of exposure; risk factor identification
Incidence density with cross-sectional design	Addresses temporality in part
Cohort longitudinal design	Addresses healthy worker/survivor effect and temporality
Case–control design	Efficient strategy for rare diseases
Validated questionnaire instrument	Allows comparability for external comparisons
Objective medical testing	Addresses reporting bias
Public health agency involvement	Access to workplace and multidisciplinary collaboration
Exposure estimation (tenure; job, area, process or task; measurements; biological exposure indices)	Exposure–response relationships for causal interpretation

incidence density of asthma diagnosis of building occupants before and during employment in an implicated building; in one damp office building investigation, the incidence rate of physician-diagnosed asthma in current building occupants increased from 1.9/1000 person-years before occupancy to 14.5/1000 person-years after occupancy (Cox-Ganser et al., 2005). Case definitions for analyses can be based on either questionnaire responses, such as symptom combinations or self-reported physician diagnoses or on objective abnormalities measured in medical testing. Epidemiologic design is commonly cross-sectional, but longitudinal studies can address the temporality of suspected causal exposures in relation to incident disease or recovery with exposure decreases or cessation.

Exposure indices added to standardized questionnaires must be customized for each workplace, with input from environmental scientists with knowledge of the workplace and processes. Historical exposure measurements or range-finding measurements from an initial visit are valuable to both designing a questionnaire and to planning exposure assessment in order to complement the questionnaire interview and medical testing. Sometimes, presuppositions about relative exposure in different plant work areas are entirely wrong and require post hoc adjustments of planned analyses. For example, in a coffee roasting, grinding and flavouring factory, the five sentinel cases of obliterative bronchiolitis were assumed by their physicians to be caused by flavouring exposure in the plant (CDC, 2013). However, combined exposure to diacetyl and its primary substitute, 2,3-pentanedione, in the areas in which unflavoured roast coffee was ground was higher than in the area in which coffee was flavoured (Bailey et al., 2015).

Unfettered access to workplaces and to historical environmental and medical measurements is a great advantage in investigating outbreaks of occupational lung disease. Such access may be difficult or impossible for clinicians or academic institutions, even when multidisciplinary expertise, time and funding is available. Some public health agencies may be able to access workplaces and records, as well as to mobilize the appropriate disciplinary and laboratory expertise. In countries with public health infrastructure for occupational health, the enlistment of public health agency involvement may be advantageous.

CHALLENGES OF OUTBREAK INVESTIGATIONS

Outbreak investigation is one part of the evidence that is usually required in order to establish new causes of occupational lung disease and to lead to preventative measures across an industry. Several limitations may exist, however, in terms of investigating outbreaks of suspected novel diseases or causes of lung disease (Table 10.3). One of the criteria for causation in epidemiological associations is strength of association, and finding statistically significant associations is sometimes limited by power. When suspected cases occur in a workforce, the investigator has no control over the number of workers potentially exposed to a causative agent. When workforces are too small or a disease is rare, as in the four fibreglass boat building establishments in which five sentinel cases of obliterative bronchiolitis occurred over a 20-year period (Cullinan et al., 2013), an outbreak investigation at the workplaces is not feasible. Undertaking an investigation that is doomed by inadequate power is a waste of resources and potentially misleading. A related limitation to workforce-based outbreak investigations is poor response rate, so that collected data are not representative of the targeted workforce. In settings in which workers are intimidated from participation in independent outbreak investigation, the findings are unlikely to be robust because of selection or participation bias. The healthy worker effect frequently affects the quantitative

TABLE 10.3
Challenges of Outbreak Investigations by Consequence

Challenge	Consequence
Small workforce	Limited power
Exposure range narrow	No internal exposure–response relationships and external comparisons necessary
Misclassification of exposure (e.g. historically inaccurate and not biologically relevant)	Diminished ability to demonstrate exposure–response measurements
Complex mixed exposures	Aetiology not apparent
Misclassification of health outcomes	Diminished ability to demonstrate exposure–response relationships
Poor response rate	Selection bias and decreased power
Affected workers leave work task	Healthy survivor bias, especially for asthma

strength of the association because former workers, who are rarely included in cross-sectional workforce investigations, may have left due to illness, as is frequently the case in occupational asthma.

Exposure assessment is often a challenge in outbreak investigations, even with a multidisciplinary team. Past exposure for long-latency diseases or diseases related to cumulative exposure is seldom able to be precisely reconstructed. Assumptions may depend on historical measurements, work processes, throughput of materials, production levels and timing of engineering controls and personal protective measures. Measurements, including biomonitoring, may not be biologically relevant to health outcomes or past exposures. We rarely have information on whether the pertinent exposure metric for health outcome is cumulative exposure, average exposure or peak exposure. Indeed, the approach to indices of peak exposure is evolving, with consideration of report of accidents, likelihood of process upset, geometric standard deviation of shift measurements and upper 95% confidence limit about the 95th percentile of the distribution, among others. Complex mixed exposures may not enable the teasing apart of suspected causal agents, such as in flavouring manufacturing, in which thousands of chemicals are intermittently present in short-term batch operations (Cumming et al., 2014). Finally, analysis of exposure–response relationships within a workforce depends on a range of exposures among the workers studied, which is not always found.

Misclassification of health outcomes can also be a challenge in outbreak investigation, and reduces the power to ascertain relationships between exposures and health responses. Oftentimes, we are blinded by textbook knowledge about the 'classic' presentation of particular diseases. An example at the advent of the microwave popcorn investigations was that the investigators thought that obliterative bronchiolitis was characterized by fixed obstruction. A decade later, three biopsy-confirmed case series documented that spirometry can be obstructive, restrictive or normal in obliterative bronchiolitis (Markopoulou et al., 2002; Ghanei et al., 2008; King et al., 2011). Accordingly, occupational lung disease was probably underestimated in the microwave popcorn industry by not including workers with pure spirometric restriction or only symptoms in case definitions. A similar example of evolving classification of indium lung disease started with interstitial pneumonia that progressed to fibrosis and finally alveolar proteinosis, resulting in fibrosis and emphysema (Cummings et al., 2012). Misclassification in hypersensitivity pneumonitis investigations occurs if the case definition requires abnormal radiologic or spirometric studies, either of which is insensitive when symptomatic workers undergo trans-bronchial biopsy for diagnosis, as in lifeguard lung (Rose et al., 1998).

OUTCOMES OF OUTBREAK INVESTIGATIONS THROUGH THE EFFORTS OF OTHERS

The intent of outbreak investigation is the recognition of new hazards and the refinement of guidance regarding risk for the purpose of prevention of disease. The outbreak investigator can maximize the quality of the investigation by addressing the limitations over which he or she has control, but the ultimate preventative outcome of outbreak investigation is seldom under the control of the investigator (Table 10.4). Rather, a quality investigation motivates others to perform ancillary work on: biological plausibility in animal or in vitro studies; replication in other work settings for hypothesis testing; follow-up for natural history; treatment in clinical trials; and studying the effectiveness of intervention. For example, several investigators pursued different workforces with exposure to synthetic flock after its initial description (Figure 10.3) (Eschenbacher et al., 1999; Atis et al., 2005; Daroowalla et al., 2005; Antao et al., 2007). Despite this body of outbreak investigations showing

TABLE 10.4
Outcomes of Outbreak Investigation and Their Importance for Impact

Outcomes Performed by Others	Importance for Impact
Experimental toxicology studies	Biological plausibility for interpreting causation and mechanism
Replication/confirmation in other workplaces and industries	Needed for interpreting causation
Exposure–response studies	Needed for interpreting causation and guidance for prevention by decreasing exposures
Natural history and clinical trials	Secondary prevention
Intervention studies	Addresses experiment and primary prevention in workplace
Public health or workforce surveillance	Identifies opportunities for prevention and demonstration of intervention adequacy
Risk assessment	Needed for regulation for prevention

(a)

(b)

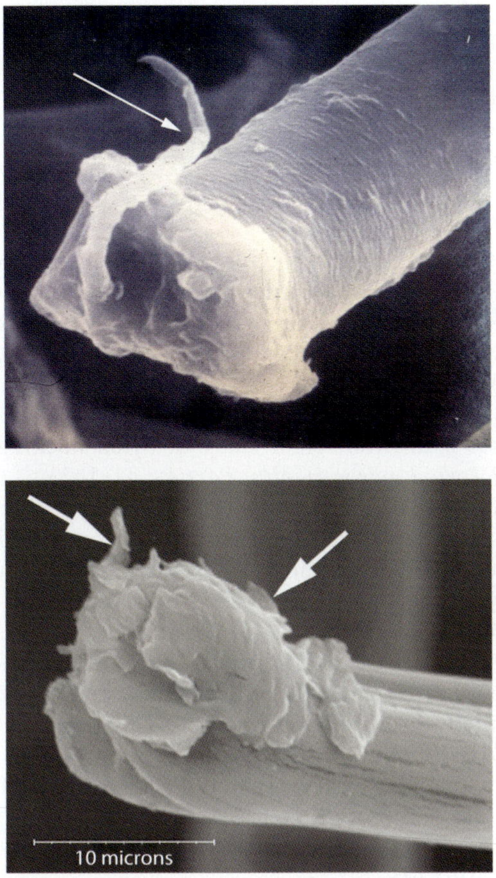

FIGURE 10.3 When nylon flock is cut, fibrils are formed (a) that break off with milling and are of respirable size. Industrial hygienists identified the respirable dust in the flock upholstery plant as nylon by the temperature at which it melted, demonstrating the utility of multidisciplinary collaboration in the flock-workers' lung outbreak investigation. (b) Potentially similar respirable dust formed at the cut end of rayon flock used in greeting card manufacture. (Reproduced from Burkhart, J. et al. 1999. *J Toxic Environ Health, Part A* 57(1):1–23. With permission; Antao, V. C. S. et al. 2007. *Am J Ind Med* 50:274–84. With permission.)

that lymphocytic bronchiolitis was a flock-related hazard, no regulation has been forthcoming for synthetic flock fibres. Respiratory risks of indoor dampness have been summarized by the US Institute of Medicine and the World Health Organization, but have so far triggered little regulation or scientific investigation on the effectiveness of remediation (Sauni et al., 2013). In part, this is because no environmental measurements have been shown to predict health risks; enforceable regulations are usually based on such measurements.

The first cross-sectional study in the sentinel microwave popcorn manufacturing facility motivated replication in other populations and by other investigators. Cases were recognized in five other microwave popcorn plants (Kanwal et al., 2006; Lockey et al., 2009), many flavouring manufacturing plants (Kim et al. 2010; Cummings et al. 2014), a diacetyl manufacturing plant supplying the chemical to flavouring manufacturers (van Rooy et al., 2009) and in downstream users of flavourings, such as cookie (Cavalcanti et al., 2012) and coffee manufacture (CDC, 2013; Bailey et al., 2015). For new agents suspected of causing occupational lung disease, such as diacetyl in artificial butter flavourings and respirable nylon flock dust, biological plausibility required animal experiments. The phenomenon of indolent onset of occupational obliterative bronchiolitis has triggered recognition of other industries that are at risk (King et al., 2011; Chen et al., 2013; Cullinan et al., 2013).

All of these further studies may become the basis of risk assessment, regulation, surveillance and consumer concern. Regulatory delays arise because of controversy regarding the science and the economic and technical feasibility. In the United States, the threat of litigation by injured workers against third-party suppliers of hazardous ingredients may motivate prevention. Workforce surveillance can be valuable in the follow-up of outbreak investigation by demonstrating whether interventions are effective. An example of post-intervention surveillance that resulted in changes in preventative approach include the study of a leisure pool with water-spray features associated with a 65% prevalence of granulomatous lung disease in lifeguards (Figure 10.4). In this instance, recurrence of disease was prevented only by replacing the chlorination system with an ozonation system (Rose et al., 1998). An example of national surveillance documenting the resolution of a many-year outbreak of interstitial lung disease is the national mortality and case reporting in Korea when humidifier disinfectants were removed from the market.

CONCLUSION

Outbreak investigation is often the basis of establishing new causes of occupational lung disease, and epidemiological characterization of work-related risks and exposure–response relationships lays the groundwork for employer guidance, preventative intervention, risk assessment, regulation and surveillance. Although a single outbreak investigation rarely achieves these outcomes by itself, it may motivate others to conduct experiments for biological plausibility, to replicate findings and to address temporality with longitudinal studies and interventions. The aggregate scientific efforts generated by outbreak investigation fulfil the criteria for causal epidemiological associations that are required for regulatory prevention and consensus among those who control the conditions of work.

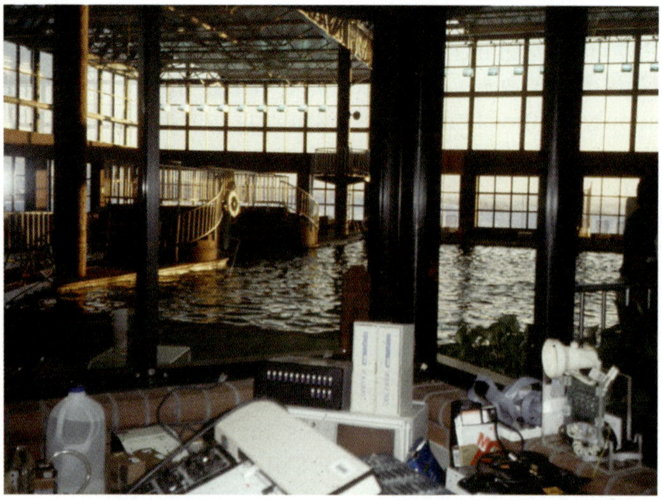

FIGURE 10.4 In this leisure pool with an outbreak of hypersensitivity pneumonitis in lifeguards, activation of the many water-spray features resulted in elevation of air endotoxin levels that distinguished this pool from other indoor pools. Ventilation upgrades after pool closure did not prevent recurrence of a second outbreak among lifeguards when the pool reopened. This second outbreak required attention to the source point of microbial contamination in the water-spray features, as demonstrated by industrial hygienists using the environmental sampling equipment shown in the foreground as water features were switched on and off. The corroded water circuits were then replaced and the chlorination system was replaced with an ozonation system in order to ensure the respiratory health of lifeguards. This outbreak investigation demonstrates the importance of interdisciplinary collaboration and follow-up in order to assess intervention effectiveness. (Photograph courtesy of Dr. Cecile Rose, National Jewish Health, Denver, Colorado.)

DISCLAIMER

The findings and conclusions in this report are those of the author and do not necessarily represent the views of the National Institute for Occupational Safety and Health, Centers for Disease Control and Prevention.

REFERENCES

Akgun, M., Araz, O., Akkurt, I., Eroglu, A., Alper, F., Saglam, L., Mirci, A. et al. 2008. An epidemic of silicosis among former denim sandblasters. *Eur Respir J* 32:1295–303.

Akgun, M., Araz, O., Ucar, E. Y., Karaman, A., Alper, F., Gorguner, M. and Kreiss, K. 2015. Silicosis appears inevitable among former denim sandblasters: A four-year follow up study. *Chest* 148(3):647–54.

Akgun, M., Gorguner, M., Meral, M., Turkyilmaz, A., Erdogan, F., Saglam, L. and Mirici, A. 2005. Silicosis caused by sandblasting of jeans in Turkey: A report of two concomitant cases. *J Occup Health* 47:346–9.

Antao, V. C. S., Piacitelli, C. A., Miller, W. E., Pinheiro, G. A. and Kreiss, K. 2007. Rayon flock: A new cause of respiratory morbidity in a card processing plant. *Am J Ind Med* 50:274–84.

Atis, S., Tutluoglu, B., Levent, E., Ozturk, C., Tunaci, A., Sahin, K., Saral, A. et al. 2005. The respiratory effects of occupational polypropylene flock exposure. *Eur Respir J* 25:110–7.

Bailey, R. L., Cox-Ganser, J. M., Duling, M. G., LeBouf, R. F., Martin, S. B., Bledsoe, T. A., Green, B. J. et al. 2015. Respiratory morbidity in a coffee processing workplace with sentinel obliterative bronchiolitis cases. *Am J Ind Med* 58:1235–45.

Burkhart, J., Piacitelli, C., Schwegler-Berry, D. and Jones, W. 1999. Environmental study of nylon flocking process. *J Toxic Environ Health, Part A* 57(1):1–23.

Cavalcanti, Z. do R., Albuquerque Filho, A. P. L., Pereira, C. A. and Coletta, E. N. 2012. Bronchiolitis associated with exposure to artificial butter flavoring in workers at a cookie factory in Brazil. *J Bras Pneumol* 38:395–9.

Centers for Disease Control and Prevention. 2002. Fixed obstructive lung disease among former workers at a microwave popcorn factory—Missouri, 2000–2002. *MMWR Morb Mortal Wkly Rep* 51:345–7.

Centers for Disease Control and Prevention. 2013. Obliterative bronchiolitis in workers in a coffee-processing facility—Texas, 2008–2013. *MMWR Morb Mortal Weekly Rep* 62(16):305–7.

Chen, C. H., Tsai, P. Y., Wang, W. C., Pan, C. H., Ho, J. J. and Guo, Y. L. 2013. Obliterative bronchiolitis in workers laying up fiberglass-reinforced plastics with polyester resin and methylethyl ketone peroxide catalyst. *Occup Environ Med* 70:675–6.

Cox-Ganser, J. M., White, S. K., Jones, R., Hilsbos, K., Storey, E., Enright, P. L., Rao, C.Y. et al. 2005. Respiratory morbidity in office workers in a water-damaged building. *Environ Health Perspect* 113:485–90.

Cullinan, P., McGavin, C. R., Kreiss, K., Nicholson, A. G., Maher, T. M., Howell, T., Banks, J. et al. 2013. Obliterative bronchiolitis in fiberglass workers: A new occupational disease? *Occup Environ Med* 70:357–9.

Cummings, K. J., Boylstein, R., Stanton, M., Piacitelli, C., Edwards, N., LeBouf, R. and Kreiss, K. 2014. Respiratory symptoms and lung function abnormalities related to work at a flavoring manufacturing facility. *Occup Environ Med* 71:539–54.

Cummings, K. J., Donat, W. E., Ettensohn, D. B., Roggli, V.L., Ingram, P. and Kreiss, K. 2010. Pulmonary alveolar proteinosis in workers at an indium processing facility. *Am J Respir Crit Care Med* 181:458–64.

Cummings, K. J., Nakano, M., Omae, K., Takeuchi, K., Chonan, T., Xiao, Y. L. Harley, R.A. et al. 2012. Indium lung disease. *Chest* 141:1512–21.

Cummings, K. J., Suarthana, E., Edwards, N., Liang, X., Stanton, M. L., Day, G. A., Saito, R. et al. 2013. Serial evaluations at an indium–tin oxide production facility. *Am J Ind Med* 56:300–7.

Daroowalla, F., Wang, M. L., Piacitelli, C., Attfield, M. D. and Kreiss, K. 2005. 'Flock workers' exposures and respiratory symptoms in five plants. *Am J Ind Med* 47:144–52.

Eschenbacher, W. L., Kreiss, K., Lougheed, D., Pransky, G. S., Day, B. and Castellan, R. M. 1999. Nylon flock-associated interstitial lung disease: Clinical pathology workshop summary. *Am J Respir Crit Care Med* 159:2003–8.

Ghanei, M., Tazelaar, H. D., Chilosi, M., Harandi, A. A., Peyman, M., Akbari, H. M. H., Shamsaei, H. et al. 2008. An international collaborative pathologic study of surgical lung biopsies from mustard gas-exposed patients. *Respir Med* 102:825–30.

Hill, A. B. 1965. The environment and disease: Association or causation? *Proc R Soc Med* 58:295–300.

Hnizdo, E., Sylvain, D., Lewis, D. M., Pechter, E. and Kreiss, K. 2004. New-onset asthma associated with exposure to 3-amino-5-mercapto-1,2,4-triazole. *J Occup Environ Med* 46(12):1246–52.

Homma, S., Miyamoto, A., Sakamoto, S., Kishi, K., Motoi, N. and Yoshimura, K. 2005. Pulmonary fibrosis in an individual occupationally exposed to inhaled indium–tin oxide. *Eur Respir J* 25:200–4.

Homma, T., Ueno, T., Sekizawa, K., Tanaka, A. and Hirata, M. 2003. Interstitial pneumonia developed in a worker dealing with particles containing indium–tin oxide. *J Occup Health* 45:137–9.

Kanwal, R., Kullman, G., Fedan, K. B. and Kreiss, K. 2011. Occupational lung disease risk and exposure to butter-flavoring chemicals after implementation of controls at a microwave popcorn plant. *Public Health Rep* 126:480–94.

Kanwal, R., Kullman, G., Piacitelli, C., Boylstein, R., Sahakian, N., Martin, S., Fedan, K. et al. 2006. Evaluation of flavorings-related lung disease risk at six microwave popcorn plants. *J Occup Environ Med* 48:149–57.

Kern, D. G., Durand, K. T. H., Crausman, R. S, Nneyeu, A., Kuhn, C. III, Vanderslice, R. R., Lougheed, M. D. et al. 1997. Chronic interstitial lung disease in nylon flocking industry workers—Rhode island, 1992–1996. *MMWR Morb Mortal Wkly Rep* 46:897–901.

Kim, K. W., Ahn, K., Yang, H. J., Lee, S., Park, J. D., Kim, W. K., Kim, J. T. et al. 2014. Humidifier disinfectant-associated children's interstitial lung disease. *Am J Respir Crit Care Med* 189(1):48–56.

Kim, T. J., Materna, B. L., Prudhomme, J. C., Fedan, K. B. Enright, P. L., Sahakian, N. M., Windham, G. C. et al. 2010. Industry-wide medical surveillance of California flavoring manufacturing workers: Cross-sectional results. *Am J Ind Med* 53:857–65.

King, M. S., Eisenberg, R., Newman, J. H., Tolle, J. J., Harrell, F. E., Nian, H., Ninan, M. et al. 2011. Constrictive bronchiolitis in soldiers returning from Iraq and Afghanistan. *N Engl J Med* 365:222–30.

Kreiss, K. 2007. Flavoring-related bronchiolitis obliterans. *Curr Opin Allergy Clin Immunol* 7:162–7.

Kreiss, K., Gomaa, A., Kullman, G., Fedan, K., Simoes, E. J. and Enright, P. L. 2002. Clinical bronchiolitis obliterans in workers at a microwave-popcorn plant. *N Engl J Med* 347:330–8.

Lockey, J. E., Hilbert, T. J., Levin, L. P., Ryan, P. H., White, K. L., Borton, E. K., Rice, C. H. et al. 2009. Airway obstruction related to diacetyl exposure at microwave popcorn production facilities. *Eur Respir J* 34:63–71.

Markopoulou, K. D., Cool, C. D., Elliot, T. L., Lynch, D. A., Newell, J. D., Hale, V. A., Brown, K. K. et al. 2002. Obliterative bronchiolitis: Varying presentations and clinicopathological correlation. *Eur Respir J* 19:20–30.

Nakano, M., Omae, K., Tanaka, A., Hirata, M., Michikawa, T., Kikuchi, Y., Yoshioka, N. et al. 2009. Causal relationship between indium compound inhalation and effects on the lungs. *J Occup Health* 51(6):513–21.

Rose, C. S., Martyny, J. W., Newman, L. S., Milton, D. K., King, T. E. Jr., Beebe, J. L., McCammon, J. B. et al. 1998. 'Lifeguard lung': Endemic granulomatous pneumonitis in an indoor swimming pool. *Am J Public Health* 88:1795–800.

Sauni, R., Verbeek, J. H., Utti, J., Jauhiainen, M., Kreiss, K. and Sigsgaard, T. 2015. Remediating buildings damaged by dampness and mould for preventing or reducing respiratory tract symptoms, infections and asthma. *Cochrane Database Syst Rev* 2015 Feb(2):CD007897. DOI:10.1002/1461859.

van Rooy, F. G., Smit, L. A., Houba, R., Zaat, V. A., Rooyackers, J. M. and Heederik, D. J. 2009. A cross-sectional study of lung function and respiratory symptoms among chemical workers producing diacetyl for food flavourings. *Occup Environ Med* 66:105–10.

Washko, R. M., Day, B., Parker, J. E., Castellan, R. M. and Kreiss, K. 2000. Epidemiologic investigation of respiratory morbidity at a nylon flock plant. *Am J Ind Med* 38:628–38.

11 Compensation and Attribution

Anthony J. Newman Taylor

CONTENTS

Statutory no-fault compensation for accidents at work and diseases caused by work exists in some form in Europe and North America, as well as Australasia and South Africa. What is compensated and how this is done differs between the different countries and in the USA. among its different states. However, the basic principle of no-fault compensation (i.e. access to compensation without the need to demonstrate negligence) is shared for accidents at work and, to a lesser extent, for diseases caused by work.

Arrangements for no-fault compensation – initially for accidents and later for diseases – date back to the late nineteenth and early twentieth centuries. The first modern 'no-fault' compensation scheme was introduced in Germany (Workers' Accident Insurance) by Bismarck, who appreciated that such a scheme would encourage social peace by ameliorating potential conflict between workers and employers. In the UK, at a time when the number of fatal accidents at work each year was approximately 5000, of which 1000 were in the mining industry, the main driver for a no-fault compensation scheme was the failure of the civil courts to provide compensation to workers – or their families – who were injured or killed at work.

During the nineteenth century, courts in both UK and USA. had accepted what was known in the UK as the 'holy trinity of defences', which provided considerable barriers to successful claims by workers. The defence of *common* employment was of particular importance and aroused considerable hostility. This defence, called the 'fellow servant rule' in the USA., was that the employer was not liable where an injury was due to the negligence of a fellow worker. In practice, this meant that an employee only had a successful claim if the employer had been personally negligent.

In companies with a large number of employees, such as mines and railways, which had the highest rates of accidental injuries and deaths, the workman or his family was left without the means to pursue a successful claim. In the UK, steps to abolish the defence of *common employment* by Act of Parliament were first taken in 1880, but it was not effectively overcome until 1897. During debates inside and outside parliament in the 1890s, Joseph Chamberlain first advanced the principle of automatic compensation by employers for accidents at work, irrespective of cause and without the need to prove negligence. He was the architect in the UK of the first Workmen's Compensation Act of 1897, whose underlying principle was to take compensation out of the courts for accidents 'arising out of and in the course of employment,' effectively overcoming the legal barriers to employees' compensation.

This principle was revolutionary in its implications: it provided the employee with the legal right to compensation at no cost to himself, and it imposed on employers a legal obligation to compensate workers for loss of earning capacity as a result of an accident at work, with the cost to be considered as a cost of production, comparable to the cost of capital depreciation. Employer liability was independent of negligence on the part of employer or employee; strict liability (i.e. liability without fault), was written into statute. William Beveridge later described the 1897 Workmen's Compensation Act as 'the pioneer scheme of social security in Britain.'

The 1897 Act only covered accidents, but the later Workmen's Compensation Act of 1906 listed six diseases for which compensation was payable: anthrax, ankylostomiasis (hookworm) and poisoning by lead, mercury, phosphorous and arsenic and their sequelae. Workers were entitled to no-fault compensation if they could establish: (a) that the disease was due to the nature of their employment; and (b) that they had been engaged in that employment at any time during the 12 months preceding the date of disablement. The Home Secretary, who was responsible for the administration of the Act, was empowered to add further diseases to the schedule. This implied the need to define criteria for how disease could be confidently attributed to occupation.

In the USA, the federal government, driven in part by the high incidence of accidents to railroad workers, took the lead in the early twentieth century in providing compensation for accidents to its workforce. The Federal Employees Act of 1908 covered federal employees engaged in hazardous work and employees of certain carriers engaged in inter-state and foreign commerce. In a speech to Congress urging its adoption, President Theodore Roosevelt said that the 'burden of accident falls upon the hapless man, his wife and children,' which was 'an outrage.' The turning point in the development of workers' compensation legislation by individual states was its adoption by Wisconsin in 1911. This had been the subject of considerable debate, with employers lobbying successfully for what has become known as 'the great trade-off': in exchange for employers providing medical and wage replacement benefits, the employee gave up the right to sue their employer. This model was adopted by the other states, although it was not until 1976 that all 50 states had some form of coverage for occupational disease as well as injury.

The development of compensation schemes in the UK and mainland Europe and in the USA have differed greatly. In the UK, and to a variable extent in Europe, diseases are in general compensated from a list of 'prescribed' diseases. In the UK the list is continually updated for diseases when there is consistent evidence for a doubling or more in the risk of the disease, in relation to an occupational exposure, in comparison to the risk of the disease in the general population. This has allowed the inclusion of diseases such as lung cancer in asbestos workers and COPD in coal miners. Statutory compensation is not given for diseases not fulfilling those criteria. In the USA, in contrast, decisions are more usually based on individual proof that the specific exposure is the likely cause of disease. This can enable the recognition of conditions not included on a prescribed list, but has the disadvantage that the burden of proof rests more with the claimant. Also, whereas in the UK and mainland Europe compensation schemes although different in coverage and funding are consistent within countries, in the USA schemes developed on a state by state basis, with the introduction of a system over time that was incomplete in geographical coverage and remains inconsistent in its specific rules.

ACCIDENTS AND DISEASES: THE PROBLEM OF SPECIFICITY

The rationale for compensation is to provide the worker with recompense for an injury or disease that would not have occurred, other than for the incident or exposure at the place of work. This implies an acceptance of causation; this is more straightforward in the case of an accident than for a disease, particularly for a disease that is also common in the general population. The problem of causation has long been a subject of disagreement and philosophical debate:

> Observation can only tell us that certain events regularly follow other events. The rest is subjective inference.
>
> **David Hume**
> *1789*

> Whenever I look at my watch and see the hand pointing to ten, I hear bells beginning to ring in the church close by; but I have no right to assume the movement of the bells is caused by the position of the hands of my watch.
>
> **Tolstoy**
> *War and Peace*

These philosophical reflections, however, do not inform the more practical need for an understanding of causation on which to base attribution* of disease to an exposure at work. For this purpose, a more recent definition proposed by Coggon and Martyn provides a more secure foundation: a cause of disease is 'something which at least in some circumstances makes a disease more likely if it is introduced and less likely if it is removed' (Coggon and Martyn, 2005).

As an example, cigarette smoking is a cause of lung cancer: the incidence of lung cancer is increased in direct proportion to the number of cigarettes smoked each day and was shown to fall in those who gave up smoking during the subsequent 10 years (Doll and Hill, 1964). These observations demonstrate the importance of cigarette smoking as a

* Attribution: The ascribing of an effect to a cause. Shorter Oxford English Dictionary.

TABLE 11.1
Hierarchy of Attribution

Cause	Example
Accident	Acute inhalation accident
Disease with specific clinical features or high specificity of association	Occupational asthma Pneumoconiosis (e.g. silica, coal, asbestos) Mesothelioma (and asbestos) Chronic beryllium disease
Inference from population studies to individual case as 'more likely than not'	Lung cancer and asbesto COPD and coalmine dust

Abbreviation: COPD: chronic obstructive pulmonary disease.

determinant of lung cancer in populations. The concern in compensation is attribution of disease to a cause in the individual case. Inference of causation in the individual case can come either from the specific features of the disease in the individual case or by inference from epidemiological studies. Examples of the former include inhalation accidents causing acute pulmonary oedema as well as pneumoconiosis in a coal miner, and of the latter, lung cancer in an asbestos worker or COPD in a coal miner. Attribution in the two former circumstances is more straightforward than in the two latter circumstances, which have to be based on inference from the results of population studies to the individual case. This gradient of inference can helpfully be considered as a hierarchy of attribution (Table 11.1).

In making an attribution on the basis of the results of studies in populations, a decision has to be made regarding the required level of proof. Statutory compensation has, in general, accepted the same level of proof as have the courts for civil compensation – 'on the balance of probabilities' or 'more likely than not'. This level of proof was succinctly encapsulated by Lord Denning in the UK: 'if the evidence is such that the tribunal can say "we think it more probable than not" the burden of proof is discharged, but if the probabilities are equal it is not' (Miller v Minister of Pensions, 1947).

Attribution of disease in the individual case therefore implies sufficient knowledge of causation to answer the following questions:

1. Is the agent a cause of disease, at least in certain defined circumstances?
2. If so, were the circumstances of the individual case such that the factor is more likely than not to have caused the disease?

Recognition of diseases not specific to occupation and their inclusion in compensation schemes has occurred in the second half of the twentieth century with the flourishing of occupational epidemiology and the translation of 'more likely than not' into the principle of 'doubling of risk' (i.e. a relative risk [RR] of >2 or an attributable fraction in the exposed of more than 50%). Early in the history of the Workmen's Compensation in the UK, in 1906 the scheme was extended from accidents to include six diseases (as noted previously), sufficiently specific to occupation to be readily attributable. The principles for the extension of coverage to include other diseases as recommended by the Samuel Committee (1907) included that these be 'so specific to the employment that causation could be assumed in the individual case.' The Samuel Committee explained the difficulty of adding a disease that was common in the population by considering bronchitis in flax workers:

> Bronchitis, for example, is a trade disease among flax-workers; a larger proportion of that class suffer from it than of other people; but it is not specific to the employment, for numbers of people who are not flax-workers contract it also. Unless there is some symptom which differentiates the bronchitis due to dust from the ordinary type, it is clearly impracticable to include it as a subject of compensation; for no one can tell, in any individual case, whether the flax-worker with bronchitis was one of the hundreds of persons in the town whose bronchitis had no connection with dust irritation, or whether he was one of the additional tens or scores of persons whose illness was due to that cause. To ask a court of law to decide would be to lay upon it an impossible task. If the workman were required to prove his case, he might be able to show that a larger percentage of his trade suffer from bronchitis than do the rest of the population, but he could never show that he himself was a unit in the excess, and not in the normal part, of that percentage. If it were the employer who was required to disprove a claim, he could rarely, if ever, show that the workman did not contract the illness through his employment, and he would be compelled to compensate not only those labourers whose bronchitis had a trade origin, but also those whose bronchitis was in no degree an industrial disease (Samuel Committee, 1907).

Returning to this problem in 1948, after the introduction of the Industrial Injuries Act of 1946, the Dale Committee (1948) came to a more generous interpretation of the new act. They stated:

> We do not regard it essential to prescription that a disease be specific to employment, provided the

> employment causes a special exposure to the risk of the disease, such risk being inherent in the conditions of that employment. We recognise that this will appreciably enlarge the range of diseases which can be considered by enabling claims for prescription to be made in relation to diseases common to general population but alleged to result from the conditions in particular occupations (Dale Committee, 1948).

The extension of prescription to diseases that were common in the population was finally clarified in the UK in 1955, when a minority report of three dissenting members of the Beney Committee highlighted the failure to prescribe Raynaud's phenomenon as evidence of the difficulty of compensating diseases that were common in the population:

> The fundamental difficulty is the inadequate cover for diseases common among the general public which may also be due to special occupational risk, e.g. chronic bronchitis (including emphysema) and rheumatic diseases. We consider that these diseases should be eligible for prescription and that the existing test requiring attribution of individual cases to the employment is a bar to their inclusion (Beney Committee, 1955).

They recommended that a disease could be added to the list of prescribed diseases where it was probable that more cases than not were occupational in origin, whether or not individual cases could be attributed to occupation. This principle has since informed the extension of coverage of diseases in the UK and allowed inclusion of diseases such as lung cancer and COPD, both of which being common in the population and, in these cases, primarily attributable to another cause: cigarette smoking.

BURDEN OF PROOF

In principle, diseases can be compensated either on the basis of 'individual proof' – the individual has to provide evidence to demonstrate attribution in his or her case (this is the position of the claimant in civil claims in the UK, where to succeed there is also the need to demonstrate negligence or breach of statutory duty) – or from a list of 'prescribed' diseases, where the evidence of causation in well-defined circumstances is sufficient to allow claimants the benefit of presumption (e.g. in the UK, causation can be presumed in, say, an individual with a diagnosed disease [lung cancer] who has been exposed to asbestos in an asbestos textile factory for more than 5 years before, or 10 years after, 1975). In practice, a combination of individual proof and a list of scheduled diseases (prescribed list in the UK) that are recognised for compensation is found in different schemes in Europe; in the USA, there is no scheduled list of diseases.

A system of listing 'prescribed' diseases provides the great advantage to the claimant that if he or she fulfils the criteria for both the disease (e.g. COPD) and occupational exposure (e.g. work underground in a coalmine for 20 years), then they are eligible for compensation without the need for medical or legal evidence. This has allowed the UK scheme to be efficient, providing claimants with more than 90% of the costs of the scheme (as opposed to personal injury claims, where claimants obtain on the average between 40% and 60% of awards), timely (decisions usually within months, not years) and more certain than the courts in their outcome. A major criticism of the system of prescription in the UK has been the length of time between the reporting of an association between a disease and occupational exposure and disease prescription. In part, this delay from initial recognition to prescription reflects the need to ensure that the evidence of association is likely to be causal and is consistent between different studies, making it unlikely that a legislative decision to prescription will need to be reversed. Unsurprisingly, such delays have been longer where the cause is non-specific (e.g. asbestos and lung cancer) than specific (e.g. asbestos and mesothelioma [vide infra]).

In all European countries including the UK, diseases are at least in part compensated through a list of scheduled diseases. There is also a European Community list but, as yet, there is no harmony between countries in adopting this list. Individual countries vary in which diseases are listed and how comprehensive is the list. Finland has an indicative list, but this is not considered exclusive, enabling individual proof in addition to the listed conditions. In Sweden, only infectious diseases are listed, with eligibility for other conditions open and based on individual proof. The UK and France are more prescriptive, generally only compensating listed diseases, although in the UK, individual proof is allowed for some conditions, such as for occupational asthma due to an identifiable cause not on the list of prescribed causes.

Eligibility of the self-employed for compensation varies between countries. Social insurance schemes, which are common in Europe, are in general more open to inclusion of the self-employed, with eligibility based on payment of insurance premiums. The UK scheme only applies to 'employed earners' and excludes the self-employed. In the USA, the self-employed are also not covered by workers' compensation.

The majority of schemes in mainland Europe are social insurance schemes with mandated funding from employers, based on the scheme introduced by Bismarck in 1884. However, increasing costs, particularly in relation to asbestos, have led several countries to supplement social insurance with government funding. In contrast to the UK, the intention of the majority of these schemes is to replace lost earnings, at least in part, because of incapacity to work, although several European schemes have also been extended to include prevention and rehabilitation. This is most developed in Germany, where employers' liability insurance constitutes an important element in the regulatory system, as well as taking a lead in prevention and rehabilitation. A 'first principle' of the German scheme is 'rehabilitation before pension', with the purpose of reintegration into the workforce to the extent that the individual's disability allows.

INDUSTRIAL INJURIES COMPENSATION IN THE UK

The current scheme for accidents at work and diseases caused by work in the UK is the Industrial Injuries Disablement Benefit Scheme (IIDB). The IIDB is a no-fault compensation scheme, funded by government out of taxation, for employed earners, which provides benefits to those disabled by accidents arising out of or in the course of employment, or one or more of a list of 'prescribed' diseases (i.e. attributable to occupation on the balance of probability).

The 1946 Industrial Injuries Scheme provided two major benefits:

1. Industrial Injuries Disablement Benefit, payable for 'loss of faculty' ('in proportion to loss of health, strength and the power to enjoy life attributable to industrial accident or prescribed disease') for:
   a. Accidents 'arising out of and in the course of employment' (an accident has been defined as 'an unlooked for mishap or untoward event which is not expected or designed' [Lord Macnaghten in Fenton v Thorley, 1903])
   b. Prescribed diseases:
      i. Which are a recognised risk to workers in an occupation or exposed to a particular agent
      ii. Where the disease can be attributed to occupation or an agent at work on the balance of probabilities (i.e. more likely than not)

   In general, attribution of a disease to a specific cause can be based on:
      i. Specific clinical features
      ii. By inference from the results of population studies to causation in the individual patient

   In the absence of any specific characteristics to distinguish a case of disease that is attributable to an occupational cause from those that would have occurred in the absence of the occupational exposure, attribution in the individual case is based on an attributable fraction of more than 50% in the exposed workforce, and therefore a RR (or odds ratio) of greater than 2, when compared to a similar population that was not exposed, which equates to 'more likely than not'. Several prescribed diseases in the UK specify the level of exposure in the workplace where epidemiological evidence indicates that the level of risk of disease is more than doubled. Typically, the terms of prescription include the duration and, in some cases, era of exposure necessary to fulfil the criterion of doubling of risk. Examples of each of these include:

   COPD: work underground in an underground coalmine for 20 or more years (IIAC Bronchitis and Emphysema, 1988)

   Lung cancer: work in an asbestos textile factory for 5 years before and for more than 10 years after 1975 (IIAC Asbestos related disease, 2005)
2. The second important benefit introduced in the 1946 Act was Special Hardship Allowance (SHA), subsequently renamed Reduced Earnings Allowance (REA). SHA, later REA, provided an earnings replacement benefit in order to enable those with occupational disease, whose health would be adversely affected by remaining in their current job, to move to other less well-paid work. It provided the means to prevent disease progression to a severe and irreversible level of disability (e.g. enabling those with Category 2 simple coal workers' pneumoconiosis to move to dust-approved conditions, at lower pay, reducing the risk of progression to disabling complicated pneumoconiosis). REA was abolished by the Thatcher government in 1990.

The pattern of current payments for the IIDB and REA in the UK reflects the industrial history of the country during the second half of the twentieth century. Accidents are most likely to occur in manufacturing, construction and mining industries with 25% of

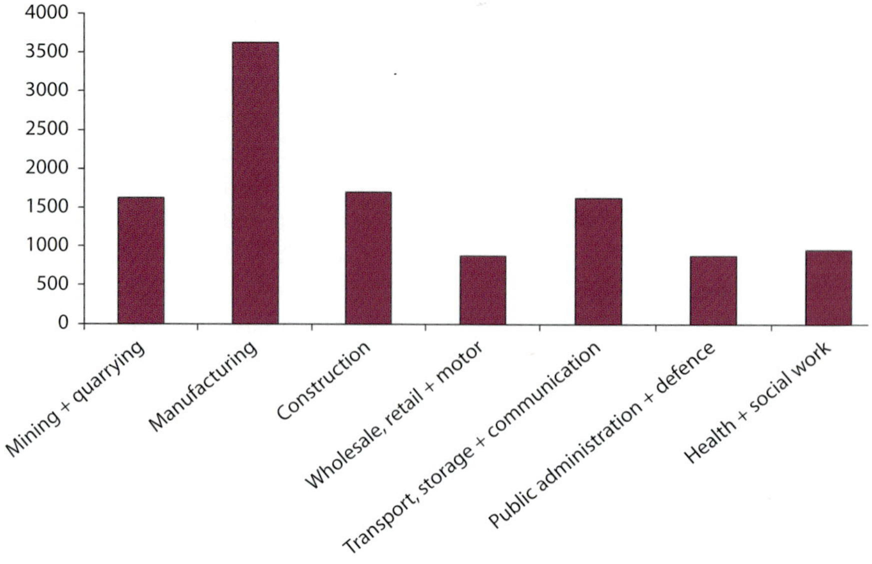

FIGURE 11.1 New Industrial Injuries Disablement Benefit Scheme and Reduced Earnings Allowance claims (>500) put into payment by industry. (From Industrial Injuries Disablement Benefit Scheme. 2007. *A Consultation Paper*. Department for Work and Pensions. London: HMSO.)

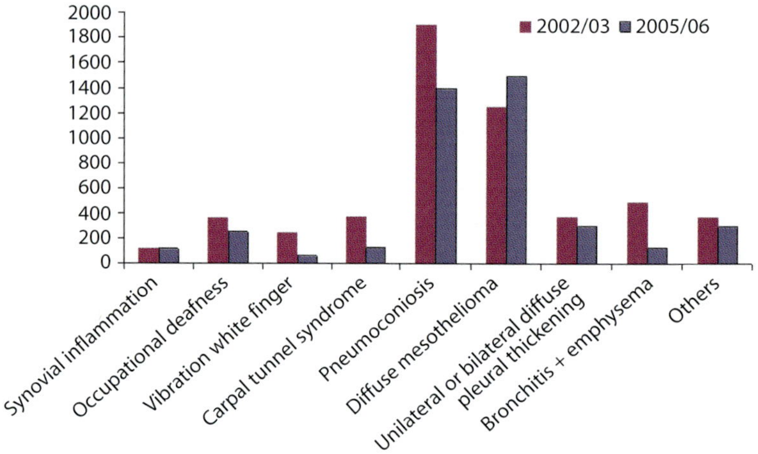

FIGURE 11.2 New prescribed disease claims put into payment by disease. (From Industrial Injuries Disablement Benefit Scheme. 2007. *A Consultation Paper*. Department for Work and Pensions. London: HMSO.)

major accidents occurring in manufacturing and some 15% in construction and in mining and quarrying. New benefit recipients for the IIDB and REA in industries with more than 500 claims in 2005/2006 are shown in Figure 11.1.

New claims for prescribed diseases are dominated by diseases associated with mining and asbestos. Some two-thirds of new benefit recipients for a prescribed disease are for pneumoconiosis or mesothelioma. The numbers of new claims for the most common prescribed diseases put into benefit in 2002/2003 and 2005/2006 are shown in Figure 11.2.

Although the incidence of pneumoconiosis is falling in the UK, the incidence of mesothelioma is increasing, and the long latency of both diseases makes it likely that they will continue to form a large proportion of the IIDB benefit recipients for many years.

THE EXAMPLE OF ASBESTOS COMPENSATION IN THE UK

Inclusion of a disease on the prescribed list follows the provision of sufficient evidence in the scientific literature to be confident of a causal association of sufficient magnitude. The history of asbestos compensation in the UK in relation to the development of scientific knowledge exemplifies this, particularly the considerably longer delays in prescription for non-specific as compared to specific diseases, which, at least in part, is because of the greater difficulty in being confident of cause and effect.

Asbestosis

Pulmonary fibrosis was first reported in the post-mortem report of an asbestos worker by Montague Murray (1899) in the UK The term 'asbestosis' was first used by Cooke (1927) reporting the case of Nellie Kershaw who died aged 33 years, having worked since the age of 13 years in asbestos factories. Increasing concerns regarding the risk of pulmonary fibrosis in asbestos workers led to a survey of the Turner and Newall factory in Rochdale, UK, by Merewether and Price (1930). They found that the prevalence of asbestosis, identified clinically, increased with increasing duration of exposure. Asbestosis was found in more than a quarter of the workforce of 363 examined and in 80% of those who had remained in employment for 20 or more years (Merewether and Price, 1930). As a consequence, in the same year, the coverage of silicosis in the Workmen's Compensation Act was extended to asbestosis. Silicosis had been included in 1918 after several years of debate in the scheme under the Workmen's Compensation (Silicosis) Act. This Act provided compensation for workmen (or their dependants) in certain specified occupations if they were certified to have been disabled by silicosis, or so disabled as to be unable to continue in their employment, or to have died from silicosis. The Act also provided for a system of regular examinations, with powers to suspend men with early signs of disease, without incapacity, in order to protect their future health. The Workmen's Compensation (Silicosis and Asbestosis) Act 1930 extended these provisions (i.e. compulsory employer liability insurance and regular medical examinations with powers of suspension) to those in certain specified occupations considered to be at particular risk of exposure to asbestos. Asbestosis continues to be compensated in the UK as a pneumoconiosis under the Industrial Injuries Act.

Mesothelioma

The association of mesothelioma with crocidolite (blue asbestos) was first described by Wagner et al. (1960). He reported 33 cases of which all but one had identifiable exposure to crocidolite in the North Western Cape Province of South Africa. The exposures identified included the mining and transport of crocidolite (ten cases), its use in insulation work (four cases) and neighbourhood exposure (18 cases). Subsequently, in the UK, cases of mesothelioma were found to cluster in areas of high asbestos usage, in shipyards (e.g. Barrow in Furness, Devonport dockyards, Belfast and Clydeside) and railway manufacture and repair (e.g. Swindon). General recognition of the causal association of the disease with asbestos is usually considered to have followed the 1964 New York Conference on the Biological Effects of Asbestos, where Selikoff (1964) described cases of mesothelioma in New Jersey insulation workers, and Newhouse and Thompson (1965) in those working and living in the vicinity of the Cape Asbestos factory in Barking, London, UK Mesothelioma was added to the list of prescribed diseases in 1968 in those exposed in their work to asbestos.

Lung Cancer

Whereas, because of the specificity, the relationships between pulmonary fibrosis and asbestos and between mesothelioma and asbestos are reasonably clear cut, this is not the case with lung cancer and asbestos. Interestingly, lung cancer in asbestos workers was prescribed as an occupational disease in Germany in 1943 during World War II. In the UK, Merewether in his report as HM Inspector of Factories in 1947, noted an excess mortality rate from lung cancer in cases of asbestosis (13.2%) as compared to cases of silicosis (1.2%). But the definitive evidence was only provided by Doll in his 1955 study of the mortality of employees of the Turner and Newall factory, all of whom had been employed before the 1931 Asbestos Regulations, which had followed the Merewether and Price report. Doll found 39 deaths, with 11 cases of lung cancer as compared to one expected (Doll, 1955). All of the cases of lung cancer occurred in men with asbestosis. In a later study of New Jersey insulators, Selikoff found the incidence of lung cancer to be some seven times the rate expected in a comparable US white male population (Selikoff et al., 1964). Subsequently an increased risk of lung cancer was also found in other populations exposed in their work to asbestos in the UK, e.g. insulation workers.

The risk of lung cancer in asbestos workers is further increased in those who also smoke. Hammond et al. (1979) reported a multiplicative interaction between asbestos and lung cancer in terms of increasing the risk of lung cancer: in a comparison to a non-smoking population not exposed to asbestos, smoking increased the risk by tenfold on average; exposure to asbestos increased the risk in non-smokers by fivefold and in smokers by 50-fold. The increased risk caused by asbestos exposure in smokers and non-smokers was therefore similar: a fivefold increase. Although there has been subsequent argument regarding the nature of the interaction, the important implication for compensation purposes is that the risk of lung cancer in workers with significant exposure to asbestos is more than doubled in both smokers and non-smokers. Smoking does not therefore need to be considered in relation to prescription.

The more contentious issue was whether the increased risk of lung cancer was limited to cases of asbestosis or whether lung cancer was an independent risk of asbestos exposure. Since 1957, lung cancer has been accepted by pneumoconiosis medical panels in the UK as a complication of asbestosis, enabling eligible dependants to claim death benefit. However, it was not until 1985 that lung cancer was prescribed in relation to asbestos exposure in those with asbestosis or diffuse pleural thickening. Subsequently, in 2006, lung cancer in the absence of asbestosis was prescribed for 'exposure to asbestos for at least 5 years before 1975 and 10 years after 1975 in: (i) workers in asbestos textile manufacture; (ii) asbestos sprayers; and (iii) asbestos insulation work, including those applying and removing asbestos-containing materials in shipbuilding.'

The striking difference in the lag period from robust scientific evidence to prescription, which were relatively short in the cases of asbestosis and mesothelioma and prolonged in the case of lung cancer, reflects the continuing problems compensation schemes in the UK (and elsewhere) face in dealing with diseases that are common in the population, such as lung cancer, as compared to diseases that are specific to occupational exposure, such as asbestosis and mesothelioma. In more recent years, such delays have been shortened. Obliterative bronchiolitis in those exposed in their work to diacetyl was prescribed in the same year as the first case was reported in the UK (Industrial Injuries Advisory Council, 2008).

Three additional pieces of UK legislation have been enacted in order to address perceived failures in common law in relation to asbestos compensation.

The Pneumoconiosis (Workmen's Compensation) Act 1979 is a state-funded scheme to provide lump sum payments to those who have developed pneumoconiosis, byssinosis, mesothelioma or lung cancer prescribed in relation to asbestos and bilateral diffuse pleural thickening for workers who are unable to recover compensation through the courts or through a private no-fault compensation scheme because their employer is no longer in business.

The Diffuse Mesothelioma Scheme (2008) provides no-fault compensation to those exposed to asbestos in the UK who are otherwise unable to obtain compensation. This includes those exposed to asbestos in the home from asbestos brought home on a worker's clothes, and the self-employed who are exposed to asbestos in their work.

The Mesothelioma Act (2014) provides substantial payments to those who develop mesothelioma and their dependants who are unable to trace an insurer for an employer who is responsible for the exposure to asbestos. The scheme is funded by a levy on insurance companies and provides a lump sum payment graded by the claimant's age. A similar scheme of lump sum compensation has since been extended to military veterans.

COMPENSATION SCHEMES IN CONTINENTAL EUROPE

Compensation schemes in continental Europe differ from the UK Industrial Injuries Scheme in a number of important ways. In general, in continental Europe, compensation for occupational injuries and disease is intended to provide at least partial earnings replacement and is part of a wider social insurance provision (Walters, 2007).

Funding has two basic models. The first, based on the German system, with self-governed sectoral associations funded by employers' contributions, provides a comprehensive system of prevention, rehabilitation and compensation. In the alternative system, also funded by contributions from employers, the state administers the scheme for compensation as part of a wider provision of social security.

Although the UK system differs in the rationale for compensation (loss of faculty and disablement, as opposed to earnings replacement) and being a standalone scheme rather than part of a comprehensive scheme that also includes prevention and rehabilitation, the UK and European schemes share important characteristics: the legacy of the industrial era is found in most systems, particularly the consequences of mining and manufacture. This is particularly the case in schemes based on lists of diseases, and in such schemes, successful claimants are likely to be predominantly male.

The different countries of Europe vary considerably in their systems of coverage for accidents and disease. In Belgium and Portugal, there are separate schemes for occupational accidents, based on private employers' insurance, with a state system for occupational diseases for industrial and commercial sector workers. In Denmark, private insurers carry the risk for occupational accidents, while occupational diseases are insured by specific funds financed by contributions from employers. In Norway and Finland, insurers carry the risk for both accidents and disease, although in Norway there is a state system and a private employers' insurance system that 'tops up' the state system. In some countries, the usual system of social insurance for incapacity resulting from occupational injury and disease, which is designed to replace lost earnings, is supplemented by additional schemes, usually resulting from agreements between trade unions, with employers to provide additional benefits for their members. In Sweden, higher pensions are available through the Labour Market Insurance scheme known as AFA Insurance.

As noted previously, all European countries have a scheduled list of compensatable diseases, although the role of the list in determining specific cases of compensation varies with different emphasis on a prescribed list in an open system of compensation. In the 'open system', each claim for an occupational disease is treated on its own merits; in Sweden, for example, the occupational disease list includes only infectious diseases, with all other conditions treated individually. At the other extreme, the French list of 112 occupational diseases appended to its Social Security Code specifies the symptoms or pathological lesions required to be present, the type of work that is known to cause the condition and the time limits for compensation claims. In theory, any disease meeting the medical, occupational and administrative criteria in the list is presumed to be occupational in origin. In other EU countries, the function of the 'list' falls somewhere between these extremes in decisions concerning the eligibility of conditions. A trend that is evident in many countries has been the increasing recourse to 'open' systems in recent years.

Whether the condition is on a list or identified individually as part of a mixed system, the process by which evidence is assessed and decisions taken as to its 'occupational' cause in most cases concerns two issues: the extent to which the disease can be ascribed to an occupational cause and the extent to which a claimant can show that they have experienced relevant exposures. The means by which the first of these issues is resolved in most countries, as in the UK, is defined in legislation or the guidance to it. Determining the recognition of occupational associations with the cause of conditions involves review of epidemiological and other scientific and medical evidence, and the achievement of broad expert agreement concerning increased risk in relation to occupational exposure. Practice in other European countries does not follow exactly the rule adopted in the UK, where decisions for prescription are based on robust epidemiological evidence of a greater than doubled risk of the disease in an exposed occupational group as compared to a comparable unexposed group or the general population. However, there are broad similarities in the approach in all countries in as far as there is emphasis on the need for robust evidence of occupational risk and agreement of expert opinion.

Current data on occupationally related ill health compared with the number of claims made for occupational disease and those claims actually 'recognised' (approved) suggest that only a minority of those whose health is affected by their work seek and are awarded compensation. Thus in any European system such claims rarely exceed 50% of the actual number of probable cases. Several explanations have been proposed for this. These include the limitations of the experience and ability of physicians to recognise occupational causes, ignorance of workers concerning both the hazards of their work and their entitlements to compensation, and the complexity of the administration of the system for compensation. It is also important to appreciate that not only does the complexity of making a claim exclude many, but the claim process itself may also have negative consequences for recovery and return to work. While one of the great virtues of 'no-fault' systems for compensation is that they act to eliminate adversarial approaches to claims, the use of experience ratings by some insurance systems destroys this advantage, since it provides a strong incentive for employers to contest claims. It is also argued that the growth in precarious employment in advanced market economies has eroded the coverage of workers' compensation systems, creating administrative difficulties, undermining the coverage and objectives of compulsory insurance and weakening processes for making claims. There can also be the difficulty of identifying the relevant exposures in long latency conditions.

As is the case in the UK, recognition of some of these problems means that reform of present systems is planned or called for in most countries. Generally, however, the main thrust of such reforms is to seek to address issues of affordability and efficiency, while at the same time dealing with perceived weaknesses in cover and redress of harm. It seems unlikely that these changes to existing systems will lead to greater access to benefits for potential claimants.

COMPENSATION SCHEMES IN THE USA

The coverage of compensation in the USA differs greatly among the various states, particularly with regards to coverage for disease. As noted earlier, unlike the UK or European model of a 'prescribed' list of diseases, the USA does not have a list of compensatable diseases. Any disease can be claimed, its attribution to work based on physicians' assessment, and argued by lawyers and adjudicated by workers' compensation arbitrators and judges. For several decades of the twentieth century, long-latency diseases were excluded in many states by the statute of limitations; in more recent times, the period of limitation has been determined as being from the time of diagnosis and of being informed that the disease was attributable to occupation.

The basic structures of workers' compensation in the USA and Canada are similar, although the basis of funding differs, being predominantly private insurance in the USA and governmental insurance in Canada. A board or commission sets the rules, an insurer provides coverage on the basis of the payroll for eligible workers and cases are adjudicated in the first instance by the insurer and subsequently, if contested, by an appeals system. Despite the original intention of avoiding litigation, legal advocacy remains part of the process, particularly in complicated or disputed appeals. Because of deadlines by which time an insurer must decide claims, many requests for compensation are initially rejected, forcing claimants to retain legal counsel and file lengthy appeals. The consequences for the worker may include uncompensated legal expenses and economic hardship.

Federal as opposed to state-based schemes in the USA include the Black Lung programme for coal miners, the Longshoremen and Harbour Workers' Compensation Program, the Federal Employees' Compensation Act, the Radiation Exposure Compensation Act and the Energy Employees Occupational Illness Compensation Program Act. In several instances, these federal programmes replace or are intended to complement state-based compensation programmes.

In the majority of states, compensation is limited to two-thirds of previous wages and coverage of medical costs. Funding of the schemes by employers, of whom the majority are insured, is intended to internalise the costs of work-related accidents and disease, providing an incentive to employers to ensure job safety and workforce health. However, risk pooling – the basis of insurance – blunts the financial consequences of accidents and diseases caused by work, diminishing the impact of such incentives.

All claims for compensation schemes that require adjudication are handled by state compensation boards. Insurers are entitled to dispute permanent disability claims. In any contested claim, the burden of proof is on the worker. This can cause considerable difficulty in substantiating the claim, particularly for conditions of long latency, where the relevant exposure occurred many years before.

Apart from federal schemes, workers' compensation varies from state to state. This is particularly the case for diseases. State schemes cover accidents without regard to fault unless self-inflicted or caused by self-intoxication. In most states, disease coverage was originally covered by schedules, which provided guidance for compensation boards and courts. However, the continuous need to update the schedules, as well as their being considered restrictive and inflexible, has led to their being generally abandoned.

Many states only compensate diseases that are 'peculiar to' or 'characteristic of' (i.e. specific to) occupation. This creates particular difficulty for conditions that have multiple causes and are of long latency, where it can be difficult to identify the particular workplace in which the relevant exposure occurred. This is especially true of respiratory diseases, such as lung cancer or COPD, which have a predominant non-occupational cause – cigarette smoking – as well as several well-recognised occupational causes, including asbestos for lung cancer and coal dust for COPD, which are compensated uncommonly in the USA This contrasts with mesothelioma caused by asbestos or chronic beryllium disease, which are more specific to occupation and therefore less contentious. Disputes often revolve around 'apportionment' when a worker has multiple causes of a disease, such as the estimated contribution of a worker's asbestos exposure and cigarette smoking to the development of lung cancer.

Workers' compensation in the USA is primarily a state responsibility that has developed in a more piecemeal manner than in the UK Its potential strengths lie in the incentives in the scheme to improve workplace health and safety through employers' insurance and rehabilitation from the responsibility for payment of medical costs. Coverage varies between the states.

COMPENSATION SCHEMES IN SOUTH AFRICA

South Africa has separate workers' compensation systems for mining and non-mining occupational lung diseases: the Occupational Diseases in Mines and Works Act and the Compensation for Occupational Injuries and Diseases Act. The reasons for the development of two systems are not well documented, but probably relate to the urgency of responding to the serious occupational lung disease epidemic in the mining industry in the late nineteenth and early twentieth centuries. Specific legislation was needed in order to provide financial support for miners who had lost earnings due to disease and disability, which resulted in the Miners' Phthisis Allowance Act of 1911 (Ehrlich, 2012). The Act covered only some lung diseases that were common in mining and was too limited to form the basis of a more general compensation statute for occupational injury and disease; this came into being in 1917 as the Workmen's Compensation Act. The mining-specific act could have been rescinded on promulgation of the general statute in

1917, but the two systems were retained. South Africa continues to have two systems, which is problematic in a number of ways. Very different benefits for the same disease are provided depending on the causative industry (Ehrlich, 2012). In general, miners are worse off financially. For example, only single lump sum payments are made in the mining system, but monthly life-long pensions are available to non-mining claimants when certified as greater than 30% impaired. Medical aid provisions are also much better for non-miners. Miners do, however, have some benefits that are not available to their non-mining colleagues: statutory biennial state-funded medical examinations and autopsy examinations are among these benefits. The autopsy examination may be unique, in that all miners who have performed risky work are entitled to a free post-mortem examination of their hearts and lungs. Listed occupational diseases found at autopsy are compensable, even if they did not contribute to the death of the miner, which is an unusual provision, as most jurisdictions stipulate that, in order to be covered, the occupational disease should have contributed to death. Inequity is not the only problem: not having a single workers' compensation act has resulted in uncertainties regarding coverage. It is not always clear, especially to submitting doctors, whether an enterprise is covered by the mining or non-mining legislation, and even whether a particular disease falls under the mining act or not. The advantages of a single system have been recognised for decades (Nieuwenhuizen Commission, 1981), but merging the two systems is not simple. There are financial considerations – the mining compensation fund may be underfunded and current mining houses are reluctant to make up a historical deficit – and miners would lose the not inconsiderable advantages of autopsies and biennial examinations. Despite these hurdles, unified compensation for occupational disease and injury is currently under serious discussion. The South African situation, although not unique, does illustrate the difficulties of bringing together long-standing systems with entrenched, but different, benefits.

COMPENSATION SCHEMES IN AUSTRALIA

Workers' compensation in Australia is the responsibility of the different states (or jurisdictions), each of which has its separate legislation and responsible agencies, in addition to a national Commonwealth Scheme. Each of the schemes is a 'no-fault' insurance-based scheme that provides benefits on the condition that the worker:

- Is an employee as defined in the law of their jurisdiction
- Has a medical condition that was diagnosed by a qualified practitioner who stated that the condition arose out of or in the course of employment
- Has suffered a financial loss, such as loss of income, or has incurred medical costs

The benefits payable under the schemes are for income replacement, the costs of medical treatment and death benefits, which include special provisions for children and income payments for dependents. In common with several European schemes, these also cover return-to-work plans, involving work-related rehabilitation and modification of workplaces and work duties.

Lump sum compensation is also paid for permanent impairment such as loss of a limb, loss of vision or hearing and pain and suffering.

Workers' compensation schemes for asbestos-related diseases vary between different Australian states and territories. There are also Commonwealth compensation schemes for asbestos-related disease due to service in the Australian Defence Force, Commonwealth employment or employment as seafarers.

ACKNOWLEDGEMENTS

I have been greatly helped in writing this chapter by review of my text and the provision of text by colleagues with knowledge of compensation schemes outside of the UK: Professor David Walters, whose review of European compensation schemes for the UK Industrial Injuries Advisory Council has been particularly informative; Professor Paul Blanc for his comments on compensation arrangements in the USA; and Professor David Rees for his text on compensation in South Africa.

REFERENCES

Beney Committee Report of the Departmental Committee appointed to review the Diseases Provisions of the National Insurance (Industrial Injuries) Act. 1955. Parliamentary Papers. Cmnd. 9548. London: HMSO.

Coggon, D. I. W. and Martyn, C. N. 2005. Time and chance: The stochastic nature of disease causation. *Lancet* 365:1434–7.

Cooke, W. E. 1927. Pulmonary asbestosis. *Br Med J* 2:1024–25.

Dale Committee Report of the Departmental Committee on Industrial Disease. 1948. Cmd. 7557. London: HMSO.

Doll, R. 1955. Mortality from lung cancer in asbestos workers. *Br J Ind Med* 12(2):81–6.

Doll, R. and Bradford Hill, A. 1964. Mortality in relation to smoking. Ten years observation of British doctors. *Br Med J* 1:1399–410.

Ehrlich, R. 2012. A century of miners' compensation in South Africa. *Am J Ind Med* 55:560–9.

Fenton v Thorley. 1903. AC 443 at 448.

Hammond, E. C., Selikoff, I. J. and Seidman, H. 1979. Asbestos exposure, cigarette smoking and death rates. *Ann NY Acad Sci* 330:473–90.

Industrial Injuries Advisory Council. 1988. *Bronchitis and Emphysema*. Cd. 379. London: HMSO.

Industrial Injuries Advisory Council. 2005. *Asbestos Related disease*. Cd. 6553. London: HMSO.

Industrial Injuries Advisory Council. 2008. *Bronchiolitis Obliterans and Food Flavouring Agents*. Cd. 7439. London: HMSO.

Industrial Injuries Disablement Benefit Scheme. 2007. *A Consultation Paper*. Department for Work and Pensions. London: HMSO.

Merewether, E. R. A. 1947. *Chief Inspector of Factories*. Annual Report of the Chief Inspector of Factories for 83-5 Parliamentary Papers 1948–9. Cd. 7621. London: HMSO.

Merewether, E. R. A. and Price, C. W. 1930. *Report on Effects of Asbestos Dust on the Lungs and Dust Suppression in the Asbestos Industry*. London: HMSO.

Miller v Minister of Pensions. 1947. 2 All. E.R. 372 at 374 KBD.

Murray, M. 1899. *Departmental Commission on Compensation for Industrial Disease*. Cd. 3495 p.14. Cd. 3496 p.127. London: HMSO.

Newhouse, M. L. and Thompson, H. 1965. Mesothelioma of pleura and peritoneum following exposure to asbestos in the London area. *Br J Ind Med* 22:261–9.

Nieuwenhuizen Commission. 1981. *The Commission of Inquiry into the Compensation for Occupational Diseases in South Africa*. Pretoria: Department of Mineral and Energy Affairs, Government Printer.

Samuel Committee. 1907. *Report of the Departmental Committee on Compensation for Industrial Diseases*. Cd. 3495. London: HMSO.

Selikoff, I. J., Cherg, J. and Hammond, E. C. 1964. Asbestos exposure and neoplasia. *JAMA* 6:142–6.

Wagner, J. C., Sleggs, C. A. and Marchand, P. 1960. Diffuse pleural mesothelioma and asbestos exposure in the North Western Cape Province. *Br J Ind Med* 17:260–71.

Walters, D. 2007. *An International Comparison of Occupational Disease and Injury Compensation Schemes*. A Research Report prepared for the Industrial Injuries Advisory Council (IIAC).

12 Principles of Prevention and Control

Dick Heederik and Remko Houba

CONTENTS

INTRODUCTION

Occupational respiratory diseases are in principle preventable. Prevention can be defined as actions that converge on changeable factors to improve the health of individuals and communities, and are aimed at eradicating, eliminating or minimizing the impact of disease or disability. Primary, secondary and tertiary preventions are distinguished: primary prevention aims to reduce the incidence of disease (public health); secondary prevention aims to reduce the prevalence of disease by shortening its duration and progression (preventative medicine); tertiary prevention aims to reduce the numbers and/or impacts of complications of disease (rehabilitation). Some also distinguish 'primordial' prevention as actions that inhibit the emergence and establishment of environmental, economic, social and behavioural conditions, cultural patterns of living, etc., known to increase the risk of disease (health promotion).

This chapter focuses on primary prevention in the work environment in relation to respiratory disease. Primary prevention has many different elements, including assessing the nature and extent of a hazard, introducing and maintaining effective control measures and increasing awareness among workers and employees. Epidemiology is often seen as the science of public health. Thus, in the work environment, occupational epidemiology plays a crucial role in assessing health hazards, controlling the adverse health impacts of hazardous exposures and evaluating the effects of changes in exposure. However, other disciplines are equally important; occupational hygiene and toxicology also contribute to understanding of the associations between exposure and disease and help to target exposure–disease associations and evaluate the effectiveness of control.

HISTORICAL CONTEXT

The modern beginnings of occupational medicine, public health and epidemiology lie in the era of the Industrial Revolution (see Chapter 1 for a broader historical overview) (Hunter, 1978). This led to major social and demographic changes over short periods of time, such as urbanization, overcrowding in old towns leading to environmental and public health problems and mass production. These changes resulted in occupational and environmental pollution (air and water pollution and refuse dumping) and regular outbreaks of infectious disease (typhus and cholera). Life in the new industrial society, with its crowded and polluted cities, required major adjustments of individuals and society, including in the first half of the nineteenth century the first public health and hygiene campaigns and, in the twentieth century, the emergence of analytical epidemiological studies. We now live in an era in which many of the basic industries have moved from developed countries to lower-income countries. With this change, large, heavily exposed occupational populations in basic industries have disappeared from most Western nations, but are present in countries that often cannot deal with the occupational and environmental health risks because of their inadequate infrastructures. Western economies have transformed into service economies in which development and production are separated and take place in different regions of the world. 'Old' exposures, such as silica exposure in mining and construction, are still present, and can even be higher because of uncontrolled mechanization, but no longer involve the large workforces from the past (Heederik and Sigsgaard, 2014). New technologies, for instance, nanotechnology and biotechnology, have led to the emergence of potential new health risks, but again, usually only for small and relatively defined worker populations. Allergic respiratory diseases such as allergic asthma and rhinitis, as well as the non-allergic forms of these respiratory diseases, resulting from exposure to irritants and toxins, have become more prominent (Heederik and Sigsgaard, 2014).

These major historical trends are directly relevant to prevention. Prevention in the work environment takes place in a complex social and political environment in which employers, employees and the government have their own and partially shared responsibilities. The roles and responsibilities of these stakeholders have undergone great changes in recent years and are complicated by the emergence of large (and sometimes illegal) immigrant workforces, workforces of temporary workers who work in one country and remain living in another and economic crises. This may result in situations in which costs and benefits are not balanced across stakeholder groups. As a result, it may be difficult to convince stakeholders that reduction or elimination of exposures with harmful effects on health is effective for preventing the occurrence of disease.

SCREENING AND EVALUATING NEW CHEMICALS

Prevention of exposure can start with the introduction of new chemicals and the evaluation of their toxic properties. Procedures for pre-product screening have been established in the European Union since 2007 through the Registration, Evaluation, Authorization and Restriction of Chemicals (REACH) regulatory framework, which also influences legislation on the introduction of new chemicals in other continents. The key objective of REACH is to promote sustainable industrial development and reduce health risks associated with the use of chemicals by encouraging the substitution of chemicals and processes that have a negative impact on health and the environment. Although REACH is not primarily aimed at the work environment, it impacts workplaces because it determines the circumstances under which workers may handle chemicals. As part of REACH, derived no-effect levels (DNELs) and exposure scenarios for different processes have to be established and health risks evaluated for exposed workers. However, several large groups of agents that are particularly relevant to respiratory disease are exempt from the REACH process:

- Enzymes used for technical applications (e.g. in detergents, textiles, etc.) require registration, but those used in food and animal feed are exempt.
- Natural substances and bulk products such as latex and wheat and rye flour are also exempted.
- Many minerals are exempt as they are 'naturally occurring chemicals not chemically modified'.
- REACH also does not cover agents that have 'no owner (producer)'; for instance, allergens from plants or animals or process-generated or combustion products, such as diesel particulates.

As part of REACH, chemicals have to be tested through a range of toxicological approaches, including animal models, in order to assess the hazard potential (Kimber et al., 1999; Arts et al., 2008). A particular concern is hazard evaluation for the sensitizing potential of chemicals. This includes testing of dermal sensitization potential, usually by the local lymph node test, which tests the ability of topically applied chemicals to induce the proliferation of lymphocytes in draining nodes (Dearman et al., 1999; Arts et al., 2008). Cytokine fingerprinting in combination with the lymph node test may measure the sensitizing potential more specifically (Dearman and Kimber, 2001). There is no a priori reason to assume that the dermal route of administration of chemicals is critical to eliciting a sensitization response, and the presence of both antigen-presenting cells and lymphocytes is not confined to the skin (Cullinan et al., 2003). However, dose–response differences for sensitization appear to exist between the dermal and the respiratory routes of exposure (Arts et al., 2006, 2008). Chemicals with a positive response in lymph node tests are considered to be sensitizing agents regardless of their mode of contact, including through inhalation (Briatico-Vangosa et al., 1994). No animal models exist to test respiratory sensitization potential. The assumption that chemicals eliciting positive responses after dermal application in animals may also cause respiratory sensitization is debatable. Depending on the outcomes of routine toxicity testing, agents have to be labelled or can only be used under certain conditions (exposure scenarios).

For chemicals regulated under REACH, the emphasis is on hazard identification using animal tests. Employers also have to derive exposure standards for agents regulated under REACH. Exposure standards can be obtained when a no-effect level (DNEL in REACH terminology) or derived minimal-effect level can be calculated. The latter assumes a minimal acceptable risk, which is an established approach for carcinogens and theoretically also for allergens (see section "The Role of Exposure Standards in Respiratory Disease Management").

Some have attempted to predict the risks of chemicals based on their structure. A quantitative structure–activity relationship model for low-molecular-weight asthmagens had promising results, and was able to identify these agents with high sensitivity and specificity (Jarvis et al., 2015).

THE ROLE OF EXPOSURE STANDARDS IN RESPIRATORY DISEASE MANAGEMENT

Although the aim of prevention is the reduction of disease burden, the point of engagement is exposure reduction. Exposure standards define a level below which workers will not develop adverse health effects in an exposed population. An exposure standard compiles and translates, through risk assessment, the available information on the relationship between exposure and response. Thus, ideally, exposure standards are health based. Sometimes, a residual risk cannot be excluded (e.g. in the case of carcinogens); in these cases, the allowable or recommended exposure can be calculated as that which infers negligible risk or the lowest that is reasonably achievable. Thus, exposure standards are not always fully health based, but can be a compromise between health risks and the levels that are practically or economically achievable. For many agents with potential adverse respiratory effects, ranging from pneumoconiosis to cancer and asthma, exposure standards have been defined. Standard setting for workplace sensitizers has only been realized for a few allergens, and the methodology for this is still a matter of debate (Rijnkels et al., 2008).

In Europe, REACH regulations place responsibility for providing safety information, including DNELs, for chemicals and chemical products on 'industry' (i.e. manufacturers and importers). A comparison of industry-derived DNELs with governmental occupational exposure limits (OELs) derived by the Swedish authorities showed that industry DNELs varied widely and were generally higher (less protective); only five DNELs were equal to or lower than the Swedish OELs for the respective materials. The choice of key studies, dose descriptors and assessment factors all seemed to contribute to these discrepancies (Schenk et al., 2015). Elsewhere, legally enforceable standard setting is a governmental regulatory activity; an example is the Occupational Safety and Health Administration (OSHA) permissible exposure limits in the United States. Nonetheless, other governmental and non-governmental agencies may make non-binding recommendations, such as those made by the US National Institute for Occupational Safety and Health (NIOSH), which are generally more health protective than the OSHA's recommendations. Such inconsistencies underscore the critical role of healthcare professionals in the selection and application of exposure standards in primary prevention.

THE ROLE OF EXPOSURE ASSESSMENT IN PREVENTION

Because workers' exposure is the point of engagement for preventative strategies, exposure assessment is crucial. First, with measurement, the exposure level can be assessed and monitored and the measured level can be compared to known exposure standards. Such a comparison makes clear the extent to which exposure may need to be reduced. Second, how exposure occurs and which tasks or activities or production process-related factors are important for determining a worker's exposure.

Usually, exposure is measured as time-weighted exposure over a full work shift. For agents with chronic effects, such as those that cause pneumoconiosis or cancer, strategies based on full work shift measurements are adequate. There are indications that occupational allergic asthma and irritant asthma can be caused by relatively short exposure peaks; for instance, the result of process spills or short-term high-exposure activities (Nieuwenhuijsen et al., 1995; Meijster et al., 2008). However, peak exposures (expressed as the number of peaks above a certain exposure level over a work shift) are highly correlated to 8-hour exposure levels, indicating that assessing peak exposures is not necessary for exposure–response studies, but may provide additional information (Meijster et al., 2008) by revealing which tasks and activities are associated with health-relevant elevated exposures. Peak exposure can be assessed by short-term or so-called real-time measurements. For some gases and dusts, continuous measurement devices exist. An alternative to short-term measurements is statistical modelling of 8-hour measurement data (Basinas et al., 2014).

SIMPLE INTERVENTION STUDIES AND COMPLEX PRAGMATIC INTERVENTIONS

Despite the existence of exposure–response relationships for many respiratory hazards, including allergens, few clear-cut examples exist of the effect of exposure reduction on disease burden. Optimally, the effects of intervention strategies and individual intervention measures should be evaluated using randomized trials or cross-over designs, but there are very few examples of the application of these in the case of respiratory hazards. Some isolated examples exist for exposure to latex, wheat flour, wood dust and silica exposure (Heilman et al., 1996; Brosseau et al., 2002; Lazovich et al., 2002; Baatjies et al., 2010, 2014; Oude Hengel et al., 2014; van Deurssen et al., 2015a,b). The Minnesota wood dust study was one of the first randomized intervention studies in this area (Brosseau et al., 2002; Lazovich et al., 2002). In this study, businesses in the intervention group were given written recommendations, technical assistance and worker training in comparison with a control group that received written recommendations only. Changes from baseline in dust concentration, dust control methods and worker behaviour were compared between the intervention arms 1 year later. At follow-up, workers in intervention workshops relative to comparison workshops reported greater awareness, increases in stage of readiness and behavioural changes consistent with dust control. The median dust concentration change in the intervention arm from baseline to follow-up was not statistically different from the change in the comparison arm. This smaller-than-expected reduction in wood dust was attributed to the challenge of conducting rigorous intervention effectiveness research in occupational settings.

Some potential problems with intervention studies in occupational settings are clearly illustrated by a study in supermarkets in South Africa (Baatjies et al., 2010, 2014). This study aimed to assess the effects of the introduction of technical and organizational measures on flour dust exposure. Some of the interventions were introduced to the control arm of the study by managers who moved during the study from supermarkets where the intervention took place to other supermarket locations, thus distorting the intervention design unintentionally. Post hoc statistical analysis of the effects of some of the intervention measures across the intervention and control groups showed a very strong effect on exposure, with one example being the use of a lid on top of a flour mixing bowl.

Sometimes, technical measures function in the laboratory, but are considered impractical by workers and are not used or are sub-optimally used after a while. This requires surveys over longer periods of time that consider not only technical, but also organizational and contextual aspects.

An intervention study has been conducted in the construction industry with the aim of reducing silica dust exposure (Oude Hengel et al., 2014; van Deurssen et al., 2015a,b). The interventions included engineering, organizational and behavioural elements at both the organizational and individual levels; a strength of the study was that changes over time and compliance with the planned interventions were closely monitored. A substantial overall reduction in dust exposure was observed related to the intervention; concrete drillers in the intervention group, for instance, used more technical dust-reduction controls, particularly water suppression. However, sensitivity analyses indicated that the observed reduction in exposure was at least partially attributable to changes in work location and in the tasks performed, again illustrating the difficulties of performing well-controlled studies under practical circumstances.

In many situations, it is not possible to complete structured interventions because companies are heterogeneous with regards to industrial processes, and as a result, multidimensional (combinations of technical and organizational) changes are appropriate in different companies in order to realize certain exposure reductions. This approach is referred to 'pragmatic' intervention studies.

Most information on the effects of interventions on exposure or disease comes from observational studies, and many have explored the effects of work tasks, cleaning and protective procedures, quality of ventilation systems and work routines on exposure in many different settings (Burdorf et al., 1994; Scheeper et al., 1995; Hollund and Moen, 1998; Alwis et al., 1999; Bulat et al., 2004; Friesen et al., 2005; Meijster et al., 2007; Schlunssen et al., 2008). Most of these studies were cross-sectional, although exposure and determinants of exposure have been measured on the individual (worker) level. Several evaluations of longer-term time trends in exposure have been published that made use of large hygiene exposure databases, which sometimes have been collected over several decades (Kromhout and Vermeulen, 2000; Creely et al., 2006). Overall, downward trends in exposure were observed over long periods of time for most of the substances explored (Galea et al., 2009; van Tongeren et al., 2009). In many studies, information regarding changes in the working environment, such as process conditions, was lacking, but factors that were commonly mentioned as being responsible for exposure reductions included the introduction of new exposure standards, responses to regulatory requirements and changes in production methods (Creely et al., 2006). Over longer periods of time, industrial processes, job titles and the tasks performed within a job title change. An observational exposure study in the baking industry did explore the effects of changes in control measures over time (Meijster et al., 2009a) and found that changes in exposure over time varied substantially between sectors and jobs. A modest increase in the use of control measures and proper work practices was reported in most sectors, especially the use of local exhaust ventilation and a decrease in the use of compressed air.

LONG-TERM TRENDS IN EXPOSURE AND DISEASE IN RELATION TO INTERVENTIONS

Most information regarding the effects of interventions and changes in industrial processes comes from longer-term studies in which trends in disease burden have been observed. However, these studies collected information on an aggregate level (industry and country) and, as a result, trends cannot be associated with specific intervention measures. As a result, relatively little is known about the effectiveness and efficacy of many possible exposure-reduction measures. A clear example involves the time trends for occupational respiratory diseases such as allergy or asthma cases from disease registry data on a national level (Creely et al., 2006). Time trends in disease occurrence from sentinel registries have the limitation that the number of cases might be accurate, but the denominator—the population at risk from which the cases arise—is not well defined and may actually change over longer periods of time. Thus, the case burden may reduce, as measured by the registry, but the actual risk for a worker might not have been reduced, despite reductions in exposure. This can be explained because the initial exposure is high and exposure reductions, although measurable, are not sufficient to lead to significant reductions in risk.

The evidence regarding the effects of exposure reduction to allergens on exposure and disease burden has recently been extensively evaluated in the form of an evidence-based approach by the European Respiratory Society (Baur et al., 2012a,b; Heederik et al., 2012). The most convincing example of the effects of intervention measures is probably that of exposure to latex allergens. Several studies explored differences in exposure levels between healthcare workers using powdered and non-powdered gloves; the most powerful study that showed that use of non-powdered gloves was associated with lower exposure was a longitudinal case cross-over intervention, which showed a tenfold reduction in aeroallergen exposure levels when non-powdered gloves were used (Heilman et al., 1996). A review of the literature in 2006 evaluated the effect of this single preventative measure on the prevalence or incidence of sensitisation and occupational asthma in eight primary prevention intervention studies published on natural rubber latex (NRL) exposure since 1990 (LaMontagne et al., 2006). All were observational studies and reported a decrease in sensitization rates, either in a cross-sectional analysis or in a longitudinal design (both prospective and retrospective) (Levy et al., 1999; Cadot et al., 2001; Liss and Tarlo, 2001; Saary et al., 2002; Jones et al., 2004). The review clearly indicated that substitution of powdered latex gloves with low-protein powder-free NRL gloves or latex-free gloves greatly reduced NRL aeroallergens, NRL sensitization and NRL-related asthma in healthcare workers. None of the studies fulfilled the strict criteria for high-quality intervention studies; these were observational studies without a randomized design and without a control group, but taken together, they support the conclusion that substitution of NRL greatly reduces NRL sensitization and the occurrence of NRL-related asthma.

In many other environments, studies have been undertaken with interventions that comprised a combination of different preventative dust control measures, as well as education and personal protective equipment, often in the context of surveillance programmes. Examples come from the baking industry (Smith, 2004), spray painters and other di-isocyanate-exposed workers (Tarlo et al., 1997, 2002), laboratory animal workers (Botham et al., 1987; Fisher et al., 1998) and the detergent industry (Juniper and Roberts, 1984; Cathcart et al., 1997; Schweigert et al., 2000). A recent study showed a clear exposure–response relationship in a plant that exclusively used encapsulated enzymes resulting in a high sensitization risk at higher exposure levels (Cullinan et al., 2000). Similarly, a study of a factory using liquid enzyme formulations also indicated that levels are still sufficiently high to cause respiratory health effects (van Rooy et al., 2009). Thus, as mentioned earlier, limitations of surveillance information should be acknowledged when interpreting longer-term trends.

PERSONAL PROTECTIVE EQUIPMENT

Eliminating or minimizing exposures at source or in the environment is considered more effective than using personal protective equipment (Weeks et al., 1991). The efficacy of respiratory personal protection requires an ongoing commitment by employers and employees to comply with a programme that includes selection, fit testing, cleaning, maintenance, storage of equipment and training, as well as medical monitoring of users. Respirators are best used as an interim measure while efforts to control exposures at source or in the environment are being implemented, when controls at these other levels are not possible or for special activities with exposures of an unexpected nature (e.g. process disturbances). Examples exist of comprehensive programmes that include the use of respirators in different industries or for different agents (Pisati et al., 1993; Fisher et al., 1998; Sjostedt et al., 1998; Sorgdrager et al., 1998; Petsonk et al., 2000; Vanhanen et al., 2000; Goodno and Stave, 2002; Fujita et al., 2007). These programmes likely contributed to disease prevention, although the contribution of respirators cannot be separated from the overall effect.

IS EXPOSURE REDUCTION FOR WORKERS WITH RESPIRATORY DISEASE USEFUL?

In most cases, exposure reduction is performed with the purpose of primary intervention for the entire population at risk. Another aim can be to reduce exposure for workers who have already developed disease in order to avoid further progression. As an example, the effect of exposure reduction as a management option in occupational asthma was systematically reviewed in comparison to complete avoidance of exposure (Vandenplas et al., 2011). This review suggested that, at a population level, a reduction of exposure was associated with a lower likelihood of improvement and recovery of asthma symptoms and a higher risk of worsening non-specific bronchial hyper-responsiveness compared with complete avoidance of exposure. However, tailor-made solutions may still be possible in individual situations. In The Netherlands, a branch-specific health surveillance system has been implemented in the baking industry based on a validated risk stratification approach (Meijer et al., 2010). As part of this system, workplace surveys are performed after the identification of newly allergic bakers; in many cases, the only option seems to be to leave the baking industry, but in individual cases, solutions are found within the bakery. The case outlined in Box 12.1 illustrates this principal.

BOX 12.1 CASE STUDY

A 53 year old baker with a working history of 35 years in that trade and an owner of his own bakery since the age of 18 developed occupational allergy to wheat flour with severe rhinoconjunctivitis, sometimes accompanied by chest symptoms. Bread production was mainly done by his two employees, but since he was also working in the bakery, he continued to have complaints due to background exposure; stopping his work would have serious socioeconomic consequences. A project was started in order to design an intervention in the bakery.

The following set of interventions was implemented, with the aim of creating a non-dusty area for pastry production. The owner could fully focus on pastry production without direct contact with wheat flour.

1. A new wall was built in the bread production area in order to isolate the flour-handling area.
2. Local exhaust ventilation was installed on dough mixers and at the workbench. As a result, there was negative pressure in the new area, preventing dust transport by air to the other areas.
3. A heater was replaced, as this device disturbed the airflow resulting from the negative pressure.
4. Storage of ingredients for bread and pastry production was separated (no cereal flours in the pastry area).
5. The transport route of wheat flour bags to the storage room was changed.
6. For scattering flour on workbenches, a non-dusty wheat flour product was introduced.
7. Working methods were slightly changed in order to prevent the transport of wheat flour out of the bread production area (leaving working jackets in the production area and cleaning equipment before transport to other areas).
8. Thorough cleaning of the bakery was performed after the construction (in order to remove all remaining wheat flour from the new non-dusty areas).

The total cost of the intervention was approximately €40,000. Fortunately, the owner had insurance that financed the interventions; the alternative would have been to stop working as a baker, which would have cost the insurance company substantially more.

The optimal intervention per individual may also depend on other factors, such as severity of the disease (more management options are available for less severe stages of disease) and age (more stringent measures might be necessary for young workers with a working life ahead as compared with workers who are close to retirement). Often, this type of intervention needs to be accompanied by regular medical check-ups.

LONG-LATENCY OCCUPATIONAL RESPIRATORY DISEASES: THE PREVENTION OF PROGRESSIVE MASSIVE FIBROSIS IN COAL WORKERS—A SUCCESSFUL PROGRAMME IN THE UK AND USA BASED ON CLEAR SCIENTIFIC EVIDENCE

In 1942, the UK Medical Research Council reported that an epidemic of progressive massive fibrosis (PMF) had followed the greatly increased levels of coal dust caused by large-scale mechanization in the 1930s in underground coal mines (Hart and Aslett, 1942).

PMF was the major cause of lung function loss and premature death in coal miners, with some 36,000 UK coal miners considered disabled by pneumoconiosis between 1931 and 1949 (Cochrane et al., 1951). The prevention of PMF was a major public health priority, which required understanding of its cause. At this time, there were three major aetiological hypotheses:

1. PMF was an atypical form of tuberculosis (TB) caused by an interaction of coal dust and *Mycobacterium tuberculosis*
2. PMF was a reaction to the silica content of coal dust
3. PMF was due to retained coal dust and a progression from simple coal workers' pneumoconiosis (CWP)

Cochrane investigated the first hypothesis in a study in south Wales. He showed that despite reductions of cases of 'open' TB in Rhondda Fach, through early identification and isolation in hospital of sputum-positive cases of TB, the incidence of PMF was no different from Aberdare, where no special measures had been taken to identify and isolate infectious TB cases (Cochrane et al., 1952).

Evidence that PMF in coal miners occurred independently of silica exposure came from a study of coal trimmers working on barges, who were exposed to coal dust not contaminated with silica. Evidence was found of simple CWP and PMF in the coal trimmers, excluding an effect of silica. Subsequently, in a study of miners and ex-miners in the Rhonnda Fach and Aberdare valleys, Cochrane showed that the most important determinant of PMF was the category of simple CWP—itself primarily determined by level of coal dust exposure—rising from 0% at Category 1% to 30% at Category 3, with an intermediate level at Category 2 (Cochrane, 1962).

Cochrane recognized that his studies of pneumoconiosis in coal workers was limited by the lack of direct exposure measurements; he had to rely on the category of simple pneumoconiosis as a surrogate for cumulative exposure. In 1952, the UK National Coal Board established the Pneumoconiosis Field Research (PFR) programme in order to investigate the relationship between pneumoconiosis and coal dust exposure in British mines. Jacobsen and his colleagues subsequently reported the results of 15 years of research of the PFR programme (Jacobsen et al., 1971). They found that the most important determinant of CWP was the level of inhaled respirable coal dust. Their exposure–response model predicted zero probability that a coal miner would develop Category 2 or greater simple CWP after 35 years of exposure to a level of 2 mg/m^3, and a 3.4% risk at a concentration of 4.3 mg/m^3. They had convincingly shown that control of CWP lay primarily in the reduction of levels of airborne respirable coal mine dust. On the basis of these results, the USA designated 2 mg/m^3 as the exposure limit over a full shift in US coal mines and the UK designated 4.3 mg/m^3 as the dust exposure limit for underground coal mines.

In the UK, regular chest radiographs of underground coal miners were instituted in parallel with the exposure limit of 4.3 mg/m^3. Those who developed Category 2 simple pneumoconiosis were relocated from the coal face to 'dust-approved conditions' in order to minimize the risk of progression to PMF. The loss of pay consequent on not working at the coal face was compensated by means of 'Special Hardship Allowance', a benefit under the UK Industrial Injuries Disablement Scheme.

These exposure limits with regular radiographic surveillance succeeded in dramatically reducing the prevalence of simple CWP and of PMF in the UK.

FUTURE DEVELOPMENTS

Often examples can be found of expert systems that can be of use in prevention. Some generic expert systems can also be used to generate and compare different control scenarios, although the precision of the exposure estimates is limited (Marquart et al., 2008; Schinkel et al., 2011). Potentially, they facilitate the rapid evaluation of the work environment, especially in small- and medium-sized enterprises where few resources are available and major budgetary constraints exist. When exposure data are available and an association between exposure and determinants has been established, the exposure can be predicted on the basis of the presence or absence of these determinants in specific workplaces. An example exists for welding fumes, with a validated web-based tool based on more than 1500 exposure measurements (Huizer et al., 2007). Other tools exist that do not estimate exposure, but support selection of exposure control options, such as control of substances hazardous to health (COSHH) Essentials from the UK (http://www.hse.gov.uk/coshh/essentials/index.htm). When sector-wide prevention strategies are being implemented, the effects of different exposure reduction scenarios on the burden of disease can be evaluated using health impact assessment models. Very few examples exist, but some have been published for the baking industry (Meijster et al., 2009b, 2011b; Warren et al., 2009) and isocyanate exposure (Wild et al., 2005). These models can be extended with cost–benefit analyses in order to support decision making (Wild et al., 2005; Meijster et al., 2011a).

REFERENCES

Alwis, U., Mandryk, J., Hocking, A. D., Lee, J., Mayhew, T. and Baker, W. 1999. Dust exposures in the wood processing industry. *Am Ind Hyg Assoc J* 60:641–6.

Arts, J. H., De Jong, W. H., van Triel, J. J., Schijf, M. A., De Klerk, A., van Loveren, H. and Kuper, C. F. 2008. The respiratory local lymph node assay as a tool to study respiratory sensitizers. *Toxicol Sci* 106:423–34.

Arts, J. H., Mommers, C. and de Heer, C. 2006. Dose–response relationships and threshold levels in skin and respiratory allergy. *Crit Rev.Toxicol* 36:219–51.

Baatjies, R., Meijster, T., Heederik, D., Sander, I. and Jeebhay, M. F. 2014. Effectiveness of interventions to reduce flour dust exposures in supermarket bakeries in South Africa. *Occup Environ Med* 71:811–8.

Baatjies, R., Meijster, T., Lopata, A., Sander, I., Raulf-Heimsoth, M., Heederik, D. and Jeebhay, M. 2010. Exposure to flour dust in South African supermarket bakeries: Modeling of baseline measurements of an intervention study. *Ann Occup Hyg* 54:309–18.

Basinas, I., Sigsgaard, T., Erlandsen, M., Andersen, N. T., Takai, H., Heederik, D., Omland, O. et al. 2014. Exposure-affecting factors of dairy farmers' exposure to inhalable dust and endotoxin. *Ann Occup Hyg* 58:707–23.

Baur, X., Aasen, T. B., Burge, P. S., Heederik, D., Henneberger, P. K., Maestrelli, P., Schlunssen, V. et al. 2012a. The management of work-related asthma guidelines: A broader perspective. *Eur Respir Rev* 21:125–39.

Baur, X., Sigsgaard, T., Aasen, T. B., Burge, P. S., Heederik, D., Henneberger, P., Maestrelli, P. et al. 2012b. Guidelines for the management of work-related asthma. *Eur Respir J* 39:529–45.

Botham, P. A., Davies, G. E. and Teasdale, E. L. 1987. Allergy to laboratory animals: A prospective study of its incidence and of the influence of atopy on its development. *Br J Ind Med* 44:627–32.

Briatico-Vangosa, G., Braun, C. L., Cookman, G., Hofmann, T., Kimber, I., Loveless, S. E., Morrow, T. et al. 1994. Respiratory allergy: Hazard identification and risk assessment. *Fundam Appl Toxicol* 23:145–58.

Brosseau, L. M., Parker, D. L., Lazovich, D., Milton, T. and Dugan, S. 2002. Designing intervention effectiveness studies for occupational health and safety: The Minnesota Wood Dust Study. *Am J Ind Med* 41:54–61.

Bulat, P., Myny, K., Braeckman, L., van Sprundel, M., Kusters, E., Doekes, G., Possel, K. et al. 2004. Exposure to inhalable dust, wheat flour and alpha-amylase allergens in industrial and traditional bakeries. *Ann Occup Hyg* 48:57–63.

Burdorf, A., Lillienberg, L. and Brisman, J. 1994. Characterization of exposure to inhalable flour dust in Swedish bakeries. *Ann Occup Hyg* 38:67–78.

Cadot, P., Tits, G., Bussels, L. and Ceuppens, J. L. 2001. Asthma and hand dermatitis to leek. *Allergy* 56:192–3.

Cathcart, M., Nicholson, P., Roberts, D., Bazley, M., Juniper, C., Murray, P. and Randell, M. 1997. Enzyme exposure, smoking and lung function in employees in the detergent industry over 20 years. Medical Subcommittee of the UK Soap and Detergent Industry Association. *Occup Med (Lond)* 47:473–8.

Creely, C., Tongeren, M. V., While, D., Soutar, A. J., Tickner, J., Agostini, M., Vocht, F. D. et al. 2006. *Trends in Inhalation Exposure: Mid 1980s Sill Present.* Norwich: Health Safety Executive.

Cochrane, A. L. 1962. The attack rate of progressive massive fibrosis. *Br J Ind Med* 19:52–64.

Cochrane, A. L, Cox, J. G. and Jarman, T. F. 1952. Pulmonary tuberculosis in the Rhonnda Fach. *BMJ* 2:843–53.

Cochrane, A. L., Fletcher, C. M., Gilson, J. C. and Hugh Jones, P. 1951. The role of the periodic examination in the prevention of coal workers pneumoconiosis. *Br J Ind Med* 8:53–61.

Cullinan, P., Harris, J. M., Newman Taylor, A. J., Hole, A. M., Jones, M., Barnes, F. and Jolliffe, G. 2000. An outbreak of asthma in a modern detergent factory. *Lancet* 356:1899–900.

Cullinan, P., Tarlo, S. and Nemery, B. 2003. The prevention of occupational asthma. *Eur Respir J* 22:853–60.

Dearman, R. J., Basketter, D. A. and Kimber, I. 1999. Local lymph node assay: Use in hazard and risk assessment. *J Appl Toxicol* 19:299–306.

Dearman, R. J. and Kimber, I. 2001. Cytokine fingerprinting and hazard assessment of chemical respiratory allergy. *J Appl Toxicol* 21:153–63.

Fisher, R., Saunders, W. B., Murray, S. J. and Stave, G. M. 1998. Prevention of laboratory animal allergy. *J Occup Environ Med* 40:609–13.

Friesen, M. C., Davies, H. W., Teschke, K., Marion, S. and Demers, P. A. 2005. Predicting historical dust and wood dust exposure in sawmills: Model development and validation. *J Occup Environ Hyg* 2:650–8.

Fujita, H., Sawada, Y., Ogawa, M. and Endo, Y. 2007. [Health hazards from exposure to ortho-phthalaldehyde, a disinfectant for endoscopes, and preventive measures for health care workers]. *Sangyo Eiseigaku Zasshi* 49:1–8.

Galea, K. S., van Tongeren, M., Sleeuwenhoek, A. J., While, D., Graham, M., Bolton, A., Kromhout, H. et al. 2009. Trends in wood dust inhalation exposure in the UK, 1985–2005. *Ann Occup Hyg* 53:657–67.

Goodno, L. E. and Stave, G. M. 2002. Primary and secondary allergies to laboratory animals. *J Occup Environ Med* 44:1143–52.

Hart P. d'.A. and Aslett A. E. 1942. *Special Report Series No 243*. London: Medical Research Council.

Heederik, D., Henneberger, P. K. and Redlich, C. A. 2012. Primary prevention: Exposure reduction, skin exposure and respiratory protection. *Eur Respir Rev* 21:112–24.

Heederik, D. and Sigsgaard, T. 2014. Work-related respiratory diseases in the European Union. In I. Annesi-Maesano, B. Lundbackand and G. Viegi (eds), *Respiratory Epidemiology*. Sheffield: European Respiratory Society. ERS Monograph. 211–222.

Heilman, D. K., Jones, R. T., Swanson, M. C. and Yunginger, J. W. 1996. A prospective, controlled study showing that rubber gloves are the major contributor to latex aeroallergen levels in the operating room. *J Allergy Clin Immunol* 98:325–30.

Hollund, B. E. and Moen, B. E. 1998. Chemical exposure in hairdresser salons: Effect of local exhaust ventilation. *Ann Occup Hyg* 42:277–82.

Huizer, D., Noy, D., Houba, R. and Kromhout, H. 2007. Development of a welding fume assistant. *TTA* 3–4:23–7.

Hunter, D. 1978. *The Diseases of Occupations*, sixth edition. Sevenoaks: Hodder and Stoughton Ltd.

Jacobsen, M., Rae, S., Walton, W. H. and Rogan, J. H. 1971. The relation between pneumoconiosis and coal dust exposure in British coal mines. In W. H. Walton (ed.), *Inhaled Particles 3*, Vol. 2. Woking, UK: Unwin Bros, 903–16.

Jarvis, J., Seed, M. J., Stocks, S. J. and Agius, R. M. 2015. A refined QSAR model for prediction of chemical asthma hazard. *Occup Med (Lond)* 65:659–66.

Jones, K. P., Rolf, S., Stingl, C., Edmunds, D. and Davies, B. H. 2004. Longitudinal study of sensitization to natural rubber latex among dental school students using powder-free gloves. *Ann Occup Hyg* 48:455–7.

Juniper, C. P. and Roberts, D. M. 1984. Enzyme asthma: Fourteen years' clinical experience of a recently prescribed disease. *J Soc Occup Med* 34:127–32.

Kimber, I., Kerkvliet, N. I., Taylor, S. L., Astwood, J. D., Sarlo, K. and Dearman, R. J. 1999. Toxicology of protein allergenicity: Prediction and characterization. *Toxicol Sci* 48:157–62.

Kromhout, H. and Vermeulen, R. 2000. Long-term trends in occupational exposure: Are they real? What causes them? What shall we do with them? *Ann Occup Hyg* 44:325–7.

Lamontagne, A. D., Radi, S., Elder, D. S., Abramson, M. J. and Sim, M. 2006. Primary prevention of latex related sensitisation and occupational asthma: A systematic review. *Occup Environ Med* 63:359–64.

Lazovich, D., Parker, D. L., Brosseau, L. M., Milton, F. T., Dugan, S. K., Pan, W. and Hock, L. 2002. Effectiveness of a worksite intervention to reduce an occupational exposure: The Minnesota Wood Dust Study. *Am J Public Health* 92:1498–505.

Levy, D., Allouache, S., Chabane, M. H., Leynadier, F. and Burney, P. 1999. Powder-free protein-poor natural rubber latex gloves and latex sensitization. *JAMA* 281:988.

Liss, G. M. and Tarlo, S. M. 2001. Natural rubber latex-related occupational asthma: Association with interventions and glove changes over time. *Am J Ind Med* 40:347–53.

Marquart, H., Heussen, H., Le Feber, M., Noy, D., Tielemans, E., Schinkel, J., West, J. et al. 2008. 'Stoffenmanager', a web-based control banding tool using an exposure process model. *Ann Occup Hyg* 52:429–41.

Meijer, E., Suarthana, E., Rooijackers, J., Grobbee, D. E., Jacobs, J. H., Meijster, T., DE Monchy, J. G. et al. 2010. Application of a prediction model for work-related sensitisation in bakery workers. *Eur Respir J* 36:735–42.

Meijster, T., Tielemans, E., De Pater, N. and Heederik, D. 2007. Modelling exposure in flour processing sectors in The Netherlands: A baseline measurement in the context of an intervention program. *Ann Occup Hyg* 51:293–304.

Meijster, T., Tielemans, E. and Heederik, D. 2009a. Effect of an intervention aimed at reducing the risk of allergic respiratory disease in bakers: Change in flour dust and fungal alpha-amylase levels. *Occup Environ Med* 66:543–9.

Meijster, T., Tielemans, E., Schinkel, J. and Heederik, D. 2008. Evaluation of peak exposures in the Dutch flour processing industry: Implications for intervention strategies. *Ann Occup Hyg* 52:587–96.

Meijster, T., van Duuren-Stuurman, B., Heederik, D., Houba, R., Koningsveld, E., Warren, N. and Tielemans, E. 2011a. Cost–benefit analysis in occupational health: A comparison of intervention scenarios for occupational asthma and rhinitis among bakery workers. *Occup Environ Med* 68:739–45.

Meijster, T., Warren, N., Heederik, D. and Tielemans, E. 2009b. Application of a dynamic population-based model for evaluation of exposure reduction strategies in the baking industry. *J Phys Conf Ser* 151:012001.

Meijster, T., Warren, N., Heederik, D. and Tielemans, E. 2011b. What is the best strategy to reduce the burden of occupational asthma and allergy in bakers? *Occup Environ Med* 68:176–82.

Nieuwenhuijsen, M. J., Sandiford, C. P., Lowson, D., Tee, R. D., Venables, K. M. and Newman Taylor, A. J. 1995. Peak exposure concentrations of dust and flour aeroallergen in flour mills and bakeries. *Ann Occup Hyg* 39:193–201.

Oude Hengel, K. M., van Deurssen, E., Meijster, T., Tielemans, E., Heederik, D. and Pronk, A. 2014. 'Relieved Working' study: Systematic development and design of an intervention to decrease occupational quartz exposure at construction worksites. *BMC Public Health* 14:760.

Petsonk, E. L., Wang, M. L., Lewis, D. M., Siegel, P. D. and Husberg, B. J. 2000. Asthma-like symptoms in wood product plant workers exposed to methylene diphenyl diisocyanate. *Chest* 118:1183–93.

Pisati, G., Baruffini, A. and Zedda, S. 1993. Toluene diisocyanate induced asthma: Outcome according to persistence or cessation of exposure. *Br J Ind Med* 50:60–4.

Rijnkels, J. M., Smid, T., van den Aker, E. C., Burdorf, A., van Wijk, R. G., Heederik, D. J., Houben, G. F. et al. 2008. Prevention of work-related airway allergies; summary of the advice from the Health Council of The Netherlands. *Allergy* 63:1593–6.

Saary, M. J., Kanani, A., Alghadeer, H., Holness, D. L. and Tarlo, S. M. 2002. Changes in rates of natural rubber latex sensitivity among dental school students and staff members after changes in latex gloves. *J Allergy Clin Immunol* 109:131–5.

Scheeper, B., Kromhout, H. and Boleij, J. S. 1995. Wood-dust exposure during wood-working processes. *Ann Occup Hyg* 39:141–54.

Schenk, L., Deng, U. and Johanson, G. 2015. Derived no-effect levels (DNELs) under the European chemicals regulation REACH—An analysis of long-term inhalation worker-DNELs presented by industry. *Ann Occup Hyg* 59:416–38.

Schinkel, J., Warren, N., Fransman, W., van Tongeren, M., McDonnell, P., Voogd, E., Cherrie, J. W. et al. 2011. Advanced REACH Tool (ART): Calibration of the mechanistic model. *J Environ Monit* 13:1374–82.

Schlunssen, V., Jacobsen, G., Erlandsen, M., Mikkelsen, A. B., Schaumburg, I. and Sigsgaard, T. 2008. Determinants of wood dust exposure in the Danish furniture industry—Results from two cross-sectional studies 6 years apart. *Ann Occup Hyg* 52:227–38.

Schweigert, M. K., Mackenzie, D. P. and Sarlo, K. 2000. Occupational asthma and allergy associated with the use of enzymes in the detergent industry—A review of the epidemiology, toxicology and methods of prevention. *Clin Exp Allergy* 30:1511–8.

Sjostedt, L., Willers, S., Orbaek, P. and Wollmer, P. 1998. A seven-year follow-up study of lung function and methacholine responsiveness in sensitized and non-sensitized workers handling laboratory animals. *J Occup Environ Med* 40:118–24.

Smith, T. A. 2004. Preventing baker's asthma: An alternative strategy. *Occup Med (Lond)* 54:21–7.

Sorgdrager, B., de Looff, A. J., de Monchy, J. G., Pal, T. M., Dubois, A. E. and Rijcken, B. 1998. Occurrence of occupational asthma in aluminum potroom workers in relation to preventive measures. *Int Arch Occup Environ Health* 71:53–59.

Tarlo, S. M., Liss, G. M., Dias, C. and Banks, D. E. 1997. Assessment of the relationship between isocyanate exposure levels and occupational asthma. *Am J Ind Med* 32:517–21.

Tarlo, S. M., Liss, G. M. and Yeung, K. S. 2002. Changes in rates and severity of compensation claims for asthma due to diisocyanates: A possible effect of medical surveillance measures. *Occup Environ Med* 59:58–62.

van Deurssen, E., Meijster, T., Oude Hengel, K. M., Boessen, R., Spaan, S., Tielemans, E., Heederik, D. et al. 2015a. Effectiveness of a multidimensional randomized control intervention to reduce quartz exposure among construction workers. *Ann Occup Hyg* 59:959–71.

van Deurssen, E. H., Pronk, A., Meijster, T., Tielemans, E., Heederik, D. and Oude Hengel, K. M. 2015b. Process evaluation of an intervention program to reduce occupational quartz exposure among Dutch construction workers. *J Occup Environ Med* 57:428–35.

van Rooy, F. G., Houba, R., Palmen, N., Zengeni, M. M., Sander, I., Spithoven, J., Rooyackers, J. M. et al. 2009. A cross-sectional study among detergent workers exposed to liquid detergent enzymes. *Occup Environ Med* 66:759–65.

van Tongeren, M., Galea, K. S., Ticker, J., While, D., Kromhout, H. and Cherrie, J. W. 2009. Temporal trends of flour dust exposure in the United Kingdom, 1985–2003. *J Environ Monit* 11:1492–7.

Vandenplas, O., Dressel, H., Wilken, D., Jamart, J., Heederik, D., Maestrelli, P., Sigsgaard, T. et al. 2011. Management of occupational asthma: Cessation or reduction of exposure? A systematic review of available evidence. *Eur Respir J* 38:804–11.

Vanhanen, M., Tuomi, T., Tiikkainen, U., Tupasela, O., Voutilainen, R. and Nordman, H. 2000. Risk of enzyme allergy in the detergent industry. *Occup Environ Med* 57:121–125.

Warren, N., Meijster, T., Heederik, D. and Tielemans, E. 2009. A dynamic population-based model for the development of work-related respiratory health effects among bakery workers. *Occup Environ Med* 66:810–7.

Weeks, J. L., Levy, B. S. and Wagner, G. R. 1991. *Preventing Occupational Disease and Injury.* Washington, DC: American Public Health Association.

Wild, D. M., Redlich, C. A. and Paltiel, A. D. 2005. Surveillance for isocyanate asthma: A model based cost effectiveness analysis. *Occup Environ Med* 62:743–9.

13 Predictive Toxicology in Occupational Lung Disease

Craig A. Poland, Raymond Agius, Sarah E. Howie and Ken Donaldson

CONTENTS

INTRODUCTION

This chapter deals with the application of toxicological approaches and concepts in order to aid in the prediction of toxicity and resultant disease in the lungs. Given the enormous range of possible exposures in the modern world, covering all possible inhalable xenobiotics is beyond the scope of this chapter, and so we will use, as exemplars, two of the most important inhaled agents that cause lung disease. We believe that the general principles that are used for predictive toxicology for these two classes will be relevant and transferable to other types of inhaled xenobiotic. The two types of xenobiotics that will be used as exemplars are:

1. Particles; this category is of course currently dominated by nanoparticles, and so they will be a major focus
2. Occupational lung sensitisers

Toxicology, at its heart, is the study of the characteristics and effects of hazardous substances, and particularly the relationship between dose and effect. However, it can be more wide ranging than a specific understanding of pathobiological processes, as it can inform multiple components of health, safety and risk in the occupational environment. For example:

- The characterisation of hazard aids risk assessment and management.
- Understanding what makes substances (particles/chemicals) harmful or not provides the potential for the design or use of safer industrial chemicals and particles.
- Understanding the mechanism of disease caused by the industrial xenobiotic provides the potential for developing biomarkers and intervening in the progression of disease.
- Overarching all of the above is the ability to construct a structure/toxicity model, hereafter referred to as a structure/activity model. Such a model, relating physicochemistry to toxicity, should allow for the rational prediction of toxic potency and mode of toxicity based solely on knowledge of the physicochemical properties of an untested xenobiotic.

For toxicological effects to arise, exogenous agents must interact with biological systems in ways that lead to disruption of normal physiological pathways and processes and redirection down pathophysiological pathways that may ultimately lead to pathological change. Such pathways, like inflammation or immune responses, can be defensive under normal circumstance, but when induced by the xenobiotic in ways that are inappropriate, exaggerated or protracted over time, may lead to tissue damage and pathological change. A primary aim of 'industrial toxicology' is the exploration and elucidation of this interface between the exogenous agent and the biological environment so as to gain an understanding

TABLE 13.1
Characteristics of Typical Pathogenic Structures in Sensitising Chemicals and Particles

Xenobiotic	Typical Pathogenic Physicochemical Structures	Relevant Pathogenic Pathways	Adverse Effect
Sensitising chemicals	Di-isocyanates	Hypersensitive immune responses	Asthma, pneumonitis
Particles	Long fibres	Inflammation	Fibrosis, cancer

of the mechanism whereby the xenobiotic initiates these pathological pathways. This must eventually be reducible to the physicochemistry of the xenobiotic in question.

Table 13.1 shows the different characteristics, pathways and pathologies for sensitising chemicals and particles, highlighting the differences between them.

In the case of occupational lung diseases, adverse effects arise after interaction of the xenobiotic with cells on the airway surface or in the interstitium, internalisation into cells or distribution to sites distal to the initial point of entry into the body at the lungs. These relationships and any adverse effect resulting from them, as mentioned above, must be determined by the morphological and chemical properties of the xenobiotic. The physicochemistry can differ widely between different forms of xenobiotic from different sources, resulting in a spectrum of toxicity and disease. However, at its heart, the toxicological response, or lack thereof, is determined by the sum of these physicochemical properties. Together, these physicochemical characteristics dictate the extent and type of toxicity and form the basis of the structure/activity relationship for the class of toxin.

It is important to draw a distinction between dose and dosimetry. The former deals classically with the mass dose or concentration dose, its distribution and its fate within the organism or cells in culture. Dosimetry deals in a more complex way with dose by considering the ways that the chemical or physical entity delivers specific 'harm' to a biological system, resulting in response. The physicochemical entities associated with a chemical or particle exposure that mediate toxicity can represent a relatively small fraction of the total amount of xenobiotic entering the biological system. For a chemical xenobiotic, there may be a requirement for bio-activation of a fraction of the chemical in order to reach a sufficiently reactive state to react with host macromolecules. In addition, there may be systems of clearance for some of the reactive chemicals before they reach their target macromolecule.

In the case of particles, the real-life particle exposure always comprises a highly heterogeneous mix of particle types, whilst only a subgroup of particles are likely to be pathogenic and much of the dust will be of low toxicity. Clearance of particles always occurs to an extent, but it is commonly seen that pathogenic particles are more likely to be retained in the lungs, increasing the period of interaction. For example, quartz kills macrophages and retains them in the inflammatory milieu it creates (Albrecht et al., 2007) and long fibres inhibit macrophage locomotion (Schinwald et al., 2012a) as well as initiating inflammation (Donaldson and Tran, 2002; Shukla et al., 2003; Donaldson et al., 2010).

STRUCTURE/ACTIVITY RELATIONSHIPS IN PARTICLE TOXICOLOGY

Predicting the toxicity of a particle and its potential impact on the human system is challenging and is typically done on the basis of toxicological testing. Such testing for the purposes of regulating substances and the setting of exposure limits, either in terms of rigorous health-based occupational exposure limits (e.g. workplace exposure limits) or more prescriptive, process-based limits, such as derived no-effect levels under Registration, Evaluation, Authorisation and restriction of CHemicals (REACH) in the EU, typically involve animal testing to international test standards (e.g. Organisation for Economic Co-operation and Development [OECD]). Such well-performed toxicological studies, especially when combined with epidemiological data, provide a solid grounding for predicting health effects in humans (with suitably applied uncertainty factors). However, such testing tends to represent the specific material under test (i.e. specific composition, size, shape, etc.), but can be read across to other materials (with justification), often of the same composition; for example, inhalation toxicity data on the specific size/crystallinity, etc., of titanium dioxide (TiO_2) being used in the consideration of alternatively sized TiO_2 particles. The difficulty here is that toxicity is not based purely on substance type (e.g. particulate TiO_2), but on the properties of the specific sample (e.g. 25 nm spherical anatase TiO_2 with a surface charge of −2 mV with no contaminants). This may seem somewhat arbitrary, but it reflects the notion that the toxicity of a substance is based on the sum of properties that may drive toxicity, and these can differ despite being two samples based on the same substance identity (e.g. chemical abstracts service [CAS] number). Considering this example of TiO_2 further, an elegant example of a marked modification in toxicity despite the same bulk composition can be found in the study by Hamilton et al. (2009). Here, the authors compared the toxicity of three forms of TiO_2 of the same bulk composition, but presented as a spherical TiO_2 nanoparticle (60–200 nm), a short fibre (0.8–4 μm) or a long fibre (15–30 μm) in mouse alveolar macrophages. They found that presenting the relatively low-toxicity TiO_2 as a long fibre structure led to a profound inflammatory response that was not observed with the shorter/non-fibrous particles of the same composition (Hamilton et al., 2009). Thus, it can be seen that considering particles based solely on their composition is unhelpful when attempting to predict possible health implications resulting from exposure. These properties that can dictate toxicity such as the reactive surface of quartz (Fubini, 1998), cause a toxicological activity such as inflammation (Donaldson et al., 2001) and cause the modification of structures such as through the passivation of a quartz surface by aluminium lactate can, in turn, modify the response (Duffin et al., 2001).

When particles are viewed not as a single entity but as a sum of different structure/activity relationships, a clearer picture emerges regarding toxic potency and the mechanisms of toxicity, also offering opportunities for modification in order to remove the structures that confer toxicity, thereby making the material inherently safer by design. Examples of structure/activity relationships are listed below and are discussed in the proceeding sections (Figure 13.1):

1. Particle size
2. Particle reactivity
3. Particle surface charge
4. Particle shape
5. Particle solubility

Particle Size

Particle size has long been known to affect toxicity, not least because of its role in determining the region of deposition in the lung and subsequent regional lung dose. However, it has also been noted in numerous studies that, when applied at the same mass dose, smaller particles (e.g. nanoparticles) elicit a more pronounced response than larger particles, despite having the same composition. An example of this differential toxicity on a mass basis of the same material can be found in the study by Renwick (2004), who instilled TiO_2 or carbon black particles into the lungs of rats and measured the inflammatory response. The author found that the larger, bulk TiO_2 sample with a mean diameter of 250 nm caused no significant response over the vehicle (saline) control, whilst instillation of the much smaller 29-nm TiO_2 caused a significant response, a response that was mirrored when comparing 260.2-nm and 14.3-nm carbon black. The driver here of the comparatively greater potency of the nano-form is not the nano-size per se, but the much larger surface area per unit mass displayed by the smaller particles (Schwarze et al., 2007). This differential could have an impact on safety, where an exposure is deemed non-harmful (e.g. below an exposure limit)

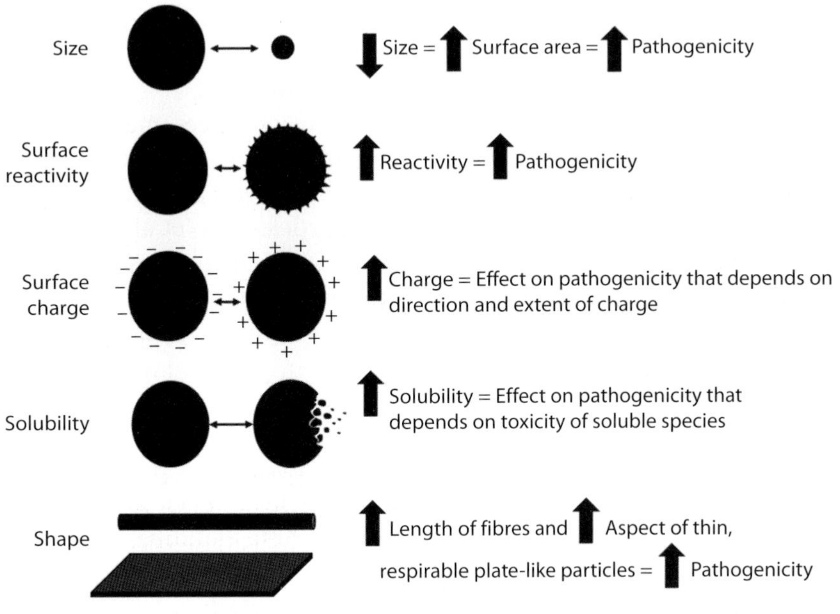

FIGURE 13.1 The main elements of a particle structure/toxicity model. A downward pointing arrow means decreasing and an upward pointing arrow denotes increasing.

based on test data for a larger-sized particle, yet the limit is used for all particle sizes (based on composition). An example of this can be seen in the recent recommended exposure limit for TiO_2 put forward by the National Institute for Occupational Safety and Health (NIOSH). In its evaluation of the evidence, the NIOSH recommended exposure limits of 2.4 mg/m^3 for fine TiO_2, yet a much lower limit of 0.3 mg/m^3 was recommended for ultrafine (including engineered nanoscale) TiO_2 of time-weighted average concentrations for up to 10 hours per day during a 40-hour work week (NIOSH, 2011). It should also be considered that whilst taking a more polarised analysis of size does show significant differences between nano-sized and larger materials, there are also spectra of toxicity within the nano-size range, and this has been observed for numerous materials (Abdelhalim, 2011, Kim et al., 2012) and modes of action (e.g. oxidative stress) (Carlson et al., 2008).

Particle Reactivity

As already mentioned, the particle surface represents the point of interaction with a biological system, and therefore the reactivity of this surface may influence the toxicity of a material. This issue of surface reactivity becomes even more important when it is considered in relation to particle surface area, as even a particle with a relatively benign surface could show toxicity due to amplification of its surface area with decreasing particle size (Duffin et al., 2007). Where particles have a combination of high surface area and high reactivity, this may lead to the formation of a 'double hazard' in terms of inflammatory potential (Duffin et al., 2007; Karlsson et al., 2009). The determinants of particle reactivity can be summarised as follows:

- The nanoparticle is contaminated with redox-active metals or other biologically active contaminant. An example of this is the presence of transition metals and resultant reactivity leading to toxicity, which has been suggested to play a substantial role in the pathogenesis of several particle-mediated diseases, including metal fume fever resulting from exposure to welding fumes (McNeilly et al., 2005). In addition to active metal components, other biologically active contaminants can be present and affect toxicity, such as poly-aromatic hydrocarbons, which have long been associated with the toxicity of diesel engine exhaust particles, as well as of other combustion-derived particles (Valavanidis et al., 2008).
- If the particle is composed primarily of a biologically active substance, such as reactive chemical groups or intrinsically photo-reactive. Whilst particles may be contaminated with biologically active components either during their production (as in the case of iron-containing crocidolite asbestos) or modified by the environment, particles may equally be intrinsically reactive due to their composition. This may be due to chemically reactive groups and/or properties such as photo-reactivity. For example, a nanomaterial composed of copper (II) oxide is likely to be redox active, which may pose a hazard, especially considering the nanomaterial's large surface area (e.g. 2 m^2/g for a 42–nm powder versus 1.5 m^2/g for a 3–μm powder), potentially meaning that the nanomaterial is far more reactive than the parent compound (Karlsson et al., 2009).

Particle Surface Charge

Different particles can present different charges (i.e. positive, negative or neutral) and different magnitudes of such charge, which can influence several factors, such as the propensity to agglomerate/aggregate, the interaction with charged molecules such as proteins and the cellular uptake. The surface charge of a particle can be readily modified, either deliberately such as via surface coatings, resulting from the environment through the adsorption of substances (e.g. proteins) (Cho et al., 2012) or through other routes such as the leaching of positively charged magnesium from the surface of chrysotile asbestos during dissolution and a resultant shift to a negative charge (Virta, 2002).

Particle surfaces mark the point of interaction with a biological environment, and it has been shown that surface charge can contribute to the toxicity of certain nanoparticle (Cho et al., 2012; Greish et al., 2012; Nagy et al., 2012), as well as for other conventional particles such as asbestos (Light and Wei, 1977a, b) and airborne particulate matter (Veronesi et al., 2002).

Particle Shape

An example of how particle shape can affect the toxicity of a particle has been given in relation to TiO_2 (Hamilton et al., 2009), building upon a considerable history of investigation into the role of fibre length on pathogenicity from the early work and development of the Stanton hypothesis (Stanton et al., 1977; Stanton et al., 1981) to more recent evaluations of nanofibers (Schinwald et al., 2012a). One such example is that of Davis et al., who compared the toxicity of long amosite asbestos to the same sample ground to shortness, and found virtually no pathology with the short form after years of inhalation exposure, but found lung cancer, fibrosis and a single mesothelioma in animals inhaling the long parent material (Davis et al., 1986). The enhanced toxicity of long fibres (i.e. presenting a fibre-type hazard) arises from the respirability of small-diameter (<3 μm) yet long-length (>15 μm) fibres that are bio-persistent (see section 'Particle Solubility') and the challenges that these present to the clearance mechanisms of the lung and pleural space. Clearance from these regions is to a large extent size restricted, being based either on the maximal particle size that an alveolar macrophage can phagocytose without hindering mobility or eliciting a pro-inflammogenic effect or, in the case of the pleural space, the maximal diameter of stomata in the parietal pleura as the route of egress to the underlying lymphatics. The threshold size at which such effects occur has recently been elucidated in mice and has been shown to be 5 μm in the case of the pleural space (reflecting the size of stomata) (Murphy et al., 2011; Schinwald et al., 2012b) and 14 μm for fibre-induced pulmonary inflammation (although hindrance of macrophage mobility was detected for as short as 5 μm) (Schinwald et al., 2012a).

Whilst the influence of shape on toxicity has primarily focused on fibres, this issue of a respirable particle (due to low aerodynamic diameter) with sufficient dimensions to hinder effective clearance and trigger inflammation is also relevant to other materials. Most recently, this has been applied to graphene-based materials that can, due to their extreme thinness, display a low aerodynamic diameter and hence be respirable, yet they can also possess a large lateral diameter that can prevent macrophage uptake and clearance (Schinwald et al., 2012c).

Particle Solubility

Particle solubility can have both positive and negative effects on a particle's propensity to cause harm. A soluble particle that does not release toxic ions or other components could result in the overall progressive reduction/removal of dose (as seen with certain bio-soluble forms of glass fibres) (Hesterberg et al., 2012) as the particle dissolves, ultimately removing any toxic stimulus (if caused) or becoming intrinsically non-toxic. Particles that are soluble but release toxic/reactive ions or other components may generate localised or even systemic toxicants and hence toxicity. This is exemplified by Zn and Cu nanoparticles in the former case, where the rapid mobilisation of toxic Cu or Zn ions in acidic phagolysosomes of alveolar macrophages in the lung following delivery to that organ elicits pulmonary inflammation (Cho et al., 2012). Evidence that some soluble nanoparticles release ions that can lead to more generalised systemic distribution with potential toxic sequelae is demonstrated by silver nanoparticles. These nanoparticles release silver ions that are found in all organs by a few days after an oral exposure, and there is long-term retention in the brain and testis (van der Zande et al., 2012). Similar widespread systemic distribution of silver nanoparticles is seen after inhalation exposure and is likely in significant part due to ionic silver (Sung et al., 2009).

Viewing a particle as a sum of its component structures and the impacts that these may have on activity, thereby interrogating the physicochemical properties of a particle for the potential to cause harm (Figure 13.1), is a useful non-testing approach for aiding in the prediction of toxicity, albeit with caveats compared to direct testing.

TESTING FOR SENSITISING CHEMICALS

A number of chemicals is known to provoke allergic reactions in the lungs following previous exposure (sensitisation) in susceptible individuals. This should not to be confused with irritant reactions that can have similar symptoms of mucus production and wheeze, but happen in any individual who inhales a sufficient quantity of a lung-toxic chemical. Allergic reactions require an individual to be immunologically sensitised (hence the term 'sensitising chemical'), following which the sensitised individual develops a specific immune response to the chemical. Subsequent exposure to even a very small amount of the sensitiser (or allergen) then triggers an allergic reaction in the sensitised individual. This reaction can be localised to the site of exposure or become systemic. In the worst cases, anaphylactic shock is induced.

The lung, like all organs, has a complex, multi-cell-type, resident immune system to protect it against infection (Gwyer Findlay and Hussell, 2012; Chen and Kolls, 2013). The composition of this resident immune system varies with the type of lung tissue. For instance, the external surfaces of the alveoli are monitored by the resident alveolar macrophages, whilst there is a complex network of macrophages and dendritic cells (Neyt and Lambrecht, 2013) in the epithelium and sub-epithelium of the trachea, bronchi and bronchioles. Mast cells are found throughout the lung tissue (Andersson et al., 2009; da Silva et al., 2014). The lungs have a lymphatic supply and are drained by the adjacent mediastinal lymph nodes in the chest cavity.

Allergic reactions can be induced by two separate immune-mediated hypersensitivity mechanisms. These result from either cross-linking of pre-existing IgE antibody molecules on the surface of mast cells (immediate hypersensitivity, also known as Type 1 hypersensitivity) or from the T-lymphocyte-induced activation of mast cells (delayed hypersensitivity, also known as contact hypersensitivity and as Type 4 hypersensitivity). IgE-induced allergy usually becomes apparent very quickly (within minutes) after exposure to the relevant sensitising chemical, whereas the T-lymphocyte-mediated reaction can take several hours to fully develop. In both cases, mast cells de-granulate at the site where the sensitising chemical is encountered (Freudenberg et al., 2009; Kambe et al., 2010; Honda et al., 2013). The major signs and symptoms of allergy are caused by the release of pro-inflammatory mediators by the mast cells. Sensitising chemicals can cause either Type 1 or Type 4 hypersensitivity allergic reactions. The responses can be localised in the skin, the gut or the lungs depending upon the route of exposure. In some individuals with Type 1 hypersensitivity, more serious systemic reactions can be seen (anaphylactic shock) if the sensitising molecules can reach the circulatory system and bind to IgE on the surfaces of mast cells in the vasculature. Allergic reactions in the lung, including those induced by sensitising chemicals, are most commonly due to Type 1 hypersensitivity and result in airway narrowing and excess mucus production, generating the signs and symptoms of asthma (Holt and Strickland, 2010).

Both Type 1 and Type 4 hypersensitivity reactions involve interactions between cells that process and present the allergen (antigen-presenting cells [APCs]) and the T lymphocytes that can specifically recognise the allergen on the surface of the APC. Normally, APCs present peptides to T lymphocytes, and any T lymphocytes that recognise peptides that are derived from self-proteins of the body are eliminated or prevented from being activated by regulatory T lymphocytes so that only peptides derived from non-self/foreign proteins initiate immune responses. This makes the nature of what is recognised by a T cell when a sensitising chemical causes an allergic reaction difficult to understand, as these chemicals are much smaller than peptides. It is currently thought that chemicals with sensitising properties can bind to self-proteins in the body and 'modify' them in such way that the configuration/charge of the modified peptides derived from these proteins can now be recognised by some T lymphocytes in some individuals (Pompeu et al., 2012; Yin et al., 2013). These T lymphocytes can then directly cause Type 4 hypersensitivity on subsequent exposure to the sensitising chemical or indirectly cause Type 1 reactions by acting as helper cells for B lymphocytes, producing IgE antibodies that can recognise the sensitising chemical directly.

Pulmonary APCs need to be previously activated by the recognition of 'danger signals' (Parker and Prince, 2011; Broggi and Granucci, 2015). Danger signals in the lung can be generated as a result of infection or, more likely, in response to a sensitising chemical by damage to adjacent tissue cells. Damaged cells release a variety of small molecules and also soluble proteins called cytokines and chemokines, which can activate and cause the migration of immune system cells. T cells are in turn activated by the recognition of antigens on the surfaces of APCs and by cytokines released by the APCs. The activated T cells release other cytokines that mediate the immune responses. APCs releasing the cytokine IL-12 are involved in inducing Type 4 hypersensitivity, which is characterised by the release of large amounts of the cytokine IFN-γ by T cells. APCs releasing the cytokine IL-10 are involved in inducing Type 1 hypersensitivity, which is characterised by the release of large amounts of IL-4, IL-5 and IL-13 by T cells.

Currently, testing of sensitising chemicals is at a crossroads. There is a need to predict which molecules might have sensitising properties, which can be done at a molecular level in the first instance (Lalko et al., 2011). However, this is unlikely to reveal the full potential of such molecules in an intact biological system. Various in vitro methods have been used, driven by a regulatory imperative to develop alternatives to in vivo testing (Vandebriel et al., 2011). These methods are becoming very sophisticated, including the use of tissue-engineering approaches in order to reconstruct the lung epithelium (Horvath et al., 2015). However, these models do not reflect the full make-up of all of the cell types in the native lung tissue. In the last few years, *ex vivo* studies using organ cultures of human lung slices in order to test sensitising chemicals have also been developed as alternatives to animal testing (Henjakovic et al., 2008; Morin et al., 2013; Lauenstein et al., 2014).

However, such approaches still fail to model the complexity of molecular and cellular interactions between the lung epithelial cells and the immune system involved in Type 1 and Type 4 hypersensitivity. Given that only some susceptible individuals will react in an allergic fashion to any sensitising chemical, testing whether or not a given molecule has sensitising properties is not simple. That these reactions depend upon previously induced immune responses means that simple in vitro assays for toxicity are unlikely to accurately predict the sensitising potential of a given chemical. It should be noted that once it has occurred, sensitisation of the immune system is systemic (i.e. the original exposure could be through skin contact, but an allergic immune response could then arise in the lungs if the same chemical was subsequently inhaled).

A number of animal models have been investigated in order to test for the allergic potential of chemicals in the lungs, with rodent models (Tarkowski et al., 2008) being the most widely used. However, the use of in vivo models makes high-throughput screening of large numbers of chemicals impractical. Various strategies have been used in order to enable rapid in vivo assessment of sensitising potential by looking for biological signatures of early events that would predict subsequent allergic outcomes. Such early events include cytokines released by damaged tissue cells and/or by APCs, which might predispose to allergy (Kimber et al., 1996). The ability of chemicals to sensitise through the skin has been exploited in order to test their sensitisation potential in the 'local lymph node assay' (Kimber et al., 2002; Tarkowski et al., 2008).

QUANTITATIVE STRUCTURE/ ACTIVITY RELATIONSHIPS AND RESPIRATORY SENSITISERS

Respiratory sensitisers present themselves to the lung either as aerosols (usually solid particles) or in the gaseous phase (usually as vapours). Although sensitisation can manifest itself in a variety of clinical syndromes, this section will limit itself to asthma, which is the most common such disease in an occupational respiratory context. The pathways whereby asthmagens bring about their adverse effects start with an interaction (usually covalent) between the xenobiotic and a host macromolecule. These interactions include those with airway cell surfaces, with the surfaces of APCs and with cell surface-bound antibodies. IgE binding is a common, important but not necessarily universal mechanism whereby respiratory sensitisers lead to occupational asthma. For many low-molecular-weight (LMW) sensitisers (i.e. those with a molecular mass of <1000 Da that behave as haptens), an early interaction is with a much larger, native 'host' molecule such as albumin, thus producing a 'complete antigen'.

The chemical structure and therefore the associated electronic properties of exogenous chemicals are thus key determinants of their toxic potential. A handful of transition metals have been associated with an occupational asthma hazard either in cationic form or else in anionic complexes whose ligands may be important factors in determining sensitising potential. However, data on metal compounds are currently too limited to permit robust generalisations (Agius et al., 1991). As regards organic LMW chemicals, qualitative observations have suggested that diamines (whether aliphatic, aromatic or secondary/heterocyclic) cause occupational asthma, while the corresponding mono-amine analogues appear not to manifest this hazard (Agius et al., 1991), thus illustrating the prospect of being able to predict immunotoxic properties. At the crudest level, the data showed how chemical groups that are capable of nucleophilic reactions such as (nitrogen-containing) amines and isocyanates or (oxygen-containing) aldehydes and di-anhydrides are associated with occupational asthma hazard. At a more sophisticated level, the data have permitted the categorisation of the putative chemical reactions mechanistically (Enoch et al., 2010).

Sufficient data arising from occupational exposures and their adverse health effects have become available concerning LMW organic sensitisers in order to use computer-based (so-called '*in silico*') models to associate the chemical structure of the xenobiotic molecules with their biological activity. These quantitative structure/activity relationships (QSARs) have found application in human respiratory immunotoxicology (Graham et al., 1997; Cunningham et al., 2005; Jarvis et al., 2005; Seed et al., 2008). QSARs can lend themselves to two purposes: the first of these is to contribute to developing and testing mechanistic hypotheses regarding why and how respiratory sensitisers bring about their adverse effects in exposed workers. The second purpose is to achieve rapid, effective and efficient prediction of the toxic hazard of novel chemicals in order to assist in the risk management and prevention of occupational lung disease.

In QSAR studies as applied to occupational asthma, the molecular substructures of confirmed occupational asthmagens have been compared with appropriate control chemicals to which workers have been exposed, but whose adverse health effects have not (so far) been shown to include occupational asthma. Some of the findings are illustrated qualitatively in Figure 13.2. Thus, from top to bottom, the columns in Figure 13.2a and 13.2b show aliphatic, heterocyclic and aromatic amines, respectively. In each pair, no evidence has been found for asthmagenicity with respect to the chemical with only one amine group (Figure 13.2a), while there is evidence for asthmagenicity in its corresponding analogue with two amine groups (Figure 13.2b). The statistical analyses have confirmed the high significance of having two or more such reactive groups per molecule, thus corroborating an

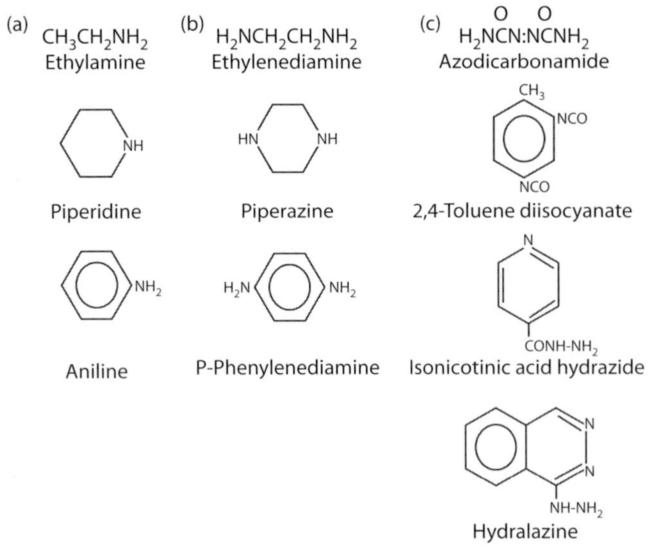

FIGURE 13.2 Chemical structures of asthmagenic chemicals contrasted with presumed non-asthmagenic ones. The chemicals shown in column (a) are examples of toxic yet not asthmagenic compounds, whilst those in columns (b) and (c) are asthmagenic. It should be noted that the asthmagens have two (or more) reactive nitrogen-containing groups, whereas those containing only one appear not to be asthmagenic.

important role for 'cross-linking' in asthmagenic sensitisation (Jarvis et al., 2005).

At the most 'user-friendly' level so far, freely available online tools permit the uploading of a chemical structure and an immediate computation of the asthma hazard index (i.e. a likelihood from 0 to 1 of the agent being asthmagenic) (Agius et al., 2005). With iteration, these QSAR techniques now achieve specificity and sensitivity values of >90% and a receiver–operator characteristic area under the curve of 0.9 (Seed and Agius, 2010). Furthermore, a data-driven QSAR approach can be usefully complemented by 'alerts' based on chemical reaction mechanisms (Enoch et al., 2012). With regards to possible 'false-positive' and 'false-negative' predictions, the greater concern probably relates to the latter. For example, morphine was not predicted as an asthmagen by Jarvis et al. (2005), perhaps because it was unique in its class and could cause asthma by direct effects on mast cell μ-receptors. However, as more data are collected and QSAR models become more sophisticated, preliminary data suggest that their predictive values are likely to increase.

The prediction of a specific asthmagenic sensitisation hazard can help both in risk management strategies (including determining the need of health surveillance and the implementation of control methods) and in clinical investigation (Moore et al., 2009; Anees et al., 2011; Pralong et al., 2012), especially when multiple putative causes need to be screened prior to challenge testing. However, the extent to which QSAR approaches and mechanistic alerts can help achieve a 'benign by design' end point remains to be determined. This difficulty arises since chemical properties such as covalent cross-linking, which are very important in industrial applications as adhesives, polymers and coatings, tend to associate very closely with sensitisation hazard. However, if knowledge of chemistry, immunotoxicology and occupational hygiene is brought together, useful mitigation of the risks associated with novel chemicals or processes may be achieved; for example, by opting for chemical analogues that are less volatile or are less reliant on cross-linking mechanistic properties for their industrial purpose.

REFERENCES

Abdelhalim, M. A. 2011. Exposure to gold nanoparticles produces cardiac tissue damage that depends on the size and duration of exposure. *Lipids Health Dis* 10:205.

Agius, R., Jarvis, J. and Seed, M. 2005. *Mechanisms of Occupational Asthma* [Online]. The University of Manchester. Available at: http://www.population-health.manchester.ac.uk/epidemiology/Coeh/research/workrelatedillhealth/asthma/.

Agius, R. M., Nee, J., McGovern, B. and Robertson, A. 1991. Structure activity hypotheses in occupational asthma caused by low molecular weight substances. *Ann Occup Hyg* 35:129–37.

Albrecht, C., Hohr, D., Haberzettl, P., Becker, A., Borm, P. J. and Schins, R. P. 2007. Surface-dependent quartz uptake by macrophages: Potential role in pulmonary inflammation and lung clearance. *Inhal Toxicol* 19(Suppl. 1):39–48.

Andersson, C. K., Mori, M., Bjermer, L., Lofdahl, C. G. and Erjefalt, J. S. 2009. Novel site-specific mast cell subpopulations in the human lung. *Thorax* 64:297–305.

Anees, W., Moore, V. C., Croft, J. S., Robertson, A. S. and Burge, P. S. 2011. Occupational asthma caused by heated triglycidyl isocyanurate. *Occup Med (Lond)* 61:65–7.

Broggi, A. and Granucci, F. 2015. Microbe- and danger-induced inflammation. *Mol Immunol* 63:127–33.

Carlson, C., Hussain, S. M., Schrand, A. M., Braydich-Stolle, L. K., Hess, K. L., Jones, R. L. and Schlager, J. J. 2008. Unique cellular interaction of silver nanoparticles: Size-dependent generation of reactive oxygen species. *J Phys Chem B* 112:13608–19.

Chen, K. and Kolls, J. K. 2013. T cell-mediated host immune defenses in the lung. *Annu Rev Immunol* 31:605–33.

Cho, W. S., Duffin, R., Thielbeer, F., Bradley, M., Megson, I. L., Macnee, W., Poland, C. A. et al. 2012. Zeta potential and solubility to toxic ions as mechanisms of lung inflammation caused by metal/metal-oxide nanoparticles. *Toxicol Sci* 126:469–77.

Cunningham, A. R., Cunningham, S. L., Consoer, D. M., Moss, S. T. and Karol, M. H. 2005. Development of an information-intensive structure–activity relationship model and its application to human respiratory chemical sensitizers. *Sar Qsar Environ Res* 16:273–85.

da Silva, E. Z., Jamur, M. C. and Oliver, C. 2014. Mast cell function: A new vision of an old cell. *J Histochem Cytochem* 62:698–738.

Davis, J., Addison, J., Bolton, R., Donaldson, K., Jones, A. and Smith, T. 1986. The pathogenicity of long versus short fibre samples of amosite asbestos administered to rats by inhalation and intraperitoneal injection. *Br J Exp Pathol* 67:415–30.

Donaldson, K. and Tran, C. L. 2002. Inflammation caused by particles and fibers. *Inhal Toxicol* 14:5–27.

Donaldson, K., Murphy, F. A., Duffin, R. and Poland, C. A. 2010. Asbestos, carbon nanotubes and the pleural mesothelium: A review and the hypothesis regarding the role of long fibre retention in the parietal pleura, inflammation and mesothelioma. *Part Fibre Toxicol* 7:5.

Donaldson, K., Stone, V., Duffin, R., Clouter, A., Schins, R. and Borm, P. 2001. The quartz hazard: Effects of surface and matrix on inflammogenic activity. *J Environ Pathol Toxicol Oncol* 20(Suppl. 1):109–18.

Duffin, R., Gilmour, P. S., Schins, R. P., Clouter, A., Guy, K., Brown, D. M., Macnee, W. et al. 2001. Aluminium lactate treatment of Dq12 quartz inhibits its ability to cause inflammation, chemokine expression and nuclear factor-kappaB activation. *Toxicol Appl Pharmacol* 176:10–7.

Duffin, R., Tran, L., Brown, D., Stone, V. and Donaldson, K. 2007. Proinflammogenic effects of low-toxicity and metal nanoparticles *in vivo* and *in vitro*: Highlighting the role of particle surface area and surface reactivity. *Inhal Toxicol* 19:849–56.

Enoch, S. J., Seed, M. J., Roberts, D. W., Cronin, M. T., Stocks, S. J. and Agius, R. M. 2012. Development of mechanism-based structural alerts for respiratory sensitization hazard identification. *Chem Res Toxicol* 25:2490–8.

Enoch, S. J., Roberts, D. W. and Cronin, M. T. 2010. Mechanistic category formation for the prediction of respiratory sensitization. *Chem Res Toxicol* 23:1547–55.

Freudenberg, M. A., Esser, P. R., Jakob, T., Galanos, C. and Martin, S. F. 2009. Innate and adaptive immune responses in contact dermatitis: Analogy with infections. *G Ital Dermatol Venereol* 144:173–85.

Fubini, B. 1998. Surface chemistry and quartz hazard. *Ann Occup Hyg* 42:521–30.

Graham, C., Rosenkranz, H. S. and Karol, M. H. 1997. Structure–activity model of chemicals that cause human respiratory sensitization. *Regul Toxicol Pharmacol* 26:296–306.

Greish, K., Thiagarajan, G., Herd, H., Price, R., Bauer, H., Hubbard, D., Burckle, A. et al. 2012. Size and surface charge significantly influence the toxicity of silica and dendritic nanoparticles. *Nanotoxicology* 6:713–23.

Gwyer Findlay, E. and Hussell, T. 2012. Macrophage-mediated inflammation and disease: A focus on the lung. *Mediators Inflamm* 2012:140937.

Hamilton, R. F., Wu, N., Porter, D., Buford, M., Wolfarth, M. and Holian, A. 2009. Particle length-dependent titanium dioxide nanomaterials toxicity and bioactivity. *Part Fibre Toxicol* 6:35.

Henjakovic, M., Martin, C., Hoymann, H. G., Sewald, K., Ressmeyer, A. R., Dassow, C., Pohlmann, G. et al. 2008. *Ex vivo* lung function measurements in precision-cut lung slices (Pcls) from chemical allergen-sensitized mice represent a suitable alternative to *in vivo* studies. *Toxicol Sci* 106:444–53.

Hesterberg, T. W., Anderson, R., Bernstein, D. M., Bunn, W. B., Chase, G. A., Jankousky, A. L., Marsh, G. M. et al. 2012. Product stewardship and science: Safe manufacture and use of fiber glass. *Regul Toxicol Pharmacol* 62:257–77.

Holt, P. G. and Strickland, D. H. 2010. Interactions between innate and adaptive immunity in asthma pathogenesis: New perspectives from studies on acute exacerbations. *J Allergy Clin Immunol* 125:963–72; quiz 973–4.

Honda, T., Egawa, G., Grabbe, S. and Kabashima, K. 2013. Update of immune events in the murine contact hypersensitivity model: Toward the understanding of allergic contact dermatitis. *J Invest Dermatol* 133:303–15.

Horvath, L., Umehara, Y., Jud, C., Blank, F., Petri-Fink, A. and Rothen-Rutishauser, B. 2015. Engineering an *in vitro* air–blood barrier by 3D bioprinting. *Sci Rep* 5:7974.

Jarvis, J., Seed, M. J., Elton, R., Sawyer, L. and Agius, R. 2005. Relationship between chemical structure and the occupational asthma hazard of low molecular weight organic compounds. *Occup Environ Med* 62:243–50.

Kambe, N., Nakamura, Y., Saito, M. and Nishikomori, R. 2010. The inflammasome, an innate immunity guardian, participates in skin urticarial reactions and contact hypersensitivity. *Allergol Int* 59:105–13.

Karlsson, H. L., Gustafsson, J., Cronholm, P. and Moller, L. 2009. Size-dependent toxicity of metal oxide particles—A comparison between nano- and micrometer size. *Toxicol Lett* 188:112–8.

Kim, T. H., Kim, M., Park, H. S., Shin, U. S., Gong, M. S. and Kim, H. W. 2012. Size-dependent cellular toxicity of silver nanoparticles. *J Biomed Mater Res A* 100:1033–43.

Kimber, I., Dearman, R. J., Basketter, D. A., Ryan, C. A. and Gerberick, G. F. 2002. The local lymph node assay: Past, present and future. *Contact Dermatitis* 47:315–28.

Kimber, I., Hilton, J., Basketter, D. A. and Dearman, R. J. 1996. Predictive testing for respiratory sensitization in the mouse. *Toxicol Lett* 86:193–8.

Lalko, J. F., Kimber, I., Dearman, R. J., Gerberick, G. F., Sarlo, K. and Api, A. M. 2011. Chemical reactivity measurements: Potential for characterization of respiratory chemical allergens. *Toxicol In Vitro* 25:433–45.

Lauenstein, L., Switalla, S., Prenzler, F., Seehase, S., Pfennig, O., Forster, C., Fieguth, H. et al. 2014. Assessment of immunotoxicity induced by chemicals in human precision-cut lung slices (Pcls). *Toxicol In Vitro* 28:588–99.

Light, W. G. and Wei, E. T. 1977a. Surface charge and asbestos toxicity. *Nature* 265:537–9.

Light, W. G. and Wei, E. T. 1977b. Surface charge and hemolytic activity of asbestos. *Environ Res* 13:135–45.

McNeilly, J. D., Jimenez, L. A., Clay, M. F., Macnee, W., Howe, A., Heal, M. R., Beverland, I. J. et al. 2005. Soluble transition metals in welding fumes cause inflammation via activation of NF-kappaB and AP-1. *Toxicol Lett* 158:152–7.

Moore, V. C., Manney, S., Vellore, A. D. and Burge, P. S. 2009. Occupational asthma to gel flux containing dodecanedioic acid. *Allergy* 64:1099–100.

Morin, J. P., Baste, J. M., Gay, A., Crochemore, C., Corbiere, C. and Monteil, C. 2013. Precision cut lung slices as an efficient tool for *in vitro* lung physio-pharmacotoxicology studies. *Xenobiotica* 43:63–72.

Murphy, F., Poland, C., Duffin, R., Al-Jamal, K., Ali-Boucetta, H. and Nunes, A. 2011. Length-dependent retention of carbon nanotubes in the pleural space of mice initiates sustained inflammation and progressive fibrosis on the parietal pleura. *Am J Pathol* 178:2587–600.

Nagy, A., Steinbruck, A., Gao, J., Doggett, N., Hollingsworth, J. A. and Iyer, R. 2012. Comprehensive analysis of the effects of CdSe quantum dot size, surface charge and functionalization on primary human lung cells. *ACS Nano* 6:4748–62.

Neyt, K. and Lambrecht, B. N. 2013. The role of lung dendritic cell subsets in immunity to respiratory viruses. *Immunol Rev* 255:57–67.

NIOSH. 2011. *Current Intelligence Bulletin 63: Occupational Exposure to Titanium Dioxide*. Atlanta, GA: National Institute for Occupational Safety and Health.

Parker, D. and Prince, A. 2011. Innate immunity in the respiratory epithelium. *Am J Respir Cell Mol Biol* 45:189–201.

Pompeu, Y. A., Stewart, J. D., Mallal, S., Phillips, E., Peters, B. and Ostrov, D. A. 2012. The structural basis of Hla-associated drug hypersensitivity syndromes. *Immunol Rev* 250:158–66.

Pralong, J. A., Seed, M. J., Cartier, A., Agius, R. M. and Labrecque, M. 2012. Is there a place for a computer based asthma hazard prediction model in clinical practice? *Occup Environ Med* 69:771–2.

Renwick, L. C. 2004. Increased inflammation and altered macrophage chemotactic responses caused by two ultrafine particle types. *Occup Environ Med* 61:442–7.

Schinwald, A., Chernova, T. and Donaldson, K. 2012a. Use of silver nanowires to determine thresholds for fibre length-dependent pulmonary inflammation and inhibition of macrophage migration *in vitro*. *Part Fibre Toxicol* 9:47.

Schinwald, A., Murphy, F., Prina-Mello, A., Poland, C., Byrne, F. and Movia, D. 2012b. The threshold length for fiber-induced acute pleural inflammation: Shedding light on the early events in asbestos-induced mesothelioma. *Toxicol Sci* 128:461–70.

Schinwald, A., Murphy, F. A., Jones, A., Macnee, W. and Donaldson, K. 2012c. Graphene-based nanoplatelets: A new risk to the respiratory system as a consequence of their unusual aerodynamic properties. *ACS Nano* 6:736–46.

Schwarze, P. E., Ovrevik, J., Hetland, R. B., Becher, R., Cassee, F. R., Lag, M. et al. 2007. Importance of size and composition of particles for effects on cells *in vitro*. *Inhal Toxicol* 19(Suppl. 1):17–22.

Seed, M. and Agius, R. 2010. Further validation of computer-based prediction of chemical asthma hazard. *Occup Med (Lond)* 60:115–20.

Seed, M. J., Cullinan, P. and Agius, R. M. 2008. Methods for the prediction of low-molecular-weight occupational respiratory sensitizers. *Curr Opin Allergy Clin Immunol* 8:103–9.

Shukla, A., Ramos-Nino, M. and Mossman, B. 2003. Cell signaling and transcription factor activation by asbestos in lung injury and disease. *Int J Biochem Cell Biol* 35:1198–209.

Stanton, M., Layard, M., Tegeris, A., Miller, E., May, M. and Morgan, E. 1981. Relation of particle dimension to carcinogenicity in amphibole asbestoses and other fibrous minerals. *J Natl Cancer Inst* 67:965–75.

Stanton, M. F., Laynard, M., Tegeris, A., Miller, E., May, M. and Kent, E. 1977. Carcinogenicity of fibrous glass: Pleural response in the rat in relation to fiber dimension. *J Natl Cancer Inst* 58:587–603.

Sung, J. H., Ji, J. H., Park, J. D., Yoon, J. U., Kim, D. S., Jeon, K. S., Song, M. Y. et al. 2009. Subchronic inhalation toxicity of silver nanoparticles. *Toxicol Sci* 108:452–61.

Tarkowski, M., Kur, B., Polakowska, E. and Jablonska, E. 2008. Comparative studies of lymph node cell subpopulations and cytokine expression in murine model for testing the potentials of chemicals to induce respiratory sensitization. *Int J Occup Med Environ Health* 21:253–62.

Valavanidis, A., Fiotakis, K. and Vlachogianni, T. 2008. Airborne particulate matter and human health: Toxicological assessment and importance of size and composition of particles for oxidative damage and carcinogenic mechanisms. *J Environ Sci Health C Environ Carcinog Ecotoxicol Rev* 26:339–62.

van der Zande, M., Vandebriel, R. J., Van Doren, E., Kramer, E., Herrera Rivera, Z., Serrano-Rojero, C. S., Gremmer, E. R. et al. 2012. Distribution, elimination and toxicity of silver nanoparticles and silver ions in rats after 28-day oral exposure. *ACS Nano* 6:7427–42.

Vandebriel, R., Callant Cransveld, C., Crommelin, D., Diamant, Z., Glazenburg, B., Joos, G., Kuper, F. et al. 2011. Respiratory sensitization: Advances in assessing the risk of respiratory inflammation and irritation. *Toxicol In Vitro* 25:1251–8.

Veronesi, B., de Haar, C., Lee, L. and Oortgiesen, M. 2002. The surface charge of visible particulate matter predicts biological activation in human bronchial epithelial cells. *Toxicol Appl Pharmacol* 178:144–54.

Virta, R. L. 2002. *Asbestos Geology, Mineralogy, Mining and Uses*, Reston, VA: U.S. Department of the Interior, U.S. Geological Survey.

Yin, L., Dai, S., Clayton, G., Gao, W., Wang, Y., Kappler, J. and Marrack, P. 2013. Recognition of self and altered self by T cells in autoimmunity and allergy. *Protein Cell* 4:8–16.

14 Genetics and Gene–Environment Interactions

William Osmond Charles Cookson

CONTENTS

OVERVIEW

Occupational lung disease results from an exuberant interaction between hostile or toxic environmental factors and the mechanisms that the lung uses to protect itself. Environmental factors are often quantifiable, but the apparatus by which they initiate disease and the host response are often poorly understood.

Genetic and genomic studies of DNA and RNA provide powerful methods for quantifying systematically the elements of host susceptibility. Importantly, the same technologies may also be of value in the discovery of previously occult microbial causes of lung disease.

This chapter will consider the sites of potential actions of genetic effects and then describe the potential application of new genomic technologies to occupational lung diseases, as well as the risk factors that are already known.

Although genomics may identify mechanisms leading to occupational lung disease, the practical use of this information is not straightforward. Even though genetic susceptibilities to occupational agents have been identified, this chapter will also consider why there has been no impetus to apply this knowledge to screening the workforce.

MECHANISMS OF HOST SUSCEPTIBILITY TO OCCUPATIONAL LUNG DISEASE

The airway epithelia must provide a barrier to a hostile environment, yet at the level of the alveoli must be thin enough to allow gasses to diffuse in and out of the blood. In common with all mucosal surfaces, including the bladder (Hilt et al., 2014), the airways are not sterile and contain a conserved microbiota (Hilty et al., 2010). The mucosal epithelium is not passive and orchestrates the interactions between the immune system and luminal contents (Turner, 2009). Host susceptibility to particular occupational exposures may therefore operate at several different levels.

Barriers to Occupational Hazards

The airway mucosa is covered by a layer of a hydrated gel of mucus, formed primarily by secreted mucins known as MUC5AC and MUC5B (Linden et al., 2008). Mucus and the goblet cells that produce it are increased in chronic airway inflammation from causes that include cigarette smoking and occupational dusts. Secretory IgA is the major immunological presence in the mucosa, and may heavily bind commensal bacteria (Pabst, 2012). Epithelial cell damage by mucosal irritants or toxins results in loss of barrier function (Turner, 2009), allowing immune responses to otherwise innocuous commensals or inhaled particles.

Genetic studies have discovered that sequence variants (polymorphisms) in the promoter of the MUC5B gene predispose carriers to idiopathic pulmonary fibrosis (Fingerlin et al., 2013), potentially through modification of the mucin barrier. The polymorphism also predicts the occurrence of fibrosis in the general population (Hunninghake et al., 2013) and is therefore of interest in workers who have developed pneumoconiosis.

Immune Recognition of Occupational Hazards

Mucosal surfaces are sites of innate and adaptive immune regulation (Blease et al., 2000; Cookson, 2004; Turner, 2009). The presence of microbial invasions is detected by pattern recognition receptors (PRRs), which identify pathogen-associated molecular patterns and damage-associated molecular patterns. Toll-like receptors are the most important major PRRs for microbial components, but many others exist (Romani, 2011).

Innate immune responses produce antimicrobial proteins and cytokines that signal the innate and adaptive immune responses. Cell-mediated immunity may be the main adaptive mechanism for defence against infections, including fungi, but antibody responses can also be protective (Blanco and Garcia, 2008).

Adaptive immunity begins with the recognition of foreign antigens, followed by specific T-cell and B-cell responses against the antigen. T cells and B cells develop their immune repertoire in response to exogenous peptides processed by antigen-presenting cells (APCs), such as dendritic cells and macrophages. Human leukocyte antigen (HLA) molecules on APCs offer these peptides in an immune synapse with T-cell and B-cell receptors. In general, HLA class II molecules (DP, DM, DOA, DOB, DQ and DR) present externally derived antigens, while HLA class I molecules (A, B and C) present antigens from within the cell (such as virus proteins). Although HLA molecules are diverse, they do not provide universal binding of all possible antigens. This leads to immune restriction, so that the strength of response to an antigenic stimulus will depend on an individual's HLA type.

Occupational diseases not only result from appropriate responses to inhaled materials, but also follow from hypersensitivity and over-activation of the inflammatory response. Cellular hypersensitivity may be exemplified by the pneumonitis in farmer's lung, whereas humoral IgE-mediated sensitivity is a feature of many forms of occupational asthma.

The temptation in these conditions is to consider that the hypersensitivity is the primary driver of the disease process, but it should not be forgotten that, in order to activate danger signals, the inhaled agents, such as fungal spores or enzymatic proteins, are likely to be causing significant damage in their own right.

Metabolic Responses to Hazards

The lungs contain enzyme systems for xenobiotic metabolism. Phase I enzymes introduce reactive or polar groups into xenobiotics, which may then be conjugated by phase II reactions. Phase I enzymes that are found in the lung include cytochrome P450 iso-enzymes (CYP1A1, CYP1B1, CYP2A6, CYP2B6, CYP2E1 and CYP3A5) (Mace et al., 1998; Castell et al., 2005). Different individuals vary substantially in the level of expression of cytochrome P450 genes (Mace et al., 1998).

Lung cells also express phase II enzymes such as epoxide hydrolase, UGT1A (glucuronyl transferase) and GST-P1 (glutathione S-transferase), which largely act as detoxifying enzymes (Mace et al., 1998; Castell et al., 2005) together with N-acetyl transferase (NAT) families (Mace et al., 1998). NAT2 is a highly polymorphic enzyme with an essential role in the inactivation of arylamines, and it is of interest that individuals with a slow acetylator phenotype are susceptible to arylamine-associated bladder cancer (Johns and Houlston, 2000).

The human respiratory system could significantly and specifically contribute to the activation and metabolism of several environmental pro-carcinogens (Mace et al., 1998), enhancing susceptibility to cancer in some individuals.

Inhaled mutagens directly damage DNA, leading eventually to tumour formation that may be synergised by other carcinogens, most notably tobacco smoke. Many pathways exist for the repair of DNA (Dietlein et al., 2014). Germline mutations or polymorphisms in DNA repair enzymes may become important risk factors for disease, as exemplified by the increased risk of lung cancer in cigarette smokers with hOGG1 (Park et al., 2004) and ERCC2/XPD polymorphisms (Feng et al., 2012), as well as the susceptibility to malignant mesothelioma caused by BAP1 mutations (Testa et al., 2011).

GENETICS AND GENOMICS

Genetic susceptibility to inhaled particles and gasses can operate at many levels, most of which have not been considered in the context of occupational lung diseases. At the same time, The Human Genome Project has driven advances in the technology for discovering not only the structure of an individual's DNA, but also for accessing the functional state of their genome.

DNA Variation

The study of genetics relates variations in DNA to variations in phenotype. DNA variations come in many forms, the most simple and common of which are single-nucleotide polymorphisms (SNPs). Approximately 150 million SNPs had been identified in the promoter variants of the human genome by 2015, and the technologies for identifying these are robust and routinely used with high throughput.

Most SNPs have no impact on genome function. Those SNPs that do alter function may do so directly, by altering the DNA code in order to cause amino acid substitutions or truncations. This type of abnormality may be called a mutation, but there is a grey area of nomenclature between rare mutations and mutations that are common enough (present in >1% of the population) to be known as a SNP.

Studies of common diseases have shown that SNPs often exert deleterious effects by altering the regions that control gene expression, as well as altering the sites that control the splicing of different exons.

Other common forms of variation include insertions and deletions (also known as indels), repeated sequences and rearrangements of DNA segments. These changes may be small or may extend over megabases of DNA.

Genetic recombination—the crossover between chromosomes that occurs during meiosis in sperm and ova—occurs at only a few sites on each chromosome, so large tracts of DNA and SNPs are consistently inherited together and remain together even in the general population. This phenomenon, known as linkage disequilibrium, allows genetic associations to be established to regions of DNA by genome-wide association studies with a few hundred thousand SNPs.

The regions of association (the local extent of linkage disequilibrium) are themselves typically several hundred thousand bases in length, so the actual genes and genetic variants that cause disease from a given locus may not be certain.

Next-generation sequencing describes the technology for sequencing the whole genome of an individual, and full genomic sequencing of multiple subjects is the gold standard for identifying rare mutations. A cheaper alternative is to limit sequencing to the genomic regions that encode for proteins, known as whole-exome sequencing (Biesecker, 2010; Ng et al., 2010).

Bioinformatics and Statistics

Given the facile ability to genotype a million SNPs or to sequence the whole genome in many different individuals, it is often assumed that genetic studies are themselves easy. The reality is different. Even robust SNP associations do not definitively identify causal variants, and there is an onus on complex functional studies to validate any reported association before applying it in a clinical or epidemiological context.

The problems are greater for whole-genome sequencing, which captures all of the genetic variation in an individual. Next-generation sequencing with the Illumina platform (the industry standard at the time of writing) typically produces 10^{8-9} fragments of sequences of a few hundred base pairs, which have to be reassembled with reference to the known human genome. The coverage of different regions may be uneven, and repetitive areas, such as those containing gene families, may be almost impossible to assemble accurately. Functional mutations have to be differentiated from variants that are present in the population, and decisions have to be made as to whether amino acid substitutions that result from mutations are likely to be harmful or benign.

RNA and Transcriptomics

DNA exerts its effects through transcription into RNA, which in turn is translated into the proteins that carry out the functions of cells. It is now technologically straightforward to measure the level of transcription of all human genes at once, either with microarrays or with direct next-generation sequencing of RNA.

The sensitivity and reproducibility of simultaneous measurements of 50,000 transcripts may be extraordinary, but this does not negate the need for carefully designed experiments in order to avoid, in the words of Sydney Brenner, 'low-input, high-throughput, no-output science'. In order to be useful, transcriptomics needs to be applied to the right tissues (often the lung and not peripheral blood), with realistic estimates of effect sizes and power corrected for all possible comparisons.

Epigenetics

Epigenetics describes the changes that affect DNA function without altering the nucleotide sequence. The importance of epigenetics was first realised during studies of X chromosome inactivation in females. In order to match gene expression with the single X chromosome of males, female cells silence one of their X chromosomes. Methylation of DNA side-chains was observed to accompany this silencing, and subsequently methylation of DNA, particularly at sequences rich in CG nucleotides (known as CpG islands), was found to be a general characteristic of inactive genes.

Epigenetic studies can therefore access states of regulation of genome function in particular cells and in response to specific stimuli (Liang and Cookson, 2014). Although there are many epigenetic markers that may be of use in systematic studies, the degree of CpG methylation at multiple sites (loci) across the genome is at the moment most easily applicable to understanding disease. CpG methylation can be measured robustly with microarrays, as well as by whole-genome bisulphite sequencing.

Epigenetic changes are strongly driven by environmental factors, as exemplified by the easy reproducibility of associations with CpG methylation status near the *F2RL3* and *GPR15* genes in current smokers (Breitling et al., 2011; Wan et al., 2012). These epigenetic approaches may well become the tool of choice for investigating workers who are at risk of occupational lung diseases.

THE MICROBIOME

This textbook contains much information about biological agents or organisms that can cause occupational lung disease either by directly damage or invasion or with a component of acute or chronic hypersensitivity. In many circumstances, the identification of the organism is unknown or inferred indirectly.

The term 'microbiome' describes all microorganisms in a particular environment together with their genes and interactions. The assemblage of microorganisms themselves is referred to as the microbiota or microbial community and can include bacteria, archaea, viruses, phage, fungi and other microbial Eukarya. The human microbiota consists of microorganisms that exist upon, within or in close proximity to the human body (Cox et al., 2013). The National Institutes of Health (NIH)-funded Human Microbiome Project has spearheaded methods for creating and interpreting high-throughput data regarding the human microbiome and for making the results available to the scientific community (Human Microbiome Project, 2012).

Of most direct utility is the huge improvement in the detection of microbiota that DNA sequencing provides over microbial cultures. Although most bacteria are not cultivated by standard methods (Staley and Konopka, 1985), the membership of complex microbial communities can be quantified and classified by DNA sequencing of the conserved bacterial 16S rRNA gene (Ahmed et al., 2007; Turnbaugh et al., 2007) and the ITS2 region in fungi (Koljalg et al., 2013).

Mycobacterial species can also be quantified through their 16S rRNA sequences (Dobner et al., 1996), and an example of the utility of 16S sequencing comes from a study of a spatially restricted outbreak of extrinsic allergic bronchiolo-alveolitis in five metal turners working in a small area of an aircraft factory (James et al., 2015). Samples of metal working fluid (MWF) from 33 machines located there and in adjacent areas of the shop floor were taken for blinded microbial community analysis. High levels of MWF contamination by members of the *Mycobacterium* genus were detected in samples from machines located in the area of the outbreak. DNA sequencing and phylogenetic analysis revealed *Mycobacterium avium* to be the dominant mycobacterial species present. This investigation shows that molecular microbial community profiling methods may be used as both a preventative monitoring method as well as a forensic tool (James et al., 2015).

The Human Microbiome Project encompasses many other tools, including 'metagenomics', in which complex microbial communities are subjected to extraction of DNA and brute force next-generation sequencing that is analysed in a way that is analogous to the study of a single genome (Handelsman et al., 1998). In the occupational context, these tools might be useful for investigating the appearance of virulence factors or the induction or toxin-inducing metabolic pathways in complex microbial mixtures either from the environment or in the lungs of workers who are at risk of disease.

KNOWN GENETIC SUSCEPTIBILITIES

The number of recognised genetic associations with occupational lung disease is surprisingly limited. Successful studies have mainly come from candidate gene studies that performed HLA typing of subjects with sensitivity to small molecules.

Chronic beryllium disease is caused by beryllium exposure in and, on occasion, outside of the workplace. It is characterised by granulomatous inflammation in the lungs (Fontenot and Maier, 2005). Susceptibility has been positively associated with HLA-DPB1*0201 and negatively associated with HLA-DPB1*0401, and it has been suggested that susceptibility is structurally conferred by HLA-DP alleles possessing a glutamic acid at the 69th position (Glu^{69}) of the β-chain (Richeldi et al., 1993).

Genetic influences on occupational asthma have been reviewed by Newman Taylor (Taylor, 2001). Most reported studies of HLA relationships have been of patients or populations exposed to low-molecular-weight chemicals.

In workers with acid anhydride exposures, positive associations have been found between HLA-DR3 and the presence of a specific IgE antibody to albumin conjugates of trimellitic anhydride (TMA), but not to the closely related phthalic anhydride (Young et al., 1995).

HLA associations have been reported with isocyanate-induced asthma (Bignon et al., 1994; Balboni et al., 1996; Jones et al., 2004) and suggest a consistent positive association with HLA-DQB*0503 and an inverse relationship with HLA-DQB*0501 (Mapp et al., 1997).

The literature also contains single reports of HLA-DR3 associations with positive skin-prick tests to ammonium hexachloroplatinate (Newman Taylor et al., 1999) and between HLA DQB1*0603 and DQB1*0302 alleles and asthma induced by western red cedar in Canadian sawmill workers (Horne et al., 2000).

HLA associations may also be found with more complex molecules. In the workplace, laboratory animal allergy (particularly rat and mouse) is a common occupational health problem. Robust association has been demonstrated between HLA-DR7 and symptomatic sensitisation to lipocalins produced by laboratory rats (Jeal et al., 2003). HLA associations have also been observed with occupational sensitivity to cow dander allergen Bos d 2 (Kauppinen et al., 2012).

These results perhaps do not do more than show that inherited HLA variation restricts an individual's ability to respond to particular small molecules. It is of interest that HLA associations to allergens in the non-industrial setting have long been recognised (Marsh et al., 1982; Hizawa et al., 1998; Moffatt et al., 2001) and that the MHC region appears to be a major asthma-susceptibility locus in genome-wide association studies (Moffatt et al., 2010), even in non-atopic subjects.

The major histocompatibility complex (MHC) is a highly complex region with extended linkage disequilibrium encompassing many genes of immune importance, and drawing a clear therapeutic message from HLA associations has been unrewarding, even in autoimmune diseases such as type I diabetes, in which tens of thousands of subjects have been studied (Thomson et al., 2007). Desensitisation is a possible therapy for occupational hypersensitivity to animal danders (Kinnunen et al., 2007).

Investigation of other candidate genes in the setting of occupational lung disease is always going to be difficult, at least because improved standards of industrial hygiene limit the numbers of workers who develop illnesses. A systemic genome-wide association study has been attempted for occupational asthma (Moffatt et al., 2010), but perhaps because of a lack of power, this study did not find any distinctive genetic effects.

GENE–ENVIRONMENT INTERACTIONS

Gene–environment interactions describe the joint influence of genetic and environmental factors on the risk of developing a human disease, and most of the genetic association studies described above do not actually fulfil this criterion. An exception may be the platinum salt allergy study described above, which suggested that HLA-DR3 susceptibility was more marked in workers with low exposure compared to those with high exposure (Newman Taylor et al., 1999).

Gene–environment interactions can be described by using different models that take into account the various ways in which genetic effects might be modified by environmental exposures (Hunter, 2005). Possible models include dominant or recessive genetic effects and whether interactions behave additively or multiplicatively. The inclusion of exposure information in association models can only be helpful if rigorous testing of genetic susceptibility to environmental hazards is to be carried out, but the numbers required for statistical power may be in the thousands (Hunter, 2005).

RISK

Despite the presence of some substantial risks (e.g. there is an odds ratio of approximately 10 for the risk of developing pulmonary berylliosis in individuals with HLA-DPB1-Glu^{69}), there has been little impetus to apply genetic screening in the workplace in part because of its low predictive value.

Ethics

The ethical considerations that have been used to justify this nihilism have been reviewed by Christiani et al. (2008). They conclude that it is difficult to evaluate the psychological and social impacts of genetic testing, especially when no specific interventions are available for carriers of the 'risk' alleles; that genetic screening assays may not have 100% sensitivity and/or specificity; that genetic traits can relate differently to different diseases; that the use of genetic screening in the workplace may lead to an increased likelihood of invasion of the privacy and confidentiality of workers; that most genetic variations distribute differently in different ethnic and racial groups and genetic screening has the potential for racial discrimination; and that concentrating on workers who are 'at risk' results in lost opportunities to prevent disease in other workers.

Genetic Risks in Populations

Genetic risk is usually considered in the context of the individual, but it should be recognised that most public health measures do not operate in this way. Patients with high blood cholesterols, for example, are routinely offered statins on the basis of population studies, even though the risk to the individual is very difficult to define.

Population-attributable risk or fraction (PARF) is widely used in order to estimate the burden of a risk factor in population surveys. When applied to genetic studies, the PARF estimates the fraction of cases that would not occur if no one in the population carried the risk allele (Kraft et al., 2009).

Use of the PARF as a measure of association does not depend on the identification of the causal allele and encapsulates not just the marginal (gene-only) association, but also any gene–environment or gene–gene interactions (Hadley and Strachan, 2009).

Genetic associations can be discovered when the underlying susceptibility alleles are common (Risch, 2000). A substantial PARF in a population of workers who are at risk would therefore encourage further interventions in order to prevent disease, even if the risk to an individual worker might be low or poorly defined.

Risk to Individuals

Because of limited study sizes, existing information on occupational lung disease has usually captured genetic variants with high per-allele odds ratios (Hemminki and Bermejo, 2007). The application of this knowledge to workers who are at risk is not widely practiced because of the poor sensitivity and specificity of particular tests and their reliability in workforces of different ancestries (Vineis et al., 2001). This has been exemplified in the negative analysis of the value of testing HLA-DPB1-Glu^{69} marker in beryllium workers (Silver and Sharp, 2006). These same issues apply to pharmacogenetic tests for adverse drug reactions, which have similarly failed to have been as widely adopted as anticipated (Goldstein et al., 2003).

The principles that have guided the consensus approach to individual risk may rapidly become outdated in a world where 'personal genomics' and genome sequencing is widely available (Blow, 2007) and routinely sold to individuals through companies such as 23andMe. It is entirely feasible that a future driver of genetic testing may come from lawsuits brought by individuals with occupational disease.

SUMMARY

It appears currently that genetic studies and their findings have had minimal impacts on the management of occupational lung diseases. This may be because investigations are often constrained by the small numbers of individuals who develop disease in any given workforce, because of a general unease about genetic screening of the workforce or because genetics only detects biological processes in which natural variation plays a part.

This state of play should be reconsidered in the light of the technological changes that are transforming human genomics.

Classical genetic approaches, in which DNA variants are matched to phenotype, will continue to be constrained by the numbers of subjects. However, genetic studies of common diseases have become successful through the embracing of international collaboration in order to build effective study sizes. Realistic cost analyses of population-attributable risks in occupational lung diseases may serve as motivators of such efforts.

Rare genetic mutations may underlie severe reactions in exposed individuals. Next-generation sequencing of the whole genomes of individuals with idiosyncratic severe reactions is likely to be informative for the patient as well as the scientific community.

Beyond genetic sequences, genomic studies of global gene expression or epigenetic changes in methylation provide flexible tools for discovering the pathways that underlie particular occupational diseases. Using these technologies, studies can encompass the full range of cells and tissues that are entrained in a disease process.

In this context, it is worth noting that occupational lung diseases can be of great value in understanding common lung diseases such as asthma, because healthy individuals can be investigated before exposure, during the prodrome and after disease has appeared. Epigenetic changes in peripheral blood appear to be strongly and reproducibly driven by environmental factors and are of particular interest.

Finally, bacteria, mycobacteria and fungi abound in the environment, and any liquid or biological powder that is aerosolised is a potential source of pulmonary infection and hypersensitivity. DNA sequencing and microbiomics are likely to transform the monitoring of workplaces for these hazards.

REFERENCES

Ahmed, S., Macfarlane, G. T., Fite, A., McBain, A. J., Gilbert, P. and Macfarlane, S. 2007. Mucosa-associated bacterial diversity in relation to human terminal ileum and colonic biopsy samples. *Appl Environ Microbiol* 73:7435–42.

Balboni, A., Baricordi, O. R., Fabbri, L. M., Gandini, E., Ciaccia, A. and Mapp, C. E. 1996. Association between toluene diisocyanate-induced asthma and DQB1 markers: A possible role for aspartic acid at position 57. *Eur Respir J* 9:207–10.

Biesecker, L. G. 2010. Exome sequencing makes medical genomics a reality. *Nat Genet* 42:13–4.

Bignon, J. S., Aron, Y., Ju, L. Y., Kopferschmitt, M. C., Garnier, R., Mapp, C., Fabbri, L. M. et al. 1994. HLA class II alleles in isocyanate-induced asthma. *Am J Respir Crit Care Med* 149:71–5.

Blanco, J. L. and Garcia, M. E. 2008. Immune response to fungal infections. *Vet Immunol Immunopathol* 125:47–70.

Blease, K., Lukacs, N. W., Hogaboam, C. M. and Kunkel, S. L. 2000. Chemokines and their role in airway hyperreactivity. *Respir Res* 1:54–61.

Blow, N. 2007. Genomics: The personal side of genomics. *Nature* 449:627–30.

Breitling, L. P., Yang, R., Korn, B., Burwinkel, B. and Brenner, H. 2011. Tobacco-smoking-related differential DNA methylation: 27K discovery and replication. *Am J Hum Genet* 88:450–7.

Castell, J. V., Donato, M. T. and Gomez-Lechon, M. J. 2005. Metabolism and bioactivation of toxicants in the lung. The *in vitro* cellular approach. *Exp Toxicol Pathol* 57(Suppl. 1):189–204.

Christiani, D. C., Mehta, A. J. and Yu, C. L. 2008. Genetic susceptibility to occupational exposures. *Occup Environ Med* 65:430–6; quiz 436, 397.

Cookson, W. 2004. The immunogenetics of asthma and eczema: A new focus on the epithelium. *Nat Rev Immunol* 4:978–88.

Cox, M. J., Cookson, W. O. and Moffatt, M. F. 2013. Sequencing the human microbiome in health and disease. *Hum Mol Genet* 22:R88–94.

Dietlein, F., Thelen, L. and Reinhardt, H. C. 2014. Cancer-specific defects in DNA repair pathways as targets for personalized therapeutic approaches. *Trends Genet* 30:326–39.

Dobner, P., Feldmann, K., Rifai, M., Loscher, T. and Rinder, H. 1996. Rapid identification of mycobacterial species by PCR amplification of hypervariable 16S rRNA gene promoter region. *J Clin Microbiol* 34:866–9.

Feng, Z., Ni, Y., Dong, W., Shen, H. and Du, J. 2012. Association of ERCC2/XPD polymorphisms and interaction with tobacco smoking in lung cancer susceptibility: A systemic review and meta-analysis. *Mol Biol Rep* 39:57–69.

Fingerlin, T. E., Murphy, E., Zhang, W., Peljto, A. L., Brown, K. K., Steele, M. P., Loyd, J. E. et al. 2013. Genome-wide association study identifies multiple susceptibility loci for pulmonary fibrosis. *Nat Genet* 45:613–20.

Fontenot, A. P. and Maier, L. A. 2005. Genetic susceptibility and immune-mediated destruction in beryllium-induced disease. *Trends Immunol* 26:543–9.

Goldstein, D. B., Tate, S. K. and Sisodiya, S. M. 2003. Pharmacogenetics goes genomic. *Nat Rev Genet* 4:937–47.

Hadley, D. and Strachan, D. P. 2009. Inference of disease associations with unmeasured genetic variants by combining results from genome-wide association studies with linkage disequilibrium patterns in a reference data set. *BMC Proc* 3(Suppl. 7):S55.

Handelsman, J., Rondon, M. R., Brady, S. F., Clardy, J. and Goodman, R. M. 1998. Molecular biological access to the chemistry of unknown soil microbes: A new frontier for natural products. *Chem Biol* 5:R245–9.

Hemminki, K. and Bermejo, J. L. 2007. Constraints for genetic association studies imposed by attributable fraction and familial risk. *Carcinogenesis* 28:648–56.

Hilt, E. E., McKinley, K., Pearce, M. M., Rosenfeld, A. B., Zilliox, M. J., Mueller, E. R., Brubaker, L. et al. 2014. Urine is not sterile: Use of enhanced urine culture techniques to detect resident bacterial flora in the adult female bladder. *J Clin Microbiol* 52:871–6.

Hilty, M., Burke, C., Pedro, H., Cardenas, P., Bush, A., Bossley, C., Davies, J. et al. 2010. Disordered microbial communities in asthmatic airways. *PLoS One* 5:e8578.

Hizawa, N., Freidhoff, L., Chiu, Y., Ehrlich, E., Luehr, C., Anderson, J., Duffy, D. et al. 1998. Genetic regulation of *Dermatophagoides pteronyssinus*-specific IgE responsiveness: A genome-wide multipoint linkage analysis in families recruited through 2 asthmatic sibs. Collaborative Study on the Genetics of Asthma (CSGA). *J Allergy Clin Immunol* 102:436–42.

Horne, C., Quintana, P. J., Keown, P. A., Dimich-Ward, H. and Chan-Yeung, M. 2000. Distribution of DRB1 and DQB1 HLA class II alleles in occupational asthma due to western red cedar. *Eur Respir J* 15:911–4.

Human Microbiome Project Consortium. 2012. A framework for human microbiome research. *Nature* 486:215–21.

Hunninghake, G. M., Hatabu, H., Okajima, Y., Gao, W., Dupuis, J., Latourelle, J. C., Nishino, M. et al. 2013. MUC5B promoter polymorphism and interstitial lung abnormalities. *N Engl J Med* 368:2192–200.

Hunter, D. J. 2005. Gene–environment interactions in human diseases. *Nat Rev Genet* 6:287–98.

James, P. L., Cannon, J., Crawford, L., D'Souza, E., Barber, C., Cowman, S., Cookson, W. O. et al. Molecular detection of *Mycobacterium avium* in aerosolised metal working fluid is linked to a localised outbreak of extrinsic allergic alveolitis in factory workers. *American Thoracic Society Annual Conference 2015*, Denver, Colorado. American Thoracic Society, A2578.

Jeal, H., Draper, A., Jones, M., Harris, J., Welsh, K., Taylor, A. N. and Cullinan, P. 2003. HLA associations with occupational sensitization to rat lipocalin allergens: A model for other animal allergies? *J Allergy Clin Immunol* 111:795–9.

Johns, L. E. and Houlston, R. S. 2000. N-acetyl transferase-2 and bladder cancer risk: A meta-analysis. *Environ Mol Mutagen* 36:221–7.

Jones, M. G., Nielsen, J., Welch, J., Harris, J., Welinder, H., Bensryd, I., Skerfving, S. et al. 2004. Association of HLA-DQ5 and HLA-DR1 with sensitization to organic acid anhydrides. *Clin Exp Allergy* 34:812–6.

Kauppinen, A., Perasaari, J., Taivainen, A., Kinnunen, T., Saarelainen, S., Rytkonen-Nissinen, M., Jeal, H. et al. 2012. Association of HLA class II alleles with sensitization to cow dander Bos d 2, an important occupational allergen. *Immunobiology* 217:8–12.

Kinnunen, T., Jutila, K., Kwok, W. W., Rytkonen-Nissinen, M., Immonen, A., Saarelainen, S., Narvanen, A. et al. 2007. Potential of an altered peptide ligand of lipocalin allergen Bos d 2 for peptide immunotherapy. *J Allergy Clin Immunol* 119:965–72.

Koljalg, U., Nilsson, R. H., Abarenkov, K., Tedersoo, L., Taylor, A. F., Bahram, M., Bates, S. T. et al. 2013. Towards a unified paradigm for sequence-based identification of fungi. *Mol Ecol* 22:5271–7.

Kraft, P., Wacholder, S., Cornelis, M. C., Hu, F. B., Hayes, R. B., Thomas, G., Hoover, R. et al. 2009. Beyond odds ratios—Communicating disease risk based on genetic profiles. *Nat Rev Genet* 10:264–9.

Liang, L. and Cookson, W. O. 2014. Grasping nettles: Cellular heterogeneity and other confounders in epigenome-wide association studies. *Hum Mol Genet* 23:R83–8.

Linden, S. K., Sutton, P., Karlsson, N. G., Korolik, V. and McGuckin, M. A. 2008. Mucins in the mucosal barrier to infection. *Mucosal Immunol* 1:183–97.

Mace, K., Bowman, E. D., Vautravers, P., Shields, P. G., Harris, C. C. and Pfeifer, A. M. 1998. Characterisation of xenobiotic-metabolising enzyme expression in human bronchial mucosa and peripheral lung tissues. *Eur J Cancer* 34:914–20.

Mapp, C. E., Balboni, A., Baricordi, R. and Fabbri, L. M. 1997. Human leukocyte antigen associations in occupational asthma induced by isocyanates. *Am J Respir Crit Care Med* 156:S139–43.

Marsh, D. G., Hsu, S. H., Roebber, M., Ehrlich-Kautzky, E., Freidhoff, L. R., Meyers, D. A., Pollard, M. K. et al. 1982. HLA-Dw2: A genetic marker for human immune response to short ragweed pollen allergen Ra5. I. Response resulting primarily from natural antigenic exposure. *J Exp Med* 155:1439–51.

Moffatt, M. F., Gut, I. G., Demenais, F., Strachan, D. P., Bouzigon, E., Heath, S., Von Mutius, E. et al. 2010. A large-scale, consortium-based genomewide association study of asthma. *N Engl J Med* 363:1211–21.

Moffatt, M. F., Schou, C., Faux, J. A., Abecasis, G. R., James, A., Musk, A. W. and Cookson, W. O. 2001. Association between quantitative traits underlying asthma and the HLA- DRB1 locus in a family-based population sample. *Eur J Hum Genet* 9:341–6.

Newman Taylor, A. J., Cullinan, P., Lympany, P. A., Harris, J. M., Dowdeswell, R. J. and Du Bois, R. M. 1999. Interaction of HLA phenotype and exposure intensity in sensitization to complex platinum salts. *Am J Respir Crit Care Med* 160:435–8.

Ng, S. B., Buckingham, K. J., Lee, C., Bigham, A. W., Tabor, H. K., Dent, K. M., Huff, C. D. et al. 2010. Exome sequencing identifies the cause of a Mendelian disorder. *Nat Genet* 42:30–5.

Pabst, O. 2012. New concepts in the generation and functions of IgA. *Nat Rev Immunol* 12:821–32.

Park, J., Chen, L., Tockman, M. S., Elahi, A. and Lazarus, P. 2004. The human 8-oxoguanine DNA N-glycosylase 1 (hOGG1) DNA repair enzyme and its association with lung cancer risk. *Pharmacogenetics* 14:103–9.

Richeldi, L., Sorrentino, R. and Saltini, C. 1993. HLA-DPB1 glutamate 69: A genetic marker of beryllium disease. *Science* 262:242–4.

Risch, N. J. 2000. Searching for genetic determinants in the new millennium. *Nature* 405:847–56.

Romani, L. 2011. Immunity to fungal infections. *Nat Rev Immunol* 11:275–88.

Silver, K. and Sharp, R. R. 2006. Ethical considerations in testing workers for the -Glu^{69} marker of genetic susceptibility to chronic beryllium disease. *J Occup Environ Med* 48:434–43.

Staley, J. T. and Konopka, A. 1985. Measurement of *in situ* activities of nonphotosynthetic microorganisms in aquatic and terrestrial habitats. *Annu Rev Microbiol* 39:321–46.

Taylor, A. N. 2001. Role of human leukocyte antigen phenotype and exposure in development of occupational asthma. *Curr Opin Allergy Clin Immunol* 1:157–61.

Testa, J. R., Cheung, M., Pei, J., Below, J. E., Tan, Y., Sementino, E., Cox, N. J. et al. 2011. Germline BAP1 mutations predispose to malignant mesothelioma. *Nat Genet* 43:1022–5.

Thomson, G., Valdes, A. M., Noble, J. A., Kockum, I., Grote, M. N., Najman, J., Erlich, H. A. et al. 2007. Relative predispositional effects of HLA class II DRB1–DQB1 haplotypes and genotypes on type 1 diabetes: A meta-analysis. *Tissue Antigens* 70:110–27.

Turnbaugh, P. J., Ley, R. E., Hamady, M., Fraser-Liggett, C. M., Knight, R. and Gordon, J. I. 2007. The Human Microbiome Project. *Nature* 449:804–10.

Turner, J. R. 2009. Intestinal mucosal barrier function in health and disease. *Nat Rev Immunol* 9:799–809.

Vineis, P., Schulte, P. and McMichael, A. J. 2001. Misconceptions about the use of genetic tests in populations. *Lancet* 357:709–12.

Wan, E. S., Qiu, W., Baccarelli, A., Carey, V. J., Bacherman, H., Rennard, S. I., Agusti, A. et al. 2012. Cigarette smoking behaviors and time since quitting are associated with differential DNA methylation across the human genome. *Hum Mol Genet* 21:3073–82.

Young, R. P., Barker, R. D., Pile, K. D., Cookson, W. O. and Taylor, A. J. 1995. The association of HLA-DR3 with specific IgE to inhaled acid anhydrides. *Am J Respir Crit Care Med* 151:219–21.

15 Respiratory Health Surveillance in the Workplace

Paul Cullinan and Joanna Szram

CONTENTS

PRINCIPLES AND DEFINITIONS

There is much—perhaps too much—discussion of the term 'surveillance' and of its distinction from related terms such as (health) 'screening' or 'health assessment' (Wagner, 1996). The arguments may usefully be circumvented by the application of two principles:

- That the chief purpose of a workplace surveillance programme should be the primary prevention of occupational disease even if it is, in part, enacted through measures that are more properly described as secondary prevention
- That any workplace programme that includes ongoing health surveillance should always incorporate ongoing hazard surveillance in the same workplace

Together, these principles should form the basis of a programme that is focused, effective, fair and conducive to a 'virtuous' circle (Figure 15.1) akin to that of good clinical audit. The recognition that an occupational disease has occurred indicates that exposure controls have failed and that further investigation is required in order to prevent future cases. Conversely, failure to adhere to these principles threatens to reduce workplace surveillance to simple 'case finding', and is probably responsible for much of the cynicism among employees, employers and even some occupational health practitioners, in which much surveillance is held.

These general principles apply particularly to occupational respiratory disease, in which surveillance is widely practised. The focus of this chapter, notwithstanding the second of the principles above, is ongoing, systematic, workplace 'health' surveillance for occupational respiratory diseases; other, broader forms of surveillance, such as regional schemes of disease notification, the inclusion of occupation on death certificates or the monitoring of sentinel events, are covered in Chapter 8. Workplace surveillance is appropriate in circumstances and for diseases where there is an established relationship between exposure and risk, but where it is not practically possible to control hazardous exposures to a level at which there is no risk, or where the exposure–risk relationship is poorly understood or is one in which there is no safe threshold. Important in the second category are diseases arising from allergic sensitisation (notably occupational asthma [OA]) and cancers. In these circumstances, many

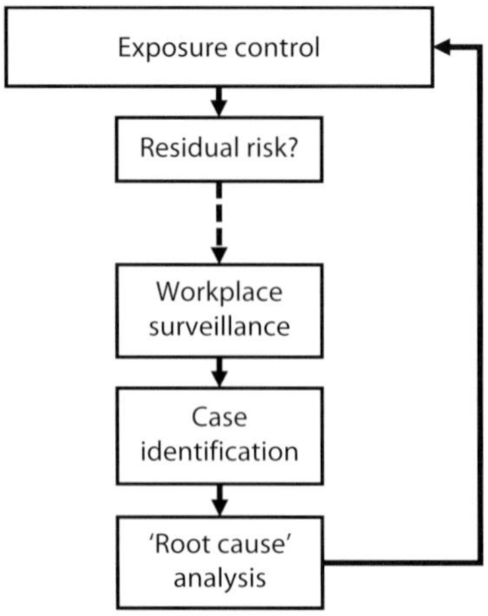

FIGURE 15.1 The inter-relationships between workplace surveillance and exposure control.

national regulatory bodies have drawn up lists of diseases or activities for which workplace surveillance is mandatory and sometimes, such as for asbestos removal work in the European Union, statutory.

A sub-category of health surveillance is preplacement 'screening', a procedure that in many jurisdictions is regulated under equality legislation. Its intended purpose is to identify, prior to exposure, individuals who may be especially susceptible or vulnerable to a workplace risk. In some circumstances the justification may be clear, even if it is still contentious; examples would include enquiry of a new employee who is hired to work as a baker as to whether they have baker's asthma acquired in a previous job, or of silicosis in an applicant for work as a stonemason. These examples relate to *existing* occupational disease and the risks from further exposure to the causative agent. Pre-employment screening for disease *susceptibility*, for traits that increase the risk of developing an occupational respiratory disease or for heightened 'vulnerability' (the extra burden that the development of an occupational disease would place on an individual who is already sick)* is more fraught with ethical—and often legal— difficulties, not least because, for the former especially, those factors that heighten individual risk tend to have low predictive power and/or are common in the population and are thus inefficient discriminatory instruments. Even where the predictive power of a susceptibility marker is higher, as is the case for Glu_{69} in chronic beryllium disease (CBD), such schemes tend to founder in a quagmire of ethical, moral and legal dispute (Silver and Sharp, 2006; Christiani et al., 2008).

* Such as one with constitutional asthma that is difficult to control who seeks work where there is a risk of OA.

All, of course, fall foul of the principle that a workplace should be made fit for all of its workers, rather than the other way around.

Similarly complex are the ethical issues inherent to ongoing health surveillance (Szram and Cullinan, 2013), since participation may be a condition of employment and thus technically involuntary. If, as above, a tenet of workplace surveillance is the primary prevention of disease, then a system that includes the identification of early cases (secondary prevention) in order to achieve this may be considered unjust to and by those who are identified in this way. Further, if a purpose of ongoing health surveillance is to identify individual workers who will be harmed by further exposure and consequently removed from or otherwise limited at their job, then it is manifest that such identification should be highly accurate, but this may be difficult to achieve.

LIMITATIONS OF WORKPLACE SURVEILLANCE

With some exceptions, workplace health surveillance is designed not to diagnose occupational disease, but to identify suggestive signals; confirmation, or otherwise, is subsequently made through more complex enquiry, which generally is not feasible across large populations of workers with (it is hoped) low rates of disease. Surveillance is only appropriate where there is an identifiable disease that may arise from the specific work activity, where there are valid techniques for its detection and—more arguably—where detection of disease leads to an intervention that will benefit the individual.

It follows that the techniques used should have high discriminant properties in both sensitivity and specificity in order to minimise the risks of false-negative and false-positive identifications, respectively. In practice, this is rarely realised, since one of these desirable features is usually achieved at the expense of the other. While it may be thought that tests of high sensitivity—likely to detect all or most possible cases—are to be preferred, this is not necessarily the case. A programme that identifies a high proportion of employees who subsequently turn out not to have the disease under scrutiny may rapidly lose its credibility with both employees and their employers.

More pragmatically, while techniques of high predictive value are clearly preferable, these too may be difficult to achieve. Many non-specific instruments used in workplace respiratory surveillance, including symptoms questionnaires and some techniques of lung function measurement, were devised and their interpretations developed in populations with rates (and ranges) of disease that are higher than in most occupational settings. Their (positive) predictive performance will thus be lower, and sometimes far lower, when they are applied in a workplace that is populated by individuals who are generally fitter and healthier than average.

The value of surveillance is more obvious for respiratory diseases of short or moderate latency, since these are more likely to be detectable during employment; the prime example is OA, but others include CBD and some forms of simple silicosis. Surveillance for diseases of moderate latency, such as many forms of pneumoconiosis, can be very difficult to organise in workforces where turnover is high; the construction industry is a good example of this. Ongoing in-employment health surveillance for diseases of very long latency is of questionable value, despite it being mandated in some jurisdictions (European Agency for Safety and Health at Work, 2009). In these instances, exposure monitoring and control, individually and collectively, are more relevant. The issue of whether post-employment surveillance for these conditions should be instituted—and who should be responsible for it—is contentious. An important example of such an approach is that of the lifelong surveillance in several European and other countries of workers who have been previously exposed to asbestos (Carton et al., 2011).

The organisation and implementation of surveillance generally fall to an occupational health service. Broadly, such services are either internal ('in-house') or provided by an external contractor; the difference has important implications. The former—and currently rarer—model has the potential advantage of a close relationship with workplace safety professionals and of more readily integrating surveillance with other elements of a primary preventative strategy. It also, in most settings, allows for readier detection of 'interval' disease that becomes apparent between two rounds of surveillance. More pragmatically, in-house services may more readily be able to follow workers with 'surveillance failure', such as those with inadequate or omitted spirometry and those who require further investigation. These are generally more difficult when occupational health is provided from a distance. Mackie, in an analysis of OA surveillance provided to the motor vehicle repair industry by an external contractor, provides a clear example of how such a system may fail at almost every step (Mackie, 2008) and of the importance of clear lines of effective communication with those who will carry out further diagnostic investigations. Finally, when surveillance is provided on a fee-for-service principle, it may have a distorting effect on which techniques are included, an explanation perhaps of the continuing use of routine spirometry in the surveillance of OA when it is demonstrably inefficient (Nicholson et al., 2010).

APPLICATIONS OF WORKPLACE SCREENING

The use of health screening at the point of employment or placement has been discussed above. There is a broader issue of screening for respiratory 'fitness to work', especially for jobs that are considered to be safety critical, such as commercial diving, firefighting, military service or, increasingly, construction. Here is not the place for a detailed discussion on this topic, since most sectors or jurisdictions have their own specific guidance and more general advice is available (Cullinan, 2011; Palmer et al., 2013). Briefly, however, the issue is not a simple one, since tests of respiratory fitness are often crude predictors of performance or are difficult to perform in an occupational health setting, or both.

Respiratory diseases for which ongoing health surveillance is commonly practised include:

- Occupational or other work-related asthma
- Silicosis and other consequences of work with respirable crystalline silica
- Coal workers' and other miners' pneumoconiosis
- CBD
- Diseases arising from work with chromates, cadmium fume, hard metals, indium–tin oxide, etc.

The rationale for these is more or less clear, since for each there is an established, exposure-related risk, the disease can demonstrably be determined to be of occupational origin at an individual level, most or at least some cases can be expected to arise during employment and there is evidence (or at any rate a well-founded belief) that early identification is of benefit to the individual.

Less specifically, and more contentiously, surveillance is also offered to a wide variety of workforces as a means of 'monitoring' their respiratory health. Such surveillance frequently includes the use of repeated spirometry, even when the evidence that lung function is materially diminished by such work is uncertain. Groups to whom this applies often include welders, construction workers (broadly defined), transport drivers and even those with exposure to unspecified 'vapours, dusts or fumes'. Lung function that is declining at a rate faster than is considered normal is a non-specific finding with several non-occupational causes, notably cigarette smoking. Attribution to workplace exposure(s) at an individual level is essentially impossible—although easier perhaps in otherwise well non-smokers—making its surveillance more properly a means of monitoring exposure controls in the workplace.

INSTRUMENTS OF WORKPLACE RESPIRATORY SURVEILLANCE

Questionnaires

Almost all respiratory surveillance programmes include a symptoms questionnaire that is usually self-completed. As a general principle, these questionnaires should – but rarely do—contain an explicit statement of the consequences of reporting symptoms; without this, the employee is put in a manifestly inequitable position. A good example is the questionnaire suggested by the UK's Health and Safety Executive (HSE) (Health and Safety Executive, 2010) for use in the surveillance of workplace asthma, which is clearly prefaced by such a statement (see Figure 15.2).

As stated earlier, questionnaires are usually adapted from ones developed in non-working populations, where their diagnostic performance may be very different. Their application to a workforce under surveillance may be unsatisfactory. In a survey of shipyard workers in Newcastle, England, responses to a questionnaire that was designed to detect current asthma were compared with individual measurements of non-specific bronchial reactivity (Stenton et al., 1993). In this way, the questionnaire was shown to have very low sensitivity (28%); its specificity was higher (73%), but the positive predictive value was poor (25%), despite a 24% prevalence of bronchial hyper-reactivity.

Some have argued that surveillance for asthma in the workplace should not be limited to classical 'OA', but rather to any types of the disease, related to work or otherwise (Wagner and Wegman, 1998). The HSE questionnaire mentioned above would be suitable for this purpose, but most surveillance has a more limited scope. There are no (English-language) questionnaires designed specifically and validated robustly for identifying *occupational* (or even work-related) asthma (Miller et al., 2003), and most rely on a series of ad hoc questions that are intended to identify symptoms that are temporally related to periods at work. A further difficulty lies in the likelihood that some workers may provide deliberately misleading (negative) responses, a behaviour that is presumably absent in the general populations in which questionnaires are usually validated. A comparison, for example, of responses from supermarket bakers to their occupational surveillance with those to identical questions posed by an external research team with a guarantee of confidentiality (Brant et al., 2005) indicated a threefold deficit in positive responses to the former. The result is a further reduction in the sensitivity of surveillance. This contrast was not present in a study of similar design set in a UK animal research facility (Allan et al., 2010), although interpretation of this finding must be tempered by a low response (60%) to the confidential survey. The apparent difference may reflect a greater sense of job security in university-employed scientists than in commercial bakers. To what extent, if any, workers report symptoms that they do *not* have—so reducing the specificity of a questionnaire—is unknown, but it is presumably small.

Further advice will be required from the company occupational health adviser if any yes box is ticked.

Since starting your present job have you had any of the following symptoms either at work or at home? (Do not include isolated colds, sore throats or flu.)

(a)	Recurring soreness of or watering of eyes	Yes ☐ No ☐
(b)	Recurring blocked or running nose	Yes ☐ No ☐
(c)	Bouts of coughing	Yes ☐ No ☐
(d)	Chest tightness	Yes ☐ No ☐
(e)	Wheeze	Yes ☐ No ☐
(f)	Breathlessness	Yes ☐ No ☐
(g)	Have you consulted your doctor about chest problems since the last questionnaire?	Yes ☐ No ☐

FIGURE 15.2 Questionnaire used in surveillance for work-related asthma in which the consequences of reported symptoms are clearly stated (Health and Safety Executive. 2010. Health questionnaire for on-going surveillance of people potentially exposed to substances that can cause occupational asthma. Available at: http://www.hse.gov.uk/asthma/samplequest3.pdf.)

Questions used in the surveillance of other respiratory diseases such as silicosis, CBD and other forms of pneumoconiosis suffer from similar deficits. They too are adapted from instruments that are designed and tested to detect non-occupational diseases in non-occupational settings, and probably have both low sensitivity and predictive value. It is not uncommon, for example, for young and otherwise fit men to develop extensive radiological evidence of silicosis while remaining, in their view, asymptomatic.

This somewhat unpromising picture should not deter the use of questionnaires in workplace respiratory surveillance. Rather, it should temper their interpretation and help to inform the points at which further action is required, depending on the sensitivity and specificity that is deemed appropriate to a particular setting.

Lung Function Testing

For better or worse, measurement of lung function is included in most programmes of occupational respiratory surveillance. It almost always takes the form of spirometry, usually—but not universally—carried out in the workplace and only rarely with direct reference to a bronchodilator, since most consider this difficult to organise in this setting. Spirometry is covered in detail in Chapter 4 and only two issues will be emphasised here. The first is that it is an insensitive indicator of disease in the more distal parts of the bronchial tree and it may appear and remain 'normal' despite fairly extensive and progressive small airways disease. Second, while it is not especially difficult to conduct spirometry, it can be difficult to conduct it well, and this is particularly so with consistency over large populations and long periods of time.

There are plenty of guidelines on spirometry that have been produced by national and international respiratory societies, but it is worth remembering that they have been developed by those whose remit is to work with communities in which the prevalence of disease is high. As with respiratory questionnaires, the guidance may not be wholly suitable for use in generally fit, low-prevalence populations in whom the predictive value of a 'positive' test result may be low(er). By way of example, it is not uncommon for occupational spirometry to record, in an employee, a 'mild restrictive defect' even when the prior likelihood of such a result is very low, as would be the case in a population of researchers undergoing surveillance for laboratory animal allergy (LAA), a condition that, if clinically apparent, would be expected to produce an obstructive picture. It is a general rule that in settings of low pre-test probability, a 'positive' screening test result is usually a 'false positive', and this is especially so when 'restriction' is a common outcome of poor-quality spirometry. The difficulty arises because the spirometer has been calibrated against a population in which restrictive disease is far from uncommon. It is for occasions such as this that special algorithms have—albeit too rarely—been developed for workplace measurements (De Matteis et al., 2015).

If spirometry is to be used in occupational surveillance, it must be of the highest quality. The American College of Occupational and Environmental Medicine has developed guidance (Townsend, 2011) specifically for use in the workplace, with detailed information on technique, common errors and quality assurance. Operator training is requisite and in some jurisdictions is mandated; if this is considered desirable, then so should be longer-term monitoring of quality. Maintaining high programme performance over time can be very difficult, especially when operators—and often spirometers—change, but it is crucial in settings where decline in lung function is the primary indicator. A system in which there is considerable 'noise' from inconsistent performance will be far less sensitive, with the consequence that workers who are developing difficulties will be detected at a later stage of their disease (see also below).

Spirometry is frequently used in the surveillance of workforces that are at risk of OA, even though it appears to be near-useless in this regard (Nicholson et al., 2010). The available evidence suggests that cases of OA detected through surveillance are very rarely, if ever, done so through abnormalities in spirometry alone, but almost always in the context of a positive response to an accompanying questionnaire. In Ontario, referrals to a specialist clinic of workers in a polyurethane foam factory suspected, through surveillance, of having OA were scrutinised (Kraw and Tarlo, 1999). The findings suggested that the surveillance questionnaire was sensitive but not specific and that spirometry had not added to the detection of asthma; most cases of 'abnormal' lung function in the absence of symptoms reflected 'inadequate workplace spirometry'. Similarly, in a UK programme of surveillance of workers in the motor vehicle repair industry (Mackie, 2008), none of the cases of OA were identified through spirometry alone. This should not, perhaps, be surprising. Asthma of any cause is reflected in variable lung function, which may be normal during asymptomatic periods. Moreover, in a working population in which the highest rate of incident disease is in newer employees—OA generally has a short latency—most at-risk workers will be fit, young and readily able to produce a set of measurements within a supposedly 'normal' range. In the description of their experience in Ontario above, the authors make the additional, wry suggestion that workers may have been more 'honest' in completing their questionnaires since they knew that an 'objective' test (spirometry) was to follow. Logically, it appears that in surveillance designed purely to detect incident OA, spirometry should be restricted to those who report characteristic symptoms on questionnaire.

The above experiences refer essentially to consideration of single measurements of lung function interpreted with reference to a 'predicted' value for an individual of the same age, sex, height and ethnicity. Even if a measurement is within the normal range of a predicted value, it does not mean necessarily that it is 'normal' for that individual. Measuring and monitoring changes in spirometry over time are more informative in the surveillance of conditions in which there is a risk of progressive decline, such as those working with crystalline silica or coal mine dust. This is not as straightforward as it may seem because the inherent non-reproducibility of spirometry is often greater than the rate of decline one would wish to detect. This has at least three important consequences: first, maintaining a high-quality spirometry programme will enhance its sensitivity in detecting excess decline in individual workers; this can be achieved or improved through the monitoring of spirometry quality and longitudinal data precision, technician training and, if necessary, a change of spirometer (Hnizdo et al., 2011). Second, a valid approach to the identification of what constitutes real decline is crucial, a process that is greatly aided by the use of software designed explicitly for this purpose (NIOSH, 2012). It is worth noting that an individual's lung function may fall at a rate that is both abnormal and clinically important while each value itself remains in the 'normal' range (see Figure 15.3) (Townsend, 2005). Third, repeated measurements made within a high-quality programme will detect significant decline sooner than will measurements made within a programme with a high degree of extraneous variability (see Figure 15.4).

Ideally, spirometry tests should be performed annually, but precision is not greatly affected if the frequency is reduced to every 2–3 years. Thus, when monitoring is applied to a stable workforce in which the toxicity of exposure is well characterised and unlikely to cause severe declines within a short period, and in which cost is a limiting factor, the interval between tests can be extended to 3 years. In settings with exposures of unknown toxicity, or in which excessive declines within short times are recognised, the frequency should be increased proportionally to the risk. Further consideration should include an individual's age, duration of exposure and the personal risk of impairment. These issues have been comprehensively reviewed elsewhere (Townsend, 2005).

As a means of secondary prevention, monitoring of spirometry provides a potential opportunity to preserve lung function through early advice on risk and lifestyle factors such as smoking, weight control and exercise; through the appropriate treatment of non-occupational respiratory conditions such as chronic obstructive pulmonary disease or asthma; and of course through the (early) identification of established and identifiable occupational lung diseases such as silicosis or coal workers' pneumoconiosis

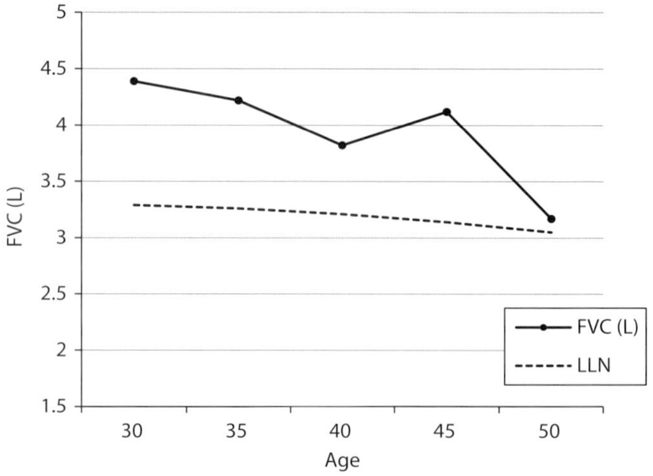

FIGURE 15.3 Longitudinal reduction in an employee's lung function that, nonetheless, remains within a 'normal' range. FVC: forced vital capacity; LLN: lower limit of normal. (Data from Townsend, M. C. 2005. *J Occup Environ Med* 47(12):1307–16.)

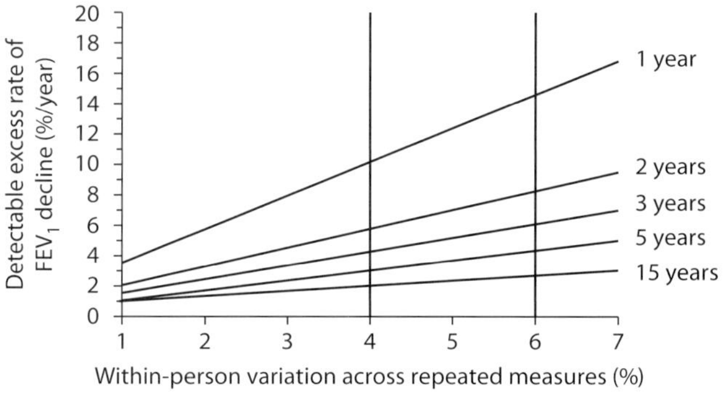

FIGURE 15.4 Detectable excess decline in FEV_1 (%/year) by relative within-employee variation and duration of follow-up (years). Two limits (within-employee variations of 4% and 6%) are depicted by vertical lines. FEV_1: forced expiratory volume in 1 second. (Adapted from Hnizdo, E. et al. 2011. *J Occup Environ Med* 53(10):1205–9.)

TABLE 15.1
Arguments for and Against Surveillance for Chronic Obstructive Pulmonary Disease in Workforces in Which the Risk is Uncertain

For	Against
Earlier identification and treatment of disease	Risk of misdiagnosis (false positives), leading to overtreatment and inaccurate health records
May improve success of smoking cessation and other lifestyle advice	Risk of individual employment loss or disruption due to incorrect occupational attribution
Access to pulmonary rehabilitation, leading to improvement in function	'Normal' lung function may provide false reassurance, with accelerated decline being missed
Identification of disease clusters directs targeted interventions in order to reduce exposure	Expense

(CWP). None of these is contentious. A more difficult issue arises, however (see Table 15.1), when excess decline in lung function is detected in a worker without known non-occupational respiratory disease who is exposed to non-specific workplace dust or fume of uncertain toxicity. Since the evidence that such exposures are harmful is generally epidemiological and so referring to 'average' employees, such evidence cannot be applied with any certainty to an individual, nor to decisions regarding the risk or otherwise of their continuing exposure (and employment). Advice on reducing exposure while maintaining employment is obviously sensible, but it is difficult to see why this should not be applied to every employee, regardless of their spirometric trajectory.

Immunology and Inflammatology

Some types of occupational respiratory disease are associated with a specific and identifiable immunological response. Most cases of OA, for example, arise through specific sensitisation to an airborne allergen in the workplace and, in many varieties, a specific IgE response of high diagnostic sensitivity can be detected through serum assay or skin-prick test. Several causes of hypersensitivity pneumonitis are associated with an IgG response, although the finding is generally of low diagnostic specificity, being more closely related to exposure than to disease. CBD is characterised by a specific lymphocyte proliferative response, the basis for the beryllium lymphocyte proliferation test upon which the diagnosis of CBD rests.

Occupational Asthma

The high diagnostic sensitivity—and in some cases specificity—of specific IgE responses in OA have led some to use them within an integrated surveillance programme. Four examples are summarised in Box 15.1.

Airway Inflammation

Measurements of immune mediators, chemicals and metals and other biomarkers in exhaled breath has seen increasing use in the diagnosis and management of asthma and some other respiratory diseases. This subject is covered in detail in Chapters 5 and 6, but there has been little effort yet put into evaluating the use of these biomarkers in a programme of workplace surveillance. A study of the value of exhaled nitric oxide measurement in the surveillance of French bakery and hairdressing employees suggests that, by itself, it is not a useful screening test for OA (Florentin et al., 2014).

Chronic Beryllium Disease

The beryllium lymphocyte proliferation test was introduced in 1989 and soon became incorporated into some workplace surveillance programmes in the USA (Stange et al., 1996; Newman et al., 2001), but not other countries (Middleton et al., 2006). The arguments for and against its use are well outlined elsewhere (Borak, 2006; Kreiss et al., 2007; Darby and Fishwick, 2011). Essentially, its proponents argue that the identification of specific beryllium sensitisation is a useful adjunct to workplace exposure control, while its detractors argue that it confers no individual benefit to an asymptomatic employee.

Tuberculosis

Some occupational groups—notably those working in certain kinds of healthcare or immigration and custodial services—are at increased risk of contracting tuberculosis (TB). This issue is covered in detail in Chapter 33 but, in brief, many countries have national and often mandatory surveillance schemes for new and continuing employees in these sectors (CDC, 2005; NICE, 2011). Methods usually include active case detection using a risk-stratified combination of symptoms enquiry, immunological tests (TB skin tests and IFN-γ assays) and chest radiography.

Silicotuberculosis

Exposure to respirable crystalline silica, even when there is no identifiable silicosis, increases the risk of pulmonary TB, especially in communities in which tuberculous infection is endemic (Corbett et al., 2000). Passive case detection, which relies on workers reporting

BOX 15.1 IMMUNOLOGICAL SURVEILLANCE FOR OCCUPATIONAL RESPIRATORY SENSITISATION/ASTHMA: FOUR EXAMPLES (SEE TEXT FOR FURTHER DETAILS)

Setting (Allergen)	Precious Metal Refining (Complex Platinum Salts)	Detergent Manufacture (Biological Enzymes)	Baking (Flour/ Enzymes)	Animal Research (Animal Proteins)
Method of Detecting Sensitisation	Skin-prick test	Skin-prick test/specific IgE	Specific IgE	Specific IgE
Purpose	Case identification and exposure control	Case identification and exposure control	Enhanced specificity of reported symptoms	Identification of source of sensitisation

- For several decades, periodic skin-prick tests with extracts of complex platinum salts have been used in the surveillance of workers in the precious metal refining sector. Platinum salts are very potent antigens and a positive skin-prick test result is strongly predictive of respiratory sensitisation, with a low rate of false-positive responses (Merget et al., 2001).
- Workers in much of the detergent industry, who are exposed to 'biological' enzymes, are routinely screened for specific sensitisation using either serum assay or skin-prick test. There is a legacy of high rates of OA in this industry and an ever-present threat of future outbreaks (Cullinan et al., 2000), particularly with the high turnover of novel enzymes of uncertain immunogenicity. Immunological screening in this case is used explicitly to aid in exposure control with, in the better factories, careful scrutiny of the circumstances surrounding each incident case (Nicholson et al., 2001).
- Bakers frequently report work-related respiratory symptoms and it can be difficult to distinguish those that indicate classical bakers' asthma from those that reflect simple irritation. The former is almost always associated with IgE sensitisation to either cereal flour or an additive enzyme, and some workplace surveillance programmes use this property iteratively in order to identify symptomatic employees who require further investigation (Brant et al., 2005).
- Researchers and technicians who work with laboratory animals frequently move between institutions. Some surveillance programmes for LAA include the collection of serum from new employees; this is stored so that, should an individual develop symptoms of LAA, their specific IgE status at employment can be checked as an indicator of where their sensitisation was acquired.

symptoms to their occupational health provider, may be insensitive where the risks are especially high, since the symptoms of pulmonary TB are often non-specific and common in miners and masons. Active case finding with chest radiography and sputum microbiology is both more sensitive and specific, but is expensive and practised in only few settings, notably parts of the mining industry in South Africa (Johns Hopkins Bloomberg School of Public Health Departments of GDEC and International Health, 2015).

It is unclear whether exposure to silica increases the risk that latent TB will progress to active disease. The American College of Occupational and Environmental Medicine recommends that at employment (and 'periodically' afterwards), every exposed worker should be offered tuberculin skin testing in order to help detect both latent and active cases of TB (Raymond and Wintermeyer, 2006). This is, however, far from universally practised, even in the United States, and is of course not appropriate for populations with high rates of active disease or universal BCG vaccination. The value of more modern immunological techniques—particularly those that measure specific IFN-γ release—is not yet established in this setting.

Radiology

Some types of occupational lung disease give rise to characteristic radiological changes within an interval that is short enough to be detectable while the affected worker is still in employment. Silicosis and CWP are two clear examples, but others would include CBD and hard metal disease. At current levels of asbestos exposure, even in countries where regulation is lax, the latency of asbestos-related diseases is generally too long for workplace radiological screening to be useful.

It is evident that in both silicosis and CWP, disease may be radiologically evident before the onset of distinctive respiratory symptoms or a measurable decline in lung function. In this sense, radiology is a more sensitive tool for use in workplace screening and, if other considerations did not apply, would be universally recommended. The matter is, of course, more complex. Where exposure controls (to respirable crystalline silica, coal mine dust, etc.) are good, then the risk of pneumoconiosis is low and a policy of routine, repeated radiology would be inefficient (since the detection rate would be extremely low), hazardous (radiology is itself not free of risk), expensive and logistically difficult, especially as fewer radiologists have sufficient training in the detection of early pneumoconiosis. Each of these factors will be weighted differently when exposure control is or has been less than adequate and the prior probability of disease is higher.

Given these ponderables, it is unsurprising that there is no universally applicable, evidence-based guidance on the use of radiology in workplace surveillance for pneumoconiosis (Health and Safety Laboratory, 2010). Where guidance is provided, it is usually based on a summative document produced for the World Health Organisation in 1996 (Wagner, 1996), but often with a more nuanced risk-based approach (Rosenman, 2011). Attempts have been made at developing algorithms that can be used to determine the clinical utility of an abnormal chest radiograph (see Figure 15.5) (Suarthana et al., 2007), but as yet they have not been validated in practice and their performance is uncertain (Nicol et al., 2015).

Low-dose computed tomography (CT) scanning of the thorax is likely to be widely used in population screening programmes for lung cancer with targeted individuals who, on the basis of their age and smoking history, are at high risk. In some countries, this has also been applied to workers with historical asbestos exposure; in France, for example, national health insurance funds provide post-retirement asbestos surveillance that includes a medical consultation and a chest CT scan every 5 years for those who were highly exposed, and every 10 years for those with lower exposure (Haute Autorité de Santé, 2010).

IS WORKPLACE SURVEILLANCE EFFECTIVE?

The chief purpose of workplace surveillance is to reduce the incidence of occupational respiratory disease. This aim might reasonably be adjusted to include a reduction in the incidence of *severe* occupational disease; for example, more advanced types of silicosis or cases of irreversible OA. No randomised trials have formally tested these aims; such trials would be difficult to organise—especially where the baseline incidence of disease is low—and, perhaps, justify. Moreover, workplace surveillance is almost always instituted or improved in a context of a wider risk-reduction programme, from which it is difficult to disentangle the effects of any one element.

One or two published experiences are, however, instructive. In 1983, new legislation in Ontario required firms using diisocyanates to control exposures and introduce mandatory surveillance comprising a questionnaire and spirometry. Employees with respiratory symptoms or reductions in spirometry were required to have a medical assessment. There was no similar legislation to provide surveillance for firms using other respiratory sensitisers. Throughout a period of evaluation, diisocyanates remained the most commonly recognised cause of compensated OA (Figure 15.6); indeed, there was an initial increase in annual claims after the introduction of the surveillance programme, consistent with an increased detection of prevalent cases (Tarlo et al., 2002). This was subsequently followed by reductions in both the proportionate and actual numbers of accepted diisocyanate-induced asthma claims.

Variable	Odds ratio	Score
Age ≥40	2.3	1.0
Current smoker	2.4	1.0
High exposure job	4.0	1.5
Construction work ≥15 years	3.4	1.5
Self-reported 'unhealthy'	2.8	1.25
FEV_1 ≤ −1 standardised residual	3.0	1.25

Total score	<3	3	3.75	4	4.25	4.75	5.25	6.25	7.5
Probability of abnormal CXR	0%	1%	2%	2.5%	3%	5%	8%	19%	45%

FIGURE 15.5 The strength of predictors for a CXR indicative of pneumoconiosis (ILO category >1/1) in workers exposed to silica. (Data from Suarthana, E. et al. 2007. *Occup Environ Med* 64(9):595–601.)

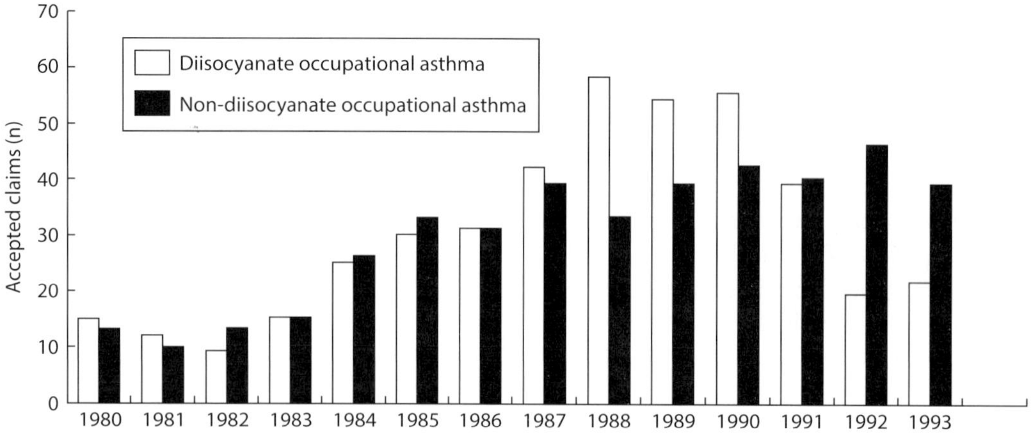

FIGURE 15.6 Accepted claims for diisocyanate-induced asthma (white columns) and other causes of OA (black columns) in Ontario by year of onset. (Adapted from Tarlo, S. M., Liss, G. M. and Yeung, K. S. 2002. *Occup Environ Med* 59(1):58–62.)

Further, in employees of companies that were known to be compliant with the programme, there was an earlier diagnosis of OA (a mean of 1.7 years after symptoms onset compared to 2.7 years for workers in companies without documented compliance). Perhaps as a consequence, indices of asthma severity at the time of diagnosis suggested milder disease in those who were diagnosed in the second period of the study.

In Germany, the potential effectiveness of a workplace surveillance programme for employees exposed to complex platinum salts in a catalyst production plant was evaluated through a small case-referent study of the 14 employees in whom skin-prick test responses to platinum salt had converted during a 5-year surveillance programme. Twelve were relocated to positions where further exposure was eliminated; in these, symptoms improved and skin-prick test reactions decreased or became negative. No point of comparison was reported, but these findings suggest that regular workplace surveillance may reduce the incidence of irreversible disease in this context (Merget et al., 2001). A Canadian study based on the compensation scheme in Quebec examined the clinical information available on 1388 workers with a history of silicosis. Employees who had been engaged in a surveillance programme were less likely to have a vital capacity below 80% of their predicted value and/or a more severe classification of chest radiographic abnormality (Infante-Rivard, 2005).

CONCLUDING REMARKS

For an activity that is so widespread (and often lucrative), it is perhaps surprising that workplace surveillance for respiratory disease remains largely unstandardised and of uncertain benefit. There is little doubt, too, that it operates under an 'inverse care law' whereby employees (or the self-employed) who are at greatest risk—working in settings or industries with poorly controlled exposures—are likely to be offered surveillance of relatively poor quality, if at all. The development of effective, efficient and fair methods of surveillance and their delivery to all workers who are at risk—particularly including those working in newly industrialising parts of the world—remain worthy challenges.

REFERENCES

Allan, K. M., Murphy, E. and Ayres, J. G. 2010. Assessment of respiratory health surveillance for laboratory animal workers. *Occup Med (Lond)* 60(6):458–63.

Borak, J. 2006. The beryllium occupational exposure limit: Historical origin and current inadequacy. *J Occup Environ Med* 48(2):109–16.

Brant, A., Nightingale, S., Berriman, J., Sharp, C., Welch, J., Newman Taylor, A. J. and Cullinan, P. 2005. Supermarket baker's asthma: How accurate is routine health surveillance? *Occup Environ Med* 62(6):395–99.

Carton, M., Bonnaud, S., Nachtigal, M., Serrano, A., Carole, C., Bonenfant, S., Coste, D. et al. 2011. Post-retirement surveillance of workers exposed to asbestos or wood dust: first results of the French national SPIRALE Program. *Epidemiol Prev* 35(5–6):315–23.

CDC. 2005. *Guidelines for Preventing the Transmission of Mycobacterium tuberculosis in Health-Care Settings*. Available at: http://www.cdc.gov/mmwr/pdf/rr/rr5417.pdf (accessed 7 July 2015).

Christiani, D. C., Mehta, A. J. and Yu, C. L. 2008. Genetic susceptibility to occupational exposures. *Occup Environ Med* 65(6):430–36.

Corbett, E. L., Churchyard, G. J., Clayton, T. C., Williams, B. G., Mulder, D., Hayes, R. J. and De Cock, K. M. 2000. HIV infection and silicosis: The impact of two potent risk factors on the incidence of mycobacterial disease in South African miners. *AIDS* 14(17):2759–68.

Cullinan, P. 2011. *Evidence-Based Guidance for the Assessment of New Employees with Asthma*. Available at: http://www.bohrf.org.uk/downloads/Evidence_based_guidance_for_the_assessment_of_new_employees_with_asthma.pdf (accessed 7 July 2015).

Cullinan, P., Harris, J. M., Newman Taylor, A. J., Hole, A. M., Jones, M., Barnes, F. and Jolliffe, G. 2000. An outbreak of asthma in a modern detergent factory. *Lancet* 356(9245):1899–900.

Darby, A. and Fishwick, D. 2011. *Beryllium: A Review of the Health Effects and the Evidence for Screening or Surveillance in Workers Exposed to Beryllium*. London, UK: HSE Books.

De Matteis, S., Atenea Iridoy, A., Shawn, A., Swann, A. and Cullinan, P. 2016. A new spirometry-based algorithm to predict occupational pulmonary restrictive impairment. *Occup Med* 66(1):50–3.

European Agency for Safety and Health at Work. 2009. Directive 2009/148/EC—Exposure to asbestos at work. Available at: https://osha.europa.eu/en/legislation/directives/2009-148-ec-exposure-to-asbestos-at-work (accessed 7 July 2015).

Florentin, A., Acouetey, D. S., Remen, T., Penven, E., Thaon, I., Zmirou-Navier, D. and Paris, C. 2014. Exhaled nitric oxide and screening for occupational asthma in two at-risk sectors: Bakery and hairdressing. *Int J Tuberc Lung Dis* 18(6):744–50.

Haute Autorité de Santé. 2010. Suivi post-professionel après exposition à l'amiante. Available at: http://www.has-sante.fr/portail/upload/docs/application/pdf/2010-05/amiante_-_suivi_post-professionnel_-_recommandations.pdf (accessed 7 July 2015).

Health and Safety Executive. 2010. Health questionnaire for on-going surveillance of people potentially exposed to substances that can cause occupational asthma. Available at: http://www.hse.gov.uk/asthma/samplequest3.pdf.

Health and Safety Laboratory. 2010. Health surveillance in silica exposed workers. Available at: http://www.hse.gov.uk/research/rrpdf/rr827.pdf (accessed 7 July 2015).

Hnizdo, E., Glindmeyer, H. W. and Petsonk, E. L. 2010. Workplace spirometry monitoring for respiratory disease prevention: A methods review. *Int J Tuberc Lung Dis* 14(7):796–805.

Hnizdo, E., Hakobyan, A., Fleming, J. L. and Beeckman-Wagner, L. A. 2011. Periodic spirometry in occupational setting: Improving quality, accuracy, and precision. *J Occup Environ Med* 53(10):1205–9.

Infante-Rivard, C. 2005. Severity of silicosis at compensation between medically screened and unscreened workers. *J Occup Environ Med* 47(3):265–71.

Johns Hopkins Bloomberg School of Public Health Departments of GDEC and International Health 2015. MINE TB: Active TB Case Finding in Mine Labour-Sending Regions. Available at: http://www.hopkinsglobalhealth.org/funding-opportunities/student-and-trainee-grants/ghefp/project-list/mine-tb-active-tb-case-finding-in-mine-labour-sending-regions/ (accessed 7 July 2015).

Kraw, M. and Tarlo, S. M. 1999. Isocyanate medical surveillance: Respiratory referrals from a foam manufacturing plant over a five-year period. *Am J Ind Med* 35(1):87–91.

Kreiss, K., Day, G. A. and Schuler, C. R. 2007. Beryllium: A modern industrial hazard. *Annu Rev Public Health* 28:259–77.

Mackie, J. 2008. Effective health surveillance for occupational asthma in motor vehicle repair. *Occup Med (Lond)* 58(8):551–55.

Merget, R., Caspari, C., Dierkes-Globisch, A., Kulzer, R., Breitstadt, R., Kniffka, A., Degens, P. et al. 2001. Effectiveness of a medical surveillance program for the prevention of occupational asthma caused by platinum salts: A nested case–control study. *J Allergy Clin Immunol* 107(4):707–12.

Middleton, D. C., Lewin, M. D., Kowalski, P. J., Cox, S. S. and Kleinbaum, D. 2006. The BeLPT: Algorithms and implications. *Am J Ind Med* 49(1):36–44.

Miller, B. G., Graham, M. K., Creely, K. S., Cowie, H. A. and Soutar, C. A. 2003. *Questionnaire Predictors of Asthma and Occupational Asthma*. London, UK: HSE Books.

Newman, L. S., Mroz, M. M., Maier, L. A., Daniloff, E. M. and Balkissoon, R. 2001. Efficacy of serial medical surveillance for chronic beryllium disease in a beryllium machining plant. *J Occup Environ Med* 43(3):231–37.

NICE. 2011. NICE Guidelines CG117. Tuberculosis: Clinical diagnosis and management of tuberculosis, and measures for its prevention and control. Available at: https://www.nice.org.uk/guidance/cg117/chapter/guidance#/preventing-infection-in-specific-settings (accessed 7 July 2015).

Nicholson, P. J., Cullinan, P., Burge, P. S. and Boyle, C. 2010. *Occupational Asthma: Prevention, Identification and Management. Systematic Review and Recommendations*. London: British Occupational Health Research Foundation.

Nicholson, P. J., Newman Taylor, A. J., Oliver, P. and Cathcart, M. 2001. Current best practice for the health surveillance of enzyme workers in the soap and detergent industry. *Occup Med (Lond)* 51(2):81–92.

Nicol, L. M., McFarlane, P. A., Hirani, N. and Reid, P. T. 2015. Six cases of silicosis: Implications for health surveillance of stonemasons. *Occup Med (Lond)* 65(3):220–25.

NIOSH. 2012. Spirometry Monitoring Technology, SPIROLA software. Available at: http://www.cdc.gov/niosh/topics/spirometry/spirola.html.

Palmer, K. T., Brown, I. and Hobson, J. 2013. *Fitness for Work*. Oxford: Oxford University Press.

Raymond, L. W. and Wintermeyer, S. 2006. Medical surveillance of workers exposed to crystalline silica. *J Occup Environ Med* 48(1):95–101.

Rosenman, K. D. 2011. Recommended Medical Screening Protocol for Silica Exposed Workers. Available at: http://www.oem.msu.edu/userfiles/file/resources/silica%20screen%20protocol.pdf.

Silver, K. and Sharp, R. R. 2006. Ethical considerations in testing workers for the -Glu69 marker of genetic susceptibility to chronic beryllium disease. *J Occup Environ Med* 48(4):434–43.

Stange, A. W., Furman, F. J. and Hilmas, D. E. 1996. Rocky flats beryllium health surveillance. *Environ Health Perspect* 104(Suppl. 5):981–86.

Stenton, S. C., Beach, J. R., Avery, A. J. and Hendrick, D. J. 1993. The value of questionnaires and spirometry in asthma surveillance programmes in the workplace. *Occup Med (Lond)* 43(4):203–6.

Suarthana, E., Moons, K. G., Heederik, D. and Meijer, E. 2007. A simple diagnostic model for ruling out pneumoconiosis among construction workers. *Occup Environ Med* 64(9):595–601.

Szram, J. and Cullinan, P. 2013. Medical surveillance for prevention of occupational asthma. *Curr Opin Allergy Clin Immunol* 13(2):138–44.

Tarlo, S. M., Liss, G. M. and Yeung, K. S. 2002. Changes in rates and severity of compensation claims for asthma due to diisocyanates: A possible effect of medical surveillance measures. *Occup Environ Med* 59(1):58–62.

Townsend, M. C. 2005. Evaluating pulmonary function change over time in the occupational setting. *J Occup Environ Med* 47(12):1307–16.

Townsend, M. C. 2011. Spirometry in the occupational health setting—2011 update. *J Occup Environ Med* 53(5):569–84.

Wagner, G. R. 1996. *Screening and Surveillance of Workers Exposed to Mineral Dust*. Geneva: WHO Press.

Wagner, G. R. and Wegman, D. H. 1998. Occupational asthma: Prevention by definition. *Am J Ind Med* 33(5):427–29.

16 Parenchymal Disease Related to Asbestos

Eduardo Algranti and Steven Markowitz

CONTENTS

INTRODUCTION

Asbestos use expanded in many countries beginning in the 1940s and peaked in many developed countries in Western Europe, North America and Australia in the 1970s and 1980s, after which it dropped dramatically. Industrializing countries began large-scale use of asbestos in the 1960s, and many of these countries still use asbestos. At present, 55 countries have banned the import and use of asbestos, and many others have applied strict regulations on its use and handling (World Health Organization, 2014a,b). However, it is still manufactured and otherwise used in several dozen countries worldwide. Furthermore, in countries that have banned or restricted the use of the fibre, exposures still occur in industrial maintenance, asbestos abatement, construction repair, renovation and demolition, rescue and firefighting and as a consequence of natural disasters, due to a large amount of asbestos being in place (Collegium Ramazzini, 2011; World Health Organization, 2014b).

Asbestos (Figure 16.1) was used in more than 3000 products. Its useful qualities (i.e. thermal resistance, high tensile strength, flexibility, resistance to acidic chemicals and relatively low cost) led to its widespread use in insulation materials, cement, roofing, flooring and other building materials, friction products, textiles, jointing materials, plastics and coatings and other products. Although many of the prior uses of asbestos have been banned or phased out, they may still be reported in contemporary cases of asbestos-related diseases.

The World Health Organization (WHO) estimates that there are currently approximately 125 million people in the world who are exposed to asbestos in the workplace (World Health Organization, 2014a). In addition, there is a large reservoir of people who are no longer exposed to asbestos but had significant exposure in the past. For example, in the United States, there are an estimated 10–15 million people who worked with asbestos in the past. According to the most recent WHO estimates, more than 107,000 people die each year from asbestos-related lung cancer, mesothelioma and asbestosis resulting from exposure at work (World Health Organization, 2006, 2014b). Approximately half of the deaths from occupational cancer are estimated to be caused by asbestos.

Worldwide asbestos production exceeded 5 million metric tons in the 1970s and subsequently dropped, slowly decreasing in recent years from 2.2 million metric tons in 2007 to 1.97 million metric tons in 2012 (International Agency for Research on Cancer, 2012; Virta, 2013). Just four countries—Russia, China, Brazil and Kazakhstan—accounted for 99% of the world's production of asbestos in 2012, all or mostly chrysotile. Canada no longer mines asbestos. Asbestos is consumed principally in ten countries, accounting for 94% of the world's consumption of asbestos in 2011, led, in order, by China, India, Russia, Brazil and Kazakhstan. China used nearly a third of all asbestos consumed worldwide in 2011—638,000 metric tons—which, to provide historical perspective, is nearly 90% of the quantity that the

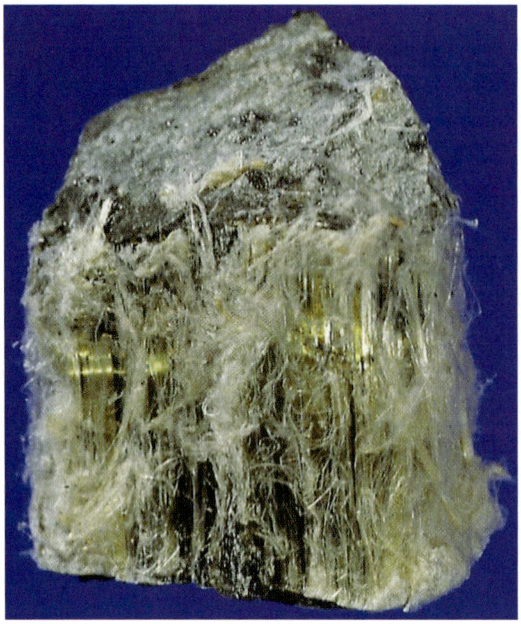

FIGURE 16.1 A sample of Quebec chrysotile asbestos showing the fibrous nature of the ore. (Courtesy of Bryan Corrin, MD.)

United States consumed in its year of peak asbestos consumption of 1973 (Virta, 2013). Much of current asbestos use is in cement and other building materials.

Asbestos has been banned in the European Union, Japan, Korea, Australia and selected other countries (Collegium Ramazzini, 2011; World Health Organization, 2014b). It is regulated in the United States, where it is also the subject of much litigation, but has not yet been banned from import or use. The consumption of asbestos in the United States reached a high of 719,000 metric tons in 1973 and was 1020 metric tons in 2012, all imported from Brazil (International Agency for Research on Cancer, 2012; Virta, 2013). Two-thirds of asbestos consumed in the United States is used in the chloralkali industry, and most of the remainder is incorporated in roofing products, with smaller amounts used in coatings and plastics (Virta, 2013). The USA also imported limited additional quantities of products that were likely to have contained asbestos in 2012, including cement products, yarn and thread, brake linings/pads and other friction products.

ASBESTOSIS

Incidence and Prevalence

Given the differing chronologies in asbestos use by industrialized and industrializing countries, the time trends in the incidence and prevalence of asbestosis differ accordingly. The prevalence of asbestosis globally also varies according to exposure intensity, occupation and industry. In Poland, during the period 1970–2001, the average incidence of asbestosis was estimated at 0.5/100,000 employees per year with an increasing trend during the study period, according to its national occupational disease registry (Wilczynska et al., 2002). In the United States, asbestosis was cited on death certificates as an underlying cause of death in 6290 deaths during the period 1999–2010, with a median of 8.0 years of potential life lost per case (Bang et al., 2014). Asbestosis mortality in the United States increased from <1 per million of the general population in 1968 to nearly 3 per million in 2003, dropping to 2.5 per million by 2010 (Center for Disease Control, 2012). In England and Wales, average annual asbestosis mortality rates increased from 0.4 per million of the general population in 1968–1972 to 1.2 per million of the general population in 2005–2008 (Hanley et al., 2011).

Asbestosis is generally lessening in prevalence and severity in industrialized countries, but it remains a current problem and is likely to persist in the future in industrializing countries where asbestos use continues (Algranti et al., 2001).

Clinical, Radiological and Physiological Features

Asbestosis is identified generally in the fifth or sixth decade of life after a variable period of exposure. It is a dose-dependent disease in at-risk subjects (Finkelstein et al., 1984; Finkelstein, 1985) and, among the various malignant and non-malignant diseases related to asbestos, asbestosis tends to require higher levels of exposure to asbestos (Helsinki Consensus, 1997). However, mild asbestosis can occur at lower levels of exposure (Helsinki Consensus, 2015). Statistical modelling for ascertaining dose–response relationships in asbestosis using a number of dose metrics explains approximately a third of the variability (Finkelstein, 1985). At present, exposure to sufficient levels of asbestos to cause asbestosis is far more likely to occur in industrializing countries that still fabricate or use new asbestos-containing products. Although asbestos exposure may frequently be occult or unknown to the worker, it is uncommon that the affected individual does not report a substantial history of exposure to asbestos or to a product that likely contained asbestos.

Asbestosis is a diffuse interstitial fibrosis that involves the respiratory bronchioles, alveolar ducts and alveoli (Craighead et al., 1982; Wright et al., 1985; Roggli et al., 2010; Hammar, 2011). It is usually diagnosed on a clinical basis, which depends principally on the finding of characteristic changes on chest imaging, a history of asbestos exposure and exclusion of other known causes of interstitial fibrosis. Its cardinal symptom of shortness of breath on exertion is caused by decreased oxygen uptake and increased inspiratory workload. Chronic non-productive cough is often associated with later stages of asbestosis. On clinical examination, the characteristic feature is the presence of fine mid-to-late inspiratory rales of dry quality at the lung bases. Rales are present in over 70% of patients with established asbestosis and can precede chest X-ray alterations (al Jarad et al., 1993). Finger clubbing is less often found: in a study of 167 patients with asbestosis, clubbing was present in 43%, with a significant upward trend as the chest X-ray profusion category increased. Finger clubbing was associated with rapid disease progression and earlier mortality (Coutts et al., 1987). These symptoms and signs are shared by other non-occupational interstitial lung diseases.

When eliciting an occupational history, the patient may not recall all past jobs or attendant exposures. The use of specific questionnaires (Bourgkard et al., 2013) and/or information derived from high-quality job exposure matrices (Hardt et al., 2014) is beneficial for estimating lifelong asbestos exposure, although a careful occupational history usually suffices.

When asbestosis is suspected and a classic setting of asbestos exposure is not reported, other sources of potential asbestos exposure should be explored. Often, workers who used asbestos-containing products in the past or who worked near others who used such products were not aware that they worked with asbestos (Rodelsperger et al., 1986; Welch et al., 1994; Burdorf et al., 2003). In these situations, workers can be either exposed directly or as bystanders (i.e. working in the vicinity of others who are personally handling asbestos-containing materials). It is well established that domestic or environmental exposures or working in the vicinity of asbestos sources are causes of asbestos-related diseases (Lilis et al., 1991; Magnani et al., 1998; Conti et al., 2014). Indeed, the number of individuals who are inadvertently exposed to asbestos may surpass the number of workers who are exposed in a typical asbestos industry (Algranti, 1998).

Mineral deposits of talc (Scancarello et al., 1996; Loyola et al., 2010), vermiculite (Amandus et al., 1987; Peipins et al., 2003) and soapstone (Bezerra et al., 2003) can be contaminated with amphibole asbestos, as these minerals share similar geological formations. Mining, milling, handicraft or other uses of these minerals can be sources of asbestos exposure.

The latency period between the onset of asbestos exposure and detection of asbestosis is typically 20–30 years, but may be shorter or longer. In general, higher exposures can lead to a shorter latency time. Latency may also depend on the presence and sensitivity of a medical surveillance programme established for the purpose of detecting pre-symptomatic disease. If surveillance is instituted according to national regulations, employer policies or union sponsorship, earlier detection of asbestosis is more likely, which, in turn, shortens observed latency.

Radiographic Imaging

On chest X-rays, asbestosis is demonstrated by the presence of irregular linear interstitial opacities, usually involving the lower-lung fields at a minimum. The classical chest X-ray signs of asbestosis in its early stages are 's'- and 't'-irregular small opacities in the lower lung fields (International Labour Organization, 2011). As the disease progresses, irregular opacities may extend to the mid- and upper-lung fields and may be accompanied by lung volume loss, blurring of the cardiac and/or the diaphragmatic contours and a thickening of the horizontal fissure. Honeycombing is a characteristic feature of advanced stages of the disease. Chronic obstructive pulmonary disease, particularly when accompanied by emphysema, smoking and ageing, can give rise to false-positive interpretations when utilizing the International Labour Organization (ILO) reading protocol (Dick et al., 1992). Figure 16.2 provides illustrations of chest X-rays with early and advanced asbestosis. Plain chest films should be interpreted according to the standard classification system for interpreting radiographs of dust-exposed workers, first created by the ILO in 1930 and now in its eighth version (International Labour Organization, 2011). The system is designed to describe findings that are related and unrelated to pneumoconiosis in a coded and reproducible way. Its use facilitates the gathering of epidemiological data and aids in the diagnostic workup of individuals by comparing a given chest X-ray with a set of standard chest radiographs that illustrate the principal components of the classification. The system of reading addresses the quality of the chest X-ray, the quantification and type of parenchymal changes (small and large opacities) and the type and extent of pleural changes (thickening and calcification), and provides a set of 29 symbols for addressing features that are related or unrelated to mineral dust exposure. The findings should be documented on an appropriate reading sheet. Physicians who use the ILO system should receive training.

Computed tomography (CT) and high-resolution CT (HRCT) are more sensitive imaging methods than plain

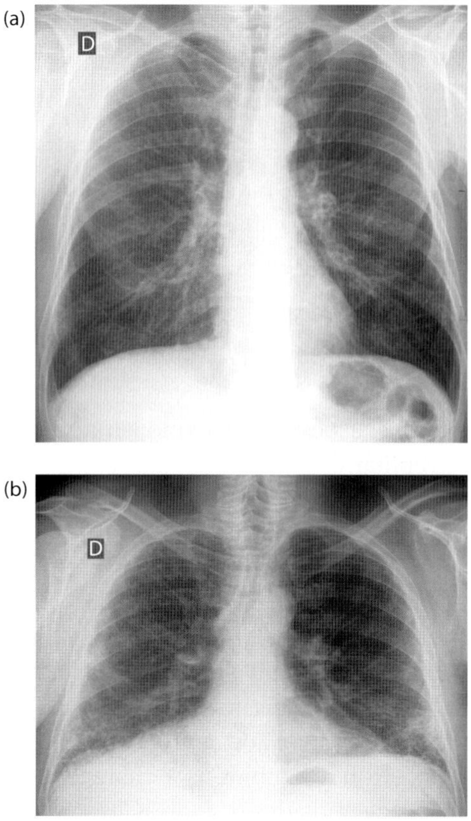

FIGURE 16.2 Chest radiography in asbestosis. (a) A bilateral lower-lobe irregular pattern is seen in individuals with early asbestosis. (b) As asbestosis progresses, the cardiac outline often becomes ill defined and irregular. Basal volume loss occurs with elevation of the diaphragm and depression of the horizontal fissure. The radiographic features are similar to idiopathic pulmonary fibrosis, but the presence of bilateral pleural plaques, sometimes calcified, may be a useful pointer to the diagnosis.

chest X-rays in the identification of asbestosis (Aberle et al., 1988; Friedman et al., 1988; Staples et al., 1989). A fifth to a quarter of cases of asbestosis and of pleural plaques are missed by the chest X-ray (Aberle et al., 1988; Staples et al., 1989; Algranti et al., 2001).

In the early phases of asbestosis, the HRCT has the advantage of better depicting the posterior lung recesses, which are obscured by the diaphragmatic domes on the chest X-ray. The HRCT findings associated with asbestosis include (Aberle et al., 1988; Akira et al., 1991; Gamsu et al., 1995):

- Sub-pleural dot-like structures
- Thickening of the interlobular septa
- Intralobular thickening
- Sub-pleural curvilinear lines
- Ground-glass opacities
- Parenchymal bands
- Traction bronchiectasis and bronchiolectasis
- Honeycombing

Figures 16.3 and 16.4 depict the main HRCT findings in asbestosis. Interstitial lines, parenchymal bands and distortion of lobules are the most common HRCT findings in asbestosis (Gamsu et al., 1995). Interlobular thickening and ground-glass opacities may not represent fibrosis in that they may indicate tissue swelling from other causes and are potentially reversible. All of these findings are not specific to asbestosis and may be found in patients with other conditions, including usual interstitial pneumonia (UIP), non-specific interstitial pneumonia (NSIP) and congestive heart failure (Staples, 1992). Due to reversible gravity-dependent shadows, CT scans should be performed in the prone position in order to avoid false interpretation. Low-dose HRCT can be used to identify findings that are compatible with asbestosis (Remy-Jardin et al., 2004).

Similarly to the ILO classification for chest X-rays, an international group of experts has developed a classification system for the standard interpretation of HRCT scans for describing dust-related diseases. Implementation of and training in this system is facilitated by the availability of a written text, standard films and a reading sheet (Kusaka et al., 2005). In a study of the inter-reader agreement using this system, there was good to moderate agreement on the main findings of asbestosis, with the exception of the presence of ground-glass opacities (Suganuma et al., 2009). This classification system is being widely used in Germany (Kraus et al., 2009) and by some groups in Japan and the United States.

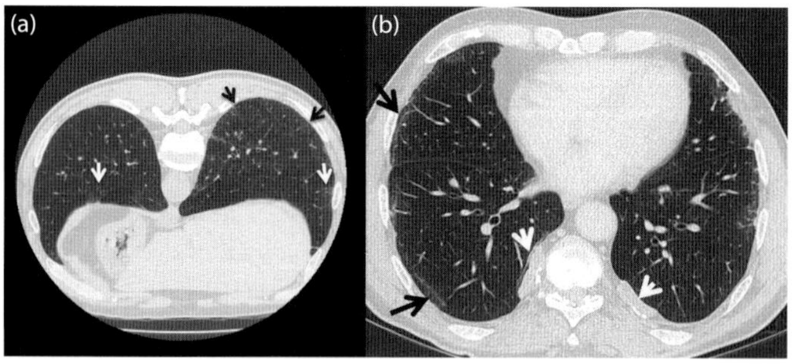

FIGURE 16.3 High-resolution computed tomography in asbestosis. (a) Scan in prone position showing subtle sub-pleural dots and interlobular septal thickening (black arrows) and sparse ground-glass opacities (white arrows). The presence of sub-pleural centrilobular dots of 'x'- and 'y'-shaped densities is seen, as opposed to tractional airway dilatation, which is a feature of early interstitial pulmonary fibrosis. (b) Sub-pleural curvilinear lines (black arrows) and pleural plaques (white arrows). The plaque on the left has a subjacent subpleural line. (Photograph courtesy of Dr. S.J. Copley, Hammersmith Hospital, London, UK.)

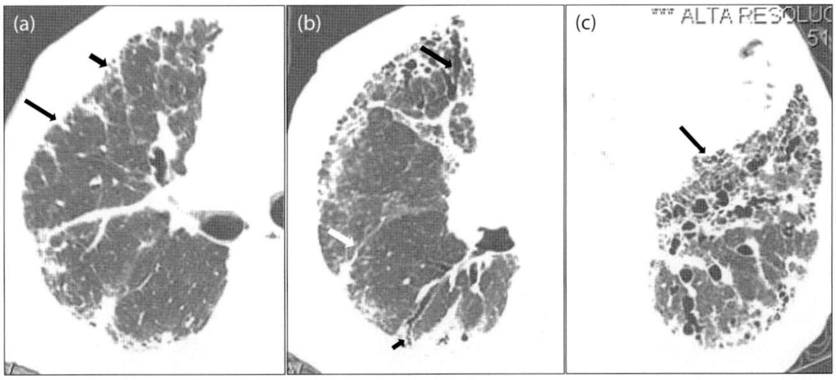

FIGURE 16.4 High-resolution computed tomography showing: (a) marked interlobular septal thickening (long arrow) and confluent dots producing pleura-based nodules (short arrow); (b) bronchiectasis (long black arrow), bronchiolectasis (short black arrow) and parenchymal band (white arrow); and (c) marked honeycombing. In advanced asbestosis, the computed tomography features are indistinguishable from interstitial pulmonary fibrosis, although the presence of coexisting pleural plaques is suggestive of asbestosis. (Photographs courtesy of Dr. Dante Escuissato, Hospital das Clínicas, Federal University of Paraná, Brazil.)

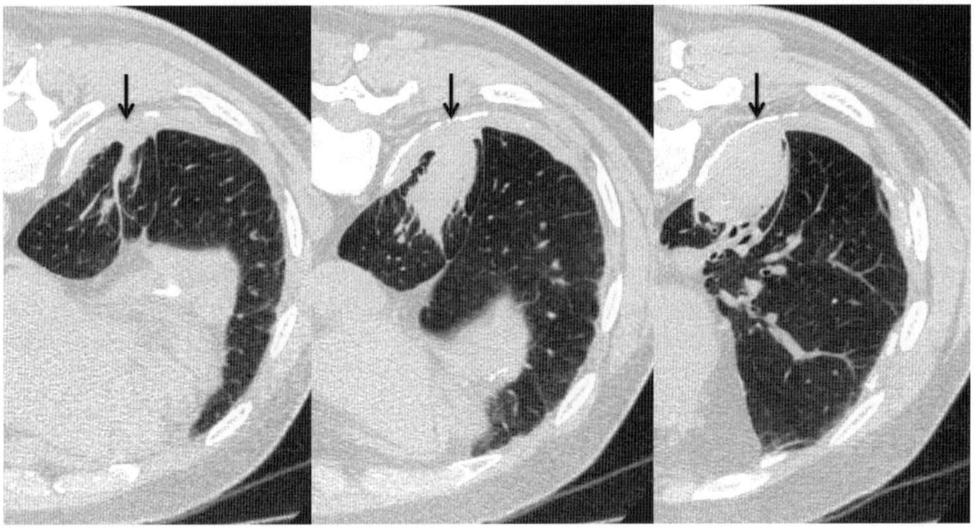

FIGURE 16.5 Upward sequence of slices of a prone high-resolution computed tomography scan showing an area of rounded atelectasis over a thick calcified pleural plaque (black arrows).

Pleural plaques are often present in cases of asbestosis, but such plaques may be easily missed on the chest X-ray if they are thin, small or not calcified. Rounded atelectasis is sometimes found in patients with pleural disease (Figure 16.4). In construction workers and former asbestos cement workers, more than 80% of cases of asbestosis also had pleural plaques on HRCT (Kishimoto et al., 2000; Algranti et al., 2001) (Figure 16.5).

Pulmonary Function Testing

Asbestosis decreases lung volumes and gas exchange in common with any diffuse interstitial fibrosis. There is an independent relationship between increased levels of exposure and both decreased forced vital capacity (FVC) (Weill et al., 1975; Algranti et al., 2001) and increasing radiological categories of profusion (Rosenstock, 1988; Miller et al., 1992). Carbon monoxide diffusing capacity (DLCO), which measures the ability of gas exchange in the lungs, is a sensitive marker that may precede overt radiographic changes and shows progressive decrements with increasing profusion scores (Orens et al., 1995; Lee et al., 2003). Functional decrements are independently intensified by smoking (Miller et al., 2013) and pleural thickening (Miller et al., 1992; Algranti et al., 2001), particularly with diffuse pleural thickening (Schwartz et al., 1990). DLCO shows a more pronounced decrement gradient along the ILO profusion scale compared

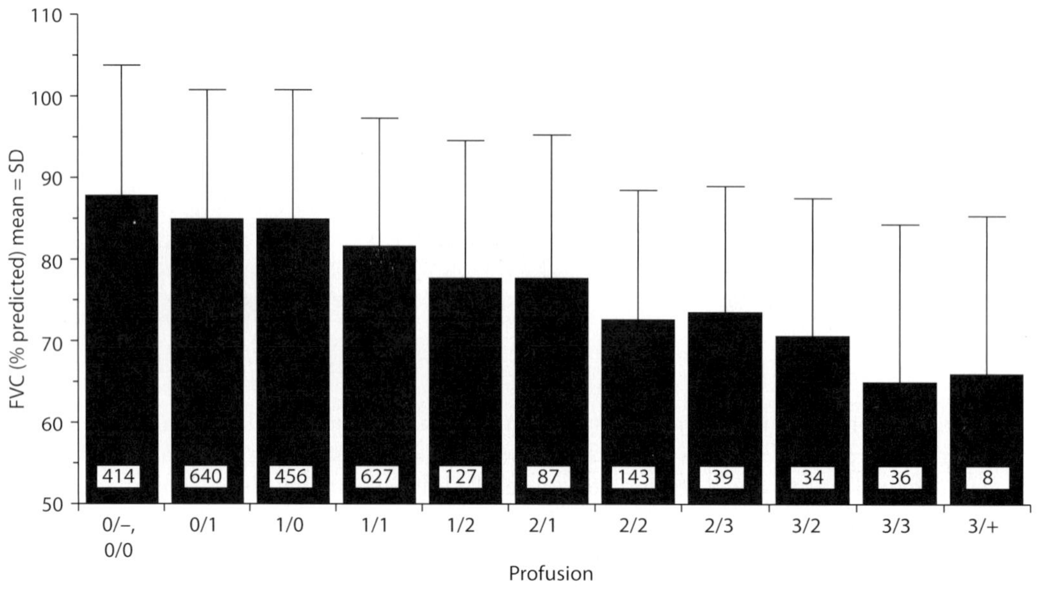

FIGURE 16.6 Forced vital capacity (FVC; percentage of predicted) versus profusion of small irregular opacities in 2611 long-term insulators irrespective of pleural thickening or smoking history. (From Miller, A. et al. 1992. *Am Rev Respir Dis* 145(2 Pt 1):263–70. Reprinted with permission of the American Thoracic Society. Copyright 2015 American Thoracic Society.)

to FVC (Miller et al., 2013) and has been shown to be the function test that best correlates with disease progression observed over time on HRCT (Nogueira et al., 2011). Figure 16.6 shows the mean percentages of predicted FVC in long-term asbestos-exposed insulators by ILO profusion score (Miller et al., 1992). Figure 16.7 shows the mean percentages of predicted DLCO by ILO profusion score in a large group of workers from various asbestos trades, including smokers and non-smokers (Miller et al., 2013).

Asbestosis is characterized by restrictive physiological dysfunction. Nevertheless, in asbestos-exposed workers, obstruction is a commonly found ventilatory defect (Algranti et al., 2001; Ohar et al., 2004). Autopsies on chrysotile miners without asbestosis showed marked changes in the small airways, including membranous bronchioles, when compared with non-exposed smoking controls (Wright et al., 1985). An analysis of lung function in 24 asbestos-exposed workers found an increased elastic recoil, smaller vital capacity, ventilation inhomogeneity and larger mid-expiratory flows with decreased peak flows at any trans-pulmonary pressure level in heavily exposed workers. This suggests that the primary lesion has a predominant peri-bronchiolar location (Jodoin et al., 1971). In non-smokers, asbestos exposure was associated with decreased airflow when compared with a reference population (Kilburn et al., 1985). A cross-sectional study involving asbestos cement workers showed significant reductions in the forced expiratory volume in 1 second (FEV_1) and FVC percentages with increasing quartiles of exposure (Algranti et al., 2001).

There are few studies of longitudinal decline in lung function among asbestos-exposed workers. Asbestos cement workers showed an accelerated decline (beyond age) in FVC and FEV_1 during a 7-year follow-up period in workers with more than 15 years of latency from first exposure (Siracusa et al., 1984) and significant accentuation of the FEV_1 decline in the higher-exposure group (Ohlson et al., 1985). Chinese asbestos manufacturing workers with asbestosis showed an accelerated decline in FVC over a 10-year observation period (Wang et al., 2010). An analysis of 502 former asbestos cement workers followed for a mean period of 9 years showed that asbestos exposure contributed to accelerated FEV_1 declines in smokers, and it was associated with lower levels of lung function at the start of follow-up (Algranti et al., 2013).

A meta-analysis of lung function in asbestos-exposed workers focusing on spirometric parameters concluded that, in the absence of radiographically apparent parenchymal disease, there are modest excesses of both restrictive and obstructive impairments (Wilken et al., 2011). Even though asbestos-induced physiological effects in the absence of radiographic changes are limited, they contribute to the development of small airways disease and accelerate FEV_1 decline when combined with smoking (Miller et al., 2010; Algranti et al., 2013).

New methods of investigation of lung inflammation, such as exhaled nitric oxide and markers in the exhaled

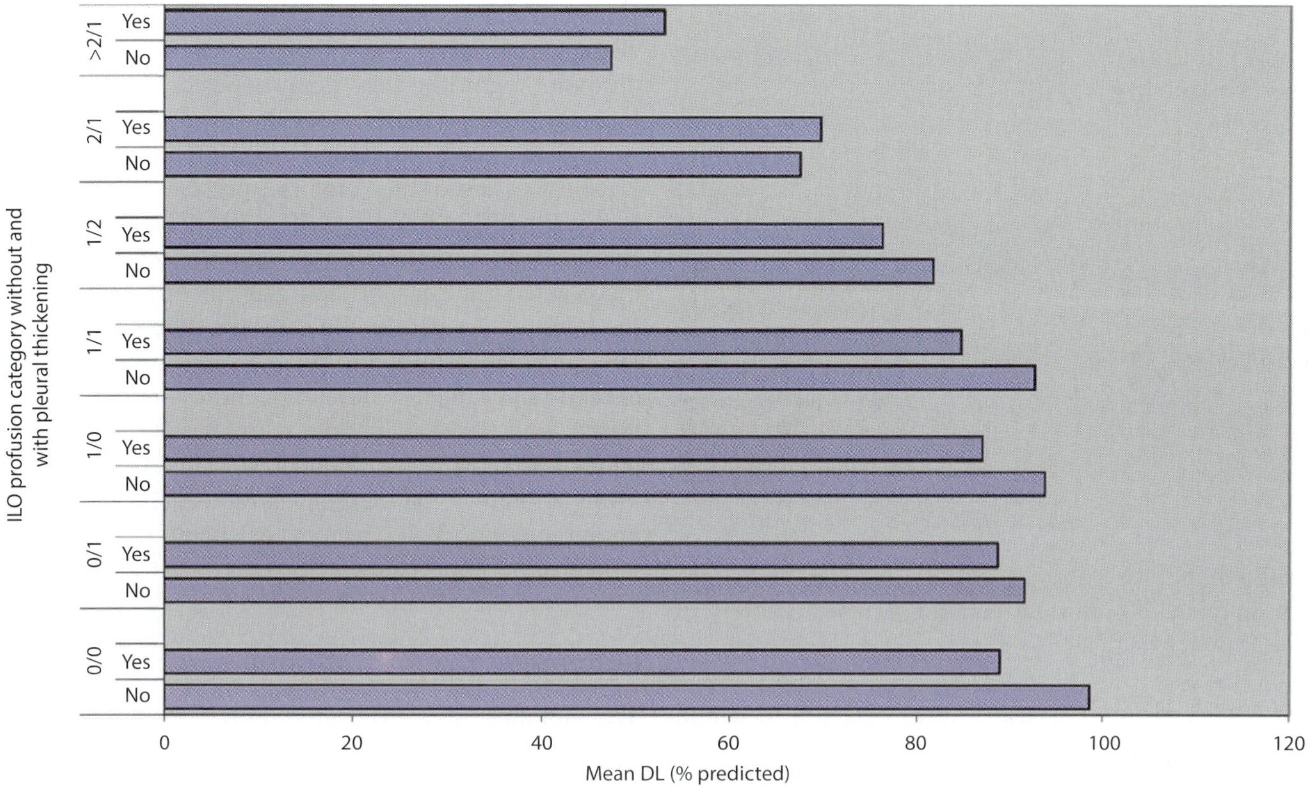

FIGURE 16.7 Diffusing capacity (DL) according to International Labour Organization (ILO) radiologic profusion category of 5003 asbestos-exposed workers. (From Miller, A., Warshaw, R. and Nezamis, J. 2013. *Am J Ind Med* 56(12):1383–93. Reprinted with permission from the *American Journal of Industrial Medicine*.)

breath condensate, are being tested. In the future, they may contribute to the assessment of inflammation (Lehtonen et al., 2007) and the early diagnosis of asbestosis (Lehtimaki et al., 2010).

Pathology

Asbestosis is a diffuse interstitial fibrosis of the lungs that is caused by asbestos exposure. It is typically diagnosed clinically, and biopsy is not required. However, under some circumstances, obtaining lung tissue for pathology review is warranted or obtained for other reasons. The clinical diagnosis of asbestosis may have some uncertainty, especially in mild cases, which can usually be resolved by examination of lung tissue, although there may be some residual uncertainty even following pathology review. Lung biopsy for disease confirmation solely for the purpose of compensation is not justified.

The histological continuum of asbestosis as it increases in severity begins with fibrosis surrounding the respiratory bronchioles (grade 1), which then extends into the alveolar ducts and alveoli (grade 2). Involvement of multiple contiguous bronchiolar units with erasure of alveoli (grade 3) alters the process from a focal one to a continuous and more disruptive fibrosis. More extensive and diffuse fibrosis and the development of honeycombing constitute severe asbestosis (grade 4). The fibrosis of asbestosis is characterized by few cells and much collagen. The fibrotic process affects the lower lobes of the lungs and may extend to the middle and upper lobes.

Diagnostic problems arise at the early grades of asbestosis, because the described histological changes are not specific to asbestos. In addition, the initial phase is composed of focal changes and the subsequent extent of fibrotic changes is variable, leading to differences of opinion concerning whether the fibrotic process is sufficiently widespread to be considered asbestosis.

Evidence of asbestos exposure in pathology specimens is required in order to meet the criteria for the pathological definition of asbestos. There are two metrics for documenting asbestos exposure in the lungs: counting asbestos bodies and counting asbestos fibres. An asbestos body consists of an iron protein coating over a translucent fibrous core and has a characteristic clubbed shape with variable segmentation along the length of the body (Figure 16.8). They are usually found in the lung interstitium (Figure 16.9) and the alveolar spaces and may be seen in sputum or bronchoalveolar lavage fluid.

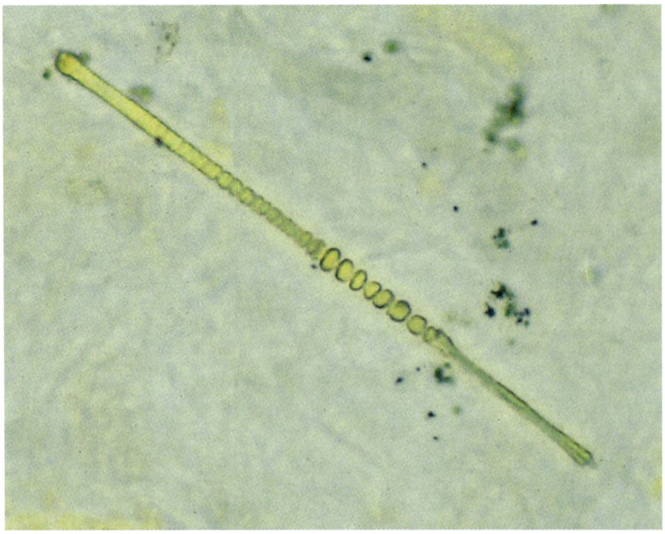

FIGURE 16.8 An asbestos body seen by light microscopy in an unstained 30-μm thick paraffin section. (Courtesy of Bryan Corrin, MD.)

Such bodies form on asbestos fibres >20 μm in length and only a small proportion of asbestos fibres form asbestos bodies. Chrysotile fibres typically do not form asbestos bodies, or form them much less commonly than with amphibole asbestos, so asbestos body counts are not reliable measures of prior chrysotile exposure.

A finding of 2 asbestos bodies per cm^2 on average in 5-μm haematoxylin–eosin- or iron-stained sections of lung tissue is considered evidence of asbestos exposure (Helsinki Consensus, 1997; Roggli et al., 2010; Oksa, 2014). Pathologists, however, disagree on the point regarding how many asbestos bodies must be found in lung sections as evidence of exposure, but it is clear that asbestosis can be present when fewer than 2 asbestos bodies per cm^2 are present (Warnock and Isenberg, 1986; Roggli et al., 2010; Hammar, 2011). Importantly, numerous lung sections need to be examined, since asbestos bodies vary in different parts of the lung. Alternatively, the asbestos fibre content of the lung may be examined in order to determine whether it exceeds the range of fibre concentrations that is found in the lung tissue of people without asbestos exposure and whose tissue fibre counts have been evaluated in the same laboratory. Laboratory methods and findings vary among laboratories—even experienced ones—so intralaboratory comparisons are required.

Diagnosis

The diagnosis of asbestosis requires evidence of a reasonable magnitude and timing of asbestos exposure, the presence of lung structural changes demonstrated by imaging or pathology evaluation and exclusion of other diseases (Helsinki Consensus, 1997). A careful and reliable occupational history of asbestos exposure suffices as aetiological evidence (Helsinki Consensus, 1997), together with characteristic radiological findings in the lungs, obviating the need for histological confirmation,

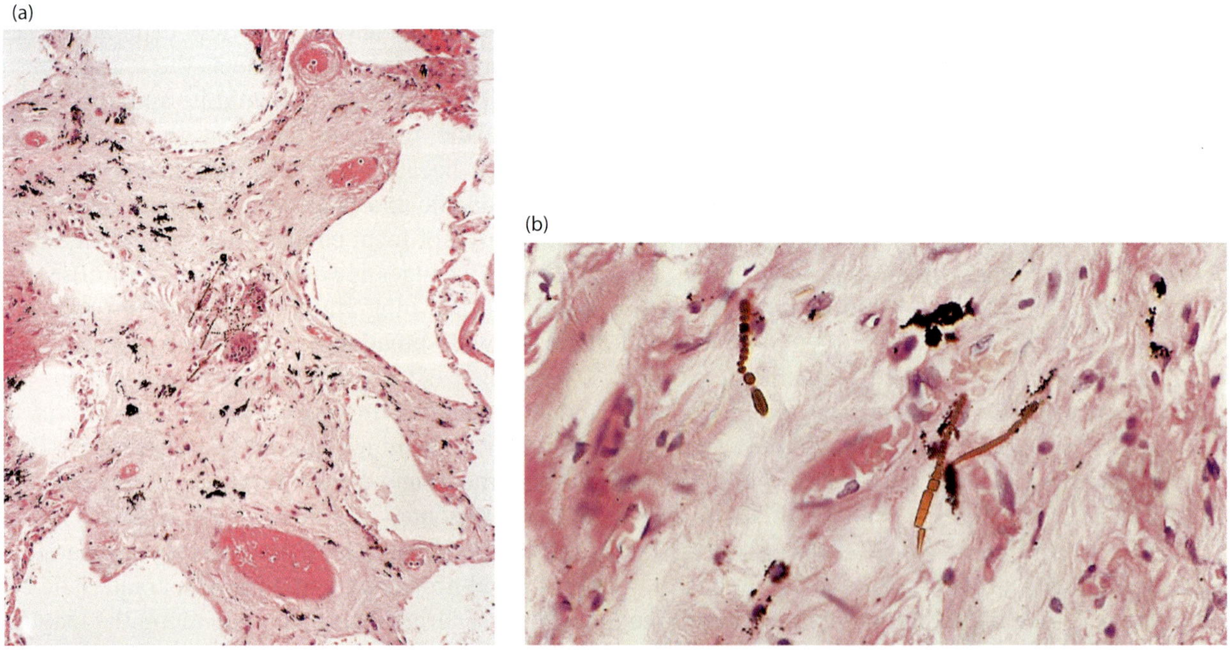

FIGURE 16.9 Asbestosis. Interstitial fibrosis is associated with many asbestos bodies in (a), which are shown in detail in (b). (Courtesy of Bryan Corrin, MD.)

especially if there is no indication for biopsy. With the development of more sensitive imaging techniques that yield very detailed lung images, the need for invasive methods is becoming less common. Additional findings, including the presence of rales, lung function impairment and pleural plaques, although not necessary, may contribute to the certainty of the diagnosis (Helsinki Consensus, 1997).

The ILO classification provides a 12-point continuous scale of radiological alterations on the chest X-ray. By definition, a chest X-ray interpreted as ILO subcategory 1/0 or more is considered abnormal; 's' and 't' irregular opacities are found in asbestosis. In cases of 1/0 parenchymal profusion, a chest CT scan may be helpful in order to obtain better-defined imaging of the chest parenchyma (Helsinki Consensus, 2015). Chest CT scans may also prove helpful in other circumstances (Helsinki Consensus, 2015): (1) in the presence of extensive pleural scarring that obscures the lung parenchyma on plain chest films; (2) in symptomatic asbestos-exposed subjects with normal chest X-rays; and (3) in asbestos-exposed subjects with functional impairment and a normal chest X-ray.

The spectrum of CT findings seen in asbestosis is noted above. Signs of definite fibrosis on HRCT include traction bronchiectasis, architectural distortion and honeycombing. In their absence, there is no established consensus on the number or combination of other CT findings that are required for a diagnosis of early asbestosis. However, CT scans that show three or more of the following findings at two or more levels are considered sufficient to be classified as cases of asbestosis: sub-pleural nodules, thickening of interlobular septa, sub-pleural curvilinear lines and ground-glass opacities (Gamsu et al., 1995).

Inspiratory dry rales are present in over 70% of asbestosis cases. Among well-trained physicians, the presence of this auscultatory sign has good inter-observer and intra-observer correlations (Workum et al., 1986).

Vital capacity is typically reduced in interstitial lung diseases but is non-specific. Patients in the early stages of asbestosis may present with normal spirometry or with evidence of small airways dysfunction. A reduced DLCO is more sensitive than a reduced FVC for identifying interstitial lung diseases (Orens et al., 1995).

As asbestos exposure in working populations declines and asbestosis becomes less frequent, a progressive decline in the positive predictive value of the available diagnostic tools can be expected. The diagnosis of asbestosis, which is always dependent on the aggregation of exposure history and numerous test results, will likely continue to be challenging in the future.

Differential Diagnosis

The clinical presentation of asbestosis is similar to other interstitial lung diseases. Dyspnoea and basal rales on lung examination of asbestotics are non-specific findings of many pulmonary and cardiac diseases. Chest image findings of irregular linear opacities, predominantly in the lower-lung fields, share similarities with interstitial pneumonias, sarcoidosis, hypersensitivity pneumonia and other pneumoconioses. Pursuing the differential diagnosis in patients who may have asbestosis is important, because selected other diseases in the differential diagnosis are potentially treatable and may have different prognoses, and because a diagnosis of asbestosis has medico-legal and compensation consequences (Gaensler et al., 1991).

Within the group of interstitial pneumonias, UIP closely resembles asbestosis. The only histological difference in the two diagnoses is the finding of asbestos bodies associated with fibrosis (Craighead et al., 1982; Roggli et al., 2010). Sub-pleural dot-like structures, curvilinear lines, mosaic perfusion and parenchymal bands are more frequently found in asbestosis, whereas intralobular branching structures, bronchiolectasis, honeycombing and masses are more commonly found in idiopathic pulmonary fibrosis (a corollary of interstitial pneumonias) (Akira et al., 2003). However, these differences are not entirely specific. The finding of pleural plaques indicates a very high likelihood of asbestosis. A study comparing HRCT findings of asbestosis with UIP and NSIP showed that asbestosis and UIP demonstrated coarser radiographic fibrosis compared to a more delicate fibrotic pattern seen in NSIP. Although asbestosis and UIP did not show clear-cut differences, asbestosis tended to be predominantly basal (Copley et al., 2003).

Asbestosis and UIP also differ in prognosis, with the latter progressing more rapidly and associated with higher mortality (Carrington et al., 1978).

Influence of Smoking

Smoking is associated with architectural changes in lung tissue. The most common findings are thickening of bronchial walls, peri-bronchiolar inflammation and fibrosis and emphysema. These changes can alter the findings of asbestosis on the chest X-ray.

Smoking produces histological lesions that affect airways and impair lung clearance. Cigarette smoke enhances the retention of asbestos fibres, especially short fibres, in the airways and lung parenchyma (Churg et al., 1992; Churg et al., 1995). Among workers who are exposed to asbestos, smokers have a higher prevalence and profusion of irregular linear opacities (Kilburn, 1981; Barnhart et al., 1990; Lilis et al., 1991). A South African study among miners examined this issue using chest X-ray results and autopsy-obtained pathology results and found an association between radiographic evidence of asbestosis and smoking, but no such relationship was found between autopsy-based findings of asbestosis and cigarette smoking (Hnizdo et al., 1988).

The evaluation of asbestosis using CT has provided new insights. Among 587 asbestos-exposed workers in various construction trades, CT scans showed that smoking was positively associated with emphysema and bronchial wall thickening and negatively associated with septal lines, sub-pleural dots or honeycombing (Vehmas et al., 2003), which are findings that are strongly associated with asbestosis (Gamsu et al., 1995). Thus, CT may be useful in differentiating architectural changes due to smoking and asbestos.

The pulmonary function of asbestotics who smoke frequently presents a mixed profile of restrictive and obstructive dysfunction. Typical smoking-related findings of ventilatory obstruction (characterized by a low FEV_1/FVC), low mid-expiratory flows and increased total lung capacity (TLC) may be offset by the decrease in lung volumes associated with the interstitial fibrosis of asbestosis. Both exposures decrease gas transfer. Thus, impairment assessment in an asbestos-exposed smoker may be challenging. High-quality HRCT scans combined with lung function studies may be useful in apportioning the relative contribution of each exposure in determining lung function decrements. CT permits the quantification of pleural and parenchymal fibrosis and emphysema, which may be used in parallel with pulmonary function results in order to approximate the relative importance of smoking and asbestos exposure in causing pulmonary compromise (Copley et al., 2007).

Management and Prognosis

Asbestosis is usually diagnosed several decades after the onset of asbestos exposure at a time when affected patients are no longer exposed to asbestos. Nonetheless, the clinician has the obligation to inform affected patients of the aetiology of their disease and to advise that they investigate their rights to compensation in a timely manner. This is especially important because such rights may be time limited once the patient has been informed that they have a condition that was caused by workplace exposures. For patients who actively work and may still be exposed to asbestos, they should be advised to cease exposure to asbestos, seeking necessary assistance to achieve this without job or financial loss to the best extent possible. In some countries, clinicians are obligated to report asbestosis cases to government authorities.

After cessation of asbestos exposure, progression of asbestosis may or may not occur, or it may be slow. Markowitz et al. followed long-term insulators (mean age, 58 years; mean duration of asbestos exposure, 35 years) with varying degrees of asbestosis and found that those with ILO category 1 asbestosis had a cumulative mortality of 2.4% from asbestosis over the 10 years following clinical evaluation (Markowitz et al., 1997). In a follow-up study of 85 asbestosis patients over 6.5 years, Oksa and colleagues found that a third showed progression of fibrosis (Oksa et al., 1998). The incidence of lung cancer was significantly greater in those who showed radiological progression (Oksa et al., 1998). At present, with the decreasing levels of exposure in many work settings, most new cases of asbestosis are expected to be of low profusion on chest X-ray with a diminished likelihood of severe fibrotic disease or death. Exceptions, however, may occur among groups of workers with uncontrolled exposure, especially in industrializing countries.

Important elements of the regular care of patients with asbestosis include: (1) impairment evaluation for compensation purposes; (2) encouragement of smoking cessation, if relevant; (3) prompt treatment of chest infections and comorbid pulmonary and cardiac diseases; (4) immunization against pneumococcal disease and yearly influenza vaccines; and (5) participation in low-dose CT screening for lung cancer. Periodic clinical examination and chest imaging studies are advised in order to monitor the progression of the disease (Levin et al., 2000).

Asbestosis patients must also be evaluated for participation in lung cancer screening programmes that use low-dose CT scanning. In the absence of a local organized screening programme, the clinician should consider referring the patient with asbestosis directly for a low-dose CT scan. A large randomized clinical trial in the United States demonstrated that high-risk groups that had annual low-dose CT scanning experienced a 20% reduction in lung cancer mortality over the ensuing years (National Lung Screening Trial Research Team et al., 2011). Given the elevated lung cancer risk of patients with asbestosis, especially among smokers and former smokers, the advent of low-dose CT scanning as an effective tool in the early detection of lung cancer represents an unprecedented opportunity to prevent lung cancer deaths among these patients (International Conference on Monitoring and Surveillance of Asbestos-Related Diseases, 2014).

National or regional registries of workers exposed to asbestos or of patients with asbestosis are required or recommended in some jurisdictions. Such registries are advantageous as a rational means of organizing surveillance programmes, notifying and communicating with asbestos-exposed workers and initiating lung cancer screening programmes (International Conference on Monitoring and Surveillance of Asbestos-Related Diseases, 2014).

REFERENCES

Aberle, D. R., Gamsu, G. and Ray, C. S. 1988. High-resolution CT of benign asbestos-related diseases: Clinical and radiographic correlation. *Am J Roentgenol* 151(5):883–91.

Akira, M., Yamamoto, S., Inoue, Y. and Sakatani, M. 2003. High-resolution CT of asbestosis and idiopathic pulmonary fibrosis. *Am J Roentgenol* 181(1):163–69.

Akira, M., Yokoyama, K., Yamamoto, S., Higashihara, T., Morinaga, K., Kita, N., Morimoto, S., Ikezoe, J. and Kozuka, T. 1991. Early asbestosis: Evaluation with high-resolution CT. *Radiology* 178(2):409–16.

al Jarad, N., Strickland, B., Bothamley, G., Lock, S., Logan-Sinclair, R. and Rudd, R. M. 1993. Diagnosis of asbestosis by a time expanded wave form analysis, auscultation and high resolution computed tomography: A comparative study. *Thorax* 48(4):347–53.

Algranti, E. 1998. Occupational lung diseases in Brazil. In J. E. Parker and D. E. Banks (eds), *Occupational Lung Disease: An International Perspective*, 105–115. London: Chapman & Hall.

Algranti, E., Mendonca, E. M., DeCapitani, E. M., Freitas, J. B., Silva, H. C. and Bussacos, M. A. 2001. Non-malignant asbestos-related diseases in Brazilian asbestos-cement workers. *Am J Ind Med* 40(3):240–54.

Algranti, E., Mendonca, E. M., Hnizdo, E., De Capitani, E. M., Freitas, J. B., Raile, V. and Bussacos, M. A. 2013. Longitudinal decline in lung function in former asbestos exposed workers. *Occup Environ Med* 70(1):15–21.

Amandus, H. E., Wheeler, R., Jankovic, J. and Tucker, J. 1987. The morbidity and mortality of vermiculite miners and millers exposed to tremolite-actinolite: Part I. Exposure estimates. *Am J Ind Med* 11(1):1–4.

Bang, K. M., Mazurek, J. M., Wood, J. M. and Hendricks, S. A. 2014. Diseases attributable to asbestos exposure: Years of potential life lost, United States, 1999–2010. *Am J Ind Med* 57(1):38–48.

Barnhart, S., Thornquist, M., Omenn, G. S., Goodman, G., Feigl, P. and Rosenstock, L. 1990. The degree of roentgenographic parenchymal opacities attributable to smoking among asbestos-exposed subjects. *Am Rev Respir Dis* 141(5 Pt 1):1102–6.

Bezerra, O. M., Dias, E. C., Galvao, M. A. and Carneiro, A. P. 2003. Talc pneumoconiosis among soapstone handicraft workers in a rural area of Ouro Preto, Minas Gerais, Brazil. *Cad Saude Publica* 19(6):1751–9.

Bourgkard, E., Wild, P., Gonzalez, M., Fevotte, J., Penven, E. and Paris, C. 2013. Comparison of exposure assessment methods in a lung cancer case–control study: Performance of a lifelong task-based questionnaire for asbestos and PAHs. *Occup Environ Med* 70(12):884–91.

Burdorf, A., Dahhan, M. and Swuste, P. 2003. Occupational characteristics of cases with asbestos-related diseases in the Netherlands. *Ann Occup Hyg* 47(6):485–92.

Carrington, C. B., Gaensler, E. A., Coutu, R. E., FitzGerald, M. X. and Gupta, R. G. 1978. Natural history and treated course of usual and desquamative interstitial pneumonia. *N Engl J Med* 298(15):801–9.

Center for Disease Control. 2012. 10 Leading Causes of Death by Age Group, United States—2012. Available at: http://www.cdc.gov/injury/wisqars/pdf/leading_causes_of_death_by_age_group_2012-a.pdf (accessed 10 March 2015).

Churg, A. and Stevens, B. 1995. Enhanced retention of asbestos fibres in the airways of human smokers. *Am J Respir Crit Care Med* 151(5):1409–13.

Churg, A., Wright, J. L., Hobson, J. and Stevens, B. 1992. Effects of cigarette smoke on the clearance of short asbestos fibres from the lung and a comparison with the clearance of long asbestos fibres. *Int J Exp Pathol* 73(3):287–97.

Collegium Ramazzini. 2011. Asbestos is still with us: Repeat call for a universal ban. *Am J Ind Med* 54:168–73.

Conti, S., Minelli, G., Manno, V., Iavarone, I., Comba, P., Scondotto, S. and Cernigliaro, A. 2014. Health impact of the exposure to fibres with fluoro-edenitic composition on the residents in Biancavilla (Sicily, Italy): Mortality and hospitalization from current data. *Ann Ist Super Sanita* 50(2):127–32.

Copley, S. J., Lee, Y. C., Hansell, D. M., Sivakumaran, P., Rubens, M. B., Newman Taylor, A. J., Rudd, R. M., Musk, A. W. and Wells, A. U. 2007. Asbestos-induced and smoking-related disease: Apportioning pulmonary function deficit by using thin-section CT. *Radiology* 242(1):258–66.

Copley, S. J., Wells, A. U., Sivakumaran, P., Rubens, M. B., Lee, Y. C., Desai, S. R., MacDonald, S. L. et al. 2003. Asbestosis and idiopathic pulmonary fibrosis: Comparison of thin-section CT features. *Radiology* 229(3):731–36.

Coutts, I. I., Gilson, J. C., Kerr, I. H., Parkes, W. R. and Turner-Warwick, M. 1987. Significance of finger clubbing in asbestosis. *Thorax* 42(2):117–9.

Craighead, J. E., Abraham, J. L., Churg, A., Green, F. H., Kleinerman, J., Pratt, P. C., Seemayer, T. A., Vallyathan, V. and Weill, H. 1982. The pathology of asbestos-associated diseases of the lungs and pleural cavities: Diagnostic criteria and proposed grading schema. Report of the pneumoconiosis committee of the college of American Pathologists and the National Institute for Occupational Safety and Health. *Arch Pathol Lab Med* 106(11):544–96.

Dick, J. A., Morgan, W. K., Muir, D. F., Reger, R. B. and Sargent, N. 1992. The significance of irregular opacities on the chest roentgenogram. *Chest* 102(1):251–60.

Finkelstein, M. M. 1985. A study of dose–response relationships for asbestos associated disease. *Br J Ind Med* 42(5):319–25.

Finkelstein, M. M. and Vingilis, J. J. 1984. Radiographic abnormalities among asbestos-cement workers. An exposure–response study. *Am Rev Respir Dis* 129(1):17–22.

Friedman, A. C., Fiel, S. B., Fisher, M. S., Radecki, P. D., Lev-Toaff, A. S. and Caroline, D. F. 1988. Asbestos-related pleural disease and asbestosis: A comparison of CT and chest radiography. *Am J Roentgenol* 150(2):269–75.

Gaensler, E. A., Jederlinic, P. J. and Churg, A. 1991. Idiopathic pulmonary fibrosis in asbestos-exposed workers. *Am Rev Respir Dis* 144(3 Pt 1):689–96.

Gamsu, G., Salmon, C. J., Warnock, M. L. and Blanc, P. D. 1995. CT quantification of interstitial fibrosis in patients with asbestosis: A comparison of two methods. *Am J Roentgenol* 164(1):63–8.

Hammar, S. P. 2011. Asbestosis. In R. F. Dodson and S. P. Hammar (eds), *Asbestos: Risk Assessment, Epidemiology, and Health Effects*. 2nd ed., 447–480. Boca Raton, FL: CRC Press.

Hanley, A., Hubbard, R. B. and Navaratnam, V. 2011. Mortality trends in asbestosis, extrinsic allergic alveolitis and sarcoidosis in England and wales. *Respir Med* 105(9):1373–9.

Hardt, J. S., Vermeulen, R., Peters, S., Kromhout, H., McLaughlin, J. R. and Demers, P. A. 2014. A comparison of exposure assessment approaches: Lung cancer and occupational asbestos exposure in a population-based case-control study. *Occup Environ Med* 71(4):282–8.

Helsinki Consensus. 1997. Asbestos, asbestosis, and cancer: The Helsinki criteria for diagnosis and attribution. *Scand J Work Environ Health* 23:311–6.

Helsinki Consensus. 2015. Asbestos, asbestosis, and cancer: The Helsinki criteria for diagnosis and attribution 2014: Recommendations. *Scand J Work Environ Health* 41:5–15.

Hnizdo, E. and Sluis-Cremer, G. K. 1988. Effect of tobacco smoking on the presence of asbestosis at postmortem and on the reading of irregular opacities on roentgenograms in asbestos-exposed workers. *Am Rev Respir Dis* 138(5):1207–12.

International Agency for Research on Cancer. 2012. *IARC Monographs on the Evaluation of Carcinogenic Risks to Humans: Volume 100c: Arsenic, Metals. Fibres and Dusts*. Geneva: WHO Press.

International Conference on Monitoring and Surveillance of Asbestos-Related Diseases. 2014. *The Helsinki Declaration on Management and Elimination of Asbestos-Related Diseases*. Espoo: Finnish Institute of Occupational Health.

International Labour Organization. 2011. Guidelines for the Use of the ILO International Classification of Radiographs of Pneumoconiosis. International Labour Office, Geneva, Switzerland.

Jodoin, G., Gibbs, G. W., Macklem, P. T., McDonald, J. C. and Becklake, M. R. 1971. Early effects of asbestos exposure on lung function. *Am Rev Respir Dis* 104(4):525–35.

Kilburn, K. H. 1981. Cigarette smoking does not produce or enhance the radiologic appearance of pulmonary fibrosis. *Am J Ind Med* 2:305–8.

Kilburn, K. H., Warshaw, R. H., Einstein, K. and Bernstein, J. 1985. Airway disease in non-smoking asbestos workers. *Arch Environ Health* 40(6):293–5.

Kishimoto, T., Morinaga, K. and Kira, S. 2000. The prevalence of pleural plaques and/or pulmonary changes among construction workers in Okayama, Japan. *Am J Ind Med* 37(3):291–5.

Kraus, T., Borsch-Galetke, E., Elliehausen, H. J., Frank, K., Hering, K. G., Hieckel, H. G., Hofmann-Preiss, K. et al. 2009. Recommendations for reporting benign asbestos-related findings in chest X-ray and CT to the accident insurances. *Pneumologie* 63(12):726–32.

Kusaka, Y., Hering, K. G. and Parker, J. E. 2005. *International Classification of HRCT for Occupational and Environmental Respiratory Diseases*. Tokyo: Springer-Verlag.

Lee, Y. C., Singh, B., Pang, S. C., de Klerk, N. H., Hillman, D. R. and Musk, A. W. 2003. Radiographic (ILO) readings predict arterial oxygen desaturation during exercise in subjects with asbestosis. *Occup Environ Med* 60(3):201–6.

Lehtimaki, L., Oksa, P., Jarvenpaa, R., Vierikko, T., Nieminen, R., Kankaanranta, H., Uitti, J. and Moilanen, E. 2010. Pulmonary inflammation in asbestos-exposed subjects with borderline parenchymal changes on HRCT. *Respir Med* 104(7):1042–9.

Lehtonen, H., Oksa, P., Lehtimaki, L., Sepponen, A., Nieminen, R., Kankaanranta, H., Saarelainen, S. , Jarvenpaa, R. Uitti, J. and Moilanen, E. 2007. Increased alveolar nitric oxide concentration and high levels of Leukotriene B(4) and 8-isoprostane in exhaled breath condensate in patients with asbestosis. *Thorax* 62(7):602–7.

Levin, S. M., Kann, P. E. and Lax, M. B. 2000. Medical examination for asbestos-related disease. *Am J Ind Med* 37(1):6–22.

Lilis, R., Miller, A., Godbold, J., Chan, E. and Selikoff, I. J. 1991. Radiographic abnormalities in asbestos insulators: Effects of duration from onset of exposure and smoking. Relationships of dyspnea with parenchymal and pleural fibrosis. *Am J Ind Med* 20(1):1–5.

Loyola, R. C., Carneiro, A. P., Silveira, A. M., La Rocca P. de F., Nascimento, M. S. and Chaves, R. H. 2010. Respiratory effects from industrial talc exposure among former mining workers. *Rev Saude Publica* 44(3):541–7.

Magnani, C., Mollo, F., Paoletti, L., Bellis, D., Bernardi, P., Betta, P., Botta, M., Falchi, M. Ivaldi, C. and Pavesi, M. 1998. Asbestos lung burden and asbestosis after occupational and environmental exposure in an asbestos cement manufacturing area: A necropsy study. *Occup Environ Med* 55(12):840–6.

Markowitz, S. B., Morabia, A., Lilis, R., Miller, A., Nicholson, W. J. and Levin, S. 1997. Clinical predictors of mortality from asbestosis in the North American insulator cohort, 1981 to 1991. *Am J Respir Crit Care Med* 156(1):101–8.

Miller, A., Lilis, R., Godbold, J., Chan, E. and Selikoff, I. J. 1992. Relationship of pulmonary function to radiographic interstitial fibrosis in 2,611 long-term asbestos insulators. An assessment of the International Labour Office profusion score. *Am Rev Respir Dis* 145(2 Pt 1):263–70.

Miller, A. and Mann, J. M. 2013. Airways disease presenting as restrictive impairment: A variant in asthma, a defining feature in World Trade Center lung disorder. *Chest* 144(6):1977–8.

Miller, A. and Rom, W. N. 2010. Does asbestos exposure (asbestosis) cause (clinical) airway obstruction (small airway disease)? *Am J Respir Crit Care* Med 182(4):444–5.

National Lung Screening Trial Research Team, Aberle, D. R., Adams, A. M., Berg, C. D., Black, W. C., Clapp, J. D., Fagerstrom, R. M. et al. 2011. Reduced lung-cancer mortality with low-dose computed tomographic screening. *N Engl J Med* 365(5):395–409.

Nogueira, C. R., Napolis, L. M., Bagatin, E., Terra-Filho, M., Muller, N. L., Silva, C. I., Rodrigues, R. T., Neder, J. A. and Nery, L. E. 2011. Lung diffusing capacity relates better to short-term progression on HRCT abnormalities than spirometry in mild asbestosis. *Am J Ind Med* 54(3):185–93.

Ohar, J., Sterling, D. A., Bleecker, E. and Donohue, J. 2004. Changing patterns in asbestos-induced lung disease. *Chest* 125(2):744–53.

Ohlson, C. G., Bodin, L., Rydman, T. and Hogstedt, C. 1985. Ventilatory decrements in former asbestos cement workers: A four year follow up. *Br J Ind Med* 42(9):612–6.

Oksa, P., Wolff, H., Vehmas, T., Pallasaho, P. and Frilander, H. 2014. *Asbestos, Asbestosis, and Cancer: Helsinki Criteria for Diagnosis and Attribution.* Helsinki: Finnish Institute of Occupational Health, 1–53.

Oksa, P., Huuskonen, M. S., Jarvisalo, J., Klockars, M., Zitting, A., Suoranta, H., Tossavainen, A., Vattulainen, K. and Laippala, P. 1998. Follow-up of asbestosis patients and predictors for radiographic progression. *Int Arch Occup Environ Health* 71(7):465–71.

Orens, J. B., Kazerooni, E. A., Martinez, F. J., Curtis, J. L., Gross, B. H., Flint, A. and Lynch, J. P. 3rd. 1995. The sensitivity of high-resolution CT in detecting idiopathic pulmonary fibrosis proved by open lung biopsy. A prospective study. *Chest* 108(1):109–15.

Peipins, L. A., Lewin, M., Campolucci, S., Lybarger, J. A., Miller, A., Middleton, D., Weis, C., Spence, M. Black, B. and Kapil, V. 2003. Radiographic abnormalities and exposure to asbestos-contaminated vermiculite in the community of Libby, Montana, USA. *Environ Health Perspect* 111(14):1753–9.

Remy-Jardin, M., Sobaszek, A., Duhamel, A., Mastora, I., Zanetti, C. and Remy, J. 2004. Asbestos-related pleuropulmonary diseases: Evaluation with low-dose four-detector row spiral CT. *Radiology* 233(1):182–90.

Rodelsperger, K., Jahn, H., Bruckel, B., Manke, J., Paur, R. and Woitowitz, H. J. 1986. Asbestos dust exposure during brake repair. *Am J Ind Med* 10(1):63–72.

Roggli, V. L., Gibbs, A. R., Attanoos, R., Churg, A., Popper, H., Cagle, P., Corrin, B. et al. 2010. Pathology of asbestosis- an update of the diagnostic criteria: Report of the asbestosis committee of the college of American Pathologists and Pulmonary Pathology Society. *Arch Pathol Lab Med* 134(3):462–80.

Rosenstock, L., Barnhart, S., Heyer, N. J., Pierson, D. J. and Hudson, L. D. 1988. The relation among pulmonary function, chest roentgenographic abnormalities, and smoking status in an asbestos-exposed cohort. *Am Rev Respir Dis* 138(2):272–7.

Scancarello, G., Romeo, R. and Sartorelli, E. 1996. Respiratory disease as a result of talc inhalation. *J Occup Environ Med* 38(6):610–4.

Schwartz, D. A., Fuortes, L. J., Galvin, J. R., Burmeister, L. F., Schmidt, L. E., Leistikow, B. N., LaMarte, F. P. and Merchant, J. A. 1990. Asbestos-induced pleural fibrosis and impaired lung function. *Am Rev Respir Dis* 141(2):321–6.

Siracusa, A., Cicioni, C., Volpi, R., Canalicchi, P., Brugnami, G., Comodi, A. R. and Abbritti, G. 1984. Lung function among asbestos cement factory workers: Cross-sectional and longitudinal study. *Am J Ind Med* 5(4):315–25.

Staples, C. A. 1992. Computed tomography in the evaluation of benign asbestos-related disorders. *Radiol Clin North Am* 30(6):1191–207.

Staples, C. A., Gamsu, G. Ray, C. S. and Webb, W. R. 1989. High resolution computed tomography and lung function in asbestos-exposed workers with normal chest radiographs. *Am Rev Respir Dis* 139(6):1502–8.

Suganuma, N., Kusaka, Y. Hering, K. G. Vehmas, T. Kraus, T. Arakawa, H. and Parker, J. E. et al. 2009. Reliability of the proposed international classification of high-resolution computed tomography for occupational and environmental respiratory diseases. *J Occup Health* 51(3):210–22.

Vehmas, T., Kivisaari, L., Huuskonen, M. S. and Jaakkola, M. S. 2003. Effects of tobacco smoking on findings in chest computed tomography among asbestos-exposed workers. *Eur Respir J* 21(5):866–71.

Virta, R. 2013. *2012 Minerals Yearbook: Asbestos.* U.S. Geological Survey. Available at http://minerals.usgs.gov/minerals/pubs/commodity/asbestos/myb1-2012-asbes.pdf

Wang, X., Wang, M., Qiu, H., Yu, I. and Yano, E. 2010. Longitudinal changes in pulmonary function of asbestos workers. *J Occup Health* 52(5):272–7.

Warnock, M. L. and Isenberg, W. 1986. Asbestos burden and the pathology of lung cancer. *Chest* 89(1):20–6.

Weill, H., Ziskind, M. M., Waggenspack, C. and Rossiter, C. E. 1975. Lung function consequences of dust exposure in asbestos cement manufacturing plants. *Arch Environ Health* 30(2):88–97.

Welch, L. S., Michaels, D. and Zoloth, S. R. 1994. The national sheet metal worker asbestos disease screening program: Radiologic findings. National sheet metal examination group. *Am J Ind Med* 25(5):635–48.

Wilczynska, U. and Szeszenia-Dabrowska, N. 2002. The incidence of asbestosis in Poland. *Med Pr* 53(5):375–9.

Wilken, D., Velasco Garrido, M., Manuwald, U. and Baur, X. 2011. Lung function in asbestos-exposed workers, a systematic review and meta-analysis. *J Occup Med Toxicol* 6:21.

Workum, P., DelBono, E. A. Holford, S. K. and Murphy, R. L. Jr. 1986. Observer agreement, chest auscultation, and crackles in asbestos-exposed workers. *Chest* 89(1):27–9.

World Health Organization. 2006. *Elimination of Asbestos-Related Diseases*. Geneva: WHO Press.

World Health Organization. 2014a. Asbestos: Elimination of Asbestos-Related Diseases Fact Sheet no. 343. Available at: http://www.who.int/mediacentre/factsheets/fs343/en/ (accessed 13 November 2014).

World Health Organization. 2014b. *Chrysotile Asbestos*. Geneva: WHO Press.

17 Asbestos-Related Non-Malignant Pleural Disease and Mesothelioma

Bill Musk, Nick H. de Klerk and Fraser J. H. Brims

CONTENTS

INTRODUCTION

The word 'asbestos' comes from a Greek adjective meaning 'inextinguishable'. Historic records suggest that asbestos has been used for over 4000 years; it became increasingly popular throughout the twentieth century due to its resistance to heat, electricity and chemical damage, its sound absorption and its tensile strength. The term 'asbestos' refers to a group of crystalline-hydrated silicate minerals that exist as fibres. Asbestos is mined from the ground, and this is still done in a number of countries, including South Africa, China, Brazil, Zimbabwe and Russia (Virta, 2008). It occurs in two forms: serpentine and amphibole. Chrysotile ('white' asbestos) is the only serpentine form, whilst amphibole asbestos has several different forms, although the major commercial uses have largely been with crocidolite ('blue') and amosite ('brown'). Chrysotile fibres are long, curly and pliable and have been mostly used to make asbestos cement, thermal insulation, fabrics and other flexible items. Amphibole fibres are short, straight and stiff with superior chemical and physical stability/durability.

Despite the recognised dangers of asbestos, which were first documented in 1899 for a board of enquiry by a British physician (Tweedale and Hansen, 1998), many industrial countries used and imported asbestos throughout most of the twentieth century, with complete bans only enacted late in the 1990s or early 2000s for many but not all countries.

Many occupations have been associated with significant asbestos exposures. The risks of asbestos-related diseases including malignant mesothelioma are substantial in those who have worked in the mining, processing and transportation of raw asbestos. The principal manufacturing industries that use or used asbestos are those producing specialised cement products, insulating materials and brake linings or applying and refitting asbestos insulation, as in ship-fitting and other dockyard work, railway carriage maintenance, building construction and demolition. Joiners, carpenters, heating engineers, boilermen, railwaymen and former (naval) servicemen have often been exposed.

Some exposure is 'para-occupational', being incurred by working alongside those applying or stripping asbestos, and frequently a detailed occupational history is required, not only regarding direct exposures, but also possible exposures around the workplace that are not necessarily directly related to the performing of an individual's tasks or jobs. A detailed history should also include possible exposure from other members in the household from dust carried home on work clothes and any history of performing renovations to homes or buildings that contained asbestos. Others remain at risk due to naturally occurring deposits such as erionite (Van Gosen et al., 2013) or because they have lived in the vicinity of asbestos mines or factories (Figure 17.1).

CIRCUMSCRIBED PLEURAL PLAQUES

Circumscribed pleural plaques (CPPs) are the most common manifestations of asbestos exposure (Hillerdal

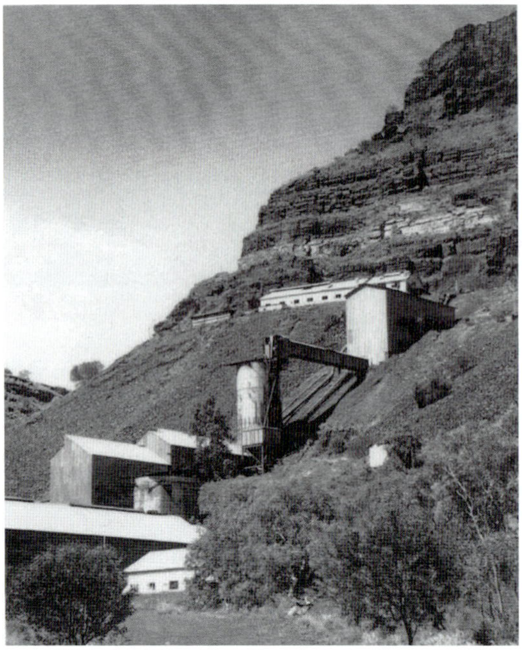

FIGURE 17.1 Mine site c. 1960 in Colonial Gorge, the second of two crocidolite asbestos mines at Wittenoom in the Pilbra region of Western Australia.

and Lindgren, 1980; Paris et al., 2009). They consist of discrete areas of hyaline pleural fibrosis with laminated collagen fibres in parallel (Craighead et al., 1982); occasionally, asbestos fibres or asbestos bodies are found within them (Sebastien et al., 1979). With the passage of time, CPPs frequently undergo dystrophic calcification, which makes them more visible radiographically (Figure 17.2). They are almost always bilateral and situated on the parietal pleura of the chest wall, diaphragm or mediastinum (most commonly posteriorly and laterally along the contours of the eighth and ninth ribs, but rarely at the apices or the costophrenic angles). They are occasionally seen in the inter-lobar fissures. If the costophrenic angle is obliterated in the presence of a CPP, it is usually taken to indicate that diffuse pleural thickening (DPT) is also present. When situated on the visceral pleura, CPPs are often associated with abnormalities in the underlying lung, with interstitial fibrotic lines radiating out and described as 'hairy plaques' radiographically (Roach et al., 2002). CPPs do not cause symphysis or even adhesion of the visceral and parietal pleural surfaces.

CPPs characteristically appear macroscopically as shiny white elevations with well-demarcated borders on the parietal pleura. They are usually multiple and up to several centimetres across. Microscopically, they consist of dense, sparsely cellular (hyaline) fibrous tissue covered with normal mesothelium (Figure 17.3). Asbestos fibres are rarely found within plaques with light microscopy, but small fibres may occasionally be seen by electron microscopy (Hillerdal and Lindgren, 1980).

It is widely accepted that CPPs form as a direct result of asbestos fibres in the pleural cavities or projecting from the visceral pleura causing irritation during respiratory movement and exciting an inflammatory response, mainly of the parietal pleura (Huggins and Sahn, 2004). It has been suggested that the fibres reach the visceral pleura by the trans-pulmonary route and enter the pleural cavity through (hypothetical) stomata in the pleural surface or (possibly) by retrograde drainage from intercostal lymphatics (Hillerdal and Lindgren, 1980). Plaques can be induced experimentally in rats

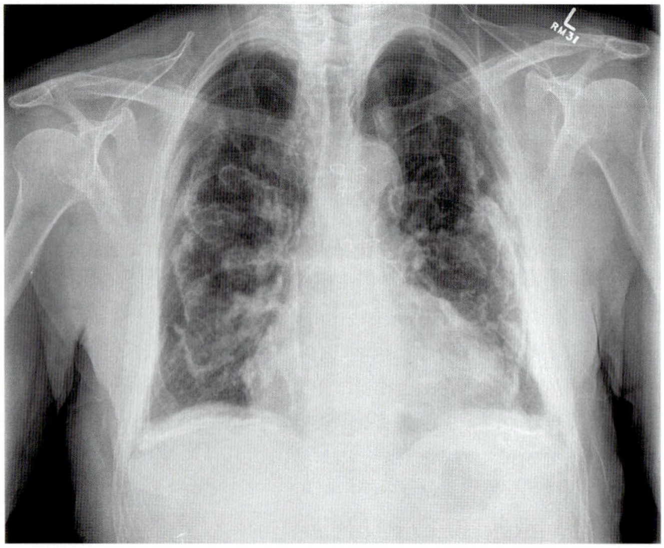

FIGURE 17.2 Calcified pleural plaques in a crocidolite asbestos miner.

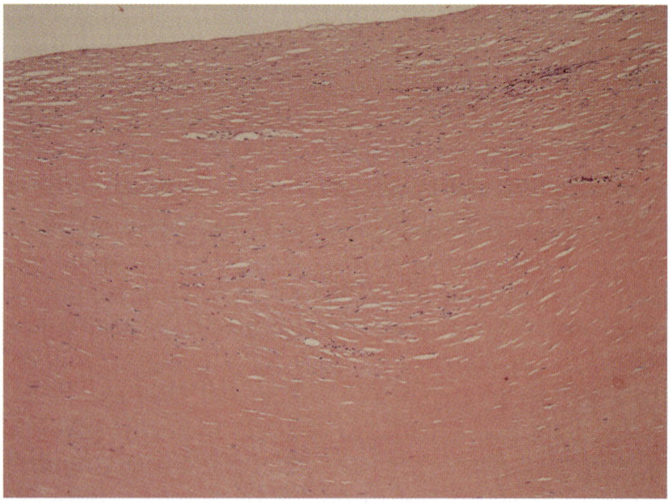

FIGURE 17.3 Pleural plaque. Hypocellular collagenous tissue demonstrating a 'basket-weave' pattern (haematoxylin and eosin ×100).

by injection of asbestos directly into the pleural cavity (Sahn and Antony, 1984).

Pleural plaques occur more commonly with increasing time since first exposure to asbestos and with greater cumulative exposure (Mastrangelo et al., 2009; Larson et al., 2012a), especially to amphibole varieties of asbestos, including Libby amphibole (Black et al., 2014; Clark et al., 2014). They are more common in urban-dwellers than people living in the country, and also in people living close to naturally occurring asbestos (or erionite) (Baris et al., 1981; Luo et al., 2003). Talc and kaolin exposure can also cause pleural plaques, although with talc this may be a result of asbestos contamination. Pleural plaques are associated with increased numbers of amphibole, but not chrysotile, fibres in the lungs (Churg, 1982). Consistent with this observation, the prevalence of plaques in dockyard workers has been shown to increase with the intensity of their estimated asbestos exposure (Sheers and Templeton, 1968; Mollo et al., 1983). An association of plaques with cigarette smoking has been suggested, but the relationship is not consistent, with just one study possibly demonstrating an association with peritoneal plaques (Andrion et al., 1983).

The natural history of CPPs following amphibole exposure is that they usually become visible on plain chest X-rays (CXR) within 10 years of asbestos exposure and do not subsequently progress in size or extent, but become more easily seen on the films due to increasing calcification (de Klerk et al., 1989). After first exposure to vermiculite contaminated with tremolite, the median time to calcification on CXR was 17.5 years (Larson et al., 2010). Initially, the calcification appears punctate, but becomes more dense (and visible) with the passage of time.

A number of small studies have demonstrated a relationship between the presence of pleural plaques and the adjusted risk of malignant pleural mesothelioma (MPM) (Hillerdal, 1994; Hillerdal and Henderson, 1997; Karjalainen et al., 1999; Pairon et al., 2013). However, this was not shown in the largest study so far published (although there was a relationship with peritoneal mesothelioma) (Reid et al., 2005).

Plain CXRs underestimate the frequency and extent of pleural plaques, as they are better seen on computed tomography (CT) scans or at post-mortem. When compared to autopsy or thoracotomy, only approximately 15% of CPPs are identified on plain postero-anterior (PA) CXRs (Ameille et al., 1993). Nevertheless, the standard PA CXR is probably still the most common means by which CPPs are identified, often as an incidental finding. Lateral and oblique views increase the likelihood of demonstrating CPPs. If of sufficient thickness, non-calcified plaques may be seen face-on as faint, sharply delineated, relatively homogeneous infiltrates. Chest CT is increasingly being used (especially since the introduction of low-dose CTs) (Brims et al., 2015) and is able to identify more subtle, smaller areas of CPPs. CT is also of value for differentiating CPPs from sub-pleural fat deposits in subjects with asbestos exposure, who often have pleural shadowing that may be confused with CPPs or DPT on plain CXR (in whom body mass index is also greater) (Friedman et al., 1990; Lee et al., 2001).

The International Labour Organization's Classification of Radiographs for the Pneumoconioses (ILO, 1980) includes a systematic means of recording the presence of benign asbestos-induced pleural diseases, which is invaluable for epidemiological purposes (but of much less value clinically). It does, however, include a convenient definition of the extent of the degree of thickening of the pleura constituting a plaque as opposed to diffuse thickening. A similar system exists for recording the presence and extent of pleural plaques on CT scans (Kusaka and Hering, 2005).

Magnetic resonance imaging (MRI) of CPPs demonstrates low signal intensity on both unenhanced and enhanced T1-weighted and T2-weighted images. This contrasts with MPM, which shows high signal intensity on proton density and T2-weighted images and homogeneous contrast enhancement in the post-contrast T1-weighted images (Armato et al., 2013).

Pleural plaques are statistically associated with minor changes in lung function, with population studies showing a minor effect on lung volumes (total lung capacity and vital capacity) (Kilburn and Warshaw, 1990; Broderick et al., 1992; Van Cleemput et al., 2001; Clin et al., 2011; Weill et al., 2011; Larson et al., 2012b). While pleural plaques alone are not physically disabling, a few countries currently compensate individuals for associated anxiety. The presence of pleural plaques in association with interstitial lung disease, pleural effusion or lung cancer is an independent indicator of asbestos exposure and raises the issue of an asbestos aetiology of the disease. This, in turn, may support a worker's compensation claim or litigation. On the other hand, the absence of plaques cannot be taken to negate an asbestos aetiology of a possible asbestos-related process.

Plaques are usually asymptomatic, although there may be an association with chest pain, with up to 53% of subjects with CPPs reporting pain (Allen et al., 2011; Park et al., 2011). The pain may have similar characteristics to angina (Mukherjee et al., 2000). Pleural friction rubs are sometimes heard in people with pleural plaques; they are usually evanescent, but may be recurrent for months/years. There is no treatment for pleural plaques.

BENIGN ASBESTOS PLEURAL EFFUSION

Benign asbestos pleural effusion (BAPE) is a term that is applied to an exudative pleural effusion occurring in subjects with asbestos exposure for which no alternative cause can be identified, and was first described in 1965 (Eisenstadt, 1965). In subjects with crocidolite exposure, it tends to occur earlier following exposure than malignant mesothelioma (MM) or DPT and is uncommon more than 25 years following exposure (Robinson and Musk, 1981; Epler et al., 1982), in marked contrast to MM (Cookson et al., 1985). Asbestos effusions are more common following amphibole exposure than chrysotile exposure and the frequency of occurrence of BAPE increases with the dose of asbestos exposure (Epler et al., 1982).

BAPE may present with exertional dyspnoea and/or pleuritic pain, or may be identified incidentally in asymptomatic individuals. The presence of fever, sweating or other constitutional symptoms raises the suspicion that some other inflammatory or neoplastic process is responsible for the effusion. BAPE may be identified clinically or by any routine imaging modality, with CT or thoracic ultrasound being more sensitive tools. As with any unexplained pleural effusion, further investigation with thoracentesis, thoracoscopy and biopsy should be considered.

There are no consistent cytological or biochemical distinguishing features of BAPE, except that it is exudative (with high protein and lactate dehydrogenase [LDH] levels) and contains inflammatory cells (neutrophils, eosinophils and lymphocytes) in varying proportions (Robinson and Musk, 1981). BAPE should not be diagnosed on the basis of a single aspiration with no specific diagnostic outcome, as repeated or more invasive diagnostic procedures may be needed before malignant cells are identified, especially in MPM. BAPE may remit and recur ipsilaterally or occur later (or synchronously) on the other side. BAPE may precede DPT in some cases (Jeebun and Stenton, 2012).

The main management issues with BAPE relate to establishing its diagnosis from the history of asbestos exposure and the exclusion of other disease processes, the management of dyspnoea by pleural aspiration or drainage and occasionally the need to perform pleurodesis in order to prevent further recurrence.

DIFFUSE PLEURAL THICKENING

DPT is a condition of more extensive, active and progressive pleural fibrosis that involves both the visceral and parietal pleura (Rudd, 2002) and usually involves obliteration of the costophrenic angles, except with Libby amphibole (Black et al., 2014; Clark et al., 2014). It was first brought to our attention by Elmes in 1966 (Elmes, 1966). DPT is less specific for asbestos exposure because other causes of exudative effusions (especially empyema, tuberculosis and haemothorax) may also cause it (Albelda et al., 1982). DPT is often unilateral and associated with bands of coarse fibrosis in the lung parenchyma. Calcification may occur in longstanding cases.

Some cases of DPT appear to follow BAPE, with a retrospective study from the United Kingdom reporting that 40% of subjects with DPT had prior BAPE (Jeebun and Stenton, 2012); among Wittenoom workers, BAPE led to much more extensive DPT (Cookson et al., 1985). It has been suggested that this is the inflammatory pathway for all cases of DPT (Mutsaers et al., 2004) (Figure 17.4). The histology of the pleural fibrosis of asbestos-induced DPT resembles fibrosis in other tissues, with excessive deposition of matrix components and destruction of normal architecture (Mutsaers et al., 2004), although Libby amphibole-induced DPT has a lamellar structure (Black et al., 2014).

DPT also appears to be more closely related to amphibole than chrysotile exposure (Churg, 1982). In asbestos cement workers, DPT was more common in those

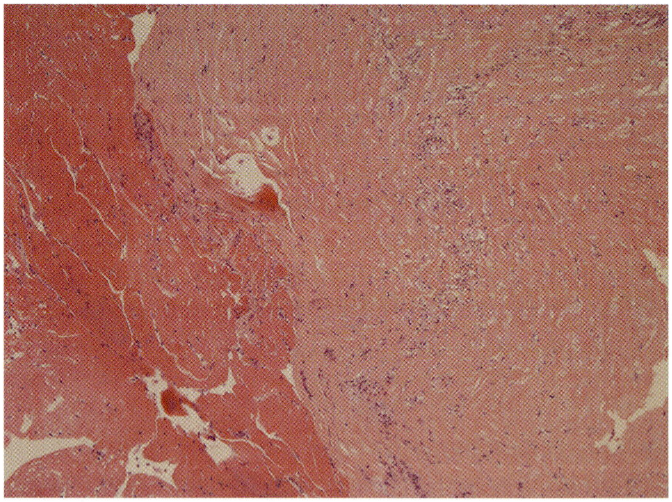

FIGURE 17.4 Organising fibrinous pleuritis. Fibrin exudate (left) undergoing organisation into fibrous tissue (right) following an asbestos-related pleural effusion (haematoxylin and eosin ×100). This is a non-specific organising process that can be seen in various other pleural inflammatory processes. It can enter the differential diagnosis for desmoplastic mesothelioma and it can be seen in association with mesothelioma, particularly if a biopsy has sampled tissue that is adjacent to malignancy, especially in the context of a clinical suspicion of mesothelioma.

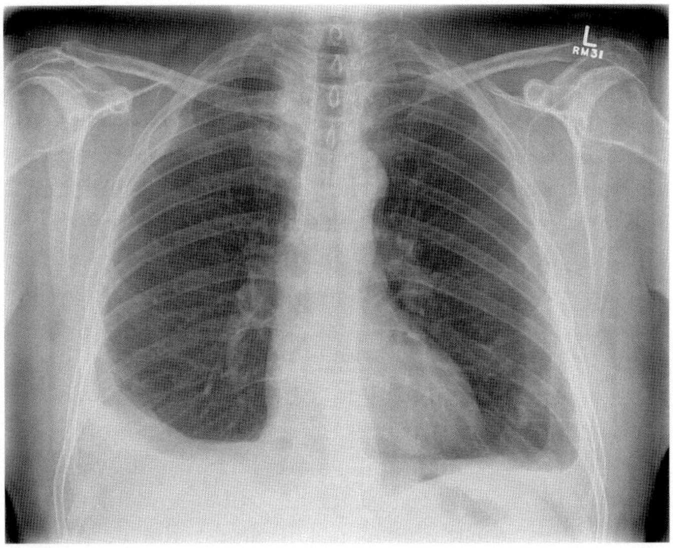

FIGURE 17.5 Diffuse pleural thickening in an ex-resident of the Wittenoom mine township.

who were more heavily exposed and also increased in incidence with increasing time since first exposure to asbestos (Rudd, 2002; Mastrangelo et al., 2009). No consistent relationship between smoking status and DPT has been demonstrated. Among Wittenoom workers, DPT appeared at a steadily increasing rate after first exposure, and progressed more rapidly in those with earlier onset (de Klerk et al., 1989) (Figure 17.5).

Beyond the plain chest radiograph, the primary aim of further imaging of DPT is differentiation from primary or secondary malignancy of the pleura (especially MPM). CT of the chest is the most practical and widely utilized modality, although improvements in spatial resolution and the use of dynamic contrast perfusion measurements continue to demonstrate the utility of MRI in the differentiation of benign from malignant disease (Horn et al., 2010; Podobnik et al., 2010). The sensitivity, specificity and diagnostic accuracy of MRI in classifying a lesion as suggestive of malignancy in one study were 100%, 95% and 95%, respectively (Boraschi et al., 1999). Evidence of chest wall invasion is highly suggestive of malignancy. Quantitative assessment of positron emission tomography (PET) discriminates between benign and malignant pleural thickening with a high negative predictive value (Kramer et al., 2004): a standardised uptake value (SUV) cut-off of 2.2 providing the best accuracy (Yildirim et al., 2009). However, infections, talc pleurodesis and uremic pleurisy may give false-positive results (Duysinx et al., 2004; Kramer et al., 2004; Kwek et al., 2004).

In contrast to CPPs, DPT may markedly reduce lung volumes, resulting in exertional dyspnoea in the absence of parenchymal fibrosis (Cotes and King, 1988; Clin et al., 2011; Weill et al., 2011). Gas transfer assessed by the single breath technique is well preserved and the transfer coefficient tends to be elevated (Cookson et al., 1983). DPT is associated with an altered ventilatory response to exercise without cardiovascular limitation or oxygen desaturation, although subjects with DPT among Wittenoom workers were at higher risk of mortality, particularly from cardiovascular disease (de Klerk et al., 1993).

Patients with DPT usually present with slowly progressive dyspnoea. The presence of any chest wall pain raises the suspicion of primary or secondary pleural malignancy, except in vermiculite-exposed subjects with DPT from occupational or environmental exposure to Libby amphibole, in whom severe chest pain is a feature of their clinical presentation (Black et al., 2014).

An increased frequency of auto-antibodies has been found in Libby amphibole-exposed workers with pleural abnormalities (Marchand et al., 2012). The significance of this finding is unclear, as Libby amphibole exposure is associated with increased auto-antibody levels, regardless of the disease from which an individual suffers (Pfau et al., 2005; Noonan et al., 2006; Pfau et al., 2014).

There is no specific therapy available for asbestos-induced DPT. Decortication is technically difficult because, unlike the pleural thickening of tuberculosis or following an empyema, there is no plane of dissection/cleavage and the underlying process of active fibrosis is not affected by surgery, so that it persists afterwards.

ROUNDED ATELECTASIS

Rounded atelectasis, sometimes referred to as 'rolled atelectasis', is a process that occurs within the lung parenchyma usually adjacent to an area of pleural thickening, in which the lung tissue appears to be drawn into the pleural or sub-pleural fibrosis. There are no consistent epidemiological data on the distribution and determinants of rounded atelectasis apart from the clinical observation of its association with other manifestations of asbestos exposure (i.e. CPP, asbestosis, DPT, etc.) and the exposure history.

It is postulated that rounded atelectasis is most likely to occur as a result of a localised, low-grade inflammatory reaction/fibrosis in the pleura involving both pleural surfaces with progressive pleural thickening and contraction of the fibrosis as it matures, drawing in the underlying lung tissue and producing a characteristic (almost diagnostic) 'comet tail' appearance radiographically (Cugell and Kamp, 2004) (Figure 17.6).

Rounded atelectasis is usually asymptomatic and found incidentally after radiographic investigation of the

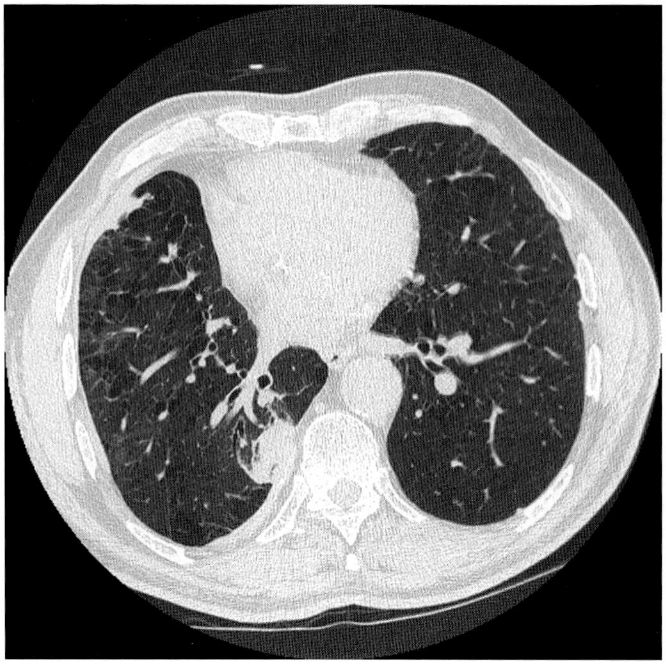

FIGURE 17.6 Rounded atelectasis in a patient exposed to asbestos in the merchant navy.

chest for other reasons. It alone is not usually associated with demonstrable abnormality on lung function testing.

While the radiographic appearances may be characteristic, the main differential diagnosis is peripheral lung cancer. Follow-up imaging is usually needed, with fluorodeoxyglucose (FDG-PET) scans usually failing to demonstrate metabolic activity, although fine-needle aspiration or other biopsy of the lesion is often carried out for reassurance and to reduce the probability of the lesion being neoplastic. After confirmation of its benign nature, no specific therapy is indicated, or available, for rounded atelectasis.

MALIGNANT MESOTHELIOMA

The entity of MM of the pleura was rare and widely doubted even by eminent pathologists (Willis, 1960) until 1960, when a pathologist from South Africa reported 33 cases of pleural malignancy in people with industrial or environmental exposure to blue asbestos (crocidolite) in the North-West Cape Province (Wagner et al., 1960). The entity of 'endothelioma of the pleura' had also been proposed, with one such case being included in the seminal report on lung cancer in asbestos workers by Doll (1955) and another described by Perry (1947).

Since the 1960s, the disease has become an epidemic in asbestos-exposed populations. Part of the initial difficulty in accepting the entity of MM was due to a number of factors: the long latent period following asbestos exposure and disease occurrence; the different potencies of the various forms of asbestos used commercially; the occurrence of MM in the peritoneal cavity as well as the pleural cavity; its heterogeneous pathological and cytological appearances; and the reluctance of an influential Australian pathologist to concede that the entity existed (Willis, 1960).

MM occurs most frequently in the pleura, but may occur in the peritoneum. The proportions have varied with different studies: early reports described a higher proportion of peritoneal to pleural MM in asbestos-exposed insulation workers in New York (Selikoff et al., 1979). In the Wittenoom workers cohort it was 14% (Berry et al., 2004; Musk et al., 2008) and in a more recent large Australian and UK study, the proportion was 7.6% (Finn et al., 2012). Data from the World Health Organisation (WHO) suggest that peritoneal MM worldwide may account for approximately 4.5% of all mesotheliomas, possibly affecting females more commonly than males (Delgermaa et al., 2011).

The true global burden of MM is unclear, largely due to variable recording and reporting methods across different countries over the previous decades. However, 88% of deaths from MM occur in high-income countries (Delgermaa et al., 2011), with almost 50,000 deaths occurring in Europe (54% of MM deaths worldwide) between 1994 and 2008 (see Figure 17.7). Australia has one of the highest per capita rates of mesothelioma worldwide (NOHSC, 2004), and deaths in Australia and New Zealand accounted for 4.6% of worldwide deaths in 2010. Debate continues as to when the peak in incidence of mesothelioma will occur in Western countries, with there being ongoing trends of increasing incidence published from a wide range of countries (Peto et al., 1995, 1999; Montanaro et al., 2003; Murayama et al., 2006; Tse et al., 2010).

MM disease rates around the world reflect the historical asbestos exposure experience of the particular community. Waves of incidence have been described that coincide with the exposure history of any population group: the first wave results from exposure in the mining, milling and transport of raw asbestos; the second wave results from the use of asbestos in industry; and the third wave results from renovations/repairs, etc., to buildings containing asbestos (Landrigan, 1991; Olsen et al., 2011; Musk et al., 2015). It is therefore of great concern that many developing nations continue to import and utilise asbestos (Brims, 2009), leading many experts to predict a continued epidemic of mesothelioma in years to come.

Hodgson and Darnton (2000) have shown that amphibole varieties of asbestos (especially crocidolite) are

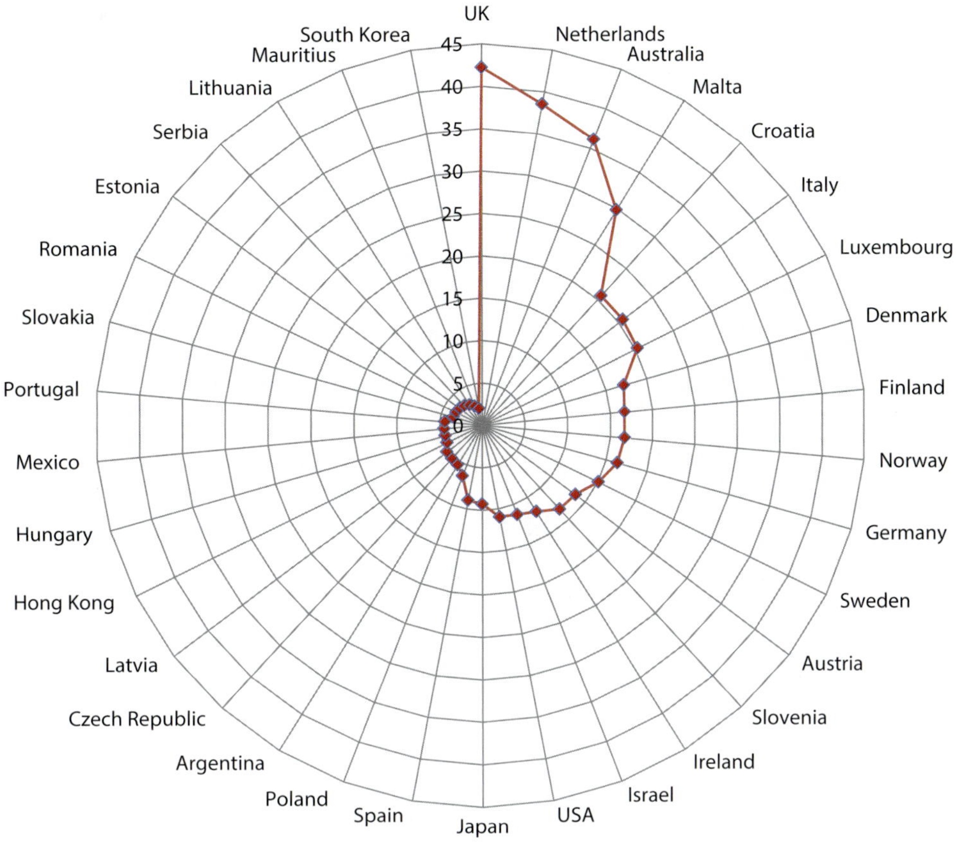

FIGURE 17.7 Male mesothelioma mortality in 2010 expressed as rate per 1 million, ASR world population aged 15–85+ years. (From WHO. 2010. World Health Organisation Mortality Database. Available at: http://www.who.int/healthinfo/statistics/mortality_rawdata/en/index.html [accessed 1 September 2014]; United Nations. 2010. World Population Prospects, the 2010 Revision. Available at: http://esa.un.org/unpd/wpp/index.htm [accessed 1 September 2014]).

much more potent than the serpentine variety (chrysotile, white asbestos) in initiating malignancy in the pleura (or peritoneum). The other commercial amphiboles (amosite, tremolite and Libby amphibole) have intermediate potencies (the suggested exposure-specific risks for crocidolite, amosite and chrysotile are 500:100:10). It has been demonstrated experimentally that durable long fibres (>5 μm) of small diameter are the most potent for inducing MM, an observation that is in accordance with epidemiological observations. The only other mineral associated with the occurrence of MM is erionite, which is not used commercially, but is responsible for endemic MM in Cappadocia (Baris et al., 1978), where environmental exposure has occurred for centuries as a result of people living in caves dug into the sides of hills. The inconsistency of information and confusion as to whether chrysotile ever causes MM can be attributed to the contamination of most chrysotile deposits in the world with an amphibole (tremolite) (Churg, 1988; McDonald et al., 1989). The risk of developing MM following asbestos exposure has no threshold and increases exponentially with increasing time since exposure, with the power of the exponent being between 3 and 4, at least for the first 30–40 years, following which it may not increase further or may fall (Berry et al., 2004).

Simian virus 40, a DNA monkey virus that contaminated poliomyelitis vaccines in the 1950s to the 1970s, has also been associated with MM (Yang et al., 2008) and is now considered to probably act as a co-carcinogen with asbestos in those who are infected (Kroczynska et al., 2006). Radiation has also been implicated as a potential cause of MM as a result of case reports and animal studies (Andersson et al., 1995; Cavazza et al., 1996; Amin et al., 2001; Travis et al., 2005; Brown et al., 2006; Teta et al., 2007). In studies of MM in Western Australia, individuals with a first- or second-degree relative with MM had an approximately twofold increase in the rate of MM, even after accounting for degree of exposure to asbestos (de Klerk et al., 2013). Germline mutations in the *BAP1* gene have been identified in families with a high incidence of MM and uveal melanoma and other cancers (Carbone et al., 2012); however, these mutations appear only to affect two high MM incidence families (Sneddon et al., 2015).

A recent genome-wide association study of common variants in MM (Cadby et al., 2013) has identified several MM candidate gene regions (Cadby et al., 2013), although further work is required in order to replicate and extend these findings.

MM first involves the parietal pleura, appearing as multiple small, grape-like nodules with gradual progression to involving the visceral pleura. The nodules coalesce to form a more continuous sheet of tumour, sometimes with considerable tumour bulk, although this is variable. Macroscopically, focal necrosis or haemorrhage may be seen. With progression, the tumour may encase the lung and other structures in the thorax as a layer of dense white tissue up to several centimetres thick, which extends into the fissures. Metastasis is a late feature of mesothelioma, but at death, tumour deposits may be widespread (Finn et al., 2012).

MM has distinctive histological subtypes: epithelioid, sarcomatoid and biphasic (a mixture of epithelioid and sarcomatoid) (see Figures 17.8–17.10). These subtypes confer distinct survival properties, with epithelioid mesothelioma generally being associated with a better prognosis (see Figure 17.11). Microscopically, MM can be difficult to differentiate from other tumours (e.g. epithelioid and adenocarcinoma; sarcomatoid and other spindle cell tumours) (Nguyen et al., 1999). More recently, the use of specific immunohistochemistry stains that, when used in batches, have good sensitivity and specificity for more reliable definition of different histologies (Wolanski et al., 1998; Segal et al., 2002), has reduced the use of electron microscopy to only very rare cases. Importantly, calretinin can identify cells as

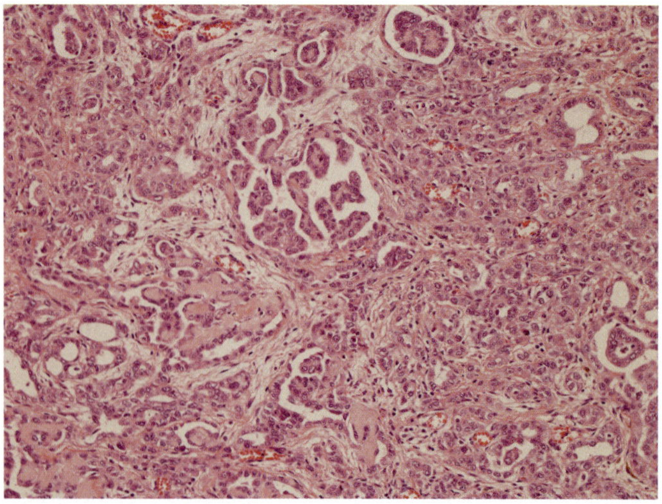

FIGURE 17.8 Epithelioid mesothelioma. Tubulopapillary architecture, as commonly seen at the well-differentiated end of the epithelioid spectrum (haematoxylin and eosin ×200).

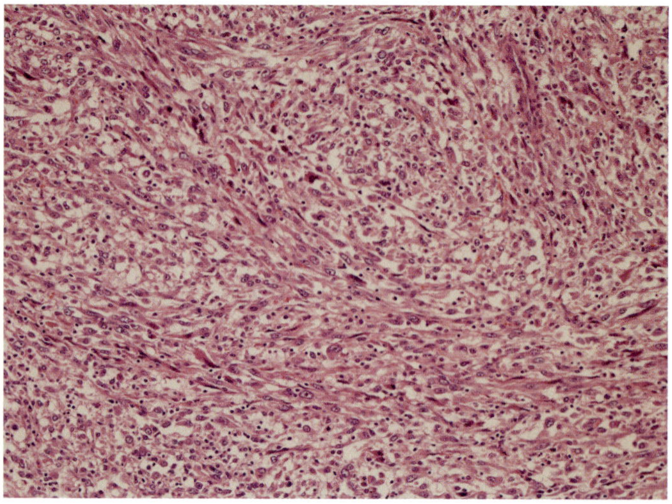

FIGURE 17.9 Sarcomatoid mesothelioma. Sarcomatoid malignancy; distinction from sarcomatoid carcinoma and sarcoma can be difficult. Sarcomatoid mesothelioma is generally strongly positive for cytokeratin, but often negative for more specific mesothelial markers; knowledge of the clinical/imaging setting is important for diagnosis (haematoxylin and eosin ×200).

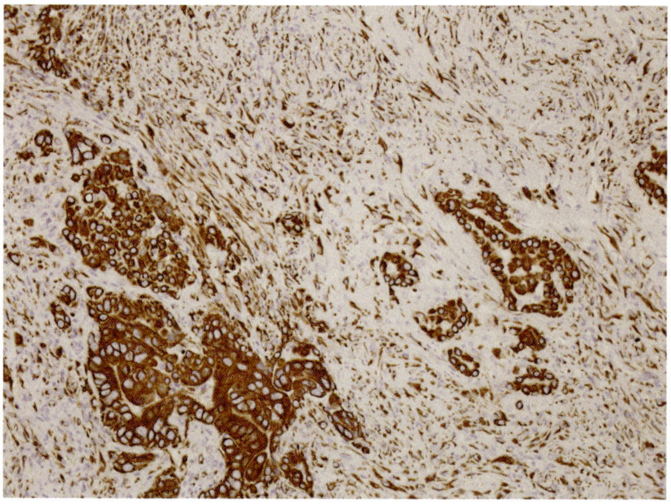

FIGURE 17.10 Biphasic mesothelioma. Combination of malignant epithelioid tubules and clusters with associated atypical spindled cells; both components demonstrate strong cytokeratin staining (cytokeratin ×200).

being of mesothelial origin, and appropriate epithelial membrane-staining antigens are highly suggestive of mesothelioma (Wolanski et al., 1998).

MM of the pleura usually presents with progressive dyspnoea, weight loss and chest wall pain. Further systemic features such as fatigue and periodic fevers may be present. There is frequently a pleural effusion and/or pleural thickening. Extra-pulmonary restriction with

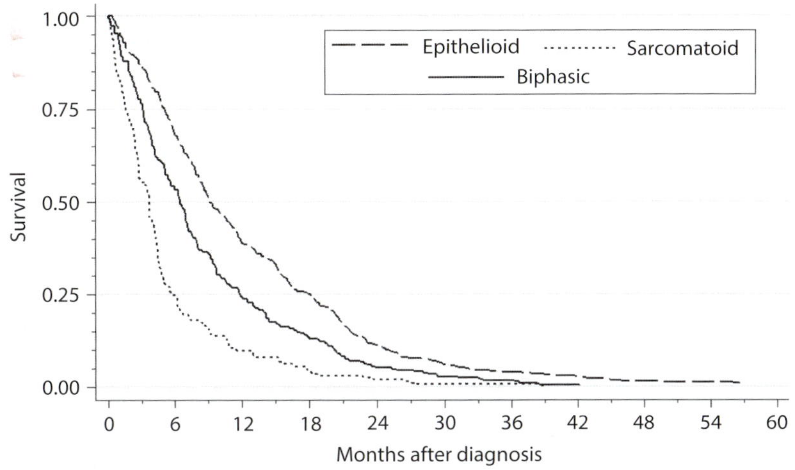

FIGURE 17.11 Survival after diagnosis—Western Australian Mesothelioma Register, 2010. The survival curves are based on 129 sarcomatoid, 360 epithelioid and 197 biphasic mesotheliomas.

ventilatory impairment may be present, as measured by a reduction in the forced expiratory volume in 1 second (FEV_1) and forced vital capacity (FVC) with a normal FEV_1:FVC ratio. Total lung capacity and gas transfer are reduced, with an increase in the diffusion constant as with DPT.

The plain CXR of pleural MM usually shows the presence of a pleural effusion or pleural thickening, which can be confirmed by CT (Figure 17.12a). MRI scans can be used, but rarely add much to CT imaging. Chest wall invasion may be seen on CT or MRI scans, thereby providing further evidence of a malignant process. PET may be used to delineate sites of greatest cellular activity in order to increase the diagnostic yield of the biopsy (Kruse et al., 2013) (Figure 17.12b).

Pathological material is necessary in order to confirm malignancy and its tissue origins. This may be accomplished by cytological examination of pleural fluid, fine-needle aspiration or biopsy of solid tumour. Recent advances in immunohistochemical stains in many cases now allow cytology alone to be sufficient to establish a definite diagnosis in an experienced laboratory (Segal et al., 2013). This avoids the need for more invasive procedures that are accompanied by significant morbidity and may delay the provision of appropriate therapy. Sarcomatoid MM is recognised to have a paucity of cell shedding into an effusion; consequently, diagnosis by effusion cytology has a low sensitivity with this histological subtype. Special immunohistochemical stains are routinely used in order to identify MM, especially for differentiating epithelioid MM from reactive mesothelial hyperplasia, adenocarcinoma and poorly differentiated squamous cell carcinoma. Electron microscopy may be useful for identifying particular

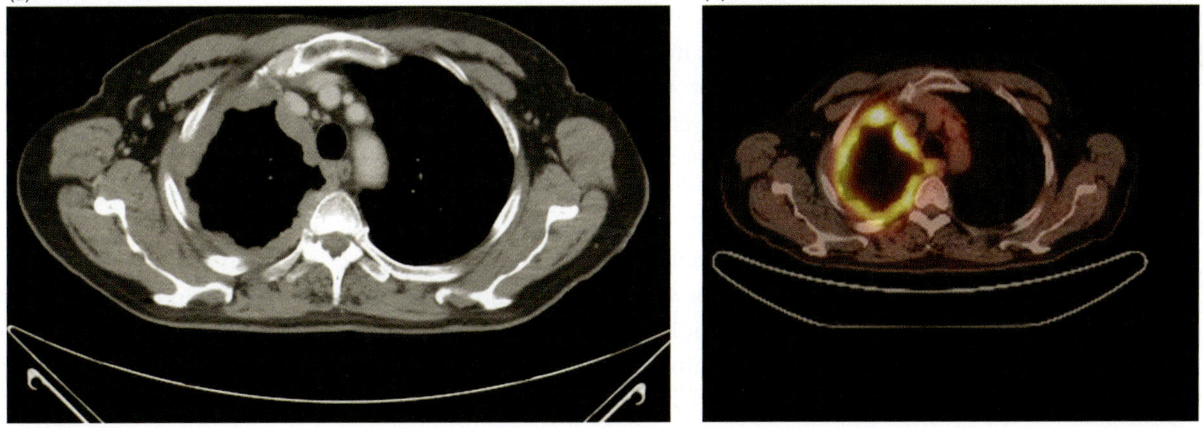

FIGURE 17.12 (a) CT and (b) FDG PET scan demonstrating malignant pleural mesothelioma in a lady whose husband was a carpenter.

ultrastructural changes, but also for distinguishing sarcomatoid MM from other spindle cell tumours and fibrosis.

Tumour markers in blood and pleural effusion fluid (e.g. mesothelin, osteopontin and fibulin-3) may be of use in order to increase the diagnostic probability of MM (Creaney et al., 2007, 2010; Pass et al., 2008, 2012; Davies et al., 2009) and possibly to monitor the response to any therapy. Tumour staging by the TNM system may be performed by CT scan (Rusch, 1995), MRI or PET.

The natural history of pleural MM is usually one of relentless increase in tumour size/bulk and resultant burden of symptoms (particularly chest wall pain, breathlessness and weight loss). Whilst these symptoms are mostly attributable to local pathology in the chest, a recent series examining 318 post-mortem results of subjects with pleural MM demonstrated a remarkably high rate of metastases both within and outside of the thoracic cavity (Finn et al., 2012). Rarely, a patient may present with metastases (Musk et al., 1991).

Currently available chemotherapy for pleural MM is never curative but is palliative, and in controlled trials, it extends survival by 2–3 months (Vogelzang et al., 2003). To date, the agents that have been shown to be most active are cisplatin and pemetrexed. Partial responses may also be seen with carbo-platinum and pemetrexed, or cisplatin and gemcitabine (Byrne et al., 1999). Single-agent chemotherapy is ineffective. Therapy should be monitored with imaging so that it can be discontinued or changed when disease progression is apparent. Advances in the understanding of cancer stem cell biology (Ghani et al., 2011; Varghese et al., 2012) and early data utilising novel immunotherapy approaches may hold promise for the future, possibly combined with existing treatment modalities (Wong et al., 2014).

Control of pleural effusions is a most important palliative objective in order to reduce breathlessness. This is best achieved by pleurodesis using talc insufflation or slurry (or another sclerosing agent) or with an indwelling pleural drainage catheter (Davies et al., 2012). Radiotherapy has limited use in the treatment of pleural MM and is usually reserved for control of pain attributable to localised areas of disease from chest wall or vertebral body invasion, deposits in biopsy tracts or occasionally to relieve compression of the superior vena cava, nerve roots or oesophagus. Prophylactic radiotherapy to biopsy sites may reduce the occurrence of tumour deposits in the biopsy wound, but is not routinely indicated following needle biopsy alone, as the risk of developing symptomatic deposits is small (Agarwal et al., 2006; Davies et al., 2008).

Surgical excision of pleural MM remains highly contentious and there is a lack of randomised controlled trials supporting its use. The only two trials published to date have failed to demonstrate any survival benefit (Treasure et al., 2011; McRonald et al., 2013), either by extrapleural pneumonectomy or by video-assisted partial pleurectomy with adjuvant chemotherapy and/or radiotherapy (Hasani et al., 2009; McRonald et al., 2013). Complications of surgery are significant and, at present, there is no established role of surgery in managing MPM (Lee, 2014).

The management of peritoneal MM is similar to that of pleural MM inasmuch that supportive and palliative measures for control of the likely malignant ascites and any pain remains paramount. Chemotherapy may be offered in this instance, although its effectiveness in this setting is extrapolated from pleural mesothelioma data (Vogelzang et al., 2003), albeit with one open-label study reporting a favourable safety profile and reasonable disease response using a pemetrexed and cisplatin regime for peritoneal mesothelioma (Janne et al., 2005). Peritonectomy or cytoreductive surgery (with or without adjuvant intraperitoneal chemotherapy) have been reported as additional treatment regimens, but there are no randomised controlled data to support this practice (Mirarabshahii et al., 2012).

For many patients, symptom palliation alone is arguably the most important aspect of the management of MM, and clinical trials are ongoing in order to establish the best timing and nature of this support (Gunatilake et al., 2014). Multidisciplinary palliative care of the terminally ill patient and his/her family/dependents is increasingly being recognised as important. Social issues include the sorting of compensation issues relating to past asbestos exposure, as this greatly concerns many patients and their families.

The prognosis of pleural MM is generally regarded as poor, with a median survival of between 9 and 12 months, although rare cases of long survival are recognised (Brims and Maskell, 2013). Previous prognostic scoring systems have mainly been based on clinical trial populations who have been accepted as being fit for attempts at surgical treatment and/or chemotherapy and consequently are not widely utilised. Population-based studies consistently confirm that non-epithelioid histology, increasing age and male gender are independent risk factors for poor outcome for pleural MM (Musk et al., 2011; Brims and Maskell, 2013). Similar factors to pleural MM have been associated with peritoneal MM prognosis (Mirarabshahii et al., 2012), which, overall, is thought to carry a slightly better prognosis as compared to pleural MM.

Genetic and immunohistochemical studies continue to provide advances in the understanding of tumour biology, but no clear validated prognostic factors for pleural MM have been identified to date. Nuclear mitotic and atypia grading systems may provide useful prognostic knowledge (Kadota et al., 2012), but require further evaluation. Biomarkers such as soluble mesothelin-related protein, osteopontin and fibulin-3 provide some limited prognostic information (Grigoriu et al., 2007; Creaney et al., 2011; Hollevoet et al., 2011; Pass et al., 2012; Creaney et al., 2014), with definite limitations. The baseline serum neutrophil-to-lymphocyte ratio might also provide prognostic information, although this needs further validation (Kao et al., 2011; Meniawy et al., 2013). Modern metabolic imaging techniques such as PET/CT can provide some prognostic information using baseline total glycolytic volumes (Nowak et al., 2010). Research to identify clinically useful prognostic factors in MPM remains a priority (Brims and Maskell, 2013).

MAN-MADE MINERAL FIBRES

The use of manufactured mineral fibres (slagwool, glasswool, rockwool, glass filaments and microfibres) as well as refractory ceramic fibres (RCFs) is increasing for industrial and domestic roles that were previously filled by asbestos. The chemical composition of the various man-made mineral fibres (MMMFs) depends on the raw materials used in their manufacture. Unlike naturally occurring fibres that have a crystalline structure, MMMFs are amorphous silicates combined with metal oxides and other additives. Some MMMFs are bioactive and may produce MM in animals by intra-cavity injection experimentally; however, there has been no epidemiological evidence of MM in cohorts of workers exposed to MMMFs (De Vuyst et al., 1995; Boillat, 1999), although industrial production of these fibres has been relatively recent.

To date, one small study has shown that workers exposed to mineral wool are more likely to have pleural plaques on plain CXRs than unexposed workers (Jarvholm et al., 1995).

REFRACTORY CERAMIC FIBRES

There has not been sufficient epidemiological evidence to demonstrate an association with MM in cohorts of workers exposed to RCFs (Boillat, 1999), although experimentally MM may be induced by RCFs in hamsters (Okayasu et al., 1999). Again, industrial production of these fibres has been relatively recent.

CARBON NANOPARTICLES

Carbon nanotubes and nanoparticulate graphene (a crystalline material with a single layer of carbon atoms in the shape of platelets), which have biomedical applications, have many physical properties that are similar to asbestos, such as an aerodynamic diameter that is in the respirable range and bio-persistence as a result of one dimension being too large to allow clearance from the lung or pleura by phagocytosis. This results in 'frustrated phagocytosis' and the capacity to incite an inflammatory reaction, with similarities to that which is induced by crocidolite, when carbon nanotubes are given to mice intrapleurally or by pharyngeal aspiration (Donaldson et al., 2010; Murphy et al., 2011, 2013). This may produce both diffuse pleural inflammation and potentially MM experimentally. The theoretical induction of MM based on animal studies of length-dependent inflammatory responses analogous to asbestos-induced MM has not been realised in animal experiments, although long-term inhalation studies have not been performed (Murphy et al., 2013).

Unintentional exposure to these particles during their manufacture or their use in biomedical applications could potentially result in pleural reactions that are similar to those resulting from asbestos exposure, although epidemiological evidence of this effect has not yet been found (Schinwald et al., 2012).

REFERENCES

Agarwal, P. P., Seely, J. M., Matzinger, F. R., Macrae, R. M., Peterson, R. A., Maziak, D. E. and Dennie, C. J. 2006. Pleural mesothelioma: Sensitivity and incidence of needle track seeding after image-guided biopsy versus surgical biopsy. *Radiology* 241:589–94.

Albelda, S. M., Epstein, D. M., Gefter, W. B. and Miller, W. T. 1982. Pleural thickening: Its significance and relationship to asbestos dust exposure. *Am Rev Respir Dis* 126:621–4.

Allen, R., Cramond, T., Lennon, D. and Waterhouse, M. 2011. A retrospective study of chest pain in benign asbestos pleural disease. *Pain Med* 12:1303–8.

Ameille, J., Brochard, P., Brechot, J. M., Pascano, T., Cherin, A., Raix, A., Fredy, M. et al. 1993. Pleural thickening: A comparison of oblique chest radiographs and high-resolution computed tomography in subjects exposed to low levels of asbestos pollution. *Int Arch Occup Environ Health* 64:545–8.

Amin, A. M. H., Mason, C. and Rowe, P. 2001. Diffuse malignant mesothelioma of the peritoneum following abdominal radiotherapy. *Eur J Surg Oncol* 27:214–5.

Andersson, M., Wallin, H., Jonsson, M., Nielsen, L. L., Visfeldt, J., Vyberg, M., Bennett, W. P. et al. 1995. Lung-carcinoma and malignant mesothelioma in patients exposed to Thorotrast—Incidence, histology and P53 status. *Int J Cancer* 63:330–6.

Andrion, A., Pira, E. and Mollo, F. 1983. Peritoneal plaques and asbestos exposure. *Arch Pathol Lab Med* 107: 609–10.
Armato, S. G. 3rd, Labby, Z. E., Coolen, J., Klabatsa, A., Feigen, M., Persigehl, T. and Gill, R. R. 2013. Imaging in pleural mesothelioma: A review of the 11th International Conference of the International Mesothelioma Interest Group. *Lung Cancer* 82:190–6.
Baris, Y. I., Sahin, A. A., Ozesmi, M., Kerse, I., Ozen, E., Kolacan, B., Altinors, M. et al. 1978. An outbreak of pleural mesothelioma and chronic fibrosing pleurisy in the village of Karain/Urgup in Anatolia. *Thorax* 33:181–92.
Baris, Y. I., Saracci, R., Simonato, L., Skidmore, J. W. and Artvinli, M. 1981. Malignant mesothelioma and radiological chest abnormalities in two villages in Central Turkey. An epidemiological and environmental investigation. *Lancet* 1:984–7.
Berry, G., de Klerk, N. H., Reid, A., Ambrosini, G. L., Fritschi, L., Olsen, N. J., Merler, E. et al. 2004. Malignant pleural and peritoneal mesotheliomas in former miners and millers of crocidolite at Wittenoom, Western Australia. *Occup Environ Med* 61:e14.
Black, B., Szeinuk, J., Whitehouse, A. C., Levin, S. M., Henschke, C. I., Yankelevitz, D. F. and Flores, R. M. 2014. Rapid progression of pleural disease due to exposure to Libby amphibole: Not your grandfather's asbestos related disease. *Am J Ind Med* 57:1197–206.
Boillat, M. A. 1999. [Synthetic mineral fibres]. *Schweiz Med Wochenschr* 129:468–74.
Boraschi, P., Neri, S., Braccini, G., Gigoni, R., Leoncini, B. and Perri, G. 1999. Magnetic resonance appearance of asbestos-related benign and malignant pleural diseases. *Scand J Work Environ Health* 25:18–23.
Brims, F. 2009. Asbestos—A legacy and a persistent problem. *J R Nav Med Serv* 95:4–11.
Brims, F. J. and Maskell, N. A. 2013a. Prognostic factors for malignant pleural mesothelioma. *Curr Respir Care Rep* 2:100–8.
Brims, F. J., Murray, C. P., de Klerk, N., Alfonso, H., Reid, A., Manners, D., Wong, P. M. et al. 2015. Ultra-low-dose chest computer tomography screening of an asbestos-exposed population in Western Australia. *Am J Respir Crit Care Med* 191:113–6.
Broderick, A., Fuortes, L. J., Merchant, J. A., Galvin, J. R. and Schwartz, D. A. 1992. Pleural determinants of restrictive lung function and respiratory symptoms in an asbestos-exposed population. *Chest* 101:684–91.
Brown, L. M., Howard, R. A. and Travis, L. B. 2006. The risk of secondary malignancies over 30 years after the treatment of non-Hodgkin lymphoma. *Cancer* 107:2741–2.
Byrne, M. J., Davidson, J. A., Musk, A. W., Dewar, J., Van Hazel, G., Buck, M., de Klerk, N. H. et al. 1999. Cisplatin and gemcitabine treatment for malignant mesothelioma: A phase II study. *J Clin Oncol* 17:25–30.
Cadby, G., Mukherjee, S., Musk, A. W., Reid, A., Garlepp, M., Dick, I., Robinson, C. et al. 2013. A genome-wide association study for malignant mesothelioma risk. *Lung Cancer* 82:1–8.
Carbone, M., Ferris, L. K., Baumann, F., Napolitano, A., Lum, C. A., Flores, E. G., Gaudino, G. et al. 2012. BAP1 cancer syndrome: Malignant mesothelioma, uveal and cutaneous melanoma, and MBAITs. *J Transl Med* 10:179.
Cavazza, A., Travis, L. B., Travis, W. D., Wolfe, J. T., Foo, M. L., Gillespie, D. J., Weidner, N. et al. 1996. Post-irradiation malignant mesothelioma. *Cancer* 77:1379–85.
Churg, A. 1982. Asbestos fibers and pleural plaques in a general autopsy population. *Am J Pathol* 109:88–96.
Churg, A. 1988. Chrysotile, tremolite, and malignant mesothelioma in man. *Chest* 93:621–8.
Clark, K. A., Flynn, J. J. 3rd, Goodman, J. E., Zu, K., Karmaus, W. J. and Mohr, L. C. 2014. Pleural plaques and their effect on lung function in Libby vermiculite miners. *Chest* 146:786–94.
Clin, B., Paris, C., Ameille, J., Brochard, P., Conso, F., Gislard, A., Laurent, F. et al. 2011. Do asbestos-related pleural plaques on HRCT scans cause restrictive impairment in the absence of pulmonary fibrosis? *Thorax* 66:985–91.
Cookson, W. O., de Klerk, N. H., Musk, A. W., Glancy, J. J., Armstrong, B. K. and Hobbs, M. S. 1985. Benign and malignant pleural effusions in former Wittenoom crocidolite millers and miners. *Aust N Z J Med* 15:731–7.
Cookson, W. O., Musk, A. W. and Glancy, J. J. 1983. Pleural thickening and gas transfer in asbestosis. *Thorax* 38:657–61.
Cotes, J. E. and King, B. 1988. Relationship of lung function to radiographic reading (ILO) in patients with asbestos related lung disease. *Thorax* 43:777–83.
Craighead, J. E., Abraham, J. L., Churg, A., Green, F. H., Kleinerman, J., Pratt, P. C., Seemayer, T. A. et al. 1982. The pathology of asbestos-associated diseases of the lungs and pleural cavities: Diagnostic criteria and proposed grading schema. Report of the Pneumoconiosis Committee of the College of American Pathologists and the National Institute for Occupational Safety and Health. *Arch Pathol Lab Med* 106:544–96.
Creaney, J., Dick, I. M., Meniawy, T. M., Leong, S. L., Leon, J. S., Demelker, Y., Segal, A. et al. 2014. Comparison of fibulin-3 and mesothelin as markers in malignant mesothelioma. *Thorax* 69:895–902.
Creaney, J., Francis, R. J., Dick, I. M., Musk, A. W., Robinson, B. W., Byrne, M. J. and Nowak, A. K. 2011. Serum soluble mesothelin concentrations in malignant pleural mesothelioma: Relationship to tumor volume, clinical stage and changes in tumor burden. *Clin Cancer Res* 17:1181–9.
Creaney, J., Olsen, N. J., Brims, F., Dick, I. M., Musk, A. W., de Klerk, N. H., Skates, S. J. et al. 2010. Serum mesothelin for early detection of the asbestos-induced cancer malignant mesothelioma. *Cancer Epidemiol Biomarkers Prev* 19:2238–46.
Creaney, J., Van Bruggen, I., Hof, M., Segal, A., Musk, A. W., de Klerk, N., Horick, N. et al. 2007. Combined CA125 and mesothelin levels for the diagnosis of malignant mesothelioma. *Chest* 132:1239–46.

Cugell, D. W. and Kamp, D. W. 2004. Asbestos and the pleura: A review. *Chest* 125:1103–17.

Davies, H. E., Mishra, E. K., Kahan, B. C., Wrightson, J. M., Stanton, A. E., Guhan, A., Davies, C. W. et al. 2012. Effect of an indwelling pleural catheter vs chest tube and talc pleurodesis for relieving dyspnea in patients with malignant pleural effusion: The TIME2 randomized controlled trial. *JAMA* 307:2383–9.

Davies, H. E., Musk, A. W. and Lee, Y. C. 2008. Prophylactic radiotherapy for pleural puncture sites in mesothelioma: The controversy continues. *Curr Opin Pulm Med* 14:326–30.

Davies, H. E., Sadler, R. S., Bielsa, S., Maskell, N. A., Rahman, N. M., Davies, R. J., Ferry, B. L. et al. 2009. Clinical impact and reliability of pleural fluid mesothelin in undiagnosed pleural effusions. *Am J Respir Crit Care Med* 180:437–44.

de Klerk, N., Alfonso, H., Olsen, N., Reid, A., Sleith, J., Palmer, L., Berry, G. et al. 2013. Familial aggregation of malignant mesothelioma in former workers and residents of Wittenoom, Western Australia. *Int J Cancer* 132:1423–8.

de Klerk, N. H., Cookson, W. O., Musk, A. W., Armstrong, B. K. and Glancy, J. J. 1989. Natural history of pleural thickening after exposure to crocidolite. *Br J Ind Med* 46:461–7.

de Klerk, N. H., Musk, A. W., Cookson, W. O., Glancy, J. J. and Hobbs, M. S. 1993. Radiographic abnormalities and mortality in subjects with exposure to crocidolite. *Br J Ind Med* 50:902–6.

Delgermaa, V., Takahashi, K., Park, E. K., Le, G. V., Hara, T. and Sorahan, T. 2011. Global mesothelioma deaths reported to the World Health Organization between 1994 and 2008. *Bull World Health Organ* 89:716–24.

De Vuyst, P., Dumortier, P., Swaen, G. M., Pairon, J. C. and Brochard, P. 1995. Respiratory health effects of man-made vitreous (mineral) fibres. *Eur Respir J* 8:2149–73.

Doll, R. 1955. Mortality from lung cancer in asbestos workers. *Br J Ind Med* 12:81–6.

Donaldson, K., Murphy, F. A., Duffin, R. and Poland, C. A. 2010. Asbestos, carbon nanotubes and the pleural mesothelium: A review of the hypothesis regarding the role of long fibre retention in the parietal pleura, inflammation and mesothelioma. *Part Fibre Toxicol* 7:5.

Duysinx, B., Nguyen, D., Louis, R., Cataldo, D., Belhocine, T., Bartsch, P. and Bury, T. 2004. Evaluation of pleural disease with 18-fluorodeoxyglucose positron emission tomography imaging. *Chest* 125:489–93.

Eisenstadt, H. B. 1965. Benign asbestos pleurisy. *JAMA* 192:419–21.

Elmes, P. C. 1966. The epidemiology and clinical features of asbestosis and related diseases. *Postgrad Med J* 42:623–35.

Epler, G. R., Mcloud, T. C. and Gaensler, E. A. 1982. Prevalence and incidence of benign asbestos pleural effusion in a working population. *JAMA* 247:617–22.

Finn, R. S., Brims, F. J., Gandhi, A., Olsen, N., Musk, A. W., Maskell, N. A. and Lee, Y. C. 2012. Postmortem findings of malignant pleural mesothelioma: A two-center study of 318 patients. *Chest* 142:1267–73.

Friedman, A. C., Fiel, S. B., Radecki, P. D. and Lev-Toaff, A. S. 1990. Computed tomography of benign pleural and pulmonary parenchymal abnormalities related to asbestos exposure. *Semin Ultrasound CT MR* 11:393–408.

Ghani, F. I., Yamazaki, H., Iwata, S., Okamoto, T., Aoe, K., Okabe, K., Mimura, Y. et al. 2011. Identification of cancer stem cell markers in human malignant mesothelioma cells. *Biochem Biophys Res Commun* 404:735–42.

Grigoriu, B. D., Scherpereel, A., Devos, P., Chahine, B., Letourneux, M., Lebailly, P., Gregoire, M. et al. 2007. Utility of osteopontin and serum mesothelin in malignant pleural mesothelioma diagnosis and prognosis assessment. *Clin Cancer Res* 13:2928–35.

Gunatilake, S., Brims, F. J., Fogg, C., Lawrie, I., Maskell, N., Forbes, K., Rahman, N. et al. 2014. A multicentre non-blinded randomised controlled trial to assess the impact of regular early specialist symptom control treatment on quality of life in malignant mesothelioma (RESPECT-MESO): Study protocol for a randomised controlled trial. *Trials* 15:367.

Hasani, A., Alvarez, J. M., Wyatt, J. M., Bydder, S., Millward, M., Byrne, M., Musk, A. W. et al. 2009. Outcome for patients with malignant pleural mesothelioma referred for trimodality therapy in Western Australia. *J Thorac Oncol* 4:1010–6.

Hillerdal, G. 1994. Pleural plaques and risk for bronchial carcinoma and mesothelioma. A prospective study. *Chest* 105:144–50.

Hillerdal, G. and Henderson, D. W. 1997. Asbestos, asbestosis, pleural plaques and lung cancer. *Scand J Work Environ Health* 23:93–103.

Hillerdal, G. and Lindgren, A. 1980. Pleural plaques: Correlation of autopsy findings to radiographic findings and occupational history. *Eur J Respir Dis* 61:315–9.

Hodgson, J. T. and Darnton, A. 2000. The quantitative risks of mesothelioma and lung cancer in relation to asbestos exposure. *Ann Occup Hyg* 44:565–601.

Hollevoet, K., Nackaerts, K., Gosselin, R., De Wever, W., Bosquee, L., De Vuyst, P., Germonpre, P. et al. 2011. Soluble mesothelin, megakaryocyte potentiating factor, and osteopontin as markers of patient response and outcome in mesothelioma. *J Thorac Oncol* 6:1930–7.

Horn, M., Oechsner, M., Gardarsdottir, M., Kostler, H. and Muller, M. F. 2010. Dynamic contrast-enhanced MR imaging for differentiation of rounded atelectasis from neoplasm. *J Magn Reson Imaging* 31:1364–70.

Huggins, J. T. and Sahn, S. A. 2004. Causes and management of pleural fibrosis. *Respirology* 9:441–7.

International Labour Office (ILO). 1980. *Guidelines for the Use of ILO International Classification of Radiographs of Pneumoconiosis*. Geneva: ILO.

Janne, P. A., Wozniak, A. J., Belani, C. P., Keohan, M. L., Ross, H. J., Polikoff, J. A., Mintzer, D. M. et al. 2005. Open-label study of pemetrexed alone or in combination with cisplatin for the treatment of patients with peritoneal mesothelioma: Outcomes of an expanded access program. *Clin Lung Cancer* 7:40–6.

Jarvholm, B., Hillerdal, G., Jarliden, A. K., Hansson, A., Lilja, B. G., Tornling, G. and Westerholm, P. 1995. Occurrence of pleural plaques in workers with exposure to mineral wool. *Int Arch Occup Environ Health* 67:343–6.

Jeebun, V. and Stenton, S. C. 2012. The presentation and natural history of asbestos-induced diffuse pleural thickening. *Occup Med* 62:266–8.

Kadota, K., Suzuki, K., Colovos, C., Sima, C. S., Rusch, V. W., Travis, W. D. and Adusumilli, P. S. 2012. A nuclear grading system is a strong predictor of survival in epitheloid diffuse malignant pleural mesothelioma. *Mod Pathol* 25:260–71.

Kao, S. C., Klebe, S., Henderson, D. W., Reid, G., Chatfield, M., Armstrong, N. J., Yan, T. D. et al. 2011. Low calretinin expression and high neutrophil-to-lymphocyte ratio are poor prognostic factors in patients with malignant mesothelioma undergoing extrapleural pneumonectomy. *J Thorac Oncol* 6:1923–9.

Karjalainen, A., Pukkala, E., Kauppinen, T. and Partanen, T. 1999. Incidence of cancer among Finnish patients with asbestos-related pulmonary or pleural fibrosis. *Cancer Causes Control* 10:51–7.

Kilburn, K. H. and Warshaw, R. 1990. Pulmonary functional impairment associated with pleural asbestos disease. Circumscribed and diffuse thickening. *Chest* 98:965–72.

Kramer, H., Pieterman, R. M., Slebos, D. J., Timens, W., Vaalburg, W., Koeter, G. H. and Groen, H. J. 2004. PET for the evaluation of pleural thickening observed on CT. *J Nucl Med* 45:995–8.

Kroczynska, B., Cutrone, R., Bocchetta, M., Yang, H., Elmishad, A. G., Vacek, P., Ramos-Nino, M. et al. 2006. Crocidolite asbestos and SV40 are cocarcinogens in human mesothelial cells and in causing mesothelioma in hamsters. *Proc Natl Acad Sci U S A* 103:14128–33.

Kruse, M., Sherry, S. J., Paidpally, V., Mercier, G. and Subramaniam, R. M. 2013. FDG PET/CT in the management of primary pleural tumors and pleural metastases. *AJR Am J Roentgenol* 201:W215–26.

Kusaka, Y. and Hering, K. G. 2005. *International Classification of HRCT for Occupational and Environmental Respiratory Diseases*. Tokyo, Japan: Springer.

Kwek, B. H., Aquino, S. L. and Fischman, A. J. 2004. Fluorodeoxyglucose positron emission tomography and CT after talc pleurodesis. *Chest* 125:2356–60.

Landrigan, P. J. 1991. A population of children at risk of exposure to asbestos in place. *Ann N Y Acad Sci* 643:283–6.

Larson, T. C., Antao, V. C., Bove, F. J. and Cusack, C. 2012a. Association between cumulative fiber exposure and respiratory outcomes among Libby vermiculite workers. *J Occup Environ Med* 54:56–63.

Larson, T. C., Lewin, M., Gottschall, E. B., Antao, V. C., Kapil, V. and Rose, C. S. 2012b. Associations between radiographic findings and spirometry in a community exposed to Libby amphibole. *Occup Environ Med* 69: 361–6.

Larson, T. C., Meyer, C. A., Kapil, V., Gurney, J. W., Tarver, R. D., Black, C. B. and Lockey, J. E. 2010. Workers with Libby amphibole exposure: Retrospective identification and progression of radiographic changes. *Radiology* 255:924–33.

Lee, Y. C. 2014. Surgical resection of mesothelioma: An evidence-free practice. *Lancet* 384:1080–1.

Lee, Y. C., Runnion, C. K., Pang, S. C., de Klerk, N. H. and Musk, A. W. 2001. Increased body mass index is related to apparent circumscribed pleural thickening on plain chest radiographs. *Am J Ind Med* 39:112–6.

Luo, S., Liu, X., Mu, S., Tsai, S. P. and Wen, C. P. 2003. Asbestos related diseases from environmental exposure to crocidolite in Da-yao, China. I. Review of exposure and epidemiological data. *Occup Environ Med* 60:35–41; discussion 41–2.

Marchand, L. S., St-Hilaire, S., Putnam, E. A., Serve, K. M. and Pfau, J. C. 2012. Mesothelial cell and anti-nuclear autoantibodies associated with pleural abnormalities in an asbestos exposed population of Libby MT. *Toxicol Lett* 208:168–73.

Mastrangelo, G., Ballarin, M. N., Bellini, E., Bicciato, F., Zannol, F., Gioffre, F., Zedde, A. et al. 2009. Asbestos exposure and benign asbestos diseases in 772 formerly exposed workers: Dose-response relationships. *Am J Ind Med* 52:596–602.

McDonald, J. C., Armstrong, B., Case, B., Doell, D., Mccaughey, W. T. E., McDonald, A. D. and Sebastien, P. 1989. Mesothelioma and asbestos fiber type—Evidence from lung-tissue analyses. *Cancer* 63:1544–7.

McRonald, F., Baldwin, D. R., Devaraj, A., Brain, K., Eisen, T., Holeman, J., Ledson, M. et al. 2013. The uniqueness of the United Kingdom Lung Cancer Screening trial (UKLS)—A population screening study. *Lung Cancer* 79:S28–9.

Meniawy, T. M., Creaney, J., Lake, R. A. and Nowak, A. K. 2013. Existing models, but not neutrophil-to-lymphocyte ratio, are prognostic in malignant mesothelioma. *Br J Cancer* 109:1813–20.

Mirarabshahii, P., Pillai, K., Chua, T. C., Pourgholami, M. H. and Morris, D. L. 2012. Diffuse malignant peritoneal mesothelioma—An update on treatment. *Cancer Treat Rev* 38:605–12.

Mollo, F., Andrion, A., Pira, E. and Barocelli, M. P. 1983. Indicators of asbestos exposure in autopsy routine. 2. Pleural plaques and occupation. *Med Lav* 74:137–42.

Montanaro, F., Bray, F., Gennaro, V., Merler, E., Tyczynski, J. E., Parkin, D. M., Strnad, M. et al. 2003. Pleural mesothelioma incidence in Europe: Evidence of some deceleration in the increasing trends. *Cancer Causes Control* 14:791–803.

Mukherjee, S., de Klerk, N., Palmer, L. J., Olsen, N. J., Pang, S. C. and William Musk, A. 2000. Chest pain in asbestos-exposed individuals with benign pleural and parenchymal disease. *Am J Respir Crit Care Med* 162:1807–11.

Murayama, T., Takahashi, K., Natori, Y. and Kurumatani, N. 2006. Estimation of future mortality from pleural malignant mesothelioma in Japan based on an age-cohort model. *Am J Ind Med* 49:1–7.

Murphy, F. A., Poland, C. A., Duffin, R., Al-Jamal, K. T., Ali-Boucetta, H., Nunes, A., Byrne, F. et al. 2011. Length-dependent retention of carbon nanotubes in the pleural space of mice initiates sustained inflammation and progressive fibrosis on the parietal pleura. *Am J Pathol* 178:2587–600.

Murphy, F. A., Poland, C. A., Duffin, R. and Donaldson, K. 2013. Length-dependent pleural inflammation and parietal pleural responses after deposition of carbon nanotubes in the pulmonary airspaces of mice. *Nanotoxicology* 7:1157–67.

Musk, A. W., de Klerk, N. H., Reid, A., Ambrosini, G. L., Fritschi, L., Olsen, N. J., Merler, E. et al. 2008. Mortality of former crocidolite (blue asbestos) miners and millers at Wittenoom. *Occup Environ Med* 65:541–3.

Musk, A. W., Dewar, J., Shilkin, K. B. and Whitaker, D. 1991. Miliary spread of malignant pleural mesothelioma without a clinically identifiable pleural tumour. *Aust N Z J Med* 21:460–2.

Musk, A. W., Olsen, N., Alfonso, H., Reid, A., Mina, R., Franklin, P., Sleith, J. et al. 2011. Predicting survival in malignant mesothelioma. *Eur Respir J* 38:1420–4.

Musk, A. W., Olsen, N., Alfonso, H., Peters, S. and Franklin, P. 2015. Pattern of malignant mesothelioma incidence and occupational exposure to asbestos in Western Australia. *Med J Aust* 203(6):251–252e 251.

Mutsaers, S. E., Prele, C. M., Brody, A. R. and Idell, S. 2004. Pathogenesis of pleural fibrosis. *Respirology* 9:428–40.

Nguyen, G. K., Akin, M. R., Villanueva, R. R. and Slatnik, J. 1999. Cytopathology of malignant mesothelioma of the pleura in fine-needle aspiration biopsy. *Diagn Cytopathol* 21:253–9.

NOHSC. 2004. *The Incidence of Mesothelioma in Australia 1999 to 2001, Australian Mesothelioma Register Report 2004. 16th Report Edition*. Canberra: National Occupational Health and Safety Commission.

Noonan, C. W., Pfau, J. C., Larson, T. C. and Spence, M. R. 2006. Nested case–control study of autoimmune disease in an asbestos-exposed population. *Environ Health Perspect* 114:1243–7.

Nowak, A. K., Francis, R. J., Phillips, M. J., Millward, M. J., Van der Schaaf, A. A., Boucek, J., Musk, A. W. et al. 2010. A novel prognostic model for malignant mesothelioma incorporating quantitative FDG-PET imaging with clinical parameters. *Clin Cancer Res* 16:2409–17.

Okayasu, R., Wu, L. and Hei, T. K. 1999. Biological effects of naturally occurring and man-made fibres: *In vitro* cytotoxicity and mutagenesis in mammalian cells. *Br J Cancer* 79:1319–24.

Olsen, N. J., Franklin, P. J., Reid, A., de Klerk, N. H., Threlfall, T. J., Shilkin, K. and Musk, B. 2011. Increasing incidence of malignant mesothelioma after exposure to asbestos during home maintenance and renovation. *Med J Aust* 195:271–4.

Pairon, J. C., Laurent, F., Rinaldo, M., Clin, B., Andujar, P., Ameille, J., Brochard, P. et al. 2013. Pleural plaques and the risk of pleural mesothelioma. *J Natl Cancer Inst* 105:293–301.

Paris, C., Thierry, S., Brochard, P., Letourneux, M., Schorle, E., Stoufflet, A., Ameille, J. et al. 2009. Pleural plaques and asbestosis: Dose– and time–response relationships based on HRCT data. *Eur Respir J* 34:72–9.

Park, E. K., Thomas, P. S., Wilson, D., Choi, H. J., Johnson, A. R. and Yates, D. H. 2011. Chest pain in asbestos and silica-exposed workers. *Occup Med* 61:178–83.

Pass, H. I., Levin, S. M., Harbut, M. R., Melamed, J., Chiriboga, L., Donington, J., Huflejt, M. et al. 2012. Fibulin-3 as a blood and effusion biomarker for pleural mesothelioma. *N Engl J Med* 367:1417–27.

Pass, H. I., Wali, A., Tang, N., Ivanova, A., Ivanov, S., Harbut, M., Carbone, M. et al. 2008. Soluble mesothelin-related peptide level elevation in mesothelioma serum and pleural effusions. *Ann Thorac Surg* 85:265–72; discussion 272.

Perry, K. M. 1947. Diseases of the lung resulting from occupational dusts other than silica. *Thorax* 2:75–120.

Peto, J., Decarli, A., La Vecchia, C., Levi, F. and Negri, E. 1999. The European mesothelioma epidemic. *Br J Cancer* 79:666–72.

Peto, J., Hodgson, J. T., Matthews, F. E. and Jones, J. R. 1995. Continuing increase in mesothelioma mortality in Britain. *Lancet* 345:535–9.

Pfau, J. C., Sentissi, J. J., Weller, G. and Putnam, E. A. 2005. Assessment of autoimmune responses associated with asbestos exposure in Libby, Montana, USA. *Environ Health Perspect* 113:25–30.

Pfau, J. C., Serve, K. M. and Noonan, C. W. 2014. Autoimmunity and asbestos exposure. *Autoimmune Dis* 2014:782045.

Podobnik, J., Kocijancic, I., Kovac, V. and Sersa, I. 2010. 3T MRI in evaluation of asbestos-related thoracic diseases—Preliminary results. *Radiol Oncol* 44:92–6.

Reid, A., de Klerk, N., Ambrosini, G., Olsen, N., Pang, S. C. and Musk, A. W. 2005. The additional risk of malignant mesothelioma in former workers and residents of Wittenoom with benign pleural disease or asbestosis. *Occup Environ Med* 62:665–9.

Roach, H. D., Davies, G. J., Attanoos, R., Crane, M., Adams, H. and Phillips, S. 2002. Asbestos: When the dust settles an imaging review of asbestos-related disease. *Radiographics* 22(Spec. No.):S167–84.

Robinson, B. W. and Musk, A. W. 1981. Benign asbestos pleural effusion: Diagnosis and course. *Thorax* 36:896–900.

Rudd, R. 2002. *Benign Pleural Disease*. London: WB Saunders and Co.

Rusch, V. W. 1995. A proposed new international TNM staging system for malignant pleural mesothelioma. From the international mesothelioma interest group. *Chest* 108:1122–8.

Sahn, S. A. and Antony, V. B. 1984. Pathogenesis of pleural plaques. Relationship of early cellular response and pathology. *Am Rev Respir Dis* 130:884–7.

Schinwald, A., Murphy, F. A., Jones, A., Macnee, W. and Donaldson, K. 2012. Graphene-based nanoplatelets: A new risk to the respiratory system as a consequence of their unusual aerodynamic properties. *ACS Nano* 6:736–46.

Sebastien, P., Billon, M. A., Dufour, G., Gaudichet, A., Bonnaud, G. and Bignon, J. 1979. Levels of asbestos air pollution in some environmental situations. *Ann N Y Acad Sci* 330:401–15.

Segal, A., Sterrett, G. F., Frost, F. A., Shilkin, K. B., Olsen, N. J., Musk, A. W., Nowak, A. K. et al. 2013. A diagnosis of malignant pleural mesothelioma can be made by effusion cytology: Results of a 20 year audit. *Pathology* 45:44–8.

Segal, A., Whitaker, D., Henderson, D. and Shilkin, K. 2002. Pathology and mesothelioma. In B. W. S. Robinson and A. P. Chabinian (eds), *Mesothelioma*. London: Martin Dunitz.

Selikoff, I. J., Hammond, E. C. and Seidman, H. 1979. Mortality experience of insulation workers in the United States and Canada, 1943–1976. *Ann N Y Acad Sci* 330:91–116.

Sheers, G. and Templeton, A. R. 1968. Effects of asbestos in dockyard workers. *Br Med J* 3:574–9.

Sneddon, S., Leon, J. S., Dick, I. M., Cadby, G., Olsen, N., Brims, F., Allcock, R. J. et al. 2015. Absence of germline mutations in BAP1 in sporadic cases of malignant mesothelioma. *Gene* 563:103–5.

Teta, M. J., Lau, E., Sceurman, B. K. and Wagner, M. E. 2007. Therapeutic radiation for lymphoma—Risk of malignant mesothelioma. *Cancer* 109:1432–8.

Travis, L. B., Fossa, S. D., Schonfeld, S. J., McMaster, M. L., Lynch, C. F., Storm, H., Hall, P. et al. 2005. Second cancers among 40576 testicular cancer patients: Focus on long-term survivors. *J Natl Cancer Inst* 97:1354–65.

Treasure, T., Lang-Lazdunski, L., Waller, D., Bliss, J. M., Tan, C., Entwisle, J., Snee, M. et al. 2011. Extra-pleural pneumonectomy versus no extra-pleural pneumonectomy for patients with malignant pleural mesothelioma: Clinical outcomes of the Mesothelioma and Radical Surgery (MARS) randomised feasibility study. *Lancet Oncol* 12:763–72.

Tse, L. A., Yu, I. T., Goggins, W., Clements, M., Wang, X. R., Au, J. S. and Yu, K. S. 2010. Are current or future mesothelioma epidemics in Hong Kong the tragic legacy of uncontrolled use of asbestos in the past? *Environ Health Perspect* 118:382–6.

Tweedale, G. and Hansen, P. 1998. Protecting the workers: The medical board and the asbestos industry, 1930s–1960s. *Med Hist* 42:439–57.

United Nations. 2010. World Population Prospects, the 2010 Revision. Available at: http://esa.un.org/unpd/wpp/index.htm (accessed 1 September 2014).

Van Cleemput, J., De Raeve, H., Verschakelen, J. A., Rombouts, J., Lacquet, L. M. and Nemery, B. 2001. Surface of localized pleural plaques quantitated by computed tomography scanning: No relation with cumulative asbestos exposure and no effect on lung function. *Am J Respir Crit Care Med* 163:705–10.

Van Gosen, B. S., Blitz, T. A., Plumlee, G. S., Meeker, G. P. and Pearson, M. P. 2013. Geologic occurrences of erionite in the United States: An emerging national public health concern for respiratory disease. *Environ Geochem Health* 35:419–30.

Varghese, S., Whipple, R., Martin, S. S. and Alexander, H. R. 2012. Multipotent cancer stem cells derived from human malignant peritoneal mesothelioma promote tumorigenesis. *PLoS One* 7:e52825.

Virta, R. 2008. *Minerals Yearbook. Asbestos (Advanced Release)*. Washington, DC: US Geological Survey.

Vogelzang, N. J., Rusthoven, J. J., Symanowski, J., Denham, C., Kaukel, E., Ruffie, P., Gatzemeier, U. et al. 2003. Phase III study of pemetrexed in combination with cisplatin versus cisplatin alone in patients with malignant pleural mesothelioma. *J Clin Oncol* 21:2636–44.

Wagner, J. C., Sleggs, C. A. and Marchand, P. 1960. Diffuse pleural mesothelioma and asbestos exposure in the North Western Cape Province. *Br J Ind Med* 17:260–71.

Weill, D., Dhillon, G., Freyder, L., Lefante, J. and Glindmeyer, H. 2011. Lung function, radiological changes and exposure: Analysis of ATSDR data from Libby, MT, USA. *Eur Respir J* 38:376–83.

WHO. 2010. World Health Organisation Mortality Database. Available at: http://www.who.int/healthinfo/statistics/mortality_rawdata/en/index.html (accessed 1 September 2014).

Willis, R. 1960. *Pathology of Tumours*. London: Butterworths.

Wolanski, K. D., Whitaker, D., Shilkin, K. B. and Henderson, D. W. 1998. The use of epithelial membrane antigen and silver-stained nucleolar organizer regions testing in the differential diagnosis of mesothelioma from benign reactive mesothelioses. *Cancer* 82:583–90.

Wong, R. M., Ianculescu, I., Sharma, S., Gage, D. L., Olevsky, O. M., Kotova, S., Kostic, M. N. et al. 2014. Immunotherapy for malignant pleural mesothelioma. Current status and future prospects. *Am J Respir Cell Mol Biol* 50:870–5.

Yang, H. N., Testa, J. R. and Carbone, M. 2008. Mesothelioma epidemiology, carcinogenesis, and pathogenesis. *Curr Treat Options Oncol* 9:147–157.

Yildirim, H., Metintas, M., Entok, E., Ak, G., Ak, I., Dundar, E. and Erginel, S. 2009. Clinical value of fluorodeoxyglucose-positron emission tomography/computed tomography in differentiation of malignant mesothelioma from asbestos-related benign pleural disease: An observational pilot study. *J Thorac Oncol* 4:1480–4.

18 Silica

David Rees and Jill Murray

CONTENTS

INTRODUCTION

Exposure to silica is still widespread. Some high-income countries have reduced exposure (Gerhardsson, 2002) and virtually eliminated the silica-associated diseases shown in Table 18.1, but silica is ubiquitous in the earth's crust and has a large number of industrial applications; consequently, silica inhalation occurs globally in many occupations. It is estimated that 1,026,000 workers in the USA in 2013 were exposed to silica at or above 25 μg/m^3 of air—a stringent but frequently cited workplace standard—and that approximately half of them had exposures above 100 μg/m^3 (OSHA, 2013)—a common standard, but one that is too high to prevent silica-associated diseases (HSE, 2005). In poorer countries, many millions are exposed, constituting approximately

TABLE 18.1
Diseases Associated with Respirable Crystalline Silica

Pneumoconiosis	Description
Chronic silicosis	Most common form of silicosis. Typically occurs after ≥15–20 years of exposure at relatively low concentrations.
Accelerated silicosis	Silicosis that manifests after less than 10 years of exposure. Associated with higher levels of exposure and more rapid disease progression.
Acute silicoproteinosis	Occurs after short-term very high exposure. Typically 1–3 years of exposure is required, but it may develop within weeks. Pathologically similar to alveolar proteinosis.
Progressive massive fibrosis	Advanced form of silicosis with radiologic or histologic lesions >10 mm.
Rheumatoid silicotic nodules (Caplan's syndrome)	Rare condition in which large lung nodules with distinct histology are found in association with rheumatoid arthritis or merely elevated rheumatoid factor.
Airways Disease	
Chronic bronchitis	Non-specific reaction to dust with chronic cough and sputum production.
Chronic obstructive pulmonary disease	The same clinical features as for chronic obstructive pulmonary disease caused by cigarette smoking.
Emphysema	Associated with silicosis and silica exposure even without the pneumoconiosis.
Mineral dust airways disease	Lesions in small airways, typically respiratory bronchioles, consisting of fibrosis, inflammation and pigment, which may lead to airflow limitation.
Mycobacterial Disease	
Pulmonary and extra-pulmonary tuberculosis	Tuberculosis rates in populations with silicosis may be ≥3-fold higher than comparable populations without the condition.
Non-tuberculous mycobacterial disease	Makes up a substantial proportion of mycobacterial infections in some populations.
Lung Cancer	Silica is an established cause of lung cancer, but relative risks are smaller than many other causes (e.g. smoking, arsenic and asbestos).
Autoimmune Diseases	
Scleroderma Systemic lupus erythematosus Rheumatoid arthritis	Small number of analytic studies, but on balance, the evidence supports an association between these diseases and silica, and less convincingly other autoimmune conditions.
Chronic Renal Disease	Inconsistent findings, but the majority of studies support an association between chronic renal disease and silica exposure.
Cardiovascular Disease	Suggestive data, but not conclusive.

11.5 million in India (Jindal, 2013) and over 2 million in Brazil (WHO, 2007). China is thought to have the largest number of people with silicosis, with 6000 new cases reported annually (Leung et al., 2012). Even with intensified prevention efforts, because of the large numbers currently exposed and the long latency of most of the conditions, silica-related diseases will present to practitioners for decades to come, albeit relatively rarely in many high-income countries.

MINERALOGY

Silica or silicon dioxide (SiO_2) occurs in crystalline and non-crystalline (amorphous) forms. The crystalline—but not amorphous—forms have an ordered and repeating pattern of silicon–oxygen tetrahedra. Both crystalline and amorphous silica occur naturally and as synthesised materials. They are sometimes referred to as free silica because they are to a large extent only SiO_2, thus being free of other elements. Because oxygen and silicon are the most abundant atoms in the earth's crust, many minerals contain SiO_2 in combination with other elements, often cations. These minerals are silicates, not silica, and are widely encountered.

Amorphous silica is considered to be of low toxicity, although studies are somewhat limited and health concerns remain (Merget et al., 2002), and the effects of amorphous silica nanoparticles are uncertain. Nevertheless, amorphous silica is not an accepted cause of the silica-related diseases in Table 18.1. Natural amorphous silicas include biogenic silica (silica in living matter; e.g. in plants and diatoms) and vitreous silica (volcanic glasses). Both biogenic and vitreous silica have industrial uses. Calcined diatomaceous earth (heated and ground deposits of skeletons of diatoms, also known as kieselguhr) and the volcanic glass perlite are used as filter aids and fillers. A number of forms of synthetic amorphous silica have commercial applications in industry, but with the exception of fused silica—a pure form of glass—amorphous silicas are treated as low-toxicity dusts in setting workplace exposure standards (GESTIS, 2015).

A number of forms (polymorphs) of crystalline silica exist. They have been described in some detail elsewhere (Appendix 1 in this edition; IARC, 1997). The major crystalline polymorphs of health concern are α-quartz, β-quartz, tridymite and cristobalite. By far the most abundant polymorph is α-quartz, which is a constituent of many soils, sands and rocks, and the usual exposure in workplaces and the environment. The percentage of α-quartz in sand and rocks varies greatly, from virtually 0% (e.g. diorites) to nearly 100% (silica sands). Because α-quartz is the overwhelmingly predominant polymorph, silica and α-quartz are often used synonymously. In this chapter, silica is used to mean free silica and not specifically α-quartz. β-quartz, tridymite and cristobalite are formed at high temperatures and occur naturally, but are also produced in industrial processes in which α-quartz or amorphous silica is heated. Examples are foundry processes, brick and ceramic manufacturing, silicon carbide production and calcining of diatomaceous earth (NIOSH, 2002). The calcining process changes some of the amorphous silica into cristobalite; calcined diatomaceous earth may contain high percentages of this hazardous material (IARC, 1997). Historically, cristobalite was considered more hazardous than quartz, but this is no longer the case (Mossman and Glenn, 2013).

The form of the silica may not be apparent to employers, employees or occupational health services: suppliers may incorrectly label raw materials and products or provide inadequate safety data sheets (Seixas, 2014); crystalline silica may be an unanticipated component of the country rock hosting an ore; or the silica may have changed during its processing. Determination of crystalline silica in bulk material or respirable dust (fine dust that can be inhaled to the gas exchanging regions of the lung, typically of <10 μm in aerodynamic diameter) may be necessary in order to clarify whether there is exposure to crystalline silica. The laboratory that is analysing samples for silica needs to know the purpose of the analysis, and interpretation of results needs to be based on what was actually measured. Some laboratories measure only α-quartz when requested to measure crystalline silica, which is appropriate in the majority of settings, but if there are other polymorphs of crystalline silica in the material, the risk will be underestimated. In addition, as with amorphous silica, measuring SiO_2 rather than the crystalline silica content in samples containing silicates will overestimate the crystalline silica risk. For these reasons, analyses should be explicitly for crystalline silica and the polymorphs included in the analyses should be known.

SOURCES OF EXPOSURE

Sources of exposure to silica are numerous because of the ubiquity of quartz and the many industrial uses of silica-containing materials. Not all exposures are hazardous, however, because the major silica-associated diseases result from inhalation of respirable crystalline silica (RCS); activities and settings in which fine dust is present in the air are important. Crystalline silica is resistant to being broken into respirable particles; consequently, force is required in order to produce RCS. Generally, the greater the mechanical forces, the more RCS. Activities in which sand, stones or rocks or materials containing them are moved, crushed, milled, processed, drilled, ground, polished, cut or collide have the potential to generate hazardous exposures. These activities take place in a large number of occupational settings, which are comprehensively described in a number of texts (Appendix 1 in this edition; IARC, 1997; NIOSH, 2002; OSHA, 2013). Table 18.2 shows the major sources of exposure. Silica is plentiful and cheap, so new applications are not uncommon and previously unidentified risky work is still documented (Table 18.3). Even in developed countries, workers may encounter very high exposures—stone restoration work in Ireland, for example. High concentrations of RCS exposure are not limited to large enterprises; one reason for this is that powerful hand-held tools that are able to generate high concentrations of respirable dust are now commonplace.

Non-Occupational and Domestic Exposures

Low levels of RCS exposure as occur in the general environment have not been linked to silica-associated

TABLE 18.2
Sources of Occupational Exposure to Respirable Crystalline Silica

Source of Exposure	Comment
General	
Moving, drilling, working, processing, crushing, milling sand, stones or rocks	
Mining and related	
Mining and milling	Country rock[a] is an important determinant of risk. Crystalline silica content may vary substantially in a mine and according to the geographic location. Coal, copper, fluorspar, gold, iron, mica, tin, tungsten and uranium are important in some regions.
Mining related	Quarrying, tunnelling, excavating and digging wells and boreholes. Country rock and mineral determines risk. Quarrying granite, sandstone, flint, quartzite, shale and slate may produce high levels of quartz. Potency of silica may be reduced in some clays.
Small-scale mining	Under-researched but exposure may be high.
Major industrial sources	
Agriculture	High levels of quartz exposure possible in farming, but silica-associated disease rarely described.
Ceramics	Manufacture and cutting, drilling, polishing, etc., of pottery, tiles, sanitary ware, table ware, bricks and refractory articles. Potency may be reduced by associated clays. Refractory materials usually have the highest crystalline silica content.
Glass manufacture	Sand is a major raw material in glass and glass fibre manufacture.
Furnace masonry	Cutting, grinding, etc., of refractory articles.
Construction	Highest number of silica-exposed workers in many countries. Cutting, grinding, drilling, etc., of concrete, tiles or bricks. Digging foundations. Cement (e.g. Portland) has little RCS, hence risk is low if exposed to cement alone.
Stone-working and monumental masonry	Making, cutting, abrasive polishing, etc., of tombstones, billiard tables, slate pencils, cladding and surfaces, including granite counter tops.
Abrasive blasting with sand (sandblasting) or siliceous material	Very high exposures common. Usually cleaning or preparation for the coating of metal pieces, but also unusual applications (e.g. sandblasting jeans and cooking pan manufacture).
Minor industrial sources	
Fillers and scourers	Fine silica used for fillers in paints, coatings, plastics, rubber, explosives, dental supplies, etc., or in scouring materials (e.g. cleaning agents and those used for polishing flour) or grinding materials.
Jewellery	Cutting, buffing, etc., of semi-precious gems and dust from casting material used by gold- and silver-smiths.
Diatomaceous earth	Calcined material contains cristobalite.
Craft work	Stone carvers, sculpture and pottery.
Manufacture of siliceous materials	Many compounds (e.g. silicon carbide and asbestos cement products). RCS may be of concern in only a small number of tasks in these workplaces.

Source: Modified with permission from the International Union against Tuberculosis and Lung Disease. Copyright The Union. Rees, D. and Murray, J. 2007. *Int J Tuberc Lung Dis* 11:474–84.

Abbreviation: RCS: respirable crystalline silica.

[a] Country rock = rock hosting the mineral being mined. Silica content varies from location to location, even within a mine.

diseases, but non-occupational exposures that are sufficient to cause disease do occur. Pneumoconiosis—not always with typical silicotic nodules—from prolonged exposure to desert dust, particularly desert storms, has been documented in China, India, Israel and Saudi Arabia (Derbyshire, 2007).

Non-occupational exposure from commercial activities taking place in residential areas has led to silicosis and tuberculosis (TB) in residents, including children. The agate and slate pencil industries in India are well-documented examples of this type of exposure (Bhagia, 2012).

TABLE 18.3
Examples of Occupational Silica Exposure from New Applications of Silica-Containing Materials, Recently Reaffirmed as Generating Very High Exposures, Shown to Occur in Previously Uncertain Settings and in Cottage Industries

Setting	Findings	Source
Sandblasting denim, Turkey	16 cases of silicosis, 2 of whom died. Average exposure duration only 3 years	Akgun et al. (2006)
Hydraulic fracturing using 'frac' sand as a proppant, USA, (11 sites)	111 RCS measurements: geometric mean (GM) = 0.122; highest = 2.76 mg/m^3	Esswein et al. (2013)
Decorative stone workers cutting new artificial stone products used for kitchen and bathroom countertops, Israel	25 patients with silicosis referred to the National Lung Transplantation Center between January 1997 and December 2010	Kramer et al. (2012)
Quartz conglomerate workers making countertops, Cadiz, Spain	Silicosis diagnosed in 46 workers. Median of only 11 years of making the countertops and median age at diagnosis of only 33 years	Pérez-Alonso et al. (2014)
Highway repair producing RCS from concrete, masonry products, etc., USA	Mean RCS concentrations from 0.007 to 1.07 mg/m^3 for seven tasks, with 69% of 52 measurements over the permissible exposure limit	Valiante et al. (2004)
Stoneworkers doing stone restoration work on national monuments, Ireland	RCS concentrations during sandstone work: 57% >0.1 mg/m^3; highest = 6 mg/m^3 (grinding with an angle grinder) RCS concentrations during granite work: 30% >0.1 mg/m^3; highest = 0.21 mg/m^3 (grinding with an angle grinder)	Healy et al. (2014)
Autopsies on platinum miners, South Africa	Five former miners diagnosed with silicosis and 25 with fibrotic nodules in lymph nodes, probably developed in platinum mining, which was formerly thought not to be a silicosis risk	Nelson and Murray (2013)
Manufacture of dental materials (e.g. impression mixtures and dental abrasives), USA	Five cases of silicosis in two dental supply factories using fillers in dental products, including calcined diatomaceous earth	de la Hoz et al. (2004)
Lung autopsy specimens from 112 Hispanic males, California, USA	Pneumoconiosis in 32% (17) of farmworkers versus 8% (4) of non-farmworkers	Schenker et al. (2009)
Cottage-industry stone carving, Brazil	Variety of minerals carved, mostly to make souvenirs. 54% of 42 stone carvers had silicosis	Antão et al. (2004)
Gold- and silver-smiths preparing moulds (using silica-rich material) and pouring metal in artisanal workshops, Central Italy	23/100 surveyed jewellery workers had silicosis (diagnosed by high high-resolution computed tomography [CT] scan)	Murgia et al. (2007)
Tatami rush matting manufacture, China	Exposure to dust from mud used in mat making. Average free-silica content of worksite dust = 25.6%. 2.6% of 661 workers had pneumoconiosis	Xiao et al. (2004)

Note: Respirable crystalline silica (RCS) concentrations are 8-hour time-weighted averages.

So-called 'hut lung', a domestically acquired pneumoconiosis of mixed aetiology, has been described in many countries. RCS contributes to the disorder in some settings; for example, in women who hand grind maize between rocks in South Africa (Grobbelaar and Bateman, 1991).

Agriculture

Overexposure to quartz occurs in farming, particularly in dry-climate regions with sandy soils (Swanepoel et al., 2010). Although convincing evidence exists that pneumoconiosis occurs in farm workers (Schenker et al., 2009), silica-associated diseases are rarely reported (Swanepoel et al., 2010). There is a number of potential explanations for the paucity of cases. Lack of awareness by practitioners combined with poor access to health-care may lead to under-diagnosis, but annual cumulative exposure may be low because of the episodic nature of RCS-generating farm work, and the low potency of farm soils is also plausible: quartz in farm soils is not freshly fractured, frequently occurs with aluminium-containing clays and may be at the larger end of the size range of RCS. More intensive case finding may reveal that farming is a more important source of silica-related diseases than currently thought.

Artisanal and Small-Scale Mining

Artisanal and small-scale mines have increased, and an estimated 20–30 million miners may work in such mines (Buxton, 2013). These mines are generally labour intensive with low levels of mechanisation; RCS generation may therefore be lower than in larger mechanised mines. However, these small mines are usually poorly regulated and hazard control is likely to be inadequate. Research is scant in this sector, but RCS levels can be high, as shown in Tanzania (Gottesfeld et al., 2015), and accelerated silicosis has been diagnosed in small-scale gold miners in China (Tse et al., 2007).

Construction

The construction industry is a very large employer globally, and some of the activities in this industry generate very high concentrations of RCS (Table 18.3). A total of 8.5 million construction workers may be exposed to silica in India (Jindal, 2013), and construction is the major industry causing silicosis in Hong Kong (Law et al., 2001). Not all construction workers are exposed to RCS; activities such as cutting, demolishing, grinding, drilling and polishing building materials containing sand or stone (concrete, bricks, tiles, cladding, counter tops, etc.) are required to generate RCS, and even though these activities are common on building sites, they may take place for short periods in a working day.

ASSESSING EXPOSURE

Occupational Exposure Limits

Occupational exposure limits (OELs) for RCS are 8-hour time-weighted averages; that is, the average exposure over a typical shift expressed as mg or μg/m^3 of air. There are several issues to consider when assessing exposures relative to OELs, as shown in Table 18.4 and as described by the British and Dutch occupational hygiene societies (BOHS, 2011). Obtaining representative workplace concentrations requires careful planning and selection of appropriate workers during periods of usual production. RCS OELs vary substantially according to their purpose. Statutory OELs are generally influenced by cost–benefit analyses, which balance the feasibility and costs of improved dust control against the benefits of reduced disease rates (HSE, 2005; OSHA, 2013), whereas non-statutory guidance OELs are less influenced by considerations that are extraneous to data on dose–response relationships. It is not surprising, therefore, that statutory RCS OELs are usually less stringent than those designed to guide practitioners; typically, statutory RCS OELs are 0.1 mg/m^3 (GESTIS, 2015)—although this is under review in some jurisdictions—but a frequently cited guidance OEL is 0.025 mg/m^3 (ACGIH, 2006). It is generally accepted that 0.1 mg/m^3 is not protective against silicosis (and hence lung cancer and TB) (HSE, 2005; ACGIH, 2006; OSHA, 2013).

Potency Factors

The disease-causing potency of RCS varies by industry. For example, Chinese pottery workers had lower silicosis risks for a given exposure than Chinese tin and tungsten miners (Chen et al., 2005). Very fine particles and freshly cut surfaces increase toxicity, whereas aged quartz, the use of wet processes and, importantly, the presence of aluminium-containing clay minerals reduce toxicity (Meldrum and Howden, 2002). Activities that produce freshly fractured, fine, dry silica that is un-associated with clays are, therefore, of particular concern—sandblasting, rock drilling, grinding and polishing of silica-containing materials and high-energy cutting are examples.

EPIDEMIOLOGY

Only epidemiological aspects of silicosis, silica-associated lung cancer and TB are covered here, because chronic obstructive pulmonary disease (COPD) and other lung conditions are dealt with elsewhere in this book.

Silicosis

Many factors influence the extent of silicosis in exposed groups, but cumulative exposure (a function of intensity and duration often expressed as mg/m^3-years), length of follow-up from first exposure and potency factors contribute. A single cumulative exposure–disease response curve will not reliably describe how much disease can be expected across different industries. Estimates of the percentage of silicosis in 11 studies at three levels of cumulative silica exposure varied considerably: from 0.4% to approximately 28% at 2 mg/m^3-years; and from 2% to 92% at 4 mg/m^3-years (OEHHA, 2005).

Cross-sectional surveys of currently exposed workers underestimate the risk of disease, as affected workers

TABLE 18.4
Interpreting Workplace Air Concentrations of Respirable Crystalline Silica Relative to Occupational Exposure Limits

Issue to Consider	Explanation
OELs vary according to purpose	Statutory OELs may be considerably less stringent than guidance OELs. Statutory limits may not be protective.
A small number of measurements may underestimate exposure	Typically, a small sample of possible RCS exposures over a working year is measured. High RCS concentrations may be undetected because the activities producing them have not been sampled and because the highest concentrations are usually less common than lower concentrations. Thus, overexposure may have occurred despite measurement data suggesting it has not.
Quantifying RCS is subject to measurement error	Respirable dust has to be captured and weighed accurately, and both are subject to measurement error. Very small amounts of RCS have to be quantified in respirable dust, often at amounts close to the level of quantification of the equipment. Experienced occupational hygienists using calibrated equipment and quality-controlled laboratories are needed for reliable measurement.
RCS OELs do not take account of the risk of pulmonary tuberculosis or COPD	RCS OELs usually aim to limit silicosis, as well as lung cancer in some instances, but not PTB or COPD. The more stringent OELs may be protective of PTB, but this is speculative.
Recent RCS concentrations may underestimate past exposure	Improved technology, substitution and legal and social pressures have lowered exposure to RCS in some industries over time.
Measuring only α-quartz may underestimate RCS exposure	When asked to quantify RCS, analytic laboratories may measure only α-quartz. This is appropriate in the majority of settings, but other polymorphs, notably cristobalite, should be measured in selected industries.

Abbreviations: OEL: occupational exposure limit; RCS: respirable crystalline silica; COPD: chronic obstructive pulmonary disease; PTB: pulmonary tuberculosis.

may have left employment or may only develop the disease long after leaving the enterprise. Cohort studies that adequately follow-up workers find higher rates of disease: 47%–77% in one review (Steenland, 2005). Defining an industry's or country's silica-related disease burden based on workplace surveys is, thus, inadequate.

Lung Cancer

Lung cancer is convincingly linked to quartz and cristobalite exposure (IARC, 2012; Liu et al., 2013; Steenland and Ward, 2014). There is uncertainty regarding whether silica exposure without silicosis causes the malignancy (Erren et al., 2009), but there is increasing evidence that silicosis is not necessary (Liu et al., 2013). The studies showing that non-silicotics are at increased risk are, however, based on the absence of *radiological* silicosis, which is an important consideration, as silicosis can be present without radiological evidence of disease (Hnizdo et al., 1993). It is, therefore, more accurate to state that the presence of radiological silicosis is not necessary in order to increase the risk of lung cancer.

The increased risk conferred by RCS is smaller than that of lung carcinogens such as arsenic and asbestos, with effect estimates being less than 2 in many studies for even the most exposed non-silicotic subgroups (IARC, 2012; Liu et al., 2013). Attribution of the malignancy to RCS in individual cases without silicosis can thus be uncertain. It is possible that RCS potency factors influence carcinogenesis as well as the silicosis-causing potential, because large studies with good exposure data have not found an association between lung cancer and exposure (Mundt et al., 2011). The risks from smoking and RCS together are more than additive in some studies in terms of increasing the risk of lung cancer (Liu et al., 2013), providing additional motivation for smoking cessation programmes in workplaces.

Tuberculosis

Silicosis substantially increases the risk of TB. The increase is typically said to be approximately three times (ATS, 1997), but it is influenced by background TB rates, HIV infection (which is a powerful determinant when combined with silicosis) (Corbett et al., 2000), workplace social factors (Rees et al., 2010) and the severity of the silicosis, with the acute form carrying a very high risk. TB rates can be very high in workers with these associated risk factors, reaching 3000–4000/100,000 in South African gold miners (Churchyard et al., 2014).

Silica exposure without silicosis has been shown to be a determinant of TB (Sherson and Lander, 1990; Hnizdo and Murray, 1998), but the relationship is less certain than for silicosis because silicosis status was determined radiologically in all but one study; undiagnosed silicosis may still explain the associations in the other studies. The study that confirmed the absence of pneumoconiosis found weak associations between TB and increasing quartiles of cumulative dust exposure, with wide 95% confidence intervals (CIs) based on only 18 cases of TB: the highest relative risk was 1.42 (95% CI 0.43–4.72) (Hnizdo and Murray, 1998). Nevertheless, an increased TB risk is likely, as it is explained by silica-induced dysfunction of macrophages (Chávez-Galán et al., 2013), which does not presuppose fibrosis in the lung, and animal studies are convincing (Pasula et al., 2009).

Neither the duration of exposure nor the cumulative dose of RCS, which increase the risk of TB above background rates, have been defined. It is assumed that OELs that are protective against silicosis will be adequate, but this is far from certain. It seems logical to assume that recurrence of TB after cure would be higher in workers with continued RCS exposure compared to those who are unexposed, but the literature is inconsistent on this issue.

Non-tuberculous pulmonary mycobacterial (NTM) disease occurs more frequently than usual in RCS-exposed individuals. *Mycobacterium kansasii, M. scrofulaceum* and *M. avium* isolates, in decreasing order of frequency, were identified in a study of South African gold miners (Corbett et al., 1999); the species will vary by locality, however (ATS, 1996). Risk factors for NTM infection include more extensive silicosis, previous TB, pre-existing radiological abnormalities and dusty work at the time of diagnosis (Corbett et al., 1999).

CLINICAL FEATURES

The clinical features of the non-specific silica-related conditions (e.g. COPD and lung cancer) are no different to those arising from other causes, except that silica-associated TB sometimes presents atypically. For this reason, only the clinical features of silicosis and aspects of TB are considered.

SILICOSIS

> The diagnosis of silicosis is based on a history of sufficient exposure, imaging findings consistent with silicosis and symptoms and signs and laboratory tests that are suggestive that another disease is not more likely. Histology is rarely required, but may be necessary in order to avoid missing a treatable condition.

The diagnostic work-up typically involves: an exposure history covering all jobs; symptoms, including those associated with TB; a physical examination with attention to features that would be unusual in silicosis (e.g. clubbing, enlarged lymph nodes, hepatomegaly, splenomegaly, rashes and inflammation of small joints); chest radiographs (high-resolution computed tomography [HRCT] scans would be usual in many developed countries); and spirometry. The diagnosis of silicosis can be made reasonably confidently without further investigation when there is a history of prolonged RCS exposure, the patient has the typical small, rounded opacities in the upper lung zones and the patient is well without systemic symptoms such as weight loss, fever or signs suggesting another disease. Patients should, however, present for re-evaluation if they develop significant symptoms, and it is advisable to review them within a few months and then within a year or so in order to confirm that the condition is consistent with the stable clinical picture of typical silicosis. Unusual features, including a short exposure history, should prompt further investigation. Review of previous chest radiographs may be helpful, and unchanged opacities over a couple of years support a diagnosis of silicosis.

Sufficient Exposure

The risk of the silica-associated diseases is a function of intensity and duration of exposure, rather than duration alone, so the occupational history should cover not only time spent in a job, but also the nature of the work, the dustiness and the use of respiratory-protective equipment. Over time, the RCS concentrations in most workplaces in high- and even middle-income countries have declined. In settings of reasonably low exposure, the silica-associated lung diseases, with the exception of TB, require prolonged exposure, typically ≥20 years. In poorly controlled settings, diseases may manifest after only a few years of exposure (Akgun et al., 2006; Mohebbi and Zubeyri, 2007). Visible dustiness can be misleading, as RCS is not visible to the naked eye—ostensibly high-risk activities may be safe and vice versa—so confirming the presence of *respirable* particles is useful. Documenting exceedance of OELs is helpful, notwithstanding the caveats in Table 18.4; historic measurements may be available in order to provide this information. The use of respiratory-protective equipment may produce a false sense of protection, as inappropriate or inadequately used respirators are commonplace. In essence, except for TB, a long duration of exposure is required unless there is evidence (on history or measurement) that work conditions were very dusty. The diseases can manifest for the first time long after exposure has ceased.

IMAGING

Acute Silicoproteinosis

Reports on the imaging features of acute silicoproteinosis are limited to small series and case reports, but the features are similar to pulmonary alveolar proteinosis (Dee et al., 1978). Areas of peri-hilar ground-glass density and/or consolidation are frequent radiographic features (Xipell et al., 1977; Dee et al., 1978). Computed tomography (CT) demonstrates areas of predominant ground-glass density and a few thickened interlobular septa with the addition of poorly defined centrilobular nodules and dependent areas of consolidation (often with punctate calcification); the latter two features may differentiate from pulmonary alveolar proteinosis (Marchiori et al., 2007). However, the 'crazy-paving' pattern (areas of geographic ground-glass density on a background of extensive thickened interlobular septa) seen in alveolar proteinosis (Godwin et al., 1988) is seen in a minority of cases. The imaging features of ground-glass density, centrilobular nodules and consolidation seen in acute silicoproteinosis are histopathological correlates of accumulation of intra-alveolar proteinaceous material (Marchiori et al., 2001). In approximately a third of the 13 patients described by Marchiori et al. (2001), minor traction bronchiectasis and pulmonary distortion were also present. An unexpected finding in this group was tracheal dilatation of uncertain aetiology. Pleural effusions and pleural thickening were also observed. Another feature that is common in acute silicoproteinosis (as opposed to alveolar proteinosis) is the presence of mediastinal and bilateral hilar lymphadenopathy, which may be calcified (Marchiori et al., 2001).

Chronic Silicosis and Progressive Massive Fibrosis (PMF)

Chronic silicosis is characterised by small (typically 3–6 mm diameter, ranging from 1 to 10 mm), rounded nodules with a posterior and upper zone predominance on chest radiography, which may calcify in up to 20% of cases (Bergin et al., 1986). Mediastinal and hilar lymph node calcification is common in silicosis; the calcification is often 'egg-shell' in morphology (referring to the peripheral distribution). This feature may predate the pulmonary parenchymal nodularity (Remy-Jardin et al., 1992). On HRCT, the nodules may be centrilobular (adjacent to the structures in the centre of the secondary pulmonary lobule) or sub-pleural and of varying size (Remy-Jardin et al., 1990). The nodules in silicosis have been reported to be more sharply defined than those of coal workers' pneumoconiosis, but may be indistinguishable due to their similar size and distribution (Oikonomou and Müller, 2003). A small percentage of nodules calcify, increasing their conspicuousness on HRCT (Remy-Jardin et al., 1992).

Radiologically, the lesions of PMF are rounded or oval, with densities of at least 1 cm in diameter (Figure 18.1a) (ILO, 2011). Upper zone predominance is the rule, and these large opacities tend to occur in the periphery of the lung and migrate centrally over time. PMF densities vary in shape and may have well- or ill-defined margins. Both unilateral and bilateral densities (either symmetrical or asymmetrical) have been described (Chong et al., 2006). The important differential diagnosis is lung cancer, particularly in the context of unilateral or asymmetrical opacities. Comparison with previous radiographs may

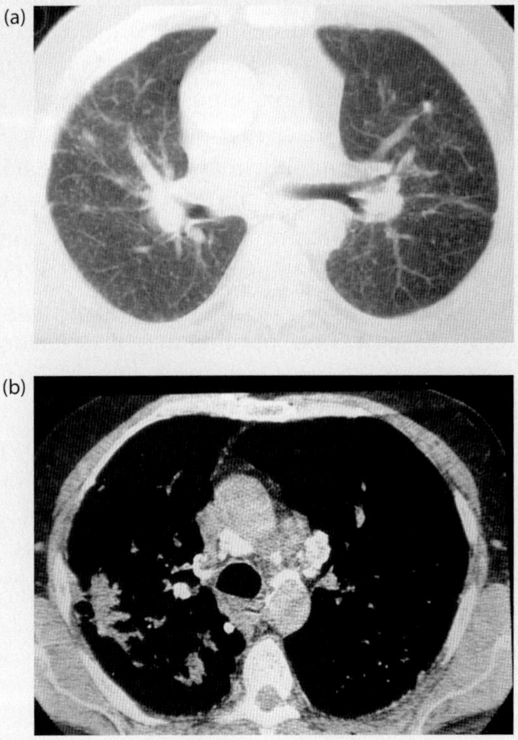

FIGURE 18.1 Computed tomography scan of an individual with complicated silicosis showing a combination of fine, small, rounded nodules in the mid-zones (a), with areas of PMF in the upper zones (not shown). (b) Computed tomography scan of an individual with complicated silicosis and PMF. Note the eggshell calcification of mediastinal lymph nodes.

be particularly helpful in demonstrating the typical peripheral to central migration and the relative stability in size over many years. In addition, there is often a background of small, nodular densities in silicosis, but occasionally this feature is absent (Chong et al., 2006). There may be indirect features of scarring and volume loss related to areas of PMF with mediastinal, tracheal and parenchymal distortion and adjacent areas of so-called paracicatricial emphysematous destruction. Cavitation has also been described, which may resolve spontaneously (Chong et al., 2006).

CT demonstrates more elegantly the conglomerate masses of PMF on a background of micronodules (which may result in irregularities in the outlines of larger densities). Surrounding paracicatricial emphysema is better demonstrated on CT than chest radiography. In addition, adjacent distortion and 'drawing in' of the extra-pleural fat is often a feature of peripheral masses (Chong et al., 2006). An upper and posterior lung distribution is frequent, although isolated lower-lobe masses are also recognised (Chong et al., 2006). A variety of calcification patterns may be seen, particularly punctate, with extensive dense calcification being less common. Avascular necrosis is a feature of large lesions, with initial areas of decreased attenuation progressing to cavitation and air–fluid levels. Infections, including TB, may complicate cavitation, but aspergillomas rarely form within PMF cavities. The imaging features of silicotuberculosis consist of the rapid progression of asymmetric nodules, consolidation and cavitation. Cavitation is the strongest predictor of TB infection, but this may also occur in the context of non-infective ischaemic necrosis in an area of PMF (Chong S et al., 2006).

The nodules of Caplan's syndrome are typically over 3 cm in diameter (ranging from 0.5 to 5 cm) and sometimes conglomerated into groups that appear suddenly. However, they commonly cavitate, and it may be difficult to differentiate radiologically between Caplan's syndrome, cavitary PMF and tuberculous infection. Other causes of a similar 'PMF'-type radiological appearance include coal workers' pneumoconiosis, talcosis, berylliosis and kaolin pneumoconiosis (Chong et al., 2006), pulmonary talc granulomatosis in intravenous drug abusers (Padley et al., 1993) and fibrotic pulmonary sarcoidosis; in the latter, the confluent fibrosis almost invariably 'streams off' the hila, in contrast to PMF (Pipavath and Godwin, 2004). Other complications that may be apparent on imaging include pulmonary arterial hypertension, right heart failure and non-tuberculous infections.

CT–function correlation studies have demonstrated a relationship between functional deficit and extent of PMF and emphysema on CT, independent of cigarette smoking and duration of silica exposure (Ooi et al., 2003). There is good correlation between the extent of radiographic and CT nodularlity in silicosis (Ooi et al., 2003); however, the main advantages of CT in individuals with suspected silicosis are increased specificity in comparison with chest radiography and the demonstration of complications (Begin et al., 1987).

A potential use of positron emission tomography (PET)/CT and magnetic resonance imaging (MRI; including diffusion-weighted MRI) in the context of complicated silicosis is to differentiate lung cancer from PMF, although false positives may occur with PET due to infection, including TB (Chung et al., 2010). Lung cancer typically returns a high signal on T2-weighted imaging, whereas PMF appears as a low signal on T2 by comparison with skeletal muscle (O'Connell and Kennedy, 2004; Chong et al., 2006).

The most common MRI appearances of PMF show iso- or high-signal intensity (bright) on T1-weighted sequences with low signal (dark) on T2 (when compared with skeletal muscle) (O'Connell and Kennedy, 2004). Areas of rim enhancement or a lack of enhancement post-gadolinium may also be seen (Jung et al., 2000).

Symptoms and Signs

Chronic silicosis, even when radiologically advanced, may be symptomless, but such patients have worked in dirty workplaces, may have smoked, have had previous TB or have other diseases due to RCS; therefore, respiratory symptoms and signs are not uncommon. A cough, with or without sputum, dyspnoea and wheezes or crackles on auscultation, is most frequently reported. The evaluation of patients who are suspected of having silicosis should include features associated with diseases in the differential diagnosis; for chronic silicosis, TB and sarcoidosis are most important, but histoplasmosis is a consideration in some parts of the world, and for PMF, lung cancer is to be considered, especially when the lesion is unilateral and newly detected radiologically. The patient's perception of their ability to meet the physical demands of his or her current job should be established, and it may be necessary to record the extent of dyspnoea in a standard manner in some jurisdictions where this contributes to grading of impairment or disability for workers' compensation. In most regions of the world, thorough questioning regarding the symptoms of TB is required at each consultation. The clinical features of accelerated silicosis are the same as for chronic silicosis, except that they may present earlier in the course of the disease. A greater proportion of patients with PMF than chronic silicosis have symptoms, signs and respiratory impairment, but even so, some are asymptomatic. Acute silicoproteinosis is rare but often fatal and should be suspected in patients who have had very high levels of exposure to fine RCS dust and who present with progressive respiratory symptoms and constitutional symptoms such as fever or weight loss.

Chest pain, clubbing, haemoptysis, fever and weight loss are unusual in uncomplicated silicosis and should prompt further investigation for potentially treatable diseases.

Lung Function Tests

Lung function tests can be normal even in radiologically advanced disease, or abnormal due to the same factors influencing symptoms. There is no specific lung function change associated with silicosis, and obstructive, restrictive or mixed patterns can be observed. Spirometry may underestimate impairment in some cases and transfer factor for carbon monoxide (TL_{CO}) should be measured in cases with discordance between dyspnoea and spirometric parameters. TL_{CO} is less useful for monitoring progression of silicosis than it is for asbestosis.

Progression

Silicosis often progresses whether or not RCS exposure continues after diagnosis. Proportions of patients whose disease advances may be very high—88% in a study of long-service South African gold miners (Hessel et al., 1988)—but is typically approximately one- to two-thirds (Mohebbi and Zubeyri, 2007) depending on factors such as nature of exposure and length of follow-up. Although one would expect continued exposure to result in more rapid progression of silicosis in higher proportions of subjects, few studies have examined this issue. Silicosis cases from a mining company entered into a Swedish case register showed greater disease progression if post-diagnosis exposure continued relative to exposure cessation (Westerholm, 1980). Continued exposure was associated with increased risk of PMF in South African gold miners (Hessel et al., 1988) and with more advanced silicosis, large opacities and TB in Brazilian gold miners (Carneiro et al., 2006). The concentration of RCS that increases the risk of progression or complications is unknown. The small number of studies in one industry means that it has not been conclusively shown that removal from further exposure will reduce progression to more advanced disease. Greater extent of radiological silicosis at diagnosis, young age at diagnosis, an initially rapid increase in the number and size of small opacities (Mohebbi and Zubeyri, 2007) and larger opacities at diagnosis (OSHA, 2013) are risk factors for progression, but there is insufficient information to predict progression with any certainty in individual cases. Sudden increases in the sizes or shapes of opacities may be signs of TB or, more rarely, rheumatoid silicotic nodules. Sudden increases are, however, difficult to define precisely, but noticeable changes within 2 years are unusual, unless past exposure has been very intense.

Laboratory Investigations

Although laboratory blood tests may be altered in silicosis, none has sufficient positive and negative predictive value to assist in making the diagnosis. Non-specific tests of inflammation such as the erythrocyte sedimentation rate and C-reactive protein may or may not be elevated, and markers of immune response are inconsistently associated with silicosis and are not specific for the disease.

TUBERCULOSIS

Especially in high-burden countries, TB should be considered at every consultation with RCS-exposed patients, irrespective of the presenting complaint. The clinical features may be the same as for TB in individuals without RCS exposure, but a more indolent form of the disease also occurs (Solomon, 2001), which can be associated with fewer symptoms than usual. These patients may well be sputum smear negative. The introduction of the Xpert® MTB/RIF assay has improved TB detection, but it has lower sensitivity in smear-negative than smear-positive cases (Steingart et al., 2013). In these circumstances, imaging becomes even more important than usual, provided the radiological features, which are frequently atypical, are recognised. Some of these features that should prompt further clinical evaluation are short latency from first RCS exposure to appearance of opacities, variability in size and shape and asymmetrical distribution of opacities, supra-clavicular opacities, regional aggregation of irregular-sized nodules and arrangement of nodules along a broncho-vascular bundle. Mediastinal lymphadenopathy and the appearance of large opacities are also of concern (Solomon, 2001; Solomon and Rees, 2010). Figure 18.2 shows florid examples of some of these features.

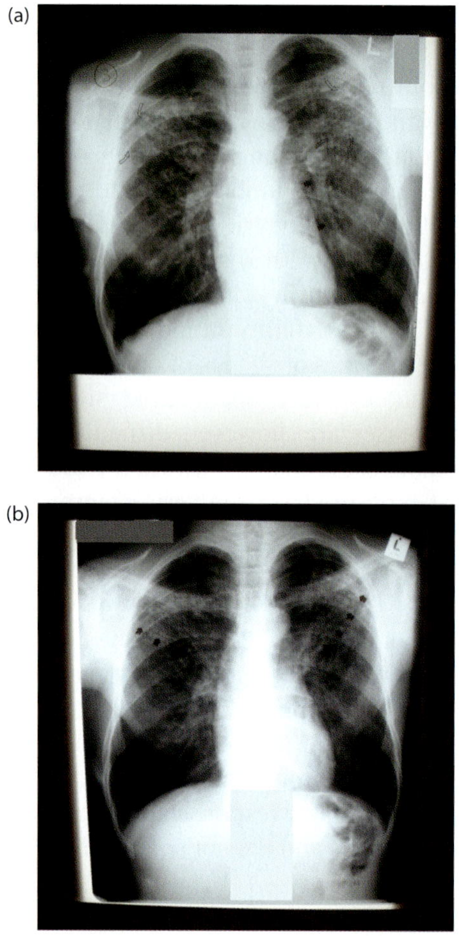

FIGURE 18.2 (a) Arrangement along the broncho-vascular bundles and variability in size of nodules in silicosis and tuberculosis. (b) Florid example of the arrangement of nodules along the broncho-vascular bundles of silicosis and tuberculosis. (From Solomon, A. and Rees, D. 2010. *Occup Health Southern Afr* 16:25–27.)

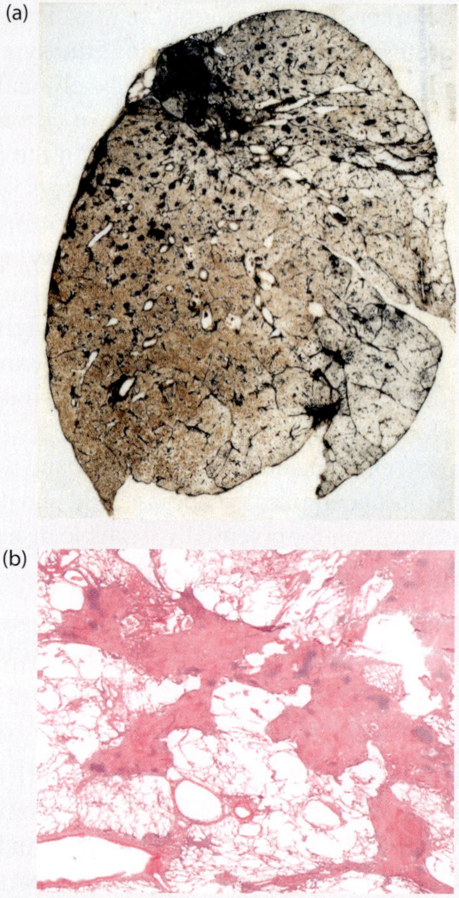

FIGURE 18.3 (a) Silicotic nodules predominate in the upper part of the lung and progressive massive fibrosis is present (paper-mounted whole-lung section). (b) Microscopy shows silicotic nodules with intervening normal lung tissue. (Courtesy of Bryan Corrin.)

PATHOLOGY AND PATHOGENESIS

Pathological Findings

Chronic silicosis is characterised by the presence of discrete, rounded, hard nodules of 3–5 mm in diameter in both upper lobes of the lung (Figure 18.3) (Craighead et al., 1988). Nodules also develop on the visceral pleura and in the peri-bronchial and hilar lymph nodes, which may be the first sites of involvement (Murray et al., 1991). Calcification of affected lymph nodes results in a characteristic eggshell radiographic appearance. Early lesions of chronic silicosis comprise aggregates of macrophages with scanty reticulin and collagen fibres; accelerated silicosis shows a predominance of these cellular lesions, and fully developed fibrotic nodules may be sparse.

The silicotic nodule has a central acellular zone of whorled collagen fibres, with dust-laden macrophages at the periphery (Figure 18.4). The presence of granulomas, giant cells and central necrosis should raise a suspicion of associated TB (Katzenstein, 2006). Silica particles are only weakly birefringent under polarised light, with any strong birefringence being due to accompanying silicates such as mica and talc. As the disease progresses, the nodules extend to involve the mid and lower zones of the lungs. With increasing duration and intensity of dust exposure, PMF develops. PMF is characterised by coalescence of the nodules to form fibrous masses ranging from one to many centimetres (Figure 18.5). The upper lobes may be

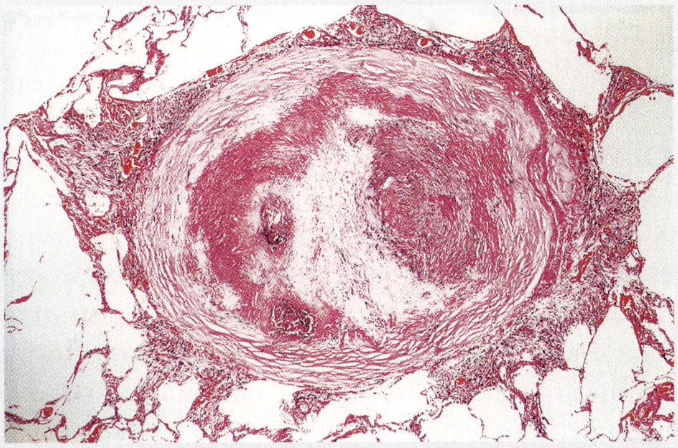

FIGURE 18.4 Silicotic nodule with central whorled collagen and a peripheral rim of dust-laden macrophages. (Courtesy of Bryan Corrin.)

(a)

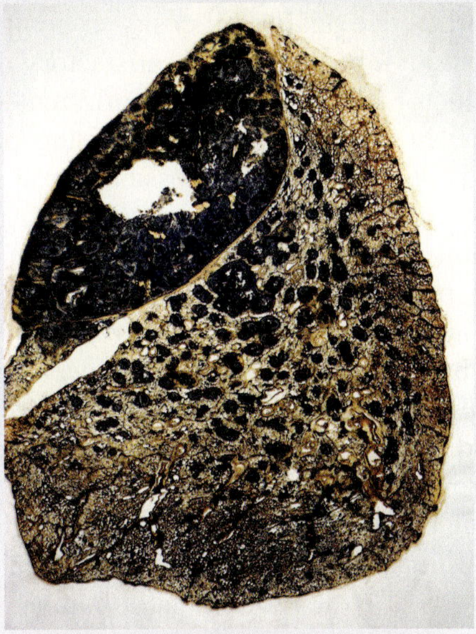

(b)

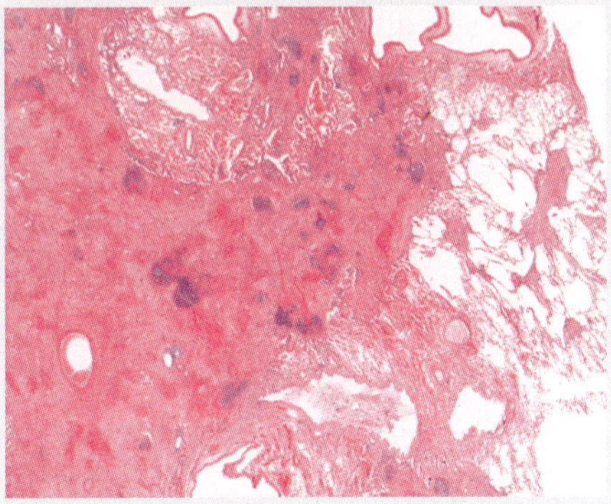

FIGURE 18.5 (a) The nodules are larger than in Figure 18.3, and many have coalesced. Progressive massive fibrosis with cavitation has destroyed most of the upper lobe (paper-mounted whole lung section). (b) Microscopy of conglomerate silicosis. (Courtesy of Bryan Corrin.)

completely replaced and the masses may obliterate the inter-lobar fissures and involve the apical regions of the lower lobes. PMF lesions may show areas of necrosis, cavitation and encapsulated necrosis, which may reflect mycobacterial infection. Cor pulmonale may be present in cases of PMF and advanced chronic silicosis (Murray et al., 1993).

Rarely, silicotic nodules may be found in the abdominal nodes, liver, spleen, peritoneum and bone marrow, but in these sites they have not been associated with any clinical disease (Slavin et al., 1985).

Acute silicoproteinosis is characterised by a lipoproteinacious material filling of the alveolar spaces. The material consists of denatured alveolar surfactant, resembling that of primary alveolar proteinosis (Craighead et al., 1988). Very fine silica particles may be seen in this exudate with the use of electron microscopy. There is minimal collagen deposition and silicotic nodules are usually absent.

Diffuse interstitial pulmonary fibrosis, pathologically resembling idiopathic pulmonary fibrosis, has occasionally been reported to occur in silica dust-exposed patients with and without nodular silicosis; however, neither the pathogenesis nor the clinical features are well understood (Arakawa et al., 2007).

Pathogenesis

The causative pathways of silica-induced fibrosis have been the subject of several recent reviews (Leung et al., 2012). Animal, in vitro and human studies have shown that reactive oxygen species may be generated directly by silica particles or as a result of uptake by macrophages. The ensuing fibro-inflammatory cascade involves the recruitment of inflammatory cells, including T cells and dendritic cells, and the release of a range of cytokines, including TNF and IL-1. Silica-induced apoptosis of macrophages releases ingested silica particles to be taken up by fresh macrophages and so triggering ongoing cycles of inflammation and fibrosis. Further elucidation of the underlying mechanisms of silicosis may result in the development of therapeutic interventions.

The mechanisms that result in increased susceptibility to mycobacterial infections in silica-exposed persons are poorly understood, but in animal models, silica reduces the ability of alveolar macrophages to kill mycobacteria (Pasula et al., 2009; Chavez-Galan et al., 2013).

TREATMENT AND MANAGEMENT

Silicosis is incurable; no treatment has been shown to be consistently effective in reducing fibrosis or preventing progression (Leung et al., 2012). Whole-lung lavage has been used to treat chronic and accelerated silicosis in China, but objective improvements in lung function and radiologic regression have not been demonstrated. Whole-lung lavage is, however, used to treat primary alveolar proteinosis and hence has been used in acute silicoproteinosis, but with limited success (Souza et al., 2010), except in isolated cases. Lung transplantation is a therapeutic modality for advanced silicosis in settings with the resources to justify its use (Singer et al., 2012).

There is no consensus that treatment of TB should be modified in patients with silicosis. Although better outcomes with extended treatment regimes have been described (Hong Kong Chest Service, 1991), the evidence is inconsistent and authoritative guidelines do not list silicosis as a reason for longer treatment. Silicosis was not a risk factor for recurrence of TB after cure in studies of South African gold miners (Cowie et al., 1989; Charalambous et al., 2008), but follow-up was short in the latter study. A modest increase in the incidence density for recurrence of silicosis (1.55, 95% CI 0.97–2.48) was shown with longer follow-up—at least 5 years (Cowie, 1995)—but increased risk of recurrence on standard regimes has not been demonstrated sufficiently to justify therapeutic changes. Higher TB case–fatality rates have been reported in both HIV-positive and -negative silicotics (Churchyard et al., 2000), but strategies specific to silicosis in order to prevent these fatalities have not been identified.

Removal from further exposure to RCS is generally recommended following the diagnosis of silicosis in order to lower the risk of progression and complications such as TB, but there is surprisingly little evidence to support this recommendation. Although discontinuation of exposure seems reasonable, it may lead to unemployment, particularly in poorer countries with inadequate social security systems and where unemployment is associated with poverty, which confers substantial health risks. Consequently, in consultation with the patient, a more flexible approach is often required. Current dust levels, the feasibility of lowering RCS concentrations in the current job, work adaptation (the more dusty tasks could be modified or reallocated) and close proximity to retirement may influence the decision. There is no evidence that removal from further exposure is urgent; continued exposure until a low-dust position becomes available may be less harmful than unemployment and may have little impact on future health.

PREVENTION

Preventing RCS diseases is possible but requires a comprehensive approach, such as described in the national programmes of the International Labour Organization (ILO)/World Health Organization (WHO) global elimination campaign. Elements of these programmes include: building political will; developing the capacity to measure and, most importantly, control RCS; appropriate OELs and stronger enforcement of them; improved case finding and surveillance programmes in order to identify silicosis-causing industries; education; and effective compensation systems that penalise workplaces that generate disease.

Controlling Exposure

The most common statutory OELs, 0.05–0.1 mg/m^3, are not protective against silicosis, so compliance with them should not be considered satisfactory dust control. Substitution of silica with less harmful materials, as has been done in abrasive blasting, scouring powders and non-silica foundry sands, is possible for some applications. However, in the majority of RCS exposure settings, substitution is unfeasible. The hierarchy of controls as routinely practised by occupational hygienists should then be applied, with the use of respirators as a last resort. It has been suggested that engineering controls in order to prevent silicosis would be cost effective in both developed and developing countries (Lahiri et al., 2005). Engineering controls may be complex and require the knowledge of experienced hygienists and engineers, but relatively simple measures have been shown to be effective (Gottesfeld et al., 2008), and a number of agencies have developed internet tools that assist companies and practitioners to select practical controls based on what has worked in similar environments. The UK's Health and Safety Executive's COSHH Essentials cover a number of silica industries (http://www.hse.gov.uk/pubns/guidance) and the Netherlands' Stoffenmanager (https://stoffenmanager.nl/) uses control banding in order to identify suitable interventions.

Respirators may appear to be an attractive solution, but in order to be effective, they must be fit-tested for individual workers, appropriate for the nature and concentration of the dust, acceptable to workers, maintained and stored appropriately and replaced at the correct intervals (ATS, 1996). A respirator programme is thus resource intensive and, over time, may cost more than engineering controls. Generally, respirators are best reserved for short-term tasks for which it is difficult to engineer satisfactory control. Not all workers can tolerate respirators. The American Thoracic Society's statement on respirator programmes guides clinicians in medically determining the suitability of respirator use (ATS, 1996).

Surveillance

Surveillance systems that identify silicosis-causing workplaces for intervention can support prevention efforts. Interventions may include medical evaluation of current and former co-workers of the sentinel cases and assessment of current exposure to RCS and workplace controls. Reporting of new cases need not be complete: even partial reporting will identify some problematic workplaces. These systems usually rely heavily on doctors to report cases. Reporter fatigue needs to countered but there is scant evidence for what works. Ensuring that officials respond to reported cases and regular communication, which acknowledges those who report and describes successful interventions, may be helpful. An alternative to doctor reporting is the use of hospital discharge records, which has been shown to be cost effective in parts of the USA (Rosenman et al., 2001), but this would not work where hospital admission is unusual.

Compensation

Workers' compensation is important for individual workers, but can also support prevention. Data can be used to identify and target disease-causing workplaces, compensation levies can be used for research on RCS controls, rebates can be given to enterprises with good RCS controls and levies increased on those without them and benefits to claimants should be sufficient to be a financial incentive for disease reduction. Consequently, clinicians should submit cases for compensation, not only for individual patients, but also to contribute to prevention.

Tuberculosis

Controlling TB requires a multifaceted programme that reduces RCS exposure, improves workers' social conditions and implements interventions that interrupt transmission or incidence, such as early identification and treatment of active disease and prevention and management of HIV.

Chemoprophylaxis, usually isoniazid prevention therapy (IPT), is recommended for preventing TB disease in individuals with silicosis or long-term silica exposure (ATS, 1997). Detailed IPT guidelines have been published (Pneumoconiosis Clinic of the Department of Health of the Government of Hong Kong SAR, 2004; de Jager et al., 2014), all of which recommend tuberculin skin testing (TST) either so that only TST-positive subjects receive IPT or a longer duration of IPT is offered—at least 36 months in South Africa (de Jager et al., 2014). Interferon-γ release assays (IGRAs) have replaced TST under certain circumstances, but are currently not recommended in resource-constrained settings (WHO, 2011). Excluding active TB is a pre-requisite for initiating IPT, and since undiagnosed TB is common in HIV-positive people with silicosis, excluding active disease should be rigorous, and sputum testing with polymerase chain reaction techniques or sputum culture has been recommended (de Jager et al., 2014). A large mass IPT trial on South African gold mines unfortunately did not improve TB control (Churchyard et al., 2014).

Smoking

The risks of lung cancer and COPD from smoking and RCS together have been found to be more than additive in some studies; smoking also increases the risk of TB and its recurrence after cure (Yen et al., 2014). Additionally, current smoking has been shown to be an important determinant of active mycobacterial disease in silicotic patients (Leung et al., 2007). Smoking cessation should therefore be an integral part of workplace programmes to prevent disease in workplaces with a RCS hazard, and individuals who have had RCS exposure should be offered support to quit.

Biological Monitoring

A number of candidate biomarkers that would indicate the presence of an adverse response to the inhalation of RCS before the onset of disease have been proposed (Gulumian et al., 2006), but so far none has been found that predicts future disease and discriminates sufficiently among other diseases.

HEALTH SURVEILLANCE

Health surveillance of workers in RCS workplaces is widely recommended, usually on placement, periodically and near exiting employment. Formerly exposed workers are less consistently covered by surveillance, even though silica-related diseases commonly present years after the last exposure, and disease prevalence is highest in groups of former workers with long follow-up (Rees and Murray, 2007). A review of recommendations for surveillance (Bradshaw et al., 2010) concluded that health questionnaires, physical examination and spirometry are generally required annually, but there was less consensus on the periodicity of chest radiographs, except that more intense or longer-duration exposure resulted in greater frequency. The American College of Occupational and Environmental Medicine recommend that workers with RCS exposure of <0.05 mg/m^3 should have a baseline evaluation, again at 1 year, then 3-yearly for the first 10 years and 2-yearly thereafter (Raymond and Wintermeyer, 2006).

Surveillance should be conducted with consideration of the context and its purpose. Typically, the stated objective of surveillance is to identify early adverse effects so that disease progression can be slowed or prevented. In order to achieve this objective, interventions must occur in workplaces upon detection of early deviations from health. If they do not, frequent surveillance—spirometry, for example—may just divert money from RCS control. In resource-constrained enterprises, the costs and benefits of surveillance versus hazard control should be evaluated, and surveillance modified accordingly. A simple diagnostic model has been developed in order to identify construction workers who are at low risk of pneumoconiosis so as to avoid unnecessary chest radiographs (Suarthana et al., 2007). The variables in the model will vary by setting, and so although such models are attractive in principle, they need to be developed for different contexts.

In high-burden countries, TB is the primary target of surveillance programmes, which need to be designed for early detection and prompt initiation of treatment. Passive case finding by asking RCS-exposed individuals about TB symptoms at every contact with a health service is the foundation of case finding. Workers knowing the benefits of early diagnosis, job protection following diagnosis and access to caring workplace services should encourage symptom reporting. Additionally, active case finding using modalities such as questionnaires and chest radiographs should be considered, especially in high-burden countries, but the resources to diagnose cases reliably and treat them need to be in place. The WHO strongly recommends that current and former RCS-exposed workers should be systematically screened for active TB (WHO, 2013). Chest radiography has been shown to improve sensitivity in TB detection, and is done as often as 6-monthly in very-high-incidence workplaces, a frequency that has been shown to detect cases with less extensive disease and to lower TB-specific mortality (Churchyard et al., 2011).

A clinical trial that showed reduced mortality from lung cancer following annual low-dose CT screening compared to screening with annual chest X-rays (NLST, 2011) has resulted in tentative recommendations for low-dose CT screening of selected high-risk individuals. It has also been recommended that people with significant RCS exposure and at least 20 pack-years of smoking should be screened for lung cancer (Steenland and Ward, 2014), but cost–benefit analyses have not been performed for silica-exposed subjects, and costs can be high, including those associated with investigating the many false positives detected during screening. It is therefore premature to recommend screening of RCS-exposed workers in most countries.

REFERENCES

Akgun, M., Mirici, A., Ucar, E. Y., Kantarci, M., Araz, O. and Gorguner, M. 2006. Silicosis in Turkish denim sandblasters. *Occup Med* 56:554–8.

Arakawa, H., Johkoh, T., Honma, K., Saito, Y., Fukushima, Y., Shida, H. and Suganuma, N. 2007. Chronic interstitial pneumonia in silicosis and mix-dust pneumoconiosis: Its prevalence and comparison of CT findings with idiopathic pulmonary fibrosis. *Chest* 131:1870–6.

ATS (American Thoracic Society). 1996. Respiratory protection guidelines. *Am J Respir Crit Care Med* 154:1153–65.

ATS (American Thoracic Society). 1997. Adverse effects of crystalline silica exposure. *Am J Respir Crit Care Med* 155:761–8.

ACGIH (American Conference of Governmental Industrial Hygienists). 2006. *Silica, Crystalline: α-Quartz and Cristobalite*. Cincinnati, OH: American Conference of Governmental Industrial Hygienists.

Antão, V. C., Pinheiro, G. A., Kavakama, J. and Terra-Filho, M. 2004. High prevalence of silicosis among stone carvers in Brazil. *Am J Ind Med* 45:194–201.

Begin, R., Bergeron, D., Samson, L., Boctor, M. and Cantin, A. 1987. CT assessment of silicosis in exposed workers. *AJR Am J Roentgenol* 148:509–14.

Bergin, C. J., Müller, N. L., Vedal, S. and Chan-Yeung, M. 1986. CT in silicosis: Correlation with plain films and pulmonary function tests. *AJR Am J Roentgenol* 146:477–83.

Bhagia, L. J. 2012. Nonoccupational exposure to silica dust. *Indian J Occup Environ Med* 16:95–100.

BOHS (British Occupational Hygiene Society), Nederlandse Vereniging voor Arbeidshygiëne. 2011. *Testing Compliance with Occupational Exposure Limits for Airborne Substances*. Derby: British Occupational Hygiene Society.

Bradshaw, L., Bowen, J., Fishwick, D. and Powell, S. 2010. *Health Surveillance in Silica Exposed Workers*. London: Health and Safety Executive.

Buxton, A. 2013. *Responding to the Challenge of Artisanal and Small-Scale Mining. How can Knowledge Networks Help*? London: International Institute for Environment and Development.

Carneiro, A. P., Barreto, S. M., Siqueira, A. L., Cavariani, F. and Forastiere, F. 2006. Continued exposure to silica after diagnosis of silicosis in Brazilian gold miners. *Am J Ind Med* 49:811–8.

Charalambous, S., Grant, A. D., Moloi, V., Warren, R., Day, J. H., van Helden, P., Hayes, R. J. et al. 2008. Contribution of reinfection to recurrent tuberculosis in South African gold miners. *Int J Tuberc Lung Dis* 12:942–8.

Chávez-Galán, L., Ramon-Luing, L. A., Bouscoulet, L. T., Pérez-Padilla, R. and Sada-Ovalle, I. 2013. Pre-exposure of *Mycobacterium tuberculosis*-infected macrophages to crystalline silica impairs control of bacterial growth by deregulating the balance between apoptosis and necrosis. *PLoS ONE* 8(11):e80971.

Chen, W., Hnizdo, E., Chen, J.-Q., Attfield, M. D., Gao, P., Hearl, F., Lu, J. et al. 2005. Risk of silicosis in cohorts of Chinese tin and tungsten miners, and pottery workers (1): An epidemiological study. *Am J Ind Med* 48:1–9.

Chong, S., Lee, K. S., Chung, M. J., Han, J., Kwon O. J. and Kim, T. S. 2006. Pneumoconiosis: Comparison of imaging and pathologic findings. *Radiographics* 26(1):59–77.

Chung, S. Y., Lee, J. H., Kim, T. H., Kim, S. J., Kim, H. J. and Ryu, Y. H. 2010. ^{18}F-FDG PET imaging of progressive massive fibrosis. *Ann Nucl Med* 24:21–7.

Churchyard, G. J., Kleinschmidt, I., Corbett, E. L., Murray, J., Smit, J. and De Cock, K. M. 2000. Factors associated with an increased case–fatality rate in HIV-infected and non-infected South African gold miners with pulmonary tuberculosis. *Int J Tuberc Lung Dis* 4:705–12.

Churchyard, G. J., Fielding, K., Roux, S., Corbett, E. L., Chaisson, R. E., De Cock, K. M., Hayes, R. J. et al. 2011. Twelve-monthly versus six-monthly radiological screening for active case-finding of tuberculosis: A randomized controlled trial. *Thorax* 66:134–9.

Churchyard, G. J., Fielding, K. L., Lewis, J. J., Coetzee, L., Corbett, E. L., Godfrey-Faussett, P., Hayes, R. J. et al. 2014. A trial of mass isoniazid preventive therapy for tuberculosis control. *N Engl J Med* 370:301–10.

Corbett, E. L., Churchyard, G. J., Clayton, T., Herselman, P., Willaims, B., Hayes, R., Mulder, D. et al. 1999. Risk factors for pulmonary mycobacterial disease in South African gold miners. A case–control study. *Am J Respir Crit Care Med* 159:94–9.

Corbett, E. L., Churchyard, G. J., Clayton, T. C., Williams, B. G., Mulder, D., Hayes, R. J. and De Cock, K. M. et al. 2000. HIV infection and silicosis: The impact of two potent risk factors on the incidence of mycobacterial disease in South African miners. *AIDS* 14:2759–68.

Cowie, R. L., Langton, M. E. and Becklake, M. R. 1989. Pulmonary tuberculosis in South African gold miners. *Am Rev Respir Dis* 139:1086–9.

Cowie, R. L. 1995. Silicotuberculsosis: Long-term outcomes after short-course chemotherapy. *Tuber Lung Dis* 76:39–42.

Craighead, J. E., Kleinerman, J., Abraham, J. L., Gibbs, A. R., Green, F. H. Y., Harley, R. A., Ruttner, J. R. et al. 1988. Diseases associated with exposure to silica and non-fibrous silicate minerals. Silicosis and Silicate Disease Committee. *Arch Pathol Lab Med* 112:673–720.

de la Hoz, R. E., Rosenman, K. and Borczuk, A. 2004. Silicosis in dental supply factory workers. *Respir Med* 98(8):791–4.

De Jager, P., Churchyard, G. J., Ismail, N., Kyaw, K. K. K., Murray, J., Nshuti, L., Rees, D. et al. 2014. Clinical guidelines on isoniazid preventive therapy for patients with silicosis in South Africa. *Occup Health Southern Afr* 20:6–11.

Dee, P., Suratt, P. and Winn, W. 1978. The radiographic findings in acute silicosis. *Radiology* 126:359–63.

Derbyshire, E. 2007. Natural minerogenic dust and human health. *Ambio* 36:73–7.

Erren, T. C., Glende, C. B., Morfeld, P. and Piekarski, C. 2009. Is exposure to silica associated with lung cancer in the absence of silicosis. A meta-analytical approach to an important public health question. *Int Arch Occup Environ Health* 82:997–1004.

Esswein, E. J., Breitenstein, M., Snawder, J., Kiefer, M. and Sieber, K. 2013. Occupational exposures to respirable crystalline silica during hydraulic fracturing. *J Occup Environ Hyg* 10:347–56.

Gerhardsson, G. 2002. The end of silicosis in Sweden—A triumph for occupational hygiene engineering. *OSH Dev* May:13–25.

GESTIS. 2015. International Limit Values. Available at: http://limitvalue.ifa.dguv.de (accessed 16 October 2015).

Godwin, J. D., Müller, N. L. and Takasugi, J. E. 1988. Pulmonary alveolar proteinosis: CT findings. *Radiology* 169:609–13.

Gottesfeld, P., Andrew, D. and Dalhoff, J. 2015. Silica exposures in artisanal small-scale gold mining in Tanzania and implications for tuberculosis prevention. *J Occup Environ Hyg* 12:647–53.

Gottesfeld, P., Nicas, M., Kephart, J., Balakrishnan, K. and Rinehart, R. 2008. Reduction of respirable silica following the introduction of water spray applications in Indian stone crusher mills. *Int J Occup Environ Health* 14:94–103.

Grobbelaar, J. P. and Bateman, E. D. 1991. Hut lung: A domestically acquired pneumoconiosis of mixed aetiology in rural women. *Thorax* 46:334–40.

Gulumian, M., Borm, P. J. A., Vallyathan, V., Castranova, V., Donaldson, K., Nelson, G. and Murray, J. 2006. Mechanistically identified suitable biomarkers of exposure, effect, and susceptibility for silicosis and coal-worker's pneumoconiosis: A comprehensive review. *J Toxicol Environ Health B Crit Rev* 9:357–95.

Healy, C. B., Coggins, M. A., van Tongeren, M., MacCalman, L. and McGowan, P. 2014. Determinants of respirable crystalline silica among stone workers involved in stone restoration work. *Ann Occup Hyg* 58:6–18.

Hessel, P. A., Sluis-Cremer, G. K., Hnizdo, E., Faure, M. H., Glyn Thomas, R. and Wiles, F. J. 1988. Progression of silicosis in relation to silica dust exposure. *Ann Occup Hyg* 32:689–96.

Hnizdo, E., Murray, J., Sluis-Cremer, G. K. and Thomas, R. G. 1993. Correlation between radiological and pathological diagnosis of silicosis: An autopsy population based study. *Am J Ind Med* 24:427–45.

Hnizdo, E. and Murray, J. 1998. Risk of pulmonary tuberculosis relative to silicosis and exposure to silica dust in South African gold miners. *Occup Environ Med* 55:496–502.

Hong Kong Chest Service/Tuberculosis Research Centre, Madras/British Medical Research Council. 1991. A controlled clinical trial of 6 and 8 months of antituberculosis chemotherapy in the treatment of patients with silicotuberculosis in Hong Kong. *Am Rev Respir Dis* 143:262–7.

HSE (Health and Safety Executive, U.K.). 2005. *Proposal for a Workplace Exposure Limit for Respirable Crystalline Silica*. Suffolk: HSE Books.

IARC (International Agency for Research on Cancer). 1997. *IARC Monographs on the Evaluation of Carcinogenic Risks to Humans. Vol. 68 Silica, Some Silicates, Coal Dust and Para-Aramid Fibrils*. Lyon: IARC.

IARC (International Agency for Research on Cancer). 2012. *IARC Monographs on the Evaluation of Carcinogenic Risks to Humans. Vol. 100C Arsenic, metals, fibres and dusts*. Lyon: IARC.

ILO (International Labour Office). 2011. *Guidelines for the Use of the ILO International Classification of Radiographs of Pneumoconioses*. Geneva: International Labour Office.

Jindal, S. K. 2013. Silicosis in India: Past and present. *Curr Opin Pulm Med* 19:163–8.

Jung, J. I., Park, S. H., Lee, J. M., Hahn, S. T. and Kim, K. A. 2000. MRI characteristics of progressive massive fibrosis. *J Thorac Imaging* 15:144–50.

Katzenstein, A. L. 2006. *Surgical Pathology of Non-Neoplastic Lung Disease,* fourth edition. Philadelphia, PA: Saunders.

Kramer, M. R., Blanc, P. D., Fireman, E., Amital, A., Guber, A., Rhahman, N. A. and Shitrit, D. 2012. Artificial stone silicosis [corrected]: Disease resurgence among artificial stone workers. *Chest* 142:419–24.

Lahiri, S., Levenstein, C., Nelson, D. I. and Rosenberg, B. J. 2005. The cost effectiveness of occupational health interventions: Prevention of silicosis. *Am J Ind Med* 48:503–14.

Law, Y. W., Leung, M. C., Leung, C. C., Yu, T. S. and Tam, C. M. 2001. Characteristics of workers attending the pneumoconiosis clinic for silicosis assessment in Hong Kong: Retrospective study. *Hong Kong Med J* 7:343–9.

Leung, C. C., Yew, W. W., Law, W. S., Tam, C. M., Leung, M., Chung, Y. W., Cheung, K. W. et al. 2007. Smoking and tuberculosis among silicotic patients. *Eur Respir* J 29:745–50.

Leung, C. C., Yu, I. T. S. and Chen, W. 2012. Silicosis. *Lancet* 379:2008–18.

Liu, Y., Steenland, K., Rong, Y., Hnizdo, E., Huang, X., Zhang, H. and Shi, T. 2013. Exposure–response analysis and risk assessment for lung cancer in relationship to silica exposure. *Am J Epidemiol* 178:1424–33.

Marchiori, E., Ferreira, A. and Müller, N. L. 2001. Silicoproteinosis: High-resolution CT and histologic findings. *J Thorac Imaging* 16:127–129.

Marchiori, E., Souza, C. A., Barbassa, T. G., Escuissato, D. L., Gasparetto, E. L. and Souza Jr, A. S. 2007. Silicoproteinosis: High-resolution CT findings in 13 patients. *AJR Am J Roentgenol* 189:1402–6.

Meldrum, M. and Howden, P. 2002. Crystalline silica: Variability in fibrogenic potency. *Ann Occup Hyg* 46(Suppl. 1):27–30.

Merget, R., Bauer, T., Küpper, H. U., Philippou, S., Bauer, H. D., Breitstadt, R. and Bruening, T. 2002. Health hazards due to inhalation of amorphous silica. *Arch Toxicol* 75:625–34.

Mohebbi, I. and Zubeyri, T. 2007. Radiological progression and mortality among silica flour packers: A longitudinal study. *Inhal Toxicol* 19:1011–7.

Mossman, B. T. and Glenn, R. E. 2013. Bioreactivity of the chrystalline silica polymorphs, quartz and cristobalite, and implications for occupational exposure limits (OELs). *Crit Rev Toxicol* 43:632–60.

Mundt, K. A., Birk, T., Parsons W., Borsch-Galetke, E., Siegmund, K., Heavner K. and Guldner, K. 2011. Respirable crystalline silica exposure–response evaluations of silicosis morbidity and lung cancer mortality in the German porcelain industry cohort. *J Occup Environ Med* 53:282–9.

Murgia, N., Muzi, G., dell'Omo, M., Sallese, D., Ciccotosto, C., Rossi, M., Scatolini, P. et al. 2007. An old threat in a new setting: High prevalence of silicosis among jewellery workers. *Am J Ind Med* 50:577–83.

Murray, J., Webster, I., Reid, G. and Kielkowski, D. 1991. The relation between fibrosis of hilar lymph glands and the development of parenchymal silicosis. *Br J Ind Med* 48:267–9.

Murray, J., Reid, G., Kielkowski, D. and de Beer, M. 1993. Cor pulmonale and silicosis: A necropsy based case-control study. *Br J Ind Med* 50:544–8.

Nelson, G. and Murray, J. 2013. Silicosis at autopsy in platinum mine workers. *Occup Med* 63:196–202.

NIOSH (National Institute for Occupational Safety and Health, U.S.A.). 2002. *Hazard Review: Health Effects of Occupational Exposure to Respirable Crystalline Silica*. Cincinnati, OH: National Institute for Occupational Safety and Health.

NLST (National Lung Screening Trial). 2011. Reduced lung-cancer mortality with low dose computed tomographic screening. *N Engl J Med* 365:395–409.

O'Connell, M. and Kennedy, M. 2004. Progressive massive fibrosis secondary to pulmonary silicosis appearance on F-18 fluorodeoxyglucose PET/CT. *Clin Nucl Med* 29:754–5.

OEHHA (Office of Environmental Health Hazard Assessment). 2005. *Silica (Chrystalline, Rrespirable).* Sacramento, California: Office of Environmental Health Hazard Assessment.

OHSA (Occupational Health and Safety Administration, U.S.A.). 2013. Proposed rule: Occupational exposure to respirable crystalline silica. *Fed Regist* 78: 56273–504.

Oikonomou, A. and Müller, N. L. 2003. Imaging of pneumoconiosis. *Imaging* 15:11–22.

Ooi, G. C., Tsang, K. W., Cheung, T. F., Khong, P. L., Ho, I. W., Ip, M. S., Tam, C. M. et al. 2003. Silicosis in 76 men: Qualitative and quantitative CT evaluation—Clinical–radiologic correlation study. *Radiology* 228:816–25.

Padley, S. P., Adler, B. D., Staples, C. A., Miller, R. R. and Muller, N. L. 1993. Pulmonarytalcosis: CT findings in three cases. *Radiology* 186 (1):125–7.

Pasula, R., Britigan, B. E., Turner J. and Martin II, W. J. 2009. Airway delivery of silica increases susceptibility to mycobacterial infection in mice: Potential role of repopulating macrophages. *J Immunol* 182:7102–9.

Pérez-Alonso, A., Córdoba-Doña, J. A., Millares-Lorenzo, J. L., Figueroa-Murillo, E., Garcia-Vadillo, C. and Romero-Morillos, J. 2014. Outbreak of silicosis in Spanish quartz conglomerate workers. *Int J Occup Environ Health* 20:26–32.

Pipavath, S. and Godwin, J. D. 2004. Imaging of interstitial lung disease. *Clin Chest Med* 25:455–65.

Pneumoconiosis Clinic of the Department of Health of the Government of Hong Kong SAR. 2004. *Guidelines on Tuberculosis Testing and Treatment of Latent TB Infection among Silicotic Patients in Hong Kong.* Available at: http://www.info.gov.hk/tb_chest/doc/Sili_LTBI_Rxguide.pdf (accessed 20 October 2015).

Raymond, L. W. and Wintermeyer, S. 2006. Medical surveillance of workers exposed to crystalline silica. *J Occup Environ Med* 48:95–101.

Rees, D. and Murray, J. 2007. Silica, silicosis and tuberculosis. *Int J Tuberc Lung Dis* 11:474–84.

Rees, D., Murray, J., Nelson, G. and Sonnenberg, P. 2010. Oscillating migration and the epidemics of silicosis, tuberculosis and HIV infection in South African gold miners. *Am J Ind Med* 53:398–404.

Remy-Jardin, M., Beuscart, R., Sault, M. C., Marquette, C. H., Remy, J. 1990. Subpleural micronodules in diffuse infiltrative lung diseases: Evaluation with thin section CT scans. *Radiology* 177:133–9.

Remy-Jardin, M., Remy, J., Farre, I. and Marquette, C. H. 1992. Computed tomographic evaluation of silicosis and coal worker's pneumoconiosis. *Radiol Clin North Am* 30:1155–76.

Rosenman, K. D., Hogan, A. and Reilly, M. J. 2001. What is the most cost-effective way to identify silica problem worksites? *Am J Ind Med* 39:629–35.

Schenker, M. B., Pinkerton, K. E., Mitchell, D., Vallyathan V., Elvine-Kreis, B. and Green, F. H. Y. 2009. Pneumoconiosis from agricultural dust exposure among young California farmworkers. *Environ Health Perspect* 117:988–94.

Seixas, N. S. 2014. Monumental hazards. *Ann Occup Hyg* 58:2–5.

Sherson, D. and Lander, F. 1990. Morbidity of pulmonary tuberculosis among silicotic and nonsilicotic foundry workers in Denmark. *J Occup Med* 32:110–5.

Singer, J. P., Chen, H., Phelan, T., Kukreja, J., Golden, J. A. and Blanc, P. D. 2012. Survival following lung transplantation for silicosis and other occupational lung diseases. *Occup Med (Lond)* 62:134–7.

Slavin, R. E., Swedo, J. L., Brandes, D., Gonzalez-Vitale, J. C. and Osornio-Vargas, A. 1985. Extrapulmonary silicosis: A clinical, morphologic, and ultrastructural study. *Hum Pathol* 16:393–412.

Solomon, A. 2001. Silicosis and tuberculosis: Part 2—A radiographic presentation of nodular tuberculosis and silicosis. *Int J Occup Environ Health* 7:54–7.

Solomon, A. and Rees, D. 2010. Back to basics—The chest radiograph in silica associated tuberculosis. *Occup Health Southern Afr* 16:25–27.

Souza, C. A., Marchiori, E., Gonçalves, L. P., Meirelles, G. P., Zanetti, G., Escuissato D. L., Capobianco, J. et al. 2010. Comparative study of clinical, pathological and HRCT findings of primary alveolar proteinosis and silicoproteinosis. *Eur J Radiol* 81:371–8.

Steenland, K. 2005. One agent, many diseases: Exposure–response data and comparative risks of different outcomes following silica exposure. *Am J Ind Med* 48:16–23.

Steenland, K. and Ward, E. 2014. Silica: A lung carcinogen. *CA Cancer J Clin* 64:63–9.

Steingart, K. R., Sohn, H., Schiller, I., Kloda, L. A., Boehme, C. C., Pai, M. and Dendukuri, N. 2013. Xpert® MTB/RIF assay for pulmonary tuberculosis and rifampicin resistance in adults. *Cochrane Database Syst Rev* 1:CD009593.

Suarthana, E., Moons, K. G. M, Heederik, D. and Meijer, E. 2007. A simple diagnostic model for ruling out pneumoconiosis among construction workers. *Occup Environ Med* 64:595–601.

Swanepoel, A. J., Rees, D., Renton, K., Swanepoel, C., Kromhout, H. and Gardiner, K. 2010. Quartz exposure in agriculture: Literature review and South African survey. *Ann Occup Hyg* 54:281–92.

Tse, L. A., Li, Z. M., Wong, T. W., Fu, Z. M. and Yu, I. T. 2007. High prevalence of accelerated silicosis among gold miners in Jiangxi, China. *Am J Ind Med* 50:876–80.

Valiante, D. J., Schill, D. P., Rosenman, K. D. and Socie, E. 2004. Highway repair: A new silicosis threat. *Am J Public Health* 94:876–80.

Westerholm, P. 1980. Silicosis. Observations on a case register, Section VIII: Dust exposure after diagnosis and risk of radiographic progression—A case-referent study. *Scand J Work Environ Health* 6(Suppl 2):43–7.

WHO (World Health Organization). The Global Occupational Health Network newsletter: Elimination of silicosis. 2007. Available at: http://www.who.int/occupational_health/publications/newsletter/gohnet12e.pdf (accessed 24 October 2014).

WHO (World Health Organization). 2011. Use of tuberculosis interferon-gamma release assays (IGRAs) in low- and middle-income countries: Policy statement. Available at: http://apps.who.int/iris/handle/10665/44759 (accessed 13 August 2013).

WHO (World Health Organization). 2013. *Systematic Screening for Active Tuberculosis. Principles and Recommendations.* Geneva: WHO Press.

Xiao, G-B., Morinaga, K., Wang, R-Y., Zhang, X. and Ma, Z-H. 2004. World at work: Manufacturing 'tatami' mats in China. *Occup Environ Med* 61:372–3.

Xipell, J. M., Ham, K. N., Price, C. G. and Thomas, D. P. 1977. Acute silicoproteinosis. *Thorax* 32:104–11.

Yen, Y-F., Yen, M-Y., Lin, Y-S., Lin, Y-P., Shih, H-C., Li, L-H., Chou, P. et al. 2014. Smoking increases risk of recurrence after successful anti-tuberculosis treatment: A population-based study. *Int J Tuberc Lung Dis* 18:492–8.

19 Coal Mine Dust Lung Disease

Robert A. Cohen, Leonard H. T. Go and Francis H. Y. Green

CONTENTS

Global energy consumption continues to grow. Because of continued dependence on fossil fuels, a large portion of this demand for energy is met by coal mining in many countries. Millions of workers around the world currently perform this physically demanding and health-endangering activity. With the proper motivation, oversight and execution, the lung diseases caused by coal mine dust are preventable. Until the necessary changes occur, however, the burden of lung disease in this population will continue to be substantial.

INTRODUCTION

Coal is a fossil fuel used primarily for energy production in both developing and developed nations. China, the United States (US), Australia, Indonesia, India, the Russian Federation and South Africa together account for nearly 90% of the world's annual output; China alone accounts for nearly 50% of the global output. Although there is intense interest in non-fossil fuel energy sources, coal is likely to remain a major fuel source due to its relative worldwide abundance and low cost of acquisition.

Mechanization of coal mining has substantially increased the productivity of mining. This in turn has resulted in a substantial decrease in the number of coal miners in some countries. However, the coal industry continues to employ millions of workers worldwide; for example, there are more than 6 million workers in the coal mine industry in China. Globally, the number of workers who continue to be exposed to the respiratory hazards of coal mining remains large, in addition to former miners who remain at risk of disease. Pulmonologists and occupational medicine physicians working in coal mining regions throughout the world will be treating workers with coal mine dust lung diseases (CMDLDs), including coal workers' pneumoconiosis (CWP), chronic obstructive pulmonary disease (COPD), diffuse dust-related fibrosis (DDF) and other respiratory diseases due to overexposure to coal mine dust for decades to come. The term CMDLD is the preferred umbrella term that includes the full range of diseases associated with coal mine dust (CMD) exposure. Historically, the term CWP has been associated with the classic features of fibrotic lung disease. It is now known that dusts in the coal mine atmosphere can cause emphysema and chronic bronchitis, as well as DDF, a form of interstitial fibrosis that may be confused with idiopathic pulmonary fibrosis (IPF). More recently, a rapidly progressive form of CMDLD has been described in US coal miners that appears to have different clinical and pathologic characteristics from classical CWP (Antao et al., 2005).

Overview of Respiratory Hazards

Coal is a predominantly carbon fossil fuel that is produced from organic matter over time through a sedimentary series. Initially, vegetative matter accumulates and may be inhibited from decaying due to acidic and anaerobic conditions in order to form peat. With application of high temperatures and pressures by the accumulation of overlying material, peat may transform into coal. With increased maturity, the coal may transition through increasing rank—lignite, sub-bituminous, bituminous and anthracite coals—with progressive hardening, transformation and increases in carbon content. Within coal is a host of non-carbon constituents, including quartz; kaolin, mica and other silicates; and metals and volatile substances. Coal dust is thus a heterogeneous mixture of substances that is predominantly carbon, exposure to which may variably promote the development of respiratory disease.

The concept of coal dust as an isolated cause of respiratory disease is essentially artificial, as the typical miner is routinely exposed to other dusts, fumes and vapours that are present in the coal mine atmosphere that may cause respiratory symptoms and disease. Silica is the most frequently considered of these other exposures, and is found in the rock strata that surround coal seams in addition to coal itself. Lung disease caused by exhaust from diesel-powered equipment and bio-aerosol exposure from water sprays may also complicate the clinical picture.

EPIDEMIOLOGY

International Prevalence Data

Radiologic Surveillance

Radiologic surveillance has been the primary tool used in public health programmes in order to identify coal workers who may have the early changes of CWP. Chest X-ray surveys have also been used to evaluate the progression of disease and prevalence of severe disease in populations of coal miners. A meta-analysis of studies published from 2001 to 2011 of radiologic CWP prevalence in China concluded that the prevalence of the disease was approximately 6% (Mo et al., 2014). In the USA, after the institution of modern dust control regulations, the Coal Workers' X-Ray Surveillance Program run by the National Institute for Occupational Safety and Health (NIOSH) reported a decline in prevalence from 6.5% in the 1970s to a low of 2.1% in the 1990s. However, CWP prevalence subsequently increased to 3.2% in the first decade of the twenty-first century without any change in the permissible exposure limits. In addition, the rate of progressive massive fibrosis (PMF) in certain coal mining states in the USA has recently increased to levels observed prior to the institution of modern dust controls (Blackley et al., 2014). Australia has had very few cases of CWP in recent decades, which is believed to be the result of strict dust exposure limits and controls. Published data of the national prevalence of radiographic CWP in other major coal mining countries are not available.

It should be noted that chest X-ray surveillance programmes may be biased. Participation bias may occur in some countries in surveillance programmes that are voluntary on the part of the miner. This may result in overestimation of CWP prevalence, as symptomatic miners may be more likely to undergo examination. There may also be under-reporting due to the healthy worker survivor effect, since most surveillance programmes focus on working miners, omitting those symptomatic workers who may have left employment due to illness and the intensive physical labour involved in mining.

Lung Function Surveillance Data

There are few reports of ongoing physiological surveillance of coal mine workers. Starting in 2005, the US NIOSH began the Enhanced Coal Workers' Health Surveillance Program, which included spirometry. Data from this study showed abnormal spirometric findings in 13.1% of 6373 miners. Notably, 12.5% of miners with International Labour Organisation (ILO) category 0 chest radiographs had abnormal spirometry results. With increasing radiographic disease, the prevalence of spirometric abnormalities increased: 24.9% of miners with ILO category 1 findings, 28.9% with categories 2 or 3 and 40% with PMF had abnormal results (Wang et al., 2013).

Pathology Studies

Autopsy prevalence studies allow for evaluation of confirmed cases of CMDLD, but they may yield higher prevalence rates of disease than radiologic studies due to the older age of the subjects and because of the higher sensitivity of pathologic examination for the findings of CMDLD (Vallyathan et al., 1996). Pathologic evaluation of lung specimens has shown a dose/response relationship between CMD exposure and emphysema (Kuempel et al., 2009) and demonstrated the association of 'non-classic' pathologic lesions with coal mining, including DDF (McConnochie et al., 1988). The US National Coal Workers' Autopsy Study was used to determine if the 2 mg/m^3 dust standard, established by the US Federal Coal Mine Health & Safety Act of 1969, had reduced the prevalence and severity of CWP (Green et al., 1989). Among mine who worked exclusively prior to the 1969 dust standard, 82.6% had coal macules, 46.3% had coal nodules, 28.2% had silicotic nodules and 10.3% had PMF. A lower prevalence was noted among miners exposed exclusively to post-1970 dust levels: 58.8% had coal macules, 15.0% had coal nodules, 8.0% had silicosis and 1.2% had PMF. These prevalence differences remained after adjustment for age, years of mining and smoking status, and were greatest for the more severe categories of CWP (Green et al., 1989). Examination of the Pathology Automation System autopsy database of South Africa from 1975 to 1997 revealed an association between the duration of coal mine exposures and the presence of CWP, silicosis and emphysema (Naidoo et al., 2005).

Exposure Assessment to Evaluate Risk

Dust Characteristics

Underground CMD is a complex mixture of particulates, which may be as little as 40% coal. Other dusts arise from the disruption of surrounding rock, which may be composed of minerals such as quartz, silicates, pyrite and calcite (National Institute for Occupational Safety and Health, 1995). Dust from high-rank coal, which is associated with higher risk of respiratory disease, has higher silica content, higher concentrations of surface free radicals when freshly fractured and more surface area for a given particle size (National Institute for Occupational Safety and Health, 1995). The size of the particulates generated influences the likelihood of the dust reaching the alveoli of the lungs, with particles smaller than 10 μm most likely to reach this region.

Workplace Characteristics

Mining methods and technologies play dominant roles in the dust exposures experienced by the coal miner, both in terms of the quantity and content of dust elaborated. Mining may be performed at the surface or underground. Surface or opencast mining entails the disruption and removal of overlying rock strata—the overburden—in order to access and extract coal relatively close to the surface. The composition of dust from surface coal mines can be highly variable, depending on the stage of the process. Surface miners usually encounter lower dust levels than underground miners. However, the risk of dust-related lung disease in surface miners exists, particularly among certain groups of workers, such as rock drillers (Halldin et al., 2015).

In contrast to surface mining, underground mining involves the use of tunnels in order to access coal seams typically 60 m or deeper underground. Modern coal preparation plants can efficiently separate coal and non-coal materials, allowing mining operations to take rock above and below coal seams for convenience, but also exposing workers to greater quantities of silica dust. Use of mechanized methods has allowed for the mining of narrower coal seams, which may expose the worker to a greater risk of lung disease (Suarthana et al., 2011). The transportation of coal within an underground mine from the coal face to the surface on swiftly moving belt lines also results in significant exposure of workers to airborne CMD. Conventional manual (non-mechanized) methods of mining remain in common use, particularly in developing countries.

Engineering controls in order to mitigate exposure to CMD are the most important measures for the control of occupational exposures. The principal methods are the controlled use of ventilation near the workface in order to remove and dilute dust, as well as suppression of dust using water sprays. The technology used to suppress airborne dust generation or ventilate an underground mine may greatly reduce the overall level of respirable dust. Personal respirators are frequently offered to miners, but are rarely used due to the increased difficulty they may pose with breathing and expectoration while performing strenuous job tasks.

Small mine size has been shown to be a risk factor for CWP in the USA. High rates of CWP as well as more severe and rapidly progressive disease in younger miners have been reported in these settings (Laney et al., 2010). The specific factors contributing to these findings are not well understood. Thin seam mining, working longer shifts with less time to expel dust between shifts and a lack of enforcement of dust controls have been suggested as possible contributing factors (Laney et al., 2010).

Job Tasks

The specific tasks performed by the worker within an underground mine may significantly modify the risk of CMDLD, with work at the coal face, including the operation of continuous mining machines, roof bolting and rock drilling, being associated most frequently with disease (Scarisbrick and Quinlan, 2002). In the USA, increased CWP prevalence has also been associated with longer work hours. Surface coal miners may be exposed to high dust levels through rock drilling and blasting, although usually not as frequently as underground miners (Halldin et al., 2015).

DISEASE MANIFESTATIONS

CWP may be defined as parenchymal lung disease that results from coal dust exposure (Churg and Green, 1998). Historically, the majority of the attention has been paid to CWP, but the manifestations of lung disease associated with CMD exposure are diverse. The development of lung disease is primarily associated with the overall quantity of CMD exposure. In addition, the nature of the coal being mined, other exposures within the mine (e.g. rock dust, diesel particulate and bio-aerosols) and host factors such as genetic predisposition to disease are contributing factors. In this section, 'classic' CWP will be discussed, followed by more recently identified entities that have strong associations with CMD exposures, which together comprise CMDLD.

Classic CWP

CWP is typically diagnosed in an individual with compatible chest radiograph findings and a history of CMD exposure for at least 10 years, although shorter work tenures may be associated with disease if the exposure was intense. The worker may be asymptomatic, with disease discovered only as part of screening for CWP. The abnormal chest imaging findings in an individual with sufficient CMD exposure may include nodular or mass-like opacities, areas of hyperlucency consistent with emphysema and architectural distortion of neighbouring anatomic structures due to loss of lung volume.

The severity of CWP radiographically is divided into 'simple' and 'complicated' disease based on the size of the opacities observed—simple CWP is composed of small opacities with any single lesion not exceeding 10 mm in diameter, while in complicated CWP there are one or more lesions equal to or greater than 10 mm in size. This is the size definition used by the ILO for radiographic PMF. It is reasonable that the same size criteria be applied to pathologic PMF. In addition to the size of the opacities, the profusion and shape of small opacities may be graded by comparison of the miner's chest radiograph to a standard set of radiographs, such as in the system of radiographic pneumoconiosis classification used by the ILO (International Labour Office, 2002).

The likelihood of developing CWP and the progression of disease is associated with numerous factors, the most important of which is believed to be cumulative CMD exposure (Hurley et al., 1982; Attfield and Seixas, 1995). The increased profusion of the small nodules of simple CWP is associated with declines in lung function (Blackley et al., 2015) and higher retained dust content in lung specimens (Ruckley et al., 1984). There are significant geographic variations of CWP prevalence, with a pattern suggesting that exposure to dust of high-rank coal, which has increased carbon content, is associated with increased risk of CWP (Bennett et al., 1979; Attfield and Seixas, 1995). The chest radiograph is a useful tool in the assessment of the severity of CWP, as the number of small opacities observed radiographically correlate well with the number of small lesions seen on pathologic specimens (Fernie and Ruckley, 1987). However, it is insensitive in the detection of the presence of early lesions of CWP. Normal radiographs were found in more than two-thirds of autopsied miners who had coal macules pathologically (Vallyathan et al., 1996). Simple CWP may progress even after cessation of dust exposure (Kimura et al., 2010).

Traditional teaching has been that simple CWP begins as small, rounded opacities that are predominantly distributed in the upper zones bilaterally, with possible later progression to involve the lower zones. However, there is a lack of published evidence to support this. Radiographic examination of active coal workers in the USA, for example, demonstrated that CWP can manifest as rounded opacities with upper zone predominance or as irregular opacities with lower zone predominance (Laney and Petsonk, 2012). This matches pathologic studies of DDF in coal miners from the UK and the USA (McConnochie et al., 1988).

PMF is the more severe form of CWP and is also referred to as complicated CWP. PMF lesions tend to be located in the upper lung zones, although there are no data reporting the frequency with which this occurs. With continued progression, the lesions are more likely to be bilaterally distributed. Severe disease may be associated with significant emphysema and architectural distortion due to fibrotic scarring.

Much like simple CWP, older age and greater cumulative dust exposure are associated with the risk of the development of PMF (Hurley et al., 1987). Higher baseline small-opacity profusion of simple CWP in a miner is also associated with increased risk of the subsequent development of PMF (Cochrane, 1962; Hurley et al., 1987). Miners with simple CWP, particularly those with higher-profusion disease, may develop PMF even after CMD exposure has ceased (Maclaren and Soutar, 1985).

Silica exposure is thought to play a significant role in the pathogenesis of at least some cases of CWP. Exposure to respirable silica dust occurs frequently in the coal mine atmosphere, with higher levels encountered in the disruption, cutting or drilling of rock strata surrounding coal seams (Isidro Montes et al., 2004). Silicosis and CWP are radiographically indistinguishable. A predominance of silicotic nodules may be found in the lung parenchyma in a significant minority of coal mine workers with CWP (Green et al., 1989). Quartz content appears to contribute to radiographic progression of disease, even when measured dust levels are low (Seaton et al., 1981).

The typical pathologic lesion of simple CWP is the coal macule, a collection of dust-laden macrophages within the wall of a respiratory bronchiole containing reticulin and collagen (Figure 19.1a). The macules are usually surrounded by enlarged airspaces consistent with centrilobular emphysema, historically called focal emphysema. Coal nodules are another lesion containing pigmented macrophages, but with a much greater degree of collagenization. Coal nodules are not confined to respiratory bronchioles and may be observed elsewhere in the lungs (Figure 19.1b). If the silica content of the dust is high, the nodules show changes of classic silicosis

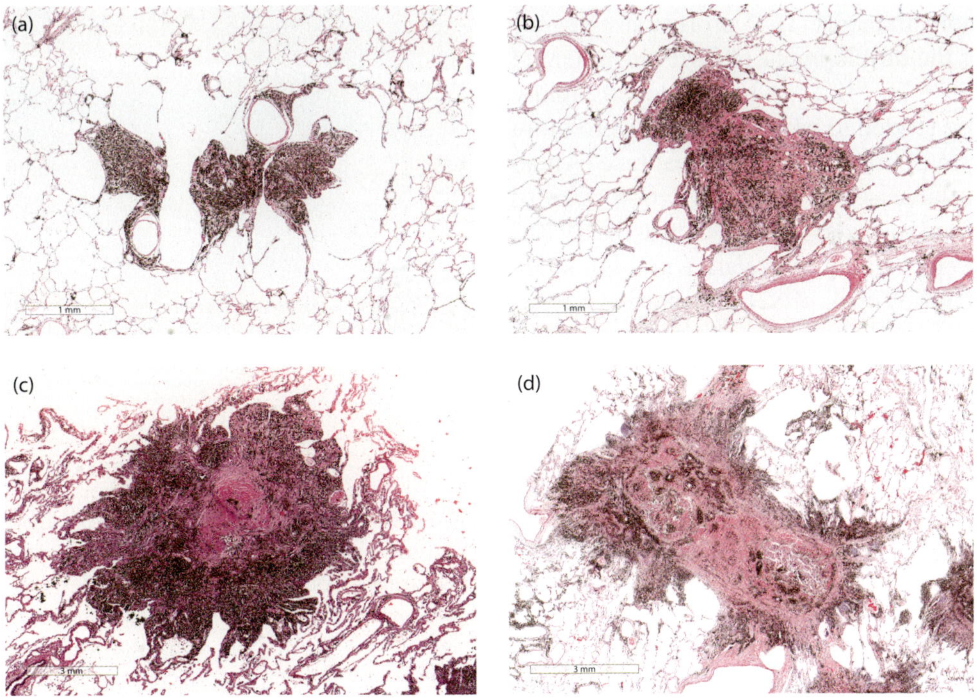

FIGURE 19.1 (a) Classic coal dust macule in the wall of a respiratory bronchiole and surrounded by a rim of centriacinar emphysema. The macule is composed of dust-containing macrophages in a reticulin stroma, with minimal fibrosis. (b) Classic coal dust nodule adjacent to a blood vessel in the interlobular septum. The nodule is composed of dust-laden macrophages within a fibrotic stroma. The emphysema adjacent is called scar emphysema. (c) A larger dust nodule with a central silicotic component. The centre is composed of concentrically arranged collagen fibres, and can be shown to contain silica with polarizing microscopy. (d) Small lesion with features of progressive massive fibrosis (PMF). In this example, the lesion has formed from the fusion of two dust nodules, one that appears silicotic. There is central necrosis with cholesterol clefts. The adjacent lung shows scar emphysema. A larger lesion of PMF is shown in Figure 19.3a.

(Figure 19.1c). Nodules tend to cluster and coalesce in order to form lesions of PMF (Figure 19.1d). PMF lesions are black fibrotic lesions with a rubbery texture. They may undergo necrosis with cavitation and become colonized by mycobacteria and fungi (Pathology Standards for Coal Workers' Pneumoconiosis, 1979).

Miners and ex-miners with category B or C PMF (with large opacities of combined diameter greater than 5 cm) have increased risk of mortality compared to non-miners (Cochrane et al., 1979) or miners with simple CWP (Carpenter et al., 1956; Yi and Zhang, 1996). Mortality risk may be modestly increased in miners with simple CWP or category A PMF compared to miners without CWP, although data are conflicting (Carpenter et al., 1956; Cochrane et al., 1979; Kuempel et al., 1995). In addition to the effect of cumulative dust exposure, a history of mining higher-rank coal is associated with increased mortality risk (Kuempel et al., 1995).

Rapidly Progressive CWP

Of great concern in the USA are reports from NIOSH reviewing data from 1996 to 2002 showing that 35% of the newly diagnosed cases of CWP were categorized as 'rapidly progressive'. This referred to radiographic progression of more than one ILO profusion category within 5 years, or the development of PMF documented after 1985 (Figure 19.2). Miners who developed rapidly progressive disease tended to be younger and were more likely to work in small mines and at the coal face (Antao et al., 2005). Similar cases of the rapid progression of CWP had been noted in Wales in the 1950s to the 1970s, and these cases were found to correlate with high silica content in CMD (Hurley et al., 1982). When using r opacities (rounded opacities 3–10 mm in diameter) on chest radiography as a surrogate marker for silicosis, there is evidence that some rapidly progressive diseases in the USA may be associated with exposure to respirable silica dust (Laney et al., 2010). However, the lack of difference in rapidly progressive CWP rates between roof bolters and coal face workers implies that silica exposure is not the only relevant factor. In one US sample, operation of continuous mining machines was the job activity that was most frequently associated with rapidly progressive CWP and PMF, despite exposures that were reported to be lower than the US permissible exposure limit for respirable CMD (Wade et al., 2011). Together, these factors raise the possibility that thin-seam mining with increased silica exposure for coal face workers and increases in silicosis underlie the increased rates of rapidly progressive disease (Attfield and Petsonk, 2007).

The pathology of rapidly progressive CWP was recently described, revealing that the pathology is

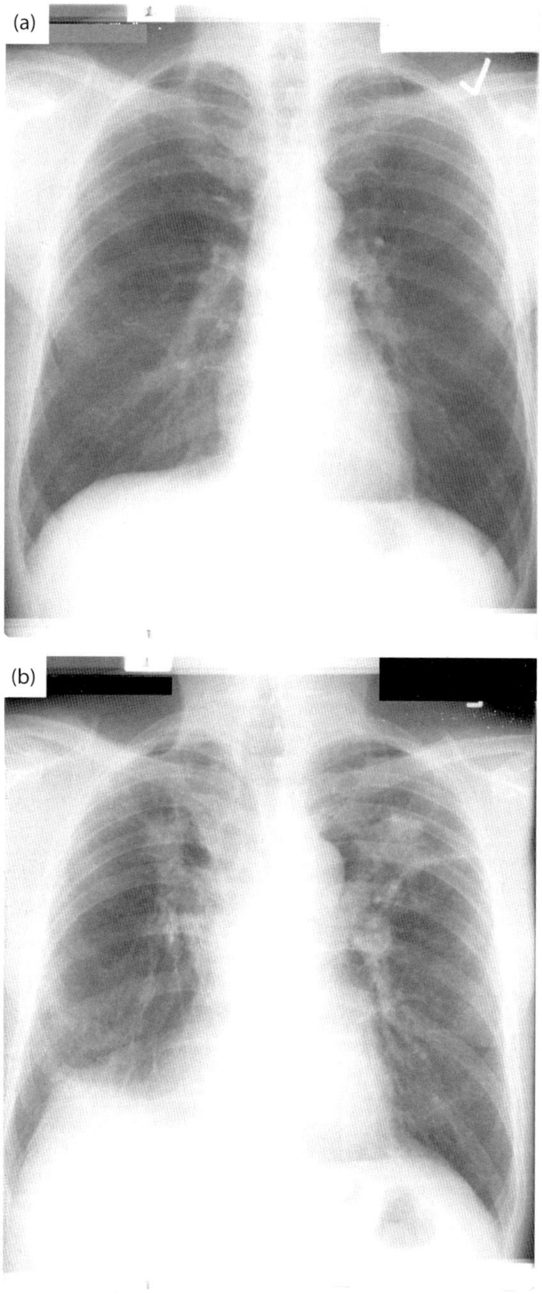

FIGURE 19.2 Development of rapidly progressive pneumoconiosis with progressive massive fibrosis in an individual coal miner from West Virginia, USA. (a) Chest radiograph performed after 19 years of coal mine employment. Note the relative lack of imaging abnormalities. (b) Chest radiograph performed after 27 years of coal mine employment. There are multiple large mass-like lesions and nodules in the bilateral upper-lung fields. Right upper lobectomy in order to evaluate a nodule had been performed 3 years prior with the finding of progressive massive fibrosis. The upper-lung field lesions were also found to be consistent with progressive massive fibrosis later on autopsy examination (see Figure 19.3c,d). The miner worked underground as a roof bolter. His coal mine dust exposure took place entirely after the enactment of dust exposure limits in the USA.

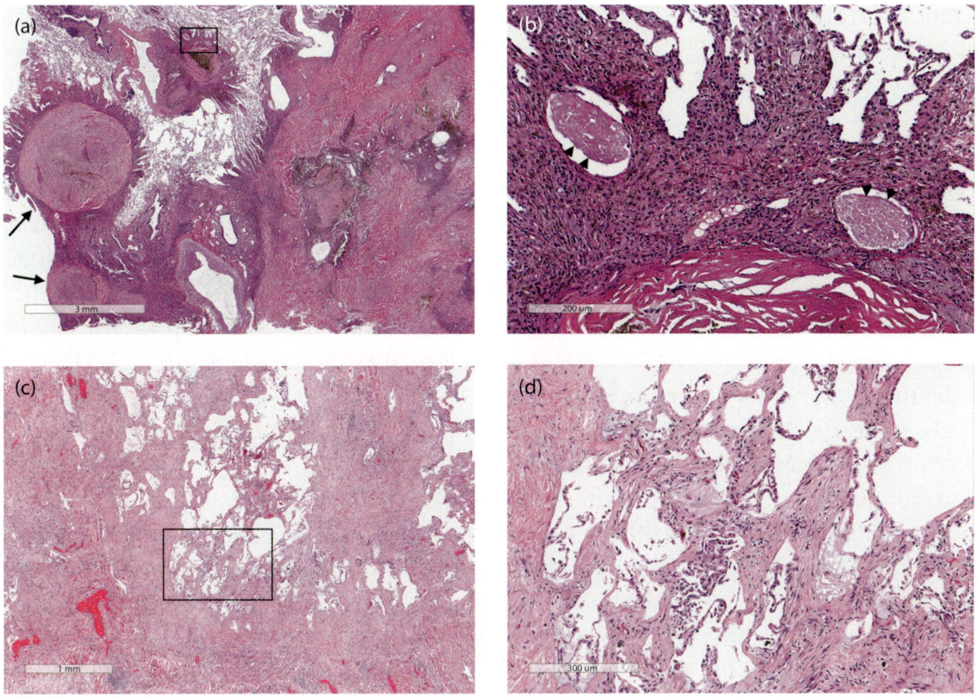

FIGURE 19.3 (a) A case of rapidly progressive coal workers' pneumoconiosis (CWP) showing silicotic nodules on the left (arrows) and a larger lesion of progressive massive fibrosis on the right. Note the relative absence of black pigment at low magnification. (b) A higher-magnification view of the boxed area shown in (a), showing the edge of a silicotic nodule with a rim of histiocytic cells containing dust, together with two foci of alveolar proteinosis (arrowheads). The latter are associated with acute and subacute silicosis. (c) Another case of rapidly progressive CWP showing confluent and interstitial fibrosis with relatively little visible pigmentation. Chest radiographs for this miner are seen in Figure 19.2. (d) Close-up of the boxed area shown in (c), showing details of the interstitial fibrosis. This pattern is strikingly similar to that seen in idiopathic pulmonary fibrosis. Almost no black pigment is seen, and polarizing microscopy (not shown) revealed large quantities of mineral dust, including silicates and silica.

distinct from the classic appearances of CWP (Cohen et al., 2016). It is characterized by less visible black carbonaceous pigment in tissue sections with greatly increased mineral dust as seen under polarized light (Figure 19.3). Subacute and mature silicosis is usually present, as well as diffuse interstitial fibrosis.

Rheumatoid CWP

Rheumatoid coal pneumoconiosis, eponymously known as Caplan's syndrome, is the association of rheumatoid arthritis with CWP in an individual (Caplan, 1953). This is a rare finding, being noted in less than 1% of autopsied miners with pneumoconiosis in North America and Japan (Honma and Vallyathan, 2002). The chest radiograph is typically notable for the finding of multiple large (0.5–5 cm), round and well-defined opacities, usually without significant presence of smaller opacities. Cavitation and calcification of these nodules may occur. The finding of lung nodules may precede the onset of joint symptoms. The nodules may become confluent and radiographically indistinguishable from PMF.

Pathologically, rheumatoid coal nodules occur on a background of mild simple CWP and show characteristic concentric light and dark bands. There is central necrosis and dust, sometimes with calcification (Honma and Vallyathan, 2002). Pulmonary tuberculosis and fungal infections need to be excluded by appropriate tests.

Accurate understanding of the prevalence of rheumatoid CWP is limited due to the relative rarity of identified cases, variability of presentation and variable presence of findings of rheumatoid arthritis at the time of chest radiographic evaluation. Historically, there has been a discrepancy between the small number of identified cases in the USA compared to the higher estimates of prevalence observed in European data.

Diffuse Dust-Related Fibrosis

Diffuse interstitial pulmonary fibrosis, although less common than nodular CWP lesions, is a recognized lesion following exposure to coal dust, silica and dusts containing a mixture of minerals (mixed-dust pneumoconiosis) (Honma and Chiyotani, 1993). Coal miners may have irregular opacities with lower-lobe predominance (Laney and Petsonk, 2012) that are consistent with pulmonary fibrosis on chest imaging. Some examiners have drawn the erroneous conclusion that the process is IPF, believing that CMD can only cause round, upper-lobe opacities and cannot result in irregular fibrotic disease. Emphysema is also associated with the finding of irregular and lower-lobe opacities in miners (Cockcroft et al., 1982, 1983).

The clinical features of DDF in coal miners (McConnochie et al., 1988; Brichet et al., 2002b) include low gas transfer rates (carbon monoxide diffusion capacity [DLCO]), hypoxaemia and a restrictive pattern on pulmonary function testing (Coultas et al., 1994; Raghu et al., 2011). It may have radiological, functional and pathological characteristics of IPF (Cockcroft et al., 1983; Coultas et al., 1994; Raghu et al., 2011), but it has a less aggressive clinical course (McConnochie et al., 1988). DDF may occur against a background of simple or complicated CWP and may show honeycomb change in the lower lobes. Histologically, the fibrosis has both pigmented and unpigmented areas (Figure 19.4) (Raghu et al., 2011) and has a lobular distribution that may resemble that of usual interstitial pneumonia. However, a joint international consensus statement on the diagnosis of IPF requires 'exclusion of other known causes of interstitial lung disease such as drug toxicities, environmental exposures, and connective tissue diseases' (Raghu et al., 2011). Consequently, the diagnosis of IPF in a heavily exposed coal miner should rarely be made without strong evidence that CMD is not a factor.

Obstructive Lung Disease

Emphysema

CMD is an important cause of emphysema (Ryder et al., 1970; Ruckley et al., 1984; Kuempel et al., 2009) and associated impairment (Kuempel et al., 2009). Centrilobular emphysema is the most common type of emphysema associated with CMD exposure and occurs in non-smoking miners (Leigh et al., 1994). The effect of cigarette smoking on emphysema is additive to the effect

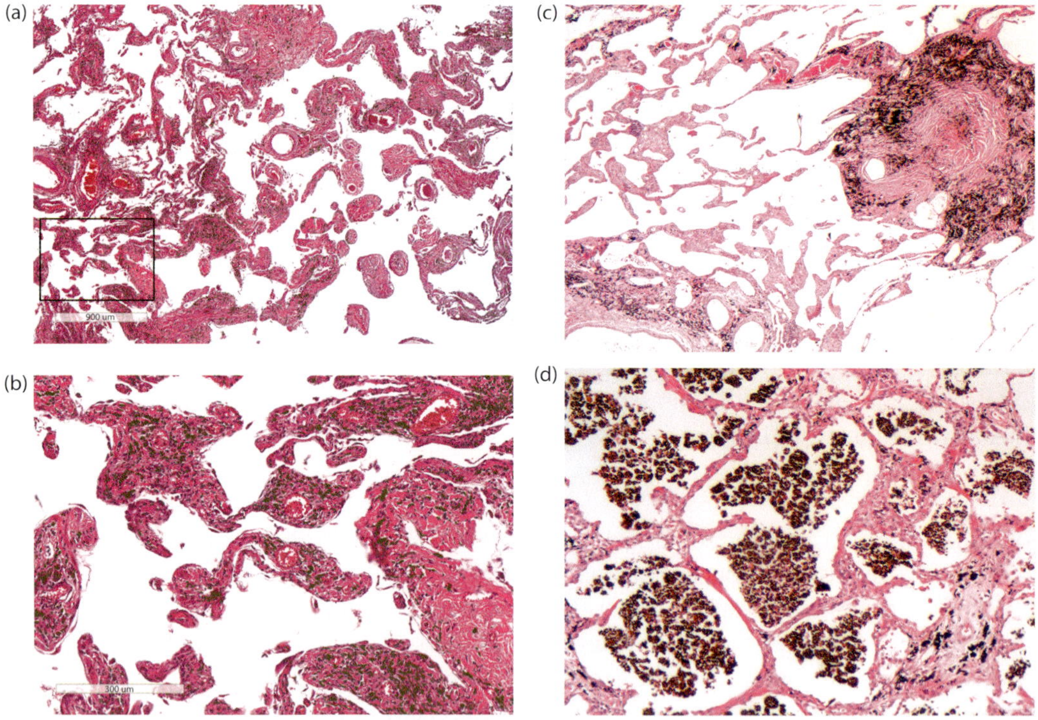

FIGURE 19.4 Examples of diffuse dust-related fibrosis in coal miners. (a) Section of a coal miner's lung taken at autopsy showing an area of diffuse interstitial fibrosis in combination with enlarged airspaces, consistent with emphysema. (b) Close-up of the boxed area shown in (a). Note the variability in pigmentation in this type of fibrosis. (c) Example of interstitial fibrosis in a coal miner's lung. On the right is a classic silicotic nodule, and to the left of the silicotic nodule is diffuse interstitial fibrosis with minimal pigmentation. (d) Interstitial fibrosis associated with macrophage accumulations in the alveoli. The macrophages contain large quantities of coal dust pigment. This pattern of disease is seen in active miners and resembles respiratory bronchiolitis and interstitial lung disease associated with cigarette smoking.

of CMD exposure (Kuempel et al., 2009). All types of emphysema, including centriacinar, panacinar and bullous emphysema, are associated with both dust exposure and cigarette smoking (Green et al., 1998). Scar emphysema is more common in coal miners. It is not possible to distinguish emphysema due to CMD from that caused by cigarette smoking.

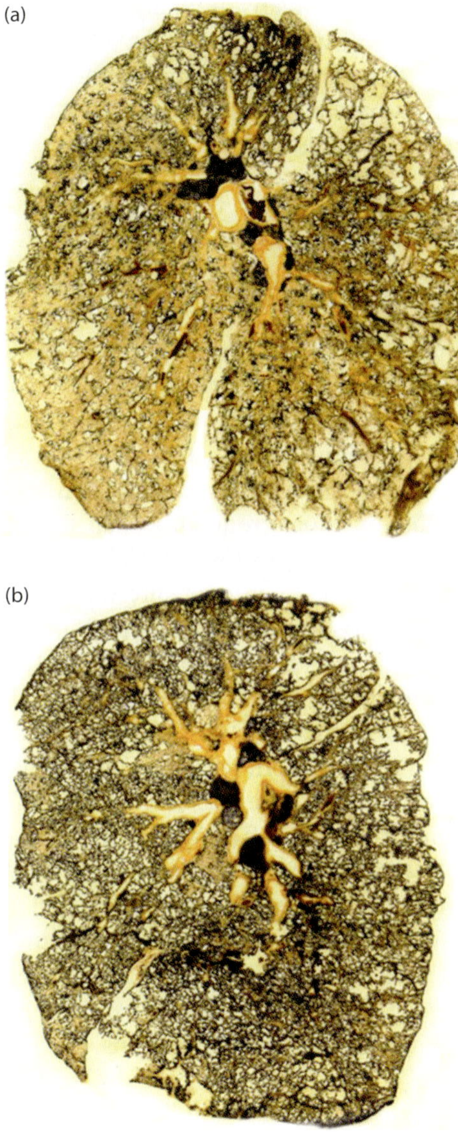

FIGURE 19.5 (a) Whole-lung section showing emphysema in a coal miner. The emphysema in the upper lobes is a combination of severe centriacinar emphysema together with panacinar emphysema. In the middle and lower zone of the upper lobe, coal dust macules with centriacinar emphysema are seen. (b) Whole-lung section showing emphysema in a coal miner. The emphysema is panacinar and involves all lobes of the lung. The interstitium is diffusely pigmented with coal mine dust; however, no classic lesions of coal workers' pneumoconiosis (CWP) are seen. The classic lesions of CWP become obscured with increasing severity of emphysema.

Emphysema severity is related to the dust content of the lungs (Cockcroft et al., 1982; Leigh et al., 1994) and cumulative lifetime exposure to CMD after adjusting for the effects of cigarette smoking, age and race (Kuempel et al., 2009). Examples of CMD-associated emphysema are shown in Figure 19.5. With increasing severity of CMD-associated emphysema, the findings of classic CWP become obscured.

Chronic Bronchitis

The presence of chronic bronchitis with chronic cough and sputum production has been strongly associated with CMD exposure. Early studies showed increasing prevalence of bronchitis associated with increased estimated coal dust exposure (Rae et al., 1970; Leigh, 1990). Mucus-producing goblet cells are increased in number within the bronchioles of miners with radiographic CWP compared to those without CWP (Naeye and Dellinger, 1972). Additionally, higher lifetime exposure to coal dust is associated with increased mucus gland size in the proximal airways (Douglas et al., 1982). A recent study of new Chinese coal miners found symptoms of chronic bronchitis to be associated with dust exposure and significant declines in forced expiratory volume in 1 second (FEV_1) (Wang et al., 1999).

Lung Function Impairment

CMD exposure is associated with impairment in lung function as measured by spirometry, even in the absence of radiographic evidence of CWP (Morgan, 1978). The examination of multiple cohorts of miners is notable for evidence of an excess lifetime risk of significant loss of lung function being attributable to dust exposure (Oxman et al., 1993). The decline in lung function may be greater in magnitude early on in a miner's tenure (Seixas et al., 1992; Carta et al., 1996; Wang et al., 2013). Supporting this is evidence that longer-tenured miners have a less rapid decline in lung function than younger miners. It has also been shown that miners are more likely to have airway hyper-reactivity than non-miners (Petsonk et al., 1995). These findings raise the possibility of a healthy worker effect in coal mining populations.

After adjusting for age and smoking status, the magnitude of decline in function is proportional to estimated cumulative CMD exposure (Love and Miller, 1982; Soutar and Hurley, 1986; Carta et al., 1996; Cowie et al., 2006). The correlation between the rate of decline in FEV_1 and cumulative CMD exposure is greater in nonsmokers (Soutar and Hurley, 1986), but is of the same order of magnitude. Data from the US National Study of Coal Workers' Pneumoconiosis showed an approximately 6–9–mL per year reduction in FEV_1 attributable to dust exposure in US miners working before 1970 when modern dust controls were mandated, and a 2–3-mL per year reduction in those after that date. Smokers in this study had a reduction of approximately 5 mL per year. In addition to being a marker for respiratory symptoms, the magnitude of FEV_1 decline is associated with increased risk of death from cardiovascular and non-malignant respiratory disease (Beeckman et al., 2001).

There has been some controversy as to whether or not simple CWP is associated with lung function impairment. However, a large body of evidence does show a significant relationship between spirometric abnormalities and the presence and severity of simple CWP detected on chest radiographs (Wang et al., 2013), although declines in lung function may actually precede the detection of the radiographic abnormalities associated with CMDLD.

The single-breath DLCO measured in miners with simple CWP may be decreased (Frans et al., 1975). Abnormalities on spirometry and of DLCO are associated with increased emphysema on chest computed tomography (CT) and profusion of small nodules on chest radiography (Gevenois et al., 1998; Akkoca Yildiz et al., 2007).

Lung Cancer

Although historically coal mining was not thought to be associated with increased risk of the development of bronchogenic lung cancer, more recent data suggest the possibility that an association exists (Hoffmann and Jöckel, 2006; Hosgood et al., 2012; Graber et al., 2014). The International Agency for Research on Cancer (IARC) last evaluated the carcinogenicity of coal dust in 1997 and concluded that there was insufficient evidence to support or refute an association (International Agency for Research on Cancer, 1997). Silica, diesel exhaust particulates and radon are present in the atmospheres of many coal mines and are all classified as carcinogenic to humans by IARC.

NON-DUST-RELATED RESPIRATORY DISEASE

Coal miners may be exposed to high concentrations of diesel exhaust particulates in underground mines. Measurements of CMD are not typically able to distinguish coal dust from diesel particulates, but up to 60% of the respirable dust in a mine using diesel-powered mechanized equipment has been found to be diesel particulates (National Institute for Occupational Safety and Health, 1995). Miners with chronic exposures to diesel engine exhaust may potentially develop respiratory symptoms and airways obstruction (Reger et al., 1982; Ames et al., 1984). Although a review of occupational data suggests an increased risk of bronchogenic lung cancer with chronic diesel exhaust exposures (Hoffmann and Jöckel, 2006), published data on the incidence of lung cancer due to diesel exhaust exposures specifically in coal miners are not available.

Water used for mine dust suppression may be contaminated with microorganisms and may exacerbate underlying lung diseases, including asthma. Other workplace exposures may exacerbate underlying asthma, and true occupational asthma has been reported as well (Nemery and Lenaerts, 1993; Gamboa et al., 1996).

DIAGNOSTIC EVALUATION

History and Physical Examination

Respiratory symptoms in a worker with possible CMDLD are non-specific and typically develop insidiously. Many miners attribute these gradually developing symptoms to ageing rather than lung disease. Coal workers with classic CWP complain of breathlessness, chronic cough and sputum production more frequently than those who do not have radiologic changes (Wang et al., 1999).

An accurate and detailed exposure history is critical to making a diagnosis of CMDLD. In addition to duration of employment as a coal worker, an understanding of the characteristics of the mine and the worker's job duties may modify the estimated risk of CMDLD substantially. The worker should be asked about the method of mining, proximity to the working face, height of the coal seam and methods of dust control, including the adequacy of ventilation and water suppression technologies in the mine. They should also be queried about the use of personal respiratory protection. Tenure in specific job roles and an estimate of the number of weekly hours worked may also be informative. The history of exposures from non-mining occupations, avocations and environmental sources must be elicited. Careful calculation of pack-years of tobacco smoke exposure is important for understanding disease causation.

The physical examination findings in a miner with CMDLD are generally non-specific. Wheezes associated with obstructive lung disease or rales attributable to pulmonary fibrosis may be heard on auscultation. Signs of pulmonary hypertension and cor pulmonale may be present in cases of advanced disease.

There are no laboratory findings specific to CMDLD. Serum angiotensin-converting enzyme levels may be elevated in CWP (Wallaert et al., 1985). Elevated levels of anti-nuclear antibodies may occur in workers with

CWP with greater frequency (Lippmann et al., 1973). Rheumatoid factor levels may also be abnormal.

Physiologic Examination

Resting and exercise pulmonary function testing are the primary means that are used in order to measure the pattern and severity of impairment due to CMDLD. Obstructive, restrictive or mixed ventilatory defects may be observed depending on the relative degree of parenchymal fibrosis, emphysema or airways disease present (Leigh et al., 1994; Miller and MacCalman, 2010). Diffusion impairment is also an important finding in CMDLD (Wang et al., 1999; Wang and Christiani, 2000). Resting pulmonary function tests may not correlate well with the severity of the miner's dyspnoea. Cardiopulmonary exercise testing (CPET) may be helpful for identifying and characterizing the underlying cause of functional impairment and dyspnoea in such cases. The alveolar–arterial oxygen gradient may widen and there may be an excessive ventilatory response to exercise associated with mismatched ventilation and pulmonary perfusion. Pulmonary hypertension may be the underlying physiologic defect in some cases (Akkoca Yildiz et al., 2007). CPET may also enable an assessment of potential confounding causes of dyspnoea, such as heart failure. It should be noted that arterial blood gases are best obtained through an indwelling arterial line within a few seconds of peak exercise in order to accurately measure the nadir PO_2 and abnormal gas exchange (Ries et al., 1983).

Imaging

The diagnosis of CMDLD is based on a detailed exposure history in combination with physiologic evaluation and chest imaging. Lung biopsy is not required for diagnosis and is employed in order to rule out other treatable diagnoses. Plain chest radiography has historically been central to the recognition of CWP, but it is limited in the detection of emphysema and airways disease.

CT of the chest is more sensitive than plain chest radiography for some abnormalities associated with CMDLD, particularly emphysema (Remy-Jardin et al., 1990b; Gevenois et al., 1998). This modality is not suitable for routine screening for CMDLD due to its expense, radiation exposure and lack of an agreed-upon international classification system. CT imaging may be most useful in the evaluation of symptomatic workers with normal or borderline chest radiographs (Bourgkard et al., 1998) or for the evaluation of radiographic lesions that are atypical of CWP.

The radiographic opacities associated with PMF may be difficult to distinguish from other lesions, with neoplasm and granulomatous infections potentially confounding or coexisting with CMDLD findings. Malignancy is the most concerning and should be distinguished from PMF, particularly when there is a paucity of background small opacities or when there is unilateral disease. Prior chest radiographs may be helpful for determining an estimate of the doubling time of growth of the lesion. Positron emission tomography (PET) scans may be of limited utility in distinguishing PMF lesions from neoplasms, as there may be significant overlap in the standardized uptake values of the two disease entities (Reichert and Bensadoun, 2009). Although pulmonary tuberculosis is associated with silica exposure, it has been observed to be variably increased in observations of coal miners (Meijers et al., 1997; Isidro Montes et al., 2004). Histoplasmosis and miliary tuberculosis may be alternative explanations of profuse small opacities.

IMAGING BOX

The radiographic diagnosis of CWP depends on the presence of typical features in the context of a significant occupational exposure to coal mine dust. CWP may be categorised by the size of the observed lesions into simple and complicated disease.

Simple CWP is characterised by small (1–5 mm typically) sub-centimetre opacities, which are frequently rounded nodules with an upper- and mid-zone predominance. Lower-zone and irregular opacities also occur in a substantial minority of cases (Laney and Petsonk, 2012). The nodules may show some calcification in approximately 10%–20% of cases (Verschakelen and Gevenois, 2006). There may be co-existing emphysema on CT densitometry, which may be due to tobacco smoking or coal mine dust inhalation (Gevenois et al., 1998). As with other pneumoconioses, CT is more sensitive and specific than chest radiography (Remy-Jardin et al., 1990; Gevenois, 1994). The earliest radiographic feature may be ill-defined tiny centrilobular nodules, which histopathologically correspond to early irregular fibrosis around the respiratory bronchioles (Akira et al., 1989). More usually, well-defined rounded micronodules are seen with a typical perilymphatic distribution in the interlobular septa, subpleural regions of the lung and around bronchovascular bundles (Remy-Jardin et al., 1992; Collins et al., 1993). When profuse, the micronodules may coalesce, particularly in the subpleural regions of the lung to form 'pseudoplaques', which are linear densities less than a centimetre in diameter. A small percentage of micronodules calcify. Sometimes, a basal reticular or honeycombing pattern similar to that seen in idiopathic pulmonary fibrosis (usual interstitial pneumonia pattern) is demonstrated (Remy-Jardin et al., 1990).

Complicated CWP occurs with continued exposure and the nodules coalesce to form conglomerate masses (*progressive massive fibrosis*). Radiographically, there are rounded, oval, or polygonal densities at least 1 cm in diameter (Figure 19.6a) (International Labour Office, 2002). An upper-zone predominance is frequently seen although mid-zone and lower-zone opacities do occur. These large opacities tend to occur in the periphery of the lung and migrate centrally over time. PMF densities vary in shape and may have well- or ill-defined margins. PMF may be unilateral or bilateral (Chong et al., 2006). The important differential diagnosis is lung cancer, particularly in the context of a unilateral opacity; comparison with previous radiographs may be particularly helpful in demonstrating the typical peripheral to central migration and the relative stability in size. Also, there is often a background of small nodular densities in CWP, but occasionally this feature is absent (Verschakelen and Gevenois, 2006). There may be indirect features of scarring and volume loss related to areas of PMF with mediastinal, tracheal and parenchymal distortion and adjacent areas of emphysematous destruction.

CT demonstrates the conglomerate masses of PMF on a background of micronodules, which may result in irregularity of the outline of larger densities. Surrounding 'scar' or paracicatricial emphysema resulting in areas of lung destruction are better demonstrated on CT than chest radiography (Figure 19.6b) (Chong et al., 2006). Also, adjacent distortion and 'drawing in' of the extrapleural fat is often a feature of peripheral masses (Figure 19.6b) (Chong et al., 2006). An upper and posterior lung distribution is frequent, although isolated lower lobe masses are also recognised (Lyons and Campbell, 1981). A variety of calcification patterns may be seen, particularly punctate, with extensive dense calcification less common. Avascular necrosis is a feature of large lesions, with initial areas of decreased attenuation progressing to cavitation and air-fluid levels. Tuberculosis infection or aspergilloma formation (resulting in intracavitary bodies) are recognised complications. Mediastinal nodal enlargement and calcification is often seen in the context of PMF and the typical eggshell distribution is commoner than punctate or diffuse dense calcification (Remy-Jardin et al., 1992).

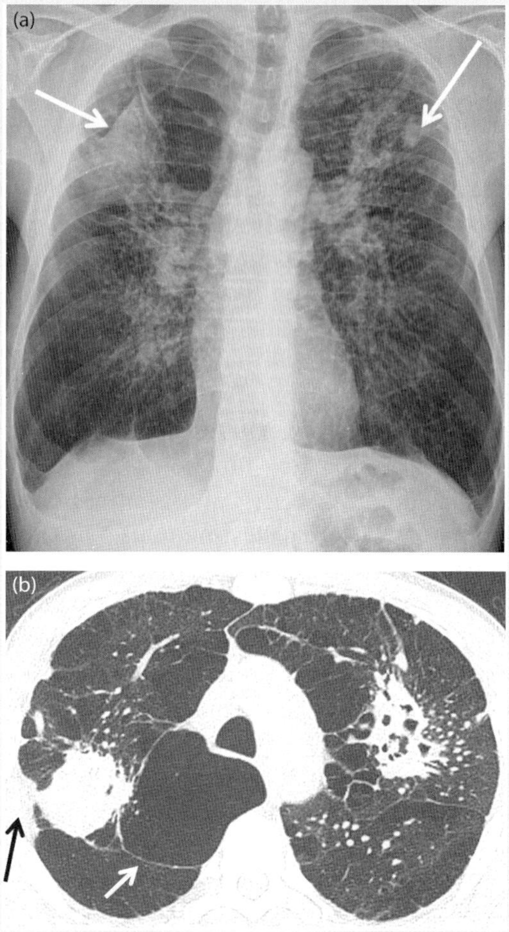

FIGURE 19.6 (a) Chest radiograph of a 67 year old male coal miner demonstrating the typical bilateral upper lobe distribution of progressive massive fibrosis (PMF) (arrows) on a background of fine nodularity consistent with complicated coal worker's pneumoconiosis. (b) Axial CT in the same individual demonstrating areas of PMF on a background of small nodules. Note the distortion and 'drawing in' of the adjacent extrapleural fat (black arrow) and the paracicatrial emphysema (white arrow). (Images courtesy of Jeffrey Kanne, MD.)

The two main patterns of emphysema demonstrated on imaging are areas of bullous destruction adjacent to areas of PMF (paracicatricial emphysema) and very subtle areas of emphysematous destruction without defined walls adjacent to ill-defined centrilobular nodules due to coal dust-laden macrophages related to respiratory bronchioles (Remy-Jardin et al., 1992). All types of emphysema, including centrilobular, panacinar, and bullous emphysema, are associated with both dust exposure and cigarette smoking, and may be seen even when nodules are not present (Green et al., 1998).

Caplan's syndrome refers to large necrobiotic nodules in individuals with rheumatoid arthritis on a background of small pneumoconiotic nodules (Caplan, 1959). The nodules of Caplan's syndrome are typically over 3 cm in diameter (range from 0.5 to 5 cm) and sometimes conglomerated into groups and may appear suddenly. The nodules commonly cavitate, and it may be difficult to differentiate radiologically between Caplan's syndrome, cavitary PMF and tuberculous infection.

Potential uses of PET/CT and MRI (including diffusion-weighted MRI) in the context of CWP are to differentiate lung cancer from PMF, although false positives may occur with PET (Chung et al., 2010). Lung cancer typically returns high signal on T2-weighted imaging, whereas PMF appears as low signal on T2 by comparison with skeletal muscle (Chong et al., 2006). Areas of rim enhancement or a lack of enhancement post-gadolinium may also be seen (Jung et al., 2000).

SUMMARY

Chest Radiography

- Small (1–5 mm diameter) rounded upper, mid-zone and posterior nodules, although in one quarter of cases lower zone and irregular opacities may occur
- Nodules may calcify (20%)
- 'Egg-shell' calcification of hilar and mediastinal lymph nodes
- Nodules may coalesce to form conglomerate masses (progressive massive fibrosis) which form in the outer lung and slowly migrate centrally over time with paracicatricial emphysema
- Caplan's syndrome results in multiple diffuse upper zone nodules 5 mm to 5 cm in diameter (appear suddenly within a few months)

NB

Volume loss and paracicatricial emphysema may differentiate PMF from complicating lung cancer (if no previous radiographs are available).

CT

- Small centrilobular or perilymphatic soft-tissue density nodules of varying size
- Nodules may coalesce to form conglomerate masses (progressive massive fibrosis) which typically form in the outer lung and slowly migrate centrally over time with adjacent paracicatricial emphysema
- Nodules may calcify
- Subpleural nodules or 'pseudoplaques'
- 'Egg-shell' calcification of mediastinal lymph nodes

MRI

May be helpful in distinguishing PMF from lung cancer due to differences in signal characteristics and enhancement post IV gadolinium.

PET/CT

Increased radio-isotope tracer uptake in PMF and mediastinal and hilar lymph nodes may result in false-positive diagnosis of lung cancer (which is usually more PET active).

MANAGEMENT

There are no specific treatments with clearly demonstrated efficacy for CMDLD. The approach to management has been focused upon treating and preventing complications, including hypoxaemia, infections, pulmonary hypertension and pneumothorax. Treatment of airflow obstruction with bronchodilators with or without inhaled corticosteroids should be considered. Cessation of the use of tobacco products, including cigarettes and smokeless tobacco, should be encouraged. Comorbid disease such as obesity and cardiovascular disease should also be addressed. Vaccinations in order to prevent pulmonary infections, including influenza and pneumococcus, are recommended. A miner with significant functional impairment should be referred to formal pulmonary rehabilitation programmes if available.

Radiographic monitoring at regular intervals is important, even in persons who are no longer exposed to CMD. The World Health Organization recommends baseline chest radiography for workers exposed to CMD, and then again at intervals of 2–5 years

(World Health Organization, 1986). Nodules that are consistent with CWP can potentially develop after cessation of dust exposure, even with baseline category 0 film (Maclaren and Soutar, 1985; Kimura et al., 2010). A significant proportion of subjects with simple CWP can progress radiographically to PMF after cessation of dust exposure, particularly in the first 10 years after removal (Kimura et al., 2010).

The impairment in pulmonary function may also worsen even after cessation of dust exposure (Bates et al., 1985; Dimich-Ward and Bates, 1994). Serial lung function measurements are recommended every 1–3 years in the USA (National Institute for Occupational Safety and Health, 1995).

In some countries, compensation for disability due to CMDLD may be available. Impairment from CMDLD may be confounded by other factors, including cardiovascular disease, smoking and obesity. In some countries, mine workers who have positive screening studies for CMDLD may be eligible for workplace removal or reassignment to areas with reduced risk of dust exposure. In practice, workers are often reluctant to take advantage of these frequently lower-paying positions and may fear repercussions from employers.

Unilateral and bilateral lung transplantation have been performed for the treatment of severe chronic respiratory failure associated with CMDLD. The clinical benefit of transplantation in this population compared to other pulmonary diseases is not well defined (Enfield et al., 2012; Hayes et al., 2012). Whole-lung lavage is hypothesized to benefit miners by the removal of CMD, as well as the possible removal of inflammatory cells and their mediators (Wilt et al., 1996). There are, however, no clinical trials or published long-term observational data to support routine utilization of this treatment.

PRIMARY PREVENTION

Role of Personal Respiratory Protection

Personal respirators may be protective of the lung health of coal mine workers when used in conjunction with environmental controls, but should not be used as a primary means of protection. There are practical barriers to their use, including their cost and the difficulty of breathing through them while performing heavy manual labour. A longitudinal study in the USA reported that greater adherence to respirator use was associated with workers who had respiratory symptoms at baseline, who were of older age and who had increased estimated dust concentrations in the workplace (Li et al., 2002), suggesting that the likelihood of use is associated with perception of risk to lung health. There is limited evidence of long-term benefit due to methodological problems, but FEV_1 levels may be higher in miners who use personal respirators (Li et al., 2002).

Role of Exposure Limits

Engineering controls utilizing ventilation, water sprays and other dust-suppression technologies in order to maintain respirable dust levels below hazardous levels of exposure are the most important public health measures for preventing CMDLD. The World Health Organization recommends a respirable CMD exposure limit of 0.5–4.0 mg/m^3 if the free-silica content is <7% of the dust (World Health Organization, 1986). Allowances above the lower limit of 0.5 mg/m^3 are made if there is epidemiological evidence of a low risk of category 1 CWP over the course of a miner's working life.

It is difficult to compare dust exposure limits between countries due to the variability in respirable dust sampling regulations, procedures and enforcement. In 2014, the USA lowered the permissible exposure limit for CMD from 2.0 to 1.5 mg/m^3 in response to concerns over increasing rates of disease. The occupational exposure limit for anthracite CMD in China is 4 mg/m^3, and it is 2.5 mg/m^3 for bituminous CMD (Liang et al., 2006).

CONCLUSION

CMDLD is entirely preventable. However, the economic equation balancing the immediate cost to industry of the equipment for dust control and suppression and future costs of compensating and treating coal workers who present years later with an insidious disease often do not favour prevention. This underscores the importance of comprehensive public health regulations with effective enforcement.

REFERENCES

Akira, M., Higasihara, T., Yokoyama, K., Yamamoto, S., Kita, N., Morimoto, S., Ikezoe, J. et al. 1989. Radiographic type p pneumoconiosis: High resolution CT. *Radiology* 171:117–23.

Akkoca Yildiz, O., Eris Gulbay, B., Saryal, S. and Karabiyikoglu, G. 2007. Evaluation of the relationship between radiological abnormalities and both pulmonary function and pulmonary hypertension in coal workers' pneumoconiosis. *Respirology* 12(3):420–6.

Ames, R. G., Hall, D. S. and Reger, R. B. 1984. Chronic respiratory effects of exposure to diesel emissions in coal mines. *Arch Environ Health* 39(6):389–94.

Antao, V.C., Petsonk, E. L., Sokolow, L. Z. et al. 2005. Rapidly progressive coal workers' pneumoconiosis in the United States: Geographic clustering and other factors. *Occup Environ Med* 62(10):670–4.

Attfield, M. D. and Petsonk, E. L. 2007. Advanced pneumoconiosis among working underground coal miners—Eastern Kentucky and Southwestern Virginia, 2006. *MMWR Morb Mortal Wkly Rep* 56(26):652–5.

Attfield, M. D. and Seixas, N. S. 1995. Prevalence of pneumoconiosis and its relationship to dust exposure in a cohort of U.S. bituminous Coal Miners and ex-miners. *Am J Ind Med* 27(1):137–51.

Bates, D. V., Pham, Q. T., Chau, N., Pivoteau, C., Dechoux, J. and Sadoul, P. 1985. A longitudinal study of pulmonary function in coal miners in Lorraine, France. *Am J Ind Med* 8(1):21–32.

Beeckman, L. A., Wang, M. L., Petsonk, E. L. and Wagner, G. R. 2001. Rapid declines in FEV_1 and subsequent respiratory symptoms, illnesses, and mortality in coal miners in the United States. *Am J Respir Crit Care Med* 163(3 Pt 1):633–9.

Bennett, J. G., Dick, J. A., Kaplan, Y. S. et al. 1979. The relationship between coal rank and the prevalence of pneumoconiosis. *Br J Ind Med* 36(3):206–10.

Blackley, D. J., Halldin, C. N. and Laney, A. S. 2014. Resurgence of a debilitating and entirely preventable respiratory disease among working coal miners. *Am J Respir Crit Care Med* 190(6):708–9.

Blackley, D. J., Laney, A. S., Halldin, C. N. and Cohen, R. A. 2015. Profusion of opacities in simple coal workers' pneumoconiosis is associated with reduced lung function. *Chest* 148(5):1292–9.

Bourgkard, E., Bernadac, P., Chau, N., Bertrand, J. P., Teculescu, D. and Pham, Q. T. 1998. Can the evolution to pneumoconiosis be suspected in coal miners? A longitudinal study. *Am J Respir Crit Care Med* 158(2):504–9.

Brichet, A., Desurmont, S. and Wallaert, B. 2002a. Coal worker's pneumoconiosis. In D. J. Hendrick, P. S. Burge, W. S. Beckett and A. Churg (eds), *Occupational Disorders of the Lung*. London: WB Saunders, 129–41.

Brichet, A., Tonnel, A. B., Brambilla, E. et al. 2002b. Chronic interstitial pneumonia with honeycombing in coal workers. *Sarcoidosis Vasc Diffuse Lung Dis* 19(3):211–9.

Caplan, A. 1953. Certain unusual radiological appearances in the chest of coal-miners suffering from rheumatoid arthritis. *Thorax* 8(1):29–37.

Carpenter, R. G., Cochrane, A. L., Clarke, W. G., Jonathan, G. and Moore, F. 1956. Death rates of miners and exminers with and without coalworkers' pneumoconiosis in South Wales. *Br J Ind Med* 13(2):102–9.

Carta, P., Aru, G., Barbieri, M. T., Avataneo, G. and Casula, D. 1996. Dust exposure, respiratory symptoms, and longitudinal decline of lung function in young coal miners. *Occup Environ Med* 53(5):312–9.

Chong, S., Lee, K. S., Chung, M. J. et al. 2006. Pneumoconiosis: Comparison of imaging and pathologic findings. *Radiographics* 26:59–77.

Chung, S. Y., Lee, J. H., Kim, T. H., Kim, S. J., Kim, H. J. and Ryu, Y.H. 2010. ^{18}F-FDG PET imaging of progressive massive fibrosis. *Ann Nucl Med* 24:21–7.

Churg, A. and Green, F. H. Y. 1998. *Pathology of Occupational Lung Disease*, second edition. Baltimore: Williams & Wilkins.

Cochrane, A. L. 1962. The attack rate of progressive massive fibrosis. *Br J Ind Med* 19(1):52–64.

Cochrane, A. L., Haley, T. J., Moore, F. and Hole, D. 1979. The mortality of men in the Rhondda Fach, 1950–1970. *Br J Ind Med* 36(1):15–22.

Cockcroft, A., Lyons, J. P., Andersson, N. and Saunders, M. J. 1983. Prevalence and relation to underground exposure of radiological irregular opacities in South Wales coal workers with pneumoconiosis. *Br J Ind Med* 40(2):169–72.

Cockcroft, A., Seal, R. M., Wagner, J. C., Lyons, J. P., Ryder, R. and Andersson, N. 1982. Post-mortem study of emphysema in coalworkers and non-coalworkers. *Lancet* 2(8298):600–3.

Cockcroft, A. E., Wagner, J. C., Seal, E. M., Lyons, J. P. and Campbell, M. J. 1982. Irregular opacities in coalworkers' pneumoconiosis—Correlation with pulmonary function and pathology. *Ann Occup Hyg* 26(1–4):767–87.

Cohen, R. A., Petsonk, E. L., Rose, C., Young, B., Regier, M., Najmuddin, A., Abraham, J. L., Churg, A. and Green, F.H.Y. 2016. Lung pathology in U.S. coal workers with rapidly progressive pneumoconiosis implicates silica and silicates. *Am J Respir Crit Care Med* 193:673–80.

Collins, L., Willing, S., Bretz, R., Harty, M., Lane, E. and Anderson, W. H. 1993. High-resolution CT in simple coal worker's pneumoconiosis. *Chest* 104: 1156–62.

Coultas, D. B., Zumwalt, R. E., Black, W. C. and Sobonya, R. E. 1994. The epidemiology of interstitial lung diseases. *Am J Respir Crit Care Med* 150(4):967–72.

Cowie, H. A., Miller, B. G., Rawbone, R. G. and Soutar, C. A. 2006. Dust related risks of clinically relevant lung functional deficits. *Occup Environ Med* 63(5):320–5.

Dimich-Ward, H. and Bates, D. V. 1994. Reanalysis of a longitudinal study of pulmonary function in coal miners in Lorraine, France. *Am J Ind Med* 25(5):613–23.

Douglas, A. N., Lamb, D. and Ruckley, V. A. 1982. Bronchial gland dimensions in coalminers: Influence of smoking and dust exposure. *Thorax* 37(10):760–4.

Enfield, K. B., Floyd, S., Barker, B. et al. 2012. Survival after lung transplant for coal workers' pneumoconiosis. *J Heart Lung Transplant* 31(12):1315–8.

Fernie, J. M. and Ruckley, V. A. 1987. Coalworkers' pneumoconiosis: Correlation between opacity profusion and number and type of dust lesions with special reference to opacity type. *Br J Ind Med* 44(4):273–7.

Frans, A., Veriter, C. and Brasseur, L. 1975. Pulmonary diffusing capacity for carbon monoxide in simple coal workers' pneumoconiosis. *Bull Physiopathol Respir (Nancy)* 11(4):479–502.

Gamboa, P. M., Jáuregui, I., Urrutia, I., Antépara, I., González, G. and Múgica, V. 1996. Occupational asthma in a coal miner. *Thorax* 51(8):867–8.

Gevenois, P.A., Pichot, E., Dargent, F., Dedeire, S., vandeWeyer, R. and De Vuyst, P. 1994. Low grade coal worker's pneumoconiosis: Comparison of CT and chest radiography. *Acta Radiol* 35:351–6.

Gevenois, P. A., Sergent, G., De Maertelaer, V., Gouat, F., Yernault, J. C. and De Vuyst, P. 1998. Micronodules and emphysema in coal mine dust or silica exposure: Relation with lung function. *Eur Respir J* 12(5):1020–4.

Graber, J. M., Stayner, L. T., Cohen, R. A., Conroy, L. M. and Attfield, M. D. 2014. Respiratory disease mortality among US coal miners; results after 37 years of follow-up. *Occup Environ Med* 71(1):30–9.

Green, F. H., Althouse, R. and Weber, K. C. 1989. Prevalence of silicosis at death in underground coal miners. *Am J Ind Med* 16(6):605–15.

Green, F. H. Y., Brower, P. S., Vallyathan, V. and Attfield, M. D. 1998. Coal mine dust exposure and type of pulmonary emphysema in coal workers. In K. Chiyotani and Y. Hosoda (eds), *Advances in the Prevention of Occupational Respiratory Diseases: Proceedings of the 9th International Conference on Occupational Respiratory Diseases, Kyoto, 13–16 October 1997.* New York, Amsterdam: Elsevier.

Halldin, C. N., Reed, W. R., Joy, G. J. et al. 2015. Debilitating lung disease among surface coal miners with no underground mining tenure. *J Occup Environ Med* 57(1):62–7.

Hayes, D. Jr., Diaz-Guzman, E., Davenport, D. L. et al. 2012. Lung transplantation in patients with coal workers' pneumoconiosis. *Clin Transplant* 26(4):629–34.

Hoffmann, B. and Jöckel, K.-H. 2006. Diesel exhaust and coal mine dust. *Ann N Y Acad Sci* 1076(1):253–65.

Honma, K. and Chiyotani, K. 1993. Diffuse interstitial fibrosis in nonasbestos pneumoconiosis—A pathological study. *Respir Int Rev Thorac Dis* 60(2):120–6.

Honma, K. and Vallyathan, V. 2002. Rheumatoid pneumoconiosis: A comparative study of autopsy cases between Japan and North America. *Ann Occup Hyg* 46(Suppl. 1):265–7.

Hosgood, H. D., Chapman, R. S., Wei, H. et al. 2012. Coal mining is associated with lung cancer risk in Xuanwei, China. *Am J Ind Med* 55(1):5–10.

Hurley, J. F., Alexander, W. P., Hazledine, D. J., Jacobsen, M. and Maclaren, W. M. 1987. Exposure to respirable coalmine dust and incidence of progressive massive fibrosis. *Br J Ind Med* 44(10):661–72.

Hurley, J. F., Burns, J., Copland, L., Dodgson, J. and Jacobsen, M. 1982. Coalworkers' simple pneumoconiosis and exposure to dust at 10 British coalmines. *Br J Ind Med* 39(2):120–7.

International Agency for Research on Cancer. 1997. Agents Classified by the IARC Monographs, Volumes 1–111. Available at: http://monographs.iarc.fr/ENG/Classification/ClassificationsAlphaOrder.pdf (accessed 31 July 2014).

International Labour Office. 2002. *Guidelines for the Use of the ILO International Classification of Radiographs of Pneumoconioses.* Geneva: International Labour Office.

Isidro Montes, I., Rego Fernández, G., Reguero, J. et al. 2004. Respiratory disease in a cohort of 2,579 coal miners followed up over a 20-year period. *Chest* 126(2):622–9.

Jung, J. I., Park, S. H., Lee, J. M. et al. 2000. MR characteristics of progressive massive fibrosis. *J Thorac Imaging* 15:144–50.

Kimura, K., Ohtsuka, Y., Kaji, H. et al. 2010. Progression of pneumoconiosis in coal miners after cessation of dust exposure: A longitudinal study based on periodic chest X-ray examinations in Hokkaido, Japan. *Intern Med* 49(18):1949–56.

Kuempel, E. D., Stayner, L. T., Attfield, M. D. and Buncher, C. R. 1995. Exposure–response analysis of mortality among coal miners in the United States. *Am J Ind Med* 28(2):167–84.

Kuempel, E. D., Vallyathan, V. and Green, F. H. Y. 2009. Emphysema and pulmonary impairment in coal miners: Quantitative relationship with dust exposure and cigarette smoking. *J Phys Conf Ser* 151:012024.

Kuempel, E. D., Wheeler, M. W., Smith, R. J., Vallyathan, V. and Green, F. H. Y. 2009. Contributions of dust exposure and cigarette smoking to emphysema severity in coal miners in the United States. *Am J Respir Crit Care Med* 180(3):257–64.

Laney, A. S. and Attfield, M. D. 2010. Coal workers' pneumoconiosis and progressive massive fibrosis are increasingly more prevalent among workers in small underground coal mines in the United States. *Occup Environ Med* 67:428–31.

Laney, A. S. and Petsonk, E. L. 2012. Small pneumoconiotic opacities on U.S. coal worker surveillance chest radiographs are not predominantly in the upper lung zones. *Am J Ind Med* 55(9):793–8.

Laney, A. S., Petsonk, E. L. and Attfield, M. D. 2010. Pneumoconiosis among underground bituminous coal miners in the United States: Is silicosis becoming more frequent? *Occup Environ Med* 67(10):652–6.

Leigh, J. 1990. 15 year longitudinal studies of FEV_1 loss and mucus hypersecretion development in coal workers in New South Wales, Australia. In *Proceedings of the VIIth International Pneumoconioses Conference Part II. U.S. Department of Health and Human Services, Public Health Service, Centers for Disease Control, National Institute for Occupational Safety and Health, DHHS (NIOSH)*, 112–21. Available at: http://www.cdc.gov/niosh/docs/90-108/ (accessed 5 December 2011).

Leigh, J., Driscoll, T. R., Cole, B. D., Beck, R. W., Hull, B. P. and Yang, J. 1994. Quantitative relation between emphysema and lung mineral content in coalworkers. *Occup Environ Med* 51(6):400–7.

Li, H., Wang, M. L., Seixas, N., Ducatman, A. and Petsonk, E. L. 2002. Respiratory protection: Associated factors and effectiveness of respirator use among underground coal miners. *Am J Ind Med* 42(1):55–62.

Liang, Y., Wong, O., Yang, L., Li, T. and Su, Z. 2006. The development and regulation of occupational exposure limits in China. *Regul Toxicol Pharmacol RTP* 46(2):107–13.

Lippmann, M., Eckert, H. L., Hahon, N. and Morgan, W. K. 1973. Circulating antinuclear and rheumatoid factors in coal miners. A prevalence study in Pennsylvania and West Virginia. *Ann Intern Med* 79(6):807–11.

Love, R. G. and Miller, B. G. 1982. Longitudinal study of lung function in coal-miners. *Thorax* 37(3):193–7.

Lyons, J. P. and Campbell, H. 1981. Relation between progressive massive fibrosis, emphysema and pulmonary dysfunction in coal worker's pneumoconiosis. *Br J Ind Med* 38:125–9.

Maclaren, W. M. and Soutar, C. A. 1985. Progressive massive fibrosis and simple pneumoconiosis in ex-miners. *Br J Ind Med* 42(11):734–40.

McConnochie, K., Green, F. H. Y., Vallyathan, V., Wagner, J. C., Seal, R. M. E. and Lyons, J. P. 1988. Interstitial fibrosis in coal workers—Experience in Wales and West Virginia. *Ann Occup Hyg* 32(Inhaled Particles VI):553–60.

Meijers, J. M., Swaen, G. M. and Slangen, J. J. 1997. Mortality of Dutch coal miners in relation to pneumoconiosis, chronic obstructive pulmonary disease, and lung function. *Occup Environ Med* 54(10):708–13.

Miller, B. G. and MacCalman, L. 2010. Cause-specific mortality in British coal workers and exposure to respirable dust and quartz. *Occup Environ Med* 67(4):270–6.

Mo, J., Wang, L., Au, W. and Su, M. 2014. Prevalence of coal workers' pneumoconiosis in China: A systematic analysis of 2001–2011 studies. *Int J Hyg Environ Health* 217(1):46–51.

Morgan, W. K. 1978. Industrial bronchitis. *Br J Ind Med* 35(4):285–91.

Naeye, R. L. and Dellinger, W. S. 1972. Coal workers' pneumoconiosis. Correlation of roentgenographic and postmortem findings. *JAMA* 220(2):223–7.

Naidoo, R. N., Robins, T. G. and Murray, J. 2005. Respiratory outcomes among South African coal miners at autopsy. *Am J Ind Med* 48(3):217–24.

National Institute for Occupational Safety and Health. 1995. *Criteria for a Recommended Standard: Occupational Exposure to Respirable Coal Mine Dust.* Cincinnati: National Institute for Occupational Safety and Health.

Nemery, B., Brasseur, L., Veriter, C. and Frans, A. 1987. Impairment of ventilatory function and pulmonary gas exchange in non-smoking coal miners. *Lancet* 2:1429–30.

Nemery, B. and Lenaerts, L. 1993. Exposure to methylene diphenyl diisocyanate in coal mines. *Lancet* 341(8840):318.

Oxman, A. D., Muir, D. C., Shannon, H. S., Stock, S. R., Hnizdo, E. and Lange, H. J. 1993. Occupational dust exposure and chronic obstructive pulmonary disease. A systematic overview of the evidence. *Am Rev Respir Dis* 148(1):38–48.

Padley, S. P., Adler, B. D., Staples, C. A. et al. 1993 Pulmonary talcosis: CT findings in three cases. *Radiology* 186:125–7.

Pathology Standards for Coal Workers' Pneumoconiosis. 1979. Report of the Pneumoconiosis Committee of the College of American Pathologists to the National Institute for Occupational Safety and Health. *Arch Pathol Lab Med* 103(8):375–432.

Petsonk, E. L., Daniloff, E. M., Mannino, D. M., Wang, M. L., Short, S. R. and Wagner, G. R. 1995. Airway responsiveness and job selection: A study in coal miners and non-mining controls. *Occup Environ Med* 52(11):745–9.

Pipavath, S. and Godwin, J. D. 2004. Imaging of interstitial lung disease. *Clin Chest Med* 25:455–65.

Rae, S., Walker, D. D. and Attfield, M. D. 1970. Chronic bronchitis and dust exposure in British coalminers. *Inhaled Part* 2:883–96.

Raghu, G., Collard, H. R., Egan, J. J. et al. 2011. An official ATS/ERS/JRS/ALAT statement: Idiopathic pulmonary fibrosis: Evidence-based guidelines for diagnosis and management. *Am J Respir Crit Care Med* 183(6):788–824.

Reger, R., Hancock, J., Hankinson, J., Hearl, F. and Merchant, J. 1982. Coal miners exposed to diesel exhaust emissions. *Ann Occup Hyg* 26(1–4):799–815.

Reichert, M. and Bensadoun, E. S. 2009. PET imaging in patients with coal workers pneumoconiosis and suspected malignancy. *J Thorac Oncol* 4(5):649–51.

Remy-Jardin, M., Beuscart, R., Sault, M. C., Marquette, C. H. and Remy, J. 1990a. Subpleural micronodules in diffuse infiltrative lung diseases: Evaluation with thin section CT scans. *Radiology* 177:133–9.

Remy-Jardin, M., Degreef, J. M., Beuscart, R., Voisin, C. and Remy, J. 1990b. Coal worker's pneumoconiosis: CT assessment in exposed workers and correlation with radiographic findings. *Radiology* 177(2):363–71.

Remy-Jardin, M., Remy, J., Farre, I. and Marquette, C. H. 1992. Computed tomographic evaluation of silicosis and coal worker's pneumoconiosis. *Radiol Clin North Am* 30:1155–76.

Ries, A. L., Fedullo, P. F. and Clausen, J. L. 1983. Rapid changes in arterial blood gas levels after exercise in pulmonary patients. *Chest* 83(3):454–6.

Ruckley, V. A., Fernie, J. M., Chapman, J. S. et al. 1984. Comparison of radiographic appearances with associated pathology and lung dust content in a group of coalworkers. *Br J Ind Med* 41(4):459–67.

Ryder, R., Lyons, J. P., Campbell, H. and Gough, J. 1970. Emphysema in coal workers' pneumoconiosis. *Br Med J* 3(5721):481–7.

Scarisbrick, D. A. and Quinlan, R. M. 2002. Health surveillance for Coal Workers' pneumoconiosis in the United Kingdom 1998–2000. *Ann Occup Hyg* 46(Suppl. 1): 254–6.

Seaton, A., Dick, J. A., Dodgson, J. and Jacobsen, M. 1981. Quartz and pneumoconiosis in coalminers. *Lancet* 2(8258):1272–5.

Seixas, N. S., Robins, T. G., Attfield, M. D. and Moulton, L. H. 1992. Exposure–response relationships for coal mine dust and obstructive lung disease following enactment of the Federal Coal Mine Health and Safety Act of 1969. *Am J Ind Med* 21(5):715–34.

Soutar, C. A. and Hurley, J. F. 1986. Relation between dust exposure and lung function in miners and ex-miners. *Br J Ind Med* 43(5):307–20.

Suarthana, E., Laney, A. S., Storey, E., Hale, J. M. and Attfield, M. D. 2011. Coal workers' pneumoconiosis in the United States: Regional differences 40 years after implementation of the 1969 Federal Coal Mine Health and Safety Act. *Occup Environ Med* 68(12):908–13.

Vallyathan, V., Brower, P. S., Green, F. H. and Attfield, M. D. 1996. Radiographic and pathologic correlation of coal workers' pneumoconiosis. *Am J Respir Crit Care Med* 154(3 Pt 1):741–8.

Verschakelen, J.A. and Gevenois, P.A. 2006. Coal worker's pneumonconiosis. In P.A. Gevenois and P. De Vuyst (eds), *Imaging of Occupational and Environmental Disorders of the Chest*. Heidelberg: Springer, 195–206.

Wade, W. A., Petsonk, E. L., Young, B. and Mogri, I. 2011. Severe occupational pneumoconiosis among West Virginian coal miners: One hundred thirty-eight cases of progressive massive fibrosis compensated between 2000 and 2009. *Chest* 139(6):1458–62.

Wallaert, B., Deflandre, J., Ramon, P. and Voisin, C. 1985. Serum angiotensin-converting enzyme in coal worker's pneumoconiosis. *Chest* 87(6):844–5.

Wang, M. L., Beeckman-Wagner, L.-A., Wolfe, A. L., Syamlal, G. and Petsonk, E. L. 2013. Lung-function impairment among US underground coal miners, 2005 to 2009: Geographic patterns and association with coal workers' pneumoconiosis. *J Occup Environ Med* 55(7): 846–50.

Wang, X., Yu, I. T., Wong, T. W. and Yano, E. 1999. Respiratory symptoms and pulmonary function in coal miners: Looking into the effects of simple pneumoconiosis. *Am J Ind Med* 35(2):124–31.

Wang, X. R. and Christiani, D. C. 2000. Respiratory symptoms and functional status in workers exposed to silica, asbestos, and coal mine dusts. *J Occup Environ Med* 42(11):1076–84.

Wilt, J. L., Banks, D. E., Weissman, D. N. et al. 1996. Reduction of lung dust burden in pneumoconiosis by whole-lung lavage. *J Occup Environ Med* 38(6):619–24.

World Health Organization. 1986. *Recommended Health-Based Limits in Occupational Exposure to Selected Mineral Dusts (Silica, Coal)*. Geneva: World Health Organization.

Yi, Q. and Zhang, Z. 1996. The survival analyses of 2738 patients with simple pneumoconiosis. *Occup Environ Med* 53(2):129–35.

20 Pneumoconiosis and Interstitial Lung Diseases Caused by Other Inorganic Dusts

Jennifer Hoyle

CONTENTS

INTRODUCTION

'Pneumoconiosis' is a generic term that is used to describe the lodgement of any inhaled dust in the lungs and its effects, excluding asthma and neoplasia. Inorganic dusts may be inhaled in their pure form or in association with other fibrogenic dusts, notably free silica in the form of quartz or cristobalite. As a result, many inorganic dusts may wrongly be considered fibrogenic because of 'contaminating' silica.

This chapter first considers metals, metalloids and their oxides in order of their atomic number, grouping together those with similar chemical properties. Minerals and man-made vitreous fibres are discussed subsequently.

METALS, METALLOIDS AND METAL OXIDES

Aluminium (Al): Atomic Number 13

Aluminium is a soft metal in common use; its chief ore is bauxite. Aluminium is used in non-ferrous alloys and has had a multitude of applications throughout industry. Aluminium powder is used in the manufacture of explosives and fireworks. Commercially available aluminium powders are coated with sodium or potassium stearate, which protects against oxidation and hydrolysis.

Reports of aluminium causing pulmonary fibrosis are relatively rare compared to the frequency with which the metal is used.

Pathology

Aluminium powder as a cause of pulmonary fibrosis is described in workers exposed to finely divided aluminium powders, in the fireworks industry (Mitchell et al., 1961) and in aluminium welders (Vallyathan et al., 1982); pulmonary alveolar proteinosis (PAP) was described in 1984 (Miller et al., 1984).

Whether aluminium oxide (as opposed to pure aluminium) is a cause of pulmonary fibrosis has been a subject of debate. An early description of interstitial lung disease in corundum (aluminium oxide) abrasive workers (Shaver and Riddell, 1947) was more probably acute silicosis. More recently (Jederlinic et al., 1990), nine workers producing aluminium oxide abrasives were reported to have developed interstitial fibrosis and honeycombing, but without asbestos bodies or silicotic nodules; again, the possibility of mixed-dust fibrosis in these workers cannot be excluded. In contrast, cross-sectional studies of Swedish aluminium welders failed to show an excess of pulmonary fibrosis (Sjogren and Ulfvarson, 1985). Thus, aluminium oxide and silicates appear to be less fibrogenic (Lindenschmidt et al., 1990) than pure aluminium or aluminium coated with other agents.

Aluminium lung disease is characterised by pulmonary nodules or ground-glass changes and, in some reports, generalised pulmonary fibrosis with more marked changes in the upper lobes (Mitchell et al., 1961). Lung tissue macroscopically has a metallic sheen on the cut surfaces and within fibrotic nodules. Microscopically, diffuse and focal fibrosis with localised infiltrates by lymphocytes are found with dense accumulations of macrophages containing metallic material. X-ray spectrometry can be used to identify aluminium particles (Vallyathan et al., 1982).

Case reports have described granulomatous reactions in people exposed to high concentrations of aluminium oxide dust, but the incidence appears to be very low (Chen et al., 1978).

Symptoms, Radiology and Lung function

Typically, symptoms include dyspnoea (Vallyathan et al., 1982), cough and sputum and a tendency to develop pneumothorax (Hull and Abraham, 2002).

Dense infiltrates are reported in the upper lobes on chest radiographs, as are both obstructed and restrictive spirometry (Figure 20.1) (Vallyathan et al., 1982; Hull and Abraham, 2002).

Prognosis

Progressive respiratory impairment and death are reported both in early and more recent case reports (Mitchell et al., 1961; Hull and Abraham, 2002).

Titanium (Ti): Atomic Number 22

Titanium is a silver transition metal with high strength and corrosion resistance. It occurs naturally as titanium

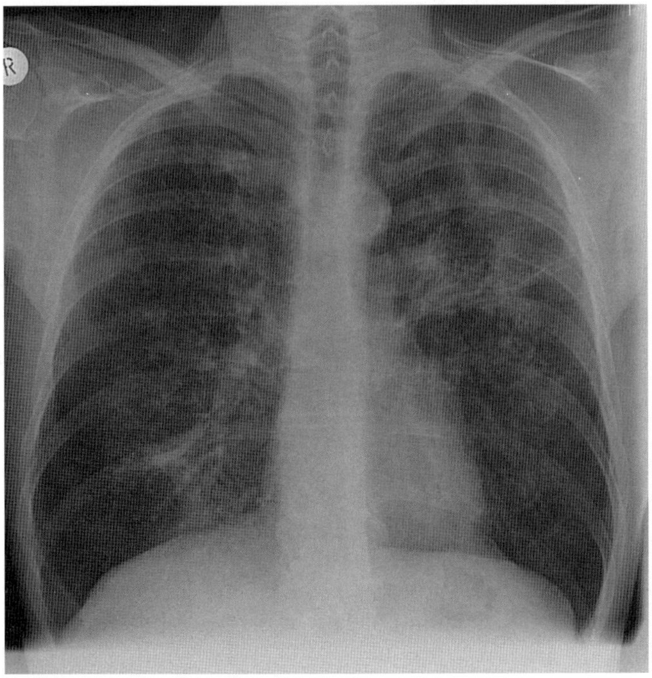

FIGURE 20.1 Aluminosis. Chest radiograph of a man who spent 20 years welding aluminium.

dioxide (TiO_2) in ilmenite; rutile and anastase are the polymorphs used in industries. TiO_2 is a white powder that is used extensively in household products including paints, cosmetics and paper, and most studies of the pulmonary toxicity of titanium are based on TiO_2 or, more rarely, titanium tetrachloride ($TiCl_4$).

Pathology

Animal and epidemiological studies of TiO_2 have produced conflicting findings. The differences might be explained by titanium manufacturing and refining processes that often involve other fibrogenic elements, including silica dust and asbestos. Other factors may include the use of synthetic rutiles in some animal studies (Nolan et al., 1987), which appear to be more biologically active than naturally occurring polymorphs, and the use of ultrafine particles, which may change the deposition characteristics of TiO_2 in the lung and thus its reactivity (Ferin et al., 1992).

Most animal studies conclude that TiO_2 is not fibrogenic (Ferin and Oberdorster, 1985), although this is not a universal finding (Lee et al., 1985). Chen and Fayerweather (1988) found no increase in chronic lung disease in a population of 1576 workers exposed to TiO_2 over a 30-year period; smaller studies, however, have described pulmonary fibrosis (Yamadori et al., 1986; Oleru, 1987), airflow obstruction and pleural abnormalities (Garabrant et al., 1987). Again, the possibility of previous or co-exposure to other minerals, including silica, cannot be excluded as a potential alternative cause.

Particles of TiO_2 are birefringent and show up brightly under Polaroid filters on lung biopsy. Most descriptions of titanium deposited in tissue report a macrophage response and some associated fibrosis of varying severity. Variations in pathology may be a result of differential particle sizes altering inhalational toxicity (Ferin et al., 1992). Animal studies indicate that TiO_2 nanoparticles are genotoxic to mice (Trouiller et al., 2009). As a result, some authorities distinguish recommended exposure limits for fine and ultrafine (including engineered nanoscale) TiO_2 based on differences in their carcinogenic potential (NIOSH, 2011). Granulomatous reactions to $TiCl_4$ (Redline et al., 1986) and TiO_2 (Maatta and Arstila, 1975) have been reported, but coexistent other disease cannot be ruled out in these cases.

$TiCl_4$ is a caustic liquid and has been associated with endobronchial polyposis and pneumonitis (Park et al., 1984).

Symptoms, Radiology and Lung Function

Small, discrete opacities similar to those in siderosis have been recorded where TiO_2 is used in the manufacture of pigments and hard metals (Schmitz-Moormann et al., 1964). There are no specific symptoms associated with TiO_2 exposure, which most texts describe as harmless, and consequently there are no specific lung function changes reported unless other minerals are present that are associated with pulmonary fibrosis.

Prognosis

TiO_2 is used extensively and is probably harmless. Lung deposition, however, and its consequences may be different when newer technologies employ particles of smaller sizes than have previously been studied.

Vanadium (V): Atomic Number 23

Vanadium is a hard, silver transition metal that is used in alloys, steel and brass. It is produced from steel smelter slag, oil fire furnace dust and as a by-product of uranium mining, and can be extracted directly from carnotite ($K_2[UO_2]_2[VO_4]_2.3H_2O$). Cross-sectional studies in vanadium pentoxide workers found no increase in pneumoconiosis or interstitial pulmonary disorders (Kiviluoto, 1980). Vanadium pentoxide is a strong irritant and exposure to its vapour causes a burning sensation in the eyes, rhinitis and cough (Sjoberg, 1950); a green–black discoloration of the tongue is described (Wyers, 1946).

Manganese (Mn): Atomic Number 25

Manganese is a metal that is used primarily to improve the quality and strength of steel. It occurs naturally as an oxide and is used in batteries, paint, ink, matches, fireworks and fertilisers.

Acute inhalation of manganese dust and fumes may cause chemical pneumonitis and fume fever (Nemery, 1990), but its main toxicity is a Parkinsonian-like syndrome (Roels et al., 1987).

Iron (Fe): Atomic Number 26 (Siderosis)

Iron is a transition metal that is associated with the naturally occurring minerals haematite, magnetite and taconite. Haematite and limonite are used as pigments in paint manufacture.

Exposure to iron and iron oxide fumes occurs when producing steel and cast iron, iron mining, crushing of iron ore and the refining, welding, cutting, grinding and finishing of iron products. While exposures to iron are very common, the reporting of siderosis itself is rare.

Pathology

Numerous animal (Harding et al., 1947; Gross et al., 1960) and human (Barrie and Harding, 1947; Koponen et al., 1980) reports indicate that iron oxide is not fibrogenic. Occasional animal studies question this belief (Stern et al., 1983).

The macroscopic appearance of the pulmonary pleura in siderosis is described as marbled and rust-brown in colour due to iron oxide deposited in lymphatics; where haematite exposure has occurred, the colour is a deep brick-red. The cut surface of the lung reveals evenly distributed grey–rust brown macules of 1–4 mm in diameter. Microscopic appearances include peri-vascular and peri-bronchiolar aggregates of dark-pigmented iron oxide in macrophages and alveolar spaces and walls.

Symptoms, Radiology and Lung Function

There are no symptoms or physical signs caused by siderosis, which is essentially a radiological disorder. Chest radiographs show small radio-dense opacities varying from 0.5 mm to approximately 2 mm in diameter with uniform distribution throughout the lungs, but without formation of conglomerates. Most changes develop after many years of exposure, but can be observed over periods as short as 3 years if exposures are high (Kleinfeld et al., 1969). Advanced disease may also include fine, dense, linear opacities in the lung parenchyma and Kerley B-lines with radio-dense but not enlarged lymph nodes (Figure 20.2).

Functional impairment is not usually described with pure siderosis unless (as is not uncommon) there is concomitant exposure to other elements such as quartz, asbestos or cristobalite, causing a mixed-dust fibrosis. This may be the case in some welders' pneumoconioses, where case reports of siderosis with significant fibrosis are found (Billings and Howard, 1993).

Prognosis

After removal from exposure, iron dust is slowly eliminated from the lungs with a gradual improvement in radiographic opacities.

Iron Oxide and Lung Cancer

Numerous studies of iron workers and miners have found an increased risk of bronchial carcinoma, but this appears to be attributable to smoking habits and exposure to known carcinogens (Duggan et al., 1970; Xu et al., 1996); there is no evidence that iron oxide itself is carcinogenic to humans.

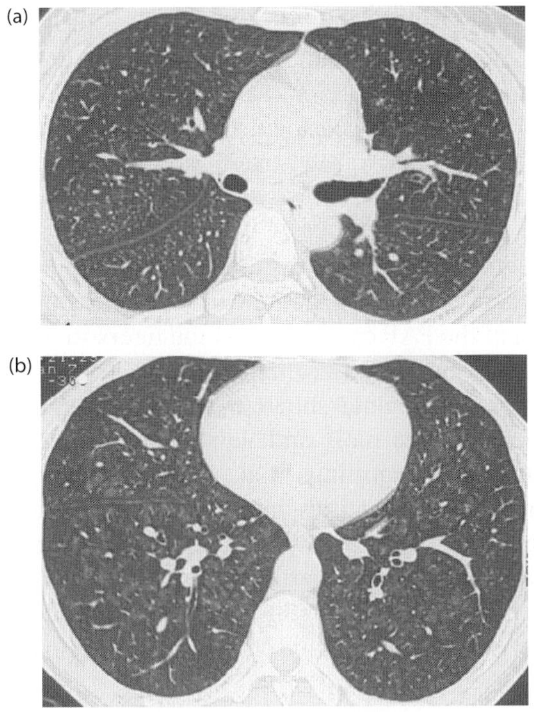

FIGURE 20.2 Siderosis. Axial high-resolution images of histopathologically proven siderosis in a welder. There are subtle, ill-defined, widespread, centrilobular nodules of ground-glass density (a) that correspond with very limited peri-bronchiolar fibrosis (b), which may not be functionally significant. Chest radiography may be normal or subtly abnormal with ill-defined, small, mid and lower zone nodules. (Images courtesy of Masanori Akira, MD, Japan.)

Chromite

Chromite (Cr_2O_3.FeO) is the mineral ore of chromium and consists of chromium and iron oxides ($FeCrO_4$). Chest radiographs of chromite miners exposed for over 8 years showed a pneumoconiosis described as very fine nodulation on chest radiograph, with nodules smaller than 1 mm in diameter. When the changes are advanced, the whole of the lung fields are involved, with a degree of sparing of the extreme apices, but no enlargement of hilar shadows (Sluis-Cremer and Du Toit, 1968). There are no physical signs or symptoms.

There are no studies directly of prognosis, but Huvinen et al. (1996) reported an increase in radiographic opacities in previous chromium mine workers, suggesting that they are more likely to persist than those in siderosis.

Nickel (Ni): Atomic Number 28

Nickel is a silvery transition metal that is often found in combination with iron in limonite or as an oxide or sulphide ore. It is commonly used in electroplating, super alloys, batteries, coins and in the steel industry. Nickel is extracted from its ores by roasting and reduction and causes skin allergy, asthma and lung cancer. Animal studies report non-specific dust pneumoconiosis with nickel oxide inhalation (Wehner et al., 1984). Small, rounded opacities of International Labour Organization (ILO) 1/0 or more on chest radiographs are described in nickel sinter plant workers, with no evidence of inflammatory or fibrogenic responses (Muir et al., 1993).

Nickel carbonyl inhalation may cause acute pulmonary oedema and acute interstitial pneumonitis (Shi, 1986).

Zirconium (Zr): Atomic Number 40 and Hafnium (Hf): Atomic Number 72

Zirconium is a transition metal that is used occasionally as an alloy agent in steel because of its strong resistance to corrosion, as a refractory agent and to make glass opaque. It has also been used in deodorant sticks and in ammunitions. Zirconium dioxide (ZrO_2) is known commercially as Zirconia and is used for polishing lenses and in thermal and electric installation, abrasives, enamels and glazes.

Zirconium occurs naturally as zircon ($ZrSiO_4$) or baddeleyite (ZrO_2). In zircon, zirconium and hafnium are geochemically associated in a ratio of 50:1; the two are only separated for use in nuclear applications. Zirconium is used in niobium tantalum alloys, which are used in atomic reactors and to line reaction vessels. Hafnium is used mainly for control rods in naval and, to a lesser extent, commercial nuclear reactors. In small amounts, it is also used in optical glass and in refractory alloys.

Zircon dust may be produced when it is processed from sand or rock; quartz dust may be a hazard during milling of the raw material and in separation processes, but is otherwise absent after processing.

Pathology

Zirconium-containing compounds are associated with non-caseating granulomata in the skin when repeatedly applied in deodorants (Neuhauser et al., 1956). Bartter et al. (1991) reported severe diffuse interstitial pulmonary fibrosis in the lower-lung fields in a man who had worked for 39 years as a lens grinder/polisher with exposure to zirconia but also to talc, asbestos, silica, zinc stearate, iron compounds and traces of other metals. Liippo et al. (1993) described granulomatous lung disease with a fulminant course, and hypersensitivity pneumonitis with granulomas has been reported in welders of nuclear fuel rods (Werfel et al., 1998).

Most cohort studies in workers who have been exposed to zirconium do not show pulmonary alterations or lung function changes (Marcus et al., 1996). Rats exposed to high concentrations of zirconium–silica dust develop radiographic shadows in the lungs; however, these do not correlate with any histological/cellular reaction on pathological examination (Kanisawa and Schroeder, 1969).

Symptoms, Radiology and Lung Function

Discrete, dense opacities ranging from ILO categories 1 to 3p have been described in men working in a factory processing zircon; these workers were also exposed to antimony, barium and titanium dust. The categories did not correlate well with duration of exposure (McCallum and Leathart, 1975).

Indium (In): Atomic Number 49

Indium is a rare post-transition metal that is used in low-melting point metal alloys and electronics. Indium tin oxide (ITO) is a sintered alloy made up mainly of indium oxide with some tin oxide, which is used in the manufacture of transparent electrodes for liquid crystal displays, touchscreens and solar cells. Indium phosphide (InP) and indium arsenide (InAs) are used in semiconductors.

Early animal studies demonstrated pulmonary damage following intra-tracheal installations of InP and ITO in hamsters (Tanaka, 2002). The first human report of interstitial pneumonia from ITO was in 2003 (Homma et al., 2003). Several subsequent studies of ITO-exposed workers suggested a strong relationship between serum indium and adverse effects on the lungs (Chonan et al., 2007; Hamaguchi et al., 2008; Nakano et al., 2009), including reports of pulmonary alveolar proteinosis (PAP) (Cummings et al., 2010).

Ten case reports of workers who produced, used or reclaimed ITO were reviewed in 2012 (Cummings et al., 2012). PAP was diagnosed in three men 1–2 years after their first exposure (with symptom onset at 6–14 months); the other cases identified pulmonary fibrosis with and without emphysema, with the appearance of interstitial lung disease at 4–13 years after the first exposure (symptom onset latency: 2–14 years).

Pathology

Histopathological features of PAP are described, including a granular, eosinophilic, intra-alveolar exudate, cholesterol clefts, particle-laden alveolar macrophages and granulomas. Unlike classical PAP, which is confined to the alveolar spaces, interstitial infiltration and fibrosis are also described, with and without emphysema. Particles can be seen in tissue on light microscopy (Cummings et al., 2012).

Symptoms, Radiology and Lung Function

Cough, breathlessness and sputum production are the most common symptoms (Homma et al., 2003; Cummings et al., 2012) with occasional digital clubbing (Chonan et al., 2007) and, rarely, haemoptysis. Symptoms are generally of insidious onset without a clear work-related pattern.

Pulmonary function tests are restrictive, with low diffusing capacity of the lung for carbon monoxide (DLCO) in most of the PAP cases; most of the interstitial lung disease (ILD) cases had normal or obstructed spirometry. Bronchoalveolar fluid shows increased cellularity with lymphocytosis in most and, less commonly, increased macrophages (Cummings et al., 2012).

Ground-glass opacities, interlobular septal thickening, traction bronchiectasis, sub-pleural disease, hilar retraction and honeycombing are described, but vary between cases. Cystic airspaces subsequent to fibrotic changes suggest developing emphysema in some (Figure 20.3).

Prognosis

Clearance from the lungs is slow, and of ten reviewed cases, lung disease progressed after being removed from exposure in eight and was fatal in two (Cummings et al., 2012).

Tin (Sn): Atomic Number 50 (Stannosis)

Tin is a crystalline silvery white metal; commercial grades of tin contain small amounts of bismuth, antimony, lead and silver as impurities. Its main uses are as a solder, tin-plated steel for food preservation, as a

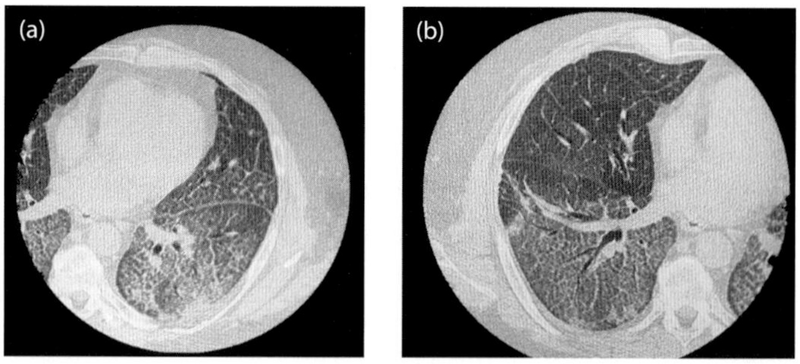

FIGURE 20.3 Indium–tin oxide. Images (a) and (b) show high-resolution computed tomography scans of a left and right lung showing bilateral ground-glass opacities, centrilobular nodules and intra-lobular and extra-lobular septal thickening. (Reprinted with permission of the American Thoracic Society. Copyright 2015, American Thoracic Society. Cummings, K. et al. 2010. *Am J Respir Crit Care Med* 181:458–64.)

specialised alloy including niobium (superconducting magnets), as a polyvinyl chloride (PVC) stabiliser (organatin) and in biocides. More recently, tin alloy associated with indium has been used in flat-screen technology (see above). The chief ore is cassiterite, a tin oxide from which tin must be recovered by smelting. The proportion of tin in crude ore is generally low and extraction procedures such as crushing and screening are unlikely to yield high exposures, although they are associated with high exposures to silicacious dust. Processes that are likely to produce tin dust or fumes include the emptying of bags of crude ore, its milling and grinding, tipping it into furnaces and chronic exposure to welding tin oxide (Giraldo et al., 2013).

Pathology

Tin oxide does not cause fibrosis in animal experiments (Robertson, 1960). Macroscopic appearances reveal numerous 1–3-mm grey–black dust molecules that are soft to the touch and not raised over the cut surface of the lung. Microscopic appearances show macrophages that contain tin oxide dust particles in the alveolar walls and spaces, peri-vascular lymphatics and interlobular septa; macules consist of dense peri-vascular and peri-bronchiolar aggregations of dust-laden macrophages. X-ray diffraction gives definitive identification; the tetragonal crystals of tin oxide exhibit strong birefringence, unlike crystals of quartz, which are poorly birefringent.

Symptoms, Radiology and Lung Function

There are no symptoms or abnormal physical signs due to the inhalation and retention of tin oxide dust. Lung function is unaffected (Robertson, 1960) unless there is coexisting disease from some other cause. Chest radiographs show numerous small and very dense opacities scattered evenly throughout the lung fields. Large, confluent opacities do not occur and the hilar shadows, although unduly thick, are of normal size (Figure 20.4).

Prognosis

Stannosis has no known effect upon health or lifespan.

Antimony (Sb): Atomic Number 51

Antimony is a metalloid occurring mainly as stibnite (Sb_2S_3). Metallic antimony is used as an alloy for lead and tin in the manufacture of lead acid batteries, solders, pewter, bullets and bearings, fire-retardant materials and microelectronics. The oxides of antimony are used in pigments, glass, rubber, paints and textiles. Antimony compounds have been used in the treatment of leishmaniasis and schistosomiasis.

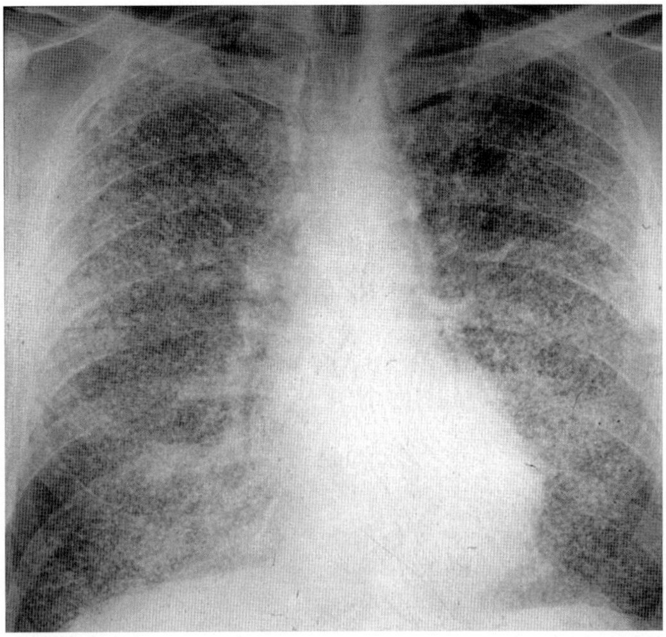

FIGURE 20.4 Stannosis. Chest radiograph of a man who worked in the UK tin industry (Cornwall).

Antimony pneumoconiosis is rare. The mining of antimony can yield high exposures to quartz; thus, antimony pneumoconiosis can be confounded by coexistent crystalline silica exposure (Potkonjak and Pavlovich, 1983), although pneumoconiosis due to the inhalation of quartz-free powdered antimony trioxide has been described (Klucik et al., 1962).

Pathology

Antimony dust particles are seen in dust-laden macrophages in alveolar walls and in perivascular regions of the lungs, but there is no fibrosis or inflammatory reaction (McCallum, 1967). The dust of antimony ore or its trioxide does not cause fibrosis of the lungs in experimental animals (Cooper et al., 1968). The biological half-life of antimony in the lungs appears to be long (>20 years).

Symptoms, Radiology and Lung Function

Orange staining of the front teeth is characteristic of exposure to antimony oxide in workers with poor oral hygiene (Potkonjak and Pavlovich, 1983). Texts vary, detailing no respiratory symptoms in some workers and non-specific respiratory symptoms including cough, wheeze, bronchitis and upper-airway inflammation in others. No abnormal physical signs or changes in lung function are associated with the radiographic changes.

Acute pulmonary oedema or acute chemical pneumonia is described rarely (Renes, 1953).

'Antimony spots' are skin pustules and eruptions on the trunk and limbs near sebaceous sweat glands, and are associated with high working temperatures (Potkonjak and Pavlovich, 1983; White et al., 1993).

Chest radiographs show numerous small, dense opacities, similar to those of siderosis, which vary from ILO category 1p to 3p. Larger component shadows are not seen, but the hilar regions may be denser than normal. The opacities appear only after 10 or more years of exposure (Potkonjak and Pavlovich, 1983).

Prognosis

There is no known detrimental effect upon health or life expectancy, but radiographic appearances persist.

Barium (Ba): Atomic Number 56 (Baritosis)

Barium is a reactive alkaline earth metal. The most important barium ore is barytes ($BaSO_4$), known as barite in the USA Barium is used as a weighting agent in muds circulated with drilling fluids in oil and gas exploration. It is also used in paints, plastics, engine compartments, friction products for automobiles and trucks, electronics, glass, ceramics and medical applications. Exposure via dust inhalation can occur during the drying and bagging of ground barytes. Barytes in some areas will contain variable and often significant quantities of free silica.

A survey of a barium plant revealed the presence of baritosis in 48% of 118 workers (Levi-Valensi et al., 1966), with an increase in risk related to the duration of employment. Pneumoconiosis in barytes miners is likely to be predominantly silicosis (Seaton et al., 1986).

Pathology

Macroscopic appearances are of discrete grey macules in the pulmonary pleura and cut surface of the lungs; if nodular changes occur, this is usually due to the presence of silica. There is no evidence of fibrosis or confluent massing, and hilar lymph nodes are not enlarged. Microscopically, the appearances are similar to those of stannosis and siderosis. X-ray diffraction or spectrographic methods can identify the mineral if needed.

Symptoms, Radiology and Lung Function

Baritosis is symptomless and causes no abnormal physical signs or changes in lung function. On chest radiography, dense, discrete, small opacities, sometimes with a star-like configuration and usually 2–4 mm in diameter, are distributed fairly evenly throughout the lung fields; they may develop after only a few months of exposure (Pancheri, 1950). Higher or longer exposures may lead to larger opacities; however, there is sometimes a lack of correlation between exposure and radiographic changes (Doig, 1976). Hilar lymph nodes may be opaque but not enlarged and Kerley B-lines are often prominent. The opacities may be difficult to distinguish from nodular silicosis (Doig, 1976).

Prognosis

Gradual clearing of the opacities occurs after exposure has ceased.

Rare Earth Metal Oxides (Lanthanides): Atomic Numbers 57–71

There are 15 metallic chemical elements—lanthanum (57) to lutetium (71)—known as the 'lanthanides'. The chemically similar elements scandium and yttrium make up the rare earth group; their uses are varied and widespread (Table 20.1).

Pathology

Lanthanides are associated with a lung disease known as 'rare earth pneumoconiosis'. This condition has been reported in workers who have been exposed to carbon arc

TABLE 20.1
Rare Earth Metals and Their Uses

Rare Earths (Lanthanides)	Exposures and Uses
Lanthanum (La)	Catalysts, carbon lighting, electrodes, ceramics with superconducting properties
Cerium (Ce)	Polishing lenses, mirrors, prisms, fireworks, cigarette lighter flints, ceramics, carbon arc electrodes
Praseodymium (Pr)	Magnets, aircraft engines, glass, lighters
Neodymium (Nd)	Laser crystals, magnets
Promethium (Pm)	Research applications (radioactive)
Samarium (Sm)	Samarium–cobalt magnets, catalysts, treatment of cancer (radioactive)
Europium (Eu)	Optoelectronics, fluorescent glass
Gadolinium (Gd)	Ceramics with superconducting properties, magnetic resonance imaging
Terbium (Tb)	Magnetic devices in computers, fuel cells
Dysprosium (Dy)	Laser crystals, computer disks
Holmium (Ho)	Laser crystals, magnets, microwave equipment
Erbium (Er)	Photographic and glass filters, lasers
Thulium (Tm)	Radiation source in portable X-rays, lasers
Ytterbium (Yb)	Source of γ-rays, nuclear medicine
Lutetium (Lu)	Metal alloys, catalysts, nuclear medicine
Scandium (Sc)	Aluminium alloys
Yttrium (Y)	Magnetic devices in computers, light-emitting diodes, cathode ray tubes

lamp fumes and among lens polishers exposed to cerium oxide powder (Waring and Watling, 1990; McDonald et al., 1995).

Case reports range from lanthanides as a cause of granulomatous lesions to progressive fibrotic lung changes that are indistinguishable from usual interstitial pneumonitis on histology (McDonald et al., 1995). Scanning electron microscopy with energy-dispersive X-ray analysis can be used for mineral particle identification (Sulotto et al., 1986). High levels of lanthanides can be found in bronchoalveolar lavage fluid and tissue many years after the cessation of exposure (Dufresne et al., 1994). A single report describes dendriform pulmonary ossification in association with rare earth pneumoconiosis (Yoon et al., 2005).

Symptoms, Radiology and Lung Function

Symptoms vary from asymptomatic chest radiographs with nodular changes to progressive breathlessness associated with fibrotic radiographic changes (Sulotto et al., 1986; McDonald et al., 1995). Various pulmonary function impairments have been described, from restrictive (Sulotto et al., 1986) to mixed restricted and obstructive disorders.

Prognosis

The few cases of rare earth pneumoconiosis in the literature suggest bio-persistence of lanthanides with little to no radiographic or clinical regression in most cases (Sulotto et al., 1986).

Bismuth (Bi): Atomic Number 83

Bismuth salts are used in medicines, glass pigments, ceramics and alloys. No cases of pneumoconiosis are reported from occupational dust exposure. A single case is described of small, metallic, punctate opacities on chest radiograph throughout the lungs and with subpleural distribution on chest tomography occurring 2 years after a bismuth-based injection (Addrizzo-Harris et al., 1997); bismuth was recovered in this case from bronchoalveolar lavage.

Uranium (U): Atomic Number 92

Uranium is a radioactive metal that is found naturally in minute quantities throughout the environment. Uranium breaks down to radon gas, which is causally associated with lung cancer. Archer et al. (1998) described a series of five uranium miners with advanced pulmonary fibrosis and little evidence of silicosis from lung biopsies, and concludes that the predominant injurious agents in these workers were α-particles from radon decay.

Further strong evidence for excess mortality due to pneumoconiosis is described in the NIOSH uranium miners health study (Roscoe et al., 1995), although confounding exposure to silica is likely to have occurred. In 2004, the National Institute of Occupational Safety and Health (NIOSH) (Pinkerton et al., 2004) again described an increased risk of mortality in uranium millers from pneumoconiosis and emphysema, but again could not estimate individual exposures to uranium, silica and vanadium and thus could not show conclusively that the deaths were due to uranium milling.

MINERALS AND PNEUMOCONIOSIS

Many minerals that are in common use do not themselves cause pneumoconiosis. Where pneumoconiosis in relation to their use is described, it is often related to contamination by silica or quartz. A summary of the radiographic changes associated with the use of the more common minerals is provided in Table 20.2; kaolin, mica and talc are exceptions to the rule and are discussed in further detail.

Kaolin (China Clay)

Kaolin is a common clay that is mainly composed of kaolinite (hydrated aluminium silicate) and is used in the manufacture of china, porcelain, paper, rubber and paints. Kaolin commonly contains varying amounts of other minerals, including quartz, feldspar and mica. Exposures can thus depend on the amount of mineral contamination, which relates to the nature of the deposit where kaolin is found and the way it is extracted.

The risk of kaolinite pneumoconiosis increases with the dryness of the material handled and cumulative years of exposure (Wagner et al., 1986).

Pathology

Two pathological patterns that are seen in china clay and stone producers are of nodular fibrosis and interstitial fibrosis (Wagner et al., 1986), with a high quartz content being associated with a nodular pattern and high kaolinite dust with interstitial fibrosis.

Symptoms, Lung Function and Radiographic Changes

Cough and dyspnoea have been reported, although the former is reported mainly in smokers (23%) (Oldham, 1983). Wagner et al. (1986) describes 13 cases of progressive massive fibrosis on chest radiography in 39 china

TABLE 20.2
Non-Fibrogenic Minerals

Mineral	Exposures and Uses	Pneumoconiosis and Radiographic Changes
Portland cement	Heated limestone (calcium oxide) ground with gypsum 'Blast furnace' cement contains blast furnace slag 'Fly-ash' cement contains 40% fly-ash Exposure occurs during manufacture	1% prevalence of small, irregular radiographic opacities and 2% pleural abnormalities are described in Portland cement workers (Abrons et al., 1997) with no pulmonary fibrosis Silicotic nodules and conglomerate masses are reported where quartz contamination is over 2% (Doerr, 1952; Prosperi and Barsi, 1957) Blast furnace slag may contain tridymite and cristobalite, increasing the risk of silicosis
Fullers earth	Clay-based fibrous silicates used to absorb oil or animal waste	Sepiolite: small opacities (mainly rounded but can be irregular) grade 0/1 to 1/1 reported in process workers (Gamble et al., 1988) Lung function decline without radiographic change is reported in Spanish sepiolite plant workers (McConnochie et al., 1993) Attapulgite: one case report of pulmonary fibrosis (Sors et al., 1979) Montmorillonite: one case report of pulmonary fibrosis (Gibbs and Pooley, 1994) Mortality studies of attapulgite millers and miners show no increase in mortality from non-malignant respiratory disease (Waxweller et al., 1988)
Gypsum ($CaSO_4.2H_2O$)	Recovered by low-temperature calcination after mining Used in cement, mortar, boarding, plaster, blocks, fertiliser and alabaster When heated, becomes plaster of Paris Large crystals are selenite	No pneumoconiosis reported from pure gypsum exposure; no lung function abnormalities Mild silicosis or mixed-dust fibrosis in gypsum miners are due to quartz contamination (Oakes et al., 1982)
Limestone ($CaCO_3$)	Calicite and aragonite ($CaCO_3$) Chalk is over 90% calcium carbonate	Exposure to limestone containing less than 1% quartz does not cause radiographic or lung function abnormalities (Bridge Davis and Nagelschmidt, 1956) If contaminated with flint or quartz, there is a risk of silicosis (Doig, 1955)
Marble, calcite ($CaCO_3$) Dolomite ($MgCO_3CaCO_3$)	Quarried, polished, sculptured and ground	White marble (99% pure) does not cause pneumoconiosis Impurities may include talc, tremolite, wollastonite, haematite and quartz ranging from 1% to 50% Marble pneumoconiosis case reports (Leikin et al., 2009) describe features of silicosis with restrictive lung disease, silicotic nodules and progressive massive fibrosis
Perlite (volcanic amorphous alumina–silicate rock; $SiO_2.Al_2O_3$)	Mined, crushed, dried and screened; used in horticulture, sandblasting and metal finishing	No evidence of pneumoconiosis in perlite workers, but where pneumoconiosis is described, other exposures have occurred (Cooper, 1975; Maxim et al., 2014)

clay ('kaolin') and china stone ('petuntse') producers, and 22 cases of simple pneumoconiosis. Radiological signs are reported after more than 5 years of exposure to kaolin in dust-drying plants (Sheers, 1964). Smoking was not related to the radiographic changes (Altekruse et al., 1984; Wagner et al., 1986). A greater loss in vital capacity has been associated with increasing radiological pneumoconiosis (Oldham, 1983).

Prognosis

There is no evidence of regression of radiological changes upon removal from exposure (Oldham, 1983).

Mica

Mica is a group of sheet minerals that is largely obtained as a by-product from the mining of other minerals, such as kaolin. It is used as a filler, added to drilling fluid and in paints. Sericite (muscovite) is a variety of mica.

An extensive literature review (Skulberg et al., 1985) reported only a few cases of respiratory disease from mica alone and inadequate animal data, concluding that pure mica is moderately toxic and may induce pneumoconiosis.

Pathology

Algranti et al. (2005) found that 52% of 44 sericite process workers had radiographic evidence of pneumoconiosis. Histology shows irregular interstitial fibrosis with mixed fibrotic lesions, macules and nodules and foreign-body giant cells containing strongly birefringent particles.

Symptoms, Radiology and Lung Function

Chest radiographic changes range from pure nodular pneumoconiosis to severe interstitial fibrosis. Most cases have rounded opacities of category 0/1 or more (Algranti et al., 2005). A mean of 17 years of exposure and 23 years of latency is described, although one case had an exposure of 1.4 years. Most publications report over 5 years of exposure before radiographic change is seen (Skulberg et al., 1985).

On spirometry, loss of forced expiratory volume in 1 second (FEV_1) and forced vital capacity (FVC) and reductions of both FEV_1 and FVC have been found, although most cases report restriction (Davies and Cotton, 1983).

Prognosis

Clinical and radiographic deterioration despite removal from exposure are described in some cases (Davies and Cotton, 1983).

Talc

Talc is a mineral composite of magnesium silicate. It is used in paints, pharmaceuticals, cosmetics and ceramics.

Pathology

Of 17 cases of talc pneumoconiosis, two were found to contain substantial quantities of quartz and several contained mica and kaolin. Tremolite fibres were found in two cases and amosite and crocidolite fibres in one; thus, 'talcosis' represents disease that is associated with a variety of minerals (Gibbs et al., 1992). Granulomatous changes, chronic interstitial lung fibrosis of varying severity (including progressive massive fibrosis) and asbestos bodies have been reported, along with birefringent dust-laden macrophages seen under polarised light. Pleural plaques and diffuse pleural thickening are also seen in talc workers (Gamble et al., 1979).

Symptoms, Radiology and Lung Function

Small, rounded and irregular opacities are described in the case literature, along with large opacities of greater than 1 cm affecting upper, middle and lower zones. Septal lines and emphysema are found in all lung zones on computed tomography, as are enlarged lymph nodes and pleural plaques (Akira et al., 2007). The changes described might be due to talc or the contaminants of the talc, such as quartz and asbestos. Associated symptoms are cough, breathlessness and sputum production.

On lung function measurement, a mixed obstructive and restrictive picture is seen, with significant decreases in FEV_1 and FVC associated with increasing dust exposure. Wild et al. (1995) report no relationship between smoking and dust effects.

Prognosis

Most texts describe progressive disease despite removal from exposure. Mortality from non-malignant respiratory disease increases with cumulative talc exposure (Wild et al., 2002).

Vermiculite

Vermiculite is a mica-like silicate that is used as a soil additive, insulating material and chemical carrier. There are no reports of vermiculite exposure alone causing respiratory disease; however, case reports of asbestosis (Howard, 2003) due to asbestos (tremolite) contamination of vermiculite have been recorded (Wright et al., 2002).

Man-Made Vitreous Fibres

Man-made vitreous fibres (MMVFs) are made from glass, rock, slag, kaolin and ceramic; the type of 'wool' produced refers to the starting material (e.g. rockwool). The MMVF group also includes refractory ceramic fibres. MMVFs are altered during manufacture by the addition of binding agents, oils, lubricants and resins, which differ between manufacturers and the requirements of the end product.

Respirable fibres can be released during the production and handling of these products; the retention times and deposition of the fibres in the respiratory tract have been studied in detail due to the similarities drawn between them and asbestos. MMVFs were found in 28 out of 112 lung samples from exposed workers (McDonald et al., 1990), but at low concentrations. The World Health Organisation (WHO, 1988) concluded that

MMVF exposure was 'possibly' carcinogenic in animal studies (category 2B) and a subsequent review (De Vuyst et al., 1995) of all evidence, and concluded that there is no firm evidence that MMVF exposure is associated with pulmonary fibrosis in humans. Contaminants in the workplace, such as asbestos, talc and silica, need to be taken into account when assessing lung disease associated with MMVFs.

REFERENCES

Abrons, H. L., Petersen, M. R., Sanderson, W. T., Engelberg, A. L. and Harber, P. 1997. Chest radiography in Portland cement workers. *J Occup Environ Med* 39:1047–54.

Addrizzo-Harris, D. J., Churg, A. and Rom, W. N. 1997. Radio-opaque punctate opacities on the chest radiograph following intravenous injection of a bismuth compound. *Thorax* 52:303–4.

Akira, M., Kozuka, T., Yamamoto, S., Sakatani, M. and Morinaga, K. 2007. Inhalational talc pneumoconiosis: Radiographic and CT findings in 14 patients. *AJR Am J Roentgenol* 188:326–33.

Algranti, E., Handar, A. M., Dumortier, P., Mendonca, E. M., Rodrigues, G. L., Santos, A. M., Mauad, T. et al. 2005. Pneumoconiosis after sericite inhalation. *Occup Environ Med* 62:e2.

Altekruse, E. B., Chaudhary, B. A., Pearson, M. G. and Morgan, W. K. 1984. Kaolin dust concentrations and pneumoconiosis at a kaolin mine. *Thorax* 39:436–41.

Archer, V. E., Renzetti, A. D., Doggett, R. S., Jarvis, J. Q. and Colby, T. V. 1998. Chronic diffuse interstitial fibrosis of the lung in uranium miners. *J Occup Environ Med* 40:460–74.

Barrie, H. J. and Harding, H. E. 1947. Argyro-siderosis of the lungs in silver finishers. *Br J Ind Med* 4:225–9.

Bartter, T., Irwin, R. S., Abraham, J. L., Dascal, A., Nash, G., Himmelstein, J. S. and Jederlinic, P. J. 1991. Zirconium compound-induced pulmonary fibrosis. *Arch Intern Med* 151:1197–201.

Billings, C. G. and Howard, P. 1993. Occupational siderosis and welders' lung: A review. *Monaldi Arch Chest Dis* 48:304–14.

Bridge Davis, S. and Nagelschmidt, G. 1956. A report on the absence of pneumoconiosis among workers in pure limestone. *Br J Ind Med* 13:6–8.

Chen, J. L. and Fayerweather, W. E. 1988. Epidemiologic study of workers exposed to titanium dioxide. *J Occup Med* 30:937–42.

Chen, W. J., Monnat, R. J. Jr., Chen, M. and Mottet, N. K. 1978. Aluminum induced pulmonary granulomatosis. *Hum Pathol* 9:705–11.

Chonan, T., Taguchi, O. and Omae, K. 2007. Interstitial pulmonary disorders in indium-processing workers. *Eur Respir J* 29:317–24.

Cooper, D. A., Pendergrass, E. P., Vorwald, A. J., Mayock, R. L. and Brieger, H. 1968. Pneumoconiosis among workers in an antimony industry. *Am J Roentgenol Radium Ther Nucl Med* 103:496–508.

Cooper, W. C. 1975. Radiographic survey of perlite workers. *J Occup Med* 17:304–7.

Cummings, K. J., Donat, W. E., Ettensohn, D. B., Roggli, V. L., Ingram, P. and Kreiss, K. 2010. Pulmonary alveolar proteinosis in workers at an indium processing facility. *Am J Respir Crit Care Med* 181:458–64.

Cummings, K. J., Nakano, M., Omae, K., Takeuchi, K., Chonan, T., Xiao, Y. L., Harley, R. A. et al. 2012. Indium lung disease. *Chest* 141:1512–21.

Davies, D. and Cotton, R. 1983. Mica pneumoconiosis. *Br J Ind Med* 40:22–7.

De Vuyst, P., Dumortier, P., Swaen, G. M., Pairon, J. C. and Brochard, P. 1995. Respiratory health effects of man-made vitreous (mineral) fibres. *Eur Respir J* 8:2149–73.

Doerr, W. 1952. [Pneumoconiosis caused by cement dust]. *Virchows Arch* 322:397–427.

Doig, A. T. 1955. Disabling pneumoconiosis from limestone dust. *Br J Ind Med* 12:206–16.

Doig, A. T. 1976. Baritosis: A benign pneumoconiosis. *Thorax* 31:30–9.

Dufresne, A., Krier, G., Muller, J. F., Case, B. and Perrault, G. 1994. Lanthanide particles in the lung of a printer. *Sci Total Environ* 151:249–52.

Duggan, M. J., Soilleux, P. J., Strong, J. C. and Howell, D. M. 1970. The exposure of United Kingdom miners to radon. *Br J Ind Med* 27:106–9.

Ferin, J. and Oberdorster, G. 1985. Biological effects and toxicity assessment of titanium dioxides: Anatase and rutile. *Am Ind Hyg Assoc J* 46:69–72.

Ferin, J., Oberdorster, G. and Penney, D. P. 1992. Pulmonary retention of ultrafine and fine particles in rats. *Am J Respir Cell Mol Biol* 6:535–42.

Gamble, J., Sieber, W. K., Wheeler, R. W., Reger, R. and Hall, B. 1988. A cross-sectional study of U.S. attapulgite workers. *Ann Occup Hyg* 32:475–81.

Gamble, J. F., Fellner, W. and Dimeo, M. J. 1979. An epidemiologic study of a group of talc workers. *Am Rev Respir Dis* 119:741–53.

Garabrant, D. H., Fine, L. J., Oliver, C., Bernstein, L. and Peters, J. M. 1987. Abnormalities of pulmonary function and pleural disease among titanium metal production workers. *Scand J Work Environ Health* 13:47–51.

Gibbs, A. E., Pooley, F. D., Griffiths, D. M., Mitha, R., Craighead, J. E. and Ruttner, J. R. 1992. Talc pneumoconiosis: A pathologic and mineralogic study. *Hum Pathol* 23:1344–54.

Gibbs, A. R. and Pooley, F. D. 1994. Fuller's earth (montmorillonite) pneumoconiosis. *Occup Environ Med* 51:644–6.

Giraldo, L. F., Bastidas, A. R., Benavides, M., Garcia, R. and Ojeda, P. 2013. Neumoconiosis ocupacional por oxido de estano. *Acta Med Colomb* 38:273–6.

Gross, P., Westrick, M. L. and McNerney, N. J. 1960. Experimental silicosis: The inhibitory effect of iron. *Dis Chest* 37:35–41.

Hamaguchi, T., Omae, K., Takebayashi, T., Kikuchi, Y., Yoshioka, N., Nishiwaki, Y., Tanaka, A. et al. 2008.

Exposure to hardly soluble indium compounds in Ito production and recycling plants is a new risk for interstitial lung damage. *Occup Environ Med* 65:51–5.

Harding, H. E., Grout, J. L. and Davies, T. A. 1947. The experimental production of X-ray shadows in the lungs by inhalation of industrial dusts; iron oxide. *Br J Ind Med* 4:223–32.

Homma, T., Ueno, T., Sekizawa, K., Tanaka, A. and Hirata, M. 2003. Interstitial pneumonia developed in a worker dealing with particles containing indium–tin oxide. *J Occup Health* 45:137–9.

Howard, T. P. 2003. Pneumoconiosis in a vermiculite end-product user. *Am J Ind Med* 44:214–7.

Hull, M. J. and Abraham, J. L. 2002. Aluminum welding fume-induced pneumoconiosis. *Hum Pathol* 33:819–25.

Huvinen, M., Uitti, J., Zitting, A., Roto, P., Virkola, K., Kuikka, P., Laippala, P. et al. 1996. Respiratory health of workers exposed to low levels of chromium in stainless steel production. *Occup Environ Med* 53:741–7.

Jederlinic, P. J., Abraham, J. L., Churg, A., Himmelstein, J. S., Epler, G. R. and Gaensler, E. A. 1990. Pulmonary fibrosis in aluminum oxide workers. Investigation of nine workers, with pathologic examination and microanalysis in three of them. *Am Rev Respir Dis* 142:1179–84.

Kanisawa, M. and Schroeder, H. A. 1969. Life term studies on the effect of trace elements on spontaneous tumors in mice and rats. *Cancer Res* 29:892–5.

Kiviluoto, M. 1980. Observations on the lungs of vanadium workers. *Br J Ind Med* 37:363–6.

Kleinfeld, M., Messite, J., Kooyman, O. and Shapiro, J. 1969. Welders' siderosis. A clinical, roentgenographic, and physiological study. *Arch Environ Health* 19:70–3.

Klucik, I., Juck, A. and Gruberova, J. 1962. [Respiratory and pulmonary lesions caused by antimony trioxide dust]. *Prac Lek* 14:363–8.

Koponen, M., Gustafsson, T., Kalliomaki, K., Kalliomaki, P. L., Moilanen, M. and Pyy, L. 1980. Dusts in a steel-making plant. Lung contamination among iron workers. *Int Arch Occup Environ Health* 47:35–45.

Lee, K. P., Trochimowicz, H. J. and Reinhardt, C. F. 1985. Pulmonary response of rats exposed to titanium dioxide (TiO_2) by inhalation for two years. *Toxicol Appl Pharmacol* 79:179–92.

Leikin, E., Zickel-Shalom, K., Balabir-Gurman, A., Goralnik, L. and Valdovsky, E. 2009. [Caplan's syndrome in marble workers as occupational disease]. *Harefuah* 148:524–6, 572.

Levi-Valensi, P., Drif, M., Dat, A. and Hadjadj, G. 1966. [Apropos of 57 cases of pulmonary baritosis. (Results of a systematic investigation in a baryta factory)]. *J Fr Med Chir Thorac* 20:443–55.

Liippo, K. K., Anttila, S. L., Taikina-Aho, O., Ruokonen, E. L., Toivonen, S. T. and Tuomi, T. 1993. Hypersensitivity pneumonitis and exposure to zirconium silicate in a young ceramic tile worker. *Am Rev Respir Dis* 148:1089–92.

Lindenschmidt, R. C., Driscoll, K. E., Perkins, M. A., Higgins, J. M., Maurer, J. K. and Belfiore, K. A. 1990. The comparison of a fibrogenic and two nonfibrogenic dusts by bronchoalveolar lavage. *Toxicol Appl Pharmacol* 102:268–81.

Maatta, K. and Arstila, A. U. 1975. Pulmonary deposits of titanium dioxide in cytologic and lung biopsy specimens. Light and electron microscopic X-ray analysis. *Lab Invest* 33:342–6.

Marcus, R. L., Turner, S. and Cherry, N. M. 1996. A study of lung function and chest radiographs in men exposed to zirconium compounds. *Occup Med (Lond)* 46:109–13.

Maxim, D., Neibo, R., McConnell E. 2014. Perlite toxicity and epidemiology—A review. *Inhal Toxicol* 26:259–70.

McCallum, R. I. 1967. Detection of antimony in process workers' lungs by X-radiation. *Trans Soc Occup Med* 17:134–8.

McCallum, R. I. and Leathart, G. L. 1975. Pneumoconiosis in zirconium process workers. *XVIII International Congress on Occupational Health*. Brighton, England. 14–19 September 1975.

McConnochie, K., Bevan, C., Newcombe, R. G., Lyons, J., Skidmore, J. W. and Wagner, J. C. 1993. A study of Spanish sepiolite workers. *Thorax* 48:370–374.

McDonald, J. C., Case, B. W., Enterline, P. E., Henderson, V., McDonald, A. D., Plourde, M. and Sebastien, P. 1990. Lung dust analysis in the assessment of past exposure of man-made mineral fibre workers. *Ann Occup Hyg* 34:427–41.

McDonald, J. W., Ghio, A. J., Sheehan, C. E., Bernhardt, P. F. and Roggli, V. L. 1995. Rare earth (cerium oxide) pneumoconiosis: Analytical scanning electron microscopy and literature review. *Mod Pathol* 8:859–65.

Miller, R. R., Churg, A. M., Hutcheon, M. and Lom, S. 1984. Pulmonary alveolar proteinosis and aluminum dust exposure. *Am Rev Respir Dis* 130:312–5.

Mitchell, J., Manning, G. B., Molyneux, M. and Lane, R. E. 1961. Pulmonary fibrosis in workers exposed to finely powdered aluminium. *Br J Ind Med* 18:10–23.

Muir, D. C., Julian, J., Jadon, N., Roberts, R., Roos, J., Chan, J., Maehle, W. et al. 1993. Prevalence of small opacities in chest radiographs of nickel sinter plant workers. *Br J Ind Med* 50:428–31.

Nakano, M., Omae, K., Tanaka, A., Hirata, M., Michikawa, T., Kikuchi, Y., Yoshioka, N. et al. 2009. Causal relationship between indium compound inhalation and effects on the lungs. *J Occup Health* 51:513–21.

Nemery, B. 1990. Metal toxicity and the respiratory tract. *Eur Respir J* 3:202–19.

Neuhauser, I., Rubin, L., Slepyan, A. H. and Weber, L. F. 1956. Granulomas of the axillas caused by deodorants. *J Am Med Assoc* 162:953–5.

NIOSH, 2011. *Current Intelligence Bulletin 63: Occupational Exposure to Titanium Dioxide*. April 2011, 2011–160.

Nolan, R. P., Langer, A. M., Weisman, I. and Herson, G. B. 1987. Surface character and membranolytic activity of rutile and anatase: Two titanium dioxide polymorphs. *Br J Ind Med* 44:687–98.

Oakes, D., Douglas, R., Knight, K., Wusteman, M. and McDonald, J. C. 1982. Respiratory effects of prolonged exposure to gypsum dust. *Ann Occup Hyg* 26:833–40.

Oldham, P. D. 1983. Pneumoconiosis in Cornish china clay workers. *Br J Ind Med* 40:131–7.

Oleru, U. G. 1987. Respiratory and nonrespiratory morbidity in a titanium oxide paint factory in Nigeria. *Am J Ind Med* 12:173–80.

Pancheri, G. 1950. [Forms of pneumoconiosis especially studied in Italy; thiopneumoconiosis and baritosis]. *Med Lav* 41:73–7.

Park, T., Dibenedetto, R., Morgan, K., Colmers, R. and Sherman, E. 1984. Diffuse endobronchial polyposis following a titanium tetrachloride inhalation injury. *Am Rev Respir Dis* 130:315–7.

Pinkerton, L. E., Bloom, T. F., Hein, M. J. and Ward, E. M. 2004. Mortality among a cohort of uranium mill workers: An update. *Occup Environ Med* 61:57–64.

Potkonjak, V. and Pavlovich, M. 1983. Antimoniosis: A particular form of pneumoconiosis. I. Etiology, clinical and X-ray findings. *Int Arch Occup Environ Health* 51:199–207.

Prosperi, G. and Barsi, C. 1957. [Pneumoconiosis in cement workers]. *Rass Med Ind Ig Lav* 26:16–24.

Redline, S., Barna, B. P., Tomashefski, J. F. Jr. and Abraham, J. L. 1986. Granulomatous disease associated with pulmonary deposition of titanium. *Br J Ind Med* 43:652–6.

Renes, L. E. 1953. Antimony poisoning in industry. *AMA Arch Ind Hyg Occup Med* 7:99–108.

Robertson, A. J. 1960. *Pneumoconiosis Due to Tin Oxide. Symposium on Industrial Pulmonary Diseases.* In E. J. King and C. M. Fletcher (Eds). Boston: Little Brown. 168–184.

Roels, H., Lauwerys, R., Buchet, J. P., Genet, P., Sarhan, M. J., Hanotiau, I., DE Fays, M. et al. 1987. Epidemiological survey among workers exposed to manganese: Effects on lung, central nervous system, and some biological indices. *Am J Ind Med* 11:307–27.

Roscoe, R. J., Deddens, J. A., Salvan, A. and Schnorr, T. M. 1995. Mortality among Navajo uranium miners. *Am J Public Health* 85:535–40.

Schmitz-Moormann, P., Hoerlein, H. and Hanefeld, F. 1964. [Lung changes in exposure to titanium dioxide dust]. *Beitr Silikoseforsch Pneumokoniose* 80:1–17.

Seaton, A., Ruckley, V. A., Addison, J. and Brown, W. R. 1986. Silicosis in barium miners. *Thorax* 41:591–5.

Shaver, C. G. and Riddell, A. R. 1947. Lung changes associated with the manufacture of alumina abrasives. *J Ind Hyg Toxicol* 29:145–57.

Sheers, G. 1964. Prevalence of pneumoconiosis in Cornish Kaolin workers. *Br J Ind Med* 21(3):218–25.

Shi, Z. C. 1986. Acute nickel carbonyl poisoning: A report of 179 cases. *Br J Ind Med* 43:422–4.

Sjoberg, S. G. 1950. Vanadium pentoxide dust; a clinical and experimental investigation on its effect after inhalation. *Acta Med Scand Suppl* 238:1–188.

Sjogren, B. and Ulfvarson, U. 1985. Respiratory symptoms and pulmonary function among welders working with aluminum, stainless steel and railroad tracks. *Scand J Work Environ Health* 11:27–32.

Skulberg, K. R., Gylseth, B., Skaug, V. and Hanoa, R. 1985. Mica pneumoconiosis—A literature review. *Scand J Work Environ Health* 11:65–74.

Sluis-Cremer, G. K. and Du Toit, R. S. 1968. Pneumoconiosis in chromite miners in South Africa. *Br J Ind Med* 25:63–7.

Sors, H., Gaudichet, A., Sebastien, P., Bignon, J. and Even, P. 1979. Lung fibrosis after inhalation of fibrous attapulgite. *Thorax* 34:695–6.

Stern, R. M., Pigott, G. H. and Abraham, J. L. 1983. Fibrogenic potential of welding fumes. *J Appl Toxicol* 3:18–30.

Sulotto, F., Romano, C., Berra, A., Botta, G. C., Rubino, G. F., Sabbioni, E. and Pietra, R. 1986. Rare-earth pneumoconiosis: A new case. *Am J Ind Med* 9:567–75.

Tanaka, A., Hoirata, M., Omura, M., Inoue, N., Ueno, T., Homma, T. and Sekizawa, K. 2002. Pulmonary toxicity of indium-tin oxide and indium phosphide after intratracheal installations into the lung of hamsters. A short communication. *J Occup Health* 44:99–102.

Trouiller, B., Reliene R., Westbrook, A., Solaimani, P., and Schiestl, R. H. 2009. Titanium dioxide nanoparticles induce DNA damage and genetic instability *in vivo* in mice. *Cancer Res* 69:8784–9.

Vallyathan, V., Bergeron, W. N., Robichaux, P. A. and Craighead, J. E. 1982. Pulmonary fibrosis in an aluminum arc welder. *Chest* 81:372–4.

Wagner, J. C., Pooley, F. D., Gibbs, A., Lyons, J., Sheers, G. and Moncrieff, C. B. 1986. Inhalation of china stone and china clay dusts: Relationship between the mineralogy of dust retained in the lungs and pathological changes. *Thorax* 41:190–6.

Waring, P. M. and Watling, R. J. 1990. Rare earth deposits in a deceased movie projectionist. A new case of rare earth pneumoconiosis? *Med J Aust* 153:726–30.

Waxweller, R. J., Zumwalde, M. S., Ness, G. O. and Brown, D. P. 1988. A retrospective cohort mortality study of males mining and milling attapulgite clay. *Am J Ind Med* 13:305–315.

Wehner, A. P., Dagle, G. E. and Busch, R. H. 1984. Pathogenicity of inhaled nickel compounds in hamsters. *IARC Sci Publ* (53):143–51.

Werfel, U., Schneider, J., Rodelsperger, K., Kotter, J., Popp, W., Woitowitz, H. J. and Zieger, G. 1998. Sarcoid granulomatosis after zirconium exposure with multiple organ involvement. *Eur Respir J* 12:750.

White, G. P., JR., Mathias, C. G. and Davin, J. S. 1993. Dermatitis in workers exposed to antimony in a melting process. *J Occup Med* 35:392–5.

World Health Organisation (WHO). 1988. International Agency for Research on Cancer (IARC) Monographs on the Evaluation of Carcinogenic Risks to Humans. Man-Made Mineral Fibres and Radon. Volume 43, 16–23 June 1987.

Wild, P., Leodolter, K., Refregier, M., Schmidt, H., Zidek, T. and Haidinger, G. 2002. A cohort mortality and nested case–control study of French and Austrian talc workers. *Occup Environ Med* 59:98–105.

Wild, P., Refregier, M., Auburtin, G., Carton, B. and Moulin, J. J. 1995. Survey of the respiratory health of the workers of a talc producing factory. *Occup Environ Med* 52:470–7.

Wright, R. S., Abraham, J. L., Harber, P., Burnett, B. R., Morris, P. and West, P. 2002. Fatal asbestosis 50 years after brief high intensity exposure in a vermiculite expansion plant. *Am J Respir Crit Care Med* 165:1145–9.

Wyers, H. 1946. Some toxic effects of vanadium pentoxide. *Br J Ind Med* 3:177–82.

Xu, Z., Brown, L. M., Pan, G. W., Liu, T. F., Gao, G. S., Stone, B. J., Cao, R. M. et al. 1996. Cancer risks among iron and steel workers in Anshan, China, part II: Case–control studies of lung and stomach cancer. *Am J Ind Med* 30:7–15.

Yamadori, I., Ohsumi, S. and Taguchi, K. 1986. Titanium dioxide deposition and adenocarcinoma of the lung. *Acta Pathol Jpn* 36:783–90.

Yoon, H. K., Moon, H. S., Park, S. H., Song, J. S., Lim, Y. and Kohyama, N. 2005. Dendriform pulmonary ossification in patient with rare earth pneumoconiosis. *Thorax* 60:701–3.

21 Occupational Lung Carcinogens

R. William Field and Rafael E. de la Hoz

CONTENTS

INTRODUCTION

Lung cancer is clearly established as one of the most important causes of morbidity and mortality, as well as the leading occupationally related cancer type (Ferlay et al., 2013). Many of the occupational factors causally related to lung cancer are amongst the most prevalent workplace exposures worldwide. The primary objective of this chapter is to provide an overview of the occupational agents and exposures listed by the International Agency for Research on Cancer (IARC) as known human lung carcinogens (IARC, 2012b). Supplementary new information, with a focus on analytic epidemiologic studies that have become available since IARC's most recent evaluations, will also be discussed.

OCCUPATIONAL LUNG CARCINOGENS: GENERAL CONSIDERATIONS

Several agents and occupational exposures are well recognized as lung carcinogens, with a body of supporting epidemiological and mechanistic scientific studies. Although these occupational lung carcinogens rarely, if ever, match the carcinogenic potency (and, other than radon, the exposure prevalence) of tobacco smoke, their contribution to the occupational burden of lung cancer morbidity and mortality is greatly enhanced by their often more than additive, if not overtly synergistic effect on tobacco carcinogenicity. In fact, the National Comprehensive Cancer Network (NCCN) guidelines recommend consideration of 'low'-radiation dose computed tomography screening beginning at age 50 for individuals with at least 20 pack-years of exposure if they have documented high radon exposure or substantial exposure to other occupational lung carcinogens, including silica, cadmium, asbestos, arsenic, beryllium, chromium, diesel fumes, nickel, coal smoke and soot (NCCN, 2014).

Multiple national and international agencies and entities strive to provide a continuously updated scientific knowledge base on carcinogens. The leading entity among them is the IARC, an agency of the World Health Organization (WHO), which assembles international working groups of experts in order to evaluate the carcinogenicity of a wide range of human exposures. This chapter focuses on those agents that are both lung carcinogens and occur in the occupational setting and are classified by IARC as 'carcinogenic to humans' (Group 1). These can be grouped into five major categories: (1) dust and fibres (asbestos, which causes both bronchogenic carcinoma and mesothelioma, is covered in Chapters 16 and 17); (2) chemicals and mixtures; (3) ionizing radiation; (4) metals; and (5) occupations and manufacturing processes not specified for the specific carcinogen involved.

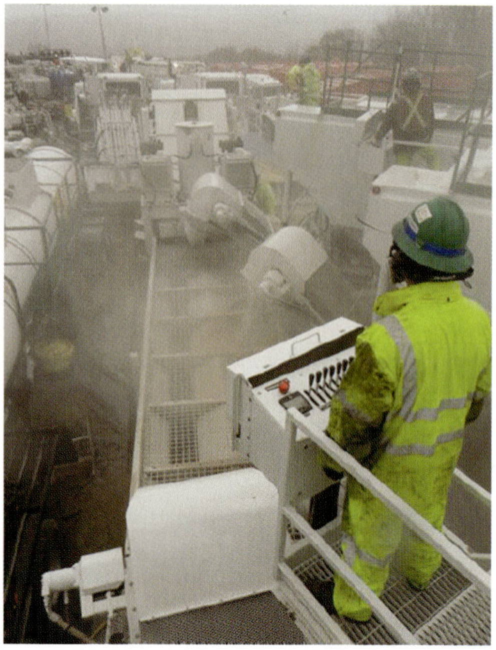

FIGURE 21.1 Silica dust generated as worker conducts sand transfer operations for hydraulic fracturing. Photo shows sand mover and transfer system. (Photo credit: NIOSH, https://www.osha.gov/dts/hazardalerts/hydraulic_frac_hazard_alert.html)

IARC GROUP 1 OCCUPATIONAL LUNG CARCINOGENS: DUST AND FIBRES

Silica Dust, Crystalline

General information (e.g. forms and potential for exposure) on silica is presented in Chapter 19. In 2012, IARC reaffirmed its 1997 decision that the scientific evidence supported the listing of crystalline silica as a known human carcinogen (Group 1) (IARC, 2012b). To date, there have been over 100 epidemiological studies examining the association between silica exposure and lung cancer due in part to the large population of workers at risk, the public health significance of silica exposure and the challenge of adjusting for confounding, coupled with silica's relatively low relative risk (RR). The major industrial settings that were relied on by IARC in order to obtain lung cancer risk estimates for silica exposure were: ceramics, diatomaceous earth, ore mining, quarries and sand and gravel operations (Figure 21.1). In its 2012 reaffirmation of the human lung carcinogenicity of silica, IARC noted that the strongest evidence supporting the lung carcinogenicity of crystalline silica was the findings of the ten pooled epidemiologic studies (Steenland et al., 2001), which reported that silica exposure was a strong predictor (i.e. exposure–response) of lung cancer ($p = 0.0001$), as well as the consistency in findings across studies. IARC also noted that numerous meta-analyses (Pelucchi et al. 2006; Erren et al. 2009; Lacasse et al., 2009) from a diverse number of industries also supported an overall effect of crystalline silica dust exposure, even though the industries and individual study designs varied.

There has been ongoing debate as to whether silicosis was an essential precursor of silica-induced lung cancer or simply an indicator of high silica exposure (Checkoway and Franzblau, 2000; Pelucchi et al., 2006; Stayner, 2007; Steenland and Ward, 2014). While the question has not been definitively answered, a 2013 cohort study that included 19,007 Chinese tungsten miners, 7663 iron miners and 7348 pottery workers, as well as detailed information on historical silica exposure and smoking, 546 lung cancer deaths and 5297 cases of silicosis, confirmed a moderate exposure–response association between silica exposure and lung cancer risk, with a higher risk for those with compared to those without silicosis. These findings strongly suggested that silicosis was not a prerequisite for silica-induced lung cancer

(Liu et al., 2013). The researchers also noted that the RR of lung cancer posed by exposure to silica was similar for smokers and non-smokers, and assessed the joint effect of silica exposure and smoking as close to multiplicative. The estimated excess lifetime risk, through to 75 years of age, was 0.51% for workers exposed from ages 20 to 65 years at 0.1 mg/m^3 of silica.

IARC GROUP 1 OCCUPATIONAL LUNG CARCINOGENS: CHEMICALS AND MIXTURES

Bis(Chloromethyl) Ether; Technical-Grade Chloromethyl Methyl Ether

Compared to silica, bis(chloromethyl) ether (BCME) has a higher RR of causing lung cancer, but a much lower population at risk of exposure. In fact, BCME is considered one of the most potent human carcinogens that is known (IARC, 2012b). IARC listed technical-grade chloromethyl methyl ether (CMME) as a Group 1 lung carcinogen along with BCME because the technical grade of CMME contains 1%–8% BCME (HSDB, 2014). While both of the chemicals were manufactured in many countries before 1976, the production of these alkylating agents and chemical intermediates has substantially decreased over time. However, even workers who continue to use these agents in a closed systems have been exposed due to failure to maintain an isolated system (Miles, 1986). Exposure to BCME has also occurred from the burning of mosquito coils containing the synergist or active ingredient octachlorodipropyl ether (Krieger et al., 2003), which is also referred to as S-2. Many countries do not permit registration of octachlorodipropyl, but workers in some countries continue to be exposed to BCME during the production and use of S-2-containing mosquito coils (Krieger et al., 2003; Zhang et al., 2015).

In determining the carcinogenicity of BCME/CMME, IARC relied in part on the findings from four retrospective cohort studies performed in the USA and UK (McCallum et al., 1983; Collingwood et al., 1987; Gowers et al., 1993; Weiss and Nash, 1997) that examined the association between occupational exposure to technical-grade CMME and lung cancer. The epidemiologic findings, as well as the finding of several case studies, convincingly demonstrated that workers exposed to CMME and/or BCME have a significantly increased risk of lung cancer, with standardized mortality ratios (SMR) frequently exceeding 30 for highly exposed workers. Duration of exposure and cumulative exposure both generally increased the lung cancer risk, as well as a general finding that higher exposures shortened the latency period. A distinctly significantly higher proportion of tumours were small-cell carcinomas. Because BCME is an alkylating agent, the mode of action is likely genotoxic.

Coal Tar Pitch

Coal tar pitch is the solid residue remaining from the distillation of coal tars, while the less viscous (i.e. liquid) by-product is referred to as coal tar. The further fractional distillation of crude coal tars yields coal tar creosotes. The National Institute for Occupational Safety and Health (NIOSH) considers coal tar pitch, coal tar and creosote to be coal tar products (NIOSH, 2011). Regardless of source material (e.g. coal composition) and distillation process, which can affect its composition, coal tars are complex hydrocarbon mixtures comprising thousands of compounds composed primarily (90%) of three- to seven-membered polycyclic aromatic hydrocarbons (PAHs) (ATSDR, 2008; IARC, 2010b; NTP, 2011a; IARC, 2012a) and are considered to be the predominant genotoxic carcinogens present in cigarette smoke, as well as other occupational exposures discussed in this chapter.

IARC indicated that there was evidence from experimental data and a finding from a human study that coal tar pitch has a genotoxic mechanism of action (IARC, 2012a). In 2009, IARC concluded—and reaffirmed in 2012 (IARC, 2012a)—that there was sufficient evidence from epidemiological studies of road pavers (Figure 21.2) and roofers to state that occupational exposures in these industries to coal tar pitch causes lung cancer in humans (IARC, 2010b). A systematic review and meta-analysis

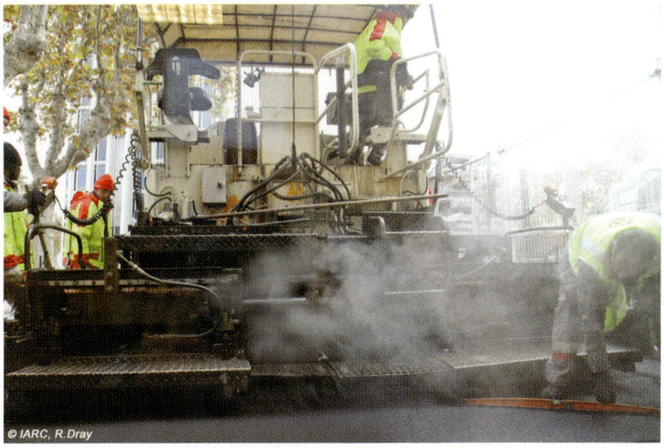

FIGURE 21.2 IARC reaffirmed in 2012 that there was sufficient evidence from epidemiologic studies of road pavers and roofers to conclude that exposures in these industries cause lung cancer in humans. (Copyright IARC, R. Dray.)

of occupational cohort studies published between 2006 and 2014 provided further quantitative support for the lung carcinogenicity of PAHs (Rota et al., 2014a).

Diesel Exhaust

Diesel exhaust contributes significantly to a broad range of occupational air pollutants, including Group 1 and Group 2 lung carcinogens, and the contribution varies by fuel type, engine type and condition, engine load, engine operation and pre-treatment (e.g. particle traps) of the exhaust (McDonald et al., 2011). Diesel exhaust contains both a gaseous component and particulate component including particles, gases, semi-volatile organic compounds (e.g. PAHs) and nitrated and oxygenated PAHs (McDonald et al., 2011; NTP, 2011b; IARC, 2013).

A 2009 review of over 300 publications reported that the highest diesel exhaust exposure was found for underground mining and construction, intermediate exposure for working in aboveground semi-enclosed areas and lowest for working outside or removed from the diesel source (Pronk et al., 2009). Other occupations with an increased risk of diesel exposure include vehicle (e.g. truck, car and bus) drivers and mechanics, airline personnel, railroad workers, ship and dock workers, toll booth attendants, construction workers, bridge and tunnel workers, garage workers, farm workers, heavy equipment operators, tunnel construction workers and firefighters (Figure 21.3).

Diesel exhaust was listed as a probable lung carcinogen (Group 2A) from 1988 (IARC, 1989) and reclassified as a Group 1 carcinogen in 2012 based primarily on occupational cohort studies of non-metal miners, workers in the trucking industry and railroad workers (IARC, 2013). A joint NIOSH and National Cancer Institute (NCI) cohort study composed of 12,315 non-metal mining workers, including quantitative exposure assessment, from eight facilities located in the US states of Missouri, New Mexico, Ohio and Wyoming found an increased SMR for lung cancer (1.26; 95% confidence interval [CI]: 1.09–1.44) as compared to the reference state populations (Attfield et al., 2012; NIOSH, 2012), and a nested case–control study within the above NIOSH/NCI cohort study provided strong evidence of a causal relationship between diesel exposure and lung cancer (Silverman et al., 2012). IARC also provided additional support for listing diesel exhaust as a Group 1 carcinogen by citing US railroad (Laden et al., 2006) and trucking industry (Garshick et al., 2012) studies and a pooled analysis of 11 case–control studies from Europe and Canada.

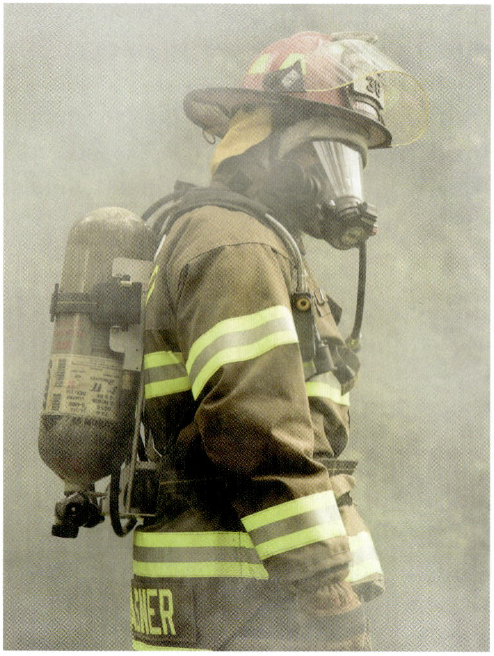

FIGURE 21.3 Some occupations like firefighters are exposed to a variety of known and suspected human lung carcinogens. (Copyright K. Reasner.)

Soot, as Found in Occupational Exposure of Chimney Sweeps

Soot is a carbonaceous by-product material with varying—and frequently unknown—composition generated by the incomplete combustion or pyrolysis of organic materials (i.e. carbon-based materials) such as waste oil, coal, paper, rubber, plastic, household waste and also some fuel oils (IARC, 2012b). Soots, which are not produced commercially, contain up to 60% black and organic carbon as well as inorganic material, chemicals, metals (e.g. arsenic, cadmium, chromium and nickel) and genotoxic (and thus carcinogenic) PAHs (IARC, 2012b).

The ratio of organic carbon to black carbon varies by source material. For example, the average organic carbon to black carbon ratio is approximately 9:1 for biomass burning, 4:1 for biofuel burning and 1:1 for diesel exhaust (EPA, 2012). Black carbon should not be confused with carbon black, which is commercially produced by the controlled combustion or thermal decomposition of acetylene, coal tar residues, natural gas and petroleum oils (Watson and Valberg, 2001; Long et al., 2013). Carbon black, which is classified by IARC as a possible human lung carcinogen (i.e. Group 2B), contains over 97% elemental carbon (IARC, 2010a; Long et al., 2013).

The link between exposure to soot in chimney sweeps and skin (i.e. scrotal) cancer was documented as early as 1775 (Pott, 1775), and chimney sweeps in particular have continued to have a high potential for exposure to soot. Other occupations with enhanced potential for soot exposure include firefighters (Figure 21.3), building demolition personnel, brick masons and helpers, heating/ventilation and air conditioning personnel, metallurgical workers and insulators. IARC relied on both a 1993 Swedish epidemiologic study (Evanoff et al., 1993) and 1995 Finnish epidemiologic study (Pukkala, 1995), which reported increased lung cancer risks for chimney sweeps with adjustment for smoking performed at the group level, in order to form the basis for the listing of soot as known human lung carcinogen (IARC, 2012b). As additional support of its classification of soot as an occupational Group 1 carcinogen, IARC cited a 2009 records linkage study of 5498 male Danish, Finnish, Norwegian and Swedish chimney sweeps that reported a standardized incidence ratio (SIR) of 1.49 (95% CI: 1.30–1.70) (Pukkala et al., 2009). A 2013 update of the 1993 Swedish study above, which included chimney sweeps employed between 1981 and 2006, as well as those included in the 1993 study (i.e. 1918–1980), provided further evidence of an increased risk of lung cancer for chimney sweeps (Hogstedt et al., 2013).

Sulphur Mustard

Sulphur mustard (i.e. bis[2-chloroethyl] sulphide), referred to as mustard gas in the military sector due to its mustard like odour, is a generally colourless chemical warfare agent that is not actually a gas, but rather acts as an aerosol liquid. Mustard gas is well known as a vesicant and bi-functional alkylating agent even at low doses (IARC, 2012b; Gupta, 2015). The potential for exposure to mustard gas includes activities related to the storage and destruction of mustard gas; construction work on military bases where mustard gas was previously released and remained as a contaminant in the soil or in excavated munitions dumps; activities in research laboratories where workers do not take the necessary precautions to prevent exposure; during fishing, when lumps of mustard gas are inadvertently caught in areas where it was historically dumped in the sea; and during armed conflicts, when it is used as a chemical warfare agent.

Mustard gas was first used as a chemical warfare agent by Germany in the First World War, by Ethiopia in 1936, during the Iran–Iraq war from 1984 to 1988 (IOM, 1993) and by Islamic State militants against Kurdish forces in 2015. While mustard gas was not used in the Second World War, the USA exposed thousands of soldiers and sailors to mustard gas during this time period in order to test clothing, equipment and anti-vesicant ointments because of the potential threat of a chemical warfare attack (IOM, 1993; NTP, 2014).

Studies performed in several cohorts of exposed veterans have not demonstrated a statistically significant causal connection between low-level, non-lethal exposures to mustard gas and lung cancer (Norman, 1975; Bullman and Kang, 1994). However, occupational epidemiological studies of mustard gas production workers in Japan (Yamakido et al., 1996), Germany (Weiss and Weiss, 1975), and the UK (Easton et al., 1988) reported elevated lung cancer rates (i.e. SMR ~1.5) for workers with a long duration of exposure. A 2011 cohort study of former workers employed from 1929 to 1945 in a mustard gas production facility in Japan (Doi et al., 2011) reported elevated RRs for lung cancer and concluded that mustard gas exposure decreased the age of occurrence of lung cancer and that risk decreased with age. Sulphur mustard has an unclear association with human laryngeal cancer.

IARC GROUP 1 OCCUPATIONAL LUNG CARCINOGENS: IONIZING RADIATION

Ionizing radiation occurs either in the form of electromagnetic rays (i.e. X-rays and γ-rays) or particles (i.e. α-particles, β-particles and neutrons). As ionizing radiation passes through tissues, it can lose energy, disrupt chemical bonds and remove electrons from molecules, ultimately resulting in radical formation (i.e. ionization). Although the following discussion will focus on lung cancer, ionizing radiation is associated with cancer of multiple organs (NRC, 2006).

Ionizing Radiation: α-Particles

IARC has classified all internalized radionuclides that emit α-particles (e.g. radon-222 decay products and plutonium-239; see below) as Group 1 carcinogens (El Ghissassi et al., 2009; IARC, 2012b). α-particles interact directly with the DNA in pulmonary epithelial cells or indirectly by producing free radicals that cause DNA breaks, gene mutations, apoptosis, chromosomal changes and genetic instability (NRC, 1999). As compared to other occupational carcinogens, including other types of radiation, α-particles directly cause a higher relative rate of double-strand DNA breaks.

Radon-222 and Its Radioactive Decay Products (α-Particles)

Radon-222 (radon) and its decay products are the most comprehensively studied occupational carcinogens (NRC,

1999). Radon, a member of the uranium-238 radioactive decay series, is a naturally occurring, invisible and odourless noble gas with a radiological half-life of 3.8 days. The long radioactive half-lives of radon's direct precursors in the uranium-238 decay series (i.e. uranium-234, thorium-230 and radium-226) provide an unlimited source of radon production in the ground (e.g. soil, rocks and groundwater).

While radon naturally occurs outdoors, it accumulates to higher concentrations in enclosed areas (e.g. mines, homes, offices and schools) (World Health Organization, 2009; Field, 2011). Two of radon's short-lived solid decay products, polonium-218 and polonium 214, rather than radon gas itself, deliver the majority of the radiation dose to the bronchial epithelium via α-decay. Inhalation and deposition of the decay products in the lung depend on the particle attachment rate of the particles to existing aerosols, particle size, tidal lung volume, respiratory rate and lung volume (NRC, 1999).

Occupational radon exposure of underground miners of uranium and of other minerals has been well documented, but the widespread potential for occupational exposure to radon is often neglected when assessing overall radiation exposure in the workplace. For example, elevated radon concentrations have been documented to occur for workers remediating radioactive contaminated sites (e.g. uranium mill sites and mill tailings), workers at underground nuclear waste repositories, radon mitigation contractors and testers, employees of natural caves, phosphate fertilizer plant workers, oil refinery workers, utility tunnel workers, subway tunnel workers, construction excavators, power plant workers (e.g. geothermal power and coal), employees of radon health mines, employees of radon balneotherapy spas, water plant operators, fish hatchery attendants, employees who come into contact with technologically enhanced sources of naturally occurring radioactive materials and agricultural exposures (e.g. ploughing) (Field and Withers, 2012). The population that is at highest risk from protracted radon exposure is in typical workplaces (e.g. offices, schools and stores) from local geologic radon sources (Barros et al., 2015).

IARC working groups in 1972, 1987 and 1988 (IARC, 2012b) concluded that radon-exposed underground haematite miners were at increased risk of lung cancer. In 1999, the US National Research Council's Biological Effects of Ionizing Radiation (BEIR) VI Committee estimated the risk posed by protracted radon exposure at lower radon concentrations from a pooled analysis of 11 cohort mortality studies of 68,000 uranium and other underground miners (i.e. tin, fluorspar and iron) in various parts of the world. Extrapolations from the pooled analyses indicated that protracted exposures of as low as 150 Bq/m^3 (4 pCi/L), a concentration frequently encountered in the residential or non-mining workplace (e.g. homes, offices and public buildings) (Barros et al., 2015), increased lung cancer risk significantly. Cohort miner studies published since the BEIR VI report continue to support the original BEIR VI projections (Schubauer-Berigan et al., 2009; Tirmarche et al., 2010; Kreuzer et al., 2015).

In addition, direct evidence of the risk posed by protracted radon exposure at the relatively lower concentrations in non-mining settings (e.g. homes, offices and schools) was obtained from pooled analyses of seven residential case–control studies in North America (Krewski et al., 2005), 13 in Europe (Darby et al., 2006) and two in China (Lubin et al., 2004). The North American, European and Chinese residential case–control studies reported pooled odds ratios of 1.08 (95% CI: 1.03–1.16), 1.11 (95% CI: 1.00–1.28) and 1.13 (95% CI: 1.01–1.36), respectively, at 100 Bq/m^3 (2.7 pCi/L). Overall, the pooled analyses exhibited a linear dose–response relationship, no evidence of a threshold and risk estimates (odds ratio: 1.12; 95% CI: 1.02–1.25) that were comparable to those extrapolated from the BEIR VI risk models for radon (NRC, 1999). The joint effect of radon and smoking is synergistic (i.e. sub-multiplicative) (NRC, 1999; Krewski et al., 2005; Darby et al., 2006). Due to the large population that is at risk for exposure, radon is the leading environmental cause of cancer mortality, is among the top ten causes of cancer mortality and is the second leading cause of lung cancer in many countries, including the United States (EPA, 2011; ICR, 2015).

Ionizing Radiation (α-Particles): Plutonium-239

Plutonium-239 is an α-emitting radionuclide with a radiological half-life of 24,110 years that is used primarily in the production of nuclear power (i.e. mixed-oxide fuel) and nuclear weapons (IARC, 2001; ATSDR, 2010). Workers involved with the mechanical or chemical processing of this man-made silvery-grey metal have the highest potential for exposure, especially from inhalation of dust contaminated with plutonium-239. Plutonium-239 is redistributed primarily to the lung, bone and liver after inhalation, and absorption follows a two-phase model of months and years (IARC, 2001; ATSDR, 2010).

Findings from the plutonium production workers at the Russian Mayak Nuclear Facility, who received much higher exposures from both external sources and inhaled plutonium than workers at similar facilities in other countries, provided the foundation for IARC's

2001 evaluation of the carcinogenicity of plutonium-239. IARC's 2012 evaluation (IARC, 2012b) that incorporated improved assessment of smoking, dosimetry and work history data (Kreisheimer et al., 2003; Shilnikova et al., 2003; Gilbert et al., 2004; Jacob et al., 2005; Sokolnikov et al., 2008) from several Mayak studies, which continued to report a statistically significant dose–response relationship between estimated lung dose and lung cancer, provided further support for the inclusion of plutonium-239 as an IARC Group 1 lung carcinogen (Kreisheimer et al., 2003; Gilbert et al., 2004; Jacob et al., 2005; Sokolnikov et al., 2008).

A more recent update of the Mayak study, which incorporated improved plutonium dose estimates and included 14,621 workers hired in the period between 1948 and 1982 and followed for at least 5 years (Gilbert et al., 2013), reported an excess relative risk (ERR) of per Gray (Gy) of 7.4 (95% CI: 5.0–11.0) for males at an attained age of 60 years, with declining ERR per Gy with increasing attained age. The researchers also reported that the combined effects of plutonium dose and smoking were greater than additive ($p < 0.001$), but less than multiplicative ($p = 0.011$).

Ionizing Radiation: X-Rays and γ-Rays

Workers with a higher potential of X-ray and γ-ray exposure include those in the following occupational areas: medical, aviation and space crews, gas and oil extraction, industrial radiography, military, mining and milling, nuclear power, nuclear weapons and research. Routine chest X-rays required by some employers and X-ray and γ-ray exposures from medical procedures that are used to assess or treat possible work-related illnesses or injuries are often neglected in calculating a yearly work-related radiation dose (Shockley et al., 2008).

IARC GROUP 1 OCCUPATIONAL LUNG CARCINOGENS: METALS

Arsenic and Inorganic Arsenic Compounds

Arsenic is a naturally occurring metalloid with widespread occurrence in food, water, air and soil (Hughes et al., 2011). Inorganic forms of arsenic, such as arsenite (AsIII) and arsenate (AsV), are linked with oxygen, chlorine and sulphur, etc., but without carbon. Occupationally, copper smelting is the largest contributor of atmospheric releases of arsenic among the mining and metals industries. Arsenic trioxide is produced from the residues produced during the treatment of other metal ores such as copper and gold. The highest occupational exposure to arsenic occurs from the use of arseniferous ores in the smelting of non-ferrous metal (IARC, 2012b).

Arsenic is used in the production of ceramics, fireworks, textiles, glassware (e.g. decolouring agents and bubble dispersants), semiconductors (e.g. high-purity arsenic metal is used in gallium–arsenic semiconductors for light-emitting diodes, cell phones and solar panels), ammunitions, solders and bearings as a hardening agent, as well as in pigment reduction (Hughes et al., 2011; IARC, 2012b; Carex Canada, 2015). An occupationally related source is the production and use of arsenic (e.g. calcium arsenate and lead arsenate) as a pesticide, herbicide, molluscicide, fungicide and growth regulator (e.g. lead arsenate). Another source of occupational exposure is from the production, use and disposal (e.g. burning and sawing) of materials (e.g. wood) that has been treated with chromated copper arsenate. Other areas with the potential for arsenic exposure include coal-fired power plants and battery assembly (IARC, 2012b).

IARC's listing of arsenic as a lung carcinogen was based primarily on over ten cohort studies of workers who had been exposed to high levels of inorganic arsenic in airborne dust employed at lead, copper and gold ore mines, as well as smelters, in the USA, the UK, Sweden, Russia and China. These studies incorporated diverse exposure metrics, including average exposure, cumulative exposure and duration of exposure (IARC, 2012b). These studies frequently reported a doubling or greater (e.g. SMR range of 2–3) in the lung cancer risk of the workers in comparison to the rates in the general population or other reference populations, with evidence of a dose–response relationship. For example, a 2008 study (Lubin et al., 2008) of over 8000 Montana copper smelter workers who were employed for at least 1 year before 1957 and followed through to 1989 reported a linear exposure–response relationship between categories of arsenic concentration and lung cancer, with a SMR for lung cancer of 1.56 (95% CI: 1.4–1.7) at a person-year-weighted mean cumulative arsenic exposure of 3.7 mg/m^3-years. These researchers also reported that the ERR for a fixed level of cumulative arsenic exposure was greater when delivered at a higher concentration and shorter duration than when delivered at a lower concentration and longer duration.

Beryllium and Beryllium Compounds

Beryllium in relation to granulomatous lung disease is addressed extensively in Chapter 24. Three IARC working groups previously reviewed the lung carcinogenicity of beryllium in 1972, 1980 and 1987, and each working group concluded that the evidence of an increased lung cancer risk was limited (IARC, 1993). However, the 1993 IARC evaluation concluded that there was sufficient evidence of increased risk based on new findings from a cohort of 9225 workers employed at seven beryllium-processing plants in the USA (Ward et al., 1992), as well as from a study of 689 individuals included in the US Beryllium Case Registry (Steenland and Ward, 1991). Both studies reported statistically significant excesses in lung cancer mortality (SMR: 1.26; 95% CI: 1.12–1.42, and SMR: 2.00; 95% CI: 1.33–2.89, respectively).

In addition to the two studies cited above that provided support for the carcinogenicity of beryllium, the most recent (2009) evaluation by IARC included a reanalysis by Schubauer-Berigan et al. (2008) of a 2001 nested case–control study of workers employed at a US beryllium-processing plant (Sanderson et al., 2001). This reanalysis was performed in part to address previous criticisms (Deubner et al., 2001; Deubner et al., 2007; Levy et al., 2007) and to adjust for the effects of birth cohort, as well as for the known differences in smoking rates by birth year. In the reanalysis, which included 142 lung cancer cases, each with five matching controls, the authors reported a significant causal relationship between average, but not cumulative, beryllium exposure and lung cancer. The IARC working group noted that the continued criticism of the nested case–control study (Deubner and Roth, 2009) did not undermine confidence in the results of the Schubauer-Berigan et al. (2008) reanalysis, especially in consideration of the publication of several articles (Hein et al., 2009; Langholz and Richardson, 2009; Wacholder, 2009) that supported the methodology that was used to select controls in Schubauer-Berigan et al.'s reanalysis.

Since IARC's latest review of beryllium (IARC, 2012b), Schubauer-Berigan et al. (2011a) reported an increased lung cancer mortality (SMR: 1.17; 95% CI: 1.08–1.28), as compared to the general population, for an extended mortality follow-up (1940–2005) of the 9199 workers employed at the seven beryllium-processing plants in Pennsylvania and Ohio, USA, which is a slightly lower rate than that reported in 1992 for the cohort of workers employed at the plants (IARC, 2012b). A second study published by Schubauer-Berigan et al. (2011b) since the last IARC review of beryllium included 5436 individuals from three of the seven beryllium-processing plants in Ohio and Pennsylvania, USA. The authors reported a 'significant and strong' increased lung cancer risk associated with mean, maximum and cumulative exposure, with an estimated 10^3 excess lifetime risk of lung cancer with a daily weighted average beryllium exposure of 0.033 mg/m^3.

Cadmium and Cadmium Compounds

The majority of refined cadmium is used in the production of nickel–cadmium batteries and, to a lesser extent, as a colour pigment (e.g. used in ceramics, plastics, glasses, enamels and art supplies), a coating (e.g. used for corrosion resistance in steel and aluminium), an alloy for heat and electrical conduction (including the use of cadmium sulphide in solar cells) and as stabilizers in order to slow the degradation of polyvinylchloride (ICA, 2015). The recycling of spent nickel–cadmium batteries reportedly accounts for 23% of the total cadmium supply (ICA, 2015). The highest potential of occupational exposure is from the inhalation of dust and fumes, especially involving the heating of cadmium-containing materials, including: welding or re-melting cadmium-coated steel; smelting zinc and lead ores; work involving solders containing cadmium (e.g. silver soldering or brazing); battery production and recycling; pigment production; plastics production; and processing, producing and handling cadmium powders (ATSDR, 2012; USGS, 2014).

Studies reporting increased risks for cadmium exposures published between 1965 and 1998 for cohorts of workers from UK copper–cadmium alloy plants, Swedish and UK nickel–cadmium battery plants, UK cadmium-processing plants and US cadmium recovery plants provided the basis for the 1993 (IARC, 1993) and 2012 (IARC, 2012b) inclusion of cadmium as a known human lung carcinogen. The 2012 IARC working group on cadmium noted that the assessment of lung cancer risk was 'constrained' by the limited number of long-term and highly exposed workers, limited exposure data and the inability to examine a range of exposures across studies (IARC, 2012b). The inability to account for co-exposures (e.g. smoking and arsenic) in some of the cohorts also presented a challenge to assessing the lung cancer risk posed by occupational cadmium exposure. The IARC working group also included the findings from a Belgian study that compared lung cancer rates in a population (n = 994) living close to one of three zinc smelters and a reference population. The study reported a statistically significantly increased risk (i.e. adjusted hazard ratio: 1.7) with a doubling of a 24-hour urinary cadmium excretion, as well as a fourfold increased lung cancer risk for residence in the high-exposure area versus the low-exposure area (Nawrot et al., 2006).

Since the 2012 IARC published review of cadmium, findings were published from two population-based case–control studies that were performed from 1979 to 1986 and 1996 to 2001 in Montreal, Canada, using job categories in order to estimate cadmium exposure. The study investigators reported a pooled odds ratio of

4.7 (95% CI: 1.5–14.3) among former or non-smokers with no observable increased risk among smokers. In addition, a 1985 cohort study of US cadmium recovery workers was reanalysed with updated mortality information (1940–2002), improved work history details and a revised cadmium exposure matrix (Thun et al., 1985). The researchers reported a significantly ($p = 0.012$) increased lung cancer risk (i.e. SMR of 3.2 for 10 mg-year/m^3 Cd) with a predicted 1/1000 excess lifetime risk of lung cancer death from an airborne exposure of approximately 2.4 mg/m^3 Cd (Park et al., 2012). In summary, based on the evidence reviewed, IARC (2012b) reaffirmed its 2000 conclusion that there was sufficient evidence of cadmium's lung carcinogenicity in humans.

Hexavalent Chromium Compounds

The primary routes of exposure to hexavalent chromium compounds are inhalation of dusts, fumes or mists containing hexavalent chrome, as well as dermal contact with chromium-containing products (IARC, 2012b). The potential for occupational exposure to hexavalent chromium compounds includes: chromate production (e.g. sodium, potassium, calcium and ammonium chromates and dichromates); chrome electroplating and plating (e.g. chromium trioxide); the production and use of chromium-containing paints and pigments (e.g. insoluble chromates of zinc and lead); welding or cutting/grinding of chromium-containing metals and alloys (e.g. high-chromium steel and stainless steel); steel smelting and welding (e.g. water-soluble alkaline chromates); leather tanning; welding or cutting on stainless steel; and glass manufacturing (IARC, 2012b; NIOSH, 2013).

In a review of cohort studies performed in numerous countries published between 1952 and 2006, the 2012 IARC working group concluded that there was sufficient evidence for the lung carcinogenicity of chromium (VI) compounds in humans based on 13 studies of workers in the chromate paint and pigment production industry, 12 studies of workers in the chromate production industry, six studies of workers in the chromium electroplating industry and 13 studies of workers in other industries (e.g. ferrochromium production, ferroalloy and stainless steel production, welders from 135 companies, aerospace, stainless steel welders from eight companies and stonemasonry) (IARC, 2012b). In a 2015 extended follow-up of a cohort of US chromium production workers, Gibbs et al. (2015) evaluated the mortality of 2354 workers who were first employed at a chromate production plant between 1950 and 1974. The lung cancer mortality rate for the cohort was significantly elevated (SMR: 1.63; 95% CI: 1.42–1.86) as compared to the reference state population's lung cancer mortality rate. When the analysis was limited to smokers, the SMR increased for each exposure quartile. Overall, cumulative chromium (VI) exposure was a significant predictor of lung cancer in a model accounting for smoking and years worked (Gibb et al., 2015). It should be noted that that exposure to hexavalent chromium dioxide also causes respiratory tract, nasal and sinus cancer (IARC, 2012b).

Nickel Compounds

Concerns regarding increased cancer rates in nickel miners working at the Mond Nickel Works in South Wales were raised by as early as 1932 (Grenfell, 1932). Occupational exposure to insoluble nickel is the predominant exposure in nickel-producing industries such as mining, refining and smelting, while exposure to soluble nickel is the predominant exposure in the wide range of nickel-using industries, including alloy and stainless steel manufacture, electroplating, ceramics, magnets, batteries, paint, stainless steel, textiles, chemicals, varnish and vacuum tubes (NTP, 2011c; IARC, 2012b; Nickel Institute, 2015).

IARC's most recent published synthesis (IARC, 2012b) of epidemiologic studies focused on the findings from workers exposed to nickel compounds produced by varying processes, and occurring at nickel refineries and smelters in Canada, Norway and the UK. Increased lung cancer risks were observed for refinery (IARC, 1990; Andersen et al., 1996; Anttila et al., 1998; Grimsrud and Peto, 2006) and nickel smelter workers in general (IARC, 1990; Anttila et al., 1998) and, more specifically, for exposure to nickel oxides (Andersen et al., 1996; Anttila et al., 1998; Grimsrud et al., 2003), nickel chloride (Grimsrud et al., 2003), nickel sulphides (Grimsrud et al., 2002), insoluble nickel compounds (Andersen et al., 1996), nickel sulphate (Anttila et al., 1998) and water-soluble nickel compounds in general (Andersen et al., 1996; Grimsrud et al., 2002, 2003, 2005). In summary, IARC concluded that there was sufficient evidence for the carcinogenicity in humans of mixtures that include nickel compounds and nickel metal (IARC, 2012b).

IARC Group 1 Lung Carcinogens: Occupations and Manufacturing Processes

Although single agents have attracted most of the attention in the lung carcinogenicity literature, even tobacco smoke is a very complex mixture, and the occurrence of multiple concurrent lung carcinogen exposures is closer to the true reality in lung cancer causation. IARC has concluded (IARC, 2012b) that there is sufficient evidence of human lung carcinogenicity for occupational exposures occurring in eight discrete occupations and manufacturing sectors for which no single specific Group 1 carcinogen has been identified.

Occupational Exposures Associated with the Acheson Process

The Acheson process, named after E. G. Acheson who invented it in 1891, is used to synthesize graphite and silicon carbide (SiC) in an electrical resistance furnace (Figure 21.4) from a mixture of silica (e.g. quartz) and carbon (e.g. petroleum coke). SiC, a green to bluish–black iridescent material with sharp crystals, is used as an abrasive (e.g. grinding wheels) and as a component of numerous other products (e.g. electronics, ceramics, boiler furnaces, tubes and valves).

There are three forms of SiC: non-fibrous, fibres and whiskers (COHCN, 2012). Exposure to non-fibrous SiC (e.g. SiC dust, SiC particles and granular SiC) can occur during the manufacturing process or when used as a synthetic abrasive materials. Even though SiC is referred to as non-fibrous, it can have fibrous particles exceeding a length of 100 μm (COHCN, 2012). SiC fibres (e.g. SiC continuous fibres and SiC ceramic fibres), a polycrystalline material, are unwanted by-product materials that are often generated during SiC crystal production at a variety of fibre lengths and diameters that meet the fibre definition of WHO (COHCN, 2012). SiC whiskers, cylindrical fibres with aspect ratios equal to or greater than 3 and diameters less than 5 μm, have a morphology that is similar to amphibole asbestos. SiC whiskers, originally developed as a substitute for asbestos, are used for a variety of applications, including sandblast nozzles, ceramic seals and other materials that require high temperature tolerance (COHCN, 2012). Exposure to SiC whiskers can occur during their manufacture, during the production, machining and finishing of composite material and as a by-product during the production of SiC for the abrasive industry (COHCN, 2012).

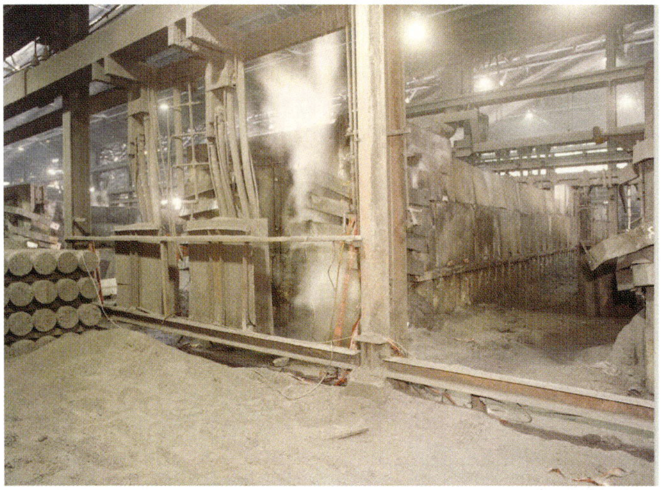

FIGURE 21.4 Acheson furnace (used to synthesize graphite and silicon carbide) exhausting smoke and gasses. (Copyright Lipsitz & Ponterio, LLC.)

The first cohort study of SiC production workers, published in 1994, reported an overall increased risk of lung cancer (SMR: 1.7; 95% CI: 1.1–2.5) (Infante-Rivard et al., 1994). A 2001 pooled study of 2620 Norwegian SiC smelter workers, with worker follow-up between 1953 and 1996, reported an overall excess risk of lung cancer (SIR: 1.9; 95% CI: 1.5–2.3) (Romundstad et al., 2001). In a 2012 follow-up cohort study of the 2001 Norwegian study (Romundstad et al., 2001), the researchers estimated the cumulative exposure to total and respirable dust, respirable quartz, cristobalite and SiC particles and SiC fibres for 1687 long-term workers employed during 1913–2003 (Bugge et al., 2012). The researchers reported that crystalline silica in the form of cristobalite increased lung cancer risk by two- to three-fold at the highest level of cumulative exposure to quartz and cristobalite compared to the general male population. Further internal analyses indicated that cristobalite was the most important occupational risk factor, but noted that exposure to SiC fibres also appeared to increase lung cancer risk (Bugge et al., 2012). Based on the evidence from human studies, IARC added occupational exposures associated with the Acheson process to the list of Group 1 lung carcinogens in 2014.

Coal Gasification, Coke Production, Iron and Steel Founding and Aluminium Production

These four industrial processes all entail a high potential for occupational exposure to PAHs, as well as to other chemical and physical hazards (IARC, 2012b). A meta-analysis of cohort studies published between 1997 and 2005 of PAH-exposed workers reported a RR of 1.51 (95% CI: 1.28–1.78) for roofers, 2.58 (95% CI: 2.28–2.92) for coal gasification, 1.58 (95% CI: 1.47–1.69) for coke production and 1.40 (95% CI: 1.31–1.49) for iron and steel foundries (Bosetti et al., 2007). A non-statistically significant summary RR of 1.03 (95% CI: 0.95–1.11) was found for aluminium production workers. The findings in the latter two industries were essentially confirmed by an updated meta-analysis by the same group, including studies published between 2006 and 2014 (Rota et al., 2014b).

Coal gasification leads to the production of a 'clean' coal gas to be used as a fuel that emits fewer sulphur and nitrogen dioxides. Besides PAHs, coal gasification potentially exposes workers to several metals, fibres, acids and aldehydes. IARC cited the epidemiologic findings from a UK and Germany study of coal gasification workers and a nested case–control study of French gas and electricity production workers as the basis for their inclusion of coal gasification as a Group 1 lung carcinogen (IARC, 2012b). Occupational exposure to coke oven emissions can occur is a variety of industries (e.g. aluminium, construction, electrical, graphite and steel). Topside oven workers generally had the highest exposures and lung cancer risks. IARC highlighted the findings of three large epidemiological studies of workers who were exposed to coal coke oven emissions, which reported an overall increased risk for lung cancer, as the basis for their inclusion of coke production as a Group 1 lung carcinogen (IARC, 2012b).

Foundries produce shaped castings from re-melted metal ingots and scrap, with some associated simple machining. Besides potential occupational exposure to PAHs, iron and steel founding involves exposures to silica, metals, ceramic fibres and chemicals such as amines and formaldehyde (IARC, 2012b). IARC listed iron and steel founding as a Group 1 lung carcinogen based on consistent findings from 13 cohort studies performed in various parts of the world and two case–control studies reporting a significantly increased risk for lung cancer for either the entire cohort or in highly exposed subgroups (IARC, 2012b).

The specific processes in aluminium production that IARC considered were its electrolytic production and casting into ingots. Workers in aluminium production are primarily exposed to PAHs, but other potential exposures exist for this and for the related anode manufacturing process (IARC, 2012b). As a basis for listing aluminium production as a Group 1 lung carcinogen, IARC noted that an increased lung cancer risk was observed in cohorts of aluminium production workers in Quebec, Canada and Sweden, as well as a similar trend with increasing cumulative exposure to benzo[a]pyrene in a cohort study performed in British Columbia, Canada.

Occupational Second-Hand Cigarette Smoke Exposure

Tobacco smoke is also quite relevant as an occupational exposure in the form of second-hand smoke. IARC established second-hand smoke as a Group 1 lung carcinogen in 2012 (IARC, 2012b) and clearly recognized the workplace as one of several relevant causally related exposure settings. A 2003 meta-analysis of data from 22 studies from worldwide locations reported a 24% increase in lung cancer risk (RR: 1.24; 95% CI: 1.18–1.29) among non-smoking workers exposed to occupational second-hand tobacco smoke and a twofold increased risk (RR: 2.01; 95% CI: 1.33–2.60) for those classified as being highly exposed compared to unexposed workers (Stayner et al., 2007). Similarly, a prospective study of occupational lung cancer risk estimated the adjusted hazard ratio for workplace second-hand tobacco smoke at 1.6 (95% CI: 1.2–2.1), slightly surpassing well-known agents such as asbestos, heavy metals and PAHs (Veglia et al., 2007).

Rubber Manufacturing Industry

Rubber manufacturing comprises a variety of processes, from raw material handling and mixing to milling, extruding and calendaring, component assembling, curing, vulcanizing, inspection and finishing. Rubber manufacturing workers are exposed to fumes with a complex chemical composition that are generated during the heating and curing of rubber compounds. Exposures include rubber dust and fumes, PAHs, solvents, phthalates and many others. The cyclohexane-soluble fraction of fumes often serves as an indicator for assessing the total particulate fume contamination (IARC, 2012b). In addition, high concentrations of nitrosamines are formed in rubber manufacturing during the vulcanizing process (Fajen et al., 1979; IARC, 1996). Furthermore, other likely potential occupational exposures include carbon black and asbestos-contaminated talc (Straif et al., 2000; IARC, 2012b).

The 2009 IARC working group concluded that there was sufficient evidence for the carcinogenicity of occupational exposures in the rubber manufacturing industry in humans based in large part on retrospective cohort mortality studies that reported increased lung cancer risks among rubber workers who were involved with mixing and milling, vulcanization and tyre-curing departments, as well as in cohorts of workers who were exposed to high concentrations of fumes and/or solvents (IARC, 2012b).

Painting

Paints are complex and highly variable mixtures that are comprised of pigments in a liquid-containing binder (resin), a volatile solvent or water and additives. The mixtures can contain chromates, lead oxide and other metals, formaldehyde, asbestos, silica, benzene, phthalates and many others. The increased use of water-based paints and the intentional reduction of some of these toxic agents in paints together have reduced the risk of adverse health outcomes related to painting. Nonetheless, painters remain potentially exposed to hundreds of hazardous chemicals (e.g. dichloromethane, diisocyanates, amines, esters, chromates, nickel, ketones, etc.) (IARC, 2012b).

Over 50 cohort and case–control studies published between 1951 and 2010 demonstrated a relatively consistent increased lung cancer risk for painters. A 2010 meta-analysis based on census reports and case–control and cohort studies published through to 2008 (Bachand et al., 2010) reported a summary lung cancer risk estimate for painters of 1.29 (95% CI: 1.10–1.51) for case–control studies and 1.22 (95% CI: 1.16–1.29) and 1.36 (95% CI: 1.34–1.41) for lung cancer incidence and mortality studies, respectively. A second large meta-analysis was also published in 2010 (Guha et al., 2010) that included over 11,000 incident lung cancer cases or deaths among painters and reported a summary lung cancer risk estimate of 1.35 (95% CI: 1.29–1.41) and of 1.35 (95% CI: 1.21–1.51) after controlling for smoking.

CONCLUSION

A fairly large group of occupational carcinogens and settings contribute to the rich array of causally related risk factors for lung cancer. The studies summarized above highlight the variability in strength of association, local and regional prevalence and relevance and secular trends related to the awareness and implementation of potentially effective exposure controls and modifications of other risk factors (e.g. smoking and diet). Much of the evidence presented in this chapter was obtained from studies performed in developed countries in the later part of the twentieth century as a result of occupational exposures related to the industrial practices that occurred in the first half of the twentieth century. Causality for some of the agents and industrial processes that have been described is likely to remain elevated for some time. This is due both to the long latency that is typical of the multistage process of lung carcinogenesis and to the lack of no-disease-effect threshold exposure levels for carcinogens. The latter means that regulated permissible occupational exposure levels still fall short of complete elimination of the exposure in question, and thus reduce, but fail to eradicate, the associated disease risk. The continued follow-up of many of the more heavily exposed worker cohorts will provide continued insights into the lung cancer risk posed by lower, protracted exposures. Study findings will also provide awareness of the risk posed to workers who are exposed to occupational lung carcinogens due to the relocation of manufacturing to countries with less stringent worker protection standards, as well as from the global process of industrialization in general.

IARC has recently added several Group 1 occupational lung carcinogens (e.g. diesel and the Acheson process), and has a long list of priority agents to review in the coming years, together with the continuing review of Group 2 lung carcinogens (see http://monographs.iarc.fr/index.php). IARC's inclusion of eight discrete occupations and manufacturing sectors for which no single specific Group 1 carcinogen has been identified highlights the complexity of the exposure settings, including mixed occupational and environmental contributions, which complicate the identification of single-agent causation. The unequivocal dominance of tobacco smoke, which is pervasive even in the workplace, in lung cancer causation, and the varying interactions between smoking and occupational carcinogens, will continue to complicate assessing the risk that is posed by occupational lung carcinogens.

REFERENCES

Andersen, A., Berge, S. R., Engeland, A. and Norseth. T. 1996. Exposure to nickel compounds and smoking in relation to incidence of lung and nasal cancer among nickel refinery workers. *Occup Environ Med* 53(10):708–13.

Anttila, A., Pukkala, E., Aitio, A., Rantanen, T. and Karjalainen, S. 1998. Update of cancer incidence among workers at a copper/nickel smelter and nickel refinery. *Int Arch Occup Environ Health* 71(4):245–50.

ATSDR. 2008. Polycyclic Aromatic Hydrocarbons (PAHs), Who Is at Risk of Exposure to PAHs? Agency for Toxic Substances and Disease Registry. Available at: http://www.atsdr.cdc.gov/csem/csem.asp?csem=13&po=7 (accessed 16 April 2016).

ATSDR. 2010. In U.S. Agency for Toxic Substances and Disease Registry (ed.), *Toxicological Profile for Plutonium*. 320 pp. Atlanta, GA: U.S. Department of Health and Human Services, Public Health Service. Available at: http://www.atsdr.cdc.gov/toxprofiles/tp143.pdf (accessed 16 April 2016).

ATSDR. 2012. In U.S. Agency for Toxic Substances and Disease Registry (ed.), *Toxicological Profile for Cadmium*. 487 pp. Atlanta, GA: U.S. Department of Health and Human Services, Public Health Service, Available at: http://www.atsdr.cdc.gov/toxprofiles/tp.asp?id=48&tid=15 (accessed 16 April 2016).

Attfield, M. D., Schleiff, P. L., Lubin, J. H., Blair A., Stewart, P. A., Vermeulen, R., Coble, J. B. et al. 2012. The diesel exhaust in miners study: A cohort mortality study with emphasis on lung cancer. *J Natl Cancer Inst* 104:869–83.

Bachand, A., Mundt, K. A., Mundt, D. J. and Carlton, L. E. 2010. Meta-analyses of occupational exposure as a painter and lung and bladder cancer morbidity and mortality 1950–2008. *Crit Rev Toxicol* 40(2):101–25.

Barros, N., Field, D. W., Steck, D. J. and Field, R. W. 2015. Comparative survey of outdoor, residential and workplace radon concentrations. *Radiat Prot Dosimetry* 163(3):325–32.

Bosetti, C., Boffetta, P. and La Vecchia, C. 2007. Occupational exposures to polycyclic aromatic hydrocarbons, and respiratory and urinary tract cancers: A quantitative review to 2005. *Ann Oncol* 18(3):431–46.

Bugge, M. D., Kjaerheim, K., Foreland, S., Eduard, W. and Kjuus, H. 2012. Lung cancer incidence among Norwegian silicon carbide industry workers: Associations with particulate exposure factors. *Occup Environ Med* 69(8):527–33.

Bullman, T. A. and Kang, H. K. 1994. The effects of mustard gas, ionizing radiation, herbicides, trauma, and oil smoke on US military personnel: The results of veteran studies. *Annu Rev Public Health* 15:69–90.

Carex Canada. 2015. Arsenic. Profiles and Estimates. Available at: http://www.carexcanada.ca/en/arsenic/ (accessed 16 April 2016).

Checkoway, H. and Franzblau, A. 2000. Is silicosis required for silica-associated lung cancer? *Am J Ind Med* 37(3):252–9.

COHCN. 2012. Silicon Carbide, Evaluation of the Carcinogenicity and Genotoxicity. Health Council of the Netherlands. Available at: http://www.gezondheidsraad.nl/sites/default/files/Siliciumcarbide201229.pdf (accessed 16 April 2016).

Collingwood, K. W., Pasternack, B. S. and Shore, R. E. 1987. An industry-wide study of respiratory cancer in chemical workers exposed to chloromethyl ethers. *J Natl Cancer Inst* 78(6):1127–36.

Darby, S., Hill, D., Deo, H., Auvinen, A., Barros-Dios, J. M., Baysson, H., Bochicchio, F. et al. 2006. Residential radon and lung cancer—Detailed results of a collaborative analysis of individual data on 7148 persons with lung cancer and 14,208 persons without lung cancer from 13 epidemiologic studies in Europe. *Scand J Work Environ Health* 32(Suppl. 1):1–83.

Deubner, D. C., Lockey, J. L., Kotin, P., Powers, M. B., Miller, F., Rogers, A. E. and Trichopoulos, D. 2001. Re: Lung cancer case–control study of beryllium workers. Sanderson WT, Ward EM, Steenland K, Petersen MR. *Am. J. Ind. Med.* 2001. 39:133–144. *Am J Ind Med* 40(3):284–8.

Deubner, D. C. and Roth, H. D. 2009. Rejoinder: Progress in understanding the relationship between beryllium exposure and lung cancer. *Epidemiology* 20(3):341–3.

Deubner, D. C., Roth, H. D. and Levy, P. S. 2007. Empirical evaluation of complex epidemiologic study designs: Workplace exposure and cancer. *J Occup Environ Med* 49(9):953–9.

Doi, M., Hattori, N., Yokoyama, A., Onari, Y., Kanehara, M., Masuda, K., Tonda, T. et al. 2011. Effect of mustard gas exposure on incidence of lung cancer: A longitudinal study. *Am J Epidemiol* 173(6):659–66.

Easton, D. F., Peto, J. and Doll, R. 1988. Cancers of the respiratory tract in mustard gas workers. *Br J Ind Med* 45(10):652–9.

El Ghissassi, F., Baan, R., Straif, K., Grosse, Y., Secretan, B., Bouvard, V., Benbrahim-Tallaa, L. et al. and WHO International Agency for Research on Cancer Monograph Working Group. 2009. A review of human carcinogens—Part D: Radiation. *Lancet Oncol* 10(8):751–2.

EPA. 2011. *Protecting People and Families from Radon, a Federal Action Plan for Saving Lives*. Washington, DC: U.S. Environmental Protection Agency, U.S. Department of Health and Human Services, U.S. Department of Agriculture, U.S. Department of Defense, U.S. Department of Energy, U.S. Department of Housing and Urban Development, U.S. Department of Interior, U.S. Department Veterans Affairs, U.S. General Services Administration.

EPA. 2012. *Report to Congress on Black Carbon. 2012.* Washington, DC: U.S. Environmental Protection Agency, Department of the Interior, Environment, and Related Agencies Appropriations Act, 2010. Office of Air Quality Planning and Standards, Office of Atmospheric Programs, Office of Radiation and Indoor Air, Office of Research and Development and Office of Transportation and Air Quality.

Erren, T. C., Glende, C. B., Morfeld, P. and Piekarski, C. 2009. Is exposure to silica associated with lung cancer in the absence of silicosis? A meta-analytical approach to an important public health question. *Int Arch Occup Environ Health* 82(8):997–1004.

Evanoff, B. A., Gustavsson, P. and Hogstedt, C. 1993. Mortality and incidence of cancer in a cohort of Swedish chimney sweeps: An extended follow up study. *Br J Ind Med* 50(5):450–9.

Fajen, J. M., Carson, G. A., Rounbehler, D. P., Fan, T. Y., Vita, R., Goff, U. E., Wolf, M. H. et al. 1979. N-nitrosamines in the rubber and tire industry. *Science* 205(4412):1262–4.

Ferlay, J., Soerjomataram, I., Ervik, M., Dikshit, R., Eser, S., Mathers, C., Rebelo, M. et al. 2013. GLOBOCAN 2012 v1.0, Cancer Incidence and Mortality Worldwide: IARC CancerBase No. 11. Available at: http://globocan.iarc.fr (accessed 16 April 2016).

Field, R. W. 2011. Radon: An overview of health effects. In J. O. Nriagu (ed.), *Encyclopedia of Environmental Health*. Burlington, ON: Elsevier, 745–53.

Field, R. W. and Withers, B. L. 2012. Occupational and environmental causes of lung cancer. *Clin Chest Med* 33(4):681–703.

Garshick, E., Laden, L., Hart, J. E., Davis, M. E., Eisen, E. A. and Smith, T. J. 2012. Lung cancer and elemental carbon exposure in trucking industry workers. *Environ Health Perspect* 120(9):1301–6.

Gibb, H. J., Lees, P. S., Wang, J. and Grace O'Leary, K. 2015. Extended followup of a cohort of chromium production workers. *Am J Ind Med* 58(8):905–13.

Gilbert, E. S., Koshurnikova, N. A., Sokolnikov, M. E., Shilnikova, N. S., Preston, D. L., Ron, E., Okatenko, P. V. et al. 2004. Lung cancer in Mayak workers. *Radiat Res* 162(5):505–16.

Gilbert, E. S., Sokolnikov, M. E., Preston, D. L., Schonfeld, S. J., Schadilov, A. E., Vasilenko, E. K. and Koshurnikova, N. A. 2013. Lung cancer risks from plutonium: An updated analysis of data from the Mayak worker cohort. *Radiat Res* 179(3):332–42.

Gowers, D. S., DeFonso, L. R., Schaffer, P., Karli, A., Monroe, C. B., Bernabeu, L. and Renshaw, F. M. 1993. Incidence of respiratory cancer among workers exposed to chloromethyl-ethers. *Am J Epidemiol* 137(1):31–4.

Grenfell, D. 1932. Parliament medical news, cancer among welsh nickel workers. *Lancet* 219(5659):375.

Grimsrud, T. K., Berge, S. R., Haldorsen, T. and Andersen, A. 2002. Exposure to different forms of nickel and risk of lung cancer. *Am J Epidemiol* 156(12):1123–32.

Grimsrud, T. K., Berge, S. R., Haldorsen, T. and Andersen, A. 2005. Can lung cancer risk among nickel refinery workers be explained by occupational exposures other than nickel? *Epidemiology* 16(2):146–54.

Grimsrud, T. K., Berge, S. R., Martinsen, J. I. and Andersen, A. 2003. Lung cancer incidence among Norwegian nickel-refinery workers 1953–2000. *J Environ Monit* 5(2):190–7.

Grimsrud, T. K. and Peto, J. 2006. Persisting risk of nickel related lung cancer and nasal cancer among Clydach refiners. *Occup Environ Med* 63(5):365–6.

Guha, N., Merletti, F., Steenland, N. K., Altieri, A., Cogliano, V. and Straif, K. 2010. Lung cancer risk in painters: A meta-analysis. *Environ Health Perspect* 118(3):303–12.

Gupta, R. 2015. *Handbook of Toxicology of Chemical Warfare Agents*. Boston, MA: Elsevier.

Hein, M. J., Deddens, J. A. and Schubauer-Berigan, M. K. 2009. Bias from matching on age at death or censor in nested case–control studies. *Epidemiology* 20(3):330–8.

Hogstedt, C., Jansson, C., Hugosson, M., Tinnerberg, H. and Gustavsson. P. 2013. Cancer incidence in a cohort of Swedish chimney sweeps, 1958–2006. *Am J Public Health* 103(9):1708–14.

HSDB. 2014. Hazardous Substances Data Bank. Available at: http://toxnet.nlm.nih.gov/cgi-bin/sis/htmlgen?HSDB (accessed 16 April 2016).

Hughes, M. F., Beck, B. D., Chen, Y., Lewis, A. S. and Thomas, D. J. 2011. Arsenic exposure and toxicology: A historical perspective. *Toxicol Sci* 123(2):305–32.

IARC. 1989. Diesel and gasoline engine exhausts and some nitroarenes. In International Agency for Research on Cancer (ed.), *IARC Monographs on the Evaluation of the Carcinogenic Risks of Chemicals to Humans*. Volume 46, Lyon, France: International Agency for Research on Cancer.

IARC. 1990. Chromium, nickel and welding. In International Agency for Research on Cancer (ed.), *IARC Monogr Eval Carcinog Risks Hum*. Volume 46, Lyon, France: International Agency for Research on Cancer .

IARC. 1993. Beryllium, cadmium, mercury, and exposures in the glass manufacturing industry. In International Agency for Research on Cancer (ed.), *IARC Monographs on the Evaluation of Carcinogenic Risks to Human*. Volume 58, Lyon, France: International Agency for Research on Cancer.

IARC. 1996. Printing processes, printing inks, carbon blacks and some nitro compounds. In International Agency for Research on Cancer (ed.), Volume 65, *IARC Monographs on the Evaluation of Carcinogenic Risks to Humans*. Lyon, France: International Agency for Research on Cancer.

IARC. 2001. Ionizing radiation, Part 2: Some internally deposited radionuclides. In International Agency for Research on Cancer (ed.), Volume 78, *IARC Monographs on the Evaluation of Carcinogenic Risks to Humans*. Lyon, France: International Agency for Research on Cancer.

IARC. 2010a. Carbon black, titanium dioxide, and talc. In International Agency for Research on Cancer (ed.), Volume 93, *IARC Monographs on the Evaluation of Carcinogenic Risks to Humans*. Lyon, France: International Agency for Research on Cancer.

IARC. 2010b. Some non-heterocyclic polycyclic aromatic hydrocarbons and some related exposures. In International Agency for Research on Cancer (ed.), *IARC Monographs on the Evaluation of Carcinogenic Risks to Humans*. Volume 92, Lyon, France: International Agency for Research on Cancer.

IARC. 2012a. Coal tar pitch. In International Agency for Research on Cancer (eds), *IARC Monographs on the Evaluation of Carcinogenic Risks to Humans*. Volume 100F, Lyon, France: International Agency for Research on Cancer.

IARC. 2012c. Arsenic, metals, fibres and dusts. In International Agency for Research on Cancer (eds), *IARC Monographs on the Evaluation of Carcinogenic Risks to Humans*. Volume 100C, Lyon, France: International Agency for Research on Cancer.

IARC. 2013. Diesel and gasoline engine exhausts and some nitroarenes. In International Agency for Research on Cancer (ed.), *IARC Monographs on the Evaluation of Carcinogenic Risks to Humans*. Volume 105, Lyon, France: International Agency for Research on Cancer.

ICA. 2015. Cadmium, Working Towards a Sustainable Future. International Cadmium Association. Available at: http://www.cadmium.org/index.php (accessed 16 April 2016).

ICR. 2015. Breathing Easier, Do You Ask Your Patients if They've Tested Their Homes for Radon? Iowa Cancer Registry. Available at: http://canceriowa.org/BreathingEasier.aspx (accessed 16 April 2016).

IOM. 1993. In Institute of Medicine (U.S.) (ed.), *Veterans at Risk: The Health Effects of Mustard Gas and Lewisite. Committee to Survey the Health Effects of Mustard Gas and Lewisite*. 448 pp. Washington, DC: National Academy Press. Available at: http://www.nap.edu/catalog/2058/veterans-at-risk-the-health-effects-of-mustard-gas-and (accessed 16 April 2016).

Infante-Rivard, C., André, D., Armstrong, B., Bouchard, P. and Thériault, G. 1994. Cohort study of silicon carbide production workers. *AJE* 140(11):1009–15.

Jacob, V., Jacob, P., Meckbach, R., Romanov, S. A. and Vasilenko, E. K. 2005. Lung cancer in Mayak workers: Interaction of smoking and plutonium exposure. *Radiat Environ Biophys* 44(2):119–29.

Kreisheimer, M., Sokolnikov, M. E., Koshurnikova, N. A., Khokhryakov, V. F., Romanow, S. A., Shilnikova, N. S., Okatenko, P. V. et al. 2003. Lung cancer mortality among nuclear workers of the Mayak facilities in the former Soviet Union. An updated analysis considering smoking as the main confounding factor. *Radiat Environ Biophys* 42(2):129–35.

Kreuzer, M., Dufey, F., Laurier, D., Nowak, D., Marsh, J. W., Schnelzer, M., Sogl, M. et al. 2015. Mortality from internal and external radiation exposure in a cohort of male German uranium millers, 1946–2008. *Int Arch Occup Environ Health* 88(4):431–41.

Krewski, D., Lubin, J. H., Zielinski, J. M., Alavanja, M., Catalan, V. S., Field, R. W., Klotz, J. B. et al. 2005. Residential radon and risk of lung cancer: A combined analysis of 7 North American case–control studies. *Epidemiology* 16(2):137–45.

Krieger, R. I., Dinoff, T. M. and Zhang, X. 2003. Octachlorodipropyl ether (S-2) mosquito coils are inadequately studied for residential use in Asia and illegal in the United States. *Environ Health Perspect* 111(12):1439–42.

Lacasse, Y., Martin, S., Gagne, D. and Lakhal, L. 2009. Dose–response meta-analysis of silica and lung cancer. *Cancer Causes Control* 20(6):925–33.

Laden, F., Hart, J. E., Eschenroeder, A., Smith, T. J. and Garshick, E. 2006. Historical estimation of diesel exhaust exposure in a cohort study of U.S. railroad workers and lung cancer. *Cancer Causes Control* 17(7):911–9.

Langholz, B. and Richardson, D. 2009. Are nested case–control studies biased? *Epidemiology* 20(3):321–9.

Levy, P. S., Roth, H. D. and Deubner, D. C. 2007. Exposure to beryllium and occurrence of lung cancer: A reexamination of findings from a nested case–control study. *J Occup Environ Med* 49(1):96–101.

Liu, Y., Steenland, K., Rong, Y., Hnizdo, E., Huang, X., Zhang, H., Shi, T. et al. 2013. Exposure–response analysis and risk assessment for lung cancer in relationship to silica exposure: A 44-year cohort study of 34,018 workers. *Am J Epidemiol* 178(9):1424–33.

Long, C. M., Nascarella, M. A. and Valberg, P. A. 2013. Carbon black vs. black carbon and other airborne materials containing elemental carbon: Physical and chemical distinctions. *Environ Pollut* 181:271–86.

Lubin, J. H., Moore, L. E., Fraumeni, J. F. Jr. and Cantor, K. P. 2008. Respiratory cancer and inhaled inorganic arsenic in copper smelters workers: A linear relationship with cumulative exposure that increases with concentration. *Environ Health Perspect* 116(12):1661–5.

Lubin, J. H., Wang, Z. Y., Boice, J. D. Jr., Xu, Z. Y., Blot, W. J., De Wang, L. and Kleinerman, R. A. 2004. Risk of lung cancer and residential radon in China: Pooled results of two studies. *Int J Cancer* 109(1):132–7.

McCallum, R., Woolley, V. and Petrie, A. 1983. Lung cancer associated with chloromethyl methyl ether manufacture: An investigation at two factories in the United Kingdom. *Br J Ind Med* 40(4):384–9.

McDonald, J. D., Campen, M. J., Harrod, K. S., Seagrave, J., Seilkop, S. K. and Mauderly, J. L. 2011. Engine-operating load influences diesel exhaust composition and cardiopulmonary and immune responses. *Environ Health Perspect* 119(8):1136–41.

Miles, J. 1986. Occupational Safety and Health Administration Department of Labor Standard Interpretation, *Some Clarifications of 29 CFR 1910.1006 and 1008.* Washington, DC. Available at: https://www.osha.gov/pls/oshaweb/owadisp.show_document?p_table=INTERPRETATIONS&p_id=19388 (accessed 16 April 2016).

Nawrot, T., Plusquin, M., Hogervorst, J., Roels, H. A., Celis, H., Thijs, L., Vangronsveld, J. et al. 2006. Environmental exposure to cadmium and risk of cancer: A prospective population-based study. *Lancet Oncol* 7(2):119–26.

NCCN. 2014. NCCN Guidelines Version 2.2014 Lung Cancer Screening. National Comprehensive Cancer Network. Available at: http://www.tri-kobe.org/nccn/guideline/lung/english/lung_screening.pdf (accessed 16 April 2016).

Nickel Institute. 2015. About Nickel. Nickel Institute. Available at: http://www.nickelinstitute.org/NickelUseInSociety/AboutNickel.aspx (accessed 16 April 2016).

NIOSH. 2011. NIOSH Pocket Guide to Chemical Hazards: Coal Tar Pitch Volatiles. National Institute for Occupational Safety and Health. Available at: http://www.cdc.gov/niosh/npg/npgd0145.html (accessed 16 April 2016).

NIOSH. 2012. Workplace Safety and Health Topics, The Diesel Exhaust in Miners Study (DEMS). National Institute for Occupational Safety and Health. Available at: http://www.cdc.gov/niosh/topics/cancer/diesel/dieselexhaustinminersstudyfull.html (accessed 16 April 2016).

NIOSH. 2013. In National Institute for Occupational Safety and Health (ed.), *Criteria for a Recommended Standard Occupational Exposure to Hexavalent Chromium.* DHHS (NIOSH) Publication Number 2013–128, 168 pp. Atlanta, GA: National Institute for Occupational Safety and Health. Available at: http://www.cdc.gov/niosh/docs/2013-128/pdfs/2013_128.pdf (accessed 16 April 2016).

Norman, J. E. Jr. 1975. Lung cancer mortality in World War I veterans with mustard-gas injury: 1919–1965. *J Natl Cancer Inst* 54(2):311–7.

NRC. 1999. Health effects of exposure to radon: BEIR VI. In National Academy of Science National Research Council, Committee on Health Effects of Exposure to Radon (eds), *BEIR*. Washington, DC: National Academy Press.

NRC. 2006. Health risks from exposure to low levels of ionizing radiation: BEIR VII, phase 2. In National Research Council National Academy of Science (ed.), *National Research Council, National Academy of Science, Committee to Assess Health Risks from Exposure to Low Levels of Ionizing Radiation, Board on Radiation Effects*, Washington, DC: National Academy Press.

NTP. 2011a. Coal tars and coal-tar pitches. In National Toxicology Program (ed.), *National Toxicology Program. Report on Carcinogens.* Research Triangle Park, NC: U.S. Department of Health and Human Services, Public Health Service.

NTP. 2011b. Diesel exhaust particulates. In National Toxicology Program (ed.), *National Toxicology Program, Report on Carcinogens*. Research Triangle Park, NC: U.S. Department of Health and Human Services, Public Health Services.

NTP. 2011c. Nickel compounds and metallic nickel substance profiles. In National Toxicology Program (ed.), *Report on Carcinogens*. Research Triangle Park, NC: U.S. Department of Health and Human Services, Public Health Service.

NTP. 2014. Mustard Gas (CAS No. 505-60-2). National Toxicology Program, Department of Health and Human Services. Available at: http://ntp.niehs.nih.gov/ntp/roc/content/profiles/mustardgas.pdf (accessed 16 April 2016).

Park, R. M., Stayner, L. T., Petersen, M. R., Finley-Couch, M., Hornung, R. and Rice, C. 2012. Cadmium and lung cancer mortality accounting for simultaneous arsenic exposure. *Occup Environ Med* 69(5):303–9.

Pelucchi, C., Pira, E., Piolatto, G., Coggiola, M., Carta, P. and La Vecchia, C. 2006. Occupational silica exposure and lung cancer risk: A review of epidemiological studies 1996–2005. *Ann Oncol* 17(7):1039–50.

Pott, P. 1775. *Chirurgical Observations: Relative to the Cataract, the Polypus of the Nose, the Cancer of the Scrotum, the Different Kinds of Ruptures, and the Mortification of the Toes and Feet.* London: Hawes, Clarke, and Collins.

Pronk, A., Coble, J. and Stewart, P. A. 2009. Occupational exposure to diesel engine exhaust: A literature review, *JESEE* 19(5):443–57.

Pukkala, E., Martinsen, J. I., Lynge, E., Gunnarsdottir, H. K., Sparen, P., Tryggvadottir, L., Weiderpass, E. et al. 2009. Occupation and cancer—Follow-up of 15 million people in five Nordic countries. *Acta Oncol* 48(5):646–790.

Pukkala, E. I. 1995. *Cancer Risk by Social Class and Occupation: A Survey of 109,000 Cancer Cases among Finns of Working Age, Contributions to Epidemiology and Biostatistics*. Basel, New York: Karger.

Romundstad, P., Andersen, A. and Haldorsen, T. 2001. Cancer incidence among workers in the Norwegian silicon carbide industry. *Am J Epidemiol* 153(10):978–86.

Rota, M., Bosetti, C., Boccia, S., Boffetta, P. and La Vecchia, C. 2014a. Occupational exposures to polycyclic aromatic hydrocarbons and respiratory and urinary tract cancers: An updated systematic review and a meta-analysis to 2014. *Arch Toxicol* 88:1479–90.

Rota, M., Bosetti, C., Boccia, S., Boffetta, P. and La Vecchia, C. 2014b. Occupational exposures to polycyclic aromatic hydrocarbons and respiratory and urinary tract cancers: An updated systematic review and a meta-analysis to 2014. *Arch Toxicol* 88(8):1479–90.

Sanderson, W. T., Ward, E. M., Steenland, K. and Petersen, M. R. 2001. Lung cancer case–control study of beryllium workers. *Am J Ind Med* 39(2):133–44.

Schubauer-Berigan, M. K., Couch, J. R., Petersen, M. R., Carreon, T., Jin, Y. and Deddens, J. A. 2011a. Cohort mortality study of workers at seven beryllium processing plants: Update and associations with cumulative and maximum exposure. *Occup Environ Med* 68(5):345–53.

Schubauer-Berigan, M. K., Daniels, R. D. and Pinkerton, L. E. 2009. Radon exposure and mortality among white and American Indian uranium miners: An update of the Colorado Plateau cohort. *Am J Epidemiol* 169(6):718–30.

Schubauer-Berigan, M. K., Deddens, J. A., Couch, J. R. and Petersen, M. R. 2011b. Risk of lung cancer associated with quantitative beryllium exposure metrics within an occupational cohort. *Occup Environ Med* 68(5):354–60.

Schubauer-Berigan, M. K., Deddens, J. A., Steenland, K., Sanderson, W. T. and Petersen, M. R. 2008. Adjustment for temporal confounders in a reanalysis of a case–control study of beryllium and lung cancer. *Occup Environ Med* 65(6):379–83.

Shilnikova, N. S., Preston, D. L., Ron, E., Gilbert, E. S., Vassilenko, E. K., Romanov, S. A., Kuznetsova, I. S. et al. 2003. Cancer mortality risk among workers at the Mayak nuclear complex. *Radiat Res* 159(6):787–98.

Shockley, V. E., Kathren, R. L. and Thomas, E. M. 2008. Reconstruction of doses from occupationally related medical X-ray examinations. *Health Phys* 95(1):107–18.

Silverman, D. T., Samanic, C. M., Lubin, J. H., Blair, A. E., Stewart, P. A., Vermeulen, R., Coble, J. B. et al. 2012. The diesel exhaust in miners study: A nested case–control study of lung cancer and diesel exhaust. *J Natl Cancer Inst* 104(11):855–68.

Sokolnikov, M. E., Gilbert, E. S., Preston, D. L., Ron, E., Shilnikova, N. S., Khokhryakov, V. V., Vasilenko, E. K. et al. 2008. Lung, liver and bone cancer mortality in Mayak workers. *Int J Cancer* 123(4):905–11.

Stayner, L. 2007. Silica and lung cancer: When is enough evidence enough? *Epidemiology* 18(1):23–4.

Stayner, L., Bena, J., Sasco, A. J., Smith, R., Steenland, K., Kreuzer, M. and Straif, K. 2007. Lung cancer risk and workplace exposure to environmental tobacco smoke. *Am J Public Health* 97(3):545–51.

Steenland, K., Mannetje, A., Boffetta, P., Stayner, L., Attfield, M., Chen, J., Dosemeci, M. et al. and International Agency for Research on Cancer. 2001. Pooled exposure–response analyses and risk assessment for lung cancer in 10 cohorts of silica-exposed workers: An IARC multicentre study. *Cancer Causes Control* 12(9):773–84.

Steenland, K. and Ward, E. 1991. Lung cancer incidence among patients with beryllium disease: A cohort mortality study. *J Natl Cancer Inst* 83(19):1380–5.

Steenland, K. and Ward, E. 2014. Silica: A lung carcinogen. *CA Cancer J Clin* 64(1):63–9.

Straif, K., Keil, U., Taeger, D., Holthenrich, D., Sun, Y., Bungers, M. and Weiland, S. K. 2000. Exposure to nitrosamines, carbon black, asbestos, and talc and mortality from stomach, lung, and laryngeal cancer in a cohort of rubber workers. *Am J Epidemiol* 152(4):297–306.

Thun, M. J., Schnorr, T. M., Smith, A. B., Halperin, W. E. and Lemen, R. A. 1985. Mortality among a cohort of U.S. cadmium production workers—An update. *J Natl Cancer Inst* 74(2):325–33.

Tirmarche, M., Harrison, J. D., Laurier, D., Paquet, F., Blanchardon, E., Marsh, J. W. and International Commission on Radiological Protection. 2010. ICRP Publication 115. Lung cancer risk from radon and progeny and statement on radon. *Ann ICRP* 40(1):1–64.

USGS. 2014. Minerals Yearbook, *Cadium*. U.S. Geological Survey, U.S. Department of the Interior. Available at: http://minerals.usgs.gov/minerals/pubs/commodity/cadmium/index.html#myb (accessed 16 April 2016).

Veglia, F., Vineis, P., Overvad, K., Boeing, H., Bergmann, M., Trichopoulou, A., Trichopoulos, D. et al. 2007. Occupational exposures, environmental tobacco smoke, and lung cancer. *Epidemiology* 18(6):769–75.

Wacholder, S. 2009. Bias in full cohort and nested case-control studies? *Epidemiology* 20(3):339–40.

Ward, E., Okun, A., Ruder, A., Fingerhut, M. and Steenland, K. 1992. A mortality study of workers at seven beryllium processing plants. *Am J Ind Med* 22(6):885–904.

Watson, A. Y. and Valberg, P. A. 2001. Carbon black and soot: Two different substances. *AIHAJ* 62(2):218–28.

Weiss, A. and Weiss, B. 1975. Carcinogenesis due to mustard gas exposure in man, important sign for therapy with alkylating agents. *Dtsch Med Wochenschr* 100:919–23.

Weiss, W. and Nash, D. 1997. An epidemic of lung cancer due to chloromethyl ethers: 30 years of observation. *J Occup Environ Med* 39 (10):1003–9.

World Health Organization. 2009. *WHO Handbook on Indoor Radon: A Public Health Perspective*. Geneva: WHO Press.

Yamakido, M., Ishioka, S., Hiyama, K. and Maeda, A. 1996. Former poison gas workers and cancer: Incidence and inhibition of tumor formation by treatment with biological response modifier N-CWS. *Environ Health Perspect* 104:3485–8.

Zhang, J., Qi, H., Sun, Y., Xie, H. and Zhou, C. 2015. Mosquito coil exposure associated with small cell lung cancer: A report of three cases. *Oncol Lett* 9(4):1667–71.

22 Cancer of the Respiratory Tract Due to Asbestos and Zeolites

Steven Markowitz

CONTENTS

LUNG CANCER

Introduction

Asbestos is universally recognized as a human lung carcinogen (International Agency for Research on Cancer, 2012; National Toxicology Program, 2014; World Health Organization, 2014a,b). All of the major asbestos fibre types—chrysotile, crocidolite, amosite, tremolite, actinolite and anthophyllite—are established as causing lung cancer, based on the cumulative scientific evidence provided by animal experiments, epidemiologic and pathology studies and mechanism-based research (International Agency for Research on Cancer, 2012; National Toxicology Program, 2014).

Asbestos was first suspected of causing human lung cancer in the 1930s, when pathologists found a rare incidental neoplasm, lung cancer, among several asbestos manufacturing workers who had died from asbestosis and had undergone autopsy in the United States and England (Figure 22.1) (Gloyne, 1935; Lynch et al., 1935). Soon thereafter, industry sponsored an animal assay at the Saranac Laboratory in upstate New York and confirmed that asbestos caused lung tumours in rodents (Castleman, 2005). The study results were suppressed, although epidemiological studies of asbestos workers were subsequently published in the 1950s, demonstrating that asbestos workers experienced excess lung cancer death rates (Doll, 1955).

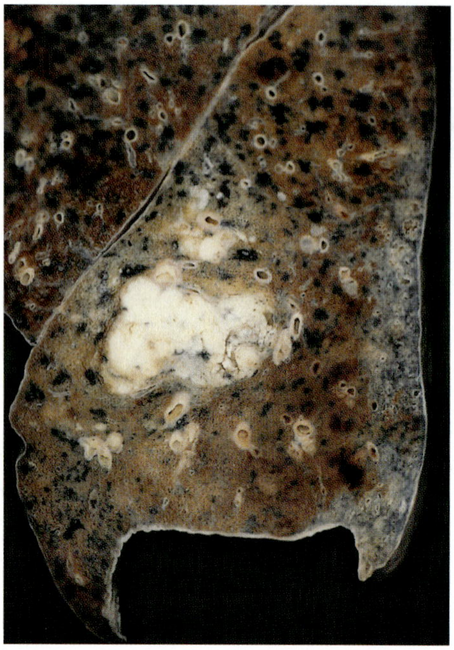

FIGURE 22.1 Asbestosis associated with carcinoma of the lung. Asbestosis is highlighted by barium sulphate impregnation and is seen as a grey sub-pleural band to the right of the picture. Although the carcinoma has arisen in the same lobe as the asbestosis, it has not arisen in an area that is obviously affected by asbestosis. (Courtesy of Bryan Corrin, MD.)

Burden of Lung Cancer Due to Asbestos

Asbestos exposure over the past 50 years has made a substantial contribution to current overall lung cancer incidence and mortality in many countries. Given the geographic distribution of the use of asbestos between 1940 and 1980 and the established latency of asbestos-related lung cancer, the countries that have been most severely affected by asbestos-related lung cancer in the recent past, and continuing to the present, are Australia, the United States, Japan, New Zealand and those in Western Europe. In studies that examine the aggregate contribution of all known occupational lung carcinogens to the overall burden of lung cancer, asbestos is responsible for more lung cancer cases than any other individual workplace carcinogen.

The World Health Organization (WHO) estimated that at least 90,000 people die from asbestos-related lung cancer each year (World Health Organization, 2006). This is nearly twice the number of deaths due to malignant mesothelioma that are estimated to occur worldwide (Driscoll et al., 2005). An earlier estimate by Tossavainen ascribed 20,000 lung cancers to prior asbestos exposure in the US, Canada, Australia, and seven countries in Europe (Tossavainen, 1997).

Lung cancer due to asbestos is generally more frequent than malignant mesothelioma, even if cases of the latter disease are far more likely to be recognized as being caused by asbestos. The under-recognition of lung cancer as being asbestos related is widely reported (Henderson et al., 2004). The ratio between the numbers or incidence rates of these two diseases varies considerably in individual studies, although a commonly used ratio of excess asbestos-related lung cancers to malignant mesothelioma is 2:1 (Henderson et al., 2004; McCormack et al., 2012). Since smoking causes lung cancer but not malignant mesothelioma and does so in a synergistic manner with asbestos exposure, differences or changes in the prevalence of smoking impact this ratio. Smoking cessation among asbestos-exposed workers is increasingly common, at least in developed countries, and will result in a lower ratio between the two diseases.

Estimating the magnitude of asbestos-related lung cancer burden is complicated due to: (1) the high but variable prevalence of cigarette smoking and other risk factors for lung cancer; (2) the variation in estimates of excess relative risk of lung cancer due to asbestos in different occupations and industries; and (3) limited knowledge about the size and extent of asbestos exposure of populations that are at risk.

Despite different approaches, accumulated studies indicate that approximately 4%–10% of lung cancers in most developed countries are due to asbestos exposure. Brown and colleagues estimated that 1937 lung cancer deaths, or 5.9% of all lung cancer deaths, in the United Kingdom were due to asbestos in 2004 (Brown et al., 2012). This estimate included 8.9% and 1.7% of lung cancer deaths among men and women, respectively, as being due to asbestos exposure. In France, Boffetta et al. recently ascribed 5.4% and 3.8% of male and female lung cancer cases and deaths, respectively, to prior asbestos exposure, translating to 1256 lung cancer deaths in 2000 (Boffetta et al., 2010). Marinaccio et al. used an ecological model and estimated that 1.6% and 3.7% of all lung cancer deaths in men in Italy between 1981 and 2000 were due to asbestos exposure, or 380–770 deaths per year (Marinaccio et al., 2008). McCormack and colleagues applied two models in order to use mesothelioma mortality to estimate asbestos-related lung cancer mortality in 20 countries and obtained a broad range of proportions of asbestos-associated lung cancer, ranging from 3.2%–5.4% in the United States to 12.2%–16.2% in the United Kingdom (McCormack et al., 2012).

Asbestos and Cell Type and Location of Lung Cancer

Asbestos causes all histologic types of lung cancer (Helsinki Consensus, 1997; Nielsen et al., 2014). Some studies have shown a predominance of adenocarcinoma, although this cell type has been increasing overall in the general population (Nielsen et al., 2014). Similarly, asbestos-related lung cancers can occur in any anatomic location in the lungs (Helsinki Consensus 1997; Nielsen et al. 2014). The current consensus is that there are no specific cell types or anatomic distributions that are distinctively associated with an asbestos aetiology (Hillerdal and Henderson, 1997; Henderson et al., 2004; Nielsen et al., 2014).

Animal Studies

All asbestos fibre types cause lung tumours in animals via multiple routes of exposure. Using standard Union for International Cancer Control samples of asbestos, Wagner et al. (1974) exposed rats to various asbestos types at approximately 10 mg/m^3 concentrations via inhalation for time periods ranging from 3 to 24 months and found elevated lung tumour percentages in exposed rats in relation to control animals for all exposure periods and for all types of asbestos tested, including amosite, crocidolite, chrysotile (Canadian and Rhodesian) and anthophyllite. Among rats exposed for 24 months, 48%–89% of the animals developed tumours, depending upon fibre type. No significant differences in potency were found among the various types of asbestos. Davis et al. performed a series of rat inhalation experiments with asbestos exposure for 12 months and showed that all types of asbestos tested (i.e. chrysotile, amosite, tremolite and crocidolite) produced elevated percentages of lung tumours, especially when 'long' fibres (>5 μm) were tested (Davis and Jones, 1988; Davis et al., 1986; Davis et al., 1991). Other studies have also shown that asbestos, including chrysotile, causes lung tumours in test animals, frequently exceeding 20% of animals (Le Bouffant et al., 1987; McConnell et al., 1991; Hesterberg et al., 1993). Coffin and colleagues instilled chrysotile or crocidolite in the trachea of rats and found that 18.3% of chrysotile-exposed rats developed lung carcinomas compared to 4.6% of crocidolite-exposed animals (Coffin et al., 1992).

The International Agency for Research on Cancer (IARC) has concluded that there is sufficient evidence in experimental animals to support the notion of the carcinogenicity of all forms of asbestos (chrysotile, crocidolite, amosite, tremolite, actinolite and anthophyllite) (International Agency for Research on Cancer, 1999; International Agency for Research on Cancer, 2012). Reviewing the subject of toxicological studies and lung cancer, Stayner and colleagues from the United States National Institute for Occupational Safety and Health concluded that 'chrysotile asbestos is at least as potent, if not more so, as the amphibole forms in the induction of lung tumors on a per-milligram basis' (Stayner et al., 1996, p. 183).

Epidemiology

IARC and others have recently reviewed over 60 epidemiologic studies of occupational exposure to asbestos and lung cancer risk (International Agency for Research on Cancer, 2012; McCormack et al., 2012; Nielsen et al., 2014). Most studies showed excess risk of lung cancer from asbestos exposure. Case–control studies generally showed lung cancer relative risks of 1.5–3.0 due to asbestos exposure, although some studies showed higher risks, especially among the more heavily exposed workers (Brownson et al., 1993; Gustavsson et al., 2002; Pintos et al., 2008). Lung cancer cases in case–control studies are usually drawn from the general population and encompass a broad range of asbestos exposures, presenting challenges for an accurate classification of exposure. However, case–control studies can advantageously control for cigarette smoking. Cohort studies of asbestos miners, insulation workers, other construction workers, asbestos manufacturing workers (including textile, friction products, gas masks, insulation products and others), cement plant workers, shipyard workers and other workers mostly demonstrate excess lung cancer risk in association with asbestos exposure in diverse settings, occupations and countries, with a broader range of excess lung cancer risk compared to the case–control studies (International Agency for Research on Cancer, 2012).

The variable level of excess risk of lung cancer among different epidemiological studies is due to a large range of factors, including study methods, data quality, reference populations, age structure of the study population, country, occupation, industry, industrial process, job tasks, calendar years, exposure intensity and duration, fibre type, fibre dimensions, smoking information, presence of other lung carcinogens and others. Stayner et al. noted that levels of lung cancer risk tended to cluster more by industry than fibre type (Stayner et al., 1996).

The best studied contrast in lung cancer risk in different exposure settings is between the Quebec mines and mills (Liddell et al., 1997) and a textile factory in South Carolina (Hein et al., 2007). Chrysotile produces a summary lung cancer relative risk of 1.37 among Quebec miners and millers (Liddell et al., 1997). It is exported to South Carolina in the United States, where the excess lung cancer risk among textile factory workers is considerably higher, at 1.96 (Hein et al., 2007). The contrast in risk is more striking when examined as the lung cancer risk per unit exposure, or the lung cancer potency factor. This is the slope of the increase in the relative risk per unit of cumulative asbestos exposure, expressed in fibres/mL-years, or K_L (US Environmental Protection Agency, 1986; Nicholson and Landrigan, 1996; Lenters et al., 2011). The lung cancer potency factor (×100) among Quebec miners and millers is 0.03 versus 1.64 among South Carolina textile workers (Lenters et al., 2011). This difference in potency is not due to amphiboles, since their use was very limited at the South Carolina plant (Elliott et al., 2012). A mineral oil hypothesis as an explanation has also been discarded (Dement et al., 1994). Nicholson and Dement have opined that the splitting of chrysotile bundles in the textile manufacturing process created thinner chrysotile fibres, which were more likely to be carcinogenic (Nicholson, 1991; Dement, 1991).

Indeed, Loomis and colleagues showed that fibre dimension differences are likely to be important in explaining differences in lung cancer potency. They found that longer (>5 μm) and thinner fibres (<0.25 μm) were most strongly related to lung cancer, although fibres of all sizes were associated with lung cancer mortality (Loomis et al., 2012). Fibres in the South Carolina textile factory tended to be longer and thinner than fibres in the Quebec mining environment (Stayner et al., 2008).

Notably, however, the lung cancer potency of asbestos at a North Carolina textile factory is considerably lower than at the South Carolina textile plant, despite similarities in type of industry and the fibre size distributions between the two plants (Dement et al., 2011; Elliott et al., 2012). Decreased data quality with resultant measurement error and the removal of ill workers from the North Carolina plant may have led to lower estimates of lung cancer mortality risk (Elliott et al., 2012).

Evaluation of the excess lung cancer risk associated with asbestos exposure is critically dependent on the quality of asbestos exposure assessment. Silverstein et al. (2009) and Lenters et al. (2011) have identified eight problem areas in asbestos exposure assessments used in epidemiological studies: (1) restriction of fibres counted by phase contrast microscopy to fibres ≥5 μm in length and >0.25 μm in width; (2) high correlations of differently sized fibres in workplaces, making separation of effects difficult; (3) variation in counts by different phase contrast microscopes; (4) variation in counting methods among laboratories and over time; (5) use of area samples in order to characterize personal exposures; (6) absent or few measurements from selected historical periods of the study site; (7) incomplete work histories; and (8) uncertain and variable conversion of fibre counts from one method (e.g. midget impinger-based dust particle counts in millions of particles per cubic foot) to another (fibre counts by phase contrast microscopy) (Henderson et al., 2004; Silverstein et al., 2009; Lenters et al., 2011). Such limitations formed an important basis for the US Environmental Protection Agency (EPA) rejecting a proposed update in asbestos risk assessment in 2008 (Johnson, 2008).

Exposure–Response and Lung Cancer Risk

Lung cancer risk increases with cumulative exposure to asbestos (Helsinki Consensus, 1997; Henderson et al., 2004; Lenters et al., 2011; van der Bij et al., 2013; Nielsen et al., 2014). Studies of sufficient size and with quantitative exposure assessments have permitted the estimation of lung cancer risk at different levels of exposure to asbestos. The slope of the resultant line that characterizes the relationship between exposure and lung cancer represents the potency of asbestos to cause lung cancer for a particular study (K_L in the published literature). These studies have principally been in asbestos textile, cement and friction products manufacturing, insulation and mining and milling. Study results vary substantially given differences in time, exposure circumstances, sample size, industry and other factors. In general, the increase in lung cancer relative risk has been found to be from 1% to 4% for each year of exposure to 1 fibre/mL (Nielsen et al., 2014). The exposure–response relationship is considered to be approximately linear (Henderson et al., 2004; Nielsen et al., 2014).

Most meta-analyses assume a linear dose–response relationship between asbestos exposure and lung cancer (Hodgson and Darnton, 2000; Lenters et al., 2011; van der Bij et al., 2013; Nielsen et al., 2014). The majority of relevant studies involved relatively heavy exposure to asbestos, and the lung cancer risk at lower levels is extrapolated from these studies, or is based on the few studies of lower levels of exposure to asbestos (van der Bij et al., 2013). A recent meta-analysis applied a non-linear meta-regression model (i.e. a natural spline model) to all available published data on exposure–response relationships at lower levels of asbestos exposure, thereby obviating the need to depend solely on extrapolating from high-level exposure results (van der Bij et al., 2013). The results demonstrated a higher level of lung cancer risk increment per fibre/mL-year for relatively low levels of asbestos exposure compared to previous meta-analyses (van der Bij et al., 2013).

As noted above, a critical source of variation and error in evaluating exposure–response relationships in asbestos is the validity of study exposure estimates. Many exposure assessments have major limitations (Silverstein et al., 2009; Lenters et al., 2011). Such constraints introduce measurement error, which often leads to underestimates of relative risk. Importantly, Lenters et al. found higher estimates of the lung cancer risk due to asbestos in studies that had higher-quality exposure assessments, which is likely to explain some of the variability in study results (Lenters et al., 2011).

Role of Asbestosis in Lung Cancer Risk

The relationship between asbestos exposure, asbestosis and lung cancer risk has long been studied and, indeed, was first raised in the 1930s when lung cancer was initially documented among workers dying from asbestosis (Gloyne, 1935; Lynch et al., 1935). The issue is complicated, because the risk and intensity of asbestosis increases with increasing asbestos exposure and because study information on the three key lung cancer risk factors—asbestos exposure, asbestosis and smoking—is incomplete in many studies. Nonetheless, it is clear that, even among never-smokers, asbestos exposure in the absence of asbestosis raises the risk of lung cancer, and that asbestosis, when present, further raises lung cancer risk.

Asbestos exposure in the absence of asbestosis increases the risk of lung cancer among a variety of different asbestos workers (Fletcher, 1972; Martischnig et al., 1977; Liddell and McDonald, 1980; Cheng and Kong, 1992; Karjalainen et al., 1994; Wilkinson et al., 1995; Finkelstein, 1997; Reid et al., 2005; Markowitz et al., 2013). The range of risk elevation in these studies is approximately 1.5–5.5. In an update of the mortality of a large North American insulator cohort, Markowitz et al. compared long-term insulators to a blue collar control group without asbestos exposure that was part of the Cancer Prevention Study II of the American Cancer Society (Markowitz et al., 2013). They found a lung cancer mortality rate ratio of 3.6 (95% confidence interval [CI]: 1.7–7.6) based on seven lung cancer deaths among long-term insulators who had never smoked and had no radiographic evidence of asbestosis (Markowitz et al., 2013).

Asbestosis, documented by chest X-rays, increases the risk of lung cancer, as observed in asbestos cement workers (Finkelstein, 1997), textile workers (Cheng et al., 1992) and miners (Sluis-Cremer et al., 1989; Reid et al., 2005). The range of elevations in the standardized mortality ratios (SMRs) for lung cancer was 194–996; these elevations were statistically significant. Control for cigarette smoking was rare in these studies, but the elevation in lung cancer risk was too high to have been caused by cigarette smoking alone (Axelson and Steenland, 1988). Controlling for cigarette smoking, Wilkinson et al. found a twofold elevation in lung cancer risk associated with asbestosis in a large British case–control study, in which cases with lung cancer had diverse sources of asbestos exposure (Wilkinson et al., 1995). Markowitz et al., updating the large North American insulator cohort, found a doubling of risk of lung cancer among insulators with asbestosis compared to insulators without asbestosis. This was true for both never-smokers and smokers. The extent of asbestos exposure was similar among the insulators with and without asbestosis, so their difference in lung cancer risk was not due to differences in asbestos exposure (Markowitz et al., 2013).

Lung Cancer and Pleural Plaques

Is the presence of pleural plaques associated with added lung cancer risk apart from its role as a marker of asbestos exposure? This issue is of practical importance, since plaques, if present, could help stratify risk, especially for lung cancer screening. Like asbestosis, the risk of asbestos-related pleural plaques increases with added exposure to asbestos, so control for asbestos exposure is needed in order to address this question. The association between pleural plaques and lung cancer has been studied with mixed results (Hillerdal et al., 1997; Henderson et al., 2004; Ameille et al., 2011). Koskinen and colleagues found a relative risk of lung cancer death of 1.2 (95% CI: 0.9–1.6) associated with the presence of pleural plaques among 17,000 Finnish construction workers after controlling for degree of asbestos exposure, occupation, chest X-ray evidence of interstitial fibrosis and age (Koskinen et al., 2002). Cullen and colleagues studied lung cancer mortality among 4060 workers with heterogeneous asbestos exposure as part of a chemoprevention trial, comparing them to 7965 heavy smokers who had not been exposed to asbestos (Cullen et al., 2005). Among a subset of workers with pleural plaques but without radiographic evidence of interstitial fibrosis, they found a lung cancer rate ratio of 1.91 (95% CI: 1.25–2.92), controlling for occupational title and years of asbestos work (Cullen et al., 2005). Markowitz et al. evaluated lung cancer mortality in 2377 long-term insulators (≥30 years of asbestos exposure) between 1981 and 2008 and found no increase in risk of lung cancer in association with pleural plaques on chest X-ray (Markowitz et al., 2013).

Conflicting study results on this issue are likely due to the inhomogeneity of asbestos exposure in the study groups and the variable ability to capture asbestos exposure through surrogates such as job title, duration of work and other measures. To the extent that pleural plaques represent a better measure of asbestos exposure than the occupational history, their presence is likely to be informative regarding an added risk of lung cancer.

Joint Effect of Asbestos Exposure and Cigarette Smoking in Lung Cancer

The joint effect of asbestos and cigarette smoking in causing lung cancer has not only been much studied in occupational health, but is also widely cited in epidemiology and public health as a classic example of causal interaction. In a classic study of North American insulators, Hammond et al. found a multiplicative effect between asbestos exposure and smoking in terms of elevating lung cancer mortality among 17,800 insulators whose deaths occurred in 1967–1976, compared to a contemporaneous blue collar cohort from the Cancer Prevention Study I of the American Cancer Society. Insulators who never smoked had a lung cancer death rate ratio of 5.2 compared to a never-smoking control group. The lung cancer mortality ratio of the smoking control group without asbestos exposure was 10.9, and the same ratio among smoking insulators was 53.2. The joint effect of asbestos and smoking was multiplicative (Hammond et al., 1979).

At least two dozen published studies have addressed the issue of the relationship between smoking and asbestos exposure in elevating lung cancer risk. Erren and colleagues reviewed 12 relevant epidemiological studies and concluded that asbestos and smoking were synergistic; that is, they produced more lung cancer cases than would be expected from simply summing their separate contributions (Erren et al., 1999). Lee reviewed 23 studies in 2001 and concluded that the joint effect of these two risk factors was compatible with a multiplicative model of risk (Lee, 2001). Liddell also examined extant studies in 2001 and reached a different conclusion; that is, that the joint effect was supra-additive but not multiplicative, and that the increase in lung cancer relative risk due to asbestos was twice as high for non-smokers as for smokers exposed to asbestos (Liddell, 2001). Central to the difficulty in studying this issue is the dearth of lung cancers among never-smokers, especially among smaller studies. Nielsen et al. reviewed the issue and concluded that the joint exposure risk was between additive and multiplicative (Nielsen et al., 2014).

Recent studies tend to confirm that the joint effect of asbestos and smoking is more than additive but less than multiplicative. Wang et al. followed 577 chrysotile asbestos manufacturing workers and 435 blue collar controls from 1972 to 2008 and found an age- and smoking-adjusted hazard ratio for lung cancer of 3.3 (95% CI: 1.6–6.9). Among non-smokers, the hazard ratio for lung cancer was 7.5 (95% CI: 0.9–62.8). Smokers from a non-asbestos-exposed control group had a lung cancer hazard ratio of 6.0. The asbestos workers who smoked had a lung cancer hazard ratio of 17.4, indicating a supra-additive effect of asbestos and smoking, although the effect did not reach statistical significance (Wang et al., 2012). Offermans et al. studied >120,000 people in the Netherlands Cohort Study and found a lung cancer hazard ratio of 1.79 (95% CI: 1.04–3.08) for never-smokers with a history of asbestos exposure. The corresponding hazard ratio among current smokers who had never been exposed to asbestos was 7.48 (95% CI: 5.55–10.08). The joint hazard ratio was 10.21 (95% CI: 7.26–14.35), suggesting a joint effect midway between additive and multiplicative (Offermans et al., 2014). Reid et al. also found a supra-additive effect among Wittenoom miners and millers (Reid et al., 2006).

The source of some of the variation in the empirical studies of the joint effect of asbestos and smoking in terms of causing lung cancer has recently been clarified. Markowitz et al. described mortality patterns from 1981 through to 2008 for 2377 North American insulators for whom information on smoking and asbestos exposure and radiographic findings of asbestosis were available (Markowitz et al., 2013). Due to lengthy follow-up of a large cohort, the study had a high number of lung cancer deaths among asbestos-exposed workers who had never smoked (n = 18). They found that the lung cancer rate ratio was 3.6 (95% CI: 1.7–7.6) for non-smoking insulators without asbestosis, 10.3 (95% CI: 8.8–12.2) among the smoking control group and 14.4 (95% CI: 10.7–19.4) among insulators who had smoked but had no asbestosis. Thus, the joint effect was largely additive in the absence of asbestosis. However, when asbestosis was present, the joint effect of asbestos and smoking was supra-additive. The lung cancer rate ratio was 7.4 (95% CI: 4.0–13.7) for non-smoking insulators with asbestosis, 10.3 (95% CI: 8.8–12.2) among the smoking control group and 36.8 (95% CI: 30.1–45.0) among insulators who had smoked and also had asbestosis (Markowitz et al., 2013).

Lung Cancer among Asbestos-Exposed Non-Smokers

Asbestos exposure alone, in the absence of cigarette smoking, causes lung cancer. Hammond et al. identified a fivefold increase in lung cancer mortality rate ratio among non-smoking long-term insulators in their study of 17,800 insulators (Hammond et al., 1979). McDonald and colleagues reported a dose-related increase in lung cancer deaths among non-smoking Quebec miners and millers (McDonald et al., 1980). Berry et al. identified mortality among 1670 asbestos factory workers between 1971 and 1980 and found a relative risk of lung cancer of 7.3 based on four lung cancers among never-smokers (Berry et al., 1985). Wang et al. followed 577 chrysotile asbestos manufacturing workers and 435 blue collar controls from 1972 to 2008 and found an overall age-adjusted lung cancer hazard ratio of 7.5 (95% CI: 0.9–62.8) among non-smoking workers (Wang et al., 2012). Markowitz et al. followed 2377 insulators from 1981 to 2008 and found a lung cancer mortality rate ratio of 5.2 (95% CI: 3.2–8.5) among non-smoking insulators based on a large number of lung cancer deaths among non-smokers (n = 18) (Markowitz et al., 2013).

Smoking Cessation and Lung Cancer Risk

Lung cancer risk following smoking cessation is of considerable public health, clinical and scientific importance, in part because lung cancer risk increases with time following asbestos exposure, but decreases in time following smoking cessation. Reid et al. followed 2935 Australian miners and millers from 1979 to 2002 and identified lung cancer incident cases. Current smokers of >1 pack per day in the study cohort had a lung cancer odds ratio (OR) of 13.2 (95% CI: 4.1–42.5). Recent quitters (<6 years) had an even higher lung cancer mortality, with an OR of lung cancer of 22.1 (95% CI: 5.6–87.0) compared to never-smokers. Thereafter, however, lung cancer risk decreased with increasing years since quitting smoking: the OR was 9.3 in ex-smokers at 6–9 years since quitting, 8.9 in ex-smokers at 10–19 years since quitting and 1.9 (95% CI: 0.50–7.2) in ex-smokers at ≥20 years since quitting (Reid et al., 2006). Frost et al. found that lung cancer mortality among 98,912 asbestos workers between 1971 and 2005 was reduced following smoking cessation, but remained possibly elevated at ≥40 years following smoking cessation (relative risk [RR]: 1.5, 95% CI: 0.8–2.8) (Frost et al., 2011). Markowitz and colleagues traced mortality among 2377 insulators from 1981 to 2008, including the nearly 60% of smoking insulators who had quit smoking. They found that lung cancer rate ratios dropped by half during the first 10 years following smoking cessation and continued to decrease thereafter. Former smoking insulators at ≥30 years following cessation had the same lung cancer risk as insulators who had never smoked cigarettes (Markowitz et al., 2013).

Fibre Type and Lung Cancer Risk

Excess lung cancer mortality has been observed in studies of workers who were exposed to all commercial types of asbestos fibres, including chrysotile. Recent examples of studies of chrysotile exposure are multiple. Wang et al. followed 577 chrysotile asbestos manufacturing workers and 435 blue collar controls from 1972 to 2008 in China and found an age- and smoking-adjusted hazard ratio of 3.31 for lung cancer (95% CI: 1.60–6.87) (Wang et al., 2012). Loomis and colleagues identified a lung cancer SMR of 1.95 (95% CI: 1.73–2.20) among North Carolina textile workers who almost exclusively used chrysotile asbestos; 277 workers died from cancer of the lung or trachea (Loomis et al., 2009). Hein et al. updated the mortality of the South Carolina textile factory cohort in which >99.9% of the asbestos used was chrysotile and found a lung cancer SMR of 1.95 (95% CI: 1.68–2.24) (Hein et al., 2007).

The relative potency of different types of asbestos in terms of causing lung cancer has been evaluated. Some meta-analyses of asbestos exposure and lung cancer studies have shown an increased potency for amphiboles relative to chrysotile in the causation of lung cancer of approximately five- to ten-fold (Hodgson and Darnton, 2000; Berman and Crump, 2008). A meta-analysis that used a different meta-regression modelling method found a non-significant three- to four-fold difference in lung cancer potency between chrysotile and amphiboles (van der Bij et al., 2013). A recent meta-analysis that factored in the quality of study exposure assessments concluded that potency differences among fibre types narrowed after taking into account quality of exposure assessment and that potency differences were inconclusive when analysis was restricted to studies with higher-quality exposure assessments (Lenters et al., 2011).

In a systematic review, Nielsen et al. (2014: 199) reviewed existing studies and concluded that 'all types of asbestos fibres are associated with lung cancer … [and] there is not sufficient evidence to derive different risk estimates for different fibre types'.

Somewhat neglected in the discussion regarding fibre type potency is the quantity of exposure to different fibre types that constitute the overall exposure of individuals. Chrysotile has been the dominant fibre type in many industries and countries, which may compensate for any differences in potency in terms of the overall contribution to cancer risk. Chrysotile, for example, has accounted for 95% or more of all asbestos used in the United States.

Fibre Dimension and Lung Cancer Risk

Animal studies have supported the assertion that longer and thinner fibres (>8 μm in length and ≤0.25 μm in width), including asbestos fibres, are more carcinogenic than shorter fibres. This has been called the 'Stanton hypothesis' (Stanton et al., 1981). These studies have involved lung tumours and also pleural or peritoneal tumours. In studies of pleural implants in rats, Stanton and colleagues found that longer and thinner (>8 μm in length and ≤0.25 μm in width) fibres of various materials produced the highest correlations with probability of pleural tumours (correlation coefficient = 0.80). However, shorter (5–8 μm) or wider (>0.25–1.5 μm) fibres were also reasonably correlated with tumour response (correlation coefficient = 0.63 and 0.68, respectively) (Stanton et al., 1981; National Institute of Occupational Safety and Health, 2011; Boulanger et al., 2014). Earlier, Pott and others injected short un-milled (94% of fibres <5 μm in length) and milled chrysotile (99.8% of fibres <5 μm in length) into the peritoneum of rats and obtained tumours in 30%–68% of animals (Pott et al., 1974). Davis et al. studied fibre length and types in the 1970s and 1980s and concluded that fibres >10 μm in length were more important for causing lung neoplasms in rats. When Davis et al. compared 'long' versus 'short chrysotile' (Canadian) fibre exposures in a rat inhalation study, they found that 48% and 18%, respectively, of the animals developed lung tumours (Davis et al., 1988). However, the 'short chrysotile' fibre dust contained 5% fibres of >5 μm in length and approximately 1% of >10 μm in length (compared to the 'long chrysotile' fibre dust, which contained 10% fibres of >5 μm and 2% of >10 μm in length), so that separation of the tumorigenic effect of shorter (≤5 μm) versus longer (>5 μm) chrysotile fibres was uncertain (Davis et al., 1988). Lipmann concluded that, since fibres of between 0.3 and 0.8 μm in width have peak retention in the lung, and given that the human alveolar macrophage is larger than the rat macrophage, asbestos fibres of >15 or 20 μm in length and >0.15 μm in width are most closely associated with lung cancer (Lippmann, 2014).

Few of the many epidemiological studies of asbestos and lung cancer risk have addressed the issue of fibre length. Indeed, there are only two epidemiological studies of asbestos-exposed workers with sufficient measurements to allow insight into the issue of fibre length (Stayner et al., 2008; Loomis et al., 2010; Elliott et al., 2012). Most epidemiological studies that have included quantitative measurements of asbestos exposure are based on the measurement of dust mass obtained by midget impingers or fibre count analyses resulting from phase contrast microscopy. The latter is typically used only to count fibres of >5 μm in length and >0.25 μm in width (so-called 'regulated fibres'), as required by regulations and dictated by feasibility.

Two relevant studies of fibre dimensions in textile mills in South and North Carolina were based on retrospective measurements of archived dust samples using transmission electron microscopy (TEM). Stayner et al. and Dement et al. reported that over 90% of the asbestos fibres in these archived samples were short or narrow (≤5 μm in length or <0.25 μm in width) and had not been counted by phase contrast microscopy in earlier studies (Stayner et al., 2008; Dement et al., 2011). They re-evaluated the relationship between TEM-based fibre measurements and lung cancer risk and concluded that the strongest association was found between lung cancer and fibres of >10 μm in length and narrower than 0.25 μm (Stayner et al., 2008; Loomis et al., 2010). However, they also found that very short and thin fibres (e.g., <1.5 μm in length and <0.25 μm in width) were associated with lung cancer risk. Fibre size categories were highly correlated in the South Carolina and North Carolina chrysotile textile factories, making it difficult to separate out the effects of fibre sizes (Stayner et al., 2008; Loomis et al., 2010; Hamra et al., 2014). Hamra et al. applied a hierarchical model to the data from the North Carolina textile factory and found that the lung cancer risk associated with different fibre length–width groups was similar (Hamra et al., 2014).

Lung fibre burden studies add limited insight into this issue. Churg and Vedal examined lung fibre burdens of 144 shipyard workers and insulators with various asbestos-related diseases. They principally found amosite in the lungs and no relationship between fibre dimensions and lung cancer risk (Churg and Vedal, 1994). Roggli and Vollmer predominantly found amosite and crocidolite in the lungs of 340 lung cancer cases collected from 1980 to 2005, but only measured fibres of >5 μm in length, so the importance of fibre length was not addressed (Roggli and Vollmer, 2008). Dodson and colleagues used TEM at 16,000- or 20,000-times magnification in order to examine the lung asbestos fibre burdens of 20 asbestos-exposed cases of lung cancer. They showed that 39%–69% of detected asbestos fibres were ≤5 μm in length, and that the majority of all fibre types—chrysotile and amphiboles—would not have been counted by phase contrast microscopy (>5 μm in length and ≥0.25 μm in width). Most counted fibres did not meet the dimensions supported by the Stanton hypothesis (≥8 μm in length and <25 μm in width), with chrysotile having the highest proportion of such short fibres (Dodson et al., 2004).

Adib and colleagues in Quebec recently used TEM in order to evaluate lung fibre burdens in 70 cases of lung cancer in the mining, maintenance, construction and other industries (Adib et al., 2013). Chrysotile and tremolite, especially fibres of <5 μm in length, were the dominant fibres seen in the lungs. Over three-quarters of the lung cancer cases had chrysotile and tremolite in the lungs, and lesser proportions had crocidolite (43%) and amosite (61%). The geometric mean fibre concentrations of chrysotile and tremolite were four-times higher than the concentration of amosite and six-times higher than that of crocidolite. The mean fibre lengths of both chrysotile and tremolite were <5 μm. Among the subset of 13 lung cancer cases whose last exposure to asbestos was ≥30 years previously, chrysotile fibres were found in all cases, with short (<5 μm) fibres outnumbering longer (≤5 μm) by at least two- to three-fold. Chrysotile fibres, especially short fibres, can remain in the lungs for long periods following exposure.

Although malignant mesothelioma differs from primary lung cancer in the site of origin, studies of fibre distribution relating to mesothelioma are highly relevant to the overall question of whether short asbestos fibres are carcinogenic. A lung fibre burden study among 73 cases of mesotheliomas in England undertaken by McDonald and colleagues showed that amphibole fibres of all lengths (<6 μm, 6–10 μm and >10 μm) were highly associated with mesothelioma. Shorter fibres were more numerous than longer fibres (McDonald et al., 2001). Suzuki and Yuen used TEM in order to measure lung fibre burden in lung, plaque and mesothelioma tissues in 168 cases of malignant mesothelioma and found that 89% of all fibres were ≤5 μm in length. Only 2.3% of all fibres met the dimensions supported by the Stanton hypothesis (≥8 μm in length and <25 μm in width). Chrysotile was the sole asbestos type that was found in the lung in 26% (31/119) of mesothelioma cases and in the mesothelioma tumour tissue in 73% (90/123) of mesothelioma cases. Only 1% of chrysotile fibres were ≥5 μm in length (Suzuki and Yuen, 2001).

In summary, the available data support the hypothesis that longer, thinner fibres have a stronger association with lung cancer than shorter, narrower fibres. Does the closer relationship between longer and thinner fibres and cancer risk signify that the observed significant associations of shorter asbestos fibres with lung cancer risk are not real or substantial? Empirical data support an association between shorter fibres and cancer (Stanton et al., 1981; Loomis et al., 2010). Animal studies demonstrate that longer and thinner fibres are more highly carcinogenic, but also show support for shorter fibres being correlated with carcinogenicity. Epidemiological studies demonstrate a statistically significant association between shorter fibres and lung cancer, although less strongly than between longer fibres and lung cancer risk. Fibre burden studies show that short fibres, especially chrysotile, are very frequently present and often outnumber longer fibres in the lung tissues of patients with a history of asbestos-related lung cancer, even many years after asbestos exposure has ceased. Short fibres, usually chrysotile, are sometimes virtually the only fibres that are found in mesothelial tissue in pleural mesothelioma cases. Current evidence does not support an assertion that there is no cancer risk associated with exposure to short asbestos fibres (Dodson et al., 2003; Dodson, 2011; Boulanger et al., 2014).

Joint Effect of Asbestos and Workplace Lung Carcinogens

Many workers who are exposed to asbestos may also work in workplaces where they are exposed to other lung carcinogens, including silica, diesel exhaust, polycyclic aromatic hydrocarbons (PAHs) and metals such as cadmium, nickel and chromium. Pastorino and colleagues obtained lifetime occupational histories of 204 lung cancer cases and 351 controls. Adjusting for smoking, they found a lung cancer relative risk of 1.9 for asbestos, of 1.6 for PAHs and, for the combined exposure to asbestos and PAHs, a relative risk of 3.3. The authors concluded that the results indicated a multiplicative joint effect (Pastorino et al., 1984). In a large population-based lung cancer case–control study in Stockholm, Gustavsson et al. took lifetime occupational histories and found that the relative risk of lung cancer for asbestos was 1.62, for combustion products was 1.67 and for the combination of asbestos and combustion products was 2.25, suggesting a joint additive effect (Gustavsson et al., 2000). In a case–control study of lung cancer in the United Kingdom, Olsson et al. found an lung cancer OR for asbestos exposure of 2.3 (95% CI: 1.3–4.3), an OR of 2.1 (95% CI: 1.0–4.3) for PAHs and an OR of 4.4 for exposure to PAHs and asbestos (95% CI: 2.2–8.9), indicating some interaction, or a supra-additive effect (Olsson et al., 2010).

Lung Fibre Burden Studies

Characterization of the concentrations and types of asbestos fibres in lung, pleura and other extrapulmonary sites has some value for the purposes of attribution and compensation for individuals, and for improving understanding of the fibre-specific aetiology and risk of asbestos-related diseases in populations. However, such characterization has numerous important scientific and technical limitations, including: (1) the absence of an accepted, widely used standard method for conducting tissue fibre counts; (2) the restriction of fibre burden studies to a limited number of individuals who may not be representative of defined asbestos-exposed populations; (3) the use of different microscopes (phase contrast microscopy, scanning electron microscopy and TEM) at varying magnifications that can detect and count different populations of fibres; (4) ranges of 'normal' fibre counts in populations without known occupational exposure to asbestos that vary among laboratories; and (5) the difficulty of inferring from an organ or tissue in which a fibre burden study is performed to the organ or tissue in which the disease occurs (Baker, 1991; Dodson and Atkinson, 2006; Dodson, 2011). An example of the latter is the applicability of lung parenchyma fibre counts to malignant mesothelioma, which originates outside of the lung. This problem exists within the lungs as well. Fibres of different dimensions and shapes deposit differently in the lungs, so that fibre concentrations in the lung parenchyma may not reflect the fibre concentration in the bronchial epithelium, where many lung cancers originate (Baker, 1991; Abraham, 1994).

An intrinsic limitation of tissue fibre burden studies is that they offer a snapshot of fibre prevalence only at the time of diagnostic biopsy or post-mortem study of an asbestos-related disease. But asbestos fibres, which were deposited in the lung and other organs over a long period of time and usually many years prior to the fibre burden analyses, are modified over time in the lung, either through division into component fibrils (chrysotile), dissolution, transport to other tissues, conversion to asbestos bodies or otherwise. Chrysotile fibres are more quickly dissolved or removed from the lung than amphibole fibres, making lung fibre burden an inadequate indicator of chrysotile exposure. Further, the critical time for cell transformation to a cancer in the lung is believed to be 10–15 years prior to the development of pulmonary symptoms, and it is the fibre profile that existed at or before this critical period that is important to carcinogenesis. These two problems—fibre count being an incomplete or inaccurate measure of exposure and fibre count characterizing fibre burdens a decade or more after critical events occurred—undermine the scientific significance of fibre burden studies.

Churg and Vedal examined the lung fibre burdens of 32 shipyard workers and insulators with lung cancer compared to eight people without an asbestos-related disease, using TEM and energy-dispersive X-ray spectroscopy (EDAX). They found higher mean concentrations of amosite and tremolite, but not chrysotile, than in controls, although the differences were not statistically significant. Mean amosite fibre length (5.7 μm) and aspect ratio (39) in lung cancer cases were not statistically significantly longer than in controls (Churg and Vedal, 1994). Roggli and Vollmer reviewed lung fibre burdens in 340 lung cancer cases from a variety of occupational backgrounds collected from 1980 to 2005. They used light microscopy and scanning electron microscopy and counted only fibres of ≥5 μm in length. All amphiboles, including tremolite, were present more frequently and at higher concentrations than chrysotile (Roggli and Vollmer, 2008).

Dodson et al. reported fibre burden analyses in 20 lung cancer cases from a variety of asbestos-using trades (Dodson et al., 2004). They used TEM and EDAX at 16,000-times or 20,000-times magnification, counting all fibres of ≥0.5 μm in length. Amphibole fibres were found in 50%–75% of cases, compared to chrysotile, which was found in 42% of cases. The mean fibre lengths of the different fibre types were similar, ranging from 4 to 7 μm, but the chrysotile fibres were much thinner than the amphibole fibres, with a geometric mean width of 0.06 μm. Indeed, Dodson et al. noted that only 1.2% of detected chrysotile fibres would have been detected by light microscopy (>5 μm in length and >0.25 μm in width). They also examined how many fibres of the different asbestos fibre types met the Stanton hypothesis threshold for most carcinogenic fibres (>8 μm in length and >0.25 μm in width) and found that chrysotile fibres of these dimensions were the most commonly detected (40%), followed by amosite (23%), crocidolite (17%) and other amphiboles (≤5%).

Adib and colleagues in Quebec reported on lung fibre burdens in 70 cases of lung cancer from mining, maintenance, construction and other industries (Adib et al., 2013). They used TEM (10,000-times magnification) and EDAX, counting fibres of >0.5 μm in length with an aspect ratio of ≥3:1. Among the lung cancer cases, chrysotile and tremolite were more commonly found than amosite and crocidolite. Three-quarters of chrysotile and tremolite fibres were <5 μm in length, and most chrysotile fibres were thin (<0.2 μm in width). Indeed, only 0.7% of chrysotile fibres were >5 μm in length and >0.2 μm in width, which is very similar to the results from Dodson et al. noted above. Among the subset of 13 lung cancer cases whose last exposure to asbestos was ≥30 years previously, chrysotile fibres were found in all cases, with short (<5 μm) fibres outnumbering longer (>5 μm) fibres by at least two- to three-fold.

In summary, lung fibre burden studies of asbestos-related lung cancer provide limited insights. Earlier studies predominantly found amphiboles, with sparse evidence of chrysotile fibres, but more recent studies using more sensitive microscopic techniques show substantial evidence of chrysotile in the lungs—principally short and/or thin fibres—even several decades after the cessation of asbestos exposure.

Threshold and Lung Cancer Risk

The current consensus is that no threshold of asbestos exposure has been demonstrated below which there is no identified risk of cancer related to asbestos (National Institute of Occupational Safety and Health-Occupational Safety and Health Administration Work

Group, 1980; Consumer Product Safety Commission, 1983; Stayner et al., 1997; World Health Organization, 2006, 2014b; van der Bij et al., 2013; Nielsen et al., 2014; United States Department of Labor Occupational Safety and Health Administration, 2014). This view is based on several lines of evidence. Current risk assessment guidelines in the United States (US Environmental Protection Agency Risk Assessment Forum, 2005) support linear extrapolation from the known dose–response curve to lower levels of exposure to DNA-reactive agents (US Environmental Protection Agency Risk Assessment Forum, 2005). Although the exact mechanisms of asbestos carcinogenesis are not known at present (Nymark et al., 2008; International Agency for Research on Cancer, 2012), asbestos fibres, including chrysotile, are genotoxic and are therefore 'DNA-reactive' (Jaurand, 1997; International Agency for Research on Cancer, 2012).

Studies of asbestos-exposed cohorts provide evidence that an exposure threshold for cancer risk is not established for asbestos. Stayner et al. evaluated alternative exposure–response models using data from a South Carolina textile factory in a study with one of the highest-quality exposure assessments available in the asbestos literature (Stayner et al., 1997; Lenters et al., 2011). The best model for lung cancer was linear on a multiplicative scale, with the best data fit obtained when the threshold was set at zero. The authors concluded that 'there was absolutely no significant evidence for a threshold in … lung cancer' (Stayner et al., 1997, p. 651). In a recent meta-analysis, van der Bij et al. used a variety of statistical models in order to examine the issue of lung cancer risk associated with relatively low exposure to asbestos and found that a natural spline model best fit the data, predicting a linear increase in lung cancer risk at low levels of exposure. They noted that no threshold for lung cancer risk due to asbestos exposure has been identified (van der Bij et al., 2013).

Nielsen and colleagues report that most relevant meta-analyses of asbestos and lung cancer have been predicated using linear dose–response relationship models, suggesting that there is no exposure threshold for lung cancer risk (Hodgson and Darnton, 2000; Lenters et al., 2011; van der Bij et al., 2013; Nielsen et al., 2014). Nielsen et al. concluded that there 'is no evidence for a no observed effect level concerning asbestos-related lung cancer' (Nielsen et al., 2014, p. 197).

There is also increasing evidence of lung cancer being attributable to relatively low levels of asbestos exposure. De Matteis et al. studied 1537 lung cancer cases from the general population in Northern Italy and found a lung cancer OR of 1.76 (95% CI: 1.42–2.18) among those deemed to have low exposure to asbestos (De Matteis et al., 2012). Gustavsson studied the occupation and smoking backgrounds of 1038 lung cancer cases in Sweden, relying on industrial hygiene expert assessment of asbestos exposure. They found that a cumulative exposure to 4 fibre/mL-years yielded an OR of 1.9 (95% CI: 1.32–2.74). They concluded that this level of risk was higher than that estimated by using a linear extrapolation from studies involving higher levels of asbestos exposure (Gustavsson et al., 2002). Hein and others evaluated mortality among 3072 workers at a South Carolina textile factory that used asbestos and found an elevated SMR (1.54; 95% CI: 1.07–2.15) for workers with <1.5 fibre/mL-years of cumulative exposure (Hein et al., 2007).

In the United States and the United Kingdom, the regulated permissible exposure level is 0.1 fibres/mL over an 8-hour period. Notably, in the United States, the Occupational Safety and Health Administration (OSHA) estimates that at this level of exposure (0.1 fibres/mL) over a 45–year working career, there is a lifetime excess of 3.4 cancers per 1000 workers, principally due to lung cancer (United States Occupational Safety and Health Administration, 1994). This accumulated amount of asbestos exposure is 4.5 fibre/mL-years, which is similar to the level of exposure described in the study by Gustavsson et al. noted above (Gustavsson et al., 2002).

Some have hypothesized that asbestos-related lung cancer only occurs among people with asbestosis, and since the latter appears to have a threshold, a threshold must also exist for asbestos-related lung cancer. However, epidemiological studies show that asbestos-related lung cancer occurs in the absence of asbestosis (see section on "Role of Asbestosis in Lung Cancer Risk"), undermining the logic of this point of view.

Latency

In general, a risk of asbestos-related lung cancer does not occur prior to 10 or more years following first exposure to asbestos (Helsinki Consensus, 1997; Henderson et al., 2004). Nielsen and colleagues concluded that a minimum latency period for asbestos and lung cancer has never been established, but that a 10-year latency is 'assumed' (Nielsen et al., 2014).

'Low Level' or Short Duration of Asbestos Exposure and Lung Cancer Risk

Studies completed in the past 10 years or so have confirmed the knowledge that lower levels of occupational exposure to asbestos cause lung cancer. Loomis and colleagues identified mortality patterns among workers at four North Carolina textile plants that almost exclusively used chrysotile asbestos and found an overall

SMR of 1.96 (95% CI: 1.73–2.20). Among workers who worked for <1 year and 1–5 years, the SMRs were 1.82 (95% CI: 1.50–2.19) and 1.86 (95% CI: 1.45–2.34), respectively (Loomis et al., 2009). Hein and others evaluated mortality among 3072 workers at a South Carolina textile factory that used chrysotile asbestos and found an elevated SMR (1.54; 95% CI: 1.07–2.15) for workers with <1.5 fibre/mL-years of cumulative exposure; there was a clear trend of increasing lung cancer risk with increasing exposure (Hein et al., 2007). Pira et al. followed 1973 Italian textile workers exposed to mixed fibre types from 1946 to 1996 and found an overall SMR of 282 (95% CI: 222–354) for lung cancer. Lung cancer risk rose with duration of employment from a SMR of 139 (based on 12 lung cancer deaths) among workers who worked for <1 year at the plant to a SMR of 250.8 among workers who worked 1– <5 years at the plant to a SMR of 530.9 among those who worked for >10 years at the plant (Pira et al., 2005). Seidman et al. studied amosite asbestos manufacturing workers in New Jersey and found a threefold increase in lung cancer deaths among workers who worked for <1 year at the plant (Seidman et al., 1979). Wang and colleagues evaluated mortality among 577 chrysotile asbestos manufacturing workers in China and found that the group with 'low-level' exposure to asbestos had a lung cancer hazard ratio of 1.94 (95% CI: 0.84–4.46), with a statistically significant trend of lung cancer risk with increasing exposure (Wang et al., 2012). Gustavsson et al. performed a population-based case–control study of 1038 lung cancer cases in Stockholm, controlling for cigarette smoking, and found an OR of 1.90 (95% CI: 1.32–2.74) for cumulative exposure to asbestos of 4 fibre/mL-years of asbestos exposure, and the risk on the lower end of the range of exposure was greater than that predicted by a linear dose–response relationship (Gustavsson et al., 2002).

Mechanism of Asbestos-Related Lung Cancer

Multiple mechanisms are likely to be involved in asbestos-related lung carcinogenesis. Excellent recent reviews are available (Nymark et al., 2008; Huang et al., 2011; International Agency for Research on Cancer, 2012). Asbestos causes a wide variety of cellular responses, some of which lead to cell transformation and cancer. Asbestos is mutagenic and genotoxic (Jaurand, 1997; Jaurand et al., 2009; Huang et al., 2011). Asbestos fibres provoke the formation of reactive oxygen species that lead to the oxidation of DNA bases and DNA strand breaks (International Agency for Research on Cancer, 1999; Nymark et al., 2008; International Agency for Research on Cancer, 2012); this is an indirect form of genotoxicity. In addition to causing oxidative stress, asbestos also alters several antioxidant pathways that restrain the cells' ability to limit the damage caused by the reactive free radicals that produce oxidative stress (Nymark et al., 2008). These cellular responses are also likely to underlie fibrogenesis. Asbestos may additionally interfere with DNA repair processes.

Asbestos directly alters mitosis during cell division, causing genetic damage in daughter cells (Toyokuni, 2009). A variety of chromosomal abnormalities caused by asbestos fibres have been described (Nymark et al., 2008). An additional carcinogenic mechanism of asbestos is the absorption of other carcinogens on the fibre surface (e.g. PAHs), which may explain the interactive effect of asbestos and smoking. Cell death (apoptosis), a mechanism for limiting the proliferation of transformed cells, is also altered by asbestos.

There is considerable non-specificity to the cellular responses to asbestos, including in the genetic changes, which appear to overlap with many of the changes found in lung cancers that are caused by cigarette smoking. Whether a distinctive molecular 'signature' will be found in lung cancers caused by asbestos is an unsettled question.

Screening for Asbestos-Related Lung Cancer

Sone et al. in 1998 and Henschke and colleagues in 1999 demonstrated that low-dose computed tomography (CT) scanning detects early-stage lung cancers in high-risk smokers (Sone et al., 1998; Henschke et al., 1999). Henschke et al. later showed that, of 302 individuals with stage 1 lung cancer who underwent surgery, 92% had a projected 10-year survival (International Early Lung Cancer Action Program Investigators et al., 2006). In 2011, the US National Cancer Institute completed a randomized controlled trial of over 53,000 people—the National Lung Screening Trial—in which the CT-screened arm experienced a 20% lung cancer mortality reduction and a 6.7% overall mortality reduction compared to the arm that underwent screening with chest radiograph (National Lung Screening Trial Research Team, 2011). These studies did not address the issue of screening people whose elevated risk of lung cancer was due to asbestos.

In 2013, the United States Preventive Services Task Force endorsed low-dose CT screening of people who are at high risk of lung cancer based on age and smoking history (US Preventive Services Task Force, 2013). The National Comprehensive Cancer Network, a collaboration of many prestigious cancer centres in the

United States, recommended low-dose CT for people aged 50 years and over who had a 20 or more pack-year history of cigarette smoking and one additional risk for lung cancer, including occupational exposure to asbestos or selected other occupational lung carcinogens (Wood, 2015). The American Association of Thoracic Surgery has similar guidelines (Jaklitsch et al., 2012).

Use of low-dose CT scanning for early lung cancer detection offers an unprecedented opportunity to detect lung cancer at an early stage in asbestos-exposed workers and to limit future lung cancer mortality due to asbestos. Occupational medicine physicians, pulmonary physicians and other occupational health professionals have an essential role in educating, organizing and promoting lung cancer screening for asbestos-exposed workers.

CANCER OF THE LARYNX

Asbestos causes cancer of the larynx (Institute of Medicine, 2006; International Agency for Research on Cancer, 2012; Oksa et al., 2014). IARC reached this conclusion after reviewing 29 relevant cohort studies, 15 case–control studies and two meta-analyses of these studies evaluating the risk of laryngeal cancer in asbestos-exposed cohorts in a wide variety of industries and countries (International Agency for Research on Cancer, 2012). Among the cohort studies, many showed statistically significant excess risks of laryngeal cancer, as well as some evidence of a dose–response relationship. Case–control studies more frequently included living cases with laryngeal cancer, rather than only deaths, and usually controlled for tobacco and alcohol consumption, which are known risk factors for laryngeal cancer. Most of these case–control studies also showed an increased risk of cancer of the larynx in association with asbestos exposure (International Agency for Research on Cancer, 2012). The United States Institute of Medicine (IOM) performed meta-analyses on the available epidemiological studies involving asbestos exposure and found a summary laryngeal cancer relative risk of 1.4 (95% CI: 1.19–1.64) among cohort studies and a relative risk of 1.18 (95% CI: 1.01–1.37) after adjusting for alcohol and tobacco consumption (Institute of Medicine, 2006). Whether there is interaction between asbestos and tobacco smoking in terms of raising laryngeal cancer risk is unclear. The reviews by the IOM and IARC have recently been updated and confirmed (Oksa et al., 2014).

The causal relationship between asbestos and laryngeal cancer is supported by the location of the larynx directly in the air passage of asbestos fibres following inhalation and the similarity between the laryngeal and bronchial epithelium, both being composed of squamous cells and both undergoing neoplastic responses to exposure to tobacco smoke. There is little evidence from animal studies that the larynx develops tumours in response to asbestos exposure (Institute of Medicine, 2006).

ZEOLITES

Zeolites comprise a hydrated aluminosilicate mineral group that has been mined and used for many commercial uses, although they have been largely replaced by synthetic non-fibrous zeolites at present (International Agency for Research on Cancer, 2012). One series within the zeolite group is erionite, which is constituted by three minerals. In health studies, erionite has been treated as a single mineral, and biological differences among its types are not known. Erionite is an elongated particle and is frequently fibrous in shape, being composed of bundles of fibrils (Van Gosen et al., 2013). Although fibrous erionite-associated disease has been identified principally in one geographic area—Turkey—erionite deposits are present in Europe, Africa, Asia and North America (International Agency for Research on Cancer, 2012), including in the western United States, where it has sometimes been used as gravel to surface unpaved roads and is found in selected recreational areas (Van Gosen et al., 2013). Knowledge regarding the human carcinogenic effect of erionite fibres is based on the epidemic of malignant mesothelioma among residents in the Cappadocia region of Turkey, where the mineral is found in soil and unpaved roads and was used as a building block material in houses.

Erionite is a human carcinogen (International Agency for Research on Cancer, 2012). It causes malignant mesothelioma (International Agency for Research on Cancer, 2012; National Toxicology Program, 2014). IARC concluded that erionite is more potent than asbestos in causing malignant mesothelioma based on human and animal studies. Erionite exposure is also associated with lung cancer, pleural plaques and calcification, pleural effusions and parenchymal pneumoconiosis (Baris and Grandjean, 2006).

The ability of erionite to cause malignant mesothelioma was first documented in the late 1970s (Baris et al., 1987). In a later account, Baris and colleagues identified causes of death among erionite-exposed residents of three Turkish villages between 1970 and 1994 (Baris et al., 1996). Over half (51.5%) of 305 deaths in one village were caused by malignant mesothelioma. Four people died from lung cancer (1.3% of all deaths), including two non-smoking women. In two other villages, 519 deaths occurred, including 184 (35.5%) from malignant mesothelioma and 14 (2.7%) from lung cancer; four lung cancer deaths occurred among nonsmoking women. Baris and Grandjean documented similar results in a subsequent prospective study of deaths in two of these villages, comparing causes of death among village residents with those of another Turkish village without erionite exposure (Baris and Grandjean, 2006). The limitations of these studies for evaluating the risk of lung cancer included the lack of risk calculations and the lack of histological confirmation of many cases of cancer (International Agency for Research on Cancer, 2012). A Turkish emigrant community from these villages who lived in Sweden was also documented to have a very high incidence of histologically confirmed malignant mesothelioma (Metintas et al., 1999).

Animal studies clearly demonstrate that erionite causes mesothelioma. Studies of rats exposed to erionite fibres by intra-pleural injection and inhalation have shown that nearly all test animals developed pleural mesotheliomas; tumours of the lung were not reported (Maltoni et al., 1982; Wagner et al., 1985).

REFERENCES

Abraham, J. L. 1994. Asbestos inhalation, not asbestosis, causes lung cancer. *Am J Ind Med* 26(6):839–42.

Adib, G., Labreche, F., De Guire, L., Dion, C. and Dufresne, A. 2013. Short, fine and WHO asbestos fibres in the lungs of Quebec workers with an asbestos-related disease. *Am J Ind Med* 56(9):1001–14.

Ameille, J., Brochard, P., Letourneux, M., Paris, C. and Pairon, J. C. 2011. Risque de cancer lie a l'aminate en presence d'asbestose ou de plaques pleurales. *Rev Mal Respir* 28:413.

Axelson, O. and Steenland, K. 1988. Indirect methods of assessing the effects of tobacco use in occupational studies. *Am J Ind Med* 13(1):105–18.

Baker, D. B. 1991. Limitations in drawing etiologic inferences based on measurement of asbestos fibres from lung tissue. *Ann N Y Acad Sci* 643:61–70.

Baris, B., Demir, A. U., Shehu, V., Karakoca, Y., Kisacik, G. and Baris, Y. I. 1996. Environmental fibrous zeolite (erionite) exposure and malignant tumors other than mesothelioma. *J Environ Pathol Toxicol Oncol* 15(2–4):183–9.

Baris, I., Simonato, L., Artvinli, M., Pooley, F., Saracci, R., Skidmore, J. and Wagner, C. 1987. Epidemiological and environmental evidence of the health effects of exposure to erionite fibres: A four-year study in the Cappadocian region of Turkey. *Int J Cancer* 39(1):10–7.

Baris, Y. I. and Grandjean, P. 2006. Prospective study of mesothelioma mortality in Turkish villages with exposure to fibrous zeolite. *J Natl Cancer Inst* 98(6):414–7.

Berman, D. W. and Crump, K. S. 2008. A meta-analysis of asbestos-related cancer risk that addresses fibre size and mineral type. *Crit Rev Toxicol* 38(Suppl. 1):49–73.

Berry, G., Newhouse, M. L. and Antonis, P. 1985. Combined effect of asbestos and smoking on mortality from lung cancer and mesothelioma in factory workers. *Br J Ind Med* 42(1):12–8.

Boffetta, P., Autier, P., Boniol, M., Boyle, P., Hill, C., Aurengo, A., Masse, R. et al. 2010. An estimate of cancers attributable to occupational exposures in France. *J Occup Environ Med* 52(4):399–406.

Boulanger, G., Andujar, P., Pairon, J. C., Billon-Galland, M. A., Dion, C., Dumortier, P., Brochard, P. et al. 2014. Quantification of short and long asbestos fibres to assess asbestos exposure: A review of fibre size toxicity. *Environ Health* 13:59.

Brown, T., Darnton, A., Fortunato, L., Rushton, L. and British Occupational Cancer Burden Study Group. 2012. Occupational cancer in Britain. Respiratory cancer sites: Larynx, lung and mesothelioma. *Br J Cancer* 107(Suppl. 1):S56–70.

Brownson, R. C., Alavanja, M. C. and Chang, J. C. 1993. Occupational risk factors for lung cancer among nonsmoking women: A case–control study in Missouri (United States). *Cancer Causes Control* 4(5):449–54.

Castleman, B. 2005. *Asbestos: Medical and Legal Aspects*, fifth edition. New York: Wolters Kluwer.

Cheng, W. N. and Kong, J. 1992. A retrospective mortality cohort study of chrysotile asbestos products workers in Tianjin 1972–1987. *Environ Res* 59(1):271–8.

Churg, A. and Vedal, S. 1994. Fibre burden and patterns of asbestos-related disease in workers with heavy mixed amosite and chrysotile exposure. *Am J Respir Crit Care Med* 150(3):663–9.

Coffin, D. L., Cook, P.M. and Creason, J.P. 1992. Relative mesothelioma induction in rats by mineral fibres: Comparison with residual pulmonary mineral fibre number and epidemiology. *Inhal Toxicol* 4:273.

Consumer Product Safety Commission (Chronic Hazard Advisory Panel on Asbestos). 1983. Report to the U.S. Consumer Product Safety Commission. U.S. Consumer Product Safety Commission Directorate for Health Sciences. Washington, D.C.

Cullen, M. R., Barnett, M. J., Balmes, J. R., Cartmel, B., Redlich, C. A., Brodkin, C. A., Barnhart, S. et al. 2005. Predictors of lung cancer among asbestos-exposed men in the β-carotene and retinol efficacy trial. *Am J Epidemiol* 161(3):260–70.

Davis, J. M. and Jones, A. D. 1988. Comparisons of the pathogenicity of long and short fibres of chrysotile asbestos in rats. *Br J Exp Pathol* 69(5):717–37.

Davis, J. M., Addison, J., McIntosh, C., Miller, B. G. and Niven, K. 1991. Variations in the carcinogenicity of tremolite dust samples of differing morphology. *Ann N Y Acad Sci* 643:473–90.

Davis, J. M., Addison, J., Bolton, R. E., Donaldson, K., Jones, A. D. and Smith, T. 1986. The pathogenicity of long versus short fibre samples of amosite asbestos administered to rats by inhalation and intraperitoneal injection. *Br J Exp Pathol* 67(3):415–30.

De Matteis, S., Consonni, D., Lubin, J. H., Tucker, M., Peters, S., Vermeulen, R. Ch., Kromhout, H. et al. 2012. Impact of occupational carcinogens on lung cancer risk in a general population. *Int J Epidemiol* 41(3):711–21.

Dement, J. M. 1991. Carcinogenicity of chrysotile asbestos: Evidence from cohort studies. *Ann N Y Acad Sci* 643:15–23.

Dement, J. M. and Brown, D. P. 1994. Lung cancer mortality among asbestos textile workers: A review and update. *Ann Occup Hyg* 38(4):525–32, 412.

Dement, J. M., Loomis, D., Richardson, D., Wolf, S. H. and Kuempel, E. D. 2011. Estimates of historical exposures by phase contrast and transmission electron microscopy for pooled exposure–response analyses of North Carolina and South Carolina, USA asbestos textile cohorts. *Occup Environ Med* 68(8):593–8.

Dodson, R. F. 2011. Analysis and relevance of asbestos burden in tissue. In R. F. Dodson and S. P. Hammar (eds), *Asbestos: Risk Assessment, Epidemiology, and Health Effects*, second edition. Boca Raton, Florida: CRC Press, 49–108.

Dodson, R. F. and Atkinson, M. A. 2006. Measurements of asbestos burden in tissues. *Ann N Y Acad Sci* 1076:281–91.

Dodson, R. F., Brooks, D. R., O'Sullivan, M. and Hammar, S. P. 2004. Quantitative analysis of asbestos burden in a series of individuals with lung cancer and a history of exposure to asbestos. *Inhal Toxicol* 16(9):637–47.

Dodson, R. F., Atkinson, M. A. and Levin, J. L. 2003. Asbestos fibre length as related to potential pathogenicity: A critical review. *Am J Ind Med* 44(3):291–7.

Doll, R. 1955. Mortality from lung cancer in asbestos workers. *Br J Ind Med* 12:81–6.

Driscoll, T., Nelson, D. I., Steenland, K., Leigh, J., Concha-Barrientos, M., Fingerhut, M. and Pruss-Ustun, A. 2005. The global burden of disease due to occupational carcinogens. *Am J Ind Med* 48(6):419–31.

Elliott, L., Loomis, D., Dement, J., Hein, M. J., Richardson, D. and Stayner, L. 2012. Lung cancer mortality in North Carolina and South Carolina chrysotile asbestos textile workers. *Occup Environ Med* 69(6):385–90.

Erren, T. C., Jacobsen, M. and Piekarski, C. 1999. Synergy between asbestos and smoking on lung cancer risks. *Epidemiology* 10(4):405–11.

Finkelstein, M. M. 1997. Radiographic asbestosis is not a prerequisite for asbestos-associated lung cancer in Ontario asbestos-cement workers. *Am J Ind Med* 32(4):341–8.

Fletcher, D. E. 1972. A mortality study of shipyard workers with pleural plaques. *Br J Ind Med* 29(2):142–5.

Frost, G., Darnton, A. and Harding, A. H. 2011. The effect of smoking on the risk of lung cancer mortality for asbestos workers in Great Britain (1971–2005). *Ann Occup Hyg* 55(3):239–47.

Gloyne, S. R. 1935. Two cases of squamous carcinoma of the lung occurring in asbestosis. *Tubercle* 2:142.

Gustavsson, P., Nyberg, F., Pershagen, G., Scheele, P., Jakobsson, R. and Plato, N. 2002. Low-dose exposure to asbestos and lung cancer: Dose–response relations and interaction with smoking in a population-based case-referent study in Stockholm, Sweden. *Am J Epidemiol* 155(11):1016–22.

Gustavsson, P., Jakobsson, R., Nyberg, F., Pershagen, G., Jarup, L. and Scheele, P. 2000. Occupational exposure and lung cancer risk: A population-based case-referent study in Sweden. *Am J Epidemiol* 152(1):32–40.

Hammond, E. C., Selikoff, I. J. and Seidman, H. 1979. Asbestos exposure, cigarette smoking and death rates. *Ann N Y Acad Sci* 330:473–90.

Hamra, G. B., Loomis, D. and Dement, J. 2014. Examining the association of lung cancer and highly correlated fibre size-specific asbestos exposures with a hierarchical Bayesian model. *Occup Environ Med* 71(5):353–7.

Hein, M. J., Stayner, L. T., Lehman, E. and Dement, J. M. 2007. Follow-up study of chrysotile textile workers: Cohort mortality and exposure–response. *Occup Environ Med* 64(9):616–25.

Helsinki Consensus. 1997. Asbestos, asbestosis, and cancer: The Helsinki criteria for diagnosis and attribution. *Scand J Work Environ Health* 23:311–6.

Henderson, D. W., Rödelsperger, K., Woitowitz, H. J. and Leigh, J. 2004. After Helsinki: A multidisciplinary review of the relationship between asbestos exposure and lung cancer, with emphasis on studies published during 1997–2004. *Pathology* 36(6):517–50.

Henschke, C. I., McCauley, D. I., Yankelevitz, D. F., Naidich, D. P., McGuinness, G., Miettinen, O. S., Libby, D. M. et al. 1999. Early lung cancer action project: Overall design and findings from baseline screening. *Lancet* 354(9173):99–105.

Hesterberg, T. W., Miiller, W. C., McConnell, E. E., Chevalier, J., Hadley, J. G., Bernstein, D. M., Thevenaz, P. et al. 1993. Chronic inhalation toxicity of size-separated glass fibres in Fischer 344 rats. *Fundam Appl Toxicol* 20(4):464–76.

Hillerdal, G. and Henderson, D. W. 1997. Asbestos, asbestosis, pleural plaques and lung cancer. *Scand J Work Environ Health* 23(2):93–103.

Hodgson, J. T. and Darnton, A. 2000. The quantitative risks of mesothelioma and lung cancer in relation to asbestos exposure. *Ann Occup Hyg* 44(8):565–601.

Huang, S. X., Jaurand, M. C., Kamp, D. W., Whysner, J. and Hei, T. K. 2011. Role of mutagenicity in asbestos fibre-induced carcinogenicity and other diseases. *J Toxicol Environ Health B Crit Rev* 14(1–4):179–245.

Institute of Medicine of the National Academies. 2006. *Asbestos: Selected Cancers*. Washington, DC: The National Academies Press.

International Agency for Research on Cancer (IARC). 1999. *IARC Monographs on the Evaluation of Carcinogenic Risks to Humans: Surgical Implants and Other Foreign Bodies*. Volume 74. Lyons, France: IARC.

International Agency for Research on Cancer. 2012. *IARC Monographs on the Evaluation of Carcinogenic Risks to Humans: Volume 100c: Arsenic, Metals, Fibres and Dusts*. Geneva: WHO Press.

International Early Lung Cancer Action Program Investigators, C. I. Henschke, Yankelevitz, D. F., Libby, D. M., Pasmantier, M. W., Smith, J. P. and Miettinen, O. S. 2006. Survival of patients with stage I lung cancer detected on CT screening. *N Engl J Med* 355(17):1763–71.

International Labour Organization. 2011. Guidelines for the use of the ILO International Classification of Radiographs of Pneumoconioses. Revised edition 2011. Geneva, Switzerland: International Labour Office.

Jaklitsch, M. T., Jacobson, F. L., Austin, J. H., Field, J. K., Jett, J. R., Keshavjee, S., MacMahon, H. et al. 2012. The American Association for Thoracic Surgery guidelines for lung cancer screening using low-dose computed tomography scans for lung cancer survivors and other high-risk groups. *J Thorac Cardiovasc Surg* 144(1):33–8.

Jaurand, M. C. 1997. Mechanisms of fibre-induced genotoxicity. *Environ Health Perspect* 105(Suppl. 5):1073–84.

Jaurand, M. C., Renier, A. and Daubriac, J. 2009. Mesothelioma: Do asbestos and carbon nanotubes pose the same health risk? *Part Fibre Toxicol* 6:16.

Johnson S. 2008. *Letter from Stephen L. Johnson, EPA Administrator to Dr. Agnes Kane, Chair of Science Advisory Board Asbestos Committee*. A. Kane (ed.).

Karjalainen, A., Anttila, S., Vanhala, E. and Vainio, H. 1994. Asbestos exposure and the risk of lung cancer in a general urban population. *Scand J Work Environ Health* 20(4):243–50.

Koskinen, K., Pukkala, E., Martikainen, R., Reijula, K. and Karjalainen, A. 2002. Different measures of asbestos exposure in estimating risk of lung cancer and mesothelioma among construction workers. *J Occup Environ Med* 44(12):1190–6.

Le Bouffant, L., Daniel, H., Henin, J. P., Martin, J. C., Normand, C., Tichoux, G. and Trolard, F. 1987. Experimental study on long-term effects of inhaled MMMF on the lungs of rats. *Ann Occup Hyg* 31(4B):765–90.

Lee, P. N. 2001. Relation between exposure to asbestos and smoking jointly and the risk of lung cancer. *Occup Environ Med* 58(3):145–53.

Lenters, V., Vermeulen, R., Dogger, S., Stayner, L., Portengen, L., Burdorf, A. and Heederik, D. 2011. A meta-analysis of asbestos and lung cancer: Is better quality exposure assessment associated with steeper slopes of the exposure–response relationships? *Environ Health Perspect* 119(11):1547–55.

Liddell, F. D. 2001. The interaction of asbestos and smoking in lung cancer. *Ann Occup Hyg* 45(5):341–56.

Liddell, F. D. and McDonald, J. C. 1980. Radiological findings as predictors of mortality in Quebec asbestos workers. *Br J Ind Med* 37(3):257–67.

Liddell, F. D., McDonald, A. D. and McDonald, J. C. 1997. The 1891–1920 birth cohort of Quebec chrysotile miners and millers: Development from 1904 and mortality to 1992. *Ann Occup Hyg* 41(1):13–36.

Lippmann, M. 2014. Toxicological and epidemiological studies on effects of airborne fibres: Coherence and public health implications. *Crit Rev Toxicol* 44(8):643–95.

Loomis, D., Dement, J., Richardson, D. and Wolf, S. 2010. Asbestos fibre dimensions and lung cancer mortality among workers exposed to chrysotile. *Occup Environ Med* 67(9):580–4.

Loomis, D., Dement, J. M., Elliott, L., Richardson, D., Kuempel, E. D. and Stayner, L. 2012. Increased lung cancer mortality among chrysotile asbestos textile workers is more strongly associated with exposure to long thin fibres. *Occup Environ Med* 69(8):564–8.

Loomis, D., Dement, J. M., Wolf, S. H. and Richardson, D. B. 2009. Lung cancer mortality and fibre exposures among North Carolina asbestos textile workers. *Occup Environ Med* 66(8):535–42.

Lynch, K. and Smith, W.A. 1935. Pulmonary asbestosis III: Carcinoma of lung in asbestos-silicosis. *Am J Cancer* 24:56.

Maltoni, C., Minardi, F. and Morisi, L. 1982. Pleural mesotheliomas in Sprague–Dawley rats by erionite: First experimental evidence. *Environ Res* 29(1):238–44.

Marinaccio, A., Scarselli, A., Binazzi, A., Mastrantonio, M., Ferrante, P. and Iavicoli, S. 2008. Magnitude of asbestos-related lung cancer mortality in Italy. *Br J Cancer* 99(1):173–5.

Markowitz, S. B., Levin, S. M., Miller, A. and Morabia, A. 2013. Asbestos, asbestosis, smoking, and lung cancer. New findings from the North American insulator cohort. *Am J Respir Crit Care Med* 188(1):90–6.

Martischnig, K. M., Newell, D. J., Barnsley, W. C., Cowan, W. K., Feinmann, E. L. and Oliver, E. 1977. Unsuspected exposure to asbestos and bronchogenic carcinoma. *Br Med J* 1(6063):746–9.

McConnell, E.E., Hall, L. and Adkins, B. 1991. Studies on the chronic toxicity (inhalation) of wollastonite in Fischer 344 rats. *Inhal Toxicol* 3:323.

McCormack, V., Peto, J., Byrnes, G., Straif, K. and Boffetta, P. 2012. Estimating the asbestos-related lung cancer burden from mesothelioma mortality. *Br J Cancer* 106(3):575–84.

McDonald, J. C., Armstrong, B. G., Edwards, C. W., Gibbs, A. R., Lloyd, H. M., Pooley, F. D., Ross, D. J. et al. 2001. Case-referent survey of young adults with mesothelioma: I. Lung fibre analyses. *Ann Occup Hyg* 45(7):513–8.

McDonald, J. C., Liddell, F. D., Gibbs, G. W., Eyssen, G. E. and McDonald, A. D. 1980. Dust exposure and mortality in chrysotile mining, 1910–75. *Br J Ind Med* 37(1):11–24.

Metintas, M., Hillerdal, G. and Metintas, S. 1999. Malignant mesothelioma due to environmental exposure to erionite: Follow-up of a Turkish emigrant cohort. *Eur Respir J* 13(3):523–6.

National Institute for Occupational Safety and Health. 2011. Current Intelligence Bulletin 62: Asbestos Fibers and Other Elongate Mineral Particles: State of the Science and Roadmap for Research. Revised Edition. DHHS (NIOSH) Publication Number 2011-159. http://www.cdc.gov/niosh/docs/2011-159/pdfs/2011-159.pdf

National Institute for Occupational Safety and Health-Occupational Safety and Health Administration

Asbestos Work Group. 1980. Recommendations: Workplace Exposure to Asbestos; Review and Recommendations. DHHS (NIOSH) Publication No. 81–103. Washington, D.C.

National Lung Screening Trial Research Team, Aberle, D. R., Adams, A. M., Berg, C. D., Black, W. C., Clapp, J. D., Fagerstrom, R. M. et al. 2011. Reduced lung-cancer mortality with low-dose computed tomographic screening. *N Engl J Med* 365(5):395–409.

National Toxicology Program. 2014. *Report on Carcinogens, Thirteenth Edition*. U.S. Department of Health and Human Services, Public Health Service. Research Triangle Park, North Carolina. http://ntp.niehs.nih.gov/pubhealth/roc/roc13/

Nicholson, W. and Landrigan, P. 1996. Asbestos: A status report. *Curr Issues Public Health* 2:118–123.

Nicholson, W. J. 1991. Comparative dose–response relationships of asbestos fibre types: Magnitudes and uncertainties. *Ann N Y Acad Sci* 643:74–84.

Nielsen, L. S., Baelum, J., Rasmussen, J., Dahl, S., Olsen, K. E., Albin, M., Hansen, N. C. and Sherson, D. 2014. Occupational asbestos exposure and lung cancer—A systematic review of the literature. *Arch Environ Occup Health* 69(4):191–206.

Nymark, P., Wikman, H., Hienonen-Kempas, T. and Anttila, S. 2008. Molecular and genetic changes in asbestos-related lung cancer. *Cancer Lett* 265(1):1–15.

Offermans, N. S., Vermeulen, R., Burdorf, A., Goldbohm, R. A., Kauppinen, T., Kromhout, H. and van den Brandt, P. A. 2014. Occupational asbestos exposure and risk of pleural mesothelioma, lung cancer, and laryngeal cancer in the prospective Netherlands Cohort Study. *J Occup Environ Med* 56(1):6–19.

Oksa, P., Wolff, H., Vehmas, T., Pallasaho, P. and Frilander, H. 2014. *Asbestos, Asbestosis, and Cancer: Helsinki Criteria for Diagnosis and Attribution*. Helsinki: Finnish Institute of Occupational Health.

Olsson, A. C., Fevotte, J., Fletcher, T., Cassidy, A., 't Mannetje, A., Zaridze, D., Szeszenia-Dabrowska, N. et al. 2010. Occupational exposure to polycyclic aromatic hydrocarbons and lung cancer risk: A multicenter study in Europe. *Occup Environ Med* 67(2):98–103.

Pastorino, U., Berrino, F., Gervasio, A., Pesenti, V., Riboli, E. and Crosignani, P. 1984. Proportion of lung cancers due to occupational exposure. *Int J Cancer* 33(2):231–7.

Pintos, J., Parent, M. E., Rousseau, M. C., Case, B. W. and Siemiatycki, J. 2008. Occupational exposure to asbestos and man-made vitreous fibres, and risk of lung cancer: Evidence from two case–control studies in Montreal, Canada. *J Occup Environ Med* 50(11):1273–81.

Pira, E., Pelucchi, C., Buffoni, L., Palmas, A., Turbiglio, M., Negri, E., Piolatto, P. G. et al. 2005. Cancer mortality in a cohort of asbestos textile workers. *Br J Cancer* 92(3):580–6.

Pott, F., Huth, F. and Friedrichs, K. H. 1974. Tumorigenic effect of fibrous dusts in experimental animals. *Environ Health Perspect* 9:313–5.

Reid, A., de Klerk, N., Ambrosini, G. L., Olsen, N., Pang, S. C., Berry, G. and Musk, A. W. 2005. The effect of asbestosis on lung cancer risk beyond the dose related effect of asbestos alone. *Occup Environ Med* 62(12):885–9.

Reid, A., de Klerk, N. H., Ambrosini, G. L., Berry, G. and Musk, A. W. 2006. The risk of lung cancer with increasing time since ceasing exposure to asbestos and quitting smoking. *Occup Environ Med* 63(8):509–12.

Roggli, V. L. and Vollmer, R. T. 2008. Twenty-five years of fibre analysis: What have we learned? *Hum Pathol* 39(3):307–15.

Seidman, H., Selikoff, I. J. and Hammond, E. C. 1979. Short-term asbestos work exposure and long-term observation. *Ann N Y Acad Sci* 330:61–89.

Silverstein, M. A., Welch, L. S. and Lemen, R. 2009. Developments in asbestos cancer risk assessment. *Am J Ind Med* 52(11):850–8.

Sluis-Cremer, G. K., Hessel, P. A. and Hnizdo, E. 1989. Factors influencing the reading of small irregular opacities in a radiological survey of asbestos miners in South Africa. *Arch Environ Health* 44(4):237–43.

Sone, S., Takashima, S., Li, F., Yang, Z., Honda, T., Maruyama, Y., Hasegawa, M. et al. 1998. Mass screening for lung cancer with mobile spiral computed tomography scanner. *Lancet* 351(9111):1242–5.

Stanton, M. F., Layard, M., Tegeris, A., Miller, E., May, M., Morgan, E. and Smith, A. 1981. Relation of particle dimension to carcinogenicity in amphibole asbestoses and other fibrous minerals. *J Natl Cancer Inst* 67(5):965–75.

Stayner, L. T., Dankovic, D. A. and Lemen, R. A. 1996. Occupational exposure to chrysotile asbestos and cancer risk: A review of the amphibole hypothesis. *Am J Public Health* 86(2):179–86.

Stayner, L., Kuempel, E., Gilbert, S., Hein, M. and Dement, J. 2008. An epidemiological study of the role of chrysotile asbestos fibre dimensions in determining respiratory disease risk in exposed workers. *Occup Environ Med* 65(9):613–9.

Stayner, L., Smith, R., Bailer, J., Gilbert, S., Steenland, K., Dement, J., Brown, D. et al. 1997. Exposure–response analysis of risk of respiratory disease associated with occupational exposure to chrysotile asbestos. *Occup Environ Med* 54(9):646–52.

Suzuki, Y. and Yuen, S. R. 2001. Asbestos tissue burden study on human malignant mesothelioma. *Ind Health* 39(2):150–60.

Tossavainen, A. 1997. *Asbestos, Asbestosis and Cancer: Exposure Criteria for Clinical Diagnosis*. Helsinki: Finnish Institute of Occupational Health.

Toyokuni, S. 2009. Mechanisms of asbestos-induced carcinogenesis. *Nagoya J Med Sci* 71(1–2):1–10.

United States Department of Labor Occupational Safety and Health Administration. 1994. Section III: Occupational Exposure to Asbestos, Summary and Explanation of Revised Standards. Available at: https://www.osha.gov/pls/oshaweb/owadisp.show_document?p_table=PREAMBLES&p_id=777 (accessed 23 June 2015).

U.S. Environmental Protection Agency Risk Assessment Forum. 2005. Guidelines for Carcinogen Risk Assessment. March, 2005. EPA/630/P-03/001F. Washington D.C.

U.S. Environmental Protection Agency (USEPA), Office of Health and Environmental Assessment. 1986. Airborne asbestos health assessment update. EPA 600/8-84/003F. U.S. Environmental Protection Agency. Research Triangle Park, North Carolina.

United States Department of Labor Occupational Safety and Health Administration. 2014. OSHA. Safety and Health Topics: Asbestos. https://www.osha.gov/SLTC/asbestos/index.html (accessed 7 October 2014).

United States Preventive Services Task Force. 2013. Lung Cancer: Screening. http://www.uspreventiveservicestaskforce.org/Page/Document/UpdateSummaryFinal/lung-cancer-screening (accessed 31 March 2016).

van der Bij, S., Koffijberg, H., Lenters, V., Portengen, L., Moons, K. G., Heederik, D. and Vermeulen, R. C. 2013. Lung cancer risk at low cumulative asbestos exposure: Meta-regression of the exposure–response relationship. *Cancer Causes Control* 24(1):1–12.

Van Gosen, B. S., Blitz, T. A., Plumlee, G. S., Meeker, G. P. and Pierson, M. P. 2013. Geologic occurrences of erionite in the United States: An emerging national public health concern for respiratory disease. *Environ Geochem Health* 35(4):419–30.

Wagner, J. C., Berry, G., Skidmore, J. W. and Timbrell, V. 1974. The effects of the inhalation of asbestos in rats. *Br J Cancer* 29(3):252–69.

Wagner, J. C., Skidmore, J. W., Hill, R. J. and Griffiths, D. M. 1985. Erionite exposure and mesotheliomas in rats. *Br J Cancer* 51(5):727–30.

Wang, X., Yano, E., Qiu, H., Yu, I., Courtice, M. N., Tse, L. A., Lin, S. et al. 2012. A 37-year observation of mortality in Chinese chrysotile asbestos workers. *Thorax* 67(2):106–10.

Wilkinson, P., Hansell, D. M., Janssens, J., Rubens, M., Rudd, R. M., Taylor, A. N. and McDonald, C. 1995. Is lung cancer associated with asbestos exposure when there are no small opacities on the chest radiograph? *Lancet* 345(8957):1074–8.

Wood, D. E. 2015. National Comprehensive Cancer Network (NCCN) Clinical Practice Guidelines for lung cancer screening. *Thorac Surg Clin* 25(2):185–9.

World Health Organization. 2006. *Elimination of Asbestos-Related Diseases*. Geneva: WHO Press.

World Health Organization. 2014b. *Chrysotile Asbestos*. Geneva: World Health Organization.

World Health Organization. 2014a. Asbestos: Elimination of Asbestos-Related Diseases Fact Sheet no. 343. Available at: http://www.who.int/mediacentre/factsheets/fs343/en/ (accessed 13 November 2014).

23 Extrinsic Allergic Alveolitis

Christopher M. Barber, David M. Hansell and Charles P. McSharry

CONTENTS

INTRODUCTION

Extrinsic allergic alveolitis (EAA) is synonymous with hypersensitivity pneumonitis and is a form of interstitial lung disease requiring previous sensitisation to an inhaled antigen. Although EAA is a commonly recognised form of interstitial lung disease (ILD), expert groups have found it challenging to produce a simple consensus definition for the condition (Girard et al., 2009). This reflects the difficulty of defining a complex disease that may have widely differing clinical features and the potential to closely mimic a range of other forms of ILD (Travis et al., 2008, 2013).

In susceptible individuals, the condition develops following repeated exposures to airborne proteins or chemicals that are predominantly encountered at work or in the home environment (Jacobs et al., 2005). The classical description of EAA comprises three different patterns of disease (acute, subacute and chronic) depending on the duration of symptoms (Fuller, 1953).

Although the main focus of this chapter is occupational EAA, domestic sources of exposure are also relevant to those who work full- or part-time from home. In a variable proportion of cases, no cause can be identified, and the disease is sometimes referred to as 'idiopathic'. Whether this truly represents a form of EAA without any cause, or more likely reflects our inability to identify the full range of responsible allergens, remains to be determined (Morell et al., 2013).

EPIDEMIOLOGY

Worldwide, the true epidemiology of occupational EAA is poorly understood, and it is likely that many cases are never recognised (Farebrother et al., 1985; Kipen et al., 1990). The incidence is likely to vary between different populations, depending on a wide range of occupational and demographic factors (Terho et al., 1987; Dalphin et al., 1993). The former include type of industry, working practises and occupational health culture, whilst the latter include climate, smoking prevalence, genetic factors and general healthcare system.

Epidemiological data from national ILD registries have confirmed that EAA (from all causes) represents approximately 2%–15% of all ILD cases, being significantly less common than idiopathic pulmonary fibrosis (IPF) and sarcoidosis amongst the general population (Thomeer et al., 2001; Xaubet et al., 2004; Kornum et al., 2008; Karakatsani et al., 2009; Kundu et al., 2014).

Specific data for occupational EAA are also available from a limited number of national reporting schemes. Although these differ in design, estimates of approximately 1–3 cases per million workers per year have been made for Australia (Elder et al., 2004), the UK (McDonald et al., 2005), Catalonia (Orriols et al., 2006) and the Czech Republic (Fenclová et al., 2009). In contrast, the estimated annual incidence in Finland has been much higher, having fallen from approximately 36 to 20 cases per million workers between 1991 and 2010 (Kanerva et al., 1994; Oksa et al., 2012). In addition to the incident data, national schemes have confirmed that EAA is a less commonly reported form of occupational lung disease than asthma. For each case of occupational EAA, there have been between 10 and 30 new cases of occupational asthma (Provencher et al., 1997).

In addition to reporting schemes, a wealth of epidemiological data has been collected from cross-sectional and longitudinal studies of cohorts of exposed workers. Together, the available evidence has confirmed certain epidemiological features of the disease. Occupational EAA occurs in both genders and is much less common in current cigarette smokers (Terho et al., 1987; Kanerva et al., 1994). The disease usually only affects a minority (often 5%–10%) of similarly exposed workers (Babbott et al., 1980; Depierre et al., 1988; Burton et al., 2012), although significantly higher attack rates have been reported (up to 52%–65%) in outbreaks of humidifier (Ganier et al., 1980) and lifeguard lung (Rose et al., 1998).

CAUSATIVE EXPOSURES

A link between agricultural dust exposure and breathing problems can be traced back many centuries. In 1555, a Swedish bishop Olaus Magnus clearly documented the hazardous nature of the fine dust that was generated by threshing crops (Rylander and Schilling, 2011). The first published description of occupational EAA came from Iceland in 1790, when Dr. Svein Pallson reported a condition termed 'hay sickness', typified by fever and cough, occurring in workers exposed to mouldy hay in winter (Eliasson, 1982). Regular case series began to appear in the medical literature in the twentieth century in workers exposed to malt (Vallery-Radot and Giroud, 1928), hay (Campbell, 1932), sugar cane (Jamison and Hopkins, 1941), pigeon excreta (Feldman and Sabin, 1948) and mushrooms (Bringhurst et al., 1959). However, it was not until the 1960s that the ground-breaking work from Jack Pepys in Britain was published, confirming that EAA in farmers was caused by an allergic response to inhaling a microbial contaminant (Pepys and Jenkins, 1965; Pepys, 1969).

Since that time, a huge range of other occupational and environmental causes of EAA has been reported, with new and unusual exposures being reported each year (Fishwick, 2012). These have generally been named after the type of worker who is at risk of the disease or by the name of the relevant exposure. In order to reach the gas exchanging regions of the lung, the causative agent must contain an aerosol with an aerodynamic diameter of less than 10 μm. The vast majority of known causes relate to the inhalation of microbial organisms contaminating either organic dusts or a water-containing mist (Table 23.1). Non-microbial causes of EAA are more limited in range due to exposure to proteins from other types of organism (Table 23.2) or working with reactive chemicals (Table 23.3).

Limited data for the most common causes of occupational EAA are available from national surveillance schemes and epidemiological surveys. In Japan, an occupational cause was responsible for 14% of all cases of EAA diagnosed in the 1980s (Yoshida et al., 1995), with

TABLE 23.1
Microbial Causes of Extrinsic Allergic Alveolitis

Name	Exposure	Antigen
Air conditioner, humidifier and ventilator lung	Contaminated water	*Thermophilic actinomycetes*
Bagassosis	Mouldy sugarcane	*Thermophilic actinomycetes*
Chacineros' lung	Dry sausage dust	*Aspergillus fumigatus* *Penicillium frequentans*
Cheese washers' lung	Mould dust	*Penicillium casei*
Chicory worker hypersensitivity pneumonitis	Chicory leaf	*Fusarium* spp.
Dog house disease	Dog bedding	*Aspergillus versicolor*
Farmers' lung	Mouldy hay	*Thermophilic actinomycetes* *Absidia* spp. *Aspergillus* spp. *Candida* spp. *Fusarium* spp. *Penicillium* spp. *Wallemia sebi*
Fertiliser workers' lung	Fertiliser	*Streptomyces albus*
Greenhouse lung	Soil	*Aspergillus* spp. *Penicillium* spp. *Cryptostroma corticale*
Hot tub lung	Contaminated water	*Mycobacterium avium* complex
Lifeguard lung	Contaminated water jets and sprays	*Pseudomonas* spp.
Maltworkers' lung	Contaminated barley	*Aspergillus clavatus*
Maple bark strippers' lung	Mouldy wood	*Cryptostroma corticale*
Machine operators' lung/metalworking fluid hypersensitivity pneumonitis	Water-based metalworking fluid	Gram-negative bacteria Environmental mycobacteria
Mushroom workers' lung	Mouldy compost and mushrooms	*Thermophilic actinomycetes* Mushroom spores
Paprika splitters' lung	Paprika	*Mucor stolonifer*
Peat moss lung	Mouldy peat	*Penicillium* and *Monocillium* spp.
Potato riddlers' lung	Mouldy hay	*Thermophilic actinomycetes* *Aspergillus* spp.
Riding school lung	Mouldy hay	*Thermophilic actinomycetes*
Salami lung	Mould on salami	*Penicillium camembertii*
Saxophone player hypersensitivity pneumonitis	Saxophone playing	*Mycobacterium chelonae/abscessus* *Fusarium* spp.
Sequoiosis	Mouldy redwood	*Graphium* spp. *Pullularia* spp.
Sewage sludge disease	Heat-treated sludge	Gram-negative bacteria
Smut lung	Japanese handicrafts	*Ustilago esculenta*
Soy sauce brewers' lung	Soy sauce fermentation	*Aspergillus oryzae*
Steam iron hypersensitivity pneumonitis	Steam ironing	*Aspergillus fumigatus* *Sphingobacterium spiritivorum*
Stipatosis	Mouldy esparto grass	*Aspergillus fumigatus*
Suberosis	Mouldy cork	*Aspergillus* spp. *Penicillium frequentans*
Tobacco workers' disease	Mouldy tobacco	*Aspergillus* spp.
Tiger nut dust (lung)	Contaminated nuts	*Junia avellaneda*
Tractor lung	Tractor cabs	*Rhizopus* spp.
Trombone players' lung		*Ulocladium botrytis* *Phoma* spp.
Wine growers' lung	Mouldy grapes	*Botrytis cinerea*
Wood pulp workers'/trimmers' disease/wood dust hypersensitivity pneumonitis	Mouldy wood	*Alternaria* spp. *Bacillus subtilis* *Mucor* spp. *Rhizopus* spp.

TABLE 23.2
Non-Microbial Organic Causes of Extrinsic Allergic Alveolitis

Name	Exposure	Antigen
Algarobba lung	Livestock feed (legume)	Algarobba (*Vicia monanthos*)
Animal handlers' lung	Rats	Serum and urine proteins
Bat lung	Bat droppings	Animal proteins
Bird breeders'/fanciers' and feather duvet lung	Chickens, pigeons, parrots, turkeys	Proteins from bloom, feather, intestine or serum
Catechin-induced hypersensitivity pneumonitis	Nebulised green tea extract	Green tea (catechin)
Coffee workers' lung	Coffee bean dust	Coffee
Fish meal workers' lung	Fish meal dust	Fish proteins
Furriers' lung	Animal fur and dander	Animal proteins
Konnyaku lung	Konnyaku food making	Konjak root flour Algae (*Huzikia fusiforme*)
Millers' lung	Grain weevils	Weevil protein
Pituitary snuff takers' lung	Snuff	Pig or ox protein
Sericulturists' lung	Silk worm larvae	Silk worm larvae proteins
Shell lung	Mollusc shells	Shell proteins

TABLE 23.3
Chemical Causes of Extrinsic Allergic Alveolitis

Name	Exposure	Antigen
Chemical workers' lung	Glue, foam, paint, plastic, resins, varnishes	HDI, MDI, TDI, TMA
Epoxy resin lung	Epoxy resin	Phthalic anhydride
Laboratory workers' lung	Pauli's reagent	Sodium diazobenzenesulphate
Pyrethrum alveolitis	Pesticide	Pyrethrum
Vineyard sprayers' lung	Mildew prevention spray	Copper sulphate

the most common causes relating to agricultural exposures (79%) and handling chemicals (17%). Farmers' lung (69%) was also the most common type of occupational EAA reported in the Czech Republic between 1992 and 2005 (Fenclová et al., 2009) and in Finland between 1991 and 2010 (Kanerva et al., 1994; Oksa et al., 2012). In the UK, however, there has been a marked shift in causation for occupational EAA over the last few decades. Between 1992 and 2001, almost all cases of occupational EAA were reported to be from agriculture, forestry and fishing (McDonald et al., 2005). More recent data from the same reporting scheme for the period 2003–2012 have demonstrated that exposure to some form of metalworking fluid has become the most common cause, accounting for approximately half of all cases (Prof Raymond Agius Manchester, personal communication).

A number of case series of EAA from all causes have also been published, and their findings are summarised in Table 23.4 (Lacasse et al., 2003; Hanak et al., 2007; Caillaud et al., 2012; Fernández Pérez et al., 2013; Mooney et al., 2013; Dobashi et al., 2014; Xu et al., 2014). Although difficult to compare, they demonstrate that where a cause can be identified, exposure to some form of avian protein is usually the most common cause. It is worth noting that these case series do not differentiate between occupational and domestic exposures, and that causative avian exposures may come from a wide range of sources (Inase et al., 2006; Chan et al., 2012).

IMMUNOPATHOGENESIS

EAA develops after a variable latent period of exposure, suggesting the development of immunological sensitisation. Lung tissue of EAA patients contains increased numbers of antigen-presenting cells (Kawanami et al., 1987), B lymphocytes and antibody-producing plasma cells (Drent et al., 1993a; McSharry, 2003) associated with alveolitis intensity and bronchoalveolar lavage (BAL) immunoglobulin concentration. IgG antibodies against known antigens may be found in the serum and in the BAL fluid and sputum of antigen-exposed, predominantly non-smoking subjects (Soda et al., 1986; McSharry et al., 2006). Smokers have a less efficient immune response (Baur et al., 1992) and the incidence of EAA in current smokers is low (Solaymani-Dodaran et al., 2007).

Lymphocyte Involvement in the Pathogenesis of EAA

Asymptomatic subjects with similar antigen exposures can also develop specific IgG antibodies, confirming that other immune pathways are necessary for the disease to develop. Studies of BAL and lung histology have confirmed the additional importance of cell-mediated immunity in EAA. The BAL cytology of acute EAA involves predominantly activated neutrophils (Hendrick et al., 1980), whereas in subacute disease, BAL shows marked lymphocytosis, moderate neutrophilia and modest increases in mast cells and eosinophils (Caillaud et al.,

TABLE 23.4
Summary of Findings from Published Case Series of Extrinsic Allergic Alveolitis (All Causes)

	Lacasse et al. (2003)	Hanak et al. (2007)	Caillaud et al. (2012)	Fernández Pérez et al. (2013)	Mooney et al. (2013)	Dobashi et al. (2014)	Xu et al. (2014)
Country	Multiple	USA	France	USA	USA	Japan	China
Period	1998–2001	1997–2002	8 years	1982–2007	2000–2010	2001–2010	2002–2011
Cases	199	85	139	142	177	165	101
Smokers	6%	2%	4%	51% (ex)	0.6%	NS	10
Male	NS	53%	65%	48%	31%	NS	M < F
Cause							
Avian	66%	34%	19%	17%	28%	52%	50%
Farming	19%	11%	80%	8%	NS	0%	?6%
Hot tub	NS	21%	NS	4%	NS	NS	1%
Mould	NS	9%	0%	11%	NS	20%	14%
None	2%	25%	0%	53%	63%	10%	28%

Abbreviation: NS: not stated in the article.

2012). EAA is associated with CD8+ and CD4+ T lymphocytic alveolitis (Yamasaki et al., 1999) with activated macrophages and multinucleate giant cell granulomata (Patel et al., 2001). The histology of chronic EAA shows fewer, poorly formed granulomata and centrilobular and bridging fibrosis with alternating normal alveoli and fibroblastic foci (Grunes and Beasley, 2013), suggesting resolving granulomata leaving residual fibrosis (Mornex et al., 1994). In subacute EAA, the lung parenchymal and BAL CD8+ cells include γΔT-cells (Raulf et al., 1994), natural killer cells (Korosec et al., 2007) and oligoclonally expanded CD8+ T lymphocytes (Facco et al., 2004) that normalise with antigen avoidance (Trentin et al., 1988; Facco et al., 2004). BAL CD4+ lymphocytes are predominantly of the T helper 1 (Th1) subset (Hirata et al., 2001) expressing the high-affinity IL-12 receptor (Yamasaki et al., 1999) that produces IFN-γ in response to IL-12 from antigen-activated macrophages (Yamasaki et al., 1999) and neutrophils (Ethuin et al., 2004). This IFN-γ in turn stimulates alveolar macrophages to produce chemokines (e.g. CXCL10 and CCL18), which, respectively, recruit CXCR3+ and CCR3+ lymphocytes and monocytes from blood into the lung in order to perpetuate granuloma formation. In EAA, the lymphocytes in BAL and lung tissue are CXCR3+ (Agostini et al., 2005). However, it is the CXCR3 and CCR3 expression on CD4 lymphocytes that correlates with the high resolution computed tomography (HRCT) alveolar and interstitial scores (Sterclova et al., 2009), suggesting that Th2 lymphocytes might be indicative of progression from subacute to chronic disease. In addition, patients with chronic EAA have higher proportions of BAL Th2 lymphocytes that produce less IFN-γ and more IL-4 in response to antigen (Barrera et al., 2008).

Immune Tolerance

Most individuals with prolonged exposure to inhaled antigens are asymptomatic and do not develop EAA, suggesting either an underlying genetic susceptibility to disease or that an additional trigger is required. Immune modulation by Th2 regulatory cells (CD4+CD25+Foxp3+; Tregs) is likely to be of key importance in maintaining tolerance to inhaled allergens and preventing the development of allergy.

Progression of EAA

Prognosis in EAA is very variable, and some individuals have a benign, non-progressive form despite evidence of immune sensitisation and long-term continued antigen exposure (Braun et al., 1979; Bourke et al., 1989). Individual determinants of susceptibility to disease progression are poorly understood, and there are no convincing genetic or epigenetic risk factors that reproducibly identify such susceptibility. There is, however, some evidence of familial clustering in patients with chronic EAA, despite patients having lived apart from their afflicted relatives for decades (Okamoto et al., 2013). In addition, there is a strikingly high incidence of severe chronic EAA among those who keep domestic pigeons in Mexico (Gaxiola et al., 2011).

The immunopathogenesis of chronic EAA is unresolved, but is associated with collateral injury to the lung and alveolar epithelium, during which the normal wound-healing repair processes cause the alveoli to be progressively obliterated and replaced with non-functional extracellular matrix (Chambers and Mercer, 2015). Histological studies of chronic EAA and IPF have found considerable overlap (Akashi et al., 2009; Morell et al., 2013), and the pathogenic pathways in both might help identify common determinants.

CLINICAL FEATURES

The clinical features of EAA are often non-specific, with a variable combination of respiratory and/or systemic symptoms. Due to this, the diagnosis is commonly missed or delayed, with symptoms being attributed to a wide range of other conditions, including viral infections, community-acquired pneumonia, asthma, chronic obstructive pulmonary disease (COPD) or an idiopathic interstitial pneumonia. EAA has no single pathognomonic diagnostic test, and a clinical diagnosis is usually made based on a history of compatible symptoms and exposure, backed up by objective findings from radiology, lung function and blood tests. In addition, difficult cases may require more invasive tests such as BAL or surgical lung biopsy. Accurately differentiating EAA from idiopathic forms of ILD can be challenging, and is improved by multidisciplinary review of cases (Travis et al., 2008; Hobbs and Lynch, 2014). Evidence that EAA is occupational in nature may come from the recognition that clinical features are work related or due to there being a known cause in the workplace.

The differing presentations seen in EAA generally reflect differing host responses to varying doses and durations of exposure, rather than the natural history of a single progressive disease. Although acute, subacute and chronic EAA are commonly used in clinical practice (Richerson et al., 1989), exact definitions for each type are less clear, and alternative classifications have been suggested (Boyd et al., 1982; Lacasse et al., 2009).

Acute EAA is typified by an abrupt onset of influenza-like symptoms that occur several hours after a heavy exposure to an allergen. Full recovery is usual, and symptoms recur within a few hours of repeated exposure. In contrast, acute symptoms may be absent in individuals who develop chronic EAA, with slowly progressive lung fibrosis. Between the extremes of acute and chronic disease are those with subacute EAA. This group is more poorly defined, as patients may have a combination of acute and chronic features, with a variable degree of recovery on cessation of exposure. Whilst the acute, subacute and chronic classification for EAA remains useful, it is clearly an oversimplification of a much more complex and variable disease. This is particularly highlighted by the severe acute idiopathic exacerbations that that have been reported in some patients with chronic fibrotic EAA (Miyazaki et al., 2008; Olson et al., 2008).

SYMPTOMS AND EXAMINATION FINDINGS

In acute occupational EAA, influenza-like symptoms occur 2–12 hours after a high-level exposure to an allergen in the workplace (Malmberg et al., 1993). Cough, chest tightness, wheeze and breathlessness usually occur, with symptoms of myalgia, arthralgia and malaise. Physical examination may reveal fever, tachycardia, increased respiratory rate and inspiratory crackles. In most cases, the symptoms are self-limiting, with clinical improvement seen over 12–24 hours and full recovery typical within a few days. In many cases, individuals do not seek medical care, taking short-term sick leave due to 'a viral illness'. A clear link to the causative exposure may not be appreciated, as symptoms may occur several hours after leaving work.

In subacute occupational disease, progressive cough and breathlessness occur over a more prolonged period, usually several weeks or months. Constitutional symptoms such as malaise, fatigue and weight loss are also common, and may predominate in certain cases. In some workers, symptoms are clearly work related, with improvements at weekends or on rest days. In others, particularly where the condition remains unrecognised, the relationship is less clear, as recovery is only apparent after longer periods away from work, such as after a 2-week holiday or prolonged sickness absence (Hodgson et al., 2001). Examination findings of breathlessness, hypoxia and inspiratory crackles may also vary with exposure and, in some cases, will have completely resolved by the time a worker is seen in secondary care. In severely affected workers, attacks of breathlessness with cyanosis occur at or after work, with some patients requiring admission to hospital.

Progressive lung fibrosis in chronic occupational disease commonly results in cough and exertional breathlessness that is not clearly work related and may be present for several years prior to diagnosis. Constitutional symptoms may be less marked or absent in these individuals. Clubbing may be present, and chest auscultation reveals fine inspiratory crackles. In severe cases, hypoxia and signs of pulmonary hypertension are also found. In some patients with chronic farmers' and bird-breeders' lung, signs of hyperinflation due to airflow obstruction and gas trapping may predominate (Lalancette et al., 1993; Remy-Jardin et al., 1993; Malinen et al., 2003).

PHYSIOLOGY

Due to the variable clinical presentation in occupational EAA, the physiological findings may also vary widely, depending on the type and severity of disease, as well as the timing of the measurements in relation to exposure.

Pulmonary function tests typically show a restrictive pattern of abnormality in EAA, with reduced values of forced expiratory volume in 1 second, forced vital capacity and total lung capacity. A reduction in carbon monoxide gas transfer is also typical, and this is a more sensitive measure of impaired gas exchange than vital capacity (Dinda et al., 1969; Barber et al., 2014). Depending on disease severity, hypoxia at rest or on exertion may be present (Schuyler, 1997), with evidence of an increased alveolar–arterial gradient (Dangman et al., 2002). In a significant proportion of workers with EAA, an obstructive pattern of lung function with gas trapping is seen due to bronchiolitis (Cordier, 2007) or emphysema (Erkinjuntti-Pekkanen et al., 1997). Increased levels of bronchial hyper-responsiveness can also be seen in 22%–50% of patients with EAA (Freedman and Ault, 1981; Mönkäre, 1984), making occupational asthma a differential diagnosis.

In many cases of subacute EAA, there is the potential for full or near-full recovery, even in those with severely abnormal lung function, hypoxia or pulmonary hypertension at the time of diagnosis (Mönkäre and Haahtela, 1987; McKeown et al., 2005). In milder cases, lung function tests show significant improvement, but remain within the normal predicted range. Following cessation of exposure, the majority of any potential improvement in gas transfer is seen by 12 months, but further gradual recovery may continue for up to 5 years (Mönkäre and Haahtela, 1987). Whilst these lung function abnormalities are non-specific, the demonstration of serial changes following cessation of exposure or in response to inhalation challenges may be very helpful in confirming a diagnosis. Variations in alveolar exhaled nitric oxide levels may, in the future, offer a more sensitive method of linking disease activity with causative exposures (Shirai et al., 2010).

Established fibrosis or emphysema in chronic EAA results in permanently impaired lung function, and the degree of physiological abnormality assists in assessing disease severity and future prognosis (Hanak et al., 2008).

BLOOD TESTS

Inflammatory Markers

The inflammatory response seen in EAA is commonly associated with peripheral blood neutrophilia and an elevation of inflammatory markers such as C-reactive protein and the erythrocyte sedimentation rate (Mönkäre, 1984; Dangman et al., 2002; Morell et al., 2008). These non-specific findings are more commonly seen in acute and subacute disease, but may also be seen in chronic EAA following acute exposure (Ohtani et al., 2005).

Specific IgG Antibodies

Although the association between EAA and the presence of specific IgG antibodies in the serum has been recognised for many decades, antibody tests alone cannot diagnose or exclude the disease. Originally, the presence of a 'precipitating antibody' was demonstrated as a visible band of antibody/antigen complex in a gel, as demonstrated in Figure 23.1 (Ouchterlony, 1949). This technique has been replaced by more standardised and sensitive laboratory techniques allowing quantification of specific IgG levels. In an individual with compatible clinical features, the presence of an elevated level of specific IgG to a known allergen in the workplace is supportive of the presence of occupational EAA. In itself, however, it is not diagnostic, as it can also be measured in up to 87% of exposed individuals without disease (Morell et al., 2008). In addition, the presence of specific IgG does not imply that EAA will occur in the future, even after decades of subsequent exposure (Cormier et al., 2004). The significance of a negative IgG test result in a symptomatic worker is dependent on the sensitivity of the test and the type of exposure, as symptoms may be due to a different condition or EAA may be due to a different antigen. Specific IgG antibodies may be present in some individuals for years after an acute attack of EAA (Mönkäre and Haahtela, 1987), but are known

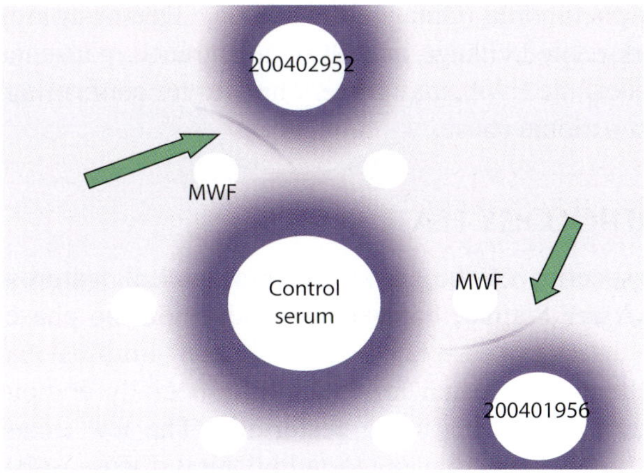

FIGURE 23.1 Confirmation of sensitisation to used metalworking fluid (MWF) samples in two workers with extrinsic allergic alveolitis. Precipitating arcs (green arrows) of the antibody/antigen complex are seen to have formed in the gel between the samples of used MWF and patient serum (nine-figure serial numbers).

to fluctuate with exposure and may be absent in chronic fibrotic disease. In a study of EAA due to avian proteins, the sensitivity of specific IgG testing was only 18% for disease with usual interstitial pneumonia (UIP) pattern fibrosis, as opposed to 85% when the biopsy showed an inflammatory pattern (Ohtani et al., 2005).

The diagnostic usefulness of these tests is further reduced by the range of antibodies that are both commercially available and have established normal ranges. In many cases, this is limited to a panel that only includes antibodies to common avian proteins and a range of microbial agents associated with agricultural exposures (Girard et al., 2009). Where standardised IgG tests are not commercially available, researchers have utilised a range of other immunological tests in order to confirm IgG sensitisation (Rodrigo et al., 2010; Tillie-LeBlond et al., 2011). In addition, antigen-induced lymphocyte proliferation studies have been used as a method of confirming cell-mediated immunity to microbiological samples taken from the home or workplace (Yoshizawa et al., 1999; Inase et al., 2006; Chiba et al., 2009).

RADIOLOGY

Although gallium scans have been recommended as non-invasive radiological tests in EAA (Hodgson et al., 2001; Dangman et al., 2002), HRCT scanning with inspiratory and expiratory images offers the most useful diagnostic information (Small et al., 1996). Whilst in some cases HRCT findings are diagnostic, in others it may be more suggestive of another disease of isolated bronchiolitis (Gaeta et al., 2013), cellular or fibrotic nonspecific interstitial pneumonia (NSIP), UIP or organising pneumonia (Ohtani et al., 2005). Demonstrating a work-related change in HRCT appearance, particularly in subacute EAA, may be very helpful for confirming an occupational cause.

RADIOLOGY FEATURES

Irrespective of the cause, the radiological features of EAA are similar, but vary depending on the phase of the disease. Acute EAA is usually self-limiting and it is therefore unusual for imaging (especially computed tomography [CT]) to be performed. The few imaging studies available have reported bilateral diffuse or basal areas of ground-glass opacity or consolidation, which rapidly resolve (Silver et al., 1989).

In the subacute phase, the chest radiograph commonly shows ground-glass opacification or fine nodularity involving the mid and lower zones (Cook et al., 1988). CT is more sensitive than chest radiography and may reveal abnormalities in the context of a normal chest X-ray (Lynch et al., 1992; Remy-Jardin et al., 1993). The HRCT features of the subacute phase typically consist of ill-defined centrilobular nodules with an upper zone distribution on a background of widespread ground-glass opacification (Figure 23.2a). Centrilobular nodules typically spare the sub-pleural regions of the lung and are of ground-glass density (Gruden et al., 1999). Ground-glass opacity is defined as a hazy increase in lung attenuation that does not obscure the vascular margins (Hansell et al., 2008). The 'black bronchus' sign (in which the segmental bronchi are more conspicuous and 'blacker' than normal) may be a useful clue that the lungs are of uniformly increased density. A mosaic attenuation pattern may also be observed with air trapping on end-expiratory images (Silver et al., 1989; Hansell and Moskovic, 1991). A mosaic attenuation pattern is defined as regional areas of differing density of the lung parenchyma, and air trapping is defined as a less than normal increase in attenuation of the lung parenchyma on end expiration. The distribution of air trapping is typically lobular and was described in 86% of patients in one series (Figure 23.2a) (Hansell et al., 1996). The combination of HRCT features is relatively specific to the subacute phase of EAA, enabling a confident and correct diagnosis in many cases (Hansell and Moskovic, 1991; Grenier et al., 1994). In smokers, the two other possible differential diagnoses to consider are desquamative interstitial pneumonitis (DIP) and respiratory bronchiolitis ILD (RB-ILD), a form of diffuse lung disease associated with heavy cigarette consumption (Lynch et al., 1995).

In the chronic phase of EAA, the radiographic findings are of fibrosis with a reticular pattern, architectural

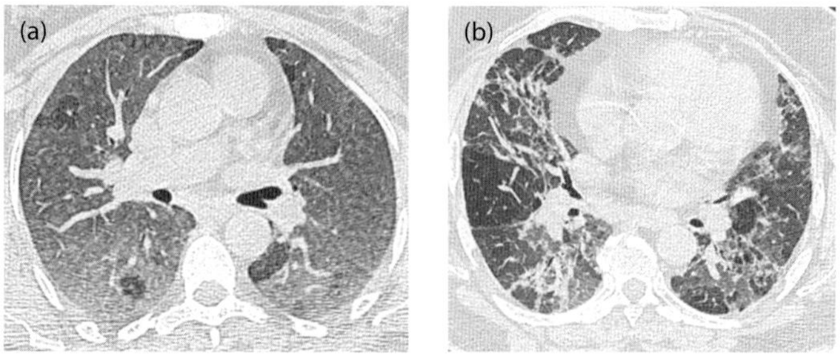

FIGURE 23.2 (a) Axial computed tomography (CT) section showing the typical features of subacute extrinsic allergic alveolitis (EAA). Note the diffuse ground-glass opacity, ill-defined centrilobular nodules and lobular areas of decreased attenuation. (b) Axial CT section showing the typical features of chronic EAA. The combination of patchy reticular pattern, ground-glass opacity and areas of decreased attenuation has given rise to the term 'head cheese' sign.

distortion and honeycombing, which commonly has a widespread distribution or mid zone predominance (Alder et al., 1992; Lynch et al., 1995). These findings are contrary to earlier studies that reported upper zone predominance based on chest radiographic findings alone (Cook et al., 1988). A lower zone and sub-pleural distribution of features may also be seen, making discrimination from IPF difficult in some instances (Lynch et al., 1995). However, in EAA, the combination of patchy or geographical areas of increased attenuation, decreased attenuation, fibrosis and relatively normal lung results in an appearance that has been likened to 'head cheese', a coarse meat pate (Figure 23.2b) (Webb, 2006). The presence of emphysema has also been described in some cases of chronic EAA (Malinen et al., 2003), although the histopathological correlate is not well described, and in some cases features may represent focal air trapping or paracicatrial emphysema (emphysema adjacent to pulmonary fibrosis), rather than the classic alveolar destruction seen in cigarette smoking. Cysts may also be a feature of subacute and chronic EAA (Franquet et al., 2003). The cysts are usually small (<15 mm in diameter) and scattered (but not with a predominant pattern), which enables differentiation from other causes of cyst that are predominant ILD such as lymphangioleiomyomatosis. The aetiology of the cysts is uncertain, but one hypothesis is that they result from partial bronchiolar obstruction by the peri-bronchiolar lymphocytic infiltrate (Franquet et al., 2003). In the majority of cases, CT enables accurate differentiation between fibrotic EAA and IPF; however, a pattern identical to UIP or NSIP may also be demonstrated (Lynch et al., 1995).

RADIOLOGY SUMMARY

Acute EAA (Unusual for Imaging to be Performed at This Stage)

Chest radiography:

- Diffuse ground-glass opacification
- Fine nodular or reticulonodular pattern

CT:

- Rarely described
- Ground-glass opacification

Subacute EAA

Chest radiography:

- May be normal (only 10% abnormal)
- Widespread ground-glass opacity
- Small, ill-defined nodules with upper zone distribution

CT:

- More sensitive than chest x-ray (CXR)
- Widespread ground-glass opacification (NB: may be difficult to recognise if very diffuse; clues are the occasional 'spared' secondary pulmonary lobule and 'black bronchus' sign)
- Small (3–4 mm diameter), ill-defined, soft-tissue density centrilobular nodules (may have upper-lobe distribution)
- Mosaic pattern (inspiratory sections)
- Air trapping (end-expiratory sections)
- Scattered lung cysts similar to lymphocytic interstitial pneumonitis (10%)

NB: similar to histopathological features, CT signs may be present to a greater or lesser extent (e.g. mainly ground-glass, profuse nodules or predominantly air trapping).

Chronic EAA

Chest radiography:

- Ground-glass opacity, reticular and honeycomb pattern
- Volume loss with pulmonary distortion
- Upper zone distribution (NB: radiographic series suggested a mainly upper zone distribution of disease; however, CT studies have subsequently demonstrated that a widespread or mid/lower CT distribution is a more frequent finding)

CT:

- Increased specificity by comparison with CXR
- Ground-glass opacification
- Reticular pattern
- Honeycombing and cysts
- Ancillary features of pulmonary fibrosis (pulmonary distortion and traction bronchiectasis—prognostically important)
- Small centrilobular nodules
- Mosaic pattern
- Air trapping on end-expiratory images
- Random or sub-pleural distribution
- Some studies describe 'emphysema'

DIFFERENTIAL DIAGNOSIS

Widespread ground-glass opacification and ill-defined centrilobular nodules: RB-ILD—knowledge of smoking history is important (nodularity usually less profuse)

Widespread ground-glass opacification—viral or pneumocystis infection, DIP
Widespread ground-glass opacification and air trapping—sarcoidosis
NSIP and UIP—may be indistinguishable; classically, EAA is more upper lobe, with less honeycombing and often demonstrating air trapping

BRONCHOALVEOLAR LAVAGE

EAA is characterised by lymphocytic inflammation, and the measurement of differential cell counts in BAL fluid may provide useful supportive diagnostic information. Samples from healthy volunteers show BAL lymphocyte levels in the region of 8%–15%, but this may be elevated to over 50% in EAA (Caillaud et al., 2012; Meyer et al., 2012). BAL lymphocytosis is not diagnostic of EAA, however, and is also be seen in a proportion of exposed workers who never develop the disease (Cormier et al., 2004). In addition, BAL lymphocytosis is also a feature of a number of other lung diseases, including sarcoidosis, connective tissue disease, organising pneumonia and miliary tuberculosis (Meyer et al., 2012). In addition to measuring differential cell counts, it is also possible to measure the ratio of $CD4^+$:$CD8^+$ lymphocytes in BAL. Although it had previously been suggested that this may be helpful for differentiating EAA from sarcoidosis (Godard et al., 1981), further work has discounted this, demonstrating that the CD4:CD8 ratio in EAA can be very variable (Caillaud et al., 2012).

The absence of an elevated lymphocyte count in an individual with suspected EAA has been suggested to effectively exclude active disease (Lacasse et al., 2008; Selman et al., 2012). This is, however, dependant on the cut-off level selected (Glazer, 2015) and the timing of the procedure in relation to exposure (Drent et al., 1993b). Variable levels of significant BAL lymphocytosis have been suggested for EAA, usually in the range of 20%–40%, with lower values expected in current smokers and those with established fibrosis (Lacasse et al., 2003; Cormier et al., 2004; Hanak et al., 2007; Morell et al., 2008; Selman et al., 2012). Nicotine has an inhibitory effect on BAL lymphocytes, which is thought to explain the low incidence of disease in current smokers. Lower levels of BAL lymphocytosis have also been demonstrated in chronic EAA with a UIP pattern of fibrosis (Ohtani et al., 2005), and a 20% cut-off level for differentiating this form of chronic EAA from IPF has been suggested (Glazer, 2015).

In some individuals, BAL lymphocytosis may persist for many years following removal of the cause, and should not therefore be taken as evidence of ongoing exposure. It may also persist despite clinical improvements, and is therefore not a reliable method of monitoring disease activity in EAA (Cormier et al., 1996).

SURGICAL BIOPSY

The diagnostic utility of HRCT, along with validated scoring systems for EAA and the increased accessibility to BAL cell differential counts, means that the majority of clinical diagnoses can be carried out without the need for biopsies (Lacasse et al., 2003; Morell et al., 2008). In certain cases, however, diagnostic uncertainty remains, and direct examination of lung tissue may be indicated (Morris and Zamvar, 2014). Small biopsy samples taken at trans-bronchial biopsy are often not diagnostic in EAA, and surgical biopsies of affected lung tissue are more helpful (Lacasse et al., 1997). The potential benefit of attaining a tissue diagnosis by video-assisted thoracoscopic surgery must be balanced against surgical risk, particularly in patients with severely impaired gas exchange (Kreider et al., 2007). How frequently surgical biopsies are performed is likely to vary between clinicians in different healthcare systems and in different countries. In a recent US cohort, 54% of EAA cases had undergone surgical biopsy (Ryerson et al., 2014), whereas in Flanders, the rate was 10% (Thomeer et al., 2001).

The histological findings in EAA, like the radiological features, are very variable. In some cases, the findings are classical, whereas in others, features may be more suggestive of NSIP, UIP, constrictive bronchiolitis or organising pneumonia (Vourlekis et al., 2002; Churg et al., 2009; Lima et al., 2009). Further detail is provided in the histopathology box (Boxes 23.1–23.4).

BOX 23.1 ACUTE DISEASE

- The lung is seldom biopsied in acute extrinsic allergic alveolitis and there are consequently few descriptions of the pathological features.
- The few reports there are describe necrotising granulomas, capillaritis, diffuse alveolar damage, neutrophilic interstitial infiltration and alveolar fibrin deposition.

BOX 23.2 SUBACUTE DISEASE

- Subacute extrinsic allergic alveolitis is characterised by poorly formed. non-necrotising granulomas accompanied by widespread lymphocytic infiltration.
- The granulomas are generally smaller and less frequent than those seen in sarcoidosis.
- No infective agents are found, but small fragments of foreign material may be present.
- Schaumann bodies may also be observed.
- Isolated giant cells with cytoplasmic clefts are frequently observed: these are suggestive of the diagnosis, but not specific.
- Knots of granulation tissue within alveoli and respiratory bronchioles are also seen.
- The granulation tissue is evidence of organisation of luminal exudates and is occasionally responsible for the accumulation of lipid-laden macrophages (endogenous lipid pneumonia).
- The granulomas resolve with time, but the diagnosis may still be suggested by the chronic inflammatory infiltrate being peribronchiolar, with airways being the portal of entry of the aetiological agent.

BOX 23.3 CHRONIC DISEASE

- Unless there is further exposure, the granulomas resolve within approximately 6 months, but the inflammation may progress to irreversible scarring, assuming either a usual interstitial pneumonia or fibrotic nonspecific interstitial pneumonia pattern.
- Cystic change may develop and, in advanced cases, the lungs show end-stage features such as honeycombing.

BOX 23.4 DIFFERENTIAL DIAGNOSIS OF EXTRINSIC ALLERGIC ALVEOLITIS

- In contrast to idiopathic pulmonary fibrosis, extrinsic allergic alveolitis (EAA) may affect the upper lobes more than the lower lobes, with central portions affected as much as the periphery.
- The fibrosis of EAA is bronchiolocentric in distribution, rather than being predominantly sub-pleural and paraseptal as in idiopathic pulmonary fibrosis.
- In contrast to sarcoidosis, the hilar lymph nodes are unaffected.
- The diffuse background interstitial inflammation is another feature distinguishing EAA.
- A further difference is the presence of knots of granulation tissue within the alveoli and respiratory bronchioles in EAA.
- The peri-bronchiolar distribution of the inflammation helps to distinguish EAA from non-specific interstitial pneumonia and lymphoid interstitial pneumonia.
- Lymphoid interstitial pneumonia may also show poorly formed granulomas, but it is characterised by a more diffuse, intense infiltrate that is seldom accompanied by any appreciable degree of fibrosis.
- The differential diagnosis also includes mycobacterial and fungal infection and adverse drug reactions.
- Although the full spectrum of microscopic changes seen in EAA permit a confident histological diagnosis, exhaustive environmental and serological investigations quite commonly fail to identify the cause.

SPECIFIC INHALATION CHALLENGE

In a minority of occupational cases, some form of challenge test may be performed in an attempt to confirm or exclude the diagnosis. Tests may be performed by comparing periods at and away from work or by specific inhalation challenge (SIC) in a hospital challenge chamber. In either case, assessing the physiological response to exposure in terms of symptoms, lung auscultation, body temperature, lung physiology, CT and inflammatory markers may provide objective confirmation of the disease. The utility of SIC is, however, limited by the availability of validated exposure protocols and the requirement for them to be carried out in specialist centres.

The SIC protocols that are available vary, but a positive test generally requires some combination of symptoms to be reported, in association with a defined fall in lung physiological parameters, a rise in inflammatory markers and elevation in body temperature

(Ohtani et al., 2005; Muñoz et al., 2014). In one large case series from Spain, SIC had a positive predictive value of 94% and a negative predictive value of 47%. The authors concluded that SIC was most useful for EAA due to avian and fungal proteins, and less helpful for other causes due to the difficulty in replicating specific exposures (Muñoz et al., 2014).

In most cases, a diagnosis of EAA can be reached without the need for SIC, but SIC may be particularly helpful in differentiating chronic EAA from idiopathic interstitial pneumonias (Ohtani et al., 2005), confirming a novel cause of EAA (Mackiewicz et al., 1999) or identifying a specific causative exposure in order to facilitate better control (Robertson et al., 2007).

DIAGNOSTIC CRITERIA

The variable clinical presentation that can be seen in EAA and the lack of a single specific diagnostic test has led to the development of a number of diagnostic criteria for the disease. As there is no agreed 'gold standard' for diagnosing EAA, it has naturally been difficult to assess their diagnostic accuracy, and the majority are therefore unvalidated. In some instances, the criteria are applicable to all EAA cases (Richerson et al., 1989; Yoshida et al., 1995; Cormier and Lacasse, 1996; Schuyler, 1997), whereas others have been specifically developed for EAA in farmers (Mönkäre, 1984; Depierre et al., 1988; Malmberg et al., 1993), bird-breeders (Morell et al., 2008) or metalworkers (Barber et al., 2014). Most include some form of scoring system based on the presence of symptoms and the results of a range of diagnostic tests. In some criteria, each element has equal value, and in others, certain features are weighted in terms of their importance. Application of the criteria may result in a definitive diagnosis of EAA or allow individuals to be classed as definite, probable or possible cases.

A prediction rule for EAA due to any cause has been developed, using international data from a number of centres, by comparing the clinical findings in cases of EAA and other ILDs (approximately 50% idiopathic interstitial pneumonias). In this study, the gold standard for diagnosis was based on BAL and HRCT findings, with pathology reviewed where available (Lacasse et al., 2003). Six significant predictors of EAA were identified, the most important being exposure to a known cause. Of the remainder, three were related to symptoms, one was related to detecting specific IgG antibodies in the blood and one was related to the presence of inspiratory crackles. The probability of EAA in a suspected case can therefore be calculated for any individual, with results ranging between 0% and 98%. This prediction rule highlights the importance of recognising exposure, as the probability of EAA varies between 98% and 62% with and without exposure to a recognised cause, if all other predictors are present. The prediction rule has been shown to work well in bird-fanciers' lung (Morell et al., 2008), but may be of more limited usefulness in suspected EAA cases in which there is no clear causative exposure or no standardised serum IgG test available.

In addition to diagnostic criteria, case definitions for EAA have also been used to facilitate outbreak investigations in lifeguards (Rose et al., 1998) and workers exposed to metalworking fluids (Barber et al., 2012). Some of these remain unvalidated (Fox et al., 1999), whereas others have been developed using consensus expert opinion (Barber et al., 2014) or biopsy data (Dangman et al., 2002) as the gold standard for diagnosis. The diagnostic approach required in an outbreak is very different to the clinical assessment of a single clinical case, as many hundreds of exposed workers may report symptoms and no standardised panel of allergen tests may be available (Burton et al., 2012). The utilisation of EAA case definitions in outbreaks helps identify affected workers and facilitates epidemiological studies in order to identify and remediate the cause.

MANAGEMENT

The management of occupational EAA should be focused on identifying the workplace exposure responsible and avoiding further contact in an attempt to prevent permanent impairment from fibrosis or emphysema. In pigeon breeders, continued exposure resulted in fourfold greater than expected lung function decline over an 18-year period (Schmidt et al., 1988). Similar data from farmers with recurrent attacks of EAA over a 14-year follow-up period demonstrated that pulmonary gas transfer was on average 20% lower than in control farmers (Erkinjuntti-Pekkanen et al., 1997).

In some cases, the likely cause is immediately apparent from the occupational history, and can easily be confirmed by a relevant specific IgG blood test. In other cases, there may be no evidence of sensitisation to the available panel of allergens, and the cause may remain obscure despite a workplace and home visit. Every effort should be made to maintain employment for those affected by EAA and to prevent further cases amongst the remaining exposed workforce. In cases where exposure cannot be avoided or the disease progresses despite cessation of exposure, the use of anti-inflammatory medication may be indicated. In selected patients with progressive fibrotic disease, lung transplantation should also be considered. In those who are not suitable for transplantation, standard palliative treatments with oxygen and opiates are indicated.

Exposure Control

Avoiding further exposure to the relevant allergen in the workplace requires consideration of the hierarchy of control measures (Ellenbecker, 1996) and is more easily achieved in some industries than others. Changes in work practice relating to hay storage have dramatically reduced the incidence of farmers' lung in Canada by preventing exposure to microbial contaminants (Cormier, 2014). In many cases, affected workers are able to remain in employment by being relocated to an unexposed area of the workplace. Alternatively, symptoms may be controlled by significantly reducing exposures through changes to work practices, improved hygiene measures, installation of local exhaust ventilation or appropriate use of respiratory-protective equipment (RPE). Challenge studies have established that the short-term use of half-face filter masks is effective in preventing symptoms in those with proven EAA (Hendrick et al., 1981). The wearing of powered helmet respirators throughout the indoor feeding seasons has also previously been shown to prevent recurrent attacks of farmers' lung (Nuutinen et al., 1987). Although wearing suitable RPE may offer an acceptable solution in some cases, other more effective exposure control measures should be used wherever possible. Prolonged use of RPE is uncomfortable, and its effectiveness is reliant on adequate training, storage and maintenance. Despite extensive hygiene measures, up to 50% of workers with occupational EAA will leave their current job due to persistent work-related symptoms and long-term health concerns (Bouchard et al., 1995; Zacharisen et al., 1998; Bracker et al., 2003).

Drug Therapy

A proportion of patients with EAA have symptoms of variable airflow obstruction and may benefit from standard asthma therapy (Kokkarinen et al., 1997). In addition, cases of chronic EAA with fixed airway disease and emphysema (Erkinjuntti-Pekkanen et al., 1998) should be treated following appropriate guidelines for COPD. Short courses of oral corticosteroids are often given to acute cases of EAA admitted to hospital with hypoxia. In this situation, corticosteroids speed recovery, but do not improve the long-term outcome (Mönkäre, 1983). In one small study of patients with acute EAA, clinical recovery at 1 month was found to be similar in those who continued in their exposure but were treated with prednisolone (at a dose of 20 mg once daily) and those who ceased further exposure (Cormier, 1994). Most patients admitted with acute or subacute occupational EAA will spontaneously improve over a period of a few days due to the avoidance of workplace exposure associated with hospital admission. A similar response to avoiding exposure and to corticosteroids can be expected in occupational EAA caused by exposure to water that is contaminated with opportunistic mycobacteria, in which treatment with anti-mycobacterial drug therapy is not usually required (Fjällbrant et al., 2013).

A therapeutic trial of immunosuppression with corticosteroids is also indicated for progressive disease where cessation of exposure has been ineffective or is not possible (Yoshizawa et al., 1999; Girard et al., 2009). Steroid-sparing agents such as azathioprine, mycophenolate and cyclophosphamide are also commonly used in progressive EAA (Lima et al., 2009; Fernández Pérez et al., 2013; Mooney et al., 2013; Cullinan et al., 2014), but there have been no controlled trials in order to establish their efficacy. Long-term usage of immunosuppression has significant potential side effects and should only be continued where there has been a clear clinical benefit. In some cases, occupational EAA progresses despite avoidance of the cause and aggressive immunosuppression (Zacharisen and Schoenwetter, 2005). Rituximab, a B-cell-depleting anti-CD20 antibody, has been used as 'rescue therapy' in this scenario (Lota et al., 2013). Results from a single case series of six patients found that rituximab therapy resulted in improved physiology in 50%, with the remainder progressing to death within 4 months (Keir et al., 2014). Patients with chronic EAA and severe life-threatening pulmonary hypertension should also be assessed for treatment with pulmonary vasodilator therapy (Koschel et al., 2010). Although antifibrotic drugs have become established in IPF (King et al., 2014; Richeldi et al., 2014), there have been no studies in chronic fibrotic EAA.

Lung Transplantation

In selected patients with progressive fibrotic EAA, lung transplantation should be considered. In a proportion of other EAA cases, the diagnosis is only recognised after histological examination of the explant. Survival post-transplant is significantly better in chronic EAA than in IPF, with 5-year survival rates in one study of 81% versus 49% (Kern et al., 2015). Recurrence post-transplantation has been described in EAA, and further allergen exposures must therefore be avoided (Kern et al., 2015). Given the better post-transplant survival in EAA, the timing of transplantation is key. It has been suggested that a transplant referral should be made in chronic EAA when predicted 3-year survival falls below 50% (Ryerson et al., 2014).

PROGNOSIS

There have not been any published studies that have directly compared prognosis in occupational disease and EAA due to other causes. In some cases, an occupational cause may equate to a good health outcome, as cases are detected early by health surveillance or during an outbreak investigation. A workplace cause may also offer the potential for complete allergen avoidance, either by elective workplace modifications (Nuutinen et al., 1987; Bracker et al., 2003) or workers having to leave employment due to uncontrolled symptoms (Zacharisen et al., 1998). In other cases, occupational EAA has resulted in a poor outcome, as a workplace cause has not been recognised early enough (Zacharisen and Schoenwetter, 2005; Cullinan et al., 2014) or workers have continued exposure due to socioeconomic pressures (Erkinjuntti-Pekkanen et al., 1997). The latter may be of particular relevance in certain industries such as farming, where an affected individual's family may have lived and worked in the same environment for many generations (Mönkäre, 1983; Bouchard et al., 1995).

The natural history of occupational EAA with ongoing exposure to the cause is very variable. In some cases, further acute episodes do not occur or are self-limiting (Braun et al., 1979; Bourke et al., 1989), whereas in others, this results in chronic airflow obstruction (Erkinjuntti-Pekkanen et al., 1997) or pulmonary fibrosis (Yoshizawa et al., 1999; Glazer, 2015). Complete cessation of exposure should prevent further episodes of acute disease and may result in a full recovery in early subacute EAA. In chronic EAA with established fibrosis or emphysema, the main aim of allergen avoidance is to stabilise disease or minimise the rate of further deterioration in lung function, rather than to attain clinical improvement. Overall, prognosis is dependant both on the ability to avoid further exposure and the degree of established fibrosis present at the time of diagnosis. In reported case series of EAA, a cause could not be identified in 2%–63% of patients (Table 23.4). The prognosis is worse in this situation (median survival of approximately 9 years versus 5 years), as measures to prevent further exposure to the cause cannot easily be undertaken (Fernández Pérez et al., 2013).

Studies have identified a wide range of factors that are associated with poor outcomes in EAA (Table 23.5), many reflecting some measure of the degree of fibrosis present. The absence of fibrosis in pathological samples has been shown to be associated with a good prognosis, with median survival of approximately 22 years. In contrast, median survival was worse for those with peribronchiolar fibrosis (11 years) or with fibrotic NSIP/UIP pattern fibrosis (2–3 years) (Churg et al., 2009).

For a given degree of radiographic fibrosis, survival is better in chronic EAA than in IPF (Mooney et al., 2013). Mortality can be predicted in chronic fibrotic lung disease using the ILD-GAP (gender age physiology) model (Ryerson et al., 2014). This model generates a score ranging from 0 to 8 based on gender, age and physiology. Predicted 3-year mortality for chronic EAA is better than in IPF and similar to that seen in idiopathic NSIP and ILD related to connective tissue disease, varying from 10% to 75% depending on the calculated score. Calculating the score may be helpful when discussing future prognosis with patients and in the timing of transplant referrals.

QUALITY OF LIFE

Health-related quality of life as measured by the Short Form-36 medical outcome survey is impaired in chronic EAA and has been found to be worse than in patients with IPF. This finding could not be accounted for by differences in age or severity of lung function impairment, but chronic EAA patients experienced more severe breathlessness and fatigue than those with IPF (Lubin et al., 2014). Whether allergen avoidance measures in chronic EAA have an additional impact on quality of life by adversely affecting the work, social or home environment remains to be confirmed (Barber et al., 2015).

CONCLUSIONS

EAA remains a fascinating and relatively poorly understood disease. It has a wide range of occupational causes and may mimic many other types of common lung disease. The main challenge for clinicians is to recognise the disease and cause early enough in order to improve clinical outcomes and protect the health of other exposed workers.

TABLE 23.5
Adverse Prognostic Features in Extrinsic Allergic Alveolitis

Demographic factors	
Current or former cigarette smoking	Ohtsuka et al. (1995); Fernández-Pérez et al. (2013); Mooney et al. (2013)
Male gender	Pérez-Padilla et al. (1993); Lima et al. (2009); Ryerson et al. (2014)
Older age	Allen et al. (1976); Lima et al. (2009); Fernández-Pérez et al. (2013); Ryerson et al. (2014)
Exposure	
Longer exposure once symptomatic	Allen et al. (1976); de Gracia et al. (1989)
No causative exposure identified	Fernández-Pérez et al. (2013)
Ongoing exposure post-diagnosis	Allen et al. (1976); Cormier and Belanger (1985); Schmidt et al. (1988); Erkinjuntti-Pekkanen et al. (1997)
Clinical	
Acute idiopathic exacerbations	Miyazaki et al. (2008); Olson et al. (2008)
Auscultatory crackles	Hanak et al. (2008); Mooney et al. (2013)
Finger clubbing	Sansores et al. (1990)
Progression despite immunosuppression	Ohtani et al. (2005); Keir et al. (2014)
Recurrence post-transplant	Kern et al. (2015)
Requirement for oxygen therapy	Mooney et al. (2013)
Physiology	
Desaturation during exercise	Lima et al. (2009)
Lower predicted forced vital capacity (FVC), total lung capacity (TLC), carbon monoxide transfer factor (TL_{CO}), oxygen saturation (SaO_2)	Hanak et al. (2008); Mooney et al. (2013)
Presence of bronchial hyper-reactivity	Mönkäre (1983)
Pulmonary hypertension (echo systolic pulmonary artery pressure [sPAP] $\geq$ 50 mm Hg)	Koschel et al. (2010)
Radiology	
Absence of mosaic pattern on HRCT	Lima et al. (2009)
Degree of honeycombing on CXR	Pérez-Padilla et al. (1993)
Presence or degree of reticulation/fibrosis on HRCT	Hanak et al. (2008); Walsh et al. (2012); Fernández Pérez et al. (2013); Mooney et al. (2013)
Severity of traction bronchiectasis	Walsh et al. (2012)
Histology	
Diffuse alveolar damage	Miyazaki et al. (2008); Olson et al. (2008)
Non-NSIP (non-specific interstitial pneumonitis) pattern	Lima et al. (2009)
Presence of fibrosis	Vourlekis et al. (2004); Fernández Pérez et al. (2013)
Usual interstitial pneumonitis (UIP) > NSIP > bronchiolar fibrosis	Churg et al. (2009)
UIP + fibrotic NSIP > bronchiolitis obliterans organising pneumonia (BOOP) + cellular NSIP	Ohtani et al. (2005)

REFERENCES

Agostini, C., Calabrese, F., Poletti, V., Marcer, G., Facco, M., Miorin, M., Cabrelle, A. et al. 2005. CXCR3/CXCL10 interactions in the development of hypersensitivity pneumonitis. *Respir Res* 6:20–7.

Akashi, T., Takemura, T., Ando, N., Eishi, Y., Kitagawa, M., Takizawa, T., Koike, M. et al. 2009. Histopathologic analysis of sixteen autopsy cases of chronic hypersensitivity pneumonitis and comparison with idiopathic pulmonary fibrosis/usual interstitial pneumonia. *Am J Clin Pathol* 131:405–15.

Alder, B. D., Padley, S., Müller, N. L., Remy Jardin, M. and Remy, J. 1992. Chronic hypersensitivity pneumonitis: High-resolution CT and radiographic features in 16 patients. *Radiology* 185:91–5.

Allen, D. H., Williams, G. V. and Woolcock, A. J. 1976. Bird breeder's hypersensitivity pneumonitis: Progress studies of lung function after cessation of exposure to the provoking antigen. *Am Rev Respir Dis* 114(3):555–66.

Babbott, F. L. Jr., Gump, D. W., Sylwester, D. L., MacPherson, B. V. and Holly, R. C. 1980. Respiratory symptoms and lung function in a sample of Vermont dairymen and industrial workers. *Am J Public Health* 70:241–45.

Barber, C. M., Burton, C. M., Hendrick, D. J., Pickering, C. A., Robertson, A. S., Robertson, W. and Burge, P. S. 2014. Hypersensitivity pneumonitis in workers exposed to metalworking fluids. *Am J Ind Med* 57(8):872–80.

Barber, C. M., Burton, C. M., Scaife, H., Crook, B. and Evans, G. S. 2012. Systematic review of respiratory case definitions in metalworking fluid outbreaks. *Occup Med (Lond)* 62(5):337–42.

Barber, C. M., Wiggans, R. E. and Fishwick, D. 2015. Impaired quality of life in chronic hypersensitivity pneumonitis. *Chest* 147(6):e230.

Barrera, L., Mendoza, F., Zuñiga, J., Estrada, A., Zamora, A. C., Melendro, E. I., Ramírez, R. et al. 2008. Functional diversity of T-cell subpopulations in subacute and chronic hypersensitivity pneumonitis. *Am J Respir Crit Care Med* 177:44–55.

Baur, X., Richter, G., Pethran, A., Czuppon, A. B. and Schwaiblmair, M. 1992. Increased prevalence of IgG-induced sensitization and hypersensitivity pneumonitis (humidifier lung) in nonsmokers exposed to aerosols of a contaminated air conditioner. *Respiration* 159:211–4.

Bouchard, S., Morin, F., Bédard, G., Gauthier, J., Paradis, J. and Cormier, Y. 1995. Farmer's lung and variables related to the decision to quit farming. *Am J Respir Crit Care Med* 152:997–1002.

Bourke, S. J., Banham, S. W., Carter, R., Lynch, P. and Boyd, G. 1989. Longitudinal course of extrinsic allergic alveolitis in pigeon breeders. *Thorax* 44:415–8.

Boyd, G., McSharry, C. P., Banham, S. W. and Lynch, P. P. 1982. A current view of pigeon fancier's lung. *Clin Allergy* 12(Suppl.):53–9.

Bracker, A., Storey, E., Yang, C. and Hodgson, M. J. 2003. An outbreak of hypersensitivity pneumonitis at a metalworking plant: A longitudinal assessment of intervention effectiveness. *Appl Occup Environ Hyg* 18(2):96–108.

Braun, S. R., doPico, G. A., Tsiatis, A., Horvath, E., Dickie, H. A. and Rankin, J. 1979. Farmer's lung disease: Long-term clinical and physiologic outcome. *Am Rev Respir Dis* 119:185–91.

Bringhurst, L. S., Byrne and R., Gershon-Cohen J. 1959. Respiratory disease of mushroom workers. *J Am Med Assoc* 171:15–8.

Burton, C. M., Crook, B., Scaife, H., Evans, G. S. and Barber, C. M. 2012. Systematic review of respiratory outbreaks associated with exposure to water-based metalworking fluids. *Ann Occup Hyg* 56(4):374–88.

Caillaud, D. M., Vergnon, J. M., Madroszyk, A., Melloni, B. M., Murris, M., Dalphin, J. C.; French Group of Environmental Immunoallergic Bronchopulmonary Diseases. 2012. Bronchoalveolar lavage in hypersensitivity pneumonitis: A series of 139 patients. *Inflamm Allergy Drug Targets* 11:15–9.

Campbell, J. M. 1932. Acute symptoms following work with hay. *Br Med J* 2:1143–44.

Chambers, R. C. and Mercer, P. F. 2015. Mechanisms of alveolar epithelial injury, repair, and fibrosis. *Ann Am Thorac Soc* 12:S16–20.

Chan, A. L., Juarez, M. M., Leslie, K. O., Ismail, H. A. and Albertson, T. E. 2012. Bird fancier's lung: A state-of-the-art review. *Clin Rev Allergy Immunol* 43(1–2):69–83.

Chiba, S., Okada, S., Suzuki, Y., Watanuki, Z., Mitsuishi, Y., Igusa, R., Sekii, T. et al. 2009. *Cladosporium* species-related hypersensitivity pneumonitis in household environments. *Intern Med* 48(5):363–67.

Churg, A., Sin, D. D., Everett, D., Brown, K. and Cool, C. 2009. Pathologic patterns and survival in chronic hypersensitivity pneumonitis. *Am J Surg Pathol* 33:1765–70.

Cook, P. G., Wells, I. P. and McGavin, C. R. 1988. The distribution of pulmonary shadowing in farmer's lung. *Clin Radiol* 39:21–7.

Cordier, J. F. 2007. Challenges in pulmonary fibrosis. 2: Bronchiolocentric fibrosis. *Thorax* 62(7):638–49.

Cormier, Y. 1994. Treatment of hypersensitivity pneumonitis (HP): Comparison between contact avoidance and corticosteroids. *Can Respir J* 1:223–8.

Cormier, Y. 2014. Hypersensitivity pneumonitis (extrinsic allergic alveolitis): A Canadian historical perspective. *Can Respir J* 21(5):277–8.

Cormier, Y. and Belanger, J. 1985. Long-term physiologic outcome after acute farmer's lung. *Chest* 87:796–800.

Cormier, Y., Israel-Assayag, E., Desmeules, M. and Lesur, O. 1996. Effect of contact avoidance or treatment with oral prednisolone on bronchoalveolar lavage surfactant protein A levels in subjects with farmer's lung. *Thorax* 51:1210–5.

Cormier, Y. and Lacasse, Y. 1996. Keys to the diagnosis of hypersensitivity pneumonitis: The role of serum precipitins, lung biopsy, and high-resolution computed tomography. *Clin Pulm Med* 3:72–7.

Cormier, Y., Letourneau, L. and Racine, G. 2004. Significance of precipitins and asymptomatic lymphocytic alveolitis: A 20-yr follow-up. *Eur Respir J* 23:523–5.

Cullinan, P., D'Souza, E., Tennant, R. and Barber, C. 2014. Lesson of the month: Extrinsic allergic (bronchiolo)alveolitis and metal working fluids. *Thorax* 69(11):1059–60.

Dalphin, J. C., Debieuvre, D., Pernet, D., Maheu, M. F., Polio, J. C., Toson, B., Dubiez, A. et al. 1993. Prevalence and risk factors for chronic bronchitis and farmer's lung in French dairy farmers. *Br J Ind Med* 50:941–4.

Dangman, K. H., Cole, S. R., Hodgson, M. J., Kuhn, C., Metersky, M. L., Schenck, P. and Storey, E. 2002. The hypersensitivity pneumonitis diagnostic index: Use of non-invasive testing to diagnose hypersensitivity pneumonitis in metalworkers. *Am J Ind Med* 42:150–62.

De Gracia, J., Morell, F., Bofill, J. M., Curull, V. and Orriols, R. 1989. Time of exposure as a prognostic factor in avian hypersensitivity pneumonitis. *Respir Med* 83(2):139–43.

Depierre, A., Dalphin, J. C., Pernet, D., Dubiez, A., Faucompre, C. and Breton, J. L. 1988. Epidemiological study of farmer's lung in five districts of the French Doubs province. *Thorax* 43:429–35.

Dinda, P., Chatterjee, S. S. and Riding, W. D. 1969. Pulmonary function studies in bird breeder's lung. *Thorax* 24(3):374–8.

Dobashi, K., Akiyama, K., Usami, A., Yokozeki, H., Ikezawa, Z., Tsurikisawa, N., Nakamura, Y. et al. 2014. Committee for Japanese Guideline for Diagnosis and Management of Occupational Allergic Diseases; Japanese Society of Allergology. 2014. Japanese Guideline for Occupational Allergic Diseases 2014. *Allergol Int* 63(3):421–42.

Drent, M., van Velzen-Blad, H., Diamant, M., Wagenaar, S. S., Hoogsteden, H. C. and van den Bosch, J. M. 1993a. Bronchoalveolar lavage in extrinsic allergic alveolitis: Effect of time elapsed since antigen exposure. *Eur Respir J* 6(9):1276–81.

Drent, M., Wagenaar, S., van Velzen-Blad, H., Mulder, P. G., Hoogsteden, H. C. and van den Bosch, J. M. 1993b. Relationship between plasma cell levels and profile of bronchoalveolar lavage fluid in patients with subacute extrinsic allergic alveolitis. *Thorax* 48:835–9.

Elder, D., Abramson, M., Fish, D., Johnson, A., McKenzie, D. and Sim, M. 2004. Surveillance of Australian workplace Based Respiratory Events (SABRE): Notifications for the first 3.5 years and validation of occupational asthma cases. *Occup Med* 54:395–9.

Eliasson, O. 1982. Farmer's lung disease: A new historical perspective from Iceland. *J Hist Med* 37:440–3.

Ellenbecker, M. J. 1996. Engineering controls as an intervention to reduce worker exposure. *Am J Ind Med* 29(4):303–7.

Erkinjuntti-Pekkanen, R., Kokkarinen, J. I., Tukiainen, H. O., Pekkanen, J., Husman, K. and Terho, E. O. 1997. Long-term outcome of pulmonary function in farmer's lung: A 14 year follow-up with matched controls. *Eur Respir J* 10(9):2046–50.

Erkinjuntti-Pekkanen, R., Rytkonen, H., Kokkarinen, J. I., Tukiainen, H. O., Partanen, K. and Terho, E. O. 1998. Long-term risk of emphysema in patients with farmer's lung and matched control farmers. *Am J Respir Crit Care Med* 158(2):662–5.

Ethuin, F., Gérard, B., Benna, J. E., Boutten, A., Gougereot-Pocidalo, M. A., Jacob, L. and Chollet-Martin, S. 2004. Human neutrophils produce interferon gamma upon stimulation by interleukin-12. *Lab Invest* 84:1363–71.

Facco, M., Trentin, L., Nicolardi, L., Miorin, M., Scquizzato, E., Carollo, D., Baesso, I. et al. 2004. T cells in the lung of patients with hypersensitivity pneumonitis accumulate in a clonal manner. *J Leukoc Biol* 75:798–803.

Farebrother, M. J., Kelson, M. C. and Heller, R. F. 1985. Death certification of farmer's lung and chronic airway diseases in different countries of the EEC. *Br J Dis Chest* 79:352–60.

Feldman, H. A. and Sabin, A. B. 1948. Pneumonitis of unknown aetiology in a group of men exposed to pigeon excreta. *J Clin Invest* 27:533.

Fenclová, Z., Pelclová, D., Urban, P., Navrátil, T., Klusácková, P. and Lebedová, J. 2009. Occupational hypersensitivity pneumonitis reported to the Czech National Registry of Occupational Diseases in the period 1992–2005. *Ind Health* 47:443–8.

Fernández Pérez, E. R., Swigris, J. J., Forssén, A. V., Tourin, O., Solomon, J. J., Huie, T. J., Olson, A. L. et al. 2013. Identifying an inciting antigen is associated with improved survival in patients with chronic hypersensitivity pneumonitis. *Chest* 144:1644–51.

Fishwick, D. 2012. New occupational and environmental causes of asthma and extrinsic allergic alveolitis. *Clin Chest Med* 33(4):605–16.

Fjällbrant, H., Akerstrom, M., Svensson, E. and Andersson, E. 2013. Hot tub lung: An occupational hazard. *Eur Respir Rev* 22(127):88–90.

Fox, J., Anderson, H., Moen, T., Gruetzmacher, G., Hanrahan, L. and Fink, J. 1999. Metal working fluid-associated hypersensitivity pneumonitis: An outbreak investigation and case–control study. *Am J Ind Med* 35:58–67.

Franquet, T., Hansell, D. M., Senbanjo, T., Remy-Jardin, M. and Müller, N. L. 2003. Lung cysts in subacute hypersensitivity pneumonitis. *J Comput Assist Tomogr* 27:475–8.

Freedman, P. M. and Ault, B. 1981. Bronchial hyperreactivity to methacholine in farmers' lung disease. *J Allergy Clin Immunol* 67(1):59–63.

Fuller, C. J. 1953. Farmer's lung: A review of present knowledge. *Thorax* 8(1):59–64.

Gaeta, M., Minutoli, F., Girbino, G., Murabito, A., Benedetto, C., Contiguglia, R., Ruggeri, P. et al. 2013. Expiratory CT scan in patients with normal inspiratory CT scan: A finding of obliterative bronchiolitis and other causes of bronchiolar obstruction. *Multidiscip Respir Med* 8(1):44.

Ganier, M., Lieberman, P., Fink, J. and Lockwood, D. G. 1980. Humidifier lung. An outbreak in office workers. *Chest* 77(2):183–7.

Gaxiola, M., Buendía-Roldán, I., Mejía, M., Carrillo, G., Estrada, A., Navarro, M. C., Rojas-Serrano, J. et al. 2011. Morphologic diversity of chronic pigeon breeder's disease: Clinical features and survival. *Respir Med* 105:608–14.

Girard, M., Lacasse, Y. and Cormier, Y. 2009. Hypersensitivity pneumonitis. *Allergy* 64:322–34.

Glazer, C. S. 2015. Chronic hypersensitivity pneumonitis: Important considerations in the work-up of this fibrotic lung disease. *Curr Opin Pulm Med* 21(2):171–7.

Godard, P., Clot, J., Jonquet, O., Bousquet, J. and Michel, F. B. 1981. Lymphocyte subpopulations in bronchoalveolar lavage of patients with sarcoidosis and hypersensitivity pneumonitis. *Chest* 80:447–52.

Grenier, P., Chevret, S., Beigelman, C., Brauner, M. W., Chastang, C. and Valeyre, D. 1994. Chronic diffuse infiltrative lung disease: Determination of the diagnostic value of clinical data, chest radiography, and CT with Bayesian analysis. *Radiology* 191:383–90.

Gruden, J. F., Webb, W. R., Naidich, D. P. and McGuiness, G. 1999. Multi-nodular disease: Anatomic localization at thin-section CT—Multireader evaluation of a simple algorithm. *Radiology* 210:711–20.

Grunes, D. and Beasley, M. B. 2013. Hypersensitivity pneumonitis: A review and update of histologic findings. *J Clin Pathol* 66:888–95.

Hanak, V., Golbin, J. M., Hartman, T. E. and Ryu, J. H. 2008. High-resolution CT findings of parenchymal fibrosis correlate with prognosis in hypersensitivity pneumonitis. *Chest* 134:133–8.

Hanak, V., Golbin, J. M. and Ryu, J. H. 2007. Causes and presenting features in 85 consecutive patients with hypersensitivity pneumonitis. *Mayo Clin Proc* 82:812–6.

Hansell, D. M., Bankier, A. A., MacMahon, H., McLoud, T. C. and Müller, N. L. 2008. Fleischner Society: Glossary of terms for thoracic imaging. *Radiology* 246;697–722.

Hansell, D. M. and Moskovic, E. 1991. High-resolution computed-tomography in extrinsic allergic alveolitis. *Clin Radiol* 43:8–12.

Hansell, D. M., Wells, A. U., Padley, S. P. and Müller, N. L. 1996. Hypersensitivity pneumonitis: Correlation of individual CT patterns with functional abnormalities. *Radiology* 199:123–8.

Hendrick, D. J., Marshall, R., Faux, J. A. and Krall, J. M. 1980. Positive "alveolar" responses to antigen inhalation provocation tests: Their validity and recognition. *Thorax* 35:415–27.

Hendrick, D. J., Marshall, R., Faux, J. A. and Krall, J. M. 1981. Protective value of dust respirators in extrinsic allergic alveolitis: Clinical assessment using inhalation provocation tests. *Thorax* 36(12):917–21.

Hirata, K., Kanazawa, H. and Kamoi, H. 2001. IV. Clinical aspects of delayed hypersensitivity in lungs: Pathophysiology of hypersensitivity disorders in clinics. *Microsc Res Tech* 53:307–12.

Hobbs, S. and Lynch, D. 2014. The idiopathic interstitial pneumonias: An update and review. *Radiol Clin North Am* 52(1):105–20.

Hodgson, M. J., Bracker, A., Yang, C., Storey, E., Jarvis, B. J., Milton, D., Lummus, Z. et al. 2001. Hypersensitivity pneumonitis in a metal-working environment. *Am J Ind Med* 39(6):616–28.

Inase, N., Ohtani, Y., Sumi, Y., Umino, T., Usui, Y., Miyake, S. and Yoshizawa, Y. 2006. A clinical study of hypersensitivity pneumonitis presumably caused by feather duvets. *Ann Allergy Asthma Immunol* 96(1):98–104.

Jacobs, R. L., Andrews, C. P. and Coalson, J. J. 2005. Hypersensitivity pneumonitis: Beyond classic occupational disease-changing concepts of diagnosis and management. *Ann Allergy Asthma Immunol* 95(2):115–28.

Jamison, C. S. and Hopkins, J. 1941. Bagassosis—A fungus disease of the lung. *New Orleans Med Surg J* 93:580–2.

Kanerva, L., Jolanki, R. and Toikkanen, J. 1994. Frequencies of occupational allergic diseases and gender differences in Finland. *Int Arch Occup Environ Health* 66(2):111–6.

Karakatsani, A., Papakosta, D., Rapti, A., Antoniou, K. M., Dimadi, M., Markopoulou, A., Latsi, P. et al. 2009. Hellenic Interstitial Lung Diseases Group. Epidemiology of interstitial lung diseases in Greece. *Respir Med* 103(8):1122–9.

Kawanami, O., Aoki, M., Miyake, H. and Mukawa, Y. 1987. Antigen-presenting Langerhans cells in the lung tissue of hypersensitivity pneumonitis patients. *Arerugi* 36:999–1005.

Keir, G. J., Maher, T. M., Ming, D., Abdullah, R., de Lauretis, A., Wickremasinghe, M., Nicholson, A. G. et al. 2014. Rituximab in severe, treatment-refractory interstitial lung disease. *Respirology* 19(3):353–9.

Kern, R. M., Singer, J. P., Koth, L., Mooney, J., Golden, J., Hays, S., Greenland, J. et al. 2015. Lung Transplantation for Hypersensitivity Pneumonitis. *Chest* 147(6): 1558–65.

King, T. E. Jr, Bradford, W. Z., Castro-Bernardini, S., Fagan, E. A., Glaspole, I., Glassberg, M. K., Gorina, E. et al. 2014. A phase 3 trial of pirfenidone in patients with idiopathic pulmonary fibrosis. *N Engl J Med* 370(22):2083–92.

Kipen, H. M., Tepper, A., Rosenman, K. and Weinrib, D. 1990. Limitations of hospital discharge diagnoses for surveillance of extrinsic allergic alveolitis. *Am J Ind Med* 17:701–9.

Kokkarinen, J. I., Tukiainen, H. O. and Terho, E. O. 1997. Asthma in patients with farmer's lung during a five-year follow-up. *Scand J Work Environ Health* 23(2): 149–51.

Kornum, J. B., Christensen, S., Grijota, M., Pedersen, L., Wogelius, P., Beiderbeck, A. and Sørensen, H. T. 2008. The incidence of interstitial lung disease 1995–2005: A Danish nationwide population-based study. *BMC Pulm Med* 8:24.

Korosec, P., Osolnik, K., Kern, I., Silar, M., Mohorcic, K. and Kosnik, M. 2007. Expansion of pulmonary $CD8^+CD56^+$ natural killer T-cells in hypersensitivity pneumonitis. *Chest* 132:1291–7.

Koschel, D. S., Kolditz, M., Höeffken, G. and Halank, M. 2010. Combined vasomodulatory therapy for severe pulmonary hypertension in chronic hypersensitivity pneumonitis. *Med Sci Monit* 16(5):CS55–7.

Kreider, M. E., Hansen-Flaschen, J., Ahmad, N. N., Rossman, M. D., Kaiser, L. R., Kucharczuk, J. C. and Shrager, J. B. 2007. Complications of video-assisted thoracoscopic lung biopsy in patients with interstitial lung disease. *Ann Thorac Surg* 83(3):1140–4.

Kundu, S., Mitra, S., Ganguly, J., Mukherjee, S., Ray, S. and Mitra, R. 2014. Spectrum of diffuse parenchymal lung diseases with special reference to idiopathic pulmonary fibrosis and connective tissue disease: An eastern India experience. *Lung India* 31(4):354–60.

Lacasse, Y., Assayag, E. and Cormier, Y. 2008. Myths and controversies in hypersensitivity pneumonitis. *Semin Respir Crit Care Med* 29(6):631–42.

Lacasse, Y., Fraser, R. S., Fournier, M. and Cormier, Y. 1997. Diagnostic accuracy of transbronchial biopsy in the diagnosis of acute farmer's lung. *Chest* 112:1459–65.

Lacasse, Y., Selman, M., Costabel, U., Dalphin, J. C., Ando, M., Morell, F., Erkinjuntti-Pekkanen, R. et al.; HP Study Group. 2003. Clinical diagnosis of hypersensitivity pneumonitis. *Am J Respir Crit Care* 168:952–8.

Lacasse, Y., Selman, M., Costabel, U., Dalphin, J. C., Morell, F., Erkinjuntti-Pekkanen, R., Mueller, N. L. et al.; HP Study Group. 2009. Classification of hypersensitivity pneumonitis: A hypothesis. *Int Arch Allergy Immunol* 149(2):161–6.

Lalancette, M., Carrier, G., Laviolette, M., Ferland, S., Rodrique, J., Bégin, R., Cantin, A. et al. 1993. Farmer's lung. Long-term outcome and lack of predictive value of bronchoalveolar lavage fibrosing factors. *Am Rev Respir Dis* 148(1):216–21.

Lima, M. S., Coletta, E. N., Ferreira, R. G., Jasinowodolinski, D., Arakaki, J. S., Rodrigues, S. C., Rocha, N. A. et al. 2009. Subacute and chronic hypersensitivity pneumonitis: Histopathological patterns and survival. *Respir Med* 103:508–15.

Lota, H. K., Keir, G. J., Hansell, D. M., Nicholson, A. G., Maher, T. M., Wells, A. U. and Renzoni, E. A. 2013. Novel use of rituximab in hypersensitivity pneumonitis refractory to conventional treatment. *Thorax* 68(8): 780–1.

Lubin, M., Chen, H., Elicker, B., Jones, K. D., Collard, H. R. and Lee, J. S. 2014. A comparison of health-related quality of life in idiopathic pulmonary fibrosis and chronic hypersensitivity pneumonitis. *Chest* 145(6): 1333–8.

Lynch, D. A., Newell, J. D., Logan, P. M., King, T. E. Jr. and Müller, N. L. 1995. Can CT distinguish hypersensitivity pneumonitis from idiopathic pulmonary fibrosis? *Am J Roentgenol* 165:807–11.

Lynch, D. A., Rose, C. S., Way, D. and King, T. E. Jr. 1992. Hypersensitivity pneumonitis: Sensitivity of high-resolution CT in a population based study. *AJR Am J Roentgenol* 159:469–72.

Mackiewicz, B., Skórska, C., Dutkiewicz, J., Michnar, M., Milanowski, J., Prazmo, Z., Krysinska-Traczyk, E. et al. 1999. Allergic alveolitis due to herb dust exposure. *Ann Agric Environ Med* 6(2):167–70.

Malinen, A. P., Erkinjuntti-Pekkanen, R. A., Partanen, P. L., Rytkönen, H. T. and Vanninen, R. L. 2003. Long-term sequelae of Farmer's lung disease in HRCT: A 14-year follow-up study of 88 patients and 83 matched control farmers. *Eur Radiol* 13(9):2212–21.

Malmberg, P., Rask-Andersen, A. and Rosenhall, L. 1993. Exposure to microorganisms associated with allergic alveolitis and febrile reactions to mold dust in farmers. *Chest* 103(4):1202–9.

McDonald, J. C., Chen, Y., Zekveld, C. and Cherry, N. M. 2005. Incidence by occupation and industry of acute work related respiratory diseases in the UK, 1992–2001. *Occup Environ Med* 62:836–42.

McKeown, P. F., Walsh, S. J. and Menown, I. B. 2005. Images in cardiology: An unusual case of right ventricular dilatation. *Heart* 91(9):1147.

McSharry, C. 2003. B lymphocytes in allergic alveolitis. *Clin Exp Allergy* 33:159–62.

McSharry, C., Dye, G. M., Ismail, T., Anderson, K., Spiers, E. M. and Boyd, G. 2006. Quantifying serum antibody in bird fanciers' hypersensitivity pneumonitis. *BMC Pulm Med* 6:16–23.

Meyer, K. C., Raghu, G., Baughman, R. P., Brown, K. K., Costabel, U., du Bois, R. M., Drent, M. et al.; American Thoracic Society Committee on BAL in Interstitial Lung Disease. 2012. An official American Thoracic Society clinical practice guideline: The clinical utility of bronchoalveolar lavage cellular analysis in interstitial lung disease. *Am J Respir Crit Care Med* 185(9):1004–14.

Miyazaki, Y., Tateishi, T., Akashi, T., Ohtani, Y., Inase, N. and Yoshizawa, Y. 2008. Clinical predictors and histologic appearance of acute exacerbations in chronic hypersensitivity pneumonitis. *Chest* 134(6):1265–70.

Mönkäre, S. 1983. Influence of corticosteroid treatment on the course of farmer's lung. *Eur J Respir Dis* 64(4):283–93.

Mönkäre, S. 1984. Clinical aspects of farmer's lung: Airway reactivity, treatment and prognosis. *Eur J Respir Dis Suppl* 137:1–68.

Mönkäre, S. and Haahtela, T. 1987. Farmer's lung—A 5-year follow-up of eighty six patients. *Clin Allergy* 17:143–51.

Mooney, J. J., Elicker, B. M., Urbania, T. H., Agarwal, M. R., Ryerson, C. J., Nguyen, M. L., Woodruff, P. G. et al. 2013. Radiographic fibrosis score predicts survival in hypersensitivity pneumonitis. *Chest* 144:586–92.

Morell, F., Roger, A., Reyes, L., Cruz, M. J., Murio, C. and Muñoz, X. 2008. Bird fancier's lung: A series of 86 patients. *Medicine (Baltimore)* 87:110–30.

Morell, F., Villar, A., Montero, M. Á., Muñoz, X., Colby, T. V., Pipvath, S., Cruz, M. J. et al. 2013. Chronic hypersensitivity pneumonitis in patients diagnosed with idiopathic pulmonary fibrosis: A prospective case–cohort study. *Lancet Respir Med* 1:685–94.

Mornex, J. F., Leroux, C., Greenland, T. and Ecochard, D. 1994. From granuloma to fibrosis in interstitial lung diseases: Molecular and cellular interactions. *Eur Respir J* 7:779–85.

Morris, D. and Zamvar, V. 2014. The efficacy of video-assisted thoracoscopic surgery lung biopsies in patients with interstitial lung disease: A retrospective study of 66 patients. *J Cardiothorac Surg* 9:45.

Muñoz, X., Sánchez-Ortiz, M., Torres, F., Villar, A., Morell, F. and Cruz, M. J. 2014. Diagnostic yield of specific inhalation challenge in hypersensitivity pneumonitis. *Eur Respir J* 44(6):1658–65.

Nuutinen, J., Terho, E. O., Husman, K., Kotimaa, M., Härkönen, R. and Nousiainen, H. 1987. Protective value of powered dust respirator helmet for farmers with farmer's lung. *Eur J Respir Dis Suppl* 152:212–20.

Ohtani, Y., Saiki, S., Kitaichi, M., Usui, Y., Inase, N., Costabel, U. and Yoshizawa, Y. 2005. Chronic bird fancier's lung: Histopathological and clinical correlation. An application of the 2002 ATS/ERS consensus classification of the idiopathic interstitial pneumonias. *Thorax* 60:665–71.

Ohtsuka, Y., Munakata, M., Tanimura, K., Ukita, H., Kusaka, H., Masaki, Y., Doi, I. et al. 1995. Smoking promotes insidious and chronic farmer's lung disease, and deteriorates the clinical outcome. *Intern Med* 34(10):966–71.

Okamoto, T., Miyazaki, Y., Tomita, M., Tamaoka, M. and Inase, N. 2013. A familial history of pulmonary fibrosis in patients with chronic hypersensitivity pneumonitis. *Respiration* 85:384–90.

Oksa, P., Palo, L., Saalo, A., Jolanki, R., Mäkinen, I. and Kauppinen, T. 2012. Ammattitaudit ja ammattitautiepäilyt 2010. Työperäisten sairauksien rekisteriin kirjatut uudet tapaukset. (Occupational diseases and suspected occupational diseases 2010). New cases registered in the Register of Occupational Diseases Finnish Institute of Occupational Health. Helsinki.

Olson, A. L., Huie, T. J., Groshong, S. D., Cosgrove, G. P., Janssen, W. J., Schwarz, M. I., Brown, K. K. et al. 2008. Acute exacerbations of fibrotic hypersensitivity pneumonitis: A case series. *Chest* 134(4):844–50.

Orriols, R., Costa, R., Albanell, M., Alberti, C., Castejon, J., Monso, E., Panades, R. et al. 2006. Members of the Malaltia Ocupacional Respiratòria (MOR) Group. Reported occupational respiratory diseases in Catalonia. *Occup Environ Med* 63:255–60.

Ouchterlony, O. 1949. Antibody-antigen reactions in gels. *Acta Pathol Microbiol Scand* 26:507–15.

Patel, A. M., Ryu, J. H. and Reed, C. E. 2001. Hypersensitivity pneumonitis: Current concepts and future questions. *J Allergy Clin Immunol* 108:661–70.

Pepys, J. and Jenkins, P. A. 1965. Precipitins (F.L.H.) test in farmer's lung. *Thorax* 20:21–35.

Pepys, J. 1969. Hypersensitivity disease of the lung due to fungi and organic dust. *Monogr Allergy* 4:1–147.

Pérez-Padilla, R., Salas, J., Chapela, R., Sánchez, M., Carrillo, G., Pérez, R., Sansores, R. et al. 1993. Mortality in Mexican patients with chronic pigeon breeder's lung compared with those with usual interstitial pneumonia. *Am Rev Respir Dis* 148(1):49–53.

Provencher, S., Labreche, F. P. and De Guire, L. 1997. Physician based surveillance system for occupational respiratory diseases: The experience of PROPULSE, Quebec, Canada. *Occup Environ Med* 54:272–6.

Raulf, M., Liebers, V., Steppert, C. and Baur, X. 1994. Increased gamma/delta-positive T-cells in blood and bronchoalveolar lavage of patients with sarcoidosis and hypersensitivity pneumonitis. *Eur Respir J* 7:140–7.

Remy-Jardin, M., Remy, J., Wallaert, B. and Müller, N. L. 1993. Subacute and chronic bird breeder hypersensitivity pneumonitis: Sequential evaluation with CT and correlation with lung function tests and bronchoalveolar lavage. *Radiology* 189(1):111–8.

Richeldi, L., du Bois, R. M., Raghu, G., Azuma, A., Brown, K. K., Costabel, U., Cottin, V. et al. 2014. Efficacy and safety of nintedanib in idiopathic pulmonary fibrosis. *N Engl J Med* 370(22):2071–82.

Richerson, H. B., Bernstein, I. L., Fink, J. N., Hunninghake, G. W., Novey, H. S., Reed, C. E., Salvaggio, J. E. et al. 1989. Guidelines for the clinical evaluation of hypersensitivity pneumonitis. Report of the Subcommittee on Hypersensitivity Pneumonitis. *J Allergy Clin Immunol* 84:839–44.

Robertson, W., Robertson, A. S., Burge, C. B., Moore, V. C., Jaakkola, M. S., Dawkins, P. A., Burd, M. et al. 2007. Clinical investigation of an outbreak of alveolitis and asthma in a car engine manufacturing plant. *Thorax* 62: 981–90.

Rodrigo, M. J., Postigo, I., Wangensteen, O., Guisantes, J. A. and Martínez, J. 2010. A new application of Streptavidin ImmunoCAP for measuring IgG antibodies against non-available commercial antigens. *Clin Chim Acta* 411(21–22):1675–8.

Rose, C. S., Martyny, J. W., Newman, L. S., Milton, D. K., King, T. E. Jr., Beebe, J. L., McCammon, J. B. et al. 1998. "Lifeguard lung": Endemic granulomatous pneumonitis in an indoor swimming pool. *Am J Public Health* 88(12):1795–800.

Ryerson, C. J., Vittinghoff, E., Ley, B., Lee, J. S., Mooney, J. J., Jones, K. D., Elicker, B. M. et al. 2014. Predicting survival across chronic interstitial lung disease: The ILD-GAP model. *Chest* 145:723–8.

Rylander, R. and Schilling, R. S. F. 2011. *Diseases Caused by Organic Dusts*. Geneva: Encyclopedia of Occupational Health and Safety, International Labour Organization.

Sansores, R., Salas, J., Chapela, R., Barquin, N. and Selman, M. 1990. Clubbing in hypersensitivity pneumonitis. Its prevalence and possible prognostic role. *Arch Intern Med* 150(9):1849–51.

Schmidt, C. D., Jensen, R. L., Christensen, L. T., Crapo, R. O. and Davis, J. J. 1988. Longitudinal pulmonary function changes in pigeon breeders. *Chest* 93(2):359–63.

Schuyler, M. 1997. The diagnosis of hypersensitivity pneumonitis. *Chest* 111:534–6.

Selman, M., Pardo, A. and King, T. E. Jr. 2012. Hypersensitivity pneumonitis: Insights in diagnosis and pathobiology. *Am J Respir Crit Care Med* 186(4):314–24.

Shirai, T., Ikeda, M., Morita, S., Asada, K., Suda, T. and Chida, K. 2010. Elevated alveolar nitric oxide concentration after environmental challenge in hypersensitivity pneumonitis. *Respirology* 15(4):721–2.

Silver, S. F., Müller, N. L., Miller, R. R. and Lefcoe, M. S. 1989. Hypersensitivity pneumonitis; evaluation with CT. *Radiology* 173:441–5.

Small, J. H., Flower, C. D., Traill, Z. C. and Gleeson, F. V. 1996. Air-trapping in extrinsic allergic alveolitis on computed tomography. *Clin Radiol* 51(10):684–8.

Soda, K., Ando, M., Shimazu, K., Sakata, T., Yoshida, K. and Araki, S. 1986. Different classes of antibody activities to *Trichosporon cutaneum* antigen in summer-type hypersensitivity pneumonitis by enzyme-linked immunosorbent assay. *Am Rev Respir Dis* 133:83–7.

Solaymani-Dodaran, M., West, J., Smith, C. and Hubbard, R. 2007. Extrinsic allergic alveolitis: Incidence and mortality in the general population. *QJM* 100:233–7.

Sterclova, M., Vasakova, M., Pavlicek, J., Metlicka, M., Krasna, E. and Striz, I. 2009. Chemokine receptors in a regulation of interstitial lung fibrosis and inflammation. *Exp Lung Res* 35:514–23.

Terho, E. O., Vohlonen, I. and Husman, K. 1987. Prevalence and incidence of chronic bronchitis and farmer's lung with respect to socioeconomic factors. *Eur J Respir Dis Suppl* 152:29–36.

Thomeer, M. J., Costabe, U., Rizzato, G., Poletti, V. and Demedts, M. 2001. Comparison of registries of interstitial lung diseases in three European countries. *Eur Respir J Suppl* 32:114s–118s.

Tillie-Leblond, I., Grenouillet, F., Reboux, G., Roussel, S., Chouraki, B., Lorthois, C., Dalphin, J. C. et al. 2011. Hypersensitivity pneumonitis and metalworking fluids contaminated by mycobacteria. *Eur Respir J* 37:640–7.

Travis, W. D., Costabel, U., Hansell, D. M., Lynch, D. A., Colby, T. V., Galvin, J. R., Brown, K. K. et al. 2013. An official American Thoracic Society/European Respiratory Society statement: Update of the international multidisciplinary classification of the idiopathic interstitial pneumonias. *Am J Respir Crit Care Med* 188:733–48.

Travis, W. D., Hunninghake, G., King, T. E. Jr., Lynch, D. A., Colby, T. V., Galvin, J. R., Brown, K. K. et al. 2008. Idiopathic nonspecific interstitial pneumonia: Report of an American Thoracic Society project. *Am J Respir Crit Care Med* 177:1338–47.

Trentin, L., Marcer, G., Chilosi, M., Zambello, R., Agostini, C., Masciarelli, M., Bizzotto, R. et al. 1988. Longitudinal study of alveolitis in hypersensitivity pneumonitis patients: An immunologic evaluation. *J Allergy Clin Immunol* 82:577–85.

Vallery-Radot, P. and Giroud, P. 1928. Sporomycosc des pelleteurs de grains. *Bull Soc Med Hop Paris* 52: 1632–45.

Vourlekis, J. S., Schwarz, M. I., Cherniack, R. M., Curran-Everett, D., Cool, C. D., Tuder, R. M., King, T. E. Jr. et al. 2004. The effect of pulmonary fibrosis on survival in patients with hypersensitivity pneumonitis. *Am J Med* 116:662–8.

Vourlekis, J. S., Schwarz, M. I., Cool, C. D., Tuder, R. M., King, T. E. and Brown, K. K. 2002. Nonspecific interstitial pneumonitis as the sole histologic expression of hypersensitivity pneumonitis. *Am J Med* 112:490–3.

Walsh, S. L., Sverzellati, N., Devaraj, A., Wells, A. U. and Hansell, D. M. 2012. Chronic hypersensitivity pneumonitis: High resolution computed tomography patterns and pulmonary function indices as prognostic determinants. *Eur Radiol* 22:1672–9.

Webb, W. R. 2006. Thin-section CT of the secondary pulmonary lobule: Anatomy and the image—The 2004 Fleischner lecture. *Radiology* 239:322–38.

Xaubet, A., Ancochea, J., Morell, F., Rodriguez-Arias, J. M., Villena, V., Blanquer, R., Montero, C. et al. 2004. Spanish Group on Interstitial Lung Diseases (SEPAR). Report on the incidence of interstitial lung diseases in Spain. *Sarcoidosis Vasc Diffuse Lung Dis* 21(1): 64–70.

Xu, J. F., Shen, L., Zhang, Y., Zhang, P., Qu, J. M. and Li, H. P. 2014. Lung biopsy-proved hypersensitivity pneumonitis without known offending antigen: Characteristics and follow-up. *Clin Respir J* 8(3):297–304.

Yamasaki, H., Ando, M., Brazer, W., Center, D. M. and Cruikshank, W. W. 1999. Polarized type 1 cytokine profile in bronchoalveolar lavage T cells of patients with hypersensitivity pneumonitis. *J Immunol* 163(6): 3516–23.

Yoshida, K., Suga, M., Nishiura, Y., Arima, K., Yoneda, R., Tamura, M. and Ando, M. 1995. Occupational hypersensitivity pneumonitis in Japan: Data on a nationwide epidemiological study. *Occup Environ Med* 52(9): 570–74.

Yoshizawa, Y., Ohtani, Y., Hayakawa, H., Sato, A., Suga, M. and Ando, M. 1999. Chronic hypersensitivity pneumonitis in Japan: A nationwide epidemiologic survey. *J Allergy Clin Immunol* 103(2 Pt 1):315–20.

Zacharisen, M. and Schoenwetter, W. 2005. Fatal hypersensitivity pneumonitis. *Ann Allergy Asthma Immunol* 95(5):484–87.

Zacharisen, M. C., Kadambi, A. R., Schlueter, D. P., Kurup, V. P., Shack, J. B., Fox, J. L., Anderson, H. A. et al. 1998. The spectrum of respiratory disease associated with exposure to metal working fluids. *J Occup Environ Med* 40:640–47.

BOX 24.3 BERYLLIUM HEALTH EFFECTS

- Two forms of beryllium lung disease are recognised: acute and chronic.
- Acute beryllium disease is now largely of historical interest, being only encountered as a result of high accidental exposure, usually above 25 µg/m^3. It represents a chemical injury, the pathology being that of diffuse alveolar damage.
- Chronic beryllium disease is characterized by granulomatous inflammation in the lung and the demonstration of beryllium sensitization in blood or lung cells. It can develop from within a few months to up to 30 years after the first exposure. Beryllium sensitization is a cell-mediated immune response to beryllium and precedes chronic beryllium disease.
- Skin effects: delayed wound healing, granulomatous nodules under the skin and allergic rash, usually to beryllium salts.
- Beryllium has been classified as a probable pulmonary carcinogen (United States Department of Labor, 1999).

et al., 2010), sensitization has been reported in workers with bystander exposure, including workers' spouses and residents of communities surrounding beryllium operations (Maier et al., 2008). The prevalence of BeS among exposed workers ranges from <1% in aluminium smelters with very low levels of exposure (Taiwo et al., 2008) to 20% in workers in highly exposed processes over time (Schuler et al., 2008).

Chronic Beryllium Disease

The proportion of workers with BeS who are subsequently diagnosed with CBD ranges from 9% to 100% in cross-sectional studies (Kreiss et al., 1989, 1993, 1996, 1997; Stange et al., 1996; Deubner et al., 2001; Henneberger et al., 2001; Kelleher et al., 2001; Newman et al., 2001; Sackett et al., 2004; Welch et al., 2004; Rosenman et al., 2005; Schuler et al., 2005). CBD develops from 10 to 20 years after the first exposure, but has been diagnosed within months of the first exposure (Henneberger et al., 2001) and up to 40 years after the last exposure (Eisenbud and Lisson, 1983). Lower levels of workplace exposure have been associated with lower risk of CBD (Kelleher et al., 2001; Van Dyke et al., 2011).

BOX 24.4 PATHOGENESIS OF CHRONIC BERYLLIUM DISEASE (FIGURE 24.1)

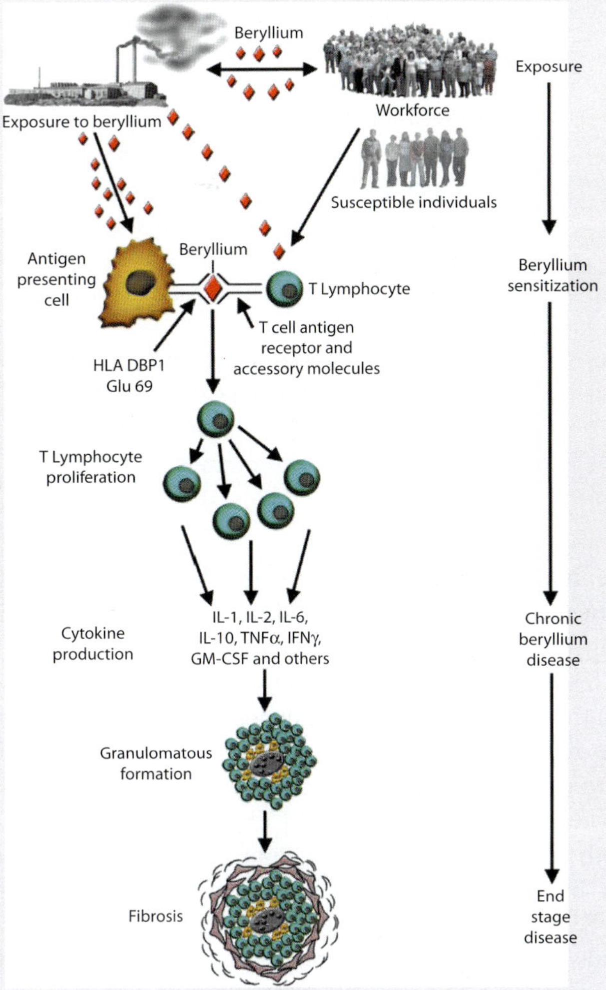

FIGURE 24.1 Diagram of the pathogenesis of chronic beryllium disease. (Adapted from Maier, L. et al. 2006. *Environmental and Occupational Medicine*, Philadelphia: Lippincott-Raven Publishers, pp. 1021–1038.)

The current exposure limits in the EU, USA and Japan, as detailed in the 'Prevention' section, are not sufficient to prevent CBD.

Genetic and Exposure Interactions

Increased frequencies of E69 are found in CBD (61%–97%) and BeS (39%–90%) cases compared with controls (30%–47%) (Richeldi et al., 1997; Wang et al., 1999, 2001; Saltini et al., 2001; Rossman et al., 2002; Maier et al., 2003; McCanlies et al., 2004; Gaede et al., 2005) (Box 24.5). While E69 functions in the development of BeS, other host and environmental factors likely impact the progression from BeS to CBD. Studies investigating

BOX 24.5 GENETIC RISK FACTORS

- *HLADPB1* Glu69 is a susceptibility marker for beryllium sensitization and chronic beryllium disease.
- Some variants of the Glu69 marker carry more risk than others.
- There is greater risk of chronic beryllium disease (CBD) and beryllium sensitization in E69-negative subjects with at least one E71 allele.
- Developing CBD requires a gene and environment interaction.
- Even seemingly trivial beryllium exposure can be sufficient to cause CBD in these genetically susceptible individuals (Van Dyke et al., 2011; Rosenman et al., 2011).

the interaction between E69 and beryllium exposure showed independent and additive effects of E69 carriage and exposure in the development of BeS and CBD (Richeldi et al., 1997; Dyke et al., 2011). A large case–control study of beryllium-exposed workers evaluated the relationship between quantitative beryllium exposure estimates in combination with E69 genotype (Van Dyke et al., 2011). Increased exposure was associated with CBD compared with control subjects; however, no exposure–response relationship was apparent for BeS, even with the inclusion of genetic risk factors. The odds of BeS and CBD were greater among carriers of a specific E69 (the non-*02 E69 alleles) and among E69 homozygotes after adjusting for beryllium exposure. Furthermore, no significant gene–environment interaction was found, and instead the findings supported the notion that both exposure and E69 contributed independently to CBD risk, with increasing higher lifetime-weighted average and cumulative exposures associated with increased CBD risk. The finding of an exposure–response relationship for CBD has implications for standard setting in the workplace.

Acute Beryllium Disease

Acute beryllium disease, a chemical pneumonitis, occurs shortly after exposure to very high levels of beryllium, typically of 25–100 $\mu g/m^3$. Historically, workers involved in the primary extraction of beryllium were exposed to very high levels of beryllium salts and to the metal, ceramic and alloy products (Lieben and Metzner, 1959), as were workers in secondary industries, such as the fluorescent lamp and light bulb industry (Hasan and Kazemi, 1974), with death observed in approximately 10% of cases (Hardy, 1965). Following the 1949 adoption of the 2 $\mu g/m^3$ 8-hour time-weighted average (TWA) permissible exposure limit and peak short-term limit of 25 $\mu g/m^3$ in the USA, cases of acute beryllium disease were markedly reduced (Eisenbud and Lisson, 1983), although occasional cases continue to be reported (Cummings et al., 2009). In 1984, an acute case was reported in a dental technician in the USA (Rom et al., 1984), and in 2004, nine cases of acute disease related to liquid metal exposures were reported in South Korea (Kim et al., 2004). Additional acute manifestations of beryllium exposure in the extraction industries included conjunctivitis, dermatitis, pharyngitis and largyngotracheobronchitis (Denardi et al., 1953).

Lung Cancer

Beryllium is recognized by the International Association for Research on Cancer as carcinogenic to humans (Group 1), but fortunately lung cancer is rare at most current-day, low-level exposures (Sanderson et al., 2001). Therefore, it will not be a focus of this chapter.

Clinical Manifestations, Evaluation and Diagnosis of BeS and CBD

BeS is an asymptomatic, cell-mediated immune response without pulmonary pathology, identified primarily through in vitro testing using the BeLPT (Jones-Williams and Williams, 1983; Newman, 1996). Usually, two abnormal blood tests are needed in order to confirm BeS (Balmes et al., 2014). Other tests, including enzyme-linked immunosorbent spot (ELISPOT) (Martin et al., 2011) or in vivo patch testing (Curtis, 1951), may also detect sensitization. BeS precedes CBD, a pathological condition that classically presents with dry cough, progressive dyspnoea on exertion, fatigue and night sweats. Anorexia and weight loss were reported in the historic cohorts (Hardy and Tabershaw, 1946), but are uncommon today. Onset of CBD symptoms is typically slow and insidious with a variable clinical course, ranging from asymptomatic patients (diagnosed based on medical surveillance with the BeLPT) to those with severe respiratory impairment and hypoxaemia (Cullen et al., 1986; Mroz et al., 2009).

Pulmonary physiology is normal in BeS, as these individuals, by definition, have no evidence of granulomatous inflammation on lung biopsy. In early CBD, lung function may also be normal. As disease worsens, restrictive, obstructive and/or gas exchange abnormalities can develop. In more recent cohorts identified through medical surveillance, the most common physiological abnormalities are mild airflow limitation (Pappas and

Newman, 1993) and slow longitudinal decline in diffusing capacity for carbon monoxide (DLCO) (Cullen et al., 1986; Mroz et al., 2009). A restrictive pattern is usually seen in advanced disease with fibrosis. Cardiopulmonary exercise testing can reveal abnormalities in early disease before alteration in static physiology, including less than expected falls in physiological dead space (higher ratio of dead space to tidal volume [VD/VT] at maximal exercise), decline in arterial partial pressure of oxygen and widening of the alveolar–arterial gradient (Pappas and Newman, 1993; Lundgren et al., 2001).

The imaging manifestations of beryllium exposure include an acute chemical pneumonitis (acute beryllium disease), acute tracheobronchitis and CBD (Box 24.6). Modern occupational safeguards have almost completely eliminated the occurrence of the acute chemical pneumonitis and tracheobronchitis associated with high-exposure conditions. Although CBD is still classified as a pneumoconiosis because it is the consequence of the inhalation of an inorganic dust, it is strictly considered a granulomatous response, and exposure does not always correlate with the severity of disease on imaging or with physiological abnormalities (Aronchick et al., 1987; Newman et al., 1994). The radiographic features of CBD are highly variable (Harris et al., 1993). In general, radiographic abnormalities are seen after the development of symptoms and physiologic impairment in CBD (Newman et al., 1994). In a study of 28 patients with pathologically proven CBD, just over 50% had an abnormal chest radiograph (Newman et al., 1994). While the spectrum of findings in CBD are similar to those of sarcoidosis (Newman et al., 1994), CBD is not usually identified incidentally on chest imaging, as is often the case in sarcoidosis. The radiographic abnormalities typically consist of either rounded nodules or small, irregular opacities with a mid to upper zone predominance (Aronchick et al., 1987). Mediastinal and hilar lymphadenopathy may be demonstrated, although almost invariably in the presence of parenchymal disease (Newman et al., 1994).

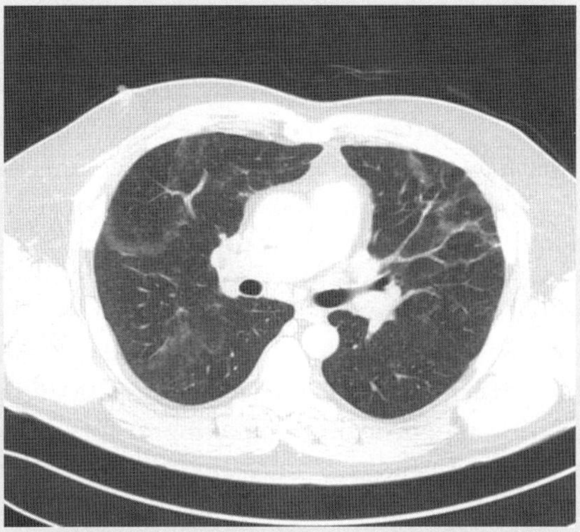

FIGURE 24.2 Computed tomography image from a recent clinically identified chronic beryllium disease case demonstrating diffuse ground-glass abnormality, poorly defined centrilobular nodules, mild interlobular septal thickening, moderate mosaic attenuation and mildly enlarged mediastinal and hilar lymph nodes.

BOX 24.6 RADIOGRAPHIC IMAGING IN CHRONIC BERYLLIUM DISEASE

- Acute interstitial pneumonitis, which is radiographically indistinguishable from other forms of chemical pneumonitis, is now rare due to exposure controls in industry.
- The imaging features of chronic beryllium disease (CBD) can be indistinguishable from pulmonary sarcoidosis.
- Mediastinal and hilar lymphadenopathy is seen almost invariably in the presence of parenchymal disease.
- Chest radiograph is often normal in earlier stages of disease. Features of CBD include upper zone small (2–5 mm), rounded nodules or irregular densities with or without mediastinal and hilar lymphadenopathy.
- HRCT may be normal in the earlier stages of disease. Features of CBD include smooth or nodular thickening of interlobular septa, small 2–5-mm nodules and/or ground-glass density with a peri-bronchovascular distribution, bronchial wall thickening and mediastinal or hilar lymphadenopathy, which may be calcified.
- Advanced disease is becoming increasingly uncommon. Computed tomography features include fibrosis comprising a reticular pattern, cysts, honeycombing, conglomerate masses (which may be calcified), architectural distortion including traction bronchiectasis and central pulmonary artery enlargement, reflecting supervening pulmonary arterial hypertension (Lynch, 2006) (Figure 24.2).

As with other diffuse interstitial lung diseases, the chest radiograph is less sensitive and specific than computed tomography (CT) for the diagnosis of CBD (Harris et al., 1993; Newman et al., 1994). High resolution CT scan (HRCT) is often normal in the earlier stages of disease (Sharma et al., 2010). Common CT features include small, soft tissue density nodules (2–5-mm diameter) with a mid- to upper-lung zone predominance bilaterally in a sub-pleural and peri-bronchovascular distribution, diffuse ground-glass opacification, smooth or nodular interlobular septal thickening and bronchial wall thickening (Daniloff et al., 1997; Naccache et al., 2003; Sharma et al., 2010), independent of smoking history (Daniloff et al., 1997). A study on inter-observer agreement for individual CT features in CBD found highest agreement for interlobular septal thickening, nodules and extent of abnormal lung, and lowest agreement for bronchial wall thickening (Daniloff et al., 1997). Mediastinal and hilar lymphadenopathy is less frequent in CBD than in sarcoidosis, being reported in only 25%–30% of patients on CT (Newman et al., 1994) and may not distort the mediastinal contour; that is, may not be visible on chest radiograph (Harris et al., 1993). The lymph nodes may be calcified. Advanced disease is becoming less common as exposures decrease. Radiographic features of advanced disease include coarse linear fibrosis and architectural distortion, which is typically most pronounced in the mid to upper zones, and conglomerate masses, bullae, cysts, coexistent areas of emphysema and spontaneous pneumothoraces may occur (Harris et al., 1993; Sharma et al., 2010). Diffuse interstitial fibrosis can also be seen. Enlargement of the central pulmonary arteries may be present, reflecting pulmonary hypertension.

Some individuals can remain asymptomatic and clinically stable with normal radiographic imaging for years, although most experience gradual worsening, with increasing respiratory symptoms and physiological decline appearing approximately 15 years from first exposure (Mroz et al., 2009). Some patients experience significant physiological impairment and radiographic progression of disease, typically those who have had the highest exposure (Sood et al., 2004). Such cases are usually identified clinically, typically from workplaces that have not been monitored and industries in which the potential for beryllium exposure was not recognized appropriately. Physiological decline can be slowed by treatment (Sood et al., 2004; Marchand-Adam et al., 2008). While it is not known whether removal from exposure will improve disease outcome, since beryllium remains in the lungs for years after exposure, it is considered medically prudent to recommend minimizing future beryllium exposure for workers with BeS and CBD.

Unlike sarcoidosis, skin involvement and extrapulmonary manifestations are not typically present in recently exposed cohorts. Skin manifestations include contact dermatitis, beryllium ulcers and dermal granulomas from skin contact with beryllium. Dermatitis was reported in workers who were exposed to beryllium salts (DeNardi et al., 1949). Chronic, non-healing ulcers and wart-like nodular granulomatous skin lesions can occur following implantation of beryllium into an abrasion or other cut in the skin; excision is required for resolution of ulcers (Van Ordstrand et al., 1950) and nodular skin lesions, although the latter may be treated with topical corticosteroids (Denardi et al., 1953). Skin patch testing has been used in order to identify the beryllium-specific immune response in individuals with normal BeLPT blood tests; however, there is a risk of inducing sensitization or exacerbating symptoms in patients who are currently exposed (Bobka et al., 1997).

It is recommended that individuals with confirmed BeS undergo a diagnostic evaluation for CBD that includes full pulmonary function tests (PFTs) (including DLCO), chest radiography and, if deemed appropriate, a bronchoscopy with bronchoalveolar lavage (BAL) and trans-bronchial biopsies. Currently, definitive diagnosis of CBD is based on: (1) evidence of BeS, usually based on a blood or BAL BeLPT and granulomatous inflammation by biopsy; or (2) abnormal BAL BeLPT and lymphocytosis without granulomatous inflammation by biopsy. The pathognomonic histopathologic lesion of CBD is the epithelioid granuloma, which is indistinguishable from the granulomas of sarcoidosis (Freiman, 1959) (Box 24.7). If a bronchoscopy cannot be obtained for medical reasons or otherwise, the diagnosis of CBD can also be made on a medically probable basis in a patient with BeS, considering the patient's exposure history, clinical course, symptoms, physiological findings and radiographic imaging (Box 24.8).

BOX 24.7 PATHOLOGICAL CHANGES

- The classic histopathological findings in chronic beryllium disease (CBD) are non-necrotizing granulomas, often including multinucleated Langerhans-type giant cells.
- These pulmonary granulomas often occur in a lymphatic/peri-bronchiolar/peri-vascular distribution.
- They are indistinguishable from those seen in sarcoidosis.
- The granulomas may be seen in lymph nodes, liver and skin, but CBD does not

typically involve the uveal tract or central nervous system (CNS).

- They are not specific, but may also be seen consequent to sensitization to less common metals such as zirconium, titanium and aluminium.
- The granulomas may range from rare and paucicellular, sometimes being indistinguishable from the findings in hypersensitivity pneumonitis, to confluent and then to fibrotic.
- Variably prominent mononuclear cell inflammation may be seen.
- Asteroid bodies and Schaumann bodies may also be seen, but are not specific for CBD.
- Figures 24.3 and 24.4 show a variety of findings that may be found in CBD.
- In contrast, acute beryllium disease is rarely observed, but may reveal diffuse alveolar damage.
- Beryllium (and/or other metals) can sometimes be detected in the granulomas when using micro-analytical methods such as secondary ion mass spectrometry or electron microscopic analytic methods, but these analyses are not required for diagnosis. Such analyses are useful for research and may, however, reveal additional potential causes of granulomatous disease when the beryllium lymphocyte proliferation test is negative or inconclusive (Freiman and Hardy, 1970; Newman, 1998; Sawter et al., 2005).

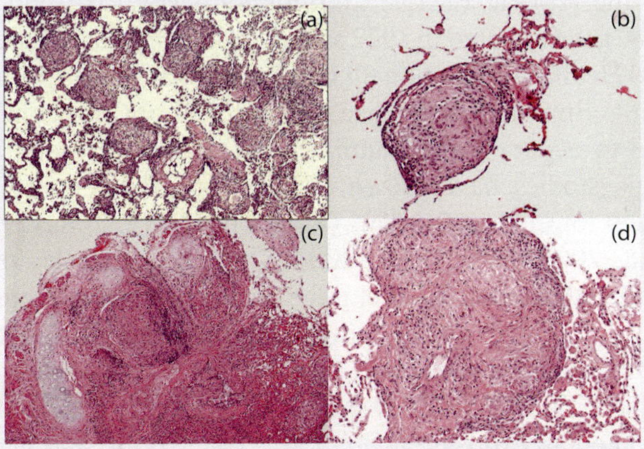

FIGURE 24.3 (a) Peri-bronchiolar distribution of non-necrotizing granulomas. (b) Isolated, interstitial, well-formed granuloma. (c) Granulomas in the bronchial wall. (d) Confluent granulomas.

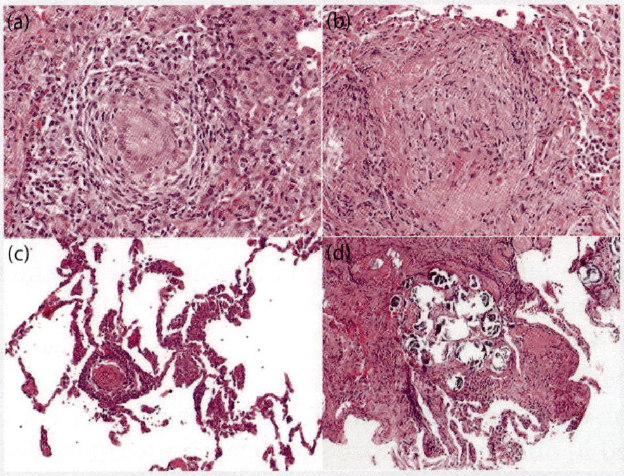

FIGURE 24.4 (a) Granuloma with prominent mononuclear infiltrates. (b) Granuloma with fibrosis. (c) Focal perivascular and interstitial mononuclear infiltration without granuloma. (d) Granulomas with many calcified bodies (Schaumann bodies).

BOX 24.8 DIFFERENTIAL DIAGNOSIS

- The differential diagnosis of chronic beryllium disease (CBD) includes pulmonary sarcoidosis, as well as other granulomatous diseases, such as hypersensitivity pneumonitis, and infections granulomatous diseases, including fungal and mycobacterial infections. From a clinical, radiological and pathological standpoint, CBD and sarcoidosis are clinically indistinguishable, hence the importance of the beryllium lymphocyte proliferation test (BeLPT).
- Beryllium disease rarely causes significant hilar lymphadenopathy in the absence of parenchymal abnormalities, unlike sarcoidosis.
- Erythema nodosum and uveitis, which are common manifestations of sarcoidosis, are not seen in CBD.
- Some patients initially diagnosed as having sarcoidosis actually have had CBD.
- Any patient thought to have sarcoidosis who has worked in any beryllium-using industries should be offered a BeLPT (Mayer et al., 2014).

Early disease may be treated with inhaled corticosteroids, along with a short-acting bronchodilator if there is mild obstructive lung disease and/or airway symptoms. Indications for systemic immunosuppressive therapy include more significant physiological impairment, particularly evidence of progressive decline, hypoxaemia, severe associated symptoms and/or evidence of secondary pulmonary hypertension or cor pulmonale. Corticosteroids are usually the first-line therapy started at 40 mg prednisone equivalent every other day or daily for 6–12 weeks following lung function response, and tapering to as low a dose as possible in order to maintain lung function. Steroid-sparing therapy is considered in order to minimize significant corticosteroid side effects. Therapy is usually continued lifelong, because disease relapses were well described with cessation of immunosuppression (Sood et al., 2004; Marchand-Adam et al., 2008). Long-term monitoring and treatment of any consequential problems is indicated, including the prevention of infections with immunization and the use of oxygen for hypoxaemia and pulmonary hypertension. Lung transplantation has been used to treat severe end-stage CBD with unknown long-term outcomes.

Biomarkers of Disease and Workplace Screening

The BeLPT, which detects a beryllium-specific, cell-mediated immune response, is used in beryllium workplace medical screening and surveillance (Box 24.9). This test is performed by culturing cells from blood or lung with beryllium salts at multiple concentrations and times. The test is interpreted as abnormal if two or more of the beryllium culture conditions show a positive response, and borderline if only one condition is elevated. Recent studies demonstrate that the positive predictive values (PPVs) of two abnormal tests for diagnosing BeS range from 96.8% to 99.7% (Stange et al., 2004; Middleton et al., 2006). Other combinations of an abnormal and borderline test, as well as three borderline tests, provide similar PPVs for BeS (Middleton et al., 2011).

The IFN-γ ELISPOT has also been studied in the diagnosis of BeS and CBD (Martin et al., 2011). The test has quick turnaround, does not utilize radioactivity and yields sensitivities and specificities of 85%–100% for CBD, with positive and negative predictive values of 81%–100%. The ELISPOT test was sensitive for detecting BeS and CBD, as all CBD individuals identified at the time of clinical evaluation had significantly increased production of IFN-γ. The peripheral blood ELISPOT may identify additional workers with BeS and help in decisions regarding who should undergo biopsy in order to confirm CBD. While the ELISPOT is not yet commercially available, in the future it may provide an alternative test option, especially in areas where the BeLPT is not feasible.

BOX 24.9 LABORATORY TESTING

As of 2014, the following laboratories in the United States provided a beryllium lymphocyte proliferation test:

1. ORISE Beryllium Testing Laboratory, Oak Ridge, TN, USA (phone: +1 865 576 3115; occ.health@orise.orau.gov)
2. Cleveland Clinic Foundation, Department of Clinical Pathology, Cleveland, OH, USA (phone: +1 216 444 2200 or +1 800 223 2273, ext. 48844 or 5576)
3. National Jewish Health, Advanced Diagnostics Laboratories, Denver, CO, USA (phone: +1 303 398 1722; deohs@njhealth.org)

There are limited sites providing the beryllium lymphocyte proliferation test outside of the USA. This includes in UK Department of Occupational and Environmental Medicine, Royal Brompton Hospital, 1b, Manresa Road, London SW3 6LR.

Prevention

In an effort to prevent acute beryllium disease and CBD in the US workplace, an occupational exposure limit (OEL) of 2 μg/m^3 as a daily-weighted average was set in 1949 by the Atomic Energy Commission (AEC) (Eisenbud, 1982) and adopted in 1972 as the US Occupational Safety and Health Association (OSHA) standard. This exposure limit eliminated acute disease, but cases of CBD continued to occur. While multiple workplace and epidemiologic studies have shown disease risk from exposures much lower than 2 μg/m^3 (Kreiss et al., 1996; Kelleher et al., 2001; Sackett et al., 2004; Schuler et al., 2005), this outdated standard has yet to be changed. A more protective and comprehensive OSHA beryllium standard is currently under development (United States Department of Labor, 2015). The US Department of Energy (DOE) has adopted an exposure action level of 0.2 μg/m^3 and mandated a Chronic Beryllium Disease Prevention Program, which includes medical surveillance with the BeLPT (United States Department of Energy, 1999). In 2009, the American Conference of Governmental Industrial Hygienists (ACGIH) recommended an exposure level of

0.05 μg/m^3 as an 8-hour TWA (ACGIH, 2009) for inhalable particles. This level was recently accepted by the Canadian Province of British Columbia (Decision on the New and Revised Occupational Exposure Limits for 2012 and Others, 2015). The Canadian Province of Quebec has adopted a limit of 0.15 μg/m^3 as an 8-hour TWA (CAREX Canada, 2014), while the United Kingdom and other European countries still use the 2.0 μg/m^3 standard. Germany is considering a new standard. The OEL in Japan is 2.0 μg/m^3 (Cherrie et al., 2011), while China's 8-hour TWA is 0.5 μg/m^3 (Ministry of Health, 2007).

Medical surveillance using the BeLPT and industrial hygiene measurements is effective for identifying sentinel cases of BeS and high-risk jobs or processes (Newman et al., 2001; Sackett et al., 2004; Stange et al., 2004; Taiwo et al., 2008). With regular surveillance, employers can make targeted changes in the workplace in order to protect workers from developing BeS and CBD while detecting BeS early and referring workers for medical testing. Serial medical surveillance has proved efficacious in identifying cases of BeS and CBD (Newman et al., 2001; Stange et al., 2004; Balmes et al., 2014). In addition to BeLPT testing, exposure reduction in the workplace should be undertaken in order to prevent BeS and CBD, and should include substitution of less hazardous materials when possible, clear material labelling, respiratory protection, skin protection and education regarding the safe handling of beryllium, as well as its health effects. Several reports on the efficacy of a comprehensive programme to prevent BeS and CBD in a beryllium manufacturing facility have been published (Cummings et al., 2007; Thomas et al., 2009, 2013; Bailey et al., 2010). The combination of increased respiratory and dermal protection, enclosure and improved ventilation of high-risk processes, dust migration control, improved housekeeping and worker and management education lower the rates of BeS and CBD. Targeted workplace training covering beryllium health effects, exposure recognition, exposure control and medical surveillance proved effective (Mayer et al., 2013) in educating workers about the risks of beryllium exposure, as approximately half of the participants changed procedures and work practices in response to the educational materials.

Regular medical follow-up for individuals identified as having BeS and CBD may prevent more severe disease. Studies have shown that soon after the development of CBD, changes in physiology are detected (Newman et al., 2005; Mroz et al., 2009). Treatment with corticosteroids was shown to be more effective in individuals who were treated before the development of lung fibrosis (Sood et al., 2004; Marchand-Adam et al., 2008).

OTHER METAL-INDUCED GRANULOMATOUS LUNG DISEASES

Cobalt–Hard Substance Lung Disease

Cobalt sintered or cemented together with tungsten carbide produces an extremely hard metal that can cause a spectrum of lung diseases, collectively termed hard metal lung disease. Asthma is the most common disease resulting from cobalt exposure, as cobalt is a sensitizer causing allergic contact dermatitis; asthma resulting from cobalt will not be further discussed in this chapter, as the focus is on the ILDs. ILD with giant cell interstitial pneumonitis (GIP) results from cobalt hard metal, and non-caseating granulomas have been reported. It is clear that cobalt exposure is critical to the development of this interstitial lung disease (Coates and Watson, 1971; Cugell et al., 1990; Nemery et al., 2001), as similar disease is noted from exposure to dust from cobalt–diamond polishing (Gheysens et al., 1985), and thus the term cobalt–hard substance lung disease (C–HSLD) is used. GIP has also been reported with cobalt alone.

While cobalt does not usually cause a granulomatous lung disease that could be confused with CBD, there are numerous similarities. As noted above, cobalt acts as a sensitizer. In addition, there is no classic exposure–response relationship, and E69 was associated with increased risk of C–HSLD in one study (Potolicchio et al., 1997). The lung disease can present acutely, subacutely or insidiously over time. Acute manifestations similar to those noted with hypersensitivity pneumonitis may be seen. Marked improvement with removal from exposure in early disease and recurrence of symptoms with return to work suggest immune mediation. More commonly, this ILD presents with subacute or chronic symptoms, without an exposure relationship noted. Similar to CBD, the physiologic and radiographic manifestations are variable, and definitive diagnosis is based on diagnostic bronchoscopy and/or biopsy.

The classic pathology is GIP, characterized by 'cannibalistic' multi-nucleated giant cells in the air spaces but not in the interstitium with a centrilobular location; the giant cells appear to be engulfing other cells such as macrophages and neutrophils. These cannibalistic cells may or may not be found on BAL, and there is no other consistent BAL pattern or CD4 to CD8 pattern. Other broader pathological features include more typical giant cells, lymphoplasmacytic infiltration of the interstitium, usual interstitial pneumonia (UIP), obliterative bronchiolitis and occasionally features of desquamative interstitial pneumonia (DIP) (Naqvi et al., 2008). While GIP defined by these broader features has also been described in seemingly unexposed patients, including housewives (Reddy et al., 1970; Sokolowski et al., 1972) and a retired non-industrial office sweeper (Menon et al., 2006), none of these cases had cannibalistic multinucleated giant cells. The addition of mineralogic analysis can reveal cobalt in the lung tissue of some GIP cases without an identified history of exposure (Lee et al., 1998). Although the American Thoracic Society (ATS)/ European Respiratory Society (ERS) revised statement removed GIP as an idiopathic pneumonia (ATS/ERS, 2002), in a recent case series, two out of 19 individuals with surgical lung biopsies demonstrated features of GIP, yet had no exposure history or retained cobalt or tungsten detected in lung tissue (Moriyama et al., 2007). These cases raise questions as to whether GIP is completely synonymous with C–HSLD (Blanc, 2007) and whether some cases of GIP might actually be idiopathic (Moriyama et al., 2007).

Radiographic features are similarly variable, including ground-glass opacities, non-specific interstitial pneumonia, a UIP pattern and cystic spaces somewhat resembling sarcoidosis (Gotway et al., 2002). Removal from exposure in early disease can result in marked improvement or remission (Nemery et al., 2001), although as disease progresses, fibrosis can develop, which is not reversible with removal from exposure. The mainstay of treatment is immunosuppressive therapy, which has resulted in clinical and radiographic improvement (Dunlop et al., 2005).

Aluminium

Aluminium has been known to cause pulmonary interstitial fibrosis, DIP and pulmonary alveolar proteinosis (Mitchell et al., 1961; Herbert et al., 1982; Miller et al., 1984; De Vuyst et al., 1986; Jederlinic et al., 1990; Kongerud and Samuelsen, 1991). In addition, there have been case reports of granulomatous lung disease attributable to aluminium. A worker exposed to aluminium powder in the aircraft industry developed non-caseating granulomas in the lung, and electron microscopy confirmed the presence of aluminium (Chen et al., 1978). Another case of granulomatous lung disease along with T-helper lymphocyte alveolitis developed in a chemist after working with aluminium powders (De Vuyst et al., 1987). Aluminium particles were identified in the granulomasm and peripheral blood cells showed abnormal lymphocyte proliferation similar to the BeLPT when challenged with aluminium salts. In 2007, Cai and colleagues reported a case of pulmonary granulomatosis in a patient who had worked in a metal reclamation facility for 15 years and was exposed to aluminium dust as well as iron, copper, zinc and nickel (Cai et al., 2007). As in the previous cases, aluminium was identified within the granulomas using scanning electron microscopy. The patient was treated with oral corticosteroids and improved. However, beryllium exposure must be excluded, as indicated in a report by Taiwo et al. of granulomatous lung disease among workers in nine aluminium smelters (Taiwo et al., 2010). The granulomatous disease was attributed to beryllium, which is a natural contaminant of bauxite, as beryllium exposures were confirmed and the workers had evidence of beryllium-specific cell-mediated immunity based on the BeLPT.

Titanium

Titanium can cause a granulomatous reaction in both the skin and the lungs. A case of granulomatous lung disease attributed to titanium was reported in a patient who had been exposed to a mix of metal dusts as a furnace feeder for an aluminium smelting company (Redline et al., 1986). In order to determine the cause of the granulomatous reaction, lymphocyte proliferation testing was performed, and while the patient's lymphocytes were challenged in vitro with metal salts—aluminium sulphate, titanium chloride, beryllium sulphate and nickel sulphate—the patient only responded to titanium chloride, on two separate occasions. Similarly, a systemic granulomatous reaction was reported in a patient with frictional wear from a titanium-containing hip prosthesis (Peoc'h et al., 1996). Symptoms resolved after removal of the replacement and treatment with corticosteroids.

Zirconium

Zirconium alloys are used in the nuclear and aerospace industries and are used as powders for polishing, foundry work and in ceramics. Zirconium is a skin sensitizer and can cause granulomatous skin disease (Rubin et al., 1956). Skin granulomas have developed after the use of deodorants containing zirconium salts (Shelley and Hauley, 1958). There have been reports of granulomatous pulmonary hypersensitivity reactions (Kotter and Zieger, 1992; Romeo et al., 1994), as well as allergic alveolitis granulomatous interstitial pneumonia in a ceramic tile glazer exposed to zirconium silicates (Liippo et al., 1993). Multisystem involvement similar to sarcoidosis has been reported in a worker exposed to grinding particles and welding fumes in the nuclear industry. The patient worked with an alloy containing tin, chromium and zirconium, and scanning electron microscopy confirmed zirconium particles within the granulomas, while beryllium could not be found (Werfel et al., 1998).

The development of pulmonary fibrosis attributable to zirconium has also been described (Bartter et al., 1991).

Copper Sulphate (Bordeaux Mixture)

Bordeaux mixture, a 1%–2.5% copper sulphate solution neutralized with hydrated lime and used to prevent mildew, was associated with lung disease among Portuguese vineyard workers (Cortez and Marques, 1969). The disease occurred in workers after years to decades of spraying. While removal from exposure improved the conditions of the workers with the acute form (Villar, 1974), onset of the other forms often occurred years after last exposure, and progression was noted to be triggered by inter-current infection. While this exposure is worth remembering, few if any additional cases have been reported since the 1970s. In contrast, a high incidence of lung cancer has been seen in vineyard sprayers (Villar, 1974; Santic et al., 2005), although the actual cause may be other exposures, such as arsenic.

WTC SARCOIDOSIS/SARCOID-LIKE GRANULOMATOUS LUNG DISEASE

While airways disease has been the most common sequelae of the WTC disaster, excess incidence of sarcoid-like lung disease has been reported in three populations: New York Fire Department Rescue Workers (FDNY; Izbicki et al., 2007), the WTC Medical Monitoring and Treatment Program (MMTP) for rescue and recovery workers (Crowley et al., 2010) and the WTC Health Registry, a voluntary cohort composed of rescue and recovery workers, volunteers, local residents and exposed children and school workers (Jordan et al., 2011). The FDNY and Registry cases were verified by pathological findings of non-caseating granulomas on biopsy, without evidence of foreign body reaction, malignancy or fungal or mycobacterial infection on culture. Thirty-five percent of the FDNY cases were identified on chest radiography performed as part of medical surveillance, while the remainder were detected during diagnostic evaluation for respiratory symptoms. Among the MMTP responders, the diagnosis was confirmed by non-caseating epithelioid granulomas or a positive Kveim test and consistent radiographic imaging. All cases were diagnosed after 9/11.

While the prevalence of sarcoidosis has been estimated to be approximately 15 per 100,000 in the United States (ATS/ERS/WASOG, 1999), the incidence of 54 per 100,000 that occurred in MMTP participants between 11 September 2003, and 11 September 2004, was notably higher. Similarly, during the first year after 9/11, the incidence rate of sarcoidosis among the FDNY was 86 per 100,000, while the average rate during the subsequent 4 years was 22 per 100,000. Pulmonary involvement was present in all FDNY and MMTP cases and all but two of the Registry cases, and the majority were symptomatic. Thirty-five percent of FDNY cases had Scadding stage 1 disease and the remaining 65% had Scadding stage 2 findings. There was a wider distribution of radiographic findings in the MMTP cases. The extra-thoracic manifestations were variable and present in 23% of FDNY cases (Izbicki et al., 2007). The extra-thoracic involvement and extent of pulmonary involvement based on Scadding staging were greater than those noted in the original FDNY sarcoidosis cases before 11 September 2001. The extra-thoracic manifestations in the MMTP cases included lymph node, skin, bone/joint/muscle and cardiac manifestations. Among the Registry cases, 44% had extra-thoracic manifestations.

The Registry study included a nested case–control study, in which work associated with the debris pile was associated with a significantly increased risk of sarcoidosis. The dust from the pile is a highly complex mixture, consisting of alkaline fragments of gypsum, glass, fiberglass, silicates, combustion products such as polycyclic aromatic hydrocarbons and metals, although metals associated with granulomatous and fibrotic lung disease, such as beryllium, zirconium and tungsten–cobalt, have not been reported (Lioy et al., 2002; Lioy and Georgopoulos, 2006). While the BeLPT was not performed in many of these workers, biomonitoring for beryllium was negative in the FDNY cohort, suggesting that there may be an as-yet unidentified triggering antigen. The heterogeneity of radiographic findings and the spectrum of pulmonary and extra-thoracic manifestations consistent with sarcoidosis raise the possibility that the exposure may have caused non-specific triggering of the innate immune system, rather than an adaptive response to a specific antigen contained in the dust.

OTHER OCCUPATIONAL/ENVIRONMENTAL EXPOSURES ASSOCIATED WITH GRANULOMATOUS INFLAMMATION

Several environmental exposures have been proposed as causative agents in sarcoidosis. The ACCESS study (A Case Controlled Etiological Study of Sarcoidosis) found association between sarcoidosis and certain occupations and exposures, including in physicians and middle/secondary school teachers, those employed in agriculture, raising birds, automotive manufacturing, insecticide manufacturing and pesticide-using industries, and in those with occupational exposure to mould and mildew and to musty odours, as well as to the use of home central air conditioning. Excess cases of sarcoidosis-like granulomatous lung disease have been reported in firefighters, as noted above and elsewhere (Kern et al., 1993; Prezant et al., 1999). A statistically significant increased risk for sarcoidosis was associated with the transportation services industry (Kucera et al., 2003), naval personnel (Gorham et al., 2004), retail trade (Kucera et al., 2003), mould and mildew exposure (Kucera et al., 2003; Rossman et al., 2008), titanium (Kucera et al., 2003), vegetable dust and organic dust exposure (Kucera et al., 2003; Barnard et al., 2005) and suppliers of building materials, hardware and gardening materials (Barnard et al., 2005). An association between silica and silicates and granulomatous lung disease has long been recognized (Hardy, 1961), including work aboard navy aircraft carriers where the grinding of silica-containing anti-skid material was performed (CDC, 1997), a diatomaceous earth plant (Rafnsson et al., 1998) and exposure to rock wool or glass wool (Drent et al., 2000). Smoking appears to have a protective effect against sarcoidosis (Newman et al., 2004). Whether some of these other exposures associated with sarcoidosis may modify the risk of CBD and the other exposure-induced granulomatous diseases discussed above is not clear at this time.

SUMMARY

Granulomatous lung disease can result from a number of occupational and environmental exposures. CBD has been the most common metal-induced granulomatous disease. The worldwide incidence is expected to decrease as additional countries, including the United States, adopt lower, more protective exposure limits in the future; however, ongoing diligence will be needed in order to continue to identify workplaces in which beryllium is present, such as in the metals and electronics recycling industry and other downstream users. Immune-mediated granulomatous lung disease from other metals, including aluminium, titanium and zirconium, occurs very infrequently, and raises the question as to why this type of response has been limited to a handful of reported cases. While this might be due to a lack of recognition of the causes of these diseases, insight into differences in pathogenesis could be helpful for controlling or preventing CBD and other diseases. In contrast, no antigen-specific response has been identified in the cases of sarcoidosis/sarcoid-like granulomatous lung disease in those exposed to the WTC dust, nor in some of the sarcoidosis cases associated with silica, mould and other exposures, raising the possibility that these exposures may have caused a non-specific triggering of the innate immune system, rather than an adaptive response, like beryllium. Elucidation of this mechanism is needed before prevention strategies can be proposed for these diseases.

REFERENCES

ACGIH, American Conference of Industrial Hygienists. 2009. Beryllium and compounds: Threshold limit values for chemical substances and physical agents and biological exposure indices. Cincinnati, OH: American Conference of Industrial Hygienists.

American Thoracic Society and European Respiratory Society. 2002. American Thoracic Society/European Respiratory Society International Multidisciplinary Consensus Classification of the Idiopathic Interstitial Pneumonias. This joint statement of the American Thoracic Society (ATS), and the European Respiratory Society (ERS) was adopted by the ATS board of directors, June 2001 and by the ERS Executive Committee, June 2001. *Am J Respir Crit Care Med* 165:277–304.

Aronchick, J. M., Rossman, M. D. and Miller, W. T. 1987. Chronic beryllium disease: Diagnosis, radiographic findings, and correlation with pulmonary function tests. *Radiology* 163:677–82.

ATS/ERS/WASOG. 1999. Statement on sarcoidosis. Joint Statement of the American Thoracic Society (ATS), the European Respiratory Society (ERS) and the World Association of Sarcoidosis and Other Granulomatous Disorders (WASOG) adopted by the ATS Board of Directors and by the ERS Executive Committee, February 1999. *Am J Respir Crit Care Med* 160:736–55.

Bailey, R. L., Thomas, C. A., Deubner, D. C., Kent, M. S., Kreiss, K. and Schuler, C. R. 2010. Evaluation of a preventive program to reduce sensitization at a beryllium metal, oxide, and alloy production plant. *J Occup Environ Med* 52:505–12.

Balmes, J. R., Abraham, J. L., Dweik, R. A., Fireman, E., Fontenot, A. P., Maier, L. A., Muller-Quernheim, J. et al. 2014. An official American Thoracic Society statement: Diagnosis and management of beryllium sensitivity and chronic beryllium disease. *Am J Respir Crit Care Med* 190:e34–59.

Barnard, J., Rose, C., Newman, L. et al. 2005. Job and industry classifications associated with sarcoidosis in A Case–Control Etiologic Study of Sarcoidosis (ACCESS). *J Occup Environ Med* 47:226–34.

Bartter, T., Irwin, R. S., Abraham, J. L. et al. 1991. Zirconium compound-induced pulmonary fibrosis. *Arch Intern Med* 151:1197–201.

Beryllium Science and Technology Association (BeST). 2016. About Beryllium. Available from: http://beryllium.eu/about-beryllium-and-beryllium-alloys/facts-and-figures/production-statistics/ (accesses 28 March 2016).

Blanc, P. D. 2007. Is giant cell interstitial pneumonitis synonymous with hard metal lung disease? *Am J Respir Crit Care Med* 176:834; author reply 834–35.

Bobka, C. A., Stewart, L. A., Engelken, G. J., Golitz, L. E. and Newman, L. S. 1997. Comparison of *in vivo* and *in vitro* measures of beryllium sensitization. *J Occup Environ Med* 39:540–7.

Cai, H. R., Cao, M., Meng, F. Q. and Wei, J. Y. 2007. Pulmonary sarcoid-like granulomatosis induced by aluminum dust: Report of a case and literature review. *Chin Med J (Engl)* 120:1556–60.

CAREX Canada. 2014. Beryllium regulations. Available at: http://www.carexcanada.ca/en/beryllium/#regulations_and_guidelines (accessed 20 September 2014).

CDC. 1997. Sarcoidosis among U.S. Navy enlisted men, 1965–1993. *MMWR Morb Mortal Wkly Rep* 46:539–43.

Chen, W. J., Monnat, R., Chen, M. and Karle-Mottet, N. 1978. Aluminum induced pulmonary granulomatosis. *Hum Pathol* 9:705–11.

Cherrie, J. W., Gorman Ng, M., Shafrir, A., Van Tongeren, M., Mistry, R., Warwick, O., Corden, C. et al. 2011. Health, socio-economic and environmental aspects of possible amendments to the EU Directive on the protection of workers from the risks related to exposure to carcinogens and mutagens at work. Beryllium and beryllium compounds. Edinburg: Institute for Occupational Medicine. p. 3.

Coates, E. O., Jr. and Watson, J. H. 1971 Diffuse interstitial lung disease in tungsten carbide workers. *Ann Intern Med* 75:709–16.

Cortez, P. J. and Marques, F. 1969. Vineyard sprayer's lung: A new occupational disease. *Thorax* 24:678–88.

Crowley, L. E., Herbert, R., Moline, J. M., Wallenstein, S., Shukla, G., Schechter, C., Skloot, G. S. et al. 2010. 'Sarcoid like' granulomatous pulmonary disease in World Trade Center disaster responders. *Am J Ind Med* 54:175–84.

Cugell, D. W., Morgan, W. K. C., Perkins, D. G. and Rubin, A. 1990. The respiratory effects of cobalt. *Arch Int Med* 150:177–83.

Cullen, M. R., Cherniack, M. G. and Kominsky, J. R. 1986. Chronic beryllium disease in the United States. *Semin Respir Med* 7:203–9.

Cummings, K. J., Deubner, D. C., Day, G. A., Henneberger, P. K., Kitt, M. M., Kent, M. S., Kreiss, K. et al. 2007. Enhanced preventive programme at a beryllium oxide ceramics facility reduces beryllium sensitisation among new workers. *Occup Environ Med* 64:134–40.

Cummings, K. J., Stefaniak, A. B., Virji, M. A. and Kreiss, K. 2009. A reconsideration of acute beryllium disease. *Environ Health Perspect* 117:1250–56.

Curtis, G. H. 1951. Cutaneous hypersensitivity due to beryllium: A study of thirteen cases. *AMA Arch Dermatol Syphilol* 64:470–82.

Daniloff, E. M., Lynch, D. A., Bucher Bartelson, B., Newell, J. D. Jr., Bernstein, S. M. and Newman, L. S. 1997. Observer variation and relationship of computed tomography to severity of beryllium disease. *Am J Respir Crit Care Med* 155:2047–56.

De Vuyst, P., Dumortier, P., Rickaert, F., Van de Weyer, R., Lenclud, C. and Yernault, J. C. 1986. Occupational lung fibrosis in an aluminium polisher. *Eur J Respir Dis* 68:131–40.

De Vuyst, P., Dumortier, P., Schandené, L., Estenne, M., Verhest, A. and Yernault, J.-C. 1987. Sarcoidlike lung granulomatosis induced by aluminum dusts. *Am Rev Respir Dis* 135:493–7.

Decision on the New and Revised Occupational Exposure Limits for 2012 and Others. 2015. Available at: http://www2.worksafebc.com/enews/rap/141219/141219.htm (accessed 9 January 2015).

DeNardi, J. M., Van Ordstrand, H. S. and Carmody, M. G. 1949. Acute dermatitis and pneumonitis in beryllium workers: Review of 406 cases in eight-year period with follow-up on recoveries. *Ohio State Med J* 45:567–75.

Denardi, J. M., Van Ordstrand, H. S., Curtis, G. H. and Zielinski, J. 1953. Berylliosis: Summary and survey of all clinical types observed in a twelve-year period. *AMA Arch Ind Hyg Occup Med* 8:1–24.

Deubner, D. C., Goodman, M. and Iannuzzi, J. 2001. Variability, predictive value, and uses of the beryllium blood lymphocyte proliferation test (BLPT): Preliminary analysis of the ongoing workforce survey. *Appl Occup Environ Hyg* 16:521–6.

Drent, M., Bomans, P. H., Van Suylen, R. J., Lamers, R. J., Bast, A. and Wouters, E. F. 2000. Association of man-made mineral fibre exposure and sarcoidlike granulomas. *Respir Med* 94:815–20.

Dunlop, P., Muller, N. L., Wilson, J., Flint, J. and Churg, A. 2005. Hard metal lung disease: High resolution CT and histologic correlation of the initial findings and demonstration of interval improvement. *J Thorac Imaging* 20:301–4.

Eisenbud, M. 1982. Origins of the standard for control of beryllium disease. *Environ Res* 27:79–88.

Eisenbud, M. and Lisson, J. 1983. Epidemiological aspects of beryllium-induced non-malignant lung disease: A 30-year update. *J Occup Med* 25:196–202.

Fireman, E., Shai, A. B., Lerman, Y., Topilsky, M., Blanc, P. D., Maier, L., Li, L. et al. 2012. Chest wall shrapnel-induced beryllium-sensitization and associated pulmonary disease. *Sarcoidosis Vasc Diffuse Lung Dis* 29:147–50.

Freiman, D. G. 1959. Pathologic changes of beryllium disease; discussion of papers by Drs. Hazard and Dudley. *AMA Arch Ind Health* 19:188–9.

Freiman, D. G. and Hardy, H. L. 1970. Beryllium disease: The relation of pulmonary pathology to clinical course and prognosis based on a study of 130 cases from the U.S. beryllium case registry. *Hum Pathol* 1:25–44.

Gaede, K. I., Amicosante, M., Schurmann, M., Fireman, E., Saltini, C. and Muller-Quernheim, J. 2005. Function associated transforming growth factor-beta gene polymorphism in chronic beryllium disease. *J Mol Med* 83:397–405.

Gheysens, B., Auwerx, J., Van den Eeckhout, A. and Demedts, M. 1985. Cobalt-induced bronchial asthma in diamond polishers. *Chest* 88:740–4.

Gorham, E. D., Garland, C. F., Garland, F. C., Kaiser, K., Travis, W. D. and Centeno, J. A. 2004. Trends and occupational associations in incidence of hospitalized pulmonary sarcoidosis and other lung diseases in Navy personnel: A 27-year historical prospective study, 1975–2001. *Chest* 126:1431–8.

Gotway, M. B., Golden, J. A., Warnock, M., Koth, L. L., Webb, R., Reddy, G. P. and Balmes, J. R. 2002. Hard metal interstitial lung disease: High-resolution computed tomography appearance. *J Thorac Imaging* 17:314–8.

Hardy, H. L. 1961. The definition of sarcoidosis. *Am Rev Respir Dis* 84(5 Pt 2):1–5.

Hardy, H. L. 1965. Beryllium poisoning: Lessons in control of man-made disease. *N Engl J Med* 273:1188–99.

Hardy, H. L. and Tabershaw, I. R. 1946. Delayed chemical pneumonitis in workers exposed to beryllium compounds. *J Ind Hyg Toxicol* 28:197–211.

Harris, K. M., McConnochie, K. and Adams, H. 1993. The computed tomographic appearances in chronic berylliosis. *Clin Radiol* 47:26–31.

Hasan, F. M. and Kazemi, H. 1974. Chronic beryllium disease: A continuing epidemiologic hazard. *Chest* 65:289–93.

Henneberger, P.K., Cumro, D., Deubner, D.D., Kent, M.S., McCawley, M. and Kreiss, K. 2001. Beryllium sensitization and disease among long-term and short-term workers in a beryllium ceramics plant. *Int Arch Occup Environ Health* 74:167–76.

Herbert, A., Sterling, G., Abraham, J. and Corrin, B. 1982. Desquamative interstitial pneumonia in an aluminum welder. *Hum Pathol* 13:694–9.

Izbicki, G., Chavko, R., Banauch, G. I., Weiden, M. D., Berger, K. I., Aldrich, T. K., Hall, C. et al. 2007. World Trade Center 'sarcoid-like' granulomatous pulmonary disease in New York City Fire Department rescue workers. *Chest* 131:1414–23.

Jederlinic, P. J., Abraham, J. L., Churg, A., Himmelstein, J. S., Epler, G. R. and Gaensler, E. A. 1990. Pulmonary fibrosis in aluminum oxide workers: Investigation of nine workers with pathologic examination and microanalysis in three of them. *Am Rev Respir Dis* 142:1179–84.

Jones-Williams, W. 1988. Beryllium disease. *Postgrad Med J* 64:511–6.

Jones-Williams, W. and Williams, W. R. 1983. Value of beryllium lymphocyte transformation tests in chronic beryllium disease and in potentially exposed workers. *Thorax* 38:41–4.

Jordan, H. T., Stellman, S. D., Prezant, D., Teirstein, A., Osahan, S. S. and Cone, J. E. 2011. Sarcoidosis diagnosed after 11 September 2001, among adults exposed to the World Trade Center disaster. *J Occup Environ Med* 53:966–74.

Kelleher, P. C., Martyny, J. W., Mroz, M. M., Maier, L. A., Ruttenber, J. A., Young, D. A. and Newman, L. S. 2001. Beryllium particulate exposure and disease relations in a beryllium machining plant. *J Occup Environ Med* 43:238–49.

Kern, D. G., Neill, M. A., Wrenn, D. S., Varone, J. C. 1993. Investigation of a unique time–space cluster of sarcoidosis in firefighters. *Am Rev Respir Dis* 148:974–80.

Kim, Y., Jee, Y., Park, J., Lee, K., Lee, S. 2004. Acute beryllium disease in liquid metal workers [Abstract]. *Eur Respir J* 24(48 Suppl.):P981.

Kongerud, J. and Samuelsen, S. O. 1991. A longitudinal study of respiratory symptoms in aluminum potroom workers. *Am Rev Respir Dis* 144:10–6.

Kotter, J. M. and Zieger, G. 1992. [Sarcoid granulomatosis after many years of exposure to zirconium, 'zirconium lung']. *Pathologe* 13:104–9.

Kreiss, K., Mroz, M. M., Newman, L. S., Martyny, J. and Zhen, B. 1996. Machining risk of beryllium disease and sensitization with median exposures below 2 mg/m^3. *Am J Ind Med* 30:16–25.

Kreiss, K., Mroz, M.M., Zhen, B., Wiedemann, H. and Barna, B. 1997. Risks of beryllium disease related to work processes at a metal, alloy, and oxide production plant. *Occup Environ Med* 54:605–12.

Kreiss, K., Newman, L. S., Mroz, M. M. and Campbell, P. A. 1989. Screening blood test identifies subclinical beryllium disease. *J Occup Med* 31:603–8.

Kreiss, K., Wasserman, S., Mroz, M. M. and Newman, L. S. 1993. Beryllium disease screening in the ceramics industry. Blood lymphocyte test performance and exposure–disease relations. *J Occup Med* 35:267–74.

Kucera, G. P., Rybicki, B. A., Kirkey, K. L., Coon, S. W., Major, M. L., Maliarik, M. J. and Iannuzzi, M. C. 2003. Occupational risk factors for sarcoidosis in African–American siblings. *Chest* 123:1527–35.

Lee, S. M., Moon, C. H., Oh, Y. B., Kim, H. Y., Ahn, Y., Ko, E. J. and Joo, J. 1998. Giant-cell interstitial pneumonia in a gas station worker. *J Korean Med Sci* 13:545–7.

Lieben, J. and Metzner, F. 1959. Epidemiological findings associated with beryllium extraction. *Am Ind Hyg Assoc J* 20:504–8.

Liippo, K. K., Anttila, S. L., Taikina-Aho, O., Ruokonen, E. L., Toivonen, S. T. and Tuomi, T. 1993. Hypersensitivity pneumonitis and exposure to zirconium silicate in a young ceramic tile worker. *Am Rev Respir Dis* 148:1089–92.

Lioy, P. J. and Georgopoulos, P. 2006. The anatomy of the exposures that occurred around the World Trade Center site: 9/11 and beyond. *Ann N Y Acad Sci* 1076:54–79.

Lioy, P. J., Weisel, C. P., Millette, J. R., Eisenreich, S., Vallero, D., Offenberg, D., Buckley, B. et al. 2002. Characterization of the dust/smoke aerosol that settled east of the World Trade Center (WTC) in lower Manhattan after the collapse of the WTC 11 September 2001. *Environ Health Perspect* 110:703–14.

Lundgren, R. A., Maier, L. A., Rose, C. S., Balkissoon, R. C. and Newman, L. S. 2001. Indirect and direct gas exchange at maximum exercise in beryllium sensitization and disease. *Chest* 120:1702–8.

Lynch, D. A. 2006. Beryllium related diseases. In *Imaging of Occupational and Environmental Disorders of the Chest*, P.A. Gevenois and P. De Vuyst (eds), São Paulo: Springer, pp. 249–56.

Maier, L., Gunn, C. and Newman, L. 2006. Beryllium disease. In: *Environmental and Occupational Medicine*, W. Rom (ed.), Philadelphia: Lippincott-Raven Publishers, pp. 1021–38.

Maier, L. A., Martyny, J. W., Liang, J. and Rossman, M. D. 2008. Recent chronic beryllium disease in residents surrounding a beryllium facility. *Am J Respir Crit Care Med* 177:1012–7.

Maier, L. A., McGrath, D. S., Sato, H., Lympany, P., Welsh, K., duBois, R., Silveira, L. et al. 2003. Influence of MHC class II in susceptibility to beryllium sensitization and chronic beryllium disease. *J Immunol* 171:6910–8.

Marchand-Adam, S., El Khatib, A., Guillon, F, Brauner, M. W., Lepage, L. V., Naccache, J-M. and Valeyre, D. 2008. Short- and long-term response to corticosteroid therapy in chronic beryllium disease. *Eur Respir J* 32:687–93.

Martin, A. K., Mack, D. G., Falta, M. T., Mroz, M. M., Newman, L. S., Maier, L. A. and Fontenot, A. P. 2011. Beryllium-specific CD4+ T cells in blood as a biomarker of disease progression. *J Allergy Clin Immunol* 128:1100–6.e1–5.

Martyny, J. W., Hoover, M. D., Mroz, M. M., Ellis, K., Maier, L. A., Sheff, K. L. and Newman, L. S. 2000. Aerosols generated during beryllium machining. *J Occup Environ Med* 42:8–18.

Mayer, A. S., Brazile, W. J., Erb, S. A., Barker, E. A., Miller, C. M., Mroz, M. M., Maier, L. M. and Van Dyke, M. V. 2013. Developing effective health and safety training materials for workers in beryllium-using industries. *J Occup Environ Med* 55:746–51.

Mayer, A. S., Hamzeh, N. and Maier, L. A. 2014. Sarcoidosis and chronic beryllium disease: Similarities and differences. *Semin Respir Crit Care Med* 35(3):316–29.

McCanlies, E. C., Ensey, J. S., Schuler, C. R., Kreiss, K. and Weston, A. 2004. The association between HLA-DPB1Glu69 and chronic beryllium disease and beryllium sensitization. *Am J Ind Med* 46:95–103.

McCanlies, E. C., Kreiss, K., Andrew, M. and Weston, A. 2003. HLA-DPB1 and chronic beryllium disease: A HuGE review. *Am J Epidemiol* 157:388–98.

Menon, B., Sharma, A., Kripalani, J. and Jain, S. 2006. Giant cell interstitial pneumonia in a 60-year-old female without hard metal exposure. *Respiration* 73:833–5.

Middleton, D. C., Lewin, M. D., Kowalski, P. J., Cox, S. S. and Kleinbaum, D. 2006. The BeLPT: Algorithms and implications. *Am J Ind Med* 49:36–44.

Middleton, D. C., Mayer, A. S., Lewin, M. D., Mroz, M. M. and Maier, L. A. 2011. Interpreting borderline BeLPT results. *Am J Ind Med* 54:205–9.

Miller, R. R., Churg, A. M., Hutcheon, M. and Lam, S. 1984. Pulmonary alveolar proteinosis and aluminum dust exposure. *Am Rev Respir Dis* 130:312–5.

Ministry of Health, People's Republic of China. 2007. Occupational exposure limits for hazardous agents in the workplace, part 1: chemical hazardous agents, GBZ 2.1-2007. http://www.moh.gov.cn/publicfiles/business/cmsresources/zwgkzt/emsrsdocument/doc3277.pdf. (accessed 2 June 2010).

Mitchell, J., Manning, G. B., Molyneux, M. and Lane, R. E. 1961. Pulmonary fibrosis in workers exposed to finely powdered aluminum. *Br J Ind Med* 18:10–20.

Moriyama, H., Kobayashi, M., Takada, T., Shimuzi, T., Terada, M., Narita, J-I., Maruyams, M. et al. 2007. Authors' response. *Am J Respir Crit Care Med* 176:834.

Moriyama, H., Kobayashi, M., Takada, T., Shimuzi, T., Terada, M., Narita, J-I., Maruyams, M. et al. 2007. Two-dimensional analysis of elements and mononuclear cells in hard metal lung disease. *Am J Respir Crit Care Med* 176:70–7.

Mroz, M. M., Maier, L. A., Strand, M., Silviera, L. and Newman, L. S. 2009. Beryllium lymphocyte proliferation test surveillance identifies clinically significant beryllium disease. *Am J Ind Med* 52:762–73.

Naccache, J. M., Marchand-Adam, S., Kambouchner, M., Guillon, F., Monnet, I., Girard, F., Brauner, M. et al. 2003. Ground-glass computed tomography pattern in chronic beryllium disease: Pathologic substratum and evolution. *J Comput Assist Tomogr* 27:496–500.

Naqvi, A. H., Hunt, A., Burnett, B. R. and Abraham, J. L. 2008. Pathologic spectrum and lung dust burden in giant cell interstitial pneumonia (hard metal disease/cobalt pneumonitis): Review of 100 cases. *Arch Environ Occup Health* 63:51–70.

Nemery, B., Verbeken, E. K. and Demedts, M. 2001. Giant cell interstitial pneumonia (hard metal lung disease, cobalt lung). *Semin Respir Crit Care Med* 22:435–48.

Newman, L. S. 1996. Significance of the blood beryllium lymphocyte proliferation test (BeLPT). *Environ Health Perspect* 104:953–6.

Newman, L. S. 1998. Metals that cause sarcoidosis. *Semin Respir Infect* 13:212–20.

Newman, L. S., Buschman, D. L., Newell, J. D. Jr. and Lynch, D. A. 1994. Beryllium disease: Assessment with CT. *Radiology* 190:835–40.

Newman, L. S., Rose, C. S., Bresnitz, E. A., Rossman, M. D., Barnard, J., Frederick, M., Terrin, M. et al. 2004. A case control etiologic study of sarcoidosis: Environmental and occupational risk factors. *Am J Respir Crit Care Med* 170:1324–30.

Newman, L., Maier, L., Martyny, J., Mroz, M., VanDyke, M. and Sackett, H. 2005. Beryllium workers' health risks. *J Occup Environ Hyg* 2:D48–50.

Newman, L. S., Mroz, M. M., Maier, L. A., Daniloff, E. M. and Balkissoon, R. 2001. Efficacy of serial medical surveillance for chronic beryllium disease in a beryllium machining plant. *J Occup Environ Med* 43:231–7.

Nilsen, A. M., Vik, R., Behrens, C., Drablos, P. A. and Espevik, T. 2010. Beryllium sensitivity among workers at a Norwegian aluminum smelter. *Am J Ind Med* 53:724–32.

Pappas, G. P. and Newman, L. S. 1993. Early pulmonary physiologic abnormalities in beryllium disease. *Am Rev Respir Dis* 148:661–6.

Peoc'h, M., Moulin, C. and Pasquier, B. 1996. Systemic granulomatous reaction to a foreign body after hip replacement. *N Engl J Med* 335:133–4.

Potolicchio, I., Mosconi, G., Forni, A., Nemery, B., Seghizzi, P. and Sorrentino, R. 1997. Susceptibility to hard metal lung disease is strongly associated with the presence of glutamate 69 in HLA-DP beta chain. *Eur J Immunol* 27:2741–3.

Prezant, D. J., Dhala, A., Goldstein, A., Janus, D., Ortiz, F., Aldrich T. K. and Kelly, K. 1999. The incidence, prevalence, and severity of sarcoidosis in New York City firefighters. *Chest* 116:1183–93.

Rafnsson, V., Ingimarsson, O., Hjalmarsson, I. and Gunnarsdottir, H. 1998. Association between exposure to crystalline silica and risk of sarcoidosis. *Occup Environ Med* 55:657–60.

Reddy, P. A., Gorelick, D. F. and Christianson, C. S. 1970. Giant cell interstitial pneumonia (GIP). *Chest* 58:319–25.

Redline, S., Barna, B. P., Tomashefski, J. F. Jr. and Abraham, J. L. 1986. Granulomatous disease associated with pulmonary deposition of titanium. *Br J Ind Med* 43:652–6.

Richeldi, L., Kreiss, K., Mroz, M. M., Zhen, B., Tartoni, P. and Saltini, C. 1997. Interaction of genetic and exposure factors in the prevalence of berylliosis. *Am J Ind Med* 4332:337–40.

Rom, W. N., Lockey, J. E., Lee, J. S., Kimball, A. C., Bang, K. M., Leaman, H., Johns, R. E. et al. 1984. Pneumoconiosis and exposures of dental laboratory technicians. *Am J Public Health* 74:1252–7.

Romeo, L., Cazzadori, A., Bontempini, L. and Martini, S. 1994. Interstitial lung granulomas as a possible consequence of exposure to zirconium dust. *Med Lav* 85:219–22.

Rosenman, K., Hertzberg, V., Rice, C., Reilly, M. J., Aronchick, J., Parker, J. E., Regovich, J. and Rossman, M. D. et al. 2005. Chronic beryllium disease and sensitization at a beryllium processing facility. *Environ Health Perspect* 113:1366–72.

Rosenman, K. D., Rossman, M., Hertzberg, V., Reilly, M. J., Rice, C., Kanterakis, E. and Monos, D. 2011. HLA class II DPB1 and DRB1 polymorphisms associated with genetic susceptibility to beryllium toxicity. *Occup Environ Med* 68:487–93.

Rossman, M. D., Stubbs, J., Lee, C. W., Argyris, E., Magira, E. and Monos, D. 2002. Human leukocyte antigen class II amino acid epitopes: Susceptibility and progression markers for beryllium hypersensitivity. *Am J Respir Crit Care Med* 165:788–94.

Rossman, M. D., Thompson, B. and Frederick, M. 2008. HLA and environmental interactions in sarcoidosis. *Sarcoidosis Vasc Diffuse Lung Dis* 25:125–32.

Rubin, L., Slepyan, A. H., Weber, L. F. and Neuhauser, I. 1956. Granulomas of the axilla caused by deodorants. *JAMA* 162:953–5.

Sackett, H. M., Maier, L. A., Silveira, L. J., Mroz, M. M., Ogden, L. G., Murphy, J. R. and Newman, L. S. 2004. Beryllium medical surveillance at a former nuclear weapons facility during cleanup operations. *J Occup Environ Med* 46:953–61.

Saltini, C., Richeldi, L., Losi, M., Amicosante, M., Voorter, C., van den Berg-Loonen, E., Dweik, R. A. et al. 2001. Major histocompatibility locus genetic markers of beryllium sensitization and disease. *Eur Respir J* 18:677–84.

Saltini, C., Winestock, K., Kirby, M., Pinkston, P. and Crystal, R. G. 1989. Maintenance of alveolitis in patients with chronic beryllium disease by beryllium-specific helper T cells. *N Engl J Med* 320:1103–9.

Sanderson, W. T., Ward, E. M., Steenland, K. and Petersen, M. R. 2001. Lung cancer case–control study of beryllium workers. *Am J Ind Med* 39:133–44.

Santic, Z., Puvacic, Z., Radovic, S. and Puvacic, S. 2005. Higher mortality risk of lungs carcinoma in vineyard sprayers. *Bosn J Basic Med Sci* 5:65–9.

Sawyer, R. T., Abraham, J. L., Daniloff, E. and Newman, L. S. 2005. Secondary ion mass spectroscopy demonstrates retention of beryllium in chronic beryllium disease granulomas. *J Occup Environ Med* 47:1218–26.

Schuler, C. R., Kent, M. S., Deubner, D.C., Berakis, M. T., McCawley, M., Henneberger, P. K., Rossman, M. D. and Kreiss, K. 2005. Process-related risk of beryllium sensitization and disease in a copper–beryllium alloy facility. *Am J Ind Med* 47:195–205.

Schuler, C. R., Kitt, M. M., Henneberger, P. K., Deubner, D. C. and Kreiss, K. 2008. Cumulative sensitization and disease in a beryllium oxide ceramics worker cohort. *J Occup Environ Med* 50:1343–50.

Sharma, N., Patel, J. and Mohammed, T. L. 2010. Chronic beryllium disease: Computed tomographic findings. *J Comput Assist Tomogr* 34:945–8.

Shelley, W. B. and Hauley, H. G. Jr. 1958. The allergic origin of zirconium deodorant granulomas. *Br J Dermatol* 70:75–101.

Sokolowski, J. W., Cordray, D. R., Cantow, E. F., Elliott, R. C. and Seal, R. B. 1972. Giant cell interstitial pneumonia. Report of a case. *Am Rev Respir Dis* 105:417–20.

Sood, A., Beckett, W. S. and Cullen, M. R. 2004. Variable response to long-term corticosteroid therapy in chronic beryllium disease. *Chest* 126:2000–7.

Stange, A. W., Furman, F. J. and Hilmas, D. E. 2004. The beryllium lymphocyte proliferation test: Relevant issues in beryllium health surveillance. *Am J Ind Med* 46:453–62.

Stange, A. W., Hilmas, D. E. and Furman, F. J. 1996. Possible health risks from low level exposure to beryllium. *Toxicology* 111:213–24.

Taiwo, O. A., Slade, M. D., Cantley, L. F., Fiellin, M. G., Wesdock, J. C., Bayer, F. J. and Cullen, M. R. 2008. Beryllium sensitization in aluminum smelter workers. *J Occup Environ Med* 50:157–62.

Taiwo, O. A., Slade, M. D., Cantley, L. F., Kirsche, S. R., Wesdock, J. C. and Cullen, M. R. 2010. Prevalence of beryllium sensitization among aluminium smelter workers. *Occup Med* 60:569–71.

Thomas, C. A., Bailey, R. L., Kent, M. S., Deubner, D. C., Kreiss, K. and Schuler, C. R. 2009. Efficacy of a program to prevent beryllium sensitization among new employees at a copper–beryllium alloy processing facility. *Public Health Rep* 124(Suppl. 1):112–24.

Thomas, C. A., Deubner, D. C., Stanton, M. L., Kreiss, K. and Schuler, C. R. 2013. Long-term efficacy of a program to prevent beryllium disease. *Am J Ind Med* 56:733–41.

United States Department of Labor. 1999. *Preventing Adverse Health Effects from Exposure to Beryllium on the Job.* Available at https://www.osha.gov/dts/hib/hib_data/hib19990902.html (accessed 28 March 2016).

United States Department of Labor. 2015. Occupational Exposure to Beryllium and Beryllium Compounds, 29 CFR 1910. Proposed Rule, 80. *Federal Register no. 152.* (7 August 2015). pp. 47566–828.

United States Department of Energy. 1999. Chronic Beryllium Disease Prevention Program 10 CFR 850. Final Rule, 64 *Federal Register no. 235.* (8 December 1999). pp. 68854–914.

USGS. 2013. Minerals: Beryllium. Available at: http://minerals.usgs.gov/minerals/pubs/commodity/beryllium/mcs-2013-beryl.pdf (accessed 10 October 2014).

Van Dyke, M. V., Martyny, J. W., Mroz, M. M., Silveira, L. J., Strand, M., Cragle, D. L., Tankersley, W. G. et al. 2011. Exposure and genetics increase risk of beryllium sensitisation and chronic beryllium disease in the nuclear weapons industry. *Occup Environ Med* 68:842–8.

Van Dyke, M. V., Martyny, J. W., Mroz, M. M., Silveira, L. J., Strand, M., Fingerlin, T. E., Sato, H. et al. 2011. Risk of chronic beryllium disease by HLA-DPB1 E69 genotype and beryllium exposure in nuclear workers. *Am J Respir Crit Care Med* 183:1680–8.

Van Ordstrand, H. S., Netherton, E. W., DeNardi, J. M. and Carmody, M. G. 1950. Beryllium skin granulomas from a broken fluorescent tube. *Cleveland Clin Q* 17:34–7.

Villar, T. G. 1974. Vineyard sprayer's lung: Clinical aspect. *Am Rev Respir Dis* 110:545–55.

Wang, Z., Farris, G. M., Newman, L. S., Shou, Y., Maier, L. A., Smith, H. N. and Marrone, B. L. 2001. Beryllium sensitivity is linked to HLA-DP genotype. *Toxicology* 165:27–38.

Wang, Z., White, P., Petrovic, M., Tatum, O. L., Newman, L. S., Maier, L. A. and Marrone, B. L. 1999. Differential susceptibilities to chronic beryllium disease contributed by different Glu69 HLA-DPB1 and -DPA1 alleles. *J Immunol* 163:1647–53.

Welch, L. S. 2012. Beryllium. In *Patty's Toxicology*, 6th Edition, E. Bingham and B. Cohrssen (eds), Hoboken, NJ: John Wiley & Sons, Inc., pp. 113–144.

Welch, L., Ringen, K., Bingham, E., Dement, J., Takaro, T., McGowan, W., Chen, A. and Quinn, P. 2004. Screening for beryllium disease among construction trade workers at Department of Energy nuclear sites. *Am J Ind Med* 46:207–18.

Werfel, U., Schneider, J., Rodelsperger, K., Kotter, J., Popp, W., Woitowitz, H. J., Zieger, G. 1998. Sarcoid granulomatosis after zirconium exposure with multiple organ involvement. *Eur Respir J* 12:750.

25 Organising Pneumonia and Other Uncommon Interstitial Disorders

Carl J. Reynolds and Paul Blanc

CONTENTS

INTRODUCTION

Attributing a disease process to a specific exposure can be difficult. Establishing causation is often complex, all the more so given the multifactorial nature of many chronic conditions. Well-studied and relatively frequent entities such as chronic obstructive pulmonary disease, ischaemic heart disease and diabetes lend themselves to epidemiologic investigation, delineating the major risk factors for disease and their relative contributions to risk at the population level. Uncommon diseases present added challenges to attribution, especially those for which the underlying pathological processes are poorly elucidated and the condition is typically considered idiopathic.

Due to their infrequency, very uncommon processes are difficult to study using standard epidemiologic techniques, even using case-referent approaches. Only infrequently are potential associations for such diseases amenable to assessments that conform to Bradford–Hill criteria or other rigorous standards of causation. In particular, the links between occupational factors and uncommon respiratory conditions are often first described in isolated case reports or limited case series. These accounts, even with their acknowledged limitations, serve to document the potential association between a disease and an exposure scenario and disseminate that information to a wider clinical and academic community.

As additional case reports appear with a similar occupational association, the initial suspicion of cause and effect can be strengthened, although this may be counterbalanced by a publication bias against the appearance of further, similar case reports due to a perceived lack of novelty in similar reports. Systematic literature reviews of multiple cases or case series and, where feasible, case-referent investigations, can serve to further support the validity of perceived causality. Animal data can also be critical, presuming that an experimental model exists for the disease process in question. The goal of this chapter is to consider relatively uncommon, generally idiopathic interstitial respiratory tract conditions in relation to potentially causative occupational exposures. In particular, we will address idiopathic pneumonias as well as certain other interstitial disease processes not typically considered as falling within the accepted canon of standard occupational lung diseases. These conditions are all related to chronic or subacute exposures that often occur over a number of years, although sometimes the duration of exposure has been only weeks or months. We will not consider here acute lung injury patterns; for example, toxic chemical-caused acute interstitial pneumonia. We also do not address chronic interstitial lung processes covered elsewhere in this text; for example, the classic pneumoconioses.

ORGANISING PNEUMONIA WITH A CRYPTOGENIC ORGANISING PNEUMONIA-LIKE PATTERN

Organising pneumonia is defined pathologically by the presence of intra-alveolar buds of granulation tissue, consisting of intermixed myofibroblasts and connective tissue (Cordier, 2000). Formerly, the term 'bronchiolitis obliterans organising pneumonia' (BOOP) was also applied to this entity, but this use has fallen out of favour. Cryptogenic organising pneumonia (COP) is a clinicopathological entity in which organising pneumonia occurs due to an unknown cause, thus being idiopathic by definition (Bradley et al., 2008). Nonetheless, there are known or suspected occupational causes of a COP-like pathological response.

The most well-established occupational cause of interstitial lung disease with a COP-like response is the chemical Acramin, also known by the trade name Ardystil (see Figures 25.1 and 25.2). In April 1992, two young women who worked at a textile factory were treated for interstitial lung disease and severe pulmonary insufficiency at the hospital of Alcoi in the Autonomous Community of Valencia, Spain (Moya et al., 1994). Their work had involved the spraying of a reactive textile dye. The illnesses were notified to the local authorities, who linked them to another case involving a young woman who had worked at the same factory and who had succumbed to respiratory failure a few months before. This prompted an investigation of all printing textile factories that used similar spraying techniques in the area of Alcoi. Eight factories with a total of 257 employees were identified. Workers were interviewed with a standardised questionnaire covering respiratory symptoms and details of employment, and each underwent a physical examination, chest radiograph, spirometry and a computed tomography (CT) chest scan. Clinical and radiological data, together with biopsy samples from 71 employees, delineated the extent of the outbreak of organising pneumonia. Altogether there were six fatal cases. Epidemiological analysis of 22 cases who met the radiological and biopsy criteria for organising pneumonia revealed that those who had worked at Factory A had the highest risk of being a case (relative risk [RR]: 24.3; 95% confidence interval [CI]: 5.7–104.4), followed by Factory B (RR: 11; 95% CI: 11.9–62.9) and only two out of 22 cases had never worked in Factories A or B. Airborne aerosols in the two factories were compared. The concentration ranged from 5 to 16 mg/m^3 (mean: 10 mg/m^3) in Factory A and from 1 to 3 mg/m^3 (mean: 2 mg/m^3) in Factory B. It was found that only in Factories A and B had the presence of an airborne chemical by the trade name Acramin FWR recently been substituted with another related compound, Acramin FWN. Subsequently, a similar outbreak was identified in Algeria (Ould Kadi et al., 1994). Unfortunately, earlier toxicology studies of Acramin FWN and FWR had been limited to ingestion and dermal application, and had not studied the effects of inhalation. Subsequent experimental studies of Acramin FWN and FWR by inhalation confirmed its respiratory tract toxicity. Although the precise mechanism remains unclear, it is suspected that the highly negatively charged long-chain molecular structure of Acramin FWN contributes to toxicity (Hoet et al., 1999).

The Ardystil story is exceptional because the magnitude of the initial outbreak did allow for classic epidemiologic study and, unfortunately, a further outbreak under similar conditions confirmed the initial observations. Finally, experimental data later gave additional support for establishing causality. In addition to Ardystil lung, however, there have also been other reports of COP-like pathology occurring in association with various occupational exposure scenarios. Each of these associations has been reported in an isolated case, and in several of these, the purported exposure was not well characterised.

A case of BOOP (the terminology used) was reported in a spice processing worker (Alleman and Darcey, 2002) whose primary responsibility was filling and operating the hopper of a misting device that sprayed spices onto potato chips. He manually transferred spice mix from sacks into the hopper and generated significant dust in the process. Unfortunately, the precise ingredients of the spice mix were unavailable to the authors, and they also were not permitted access to the workplace, such that the nature of the exposure could not be further characterised. In another case report, a cleaner was reported to have developed severe dyspnoea, cough and fever, requiring hospitalisation, 2 weeks after a cleaning agent spill at work that resulted in benzalkonium compound vapour inhalation. In addition to BOOP (and of unknown significance), the cleaner was also diagnosed with myeloperoxidase deficiency (Stefano et al., 2003). Massive exposure to acetic acid steam resulting from an explosion in a chemical factory was described as resulting in delayed-onset BOOP in a 34 year old chemical worker (Sheu et al., 2008). In another irritant-related case, accidental exposure to hydrogen sulphide fume in an oil refinery worker resulted in a chemical pneumonitis with persistent right lower-lobe consolidation; a

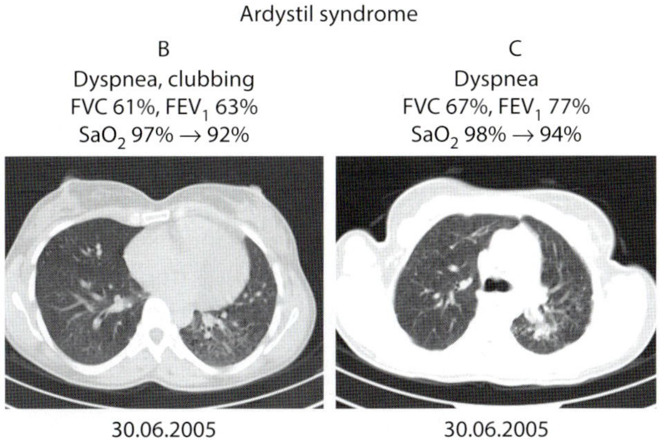

FIGURE 25.1 Chest computed tomography image of Acramin (Ardystil) dye-associated organising pneumonia. FVC: forced vital capacity; FEV$_1$: forced expiratory volume in 1 second. (Courtesy of Dr. Benoit Nemery.)

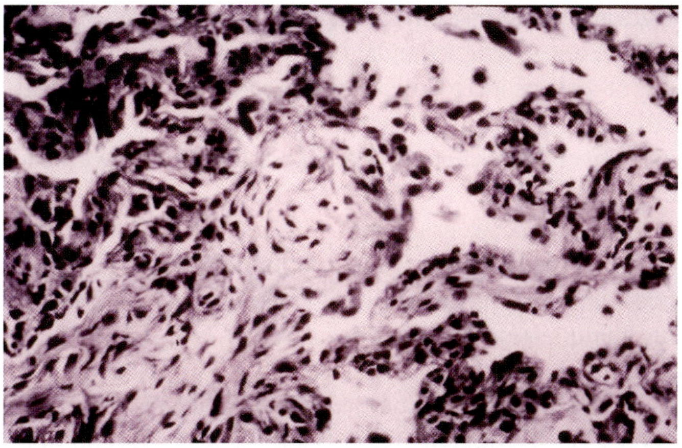

FIGURE 25.2 Cryptogenic organising pneumonia pattern in a lung biopsy of an Acramin (Ardystil) dye-exposed worker. Haematoxylin and eosin staining, magnification ×250. (Courtesy of Dr. Anthony Newman-Taylor.)

lung biopsy was reported to show diffuse alveolar damage with organising pneumonia (Doujaiji and Al-Tawfiq, 2010). A case of COP developing following exposure to ortho-phenylenediamine was described in a 29 year old laboratory worker. The patient worked with ortho-phenylenediamine for 6 months before developing episodes of fever, productive cough, dyspnoea and radiographic pulmonary infiltrates. A specific inhalation challenge with ortho-phenylenediamine with pre- and post-CT imaging supported the diagnosis (Sanchez-Ortiz et al., 2011). In another case report, a 58 year old man was reported to have developed BOOP after 3 months of exposure to heated electrostatic polyester powder paint. Mineralogical analysis indicated the presence of titanium dioxide nanoparticles in both the paint and in a lung biopsy, and this was posited to be the causal agent (Cheng et al., 2012). Finally, organising pneumonia temporally associated with gold dust inhalation was reported in a 47 year old restorer of religious art. He presented with a 3-week history of asthenia, myalgia, dry cough and fever, which responded to systemic corticosteroids (Ribeiro et al., 2011).

This heterogeneous series underscores the challenges in interpreting the case report literature as it pertains to an idiopathic parenchymal lung disease such as COP. Some of the cases (e.g. following irritant inhalation) seem more consistent with a bronchiolitis obliterans response similar to the well-established pattern following nitrogen dioxide inhalation, rather than a COP-like pattern. Other cases seem consistent with a chemically caused extrinsic alveolitis. Because the medicinal use of gold is associated with pneumonitis (Tomioka and King, 1997), the case of organising pneumonia linked with gold dust inhalation (likely to be a rare exposure scenario) may have the greatest biological plausibility among this group of individual reports. Nonetheless, the precedent of the Ardystil lung syndrome argues for continued vigilance for occupational exposures that may induce a COP-like pathological response. Further, it has been argued that polymers with natively charged functionality may be particularly suspect, and that this structure–function relationship may explain the recent outbreak of chemically associated severe lung injury to a disinfectant used in humidifiers in Korea (although this episode was not characterised by a COP-like pattern) (Nemery and Hoet, 2015).

OTHERWISE IDIOPATHIC PULMONARY FIBROSIS

Idiopathic pulmonary fibrosis (IPF) is a diagnosis of exclusion. It is made in the presence on high-resolution CT scan of a pattern consistent with usual interstitial pneumonitis (UIP) or its confirmation by biopsy. The diagnosis requires that known causes of interstitial lung disease (such as drug toxicity, connective tissue disease and domestic and occupational or environmental exposures) be excluded (Travis et al., 2013).

In practice, a known cause of fibrosis that would exclude IPF may be missed. For example, Monso et al. (1991) studied the lung dust content in IPF with scanning electron microscopy and energy-dispersive X-ray analysis in 25 patients with a previous pathological diagnosis of IPF (using optical microscopy) and 25 normal lung controls. They identified a significant asbestos fibre burden in two of the cases (8%), leading to an alternative diagnosis of asbestosis. It is known that a variety of exposures can be associated with a UIP pathological pattern of response, including asbestos. Notably, extrinsic alveolitis, which can be occupational or environmental, is also prone to misdiagnosis as IPF (Morell et al., 2013; Kern et al., 2015). Extrinsic alveolitis is covered extensively elsewhere in this text and will not be considered further here.

Individual case assessment can identify misdiagnosed IPF, but beyond this clinical approach, there have also been a series of epidemiologic investigations addressing the question of a broader association between occupational factors and otherwise idiopathic fibrotic lung disease (Taskar and Coultas, 2006). To date, there have been 13 case-referent studies yielding a substantial body of literature on this topic (Scott et al., 1990; Iwai et al., 1994; Hubbard et al., 1996; Mullen et al., 1998, 2000; Baumgartner et al., 2000; Miyake et al., 2005; Gustafson et al., 2007; Pinheiro et al., 2008; García-Sancho Figueroa et al., 2010; Awadalla et al., 2012; Ekstrom et al., 2014). Six have reported significant associations with metal dust exposure (Scott et al., 1990; Iwai et al., 1994; Hubbard et al., 1996, 2000; Miyake et al., 2005; Pinheiro et al., 2008), four with wood dust (Hubbard et al., 1996; Gustafson et al., 2007; Pinheiro et al., 2008; Awadalla et al., 2012) and two with stone dust (Mullen et al., 1998; Baumgartner et al., 2000). Collectively, these studies are limited by the use of self-reported workplace exposure information, which is vulnerable to recall bias and confounding, as well as a failure to collect cumulative exposure data, a data gap that precludes investigation of dose–response relationships. Nonetheless, taken together, these studies do provide strong evidence for an association between IPF and occupational exposures to metal, wood and stone dust.

OTHER FIBROTIC PARENCHYMAL LUNG RESPONSES TO INORGANIC INHALANTS

There are several unusual fibrotic lung conditions associated with inorganic inhalants. These can be characterised by pathological abnormalities that are difficult to distinguish from the UIP pattern of IPF, although the same exposures can also be manifested with other lung pathological patterns of response. These inhalants include rare earth pneumoconiosis, plutonium-associated fibrosis and indium–tin oxide (ITO)-associated fibrosis.

Rare earth pneumoconiosis is a term applied to a homogenous category of exposure (rare earth elements), but subsumes a heterogeneous group of parenchymal pulmonary pathologies, including diffuse fibrosis. Exposure of photoengravers to carbon arc lamp fume features prominently in the early rare earth pneumoconiosis case report literature. The earliest report described a case in which infiltrates documented by chest radiograph developed in a worker in the photographic department of a German printing plant. The worker was known to have been exposed to carbon arc lamp fume for several years, which prompted analysis of workroom flue dust. This dust was found to contain large amounts of rare earth elements. Examination of 67 men working under similar conditions demonstrated that radiographic changes were correlated with years of exposure to carbon dusts (Heuck and Hoschek, 1968).

Interstitial lung fibrosis and restrictive lung function were reported in five reproduction photographers with more than a decade each of exposure to carbon arc lamp fume. X-ray microanalysis and electron diffraction revealed the presence of rare earth minerals (mainly cerium compounds), supporting a diagnosis of cerium pneumoconiosis (Vogt et al., 1986). A 58 year old man who worked for 46 years in a photoengraving laboratory and was exposed to smoke emitted from carbon arc lamps presented with a 2 year history of progressive dyspnoea and minimally productive cough, a single case that was described in two separate publications (Sabbioni et al., 1982; Vocaturo et al., 1983). Chest radiography showed reticulonodular shadowing and cardiomegaly. An ECG showed signs of right ventricular hypertrophy, and cardiac catheterisation revealed pulmonary hypertension. Pulmonary function testing revealed obstruction and a reduced diffusing capacity for carbon monoxide (DL_{CO}). Lung biopsy showed peri-bronchiolar infiltrates and foci of sclerotic thickening of the connective septal tissue. The weight in ng/g of rare earth elements and thorium were determined using neutron activation analysis for the patient and for 11 controls who lived in the same district of North Italy but did not have occupational exposure: the patient had elevated levels of rare earth elements in the tissue compared to regional controls. Although thorium (a rare earth co-contaminant) was also elevated, its concentration was two orders of magnitude lower than the maximal permissible concentration for occupational exposure to natural thorium-232, suggesting that the rare earths but not thorium were related to the pulmonary fibrosis observed. A case of pulmonary fibrosis has also been described in another photoengraver with 13 years exposure who presented 17 years after his exposure ended (Sulotto et al., 1986).

A 60 year old man was described as having diffuse interstitial lung fibrosis secondary to a distant 12 year exposure to rare earth dusts that occurred during work as a movie projectionist with arc lamp fume exposure. Rare earths were present in significantly higher concentrations in the lung biopsy of this patient when compared to controls; there was an absence of any other identifiable cause for lung fibrosis (Porru et al., 2001). Waring and Watling (1990) described abnormally high tissue concentrations of rare earth elements in another movie projectionist with 25 years of occupational exposure to carbon arc lamp fume without the occurrence of respiratory disease, but also enumerated 21 cases of rare earth pneumoconiosis. McDonald et al. (1995) described a patient with 35 years of exposure to rare earth materials in the course of his work as an optical lens grinder who presented with progressive dyspnoea with an interstitial pattern on chest radiograph. On biopsy, rare earth elements were documented to have accumulated and the histological pattern was indistinguishable from UIP on lung biopsy.

Dendriform pulmonary ossification has been described in association with rare earth pneumoconiosis (Yoon et al., 2005). A 38 year old man presented with a non-productive cough of several months of duration. He had a history of working for 3 years as a polisher at a crystal factory 20 years previously. He recalled that his workplace had been poorly ventilated and heavily contaminated with greenish polishing powder. A chest radiograph showed reticulonodular shadowing. A CT chest scan showed diffuse, tiny, circular or bead-like densities with branching structures in the interlobular septum, including the sub-pleural region. There were also emphysematous changes and the bone windows showed a branching, twig-like ossified mass in the right lower lobe and a few dot-like ossifications in both lower lobes. An open lung biopsy showed organising pneumonia, interstitial fibrosis, peripheral emphysema, dendriform pulmonary ossification and the presence of particulate matter. Analytic transmission electron microscopy with energy-dispersive X-ray analysis demonstrated the presence of cerium oxide and lanthanum, with cerium and lanthanum both being rare earth elements. Particles other than rare earth metals, such as quartz, feldspar, mica, kaolinite, halloysite, talc and TiO_2, were also present, but were detected only infrequently. Other cases of rare earth pneumoconiosis have been reported among cerium rare earth processors (Nappée et al., 1972; Husain et al., 1980) and in glass polishers, an occupation that uses cerium-containing rouge (Le Magrex, 1979).

In addition to the literature summarised above, there has also been an additional study based on bronchoalveolar lavage (BAL) analytes from a referral laboratory in France. This study found that seven out of 416 otherwise non-characterised cases of occupational lung disease manifested elevated BAL cerium (Pairon et al., 1994). Among these, two were photoengravers and three were glass or metal polishers. Further details for one of these cases, who had also worked as a part-time projectionist, were provided in a separate case report (Pairon et al., 1995).

As noted earlier, thorium does not appear to be a confounder explaining rare earth pneumoconiosis, but inhaled radionuclides have otherwise been implicated in occupational pulmonary fibrosis. This has been shown best by Newman et al. in a retrospective study of nuclear weapons workers that estimated the absorbed radioactive dose to the lung with an internal dosimetry model (Newman et al., 2005). The study population comprised 326 plutonium-exposed workers and 194 unexposed referents. The severity of chest radiograph interstitial abnormalities between the two groups was compared using the profusion scoring system. There was a significantly higher proportion of abnormal chest radiographic profusion scores (by International Labour Organization scoring) among plutonium-exposed workers (17.5%) than among the referent population (7.2%). In this study, lung doses of 10 Sieverts (Sv) or greater conferred a 5.3-fold increased risk (95% CI: 1.22–3.4) of having an abnormal radiograph consistent with pulmonary fibrosis (controlling for the potentially confounding effects of age, smoking and asbestos exposure).

An emerging disease process in this group is interstitial pneumonia from exposure to ITO (Homma et al., 2003, 2005; Lison et al., 2009; Cummings et al., 2010, 2012, 2013; Lison and Delos, 2010; Long Xiao et al., 2010; Tanaka et al., 2010; Omae et al., 2011). ITO is a sintered material composed of indium oxide and tin oxide and used in the making of thin-film transistor liquid crystal displays for televisions and computers. An early report (Homma et al., 2003) described a prototypical case involving a 27 year old man who had worked for 3 years in a Japanese metal processing factory as an operator of a wet surface grinder. He presented with 10 months of increasing dry cough, night sweats, progressive breathlessness, anorexia and weight loss. He had digital clubbing and was hypoxaemic on room air. Chest CT demonstrated sub-pleural honeycombing and diffuse ground-glass opacities; lung biopsy found interstitial pneumonia and numerous fine particles within the alveolar macrophages and the alveolar spaces. The co-locating presence of indium and tin was demonstrated with X-ray energy spectrometry. In addition, the patient was found to have a high serum indium level (290 μg/L), approximately 3000-fold above a referent value (0.1 μg/L). Treatment with prednisolone was initiated, but the patient succumbed to his illness. The same group described a similar, although less severe, case 2 years later (Homma et al., 2005) in a 30 year old engineer from the same metal plant. A follow-up study of 115 workers at the same manufacturing plant identified 14 individuals with features of interstitial fibrosis on chest CT (Chonan and Taguchi, 2004). Experimental studies using rodents confirmed the pulmonary toxicity of ITO, as well as its constituent metallurgic components (Lison and Delos, 2010; Tanaka et al., 2010).

Since these initial reports of an IPF-like response, cases of pulmonary alveolar proteinosis (PAP), including one fatality, have been reported among workers at a US facility producing ITO (Cummings et al., 2010). The first patient described, a 49 year old non-smoker, noted the onset of dyspnoea after working for 9 months as a hydrogen furnace operator in a poorly ventilated room where he was exposed to ITO fumes. A high-resolution CT scan demonstrated extensive ground-glass opacities, centrilobular nodules and intralobular and inter-lobular septal thickening. The DL_{CO} was markedly reduced (37% predicted) and the PaO_2 was 59 mmHg. BAL demonstrated predominance of vacuolated macrophages and lymphocytes. Subsequent lung biopsy revealed proteinaceous material and globules that were positive upon periodic acid-Schiff stain, consistent with PAP. Scanning electron microscopy and energy-dispersive X-ray analysis identified the particles within the proteinaceous material as primarily indium. The patient was treated with oral steroids and segmental then whole-lung lavage, but succumbed to respiratory failure 6 years after presentation. A second patient, a 39 year old smoker, had a similar presentation and also had biopsy-proven PAP and indium was confirmed present at 29.3 μg per gram of lung tissue using inductively coupled plasma mass spectrometry.

A subsequent review of ten cases from three countries (Japan, the USA and China) of indium lung disease, of whom seven were categorised as having interstitial lung disease (ILD) and three PAP, reported common pulmonary histological features of intra-alveolar exudate typical of alveolar proteinosis (n = 9), cholesterol clefts and granulomas (n = 10) and fibrosis (n = 9) (Cummings et al., 2012). The PAP-classified cases had presented with a shorter latency from first exposure (1–2 years) compared to those diagnosed as having ILD cases (4–13 years), suggesting a time-related spectrum of response and disease progression. Workplace surveillance in a US ITO production facility found that spirometric abnormalities were frequent even in asymptomatic workers (14 out of 45 screened; 31%) (Cummings et al., 2013). The experience with rare earth pneumoconiosis, radionuclides and ITO-induced lung disease underscores the point that unusual interstitial disease, even if attributed to a discrete cause, still can have multiple pathological manifestations. Further, such exposures may also contribute to disease being misidentified as due to other causes or simply labelled as idiopathic.

In addition to rare earths and ITO, metals as a group have been associated epidemiologically with otherwise idiopathic interstitial fibrosis, as noted previously. Among this group, aluminium constitutes one distinct metallic exposure that warrants specific mention. A 1990 cases series of nine workers with aluminium oxide exposure in abrasives manufacturing implicated this as the cause of fibrosis, which was biopsy established in three cases, along with aluminium oxide detected in the tissue (Jederlinic et al., 1990). More recently, a single case of fibrosis with UIP-like features and tissue detection of aluminium was reported in a worker with extensive exposure to dust from an aluminium trihydrate polymer that is widely used in countertops (Raghu et al., 2015a). The simultaneous publication of a rebuttal from the manufacture underscores the potential contentiousness of such reports (Gannon and Rickard, 2015); follow-up correspondence on the topic extended the debate (McKeever et al., 2015; Raghu et al., 2015b).

PARENCHYMAL LUNG RESPONSES TO SYNTHETIC FIBRES

As opposed to the fibrotic lung responses to the inorganic dusts and fumes summarised in the preceding sections, other patterns of idiopathic pneumonia can be associated with the inhalation of synthetic fibres, particularly those that are generically categorised as flock. Flock is a powder-like material composed of very short fibres (0.2–5 mm) used in various industrial applications, including as a covering on adhesive-coated fabrics in order to produce a velvety surface. Flock is manufactured by cutting nylon, rayon, polyester and other synthetic fibres and filaments. There are two main flock cutting means employed. On is 'guillotine' cutting, which produces fibres of a precisely defined length and is the most common method use industrially. The second is 'rotary' cutting, which generates fibres of less-precisely defined length that may be more prone to the production of particles with adverse respiratory effects (Kern et al., 1998).

In retrospect, the initial case series of what was later recognised to be nylon flock workers' lung originated in a manufacturing plant in Ontario, Canada, where flock was produced using rotary cutters (Lougheed et al., 1995). That outbreak, however, was mis-attributed to mould exposure and pathologically classified as another idiopathic interstitial disease, desquamative interstitial pneumonia (DIP). Subsequent follow-up of this cohort in order to study the natural history of flock workers' lung

(Turcotte et al., 2013) found three main patterns after exposure cessation: complete resolution (of symptoms and radiographic and pulmonary function test abnormalities); stable persistence of symptoms and radiographic and pulmonary function test abnormalities; and a progressive decline in pulmonary function preceding death from respiratory failure and secondary pulmonary hypertension. Low baseline diffusing capacity (DL_{CO}), a marker of interstitial disease, was associated with the persistence and progression of disease.

Kern et al. (1998) described two cases of interstitial lung disease in a nylon flocking plant (Microfibres, Inc., in Rhode Island), which prompted a case-finding survey and retrospective cohort study. The index case, a 34 year old previously asymptomatic textile worker, developed work-related dyspnoea that initially resolved on holidays, then progressed over time to fixed exertional dyspnoea and chronic dry cough. Pulmonary function testing showed a moderate restrictive deficit and a reduced DL_{CO} (29% of predicted). Chest CT imaging showed diffuse, striking ground-glass opacities and patchy areas of consolidation, predominantly in the lower lobes. The patient was presumptively diagnosed with extrinsic alveolitis, removed from the work and treated with glucocorticosteroids to good effect. A second case, aged 28, who had worked at the same manufacturing plant, presented with chronic cough, dyspnoea and pleuritic chest pain. He also manifested with restrictive lung function, a reduced DL_{CO} and had a chest CT demonstrating diffuse micro-nodular densities and patchy, mild ground-glass opacities. Trans-bronchial biopsy revealed a dense lymphocytic infiltrate, and a subsequent open lung biopsy found diffuse interstitial lung disease characterised by bronchiolocentric nodular and diffuse interstitial fibrosis without granulomas. In this case, too, a presumptive diagnosis of extrinsic alveolitis was initially made.

These diagnoses were later revised in favour of a new entity: flock-related interstitial lung disease (flock workers' lung). When a case definition of abnormal BAL cellularity, restrictive lung function and chest CT showing diffuse ground-glass opacity or micro-nodularity was applied to current and former workers from the same plant, eight additional cases of flock workers' lung were identified. All improved with removal from further exposure. A further five cases, bringing the total to 19, were eventually reported (Kern et al., 2000). In a field investigation, the US National Institute for Occupational Safety and Health (NIOSH) identified the presence of respirable-sized nylon particulates in bulk samples of rotary-cut flock and in workroom air in this manufacturing process, consistent with inhalation of these fibres being causally related to the observed respiratory syndrome (Burkhart et al., 1999).

In addition to nylon-associated flock workers' lung, other similar outbreaks of disease have been linked to inhalational exposure to polypropylene, polyethylene and rayon synthetic textile fibres similarly cut into very fine particles using rotary cutters. This lends support to the presumption that the physical characteristics of synthetic fibre flock, rather than its chemical make-up, drive the pathophysiology of this condition.

Atis et al. (2005) carried out a cross-sectional study at a plant in Turkey comparing 50 polypropylene flock workers with 45 controls. Flock workers worked amidst visible clouds of dust for 8 hours per day, 6 days a week. They used rotary cutters in two small rooms with inadequate ventilation and they did not use respiratory-protective equipment. All workers with direct exposure to polypropylene flock ($n = 58$) were invited to participate and 50 agreed, forming the study group. Control group members were randomly sampled from workers at the plant who did not have direct exposure to polypropylene flock. Eligibility criteria required that the participants had worked in the same part of the factory for at least 3 years. All subjects completed a respiratory questionnaire and underwent a range of tests. Work-related respiratory symptoms were reported in 26% of the exposed subjects and in 13.3% of the controls, a difference that was not statistically significant. Logistic regression analysis showed that the risk of respiratory symptoms increased 3.6-fold in polypropylene flock workers when compared to controls (odds ratio: 3.6; 95% CI: 1.07–12.02). Multivariate analyses controlling for age, sex and tobacco use showed that being a worker in the polypropylene flock industry ($p = 0.001$) and the duration of work in years ($p = 0.03$) were predictive factors for impairment of pulmonary function. High-resolution CT scans (done in only ten participants) revealed diffuse ground-glass attenuation in two subjects, focal ground-glass appearance in one subject and bronchial thickening in four subjects. In addition to this cohort from Turkey, there has also been a separately reported case series from Spain of lung disease among polyethylene (as opposed to polypropylene) flock workers, showing CT abnormalities in three out of 15 workers and, in the most affected patient, follicular bronchiolitis on lung biopsy (Barroso et al., 2002).

Employee concern at a US plant using a greeting card manufacture process in which rayon flock was used prompted a cross-sectional survey that included an environmental evaluation, standardised questionnaire, spirometry, DL_{CO} testing and methacholine challenge testing (Antao et al., 2007). Of 239 completed questionnaires, 47 reported the cleaning of flocking equipment with compressed air (35 of these were also flock workers). Dust and fibre samples were largely below detection limits, but peaks were observed when cleaning with compressed air was carried out. Workers who cleaned for 1 or more hours per week using compressed air had a higher symptom prevalence of eye, nasal and throat irritation, sinus symptoms, chronic cough and medically diagnosed asthma. Although no statistically significant relationship was observed between flock exposure and spirometry results or methacholine challenge testing, the number of years of exposure to flock was significantly associated with abnormally low alveolar volume (VA).

DESQUAMATIVE INTERSTITIAL PNEUMONIA

DIP is characterised by the accumulation of numerous pigmented macrophages within the most distal air spaces of the lung and, sometimes, the presence of giant cells. DIP is usually associated with smoking, but is also recognised to occur in non-smokers, prompting further investigations into its causes (Godbert et al., 2013). Scanning electron microscopy and energy-dispersive X-ray analysis of 62 biopsy-proven cases of DIP found that tissue levels of inorganic particles were markedly higher in these cases than in controls (Abraham and Hertzberg, 1981).

Notably, a DIP-like pattern has been reported in association with several occupational exposures, but all at the case report level. Two cases have been reported in aluminium welders. One was a case of DIP in a 35 year old (Herbert et al., 1982) who presented with a 2-month history of exertional dyspnoea and a slight cough having worked as an electric arc welder for 16 years with exposure to aluminium, magnesium and other metal fumes. He manifested a restrictive pulmonary deficit in terms of a reduced DL_{CO} on lung function testing. Initially diagnosed with a pulmonary embolism, a subsequent lung biopsy showed diffuse chronic interstitial fibrosis, which was predominantly desquamative, but also had areas of patchy mural fibrosis. There were numerous intra-alveolar cells with abundant cytoplasm and vesicular nuclei containing refractive, but not birefringent brown particles that stained positive with Prussian blue. Transmission electron microscopy and energy-dispersive X-ray analysis showed substantial aluminium dust tissue burden. A second case was reported in a 57 year old aluminium welder with a 2-month history of progressive dyspnoea, dry cough, decreased exercise tolerance and hypoxia. For 5 years prior to presentation, he had worked as an aluminium welder, which involved grinding aluminium. A chest CT scan revealed bilateral ground-glass opacities in the upper- and mid-lung zones. Pulmonary function testing demonstrated a moderate restrictive ventilatory deficit with a severe impairment in DL_{CO}. Predominant macrophages were seen on BAL. The diagnosis of DIP was made on the basis of open lung biopsy (Chelvanathan et al., 2011). An association between occupational dust exposure and DIP has been also been observed in a drywall construction worker exposed to chrysotile asbestos fibres (Freed et al., 1991), and single cases have been reported following exposure to fire extinguisher powder, diesel fumes, beryllium and copper dust (Craig et al., 2004) and solder fume (Moon et al., 1999). A further case has been described in a 28 year old never-smoker who served in the US Navy and was involved in sanding ships for 18 months, but the specific exposure was not elucidated (Safdar and Mitchell, 2011). Although hard metal lung disease due to tungsten carbide–cobalt can have elements of desquamation, the hallmark of its pathology is the presence of giant cells. Because giant cell pneumonia is considered to be due to hard metal until proven otherwise, newer guidelines have removed this condition from consideration among otherwise idiopathic pneumonias, despite the fact that cases without apparent exposure to this causal agent have been reported (Blanc, 2007). Hard metal lung disease is discussed in greater depth elsewhere in this text.

As noted, DIP is usually associated with cigarette smoke exposure, and is along a histologic spectrum of responses that also includes respiratory bronchiolitis interstitial lung disease (RB-ILD). Both RB-ILD and DIP are characterised by macrophage accumulation, with the distinction between them dependent on the extent and distribution of this process (and also reflected by the pattern of disease on high-resolution computed tomography [HRCT]). In recent guidelines, the term 'smoking-related interstitial lung disease' has been used to refer to both of these conditions (Travis et al., 2013).

Despite the dominance of smoking for RB-ILD, a small number of cases due to occupational exposures—predominantly work-related second-hand smoking—have been reported. A clinicopathological review of ten specimens identified as having a histopathological pattern of RB-ILD (Moon et al., 1999) identified one case who was a never-smoker but who had occupational exposure to solder fume. This patient was a 35 year old female who had a high-resolution CT scan that favoured a diagnosis of DIP, a restrictive ventilatory defect and a reduced DL_{CO} (59% of predicted). A larger clinicopathological review of 109 specimens with a histopathological pattern of RB-ILD found two cases among apparent never-smokers (Fraig et al., 2002). One had substantial non-occupational second-hand smoke exposure, while the other (a 77 year old male who reported minimal exposure to smoking, having had only a 3 year history of intermittent smoking 54 years previously) reported a potentially significant occupational history, having worked as a mechanic in an environment with diesel fume and fiberglass dust. Another case of RB-ILD was reported in a 52 year old man with a 30-pack-year smoking history and a 40 year history of work repairing diesel engines (Canessa et al., 2004). The authors suggested that the patient's RB-ILD was due to both smoking and occupational exposure, but did not describe the occupational exposures in detail or provide evidence for such exposures being causal. Another case describes a 54 year old non-smoker with an 8 year history of heavy occupational exposure to second-hand cigarette smoke during her work as a waitress (Woo et al., 2007). A chest radiograph showed diffusely scattered small micronodules bilaterally, and a high-resolution CT scan showed evenly distributed ill-defined centrilobular nodules and ground-glass opacities throughout both lung fields. A lung biopsy was obtained, showing a respiratory bronchiolitis pattern with the accumulation of pigment-laden macrophages within the alveolar spaces, consistent with RB-ILD.

These case reports do not take away from the dominance of direct cigarette smoking in the aetiology of both DIP and RB-ILD. Nonetheless, they do raise the possibility that occupational factors can come into play and should be considered for both conditions.

OTHER UNUSUAL OCCUPATIONAL INTERSTITIAL LUNG DISEASES

Lipoid Pneumonia

Mineral oils are used in coolants, cutting oils or lubricants in several industrial processes and often give rise to respirable aerosolised mists. Although lipoid pneumonia is generally approached as being related to self-medication misadventure, work-related lipoid pneumonia due to mineral oil aerosols and related inhalation exposures is a well-established phenomenon.

Cullen et al. (1981) reported five out of nine tandem mill operators exposed to mineral oils being referred for evaluation of respiratory complaints prompting examination. Exercise studies revealed that the workers' exercise was limited by ventilation and arterial oxygen desaturation before reaching a submaximal heart rate, and bronchoscopy, lavage and biopsy revealed evidence of lipoid pneumonia. Assessment of the mill revealed levels of respirable oil mist as measured by personal samplers to be below the maximal acceptable levels and the authors speculated that an absence of similar case series may be due to either an unidentified peculiarity of the work process at that particular mill or workers voluntarily removing themselves from the workplace before the development of pronounced radiographic and functional changes.

At the case report level, lipoid pneumonia has been described for a variety of occupations in which oils are sprayed. A 59 year old workman is reported to have developed lipoid pneumonia after 5 years of massive exposure to aerosolised new car paraffin coating as a result of hot water cleaning using a compressed air jet in a small workshop without ventilation or respiratory-protective equipment (Pujol et al., 1990). A chest CT showed diffuse interstitial disease; trans-bronchial biopsy showed mixed alveolitis, including alveolar macrophages with abnormal cytoplasmic vacuoles. An open lung biopsy was performed, showing interstitial pneumonitis with fibrosis with electron microscopy, demonstrating alveolar macrophages with features of paraffin-laden cytoplasmic vacuoles. Cases of occupational lipoid pneumonia have also been reported in professional painters as a consequence of workplace exposure to paraffins and oily sprays, including oil entrained in an air-supplied respirator (Carby and Smith, 2000; Abad Fernandez et al., 2003). Other reports of occupational lipoid pneumonia include a cash register repairman with a 17 year history of regularly spraying machines for lubrication with a naphtha solvent and later a grade-10 liquid petrolatum (Proudfit et al., 1950) and a 30 year old aircraft mechanic developing lipoid pneumonia after employing the use of a spray to clean aircraft engines that was composed of one-half kerosene and one-half cleansing agent, which was composed of 50% vegetable oil soap (Foe and Bigham, 1954).

Finally, a 24 year old developing lipid pneumonia not as a result of oil being sprayed, but following inhalation of burning fat fume has been reported (Oldenburger et al., 1972). Another oil combustion product inhalation scenario has been described as a cause of dendriform pulmonary ossification in three patients, two of whom were exposed occupationally (Martinez and Ramos, 2008). (This rare pathological response was noted earlier in the context of rare earth pneumoconiosis.) The first hydrocarbon-exposed patient worked for 2 years burning hospital waste in an incineration oven, where he was exposed to diesel oil fume in an environment with limited ventilation. The patient did not have respiratory symptoms at the time, but 22 years after the end of exposure, radiographic changes were detected. The second patient had a history of sleeping for 4 hours every other night inside a turned-off metallurgy oven for 8 months. The oven used kerosene as a combustion fuel. Fifteen years after the end of exposure, the patient developed wheezing episodes that were initially treated as asthma, until chest CT findings led to a biopsy and tissue diagnosis.

Airway-Centred Interstitial Fibrosis

Airway-centred interstitial fibrosis is a rare histopathological pattern that has been described in small retrospective case series. The initial case series of this entity (Yousem and Dacic, 2002) reported ten patients with a similar histological appearance to hypersensitivity pneumonitis, but without interstitial granulomas, who had a striking centrilobular and bronchiolocentric concentration of chronic inflammatory cell infiltrates. No identifiable cause could be found for the cases and, at a mean follow-up of 4 years, a third had died from their respiratory disease, and over half had persistent or progressive disease, suggesting a more aggressive disease process than hypersensitivity pneumonitis. A later series (Churg et al., 2004) described 12 patients with small airway-centred interstitial fibrosis. The histopathology differed from the original series in terms of fibrosis around the large airways and microscopic evidence of fibrosis around the small airways, suggesting interstitial fibrosis, also being present. The patients presented with chronic cough and progressive dyspnoea. Seven of the patients were never-smokers, and eight had possible occupational or environmental exposures, including to wood smoke, birds, cotton or chalk dust. Chest radiographs for the patients were always abnormal, and the most common pattern seen was diffuse reticulonodular infiltrates with central predominance, thickening of the bronchial walls and small central ring shadows. CT scans were available in five patients, and the main abnormalities seen were peri-bronchovascular interstitial thickening and traction bronchiectasis with thickened airway walls and surrounding fibrosis.

A further single case of airway-centred interstitial fibrosis in a patient with exposure to cleaning product has been reported (Serrano et al., 2006). A 51 year old cleaner presented to the outpatient department of a Spanish hospital with dry cough and progressive dyspnoea. A chest radiograph showed a basal reticulonodular shadowing pattern. Lung function testing showed a restrictive ventilatory defect and diffusing capacity was reduced (47% predicted). The patient was an ex-smoker with a 10-pack-year history, as well as multiple medical comorbidities. In her work as a cleaner, she washed floors in a poorly ventilated area over a 4 year period using a cleaning solution that contained 25% hydrochloric acid, 55% sodium hydroxide (pH 14), surfactants and glycols. Despite treatment with high-dose glucocorticosteroids, she had a progressive decline in her forced vital capacity and diffusing capacity.

Eosinophilic Pneumonia

Shorr et al. (2004) reported a case series of patients with acute eosinophilic pneumonia (AEP). Eighteen patients were identified among 183,000 military personnel deployed in or near Iraq during the 13-month study period of March 2003 to March 2004. The case definition required patients to report a febrile illness followed by the development of respiratory symptoms such as cough, dyspnoea or both. Symptoms had to be present for less than 1 month and the patient had to have infiltrates on chest radiograph. Patients with evidence of pulmonary eosinophilia based on either BAL or lung biopsy were classified as definite cases of AEP (n = 7). Patients who did not undergo BAL or biopsy, but who developed peripheral eosinophilia (total eosinophil count >250 cells × 10^3/mL; percentage of eosinophils ≥10% of differential cell count) were categorised as probable cases of AEP (n = 11). All cases were extensively investigated for parasite infection and other infective pathologies, as well as autoimmune conditions associated with pulmonary eosinophilia. Two patients died. A standardised questionnaire was administered to cases and a sample of 72 controls. Controls were military personal without AEP recruited from the respective military units of the two patients who had died. All cases used tobacco, with 78% recently beginning to smoke. All but one reported significant exposure to fine airborne sand or dust. Compared with the control group, a higher proportion of cases smoked (100% vs. 67%) and had recently started smoking (78% vs. 3%). Fine airborne sand or dust exposure was similar between the two groups (94% vs. 97%). The authors speculated that the combination of new-onset smoking and dust exposure may have been causative. A second case series of 44 military personnel with AEP associated with smoking has also been reported (Sine et al., 2011). In addition, AEP has also been reported in conjunction with smoking and firework fume inhalation (Hirai et al., 2000), indoor renovation work, gasoline tank cleaning, explosion of a tear gas bomb (Philit et al., 2002) and in a fireman with exposure to high concentrations of dust from the World Trade Center during rescue efforts following the 11 September 2001, terrorist attack (Rom et al., 2002).

Anthracofibrosis

Anthracofibrosis is defined as narrowing of the bronchial lumen associated with black pigmentation (anthracosis) of the overlying mucosa. It is typically seen in the presence of active tuberculosis (TB) infection and the absence of pneumoconiosis. Several case series, however, have described anthracofibrosis occurring in the absence of TB in patients with occupational and environmental dust exposures. In one report (Naccache et al., 2008), three cases of anthracofibrosis occurred in patients with no exposure to TB. Based on occupational histories and mineralogical microanalysis using transmission electron microscopy, the authors attributed this to mixed mineral dusts containing free crystalline silica and other silicate exposures. One of the patients was previously a forklift driver at a foundry and a solderer at a metallurgy plant with exposure to aluminium and silica, one was a bricklayer with silica and asphalt exposure and one was a stonemason with silica exposure. Wynn et al. (2008) reported a series of seven patients who all presented in a manner that raised the suspicion of lung cancer, prompting bronchoscopy and subsequent diagnosis of anthracofibrosis. Six of the seven cases had no exposure to TB, but did potentially have causal occupational exposures. Three patients were exposed to tile dust, and of these, two worked at a tile-making factory and one was a tiler. Two had previously worked as coal miners and one had been exposed to asbestos, coal and flour dust in his work as an engineer. Sigari and Mohammadi (2009) report a series of 487 patients in Iran with anthracosis and 291 with anthracofibrosis. Almost half of the patients were female non-smokers, and it was suggested that the condition was mostly caused by domestic wood fires used for cooking (which can be considered a non-salaried occupational exposure). Male patients included farmers, manual workers, miners and bakers. Kim et al. (2009) describe 333 patients in Korea with anthracofibrosis diagnosed between 1998 and 2004, of which two-thirds had no exposure to pulmonary TB. All patients had long-term exposure to biomass smoke, all male patients were farmers and all female patients were housewives (again, relevant to non-salaried employment).

Non-Specific Interstitial Pneumonia and Acute Lymphocytic Pneumonia

Occupationally associated non-specific interstitial pneumonia (NSIP) has been described in two case reports. The first was a 50 year old smoker (20-pack-year history) and curry sauce factory worker with a 13 year history of exposure to curry powder dust containing a mix of ground spices and pepper (Ando et al., 2006). Chest CT revealed multiple irregular consolidations, along with bronchovascular bundles and biapical cystic airspaces. A lung biopsy showed a cellular and fibrosing NSIP pattern. Lymphocyte stimulation tests using the patient's peripheral blood lymphocytes were positive for curry powder, ground black pepper and ground white pepper, which were used at the factory. The patient was treated with azathioprine and prednisolone, but went on to develop bilateral pneumothoraces and succumbed due to ventilatory failure. The second case report was of a 62 year old hospital pharmacist with clozapine dust exposure as a result of crushing up to 5000 clozapine tablets per month in a small, poorly ventilated room. Symptoms and radiological signs resolved fully with cessation of exposure (Lewis et al., 2012). There has been only a single case report of what was categorised as 'acute lymphocytic pneumonia' (Schauble and Rich, 1994), involving a 36 year old asymptomatic crematorium worker with 6 years of heavy dust exposure on the job, who participated in a research programme as a healthy volunteer and was incidentally found to have lymphocytosis on BAL.

NANOPARTICLES

It is appropriate to conclude with consideration of engineered nanoparticles, since this relatively new group of occupational exposures has raised considerable concern over potential adverse respiratory tract effects. Longstanding sources of very fine particles that are by-products of industrial processes rather than intentionally engineered materials are capable of causing a number of adverse respiratory effects; for example, welding fumes. Moreover, there are animal experimental models in which certain classes of engineered nanoparticles (particularly nanotubules) can induce pulmonary pathological changes. In contradistinction to these experimental animal data, the human experience to date, even at the case report level, has not implicated novel, engineered nanoparticles in the causation of any of the interstitial lung diseases we have considered in the preceding sections. A widely cited case series of seven female factory workers in China with heavy exposure to nanoparticles of a polycrylic ester linked to pleural effusions has been raised as being the first report of such an effect (Song et al., 2009). In this case series, lung biopsy analysis (available for two of the seven workers) showed non-specific pulmonary inflammation and pleural foreign-body granulomas. Transmission electron microscopy demonstrated the presence of nanoparticles in the cytoplasm and nucleoplasm of pulmonary epithelial and mesothelial cells. The predominant site of pathophysiological effect was the pleura. Although this episode of toxic nanoparticle pleuritis does not fit well into any of the categories of unusual interstitial disease that we have addressed, this outbreak nonetheless reminds us that we must remain vigilant for emerging occupational associations with respiratory diseases across a wide spectrum of conditions. The label of 'idiopathic' should never be taken at face value.

REFERENCES

Abad Fernández, A., de Miguel Díez, J., López Vime, R., Gómez Santos, D., Nájera Botello, L. and Jara Chinarro, B. 2003. Lipoid pneumonia related to workplace exposure to paint. *Arch Bronconeumol* 39(3):133–5.

Abraham, J. L. and Hertzberg, M. A. 1981. Inorganic particulates associated with desquamative interstitial pneumonia. *Chest*,80(1 Suppl.):67–70.

Alleman, T. and Darcey, D. J. 2002. Case report: Bronchiolitis obliterans organizing pneumonia in a spice process technician. *J Occup Environ Med* 44(3):215–6.

Ando, S., Arai, T., Inoue, Y., Kitaichi, M. and Sakatani, M. 2006. NSIP in a curry sauce factory worker. *Thorax* 61(11):1012–3.

Antao, V. C. S., Piacitelli, C. A., Miller, W. E., Pinheiro, G. A. and Kreiss, K. 2007. Rayon flock: A new cause of respiratory morbidity in a card processing plant. *Am J Ind Med* 50(4):274–84.

Atis, S., Tutluoglu, B., Levent, E., Ozturk, C., Tunaci, A., Sahin, K., Saral, A. et al. 2005. The respiratory effects of occupational polypropylene flock exposure. *Eur Respir J* 25(1):110–7.

Awadalla, N. J., Hegazy, A., Elmetwally, R. A. and Wahby, I. 2012. Occupational and environmental risk factors for idiopathic pulmonary fibrosis in Egypt: A multicenter case–control study. *Int J Occup Environ Med* 3(3):107–16.

Barroso, E., Ibáñez, M. D., Aranda, F. I. and Romero, S. 2002. Polyethylene flock-associated interstitial lung disease in a Spanish female. *Eur Respir J* 20(6):1610–2.

Baumgartner, K. B., Samet, J. M., Coultas, D. B., Stidley, C. A., Hunt, W. C., Colby, T. V. and Waldron, J. A. 2000. Occupational and environmental risk factors for idiopathic pulmonary fibrosis: A multicenter case–control study. Collaborating centers. *Am J Epidemiol* 152(4):307–15.

Blanc, P. D. 2007. Is giant cell interstitial pneumonitis synonymous with hard metal lung disease? *Am J Respir Crit Care Med* 176(8):834; author reply 834–5.

Bradley, B., Branley, H. M., Egan, J. J., Greaves, M. S., Hansell, D. M., Harrison, N. K., Hirani, N. et al. 2008. Interstitial lung disease guideline: The British Thoracic Society in collaboration with the Thoracic Society of Australia and New Zealand and the Irish Thoracic Society. *Thorax* 63(Suppl. 5):v1–58.

Burkhart, J., Piacitelli, C., Schwegler-Berry, D. and Jones, W. 1999. Environmental study of nylon flocking process. *J Toxicol Environ Health A* 57(1):1–23.

Canessa, P. A., Prattic, L., Bancalari, L., Fedeli, F., Bacigalupo, B. and Silvano, S. 2004. Respiratory bronchiolitis associated with interstitial lung disease. *Monaldi Arch Chest Dis* 61(3):174–6.

Carby, M. and Smith, S. R. 2000. A hazard of paint spraying. *Lancet* 355(9207):896.

Chelvanathan, A., Drost, N. and Cutz, J.-C. 2011. Desquamative interstitial pneumonia in an aluminum welder: A case report (Abstract). *Chest* 140(4 Meeting Abstracts):129A.

Cheng, T.-H., Ko, F.-C., Chang, J.-L. and Wu, K.-A. 2012. Bronchiolitis obliterans organizing pneumonia due to titanium nanoparticles in paint. *Ann Thorac Surg* 93(2):666–9.

Chonan, T. and Taguchi, O. 2004. The incidence of interstitial pneumonia patients in an ITO sputtering targets producing factory. *Nihon Kokyuki Gakkai Zasshi* 42:185.

Churg, A., Myers, J., Suarez, T., Gaxiola, M., Estrada, A., Mejia, M. and Selman, M. 2004. Airway-centered interstitial fibrosis: A distinct form of aggressive diffuse lung disease. *Am J Surg Pathol* 28(1):62–8.

Cordier, J. F. 2000. Organising pneumonia. *Thorax* 55(4):318–28.

Craig, P. J., Wells, A. U., Doffman, S., Rassl, D., Colby, T. V., Hansell, D. M., Bois, R. M. D. et al. G. 2004. Desquamative interstitial pneumonia, respiratory bronchiolitis and their relationship to smoking. *Histopathology* 45(3):275–82.

Cullen, M. R., Balmes, J. R., Robins, J. M. and Smith, G. J. 1981. Lipoid pneumonia caused by oil mist exposure from a steel rolling tandem mill. *Am J Ind Med* 2(1):51–8.

Cummings, K. J., Donat, W. E., Ettensohn, D. B., Roggli, V. L., Ingram, P. and Kreiss, K. 2010. Pulmonary alveolar proteinosis in workers at an indium processing facility. *Am J Respir Crit Care Med* 181(5):458–64.

Cummings, K. J., Nakano, M., Omae, K., Takeuchi, K., Chonan, T., Long Xiao, Y., Harley, R. A. et al. 2012. Indium lung disease. *Chest* 141(6):1512–21.

Cummings, K. J., Suarthana, E., Edwards, N., Liang, X., Stanton, M. L., Day, G. A., Saito, R. et al. 2013. Serial evaluations at an indium–tin oxide production facility. *Am J Ind Med* 56(3):300–7.

Doujaiji, B. and Al-Tawfiq, J. A. 2010. Hydrogen sulfide exposure in an adult male. *Ann Saudi Med* 30(1):76 80.

Ekstrom, M., Gustafson, T., Boman, K., Nilsson, K., Tornling, G., Murgia, N. and Torén, K. 2014. Effects of smoking, gender and occupational exposure on the risk of severe pulmonary fibrosis: A population-based case–control study. *BMJ Open* 4(1):e004018.

Foe, R. B. and Bigham, R. S. 1954. Lipid pneumonia following occupational exposure to oil spray. *J Am Med Assoc* 155(1):33–4.

Fraig, M., Shreesha, U., Savici, D. and Katzenstein, A.-L. A. 2002. Respiratory bronchiolitis: A clinicopathologic study in current smokers, ex-smokers, and never-smokers. *Am J Surg Pathol* 26(5):647–53.

Freed, J. A., Miller, A., Gordon, R. E., Fischbein, A., Kleinerman, J. and Langer, A. M. 1991. Desquamative interstitial pneumonia associated with chrysotile asbestos fibres. *Br J Ind Med* 48(5):332–7.

Gannon, P. and Rickard, R. W. 2015 Pulmonary fibrosis associated with aluminum trihydrate (Corian) dust (Letter; 'Dupont, the manufacturer of Coauan, replies'). *N Engl J Med* 371: 2156–7.

García-Sancho Figueroa, M. C., Carrillo, G., Pérez-Padilla, R., Fernández-Plata, M. R., Buendía-Roldán, I., Vargas, M. H. and Selman, M. 2010. Risk factors for idiopathic pulmonary fibrosis in a Mexican population. A case–control study. *Respir Med* 104(2):305–9.

Godbert, B., Wissler, M.-P. and Vignaud, J.-M. 2013. Desquamative interstitial pneumonia: An analytic review with an emphasis on aetiology. *Eur Respir Rev* 22(128):117–23.

Gustafson, T., Dahlman-Höglund, A., Nilsson, K., Ström, K., Tornling, G. and Torén, K. 2007. Occupational exposure and severe pulmonary fibrosis. *Respir Med* 101(10):2207–12.

Herbert, A., Sterling, G., Abraham, J. and Corrin, B. 1982. Desquamative interstitial pneumonia in an aluminum welder. *Hum Pathol* 13(8):694–9.

Heuck, F. and Hoschek, R. 1968. Cer-pneumoconiosis. *Am J Roentgenol Radium Ther Nucl Med* 104(4):777–83.

Hirai, K., Yamazaki, Y., Okada, K., Furuta, S. and Kubo, K. 2000. Acute eosinophilic pneumonia associated with smoke from fireworks. *Intern Med* 39(5):401–3.

Hoet, P. H., Gilissen, L. P., Leyva, M. and Nemery, B. 1999. *In vitro* cytotoxicity of textile paint components linked to the 'ardystil syndrome'. *Toxicol Sci* 52(2):209–16.

Homma, S., Miyamoto, A., Sakamoto, S., Kishi, K., Motoi, N. and Yoshimura, K. 2005. Pulmonary fibrosis in an individual occupationally exposed to inhaled indium–tin oxide. *Eur Respir J* 25(1):200–4.

Homma, T., Ueno, T., Sekizawa, K., Tanaka, A. and Hirata, M. 2003. Interstitial pneumonia developed in a worker dealing with particles containing indium–tin oxide. *J Occup Health* 45(3):137–9.

Hubbard, R., Cooper, M., Antoniak, M., Venn, A., Khan, S., Johnston, I., Lewis, S. et al. 2000. Risk of cryptogenic fibrosing alveolitis in metal workers. *Lancet* 355(9202):466–7.

Hubbard, R., Lewis, S., Richards, K., Britton, J. and Johnston, I. 1996. Occupational exposure to metal or wood dust and aetiology of cryptogenic fibrosing alveolitis. *Lancet* 347(8997):284–9.

Husain, M. H., Dick, J. A. and Kaplan, Y. S. 1980. Rare earth pneumoconiosis. *J Soc Occup Med* 30(1):15–9.

Iwai, K., Mori, T., Yamada, N., Yamaguchi, M. and Hosoda, Y. 1994. Idiopathic pulmonary fibrosis. Epidemiologic approaches to occupational exposure. *Am J Respir Crit Care Med* 150(3):670–5.

Jederlinic, P. J., Abraham, J. L., Churg, A., Himmelstein, J. S., Epler, G. R. and Gaensler, E. A. 1990. Pulmonary fibrosis in aluminum oxide workers. Investigation of nine workers, with pathologic examination and microanalysis in three of them. *Am Rev Respir Dis* 142(5):1179–84.

Kern, D. G., Crausman, R. S., Durand, K. T., Nayer, A. and Kuhn, C. 1998. Flock worker's lung: Chronic interstitial lung disease in the nylon flocking industry. *Ann Intern Med* 129(4):261–72.

Kern, D. G., Kuhn, C., Ely, E. W., Pransky, G. S., Mello, C. J., Fraire, A. E. and Mller, J. 2000. Flock worker's lung: Broadening the spectrum of clinicopathology, narrowing the spectrum of suspected etiologies. *Chest* 117(1):251–9.

Kern, R. M., Singer, J. P., Koth, L., Mooney, J., Golden, J., Hays, S., Greenland, J. et al. 2015. Lung transplantation for hypersensitivity pneumonitis. *Chest* 147(6):1558–65.

Kim, Y. J., Jung, C. Y., Shin, H. W. and Lee, B. K. 2009. Biomass smoke induced bronchial anthracofibrosis: Presenting features and clinical course. *Respir Med* 103(5):757–65.

Le Magrex, L. 1979. Pneumoconiose et cerium [Pneumoconiosis and cerium]. *Arch Malad Prof* 40:1–2.

Lewis, A., Gibbs, A. and Hope-Gill, B. 2012. Probable occupational pneumonitis caused by inhalation of crushed clozapine. *Occup Med (Lond)* 62(5):385–7.

Lison, D. and Delos, M. 2010. Pulmonary alveolar proteinosis in workers at an indium processing facility. *Am J Respir Crit Care Med* 182(4):578; author reply 578–9.

Lison, D., Laloy, J., Corazzari, I., Muller, J., Rabolli, V., Panin, N., Huaux, F. et al. 2009. Sintered indium–tin-oxide (ITO) particles: A new pneumotoxic entity. *Toxicol Sci* 108(2):472–81.

Lougheed, M. D., Roos, J. O., Waddell, W. R. and Munt, P. W. 1995. Desquamative interstitial pneumonitis and diffuse alveolar damage in textile workers. Potential role of mycotoxins. *Chest* 108(5):1196–200.

Martinez, J. A. B. and Ramos, S. G. 2008. Inhalation of hydrocarbon combustion products as a cause of dendriform pulmonary ossification. *Med Hypotheses* 71(6):981–2.

McDonald, J. W., Ghio, A. J., Sheehan, C. E., Bernhardt, P. F. and Roggli, V. L. 1995. Rare earth (cerium oxide) pneumoconiosis: Analytical scanning electron microscopy and literature review. *Mod Pathol* 8(8):859–65.

McKeever, R., Okaneku, J. and LaSala, G. S. 2015. More on pulmonary fibrosis associated with aluminum trihydrate (Corian) dust (Letter). *N Engl J Med* 371:973.

Miyake, Y., Sasaki, S., Yokoyama, T., Chida, K., Azuma, A., Suda, T., Kudoh, S. et al. 2005. Occupational and environmental factors and idiopathic pulmonary fibrosis in Japan. *Ann Occup Hyg* 49(3):259–65.

Monso, E., Tura, J., Pujadas, J., Morell, F., Ruiz, J. and Morera, J. 1991. Lung dust content in idiopathic pulmonary fibrosis: A study with scanning electron microscopy and energy dispersive X ray analysis. *Br J Ind Med* 48(5):327–31.

Moon, J., du Bois, R. M., Colby, T. V., Hansell, D. M. and Nicholson, A. G. 1999. Clinical significance of respiratory bronchiolitis on open lung biopsy and its relationship to smoking related interstitial lung disease. *Thorax* 54(11):1009–14.

Morell, F., Villar, A., Montero, M. Á., Muoz, X., Colby, T. V., Pipvath, S., Cruz, M.-J. et al. 2013. Chronic hypersensitivity pneumonitis in patients diagnosed with idiopathic pulmonary fibrosis: A prospective case–cohort study. *Lancet Respir Med* 1(9):685–94.

Moya, C., Anto, J. M. and Newman Taylor, A. J. 1994. Outbreak of organising pneumonia in textile printing sprayers. Collaborative Group for the Study of Toxicity in Textile Aerographic Factories. *Lancet* 344(8921):498–502.

Mullen, J., Hodgson, M. J., DeGraff, C. A. and Godar, T. 1998. Case–control study of idiopathic pulmonary fibrosis and environmental exposures. *J Occup Environ Med* 40(4):363–7.

Naccache, J.-M., Monnet, I., Nunes, H., Billon-Galland, M.-A., Pairon, J.-C., Guillon, F. and Valeyre, D. 2008. Anthracofibrosis attributed to mixed mineral dust exposure: Report of three cases. *Thorax* 63(7):655–7.

Nappée, J., Bobrie, J. and Lambard, D. 1972. Pneumoconiose au cerium [Pneumoconiosis due to cerium]. *Arch Mal Prof* 33(1):13–8.

Nemery, B. and Hoet, P. H. 2015. Humidifier disinfectant-associated interstitial lung disease and the Ardystil syndrome. *Am J Respir Crit Care Med* 191(1):116–7.

Newman, L. S., Mroz, M. M. and Ruttenber, A. J. 2005. Lung fibrosis in plutonium workers. *Radiat Res* 164(2):123–31.

Oldenburger, D., Maurer, W. J., Beltaos, E. and Magnin, G. E. 1972. Inhalation lipoid pneumonia from burning fats. A newly recognized industrial hazard. *JAMA* 222(10):1288–9.

Omae, K., Nakano, M., Tanaka, A., Hirata, M., Hamaguchi, T. and Chonan, T. 2011. Indium lung—Case reports and epidemiology. *Int Arch Occup Environ Health* 84(5):471–7.

Ould Kadi, F., Mohammed-Brahim, B., Fyad, A., Lellou, S. and Nemery, B. 1994. Outbreak of pulmonary disease in textile dye sprayers in Algeria. *Lancet* 344(8927):962–3.

Pairon, J. C., Roos, F., Iwatsubo, Y., Janson, X., Billon-Galland, M. A., Bignon, J. and Brochard, P. 1994. Lung retention of cerium in humans. *Occup Environ Med* 51(3):195–9.

Pairon, J. C., Roos, F., Sébastien, P., Chamak, B., Abd-Alsamad, I., Bernaudin, J. F., Bignon, J. et al. 1995. Biopersistence of cerium in the human respiratory tract and ultrastructural findings. *Am J Ind Med* 27(3):349–58.

Philit, F., Etienne-Mastroïanni, B., Parrot, A., Guérin, C., Robert, D. and Cordier, J.-F. 2002. Idiopathic acute eosinophilic pneumonia: A study of 22 patients. *Am J Respir Crit Care Med* 166(9):1235–9.

Pinheiro, G. A., Antao, V. C., Wood, J. M. and Wassell, J. T. 2008. Occupational risks for idiopathic pulmonary fibrosis mortality in the United States. *Int J Occup Environ Health* 14(2):117–23.

Porru, S., Placidi, D., Quarta, C., Sabbioni, E., Pietra, R. and Fortaner, S. 2001. The potential role of rare earths in the pathogenesis of interstitial lung disease: A case report of movie projectionist as investigated by neutron activation analysis. *J Trace Elem Med Biol* 14(4):232–6.

Proudfit, J. P., Van Ordstrand, H. S. and Miller, C. W. 1950. Chronic lipid pneumonia following occupational exposure. *Arch Ind Hyg Occup Med* 1(1):105–11.

Pujol, J. L., Barnon, G., Bousquet, J., Michel, F. B. and Godard, P. 1990. Interstitial pulmonary disease induced by occupational exposure to paraffin. *Chest* 97(1):234–6.

Raghu G., Collins, B. F., Xia, D., Schmidt, R. and Abraham, J. L. 2015a. Pulmonary fibrosis associated with aluminum trihydrate (Corian) dust (Letter). *N Engl J Med* 371:2154–6.

Raghu, G., Xia, D. and Abraham, J. L. 2015b. More on pulmonary fibrosis associated with aluminum trihydrate (Corian) dust (Letter). *N Engl J Med* 371:973–4.

Ribeiro, P. A., Giro, F. and Henriques, P. 2011. A rich and blessed professional illness—Organizing pneumonia due to gold dust. *Rev Port Pneumol* 17(4):182–5.

Rom, W. N., Weiden, M., Garcia, R., Yie, T. A., Vathesatogkit, P., Tse, D. B., McGuinness, G. et al. 2002. Acute eosinophilic pneumonia in a New York City firefighter exposed to World Trade Center dust. *Am J Respir Crit Care Med* 166(6):797–800.

Sabbioni, E., Pietra, R., Gaglione, P., Vocaturo, G., Colombo, F., Zanoni, M. and Rodi, F. 1982. Long-term occupational risk of rare-earth pneumoconiosis. A case report as investigated by neutron activation analysis. *Sci Total Environ* 26(1):19–32.

Safdar, M. and Mitchell, J. L. J. B. 2011. Smoking related lung disease in a non-smoker. *Am J Respir Crit Care Med* 183:A5663.

Sanchez-Ortiz, M., Cruz, M., Viladrich, M., Morell, F. and Muñoz, X. 2011. Cryptogenic organizing pneumonia due to ortho-phenylenediamine. *Respir Med CME* 4(4):164–5.

Schauble, T. L. and Rich, E. A. 1994. Lymphocytic alveolitis in a crematorium worker. *Chest* 105(2):617–9.

Scott, J., Johnston, I. and Britton, J. 1990. What causes cryptogenic fibrosing alveolitis? A case–control study of environmental exposure to dust. *BMJ* 301(6759): 1015–7.

Serrano, M., Molina-Molina, M., Ramrez, J., Snchez, M. and Xaubet, A. 2006. Airway-centered interstitial fibrosis related to exposure to fumes from cleaning products. *Arch Bronconeumol* 42(10):557–9.

Sheu, B.-F., Lee, C.-C., Young, Y.-R., Li, L.-F. and Chang, S.-S. 2008. Delayed-onset bronchiolitis obliterans with organising pneumonia associated with massive acetic acid steam inhalation. *Thorax* 63(6):570.

Shorr, A. F., Scoville, S. L., Cersovsky, S. B., Shanks, G. D., Ockenhouse, C. F., Smoak, B. L., Carr, W. W. et al. 2004. Acute eosinophilic pneumonia among us military personnel deployed in or near Iraq. *JAMA* 292(24):2997–3005.

Sigari, N. and Mohammadi, S. 2009. Anthracosis and anthracofibrosis. *Saudi Med J* 30(8):1063–6.

Sine, C., Allan, P., Haynes, R., Scoville, S., Shuping, E., Hultman, A. and Osborn, E. 2011. Case series of 44 patients with idiopathic acute eosinophilic pneumonia in the deployed military setting (Abstract). *Chest* 140(4):675A.

Song, Y., Li, X. and Du, X. 2009. Exposure to nanoparticles is related to pleural effusion, pulmonary fibrosis and granuloma. *Eur Respir J* 34(3):559–67.

Stefano, F. D., Verna, N., Giampaolo, L. D., Boscolo, P. and Gioacchino, M. D. 2003. Cavitating BOOP associated with myeloperoxidase deficiency in a floor cleaner with an incidental heavy exposure to benzalkonium compounds. *J Occup Health* 45(3):182–4.

Sulotto, F., Romano, C., Berra, A., Botta, G. C., Rubino, G. F., Sabbioni, E. and Pietra, R. 1986. Rare-earth pneumoconiosis: A new case. *Am J Ind Med* 9(6):567–5.

Tanaka, A., Hirata, M., Homma, T. and Kiyohara, Y. 2010. Chronic pulmonary toxicity study of indium–tin oxide and indium oxide following intratracheal instillations into the lungs of hamsters. *J Occup Health* 52(1):14–22.

Taskar, V. S. and Coultas, D. B. 2006. Is idiopathic pulmonary fibrosis an environmental disease? *Proc Am Thorac Soc* 3(4):293–8.

Tomioka, R. and King, T. Jr. 1997. Gold-induced pulmonary disease: Clinical features, outcome, and differentiation from rheumatoid lung disease. *Am J Respir Crit Care Med* 155(3):1011–20.

Travis, W. D., Costabel, U., Hansell, D. M., King, T. E. Jr., Lynch, D. A., Nicholson, A. G., Ryerson, C. J. et al. 2013. An official American Thoracic Society/European Respiratory Society statement: Update of the international multidisciplinary classification of the idiopathic interstitial pneumonias. *Am J Respir Crit Care Med* 188(6):733–48.

Turcotte, S. E., Chee, A., Walsh, R., Grant, F. C., Liss, G. M., Boag, A., Forkert, L. et al. 2013. Flock worker's lung disease: Natural history of cases and exposed workers in Kingston, Ontario. *Chest* 143(6):1642–8.

Vocaturo, G., Colombo, F., Zanoni, M., Rodi, F., Sabbioni, E. and Pietra, R. 1983. Human exposure to heavy metals. Rare earth pneumoconiosis in occupational workers. *Chest* 83(5):780–3.

Vogt, P., Spycher, M. A. and Rü ttner, J. R. 1986. Pneumokoniose durch 'Seltene Erden' (Cer-Pneumokoniose). [Pneumoconiosis caused by 'rare earths' (cer-pneumoconiosis)]. *Schweiz Med Wochenschr* 116(38):1303–8.

Waring, P. M. and Watling, R. J. 1990. Rare earth deposits in a deceased movie projectionist. A new case of rare earth pneumoconiosis? *Med J Aust* 153(11–12):726–30.

Woo, O. H., Yong, H. S., Oh, Y.-W., Lee, S. Y., Kim, H. K. and Kang, E.-Y. 2007. Respiratory bronchiolitis-associated interstitial lung disease in a nonsmoker: Radiologic and pathologic findings. *AJR Am J Roentgenol* 188(5):W412–4.

Wynn, G. J., Turkington, P. M. and O'Driscoll, B. R. 2008. Anthracofibrosis, bronchial stenosis with overlying anthracotic mucosa: Possibly a new occupational lung disorder: A series of seven cases from one UK hospital. *Chest* 134(5):1069–73.

Xiao, YL, Cai, H. R., Wang, Y. H., Meng, F. Q. and Zhang, D. P. 2010. Pulmonary alveolar proteinosis in an indium-processing worker. *Chin Med J (Engl)* 123(10): 1347–50.

Yoon, H. K., Moon, H. S., Park, S. H., Song, J. S., Lim, Y. and Kohyama, N. 2005. Dendriform pulmonary ossification in patient with rare earth pneumoconiosis. *Thorax* 60(8):701–3.

Yousem, S. A. and Dacic, S. 2002. Idiopathic bronchiolocentric interstitial pneumonia. *Mod Pathol* 15(11):1148–53.

26 Work-Related Asthma
Occupational Asthma and Work-Exacerbated Disease

Olivier Vandenplas and Hille Suojalehto

CONTENTS

INTRODUCTION

The term 'work-related asthma' (WRA) encompasses occupational asthma (OA), which is asthma caused by a specific agent at the workplace, and work-exacerbated asthma (WEA), which describes pre-existing or coincident asthma exacerbated by non-specific stimuli at the workplace (Malo and Vandenplas, 2011). The American College of Chest Physicians has proposed the following definition of OA (Tarlo et al., 2008):

> Occupational asthma refers to de novo asthma or the recurrence of previously quiescent asthma … induced by either sensitization to a specific substance (e.g. an inhaled protein [high-molecular-weight (HMW) protein of more than 10 kDa] or a chemical at work [low-molecular-weight (LMW) agent]), which is termed sensitizer-induced OA [or 'immunologic/allergic OA' or 'OA with latency'], or by exposure to an inhaled irritant at work, which is termed irritant-induced OA [or 'non-immunologic/non-allergic OA' or 'OA without latency'].

SENSITIZER-INDUCED ASTHMA

Epidemiology

Estimates of the frequency of OA have been derived from cross-sectional and longitudinal studies of high-risk workforces, occupational disease registries, voluntary notification programmes and population-based surveys. A pooled analysis of data published up to 2007 indicated that 17.6% of all adult-onset asthma is attributable to workplace exposures (Toren and Blanc, 2009).

Cross-sectional surveys of workforces exposed to sensitizing agents report highly variable prevalence rates of OA, but these estimates are critically affected by the criteria that are used in order to identify the disease and by selection biases. Prospective cohort studies report incidence rates ranging from 1.8 to 4.1 cases of OA per 100 person-years among workers exposed to laboratory animals (Cullinan et al., 1999), wheat flour (Cullinan et al., 2001) or latex gloves (Archambault et al., 2001). Incidence rates derived from notification schemes and compensation statistics in various countries range from 24 to 174 new cases per million workers per year (Karjalainen et al., 2000; Reinisch et al., 2001; Ameille et al., 2003; McDonald et al., 2005; Piipari and Keskinen, 2005; Orriols et al., 2010; Vandenplas et al., 2011). Differences from one country to another may result from geographical patterns of industrial activity, as well as heterogeneity in diagnostic criteria and data collection procedures. The European Community Respiratory Health Survey II provided higher estimates of 250–478 incident cases of work-attributable asthma per million people per year (Karjalainen et al., 2001; Kogevinas et al., 2007). These data suggest that the disease remains largely unrecognized, although population surveys are affected by the lack of confirmation of OA through objective tests.

Pathophysiology

HMW agents induce OA via IgE-associated mechanisms. Specific IgE antibodies have also been detected in disease caused by some LMW agents, including acid anhydrides, platinum salts and reactive dyes (Maestrelli et al., 2009). These chemicals are non-immunogenic in their native state, but are thought to act as haptens and to undergo nucleophilic addition reactions with proteins that are present in the airways in order to form an immunogenic protein–hapten conjugate. However, many chemicals (e.g. plicatic acid) cause asthma, with clinical and pathological features similar to atopic disease without detectible specific IgE production or IgE receptors. Exposure to occupational agents can also induce antigen-specific IgG responses; titres of specific IgG antibodies can be related to the level of exposure, but their role is not fully understood (Pronk et al., 2007). The respiratory tract is considered the main route and site of sensitization to occupational agents, but the evidence of the skin being a route of respiratory sensitization is increasing (Redlich, 2010).

IgE-associated allergic airway inflammation caused by occupational agents is similar to allergic asthma unrelated to work (Lummus et al., 2011). Histamine, cysteinyl leukotrienes and prostaglandins are released by mast cells and basophils after IgE cross-bridging by the antigen. Allergens engage and activate antigen-presenting cells, which break allergens down into antigenic peptides. These peptides are presented to T lymphocytes which can differentiate into several subtypes. The essential cascade of allergic inflammation includes T-helper 2 (Th2) cells releasing cytokines, activation of B lymphocytes, promotion of IgE synthesis, cross-linking of antigen and IgE in mast cells and recruitment and activation of eosinophils and other inflammatory cells. Pro-inflammatory Th1 cells, Th17 cells and inhibitory T-regulatory cells also contribute to the inflammation.

Knowledge of the pathophysiological mechanisms of LMW-induced asthma is limited, and mainly based on isocyanate-induced asthma studies. In these patients, both Th1- and Th2-type inflammatory processes are involved (Maestrelli et al., 2009; Fisseler-Eckhoff et al., 2011). In vitro studies suggest that isocyanates stimulate non-adaptive immune responses; repetitive antigenic stimulation of peripheral blood mononuclear cells from patients enhanced the synthesis of TNF-α and monocyte chemoattractant protein 1 (Lummus et al., 1998). Isocyanates also up-regulated immune pattern-recognition monocytes and increased monocyte/macrophage-regulating chemokines (Wisnewski et al., 2008). In addition, altered expressions of genes involved in detoxification, oxidative stress, cytokine signalling and apoptosis were detected in macrophages derived from THP-1 human cell lines exposed to isocyanates (Verstraelen et al., 2008). Several studies suggest that isocyanates induce oxidative stress and have marked effects on glutathione, a major antioxidant in airway fluid (Wisnewski et al., 2015).

Epithelial cells interact directly with the environment and are thus susceptible to any damaging effects of inhaled occupational agents. Some agents (enzymes) are capable of disrupting epithelial cell tight junctions and damaging the epithelial barrier, affecting cell-to-cell and cell-to-matrix interactions, while others (isocyanates and anhydrides) are intrinsically cytotoxic (Wisnewski et al., 2002; Tai et al., 2006). Airway wall remodelling is similar in OA and non-OA (Frew et al., 1995). A reduction of sub-epithelial fibrosis, and in markers of ongoing inflammation and non-specific hyper-responsiveness, have been detected after cessation of workplace exposure (Saetta et al., 1995; Maghni et al., 2004; Piirilä et al., 2008; Carlsten et al., 2013).

Risk Factors

Environmental Risk Factors

Over 400 agents or processes have been reported to cause OA, and several new agents are identified annually, although only a few account for the majority of cases (Quirce and Bernstein, 2011; Vandenplas, 2011). The principal causal agents and related occupations or industries are listed in Table 26.1. More comprehensive lists are available (e.g. http://www.asthme.csst.qc.ca and http://www.asmanet.com).

The risk of developing OA and allergy increases with increasing exposure to occupational agents (Jones, 2008). Studies with both HMW and LMW agents have shown positive dose–response relationships between exposure and sensitization (Heederik et al., 2012). Individual susceptibility factors, such as genotype and timing of exposure, influence these relationships (Cullinan et al., 1999; Jones, 2008). The mode of exposure (i.e. different isoforms or physical forms of occupational agents) also has an effect on sensitization and specific airway reactivity (Vandenplas et al., 1993; Ye et al., 2006), and dermal exposure to certain agents probably increases the risk of OA (Redlich, 2010; Heederik et al., 2012). Smoking is a significant risk factor for developing occupational sensitization to several occupational agents, but reports of the relationship between smoking and OA are contradictory (Siracusa et al., 2006; Nicholson et al., 2010).

TABLE 26.1
Principal Agents Causing Sensitizer-Induced Occupational Asthma

Agent		Occupation/Industry
High-Molecular-Weight Agents		
Cereals, flour	Wheat, rye, barley, buckwheat	Flour mills, bakers, pastry makers
Latex	–	Healthcare workers, laboratory technicians
Animals	Mice, rats, cows, seafood	Laboratory workers, farmers, seafood processing
Enzymes	α-amylase, maxatase, alcalase, papain, bromelain, pancreatin	Baking product production, bakers, detergent production, pharmaceutical industry, food industry
Low-Molecular-Weight Agents		
Isocyanates	Toluene diisocyanate, methylene diphenyl-diisocyanate, hexamethylene diisocyanate	Polyurethane production, plastic industry, moulding, spray painters
Metals	Chromium, nickel, cobalt, platinum	Metal refinery, metal alloy production, electroplating, welding
Biocides	Aldehydes, quaternary ammonium compounds	Healthcare workers, cleaners
Persulfate salts	–	Hairdressers
Acid anhydrides	Phthalic, trimellitic, maleic, tetrachlorophthalic	Epoxy resin workers
Reactive dyes	Reactive black 5, pyrazolone derivatives, vinyl sulphones, carmine	Textile workers, food industry workers
Woods	Red cedar, iroko, obeche, oak and others	Sawmill workers, carpenters, cabinet and furniture makers

Individual Risk Factors

Atopy is consistently shown to increase the risk of developing OA to many HMW agents, but the association with OA from LMW agents is controversial (Nicholson et al., 2010). Pre-exposure sensitization to common environmental allergens that are capable of causing cross-reactivity (e.g. pets in laboratory animal workers) may be a stronger predictor of OA than atopy (Gautrin et al., 2001b). Occupational rhinitis is a risk factor for the development of OA, particularly with HMW agents. In a study of the Finnish register of occupational diseases, occupational rhinitis had a relative risk of 4.8 (95% confidence interval [CI]: 4.3–5.3) for the development of OA over 8 years of follow-up (Karjalainen et al., 2003). In laboratory animal workers, the relative risk for developing asthma symptoms was 7.4 (95% CI: 3.3–6.6) among those with allergy symptoms in 11 years of follow-up (Elliott et al., 2005). However, the predictive value of work-related nasal symptoms was only 11% for the development of OA in a follow-up period of 2.5–3.5 years among apprentices exposed to laboratory animals (Gautrin et al., 2001a). Prospective cohort studies of apprentices entering workplaces with occupational sensitizers have shown that non-specific bronchial hyper-responsiveness (NSBHR) at the start of the exposure was associated with an increased risk of OA (Gautrin et al., 2008).

Studies of genetic factors in OA have shown significant associations for specific occupational agents such as isocyanates, red cedar, acid anhydrides, platinum salts, latex and laboratory animals with certain human leucocyte antigen class II molecules (Bernstein, 2011). Genes associated with Th2 cell differentiation or protection against oxidative stress, such as those coding glutathione-S transferase and N-acetyl transferase, have been associated with an increased risk of OA. Currently, the diagnostic value of genetic testing is limited.

Diagnosis

The diagnosis of sensitizer-induced OA is based on the presence of bronchial asthma and an association with the workplace; the key elements are in the clinical history, immunologic tests, pulmonary function testing (including serial measurements of peak expiratory flow [PEF]) and specific and non-specific bronchial challenges (Tarlo et al., 2008; Baur et al., 2012). The assessment of airway inflammation (induced sputum and fractional exhaled nitric oxide [FeNO]) may complement the diagnosis. Diagnostic tests should preferably be performed when the patient is still working and exposed to the suspected agent. Each test has limitations (Table 26.2), and by combining several tests, the likelihood of a correct diagnosis increases, although the evidence for this is limited (Beach et al., 2007). Specific inhalation challenge (SIC) is regarded as the most reliable test for diagnosing OA; the sensitivities and specificities of diagnostic tests compared to SIC are shown in Table 26.3.

Clinical History

Symptoms of dyspnoea, wheezing, chest tightness, cough and sputum production are similar to those in asthma unrelated to work, but their occurrence is modulated by the work-related exposure. Symptoms typically improve during times away from work, such as weekends or holidays, and worsen at work. In some cases, the symptoms may occur after work, in the evenings or nights, and improvement may require several days away from exposure. The latency between first exposure and the beginning of symptoms varies; most commonly, it is between a few weeks and a few years (Malo et al., 1992). When the duration of symptomatic occupational exposure increases, it becomes less likely that symptoms will resolve when the patient is away from work (Maestrelli et al., 2012). Thus, it is useful to enquire into the temporal relationship of symptoms and work exposure during the early period of symptoms. Asthma symptoms are commonly accompanied and often preceded by nasal and conjunctival symptoms (Malo et al., 1997). The clinical history has a high sensitivity but low specificity in the diagnosis of OA (Nicholson et al., 2010), being reported to be positive in 90% of OA patients confirmed by SIC, but also in 54% of those with non-WRA (Malo et al., 1991; Tarlo et al., 1995; Vandenplas et al., 2005). Thus, the diagnosis of OA should not be based on a clinical history alone.

Exposure Assessment

A detailed work exposure history enables the determination of likely exposure to known causes of OA. Patients should be asked to describe precisely their work tasks, activities and exposures related to their work or caused by other workers and factors in the same environment. The use of respiratory (and dermal) protection and the patient's perception of any ventilation system should be assessed. Material safety datasheets of industrial materials or chemicals provide information on the hazardous effects of a product and its constituents, although the data may be incomplete (Bernstein, 2002). Industrial hygiene reports of previous air sampling in the workplace may provide information on the exposure levels of the occupational agents. Permissible air level standards for occupational agents are usually not set in order to prevent sensitization, and exposure to an occupational agent below these standards may cause OA.

TABLE 26.2
Advantages and Limitations of the Diagnostic Tests Used in the Investigation of Occupational Asthma

Diagnostic Tests	Advantages and Limitations
Immunologic tests	Easy to perform
	Low cost
	Commercial extracts are available (skin-prick tests or specific IgE for high-molecular-weight agents)
	Lack of standardization for the majority of occupational allergens, except for latex
	Measurement of specific IgE available for some low-molecular-weight agents, but low sensitivity
	Identify sensitization, but not the disease itself
Peak expiratory flow monitoring	Low cost
	Lung function is measured in a realistic exposure
	Requires the workers' collaboration
	Low adherence
	Possible falsification of results
	Ideally requires 3 weeks or 2 weeks at and away from work, which is not always possible for the workers
	Impossible to perform when the worker has already been removed from exposure
	No standardized method for interpreting the results
	Interpretation of the results requires experience
Specific-inhalation challenges in the laboratory	Confirmation of the diagnosis of occupational asthma when the test is positive
	False-negative tests are possible
	Costly
	Available in a small number of centres worldwide
Specific-inhalation challenges at the workplace	Excludes diagnosis if negative when performed in the usual work conditions
	Requires usual work conditions
	Costly
Assessment of non-specific bronchial hyper-responsiveness	Simple
	Low cost
	Confirms the diagnosis of asthma
	Low specificity for diagnosis of occupational asthma. The absence of non-specific bronchial hyperresponsiveness does not exclude the diagnosis of occupational asthma
Sputum cell counts	Impossible to falsify
	Brings additional evidence to the diagnosis of occupational asthma
	Costly
	Not widely available
	Cannot be obtained from all individuals
	Does not enable confirmation or exclusion of the diagnosis of occupational asthma by itself
Fractional exhaled nitric oxide	Easy to perform
	Inconsistent results
	Difficult to interpret
	Affected by many different factors

Immunologic Assessment

Skin-prick tests (SPTs) and the determination of specific IgE antibodies are useful for demonstrating sensitization to most HMW and some LMW occupational agents (Moscato et al., 2012), but are not sufficient for making a diagnosis of OA without additional lung function measurements (Nicholson et al., 2010).

Commercial SPT extracts and specific IgE tests are available for several HMW and some LMW (e.g. acid anhydrides and isocyanates) occupational agents. There is a lack of standardization for most of these tests, and the allergenic potency of SPT extracts may vary significantly (van Kampen et al., 2013). Patients may also be tested with laboratory-made SPT extracts and IgE tests, in which case, control tests in non-exposed subjects are required in order to confirm positive findings (Moscato et al., 2012). LMW allergens require conjugation to an appropriate carrier molecule such as human serum albumin for testing. SPTs to acid anhydrate conjugates have been shown to be biologically relevant (Kristiansson et al., 2003), whereas isocyanate conjugates appear to be very diverse, which may cause differences in their antigenicity (Campo et al., 2007). Recently, studies using allergenic molecular-based diagnosis and multiplex microarray technology have identified specific molecules related to OA caused by HMW agents (Pahr et al., 2012).

PEF Monitoring

PEF recordings are performed throughout the day on days at work and off work every 2 hours or at least four times a day when workers are in their usual jobs (Nicholson et al., 2010). At each time point, three measures (all within 20 L/minute) are recorded in a diary, and information regarding frequency of symptoms, medication use and work tasks is also collected. Forced expiratory volume in 1 second (FEV_1) and other airway indices can also be measured, but have not been shown to be more accurate than PEF recordings in the diagnosis (Moore et al., 2009). Inhaled steroid treatment should be withheld or remain unchanged during the period of measurement. Diagnostic performance falls when recordings are shorter (Nicholson et al., 2010), and a minimum duration of 3 weeks or 2 weeks at work and 2 weeks off work is recommended (Tarlo et al., 2008; Fishwick et al., 2012). In a specialist clinic, approximately 70% of patients can produce acceptable recordings (Nicholson et al., 2010).

There is no single universally accepted technique for evaluating PEF recordings. These recordings can be plotted and visually interpreted in order to detect a pattern of worsening during working periods compared to periods off work (Figure 26.1). When this evaluation is performed by 'experts', there is a relatively good agreement with SIC (Cote et al., 1993). A computer-generated discriminant analysis (OASYS-2; OASYS Research Group, Midland Thoracic Society, Birmingham, UK) based on pattern recognition calculates a work–effect index and grades recordings as positive, equivocal or negative. This method has given relatively good agreement with expert visual interpretation on plotted graphics (Baldwin et al., 2002).

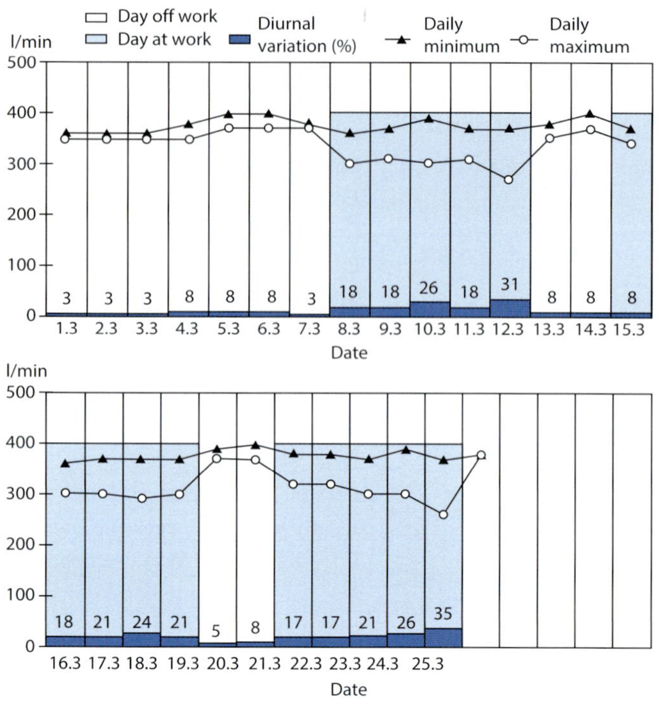

FIGURE 26.1 Peak expiratory flow monitoring curves showing increased daily variation during workdays.

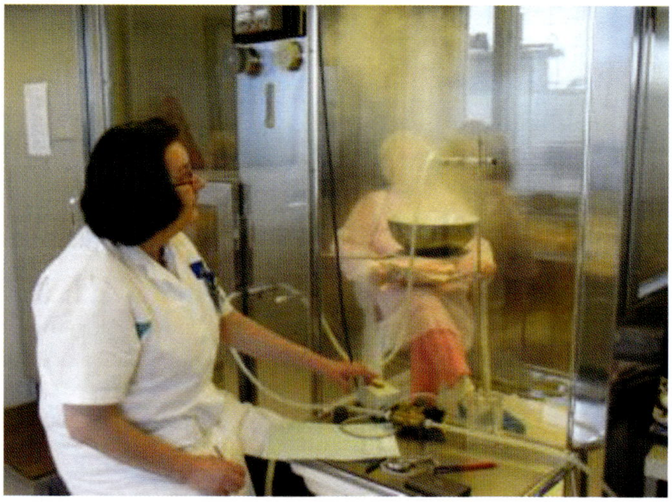

FIGURE 26.2 Specific inhalation challenge with flour in the challenge chamber supervised by a nurse.

Specific Inhalation Challenge

SIC is useful for confirming the diagnosis and the causative agent of OA, and is the best available method for determining the sensitizing potential of a formerly unrecognized occupational agent (Vandenplas et al., 2014a). It is safe when performed in specialized centres by trained personnel.

During SIC, gradually increasing exposures to the agent that is suspected of causing OA are delivered in an enclosed challenge room (Figure 26.2) or using a closed-circuit device (Vandenplas et al., 2014a). The concentration of the agent should be based on the estimated level in the workplace and be within permissible levels. The duration of exposure on each day generally varies from a few minutes to an hour. Symptoms and lung function (primarily FEV_1) are monitored for at least 6–8 hours. In addition, NSBHR and, where feasible, sputum eosinophils and FeNO are observed. A challenge to an inert control substance with similar monitoring is performed on a separate day before any test with the occupational agent. SIC is considered positive when there is a sustained fall of FEV_1 of at least 15% from the pre-challenge value and a fluctuation in FEV_1 of less than 10% during the control day. Typical patterns of asthmatic response are early (onset during or within a few minutes after challenge and recovery within 2 hours), late (onset after 2 hours following challenge) or dual (combination of early and late). NSBHR, sputum eosinophils and FeNO may increase the sensitivity of the test and clarify an equivocal reaction. In the case of a negative test, the challenge can be repeated on the next day, but it is unclear how long a patient should be tested until a SIC can be considered negative. A long period away from exposure before SIC may cause a false-negative result, in which case an increased duration of challenge exposure may be needed in order to detect a positive reaction (Lemiere et al., 1996). False-positive results may be due to irritant reactions.

Workplace Challenge

Workplace challenge involves serial FEV_1 measurements under the supervision of a technician before and throughout a work shift. This test should also include a control day without occupational exposure. Positive workplace challenges were detected in 22% of workers with highly suggestive medical histories for OA and negative SIC (Rioux et al., 2008). The test may be recommended if SIC is equivocal or not feasible (Baur et al., 2012).

Non-Specific Bronchial Hyper-Responsiveness

The specificity of a single NSBHR test for OA is low (Table 26.3), and OA cannot be ruled out in patients without hyper-responsiveness (Baur et al., 2012). In a recent study, NSBHR was detected more often in patients with non-OA than with OA (Malo et al., 2011). Serial NSBHR tests, including measurements during a period of work exposure and repeated measurement during a period away from work for 10–14 days, can be used as an additional approach to documenting functional airway changes related to work exposures (Tarlo et al., 2008).

In SIC, an increase in post-challenge NSBHR is associated with a positive reaction; a significant increase in NSBHR has a >90% predictive value for the development of an asthmatic reaction in subsequent challenges (Vandenplas et al., 1996; Sastre et al., 2003). A significant increase in NSBHR indicates a need for additional challenge in the case of a negative FEV_1 result and supports a positive response when the FEV_1 reaction is equivocal (Vandenplas et al., 2014a).

TABLE 26.3
Pooled Estimates of Sensitivity and Specificity of Immunological Tests, Airway Hyper-Responsiveness and Peak Expiratory Flow Monitoring Compared to Specific Inhalation Challenge

Diagnostic Test	Sensitivity	Specificity
Immunological Tests		
Skin-prick tests of HMW agents	81 (70–88)	60 (42–75)
Skin-prick tests of LMW agents	73 (60–83)	86 (77–92)
Specific IgE antibodies of HMW agents	74 (58–94)	82 (58–94)
Specific IgE antibodies of LMW agents	31 (23–41)	89 (85–92)
Airway Hyper-Responsiveness		
Single test of HMW agents	79 (35–72)	51 (35–67)
Single test of LMW agents	67 (58–74)	64 (56–71)
Serial test of LMW agents	68 (43–85)	66 (41–84)
Serial test of various agents	50 (36–65)	67 (53–78)
Serial PEF Monitoring		
Various agents	64 (43–80)	77 (67–85)

Abbreviations: HMW: high-molecular-weight; LMW: low-molecular-weight; PEF: peak expiratory flow.

Source: Adapted from Beach, J. et al. 2005. *Diagnosis and Management of Work-Related Asthma*. Summary, Evidence Report/Technology Assessment: Number 129 AHRQ Publication Number 06-E003-1, October 2005 Agency for Healthcare Research and Quality, Rockville, MD. http://www.ahrq.gov/clinic/epcsums/asthworksum.htm.

Note: Data presented as % (95% confidence intervals).

Induced Sputum Cell Counts

In patients with OA, worsening of asthma symptoms has been associated with an increase in eosinophilic airway inflammation and a decrease after removal of exposure (Lemiere et al., 1999, 2010). The addition of sputum cytology to serial PEF recordings improves the diagnosis of OA (Girard et al., 2004). An increase in sputum eosinophils has been observed after positive SICs to HMW and LMW agents, whereas negative test reactions have not usually induced sputum eosinophilia (Lemiere et al., 2001; Quirce et al., 2010). Moreover, an increase in sputum eosinophils of >3% after negative challenge predicts the development of an asthmatic reaction in subsequent challenges (Vandenplas et al., 2009). The best timing for sputum collection is likely to be 7–24 hours after exposure (Obata et al., 1999). In SIC, sputum eosinophilia may help to interpret equivocal results and indicate the need for additional challenges (Vandenplas et al., 2014a). However, sputum eosinophilia is not detected in all subjects with OA, and thus its absence does not exclude the diagnosis (Obata et al., 1999). An increase in sputum neutrophil count may occur after exposure to some occupational agents such as isocyanates, but has not been validated in the diagnosis of OA (Park et al., 1999).

Fractional Exhaled Nitric Oxide

FeNO, a surrogate marker of eosinophilic airway inflammation, is a simple and easy measurement providing immediate results, but it is sensitive to confounding factors, including smoking, atopy and inhaled corticosteroid treatment (Quirce et al., 2010). Some studies have shown significant increases in the levels of FeNO after positive SIC reactions, but the data are conflicting, and the role of FeNO in the diagnosis of OA has not been established clearly. SIC studies have shown that the level of FeNO is increased at 24 hours after exposure; an increase seems to be more prominent in positive tests with HMW agents than LMW agents (Lemiere et al., 2014). A significant increase in the level of FeNO may be helpful in the interpretation of equivocal SIC results, indicating the need for additional challenges, especially if induced sputum samples are not achievable (Vandenplas et al., 2014a).

Outcome and Management

Asthma symptoms and functional impairment may persist for many years after avoidance of occupational exposure, and OA may become a chronic condition similar to non-OA (Fishwick et al., 2012). A meta-analysis of outcomes in OA patients after the cessation of exposure to the occupational agent revealed rates of complete symptomatic recovery of between 0% and 100%, with a pooled estimate of 32% (Rachiotis et al., 2007). Several host and workplace factors influence the prognosis of OA (Beach et al., 2007; Tarlo et al., 2008; Nicholson et al., 2010; Maestrelli et al., 2012). A worse outcome is associated with lower lung volumes, higher NSBHR or a stronger asthmatic response to SIC at the time of the diagnosis. Similarly, longer symptomatic exposure and older age predict a worse outcome, emphasizing the importance of an early diagnosis of OA. In contrast, atopy or smoking at the time of the diagnosis are not related to outcome.

Complete removal from occupational exposure is recommended (Tarlo et al., 2008; Baur et al., 2012), but is associated with a high rate of unemployment and loss of income (de Groene et al., 2011; Vandenplas et al., 2012). Reduction of exposure to the causal agent can be considered an alternative to complete avoidance, although this approach seems to be less beneficial than complete cessation (Baur et al., 2012). Respiratory-protective equipment can result in an improvement of asthma symptoms or prevent symptoms in some but not all workers, but is not considered a safe approach, especially in the long term or in patients with severe asthma.

Asthma medication for patients with OA should be adapted to the level of asthma control, as in the management of non-OA patients. There is insufficient evidence that treatment with inhaled corticosteroids and long-acting β_2 agonists prevents long-term deterioration in workers who remain exposed to the causative agent, and these are not recommended as alternatives to exposure cessation (Vandenplas et al., 2012). Monoclonal anti-IgE antibody treatment has improved asthma control in some OA patients with continuing exposure (Moscato, 2014). Similarly, allergen-specific immunotherapy has been tested for a few sensitizing occupational agents, such as latex, flour and laboratory animals. Further studies with these therapies are needed before they can be recommended for OA.

Socioeconomic Impact

Follow-up studies in various countries have consistently reported that OA is associated with a high rate of prolonged unemployment (14%–69%) (Vandenplas, 2008; Miedinger et al., 2010). The lowest rates of unemployment have been reported in Finland (14%) (Piirilä et al., 2005) and Quebec, Canada (25%) (Dewitte et al., 1994), where effective retraining programmes are available. Overall, 44%–74% of workers with OA suffer a substantial loss of work-related income (Vandenplas, 2008). The financial consequences are more pronounced in workers who completely avoid exposure to the causative agent, which may account for the finding that a third of patients remain in exposed jobs. Worse socioeconomic outcomes are associated with change of employer, employment in small-sized firms, unskilled jobs, a low level of education, older age, younger age, a low number of economically dependent persons and a LMW causal agent (Blanc et al., 2013). Asthma severity has been detected as an important determinant only in areas (Finland and Quebec) with good socioeconomic support for workers with OA (Piirilä et al., 2005; Malo et al., 2008). It has been estimated that patients with OA use more healthcare resources than patients with non-WRA (Lemiere et al., 2007). In the UK, the total lifetime cost of a new case of OA was estimated to be between £25 million and £27 million (Ayres et al., 2011).

OA is associated with an adverse impact on mental wellbeing (Yacoub et al., 2007; Miedinger et al., 2011) and quality of life (Malo et al., 1993). After removal from exposure, the quality of life of OA patients was slightly worse than patients with non-OA matched for asthma severity.

Prevention

Reductions in exposure can reduce the risk of immunologic sensitization and asthma (Beach, 2005; Nicholson et al., 2010; Heederik et al., 2012). The best evidence for this approach is the substitution of powdered natural rubber latex gloves with non-powdered gloves, which greatly reduced sensitization and asthma in healthcare workers (LaMontagne et al., 2006). Complete elimination of exposure is the preferred primary preventative approach to reducing the burden of disease; if elimination is not possible, exposure reduction is the second-best option (Heederik et al., 2012). Respiratory-protective equipment can substantially reduce exposure to causative agents, but only when selected correctly, worn properly and maintained and stored safely. Such equipment can be used in conjunction with other measures when exposure control is not otherwise possible, or as an interim measure while other controls are implemented. Although the evidence is limited, minimizing skin exposure to asthma-inducing agents may be helpful.

Pre-placement screening can identify workers with individual risk factors such as atopy, pre-existing asthma and NSBHR, which may increase the risk of OA, but their predictive values are too poorly discriminating to be useful in screening and excluding susceptible workers from exposed jobs (Nicholson et al., 2010; Wilken et al., 2012). Instead, these workers should be given appropriate counselling and improved exposure control in the workplace.

Periodic health surveillance combined with exposure reduction has been effective for several occupational agents (Liss, 2012). A few studies have indicated that surveillance can detect asthma at an earlier stage of the disease and that asthma prognosis is improved in these workers (Tarlo et al., 2002). Questionnaires for detecting work-related respiratory symptoms, including rhinitis, are the main tools for OA surveillance, although they underestimate the prevalence of asthmatic symptoms (Nicholson et al., 2010). Spirometry does not appear to identify OA cases that would not be detected by a questionnaire alone. In contrast, identification of IgE-mediated sensitization has been shown to have a high predictive value for the development of OA to some agents. Surveillance of OA is covered in more detail in Chapter 15.

IRRITANT-INDUCED ASTHMA

The term 'irritant-induced asthma' (IIA) has been introduced to describe the development of asthma symptoms, NSBHR and airway inflammation induced by irritant mechanisms, as opposed to OA caused by immunologic mechanisms and leading to specific bronchial hypersensitivity to a workplace agent. In 1985, Brooks and co-workers introduced the term 'reactive airways dysfunction syndrome' (RADS) in order to describe the sudden onset of asthma within a few hours of a single high-level exposure to irritant substances (Brooks et al., 1985). Tarlo and Broder later proposed the term IIA in order to characterize workers who develop asthma after either single or multiple high-level irritant exposures (Tarlo and Broder, 1989). It is now widely acknowledged that various clinical phenotypes should be distinguished within the wide spectrum of irritant-related asthma: (1) acute-onset IIA or RADS, characterized by the rapid onset of asthma within a few hours of a single exposure to a very high level of irritant substance; (2) asthma that develops in workers with a history of multiple symptomatic high-level exposures to irritants; and (3) asthma occurring with a delayed onset after chronic exposure to moderate levels of irritants ('low-dose RADS', 'not-so-sudden IIA' or 'IIA with latency', respectively) (Vandenplas et al., 2014b).

Epidemiology

There is scarce information on the global impact of irritant exposures on the development of asthma. Surveillance programmes of WRA in various countries indicated that clinically identified RADS and IIA account for 5%–18% of all notified cases (Gautrin et al., 2006). A number of longitudinal (Kogevinas et al., 2007) and cross-sectional (Medina-Ramon et al., 2005; Delclos et al., 2007; Vizcaya et al., 2011; Lillienberg et al., 2013) studies documented an increased risk of asthma in individuals with a history of accidental high exposure to irritant products. A longitudinal study of the World Trade Center disaster, including rescue and recovery workers with intense dust exposure and individuals without dust exposure, showed an increased risk of new-onset asthma in the follow-up period of 5–6 years, particularly in the first months after the event (Brackbill et al., 2009). Longitudinal workforce-based studies have provided evidence that multiple high-level exposures ('gassings') to chlorine in metal production workers (Gautrin et al., 1999) and ozone or sulphur dioxide in pulp mill workers (Olin et al., 2004; Andersson et al., 2006) were associated with an increased risk of asthma. The most persuasive evidence supporting the role of chronic moderate irritant exposure in the development of asthma is provided by epidemiologic studies of workers exposed to cleaning agents (Siracusa et al., 2013). The frequent use of bleach (hypochlorite), ammonia and degreasing sprays has been consistently associated with asthma among workers exposed to cleaning agents (Medina-Ramon et al., 2005; Mirabelli et al., 2007; Vizcaya et al., 2011), although the mechanisms responsible have not been clarified, since cleaning materials typically contain a wide variety of ingredients, some of which are respiratory irritants, while others are potential airway sensitizers.

Pathophysiology

Several factors may influence the pulmonary response to irritants, such as the intensity of exposure, physical properties (such as vapour pressure and solubility) and the chemical reactivity (Brooks and Bernstein, 2011). The resulting biological effect will depend on the deposition of the irritant in the upper and/or lower airways. Water-soluble irritants and particles of aerodynamic diameter larger than 5 μm are predominantly deposited in the upper respiratory tract and proximal airways. Water-insoluble agents and particles of 0.5–5 μm can reach the distal airways and alveoli, often without causing much sensory irritation.

IIA is related to bronchial epithelial cell injury, resulting in pro-inflammatory responses, neurogenic inflammation due to stimulation of nerve endings, increased lung permeability and remodelling of the airway epithelium, although the ultimate pathogenic mechanisms remain largely speculative (Brooks and Bernstein, 2011). Upon tissue injury, alarmins are rapidly secreted by stimulated epithelial cells and leukocytes, as well as necrotic cells. Once released, these multifunctional molecules promote the activation of innate immune cells and the recruitment and activation of antigen-presenting cells engaged in tissue repair and host defence (Chan et al., 2012). Chemical irritants can also directly activate sensory nerves either by stimulation of solitary chemosensory cells or by directly stimulating chemoreceptors, most importantly transient receptor potential channels (Bautista et al., 2013). Stimulated sensory nerve endings may release tachykinin neuropeptides such as substance P, neurokinin A and calcitonin gene-related peptide, triggering airway neurogenic inflammation characterized by plasma protein extravasation, vasodilatation, bronchoconstriction and increased mucus secretion.

Bronchial biopsies in subjects with acute-onset IIA have revealed epithelial desquamation, inflammatory changes with predominance of lymphocytes, airway remodelling and collagen deposition in the bronchial wall (Gautrin et al., 1994; Takeda et al., 2009). Similar changes have been described in animal models (White and Martin, 2010). Interestingly, a murine model of exposure to chlorine demonstrated acute and transient neutrophilic inflammation in lung tissue and airways and an increase in pro-inflammatory cytokines, while NSBHR to methacholine persisted for at least 28 days (Jonasson et al., 2013). Two human studies provided information on the long-term outcomes of airway inflammation and remodelling in a large series of subjects with acute-onset IIA (Malo and Chan-Yeung, 2009; Takeda et al., 2009). Both showed inflammatory and remodelling profiles that did not differ from what is seen in allergic OA after removal from exposure, with an increase of eosinophils in some patients or neutrophils in others. However, the basement membrane demonstrated a significantly increased thickness (sub-epithelial fibrosis) in patients with IIA compared to healthy subjects and subjects with non-IIA. Altogether, the pathological changes observed during the acute phase resemble a toxic mechanism, while the long-term phase is similar to allergic OA.

Risk Factors

The environmental and host factors that determine the initiation and persistence of IIA remain largely unknown. There is some evidence that the concentration and duration of exposure may have a substantial impact on the development of IIA; a dose–response relationship between the level of exposure assessed qualitatively by industrial hygienists and the prevalence of NSBHR has been documented in subjects who had been exposed to a spill of acetic acid (Kern, 1991). In a follow-up survey of pulp mill workers exposed to high levels of chlorine, the severity of gassing incidents, as evidenced by hospital emergency room visits, was a more significant risk factor for the persistence of NSBHR than was the number of incidents (Bherer et al., 1994). The available information indicates that the development of IIA related to high-level exposures is not associated with smoking and atopy (Kern, 1991; Bherer et al., 1994).

Diagnosis

In every suspected case of IIA, the presence of asthma should be substantiated by spirometry, demonstrating airflow limitation with a significant bronchodilator response or NSBHR to methacholine/histamine. In the differential diagnosis, other conditions, such as vocal cord dysfunction, hyperventilation syndrome and multiple chemical sensitivity syndrome, should be carefully considered, especially since these disorders may also result from inhalation accidents and exposure to irritants in the workplace (Tarlo et al., 2008).

Acute-onset IIA is characterized by the onset of asthma symptoms within 24 hours of a single, most often accidental, high-level exposure to irritant substances in subjects without pre-existing asthma. This clinical phenotype is the most definitive form of asthma induced by respiratory irritants (Tarlo et al., 2008; Malo and Vandenplas, 2011).

A wide variety of exposures have been associated with the development of acute-onset IIA (Table 26.4) (Shakeri et al., 2008; Baur, 2013). It is expected that IIA may be induced by any high-level exposure to fumes, gases, sprays or even dusts that have irritating properties. Typically, the exposure is caused by spills of volatile compounds, accidental release of irritants under pressure, accidental fires with the release of complex mixtures of thermal degradation products or inadvertent reduction of ventilation rate in a confined space (Brooks and Bernstein, 2011).

TABLE 26.4
Examples of Exposures Causing Acute-Onset Irritant-Induced Asthma

Exposure	Examples
Gases	Chlorine (e.g. released by mixing sodium hypochlorite with acids), chloramines (released by mixing sodium hypochlorite with ammonia) sulphur dioxide, nitrogen oxides, dimethyl sulphate
Acids	Acetic, hydrochloric, hydrofluoric and hydrobromic acids
Alkalis	Ammonia, calcium oxide (lime), hydrazine
Biocides	Formalin, ethylene oxide, fumigating agents, insecticides (sodium methyldithiocarbamate, dichlorvos)
Halogenated derivatives	Bromochlorodifluoromethane (fire extinguisher), trifluoromethane, chlorofluorocarbons (thermal degradation products of freons), orthochlorobenzylidene malonitrile (tear gas), uranium hexafluoride, hydrogen and carbonyl fluoride
Solvents	Perchloroethylene
Fumes	Diesel exhaust, paint fumes, urea fumes, fire smoke, fumes of iodine and aluminium iodide, diethylaminoethanol (corrosion inhibitor)
Sprays	Various paints (not specified), floor sealant (aromatic hydrocarbons)
Dusts	World Trade Center alkaline dust, calcium oxide (lime)
Potential sensitizers	Isocyanates, phthalic anhydride

The diagnosis of acute-onset IIA can usually be established with a high level of confidence based on the retrospective documentation of a close temporal relationship between an inhalation incident and the acute onset of asthma symptoms. Stringent clinical and functional criteria for the diagnosis of acute-onset IIA have been proposed: (1) absence of pre-existing respiratory disorder, asthma symptomatology or a history of asthma in remission, and exclusion of conditions that can simulate asthma; (2) onset of asthma within minutes to hours and less than 24 hours after a single exposure to an irritant vapour, gas, fume or smoke in very high concentrations; (3) presence of airflow limitation with a significant bronchodilator response or NSBHR to histamine/methacholine; and (4) exclusion of another pulmonary disorder that explains the symptoms and findings (Brooks et al., 1985; Tarlo et al., 2008; Vandenplas et al., 2014b). However, some case series (Kern, 1991; Cone et al., 1994) and the 'World Trade Center asthma syndrome' (Prezant et al., 2002; Banauch et al., 2003) indicate that the symptoms leading to a diagnosis of asthma may develop insidiously over a few days to months after a massive exposure.

In subjects with a history of multiple high-level exposures, the clinical picture may be very similar to acute-onset IIA, with symptoms occurring shortly after one severe inhalation incident. In other subjects with repeated high-level exposures, the onset of symptoms may be more insidious. IIA has been documented after repeated high-level exposures ('puffs' or 'gassings') to irritant substances, mainly chlorine, SO_2 and ozone (Table 26.4) (Tarlo and Broder, 1989; Bherer et al., 1994; Chan-Yeung et al., 1994; Gautrin et al., 1999; Olin et al., 2004; Andersson et al., 2006). The causal relationship of this phenotype can be supported by the documentation of repeated symptomatic inhalation accidents requiring medical care or reports to occupational health services. In such settings in which the onset of symptoms is less abrupt than in the classical description of Brooks and co-workers, the term 'subacute IIA' would be more appropriate.

Other types of asthma attributed to chronic, moderate irritant exposures at work can only be considered as 'possible' IIA, since the causal relationship cannot be ascertained with certainty on an individual basis. Distinguishing the phenotypes of IIA attributed to repeated, 'moderate'-level exposures from WEA, from coincidental asthma that is not work-related or even from immunologic OA is difficult on a clinical basis, and there are no specific diagnostic tests. In such settings, causality can only be inferred from epidemiological studies documenting an excess risk of asthma in similar work environments.

There are some clinical features that clearly distinguish acute and subacute IIA from allergic OA. Subjects with IIA induced by high-level exposures do not develop WRA symptoms after re-exposure to a low concentration of the irritant that initiated the symptoms, since they are not 'sensitized' to the offending agent. Nevertheless, the development of specific bronchial hypersensitivity (i.e. sensitizer-induced OA) has been documented in rare cases in which the single accidental exposure had been to a low-molecular-weight sensitizer (Moller et al., 1986). On the other hand, known sensitizers may induce IIA through irritant mechanisms when inhaled at very high concentrations (Table 26.4) (Palczynski et al., 1994; Lemière et al., 1996; Vandenplas et al., 2004). In such instances, SICs with the suspected agent may be useful for distinguishing IIA from sensitizer-induced OA. Notably, subjects with acute-onset IIA may experience worsening of their asthma symptoms at work because their newly acquired NSBHR makes them more susceptible to various irritant stimuli at or outside work. Finally, unlike sensitizer-induced OA, acute-onset IIA does not require a latency period of exposure—during which the subject becomes immunologically sensitized—before the occurrence of asthma. Nevertheless, a latency period without symptoms can be present when IIA occurs after multiple high-level exposures to irritants.

Outcome and Management

Few follow-up studies of patients with IIA are available. Among 51 pulp mill workers who had experienced shortness of breath for more than 1 month after a chlorine gassing episode, a follow-up assessment at 18–24 months after the inhalation incident documented the presence of significant NSBHR in 57% of them and airway obstruction in 31% (Bherer et al., 1994). Assessment of 19 out of the 29 workers with NSBHR 12 months later revealed that six (32%) of them showed a significant improvement in NSBHR, including five subjects for whom the level of responsiveness to methacholine was no longer in the asthmatic range (Malo et al., 1994). These data indicate that NSBHR can improve over several years after an acute symptomatic inhalation accident. Among 35 subjects with acute-onset IIA who were reassessed after a mean interval of 14 years (range: 4–24 years), all reported respiratory symptoms and 68% were treated with inhaled corticosteroids (Malo et al., 2009). Only 17% of subjects had normal spirometry values and NSBHR at follow-up. Sputum eosinophil count was >2% in 22% of the subjects. The clinical and functional outcomes of acute-onset IIA seem to be similar to those in subjects with sensitizer-induced OA after cessation of exposure to the causal agent.

The published data on the management of IIA are mainly case reports of acute-onset IIA. Workers who have had a high-level irritant exposure should be assessed as early as possible in order to determine the presence of airflow limitation or NSBHR. Based on animal studies and a few case reports (Lemière et al., 1997; Demnati et al., 1998), it seems that treatment with systemic and/or inhaled steroids after the accident has a beneficial effect, but the optimal duration and dose of this treatment are still uncertain. Unless their asthma is severe, patients with IIA who are not sensitized to workplace agents can often continue to work in the same environment with appropriate asthma management and measures to prevent a further unintentional high-level exposure to irritants (Tarlo, 2003).

Prevention

The prevention of IIA relies mainly on measures that prevent exposure of workers to the levels of irritant that can cause asthma (Tarlo and Liss, 2010). Such measures include elimination of airborne irritant products where possible and control of exposures to safe levels by measures such as containment, adequate ventilation and, as a final option, use of respiratory-protective equipment. Exposure level monitoring with alarm systems may also be appropriate in some settings in which levels of potential respiratory irritants may exceed recommended levels. Educational programmes should be implemented in order to ensure safe handling of chemicals, the effective use of personal protective equipment and measures to take in the event of an accident at work.

WORK-EXACERBATED ASTHMA

The definition of WEA proposed by an American Thoracic Society Task Force (Henneberger et al., 2011) includes four criteria:

- Pre-existing or concurrent asthma: the onset of asthma may have occurred either before or during employment at the worksite of interest, but was not due to specific exposures within that worksite.
- Documentation of asthma exacerbation temporally associated with work, based either on self-reported symptoms or increased medication use relative to work, or on more objective indicators such as work-related patterns of serial PEF.
- Conditions exist that can exacerbate asthma.
- Asthma caused by work (OA) is unlikely.

Epidemiology

The reported prevalence rates of WEA are largely influenced by the definition used and the population in which the condition has been investigated. A recent systematic review of the literature indicated that 21.5% of cases of asthma could be exacerbated by conditions at the workplace (Henneberger et al., 2011).

Pathophysiology

The pathophysiological mechanisms and risk factors involved in WEA remain largely unknown. The occupational agents associated with the occurrence of WEA are likely to have irritant properties. Clinical and epidemiological studies identified a wide variety of exposures associated with WEA, including mineral and organic dusts, chemicals (i.e. ammonia, cleaning agents, paints, glues and pesticides), indoor air pollutants and secondhand smoke (Tarlo et al., 2000; Saarinen et al., 2003; Goe et al., 2004; Berger et al., 2006; Lemiere et al., 2012; Henneberger et al., 2014). Physical factors, such as abnormal temperature (Saarinen et al., 2003) and physical exertion (Saarinen et al., 2003) or emotional stress (Tarlo et al., 2000; Berger et al., 2006) have also been reported as causing WEA. A non-eosinophilic phenotype of asthma based on sputum cell analysis seems to be more frequent in subjects with WEA than in those with OA (Girard et al., 2004; Lemiere et al., 2013). Although some individual predisposing factors have been suggested for OA, no specific risk factors have been clearly identified for WEA.

Diagnosis

WEA should be suspected in patients who complain of a worsening of their symptoms or who require an increase of their asthma medication when at work (Tarlo et al., 2008). The diagnosis of asthma needs to be confirmed through spirometry or measurement of NSBHR, since a substantial proportion of subjects who experience asthma-like symptoms at work fail to demonstrate objective evidence of asthma (Chiry et al., 2009). The diagnosis of WEA relies on the documentation of a relationship between workplace exposure and the occurrence of asthma exacerbations with emergency visits or hospitalizations, or an increase in the severity of asthma symptoms and the need for asthma medications during periods at work. In addition, the possibility of OA should be carefully ruled out.

Workers with WEA are often difficult to differentiate from asthmatic subjects with OA, especially in cases who report a new onset of asthma while in the current workplace. In the few studies that compared workers with WEA to adults with non-WRA, the clinical characteristics of these two populations did not differ greatly. Some studies reported that workers with WEA tended to be older, more frequently smokers and more often treated with inhaled corticosteroids (Henneberger et al., 2011; Lemiere et al., 2013). The timing of asthma onset with respect to the start of employment at the workplace of interest does not differentiate WEA from OA. For example, only 7% of subjects with WEA defined by the presence of WRA symptoms and a negative SIC had asthma before employment, while 20% of those with a positive SIC reported a diagnosis of asthma that predated the employment (Larbanois et al., 2002).

Serial PEF monitoring can show increased variability during periods at work compared to periods away from work in subjects with a diagnosis of WEA based on a negative SIC result (Chiry et al., 2007). Although the PEF variability is greater in subjects with OA than with WEA, the difference in the magnitude of PEF variability does not enable the differentiation of WEA from OA in clinical practice (Chiry et al., 2007). A negative SIC with the suspected agents in the laboratory or at the workplace strongly supports the diagnosis of WEA, although false-negative tests can occur and the facilities for performing these tests are not widely available (Vandenplas et al., 2014a).

Outcome and Management

Although there is convincing evidence that persistent exposure to the causal agent is detrimental for workers with OA, the respiratory health impact of continuing exposure to the offending work environment currently remains unknown for WEA. There is some evidence that workers with OA show a greater improvement in lung function, NSBHR and asthma control than subjects with WEA when removed from exposure (Lemiere et al., 2006; Lemiere et al., 2013). Although there is limited evidence concerning the management of WEA, existing guidelines have advised minimizing exposures to asthma triggers at work and optimizing standard pharmacological treatment of asthma (e.g. pharmacological treatment and avoidance of symptom triggers) (Tarlo et al., 2008; Henneberger et al., 2011).

Socioeconomic Impact

There is accumulating evidence that WEA exerts a large socioeconomic impact on workers and society by inducing substantial disruption of work and using a large amount of healthcare resources. The few available studies indicate that WEA is associated with high rates of job changes, prolonged unemployment (30%–50%) and losses of earnings that are similar to those reported in OA (Henneberger et al., 2011). In a recent cohort study conducted in tertiary clinics in Quebec, Canada, Lemiere et al. found that the healthcare-related costs were similar between WEA and OA, but tenfold greater than the costs related to non-WRA in the year preceding the diagnostic assessment (Lemiere et al., 2013). Although the cost of OA decreased significantly after the diagnosis was made and the patients were removed from exposure, the cost of WEA following the diagnosis did not decrease significantly.

REFERENCES

Ameille, J., Pauli, G., Calastreng-Crinquand, A., Vervloet, D., Iwatsubo, Y., Popin, E., Bayeux-Dunglas, M. C. et al. 2003. Reported incidence of occupational asthma in France, 1996–99: The ONAP programme. *Occup Environ Med* 60:136–41.

Andersson, E., Knutsson, A., Hagberg, S., Nilsson, T., Karlsson, B., Alfredsson, L. and Toren, K. 2006. Incidence of asthma among workers exposed to sulphur dioxide and other irritant gases. *Eur Respir J* 27:720–5.

Archambault, S., Malo, J. L., Infante-Rivard, C., Ghezzo, H. and Gautrin, D. 2001. Incidence of sensitization, symptoms and probable occupational rhinoconjunctivitis and asthma in apprentices starting exposure to latex. *J Allergy Clin Immunol* 107:921–3.

Ayres, J. G., Boyd, R., Cowie, H. and Hurley, J. F. 2011. Costs of occupational asthma in the UK. *Thorax,* 66:128–33.

Baldwin, D. R., Gannon, P., Bright, P., Newton, D. T., Robertson, A., Venables, K., Graneek, B. et al. 2002. Interpretation of occupational peak flow records: Level of agreement between expert clinicians and Oasys-2. *Thorax* 57:860–4.

Banauch, G. I., Alleyne, D., Sanchez, R., Olender, K., Cohen, H. W., Weiden, M., Kelly, K. J. et al. 2003. Persistent hyperreactivity and reactive airway dysfunction in firefighters at the World Trade Center. *Am J Respir Crit Care Med* 168:54–62.

Baur, X. 2013. A compendium of causative agents of occupational asthma. *J Occup Med Toxicol* 8:15.

Baur, X., Sigsgaard, T., Aasen, T. B., Burge, P. S., Heederik, D., Henneberger, P., Maestrelli, P. et al. 2012. Guidelines for the management of work-related asthma. *Eur Respir J* 39:529–45.

Bautista, D. M., Pellegrino, M. and Tsunozaki, M. 2013. TRPA1: A gatekeeper for inflammation. *Annu Rev Physiol* 75:181–200.

Beach, J., Rowe, B. H., Blitz, S. et al. 2005. *Diagnosis and Management of Work-Related Asthma.* Summary, Evidence Report/Technology Assessment: Number 129 AHRQ Publication Number 06-E003-1, October 2005 Agency for Healthcare Research and Quality, Rockville, MD. http://www.ahrq.gov/clinic/epcsums/asthworksum.htm

Beach, J., Russell, K., Blitz, S., Hooton, N., Spooner, C., Lemiere, C., Tarlo, S. M. et al. 2007. A systematic review of the diagnosis of occupational asthma. *Chest* 131:569–78.

Berger, Z., Rom, W. N., Reibman, J., Kim, M., Zhang, S., Luo, L. and Friedman-Jimenez, G. 2006. Prevalence of workplace exacerbation of asthma symptoms in an urban working population of asthmatics. *J Occup Environ Med* 48:833–9.

Bernstein, D. I. 2011. Genetics of occupational asthma. *Curr Opin Allergy Clin Immunol* 11:86–9.

Bernstein, J. A. 2002. Material safety data sheets: Are they reliable in identifying human hazards? *J Allergy Clin Immunol* 110:35–8.

Bherer, L., Cushman, R., Courteau, J. P., Quevillon, M., Cote, G., Bourbeau, J., L'Archeveque, J. et al. 1994. Survey of construction workers repeatedly exposed to chlorine over a three to six month period in a pulpmill: II. Follow up of affected workers by questionnaire, spirometry and assessment of bronchial responsiveness 18–24 months after exposure ended. *Occup Environ Med* 51:225–8.

Blanc, P. D., Harber, P., Lavoie, K. and Vandenplas, O. 2013. Impairment and disability evaluations: I. Psychosocial, economic and medico-legal aspects. In J. L. Malo, M. Chan Yeung and D. I. Bernstein (eds), *Asthma in the Workplace.* Boca Raton, FL: CRC Press, pp. 163–181.

Brackbill, R. M., Hadler, J. L., Digrande, L., Ekenga, C. C., Farfel, M. R., Friedman, S., Perlman, S. E. et al. 2009. Asthma and posttraumatic stress symptoms 5–6 years following exposure to the World Trade Center terrorist attack. *JAMA* 302:502–16.

Brooks, S. M. and Bernstein, I. L. 2011. Irritant-induced airway disorders. *Immunol Allergy Clin North Am* 31:747–68, vi.

Brooks, S. M., Weiss, M. A. and Bernstein, I. L. 1985. Reactive airways dysfunction syndrome (RADS). Persistent asthma syndrome after high level irritant exposures. *Chest* 88:376–84.

Campo, P., Wisnewski, A. V., Lummus, Z., Cartier, A., Malo, J. L., Boulet, L. P. and Bernstein, D. I. 2007. Diisocyanate conjugate and immunoassay characteristics influence detection of specific antibodies in HDI-exposed workers. *Clin Exp Allergy* 37:1095–102.

Carlsten, C., Dybuncio, A., Pui, M. M. and Chan-Yeung, M. 2013. Respiratory impairment and systemic inflammation in cedar asthmatics removed from exposure. *PLoS One* 8:e57166.

Chan, J. K., Roth, J., Oppenheim, J. J., Tracey, K. J., Vogl, T., Feldmann, M., Horwood, N. et al. 2012. Alarmins: Awaiting a clinical response. *J Clin Invest* 122:2711–9.

Chan-Yeung, M., Lam, S., Kennedy, S. M. and Frew, A. 1994. Persistent asthma after repeated exposure to high concentrations of gases in pulpmills. *Am J Respir Crit Care Med* 149:1676–80.

Chiry, S., Boulet, L. P., Lepage, J., Forget, A., Begin, D., Chaboillez, S., Malo, J. L. et al. 2009. Frequency of work-related respiratory symptoms in workers without asthma. *Am J Ind Med* 52:447–54.

Chiry, S., Cartier, A., Malo, J. L., Tarlo, S. M. and Lemiere, C. 2007. Comparison of peak expiratory flow variability between workers with work-exacerbated asthma and occupational asthma. *Chest* 132:483–8.

Cone, J. E., Wugofski, L., Balmes, J. R., Das, R., Bowler, R., Alexeeff, G. and Shusterman, D. 1994. Persistent respiratory health effects after a metam sodium pesticide spill. *Chest* 106:500–8.

Cote, J., Kennedy, S. and Chan-Yeung, M. 1993. Quantitative versus qualitative analysis of peak expiratory flow in occupational asthma. *Thorax* 48:48–51.

Cullinan, P., Cook, A., Gordon, S., Nieuwenhuijsen, M. J., Tee, R. D., Venables, K. M., McDonald, J. C. et al. 1999. Allergen exposure, atopy and smoking as determinants of allergy to rats in a cohort of laboratory employees. *Eur Respir J* 13:1139–43.

Cullinan, P., Cook, A., Nieuwenhuijsen, M. J., Sandiford, C., Tee, R. D., Venables, K. M., McDonald, J. C. et al. 2001. Allergen and dust exposure as determinants of work-related symptoms and sensitization in a cohort of flour-exposed workers; a case-control analysis. *Ann Occup Hyg* 45:97–103.

de Groene, G. J., Pal, T. M., Beach, J., Tarlo, S. M., Spreeuwers, D., Frings-Dresen, M. H., Mattioli, S. et al. 2011. Workplace interventions for treatment of occupational asthma. *Cochrane Database Syst Rev* (5):CD006308.

Delclos, G. L., Gimeno, D., Arif, A. A., Burau, K. D., Carson, A., Lusk, C., Stock, T. et al. 2007. Occupational risk factors and asthma among health care professionals. *Am J Respir Crit Care Med* 175:667–75.

Demnati, R., Fraser, R., Martin, J. G., Plaa, G. and Malo, J. L. 1998. Effects of dexamethasone on functional and pathological changes in rat bronchi caused by high acute exposure to chlorine. *Toxicol Sci* 45:242–6.

Dewitte, J. D., Chan-Yeung, M. and Malo, J. L. 1994. Medicolegal and compensation aspects of occupational asthma. *Eur Respir J* 7:969–80.

Elliott, L., Heederik, D., Marshall, S., Peden, D. and Loomis, D. 2005. Progression of self-reported symptoms in laboratory animal allergy. *J Allergy Clin Immunol* 116:127–32.

Fishwick, D., Barber, C. M., Bradshaw, L. M., Ayres, J. G., Barraclough, R., Burge, S., Corne, J. M. et al. 2012. Standards of care for occupational asthma: An update. *Thorax* 67:278–80.

Fisseler-Eckhoff, A., Bartsch, H., Zinsky, R. and Schirren, J. 2011. Environmental isocyanate-induced asthma: Morphologic and pathogenetic aspects of an increasing occupational disease. *Int J Environ Res Public Health* 8:3672–87.

Frew, A. J., Chan, H., Lam, S. and Chan-Yeung, M. 1995. Bronchial inflammation in occupational asthma due to western red cedar. *Am J Respir Crit Care Med* 151:340–4.

Gautrin, D., Bernstein, I. L., Brooks, S. M. and Henneberger, P. K. 2006. Irritant-induced asthma and reactive airways dysfunction syndrome. In I. L. Bernstein, M. Chan-Yeung, J. L. Malo and D. I. Bernstein (eds), *Asthma in the Workplace*, third edition. New York, NY: Taylor & Francis, pp. 305–324.

Gautrin, D., Boulet, L. P., Boutet, M., Dugas, M., Bherer, L., L'Archeveque, J., Laviolette, M. et al. 1994. Is reactive airways dysfunction syndrome a variant of occupational asthma? *J Allergy Clin Immunol* 93:12–22.

Gautrin, D., Ghezzo, H., Infante-Rivard, C., Magnan, M., L'Archeveque, J., Suarthana, E. and Malo, J. L. 2008. Long-term outcomes in a prospective cohort of apprentices exposed to high-molecular-weight agents. *Am J Respir Crit Care Med* 177:871–9.

Gautrin, D., Ghezzo, H., Infante-Rivard, C. and Malo, J. L. 2001a. Natural history of sensitization, symptoms and occupational diseases in apprentices exposed to laboratory animals. *Eur Respir J* 17:904–8.

Gautrin, D., Infante-Rivard, C., Ghezzo, H. and Malo, J. L. 2001b. Incidence and host determinants of probable occupational asthma in apprentices exposed to laboratory animals. *Am J Respir Crit Care Med* 163:899–904.

Gautrin, D., Leroyer, C., Infante-Rivard, C., Ghezzo, H., Dufour, J. G., Girard, D. and Malo, J. L. 1999. Longitudinal assessment of airway caliber and responsiveness in workers exposed to chlorine. *Am J Respir Crit Care Med* 160:1232–7.

Girard, F., Chaboillez, S., Cartier, A., Cote, J., Hargreave, F. E., Labrecque, M., Malo, J. L. et al. 2004. An effective strategy for diagnosing occupational asthma: Use of induced sputum. *Am J Respir Crit Care Med* 170:845–50.

Goe, S. K., Henneberger, P. K., Reilly, M. J., Rosenman, K. D., Schill, D. P., Valiante, D., Flattery, J. et al. 2004. A descriptive study of work aggravated asthma. *Occup Environ Med* 61:512–7.

Heederik, D., Henneberger, P. K. and Redlich, C. A. 2012. Primary prevention: Exposure reduction, skin exposure and respiratory protection. *Eur Respir Rev* 21:112–24.

Henneberger, P. K., Liang, X., London, S. J., Umbach, D. M., Sandler, D. P. and Hoppin, J. A. 2014. Exacerbation of symptoms in agricultural pesticide applicators with asthma. *Int Arch Occup Environ Health* 87:423–32.

Henneberger, P. K., Redlich, C. A., Callahan, D. B., Harber, P., Lemiere, C., Martin, J., Tarlo, S. M. et al. 2011. An official American Thoracic Society statement: Work-exacerbated asthma. *Am J Respir Crit Care Med* 184:368–78.

Jonasson, S., Koch, B. and Bucht, A. 2013. Inhalation of chlorine causes long-standing lung inflammation and airway hyperresponsiveness in a murine model of chemical-induced lung injury. *Toxicology* 303:34–42.

Jones, M. G. 2008. Exposure–response in occupational allergy. *Curr Opin Allergy Clin Immunol* 8:110–4.

Karjalainen, A., Kurppa, K., Martikainen, R., Klaukka, T. and Karjalainen, J. 2001. Work is related to a substantial portion of adult-onset asthma incidence in the Finnish population. *Am J Respir Crit Care Med* 164:565–8.

Karjalainen, A., Kurppa, K., Virtanen, S., Keskinen, H. and Nordman, H. 2000. Incidence of occupational asthma by occupation and industry in Finland. *Am J Ind Med* 37:451–8.

Karjalainen, A., Martikainen, R., Klaukka, T., Saarinen, K. and Uitti, J. 2003. Risk of asthma among Finnish patients with occupational rhinitis. *Chest* 123:283–8.

Kern, D. G. 1991. Outbreak of the reactive airways dysfunction syndrome after a spill of glacial acetic acid. *Am Rev Respir Dis* 144:1058–64.

Kogevinas, M., Zock, J. P., Jarvis, D., Kromhout, H., Lillienberg, L., Plana, E., Radon, K. et al. 2007. Exposure to substances in the workplace and new-onset asthma: An international prospective population-based study (ECRHS-II). *Lancet* 370:336–41.

Kristiansson, M. H., Lindh, C. H. and Jonsson, B. A. 2003. Determination of hexahydrophthalic anhydride adducts to human serum albumin. *Biomarkers* 8:343–59.

Lamontagne, A. D., Radi, S., Elder, D. S., Abramson, M. J. and Sim, M. 2006. Primary prevention of latex related sensitisation and occupational asthma: A systematic review. *Occup Environ Med* 63:359–64.

Larbanois, A., Jamart, J., Delwiche, J. P. and Vandenplas, O. 2002. Socio-economic outcome of subjects experiencing asthma symptoms at work. *Eur Respir J* 19:1107–13.

Lemière, C., Begin, D., Camus, M., Forget, A., Boulet, L. P. and Gerin, M. 2012. Occupational risk factors associated with work-exacerbated asthma in Quebec. *Occup Environ Med* 69:901–7.

Lemière, C., Boulet, L. P., Chaboillez, S., Forget, A., Chiry, S., Villeneuve, H., Prince, P. et al. 2013. Work-exacerbated asthma and occupational asthma: Do they really differ? *J Allergy Clin Immunol* 131:704–10.

Lemière, C., Cartier, A., Dolovich, J., Chan-Yeung, M., Grammer, L., Ghezzo, H., L'Archeveque, J. et al. 1996. Outcome of specific bronchial responsiveness to occupational agents after removal from exposure. *Am J Respir Crit Care Med* 154:329–33.

Lemière, C., Chaboillez, S., Malo, J. L. and Cartier, A. 2001. Changes in sputum cell counts after exposure to occupational agents: What do they mean? *J Allergy Clin Immunol* 107:1063–8.

Lemière, C., Chaboillez, S., Welman, M. and Maghni, K. 2010. Outcome of occupational asthma after removal from exposure: A follow-up study. *Can Respir J* 17:61–6.

Lemière, C., Forget, A., Dufour, M. H., Boulet, L. P. and Blais, L. 2007. Characteristics and medical resource use of asthmatic subjects with and without work-related asthma. *J Allergy Clin Immunol* 120:1354–9.

Lemière, C., Malo, J. L., Boulet, L. P. and Boutet, M. 1996. Reactive airways dysfunction syndrome induced by exposure to a mixture containing isocyanate: Functional and histopathologic behaviour. *Allergy* 51:262–5.

Lemière, C., Malo, J. L. and Boutet, M. 1997. Reactive airways dysfunction syndrome due to chlorine: Sequential bronchial biopsies and functional assessment. *Eur Respir J* 10:241–4.

Lemière, C., Pelissier, S., Chaboillez, S. and Teolis, L. 2006. Outcome of subjects diagnosed with occupational asthma and work-aggravated asthma after removal from exposure. *J Occup Environ Med* 48:656–9.

Lemière, C., Pizzichini, M. M., Balkissoon, R., Clelland, L., Efthimiadis, A., O'Shaughnessy, D., Dolovich, J. et al. 1999. Diagnosing occupational asthma: Use of induced sputum. *Eur Respir J* 13:482–8.

Lemière, C., NGuyen, S., Sava, F., D'Alpaos, V., Huaux, F. and Vandenplas, O. 2014. Occupational asthma phenotypes identified by increased fractional exhaled nitric oxide after exposure to causal agents. *J Allergy Clin Immunol* 134:1063–7.

Lillienberg, L., Andersson, E., Janson, C., Dahlman-Hoglund, A., Forsberg, B., Holm, M., Glslason, T. et al. 2013. Occupational exposure and new-onset asthma in a population-based study in Northern Europe (RHINE). *Ann Occup Hyg* 57:482–92.

Liss, G. M., Tarlo, S. M., Labrecque, M. and Malo, J. L. 2006. Prevention and surveillance. In I. L. Bernstein, M. Chang-Yeung, J. L. Malo and D. I Bernstein (eds), *Asthma in the Workplace*, third edition. New York, NY: Taylor & Francis. pp. 150–62.

Lummus, Z. L., Alam, R., Bernstein, J. A. and Bernstein, D. I. 1998. Diisocyanate antigen-enhanced production of monocyte chemoattractant protein-1, IL-8 and tumor necrosis factor-alpha by peripheral mononuclear cells of workers with occupational asthma. *J Allergy Clin Immunol* 102:265–74.

Lummus, Z. L., Wisnewski, A. V. and Bernstein, D. I. 2011. Pathogenesis and disease mechanisms of occupational asthma. *Immunol Allergy Clin North Am* 31:699–716, vi.

Maestrelli, P., Boschetto, P., Fabbri, L. M. and Mapp, C. E. 2009. Mechanisms of occupational asthma. *J Allergy Clin Immunol* 123:531–42; quiz 543–4.

Maestrelli, P., Schlunssen, V., Mason, P. and Sigsgaard, T. 2012. Contribution of host factors and workplace exposure to the outcome of occupational asthma. *Eur Respir Rev* 21:88–96.

Maghni, K., Lemiere, C., Ghezzo, H., Yuquan, W. and Malo, J. L. 2004. Airway inflammation after cessation of exposure to agents causing occupational asthma. *Am J Respir Crit Care Med* 169:367–72.

Malo, J. L., Boulet, L. P., Dewitte, J. D., Cartier, A., L'Archeveque, J., Cote, J., Bedard, G. et al. 1993. Quality of life of subjects with occupational asthma. *J Allergy Clin Immunol* 91:1121–7.

Malo, J. L., Cardinal, S., Ghezzo, H., L'Archeveque, J., Castellanos, L. and Maghni, K. 2011. Association of bronchial reactivity to occupational agents with methacholine reactivity, sputum cells and immunoglobulin E-mediated reactivity. *Clin Exp Allergy* 41:497–504.

Malo, J. L., Cartier, A., Boulet, L. P., L'Archeveque, J., Saint-Denis, F., Bherer, L. and Courteau, J. P. 1994. Bronchial hyperresponsiveness can improve while spirometry plateaus two to three years after repeated exposure to chlorine causing respiratory symptoms. *Am J Respir Crit Care Med* 150:1142–5.

Malo, J. L. and Chan-Yeung, M. 2009. Agents causing occupational asthma. *J Allergy Clin Immunol* 123:545–50.

Malo, J. L., Ghezzo, H., D'Aquino, C., L'Archeveque, J., Cartier, A. and Chan-Yeung, M. 1992. Natural history of occupational asthma: Relevance of type of agent and other factors in the rate of development of symptoms in affected subjects. *J Allergy Clin Immunol* 90:937–44.

Malo, J. L., Ghezzo, H., L'Archeveque, J., Lagier, F., Perrin, B. and Cartier, A. 1991. Is the clinical history a satisfactory means of diagnosing occupational asthma? *Am Rev Respir Dis* 143:528–32.

Malo, J. L., L'Archeveque, J., Castellanos, L., Lavoie, K., Ghezzo, H. and Maghni, K. 2009. Long-term outcomes of acute irritant-induced asthma. *Am J Respir Crit Care Med* 179:923–8.

Malo, J. L., L'Archeveque, J. and Ghezzo, H. 2008. Direct costs of occupational asthma in Quebec between 1988 and 2002. *Can Respir J* 15:413–6.

Malo, J. L., Lemière, C., Desjardins, A. and Cartier, A. 1997. Prevalence and intensity of rhinoconjunctivitis in subjects with occupational asthma. *Eur Respir J* 10:1513–5.

Malo, J. L. and Vandenplas, O. 2011. Definitions and classification of work-related asthma. *Immunol Allergy Clin North Am* 31:645–62.

McDonald, J. C., Chen, Y., Zekveld, C. and Cherry, N. M. 2005. Incidence by occupation and industry of acute work related respiratory diseases in the UK, 1992–2001. *Occup Environ Med* 62:836–42.

Medina-Ramon, M., Zock, J. P., Kogevinas, M., Sunyer, J., Torralba, Y., Borrell, A., Burgos, F. et al. 2005. Asthma, chronic bronchitis and exposure to irritant agents in occupational domestic cleaning: A nested case–control study. *Occup Environ Med* 62:598–606.

Miedinger, D., Lavoie, K. L., L'Archeveque, J., Ghezzo, H., Zunzunuegui, M. V. and Malo, J. L. 2011. Quality-of-life, psychological and cost outcomes 2 years after diagnosis of occupational asthma. *J Occup Environ Med* 53:231–8.

Miedinger, D., Malo, J. L., Ghezzo, H., L'Archeveque, J. and Zunzunegui, M. V. 2010. Factors influencing duration of exposure with symptoms and costs of occupational asthma. *Eur Respir J* 36:728–34.

Mirabelli, M. C., Zock, J. P., Plana, E., Anto, J. M., Benke, G., Blanc, P. D., Dahlman-Hoglund, A. et al. 2007. Occupational risk factors for asthma among nurses and related healthcare professionals in an international study. *Occup Environ Med* 64:474–9.

Moller, D. R., McKay, R. T., Bernstein, I. L. and Brooks, S. M. 1986. Persistent airways disease caused by toluene diisocyanate. *Am Rev Respir Dis* 134:175–6.

Moore, V. C., Parsons, N. R., Jaakkola, M. S., Burge, C. B., Pantin, C. F., Robertson, A. S. and Burge, P. S. 2009. Serial lung function variability using four portable logging meters. *J Asthma* 46:961–6.

Moscato, G. 2014. Specific immonutherapy and biologicam treatments for occupational allergy. *Curr Opin Allergy Clin Immunol* 14:576–81.

Moscato, G., Pala, G., Barnig, C., De Blay, F., Del Giacco, S., Folletti, I., Heffler, E. et al. 2012. EAACI consensus statement for investigation of work-related asthma (WRA) in non-specialized centres. *Allergy* 67:491–501.

Nicholson, P., Cullinan, P., Burge, P. and Boyle, C. 2010. *Occupational Asthma: Prevention, Identification* and *Management: Systematic Review* and *Recommendations*. London: British Occupational Health Research Foundation.

Obata, H., Dittrick, M., Chan, H. and Chan-Yeung, M. 1999. Sputum eosinophils and exhaled nitric oxide during late asthmatic reaction in patients with western red cedar asthma. *Eur Respir J* 13:489–95.

Olin, A. C., Andersson, E., Andersson, M., Granung, G., Hagberg, S. and Toren, K. 2004. Prevalence of asthma and exhaled nitric oxide are increased in bleachery workers exposed to ozone. *Eur Respir J* 23:87–92.

Orriols, R., Isidro, I., Abu-Shams, K., Costa, R., Boldu, J., Rego, G. and Zock, J. P. 2010. Reported occupational respiratory diseases in three Spanish regions. *Am J Ind Med* 53:922–30.

Pahr, S., Constantin, C., Mari, A., Scheiblhofer, S., Thalhamer, J., Ebner, C., Vrtala, S. et al. 2012. Molecular characterization of wheat allergens specifically recognized by patients suffering from wheat-induced respiratory allergy. *Clin Exp Allergy* 42:597–609.

Palczynski, C., Gorski, P. and Jakubowski, J. 1994. The case of TDI-induced reactive airway dysfunction syndrome with the presence of specific IgE antibodies. *Allergol Immunopathol (Madr)* 22:80–2.

Park, H., Jung, K., Kim, H., Nahm, D. and Kang, K. 1999. Neutrophil activation following TDI bronchial challenges to the airway secretion from subjects with TDI-induced asthma. *Clin Exp Allergy* 29:1395–401.

Piipari, R. and Keskinen, H. 2005. Agents causing occupational asthma in Finland in 1986–2002: Cow epithelium bypassed by moulds from moisture-damaged buildings. *Clin Exp Allergy* 35:1632–7.

Piirilä, P. L., Keskinen, H. M., Luukkonen, R., Salo, S. P., Tuppurainen, M. and Nordman, H. 2005. Work, unemployment and life satisfaction among patients with diisocyanate induced asthma—A prospective study. *J Occup Health* 47:112–8.

Piirilä, P. L., Meuronen, A., Majuri, M. L., Luukkonen, R., Mäntylä, T., Wolff, H. J., Nordman, H. et al. 2008. Inflammation and functional outcome in diisocyanate-induced asthma after cessation of exposure. *Allergy* 63:583–91.

Prezant, D. J., Weiden, M., Banauch, G. I., McGuinness, G., Rom, W. N., Aldrich, T. K. and Kelly, K. J. 2002. Cough and bronchial responsiveness in firefighters at the World Trade Center site. *N Engl J Med* 347:806–15.

Pronk, A., Preller, L., Raulf-Heimsoth, M., Jonkers, I. C., Lammers, J. W., Wouters, I. M., Doekes, G. et al. 2007. Respiratory symptoms, sensitization and exposure response relationships in spray painters exposed to isocyanates. *Am J Respir Crit Care Med* 176:1090–7.

Quirce, S. and Bernstein, J. A. 2011. Old and new causes of occupational asthma. *Immunol Allergy Clin North Am* 31:677–98, v.

Quirce, S., Lemiere, C., De Blay, F., Del Pozo, V., Gerth van Wijk, R., Maestrelli, P., Pauli, G. et al. 2010. Noninvasive methods for assessment of airway inflammation in occupational settings. *Allergy* 65:445–59.

Rachiotis, G., Savani, R., Brant, A., MacNeill, S. J., Newman Taylor, A. and Cullinan, P. 2007. Outcome of occupational asthma after cessation of exposure: A systematic review. *Thorax* 62:147–52.

Redlich, C. A. 2010. Skin exposure and asthma: Is there a connection? *Proc Am Thorac Soc* 7:134–7.

Reinisch, F., Harrison, R. J., Cussler, S., Athanasoulis, M., Balmes, J., Blanc, P. and Cone, J. 2001. Physician reports of work-related asthma in California, 1993–1996. *Am J Ind Med* 39:72–83.

Rioux, J. P., Malo, J. L., L'Archeveque, J., Rabhi, K. and Labrecque, M. 2008. Workplace-specific challenges as a contribution to the diagnosis of occupational asthma. *Eur Respir J* 32:997–1003.

Saarinen, K., Karjalainen, A., Martikainen, R., Uitti, J., Tammilehto, L., Klaukka, T. and Kurppa, K. 2003. Prevalence of work-aggravated symptoms in clinically established asthma. *Eur Respir J* 22:305–9.

Saetta, M., Maestrelli, P., Turato, G., Mapp, C. E., Milani, G., Pivirotto, F., Fabbri, L. M. et al. 1995. Airway wall remodeling after cessation of exposure to isocyanates in sensitized asthmatic subjects. *Am J Respir Crit Care Med* 151:489–94.

Sastre, J., Fernandez-Nieto, M., Novalbos, A., De Las Heras, M., Cuesta, J. and Quirce, S. 2003. Need for monitoring nonspecific bronchial hyperresponsiveness before and after isocyanate inhalation challenge. *Chest* 123:1276–9.

Shakeri, M. S., Dick, F. D. and Ayres, J. G. 2008. Which agents cause reactive airways dysfunction syndrome (RADS)? A systematic review. *Occup Med (Lond)* 58:205–11.

Siracusa, A., Folletti, I. and Moscato, G. 2013. Non-IgE-mediated and irritant-induced work-related rhinitis. *Curr Opin Allergy Clin Immunol* 13:159–66.

Siracusa, A., Marabini, A., Folletti, I. and Moscato, G. 2006. Smoking and occupational asthma. *Clin Exp Allergy* 36:577–84.

Tai, H. Y., Tam, M. F., Chou, H., Peng, H. J., Su, S. N., Perng, D. W. and Shen, H. D. 2006. Pen ch 13 allergen induces secretion of mediators and degradation of occludin protein of human lung epithelial cells. *Allergy* 61:382–8.

Takeda, N., Maghni, K., Daigle, S., L'Archeveque, J., Castellanos, L., Al-Ramli, W., Malo, J. L. et al. 2009. Long-term pathologic consequences of acute irritant-induced asthma. *J Allergy Clin Immunol* 124:975–81.e1.

Tarlo, S. M. 2003. Workplace irritant exposures: Do they produce true occupational asthma? *Ann Allergy Asthma Immunol* 90:19–23.

Tarlo, S. M., Balmes, J., Balkissoon, R., Beach, J., Beckett, W., Bernstein, D., Blanc, P. D. et al. 2008. Diagnosis and management of work-related asthma: American College of Chest Physicians Consensus Statement. *Chest* 134:1S–41S.

Tarlo, S. M. and Broder, I. 1989. Irritant-induced occupational asthma. *Chest* 96:297–300.

Tarlo, S. M., Leung, K., Broder, I., Silverman, F. and Holness, D. L. 2000. Asthmatic subjects symptomatically worse at work: Prevalence and characterization among a general asthma clinic population. *Chest* 118:1309–14.

Tarlo, S. M., Liss, G., Corey, P. and Broder, I. 1995. A workers' compensation claim population for occupational asthma. Comparison of subgroups. *Chest* 107:634–41.

Tarlo, S. M. and Liss, G. M. 2010. Prevention of occupational asthma. *Curr Allergy Asthma Rep* 10:278–86.

Tarlo, S. M., Liss, G. M. and Yeung, K. S. 2002. Changes in rates and severity of compensation claims for asthma due to diisocyanates: A possible effect of medical surveillance measures. *Occup Environ Med* 59:58–62.

Toren, K. and Blanc, P. D. 2009. Asthma caused by occupational exposures is common—A systematic analysis of estimates of the population-attributable fraction. *BMC Pulm Med* 9:7.

Vandenplas, O. 2008. Socioeconomic impact of work-related asthma. *Expert Rev Pharmacoeconomics Outcome Res* 8:395–400.

Vandenplas, O. 2011. Occupational asthma: Etiologies and risk factors. *Allergy Asthma Immunol Res* 3:157–67.

Vandenplas, O., Cartier, A., Lesage, J., Cloutier, Y., Perreault, G., Grammer, L. C., Shaughnessy, M. A. et al. 1993. Prepolymers of hexamethylene diisocyanate as a cause of occupational asthma. *J Allergy Clin Immunol* 91:850–61.

Vandenplas, O., D'Alpaos, V., Heymans, J., Jamart, J., Thimpont, J., Huaux, F., Lison, D. et al. 2009. Sputum eosinophilia: An early marker of bronchial response to occupational agents. *Allergy* 64:754–61.

Vandenplas, O., Delwiche, J. P., Jamart, J. and Van De Weyer, R. 1996. Increase in non-specific bronchial hyperresponsiveness as an early marker of bronchial response to occupational agents during specific inhalation challenges. *Thorax* 51:472–8.

Vandenplas, O., Dressel, H., Nowak, D., Jamart, J. and ERS Task Force on the Management of Work-related Asthma. 2012. What is the optimal management option for occupational asthma? *Eur Respir Rev* 21:97–104.

Vandenplas, O., Fievez, P., Delwiche, J. P., Boulanger, J. and Thimpont, J. 2004. Persistent asthma following accidental exposure to formaldehyde. *Allergy* 59:115–6.

Vandenplas, O., Ghezzo, H., Munoz, X., Moscato, G., Perfetti, L., Lemiere, C., Labrecque, M. et al. 2005. What are the questionnaire items most useful in identifying subjects with occupational asthma? *Eur Respir J* 26:1056–63.

Vandenplas, O., Lantin, A. C., D'Alpaos, V., Larbanois, A., Hoet, P., Vandeweerdt, M., Thimpont, J. et al. 2011. Time trends in occupational asthma in Belgium. *Respir Med* 105:1364–72.

Vandenplas, O., Suojalehto, H., Aasen, T. B., Baur, X., Burge, P. S., De Blay, F., Fishwick, D. et al. 2014a. Specific inhalation challenge in the diagnosis of occupational asthma: Consensus statement. *Eur Respir J* 43:1573–87.

Vandenplas, O., Wiszniewska, M., Raulf, M., De Blay, F., Gerth van Wijk, R., Moscato, G., Nemery, B. et al. 2014b. EAACI position paper: Irritant-induced asthma. *Allergy* 69:1141–53.

van Kampen, V., De Blay, F., Folletti, I., Kobierski, P., Moscato, G., Olivieri, M., Quirce, S. et al. 2013. Evaluation of commercial skin prick test solutions for selected occupational allergens. *Allergy* 68:651–8.

Verstraelen, S., Wens, B., Hooyberghs, J., Nelissen, I., Witters, H., Schoeters, G., Cauwenberge, P. V. et al. 2008. Gene expression profiling of *in vitro* cultured macrophages after exposure to the respiratory sensitizer hexamethylene diisocyanate. *Toxicol In Vitro* 22:1107–14.

Vizcaya, D., Mirabelli, M. C., Anto, J. M., Orriols, R., Burgos, F., Arjona, L. and Zock, J. P. 2011. A workforce-based study of occupational exposures and asthma symptoms in cleaning workers. *Occup Environ Med* 68:914–9.

White, C. W. and Martin, J. G. 2010. Chlorine gas inhalation: Human clinical evidence of toxicity and experience in animal models. *Proc Am Thorac Soc* 7:257–63.

Wilken, D., Baur, X., Barbinova, L., Preisser, A., Meijer, E., Rooyackers, J. and Heederik, D. 2012. What are the benefits of medical screening and surveillance? *Eur Respir Rev* 21:105–11.

Wisnewski, A. V., Liu, J. and Colangelo, C. M. 2015. Glutathione reaction products with a chemical allergen, methylene-diphenyl diisocyanate, stimulate alternative macrophage activation and eosinophilic airway inflammation. *Chem Res Toxicol* 28:729–37.

Wisnewski, A. V., Liu, Q., Liu, J. and Redlich, C. A. 2008. Human innate immune responses to hexamethylene diisocyanate (HDI) and HDI-albumin conjugates. *Clin Exp Allergy* 38:957–67.

Wisnewski, A. V., Liu, Q., Miller, J. J., Magoski, N. and Redlich, C. A. 2002. Effects of hexamethylene diisocyanate exposure on human airway epithelial cells: *In vitro* cellular and molecular studies. *Environ Health Perspect* 110:901–7.

Yacoub, M. R., Lavoie, K., Lacoste, G., Daigle, S., L'Archeveque, J., Ghezzo, H., Lemiere, C. et al. 2007. Assessment of impairment/disability due to occupational asthma through a multidimensional approach. *Eur Respir J* 29:889–96.

Ye, Y. M., Kim, C. W., Kim, H. R., Kim, H. M., Suh, C. H., Nahm, D. H., Park, H. S. et al. 2006. Biophysical determinants of toluene diisocyanate antigenicity associated with exposure and asthma. *J Allergy Clin Immunol* 118:885–91.

27 Work-Related Upper Respiratory Tract Conditions

Ryan F. Hoy

CONTENTS

The upper respiratory tract comprises the nose, nasal cavity, sinuses, mouth, pharynx and larynx, and provides vital functions of air conditioning, phonation and sensation (taste, smell and irritation). The upper respiratory tract protects the lower respiratory tract through mechanisms including:

- Nasal hairs, which capture large dust particles as they enter the respiratory tract.
- The trigeminal nerve, which provides the sensation of irritation in the nose, serving as an immediate 'warning effect' when exposed to potentially harmful substances with irritant properties, such as ammonia and sulphur dioxide.
- Mucous lining the upper airway, which traps particles that come into contact with the walls by impaction (Shusterman, 2002). Mucociliary clearance removes these particles by expectoration or swallowing.
- The cough reflex, which can be triggered by stimulation of receptors in the larynx following inhalation of chemical and mechanical irritants, causing rapid clearance of air through the upper respiratory tract (Chung and Pavord, 2008).
- The 'glottic closure reflex', which induces rapid closure of the glottic aperture in the larynx in order to protect the lower airway from aspiration of foreign material, but this can also be triggered by chemical stimulation of the superior laryngeal nerve.

Occupational air pollutants that primarily affect the upper rather than lower respiratory tract include large

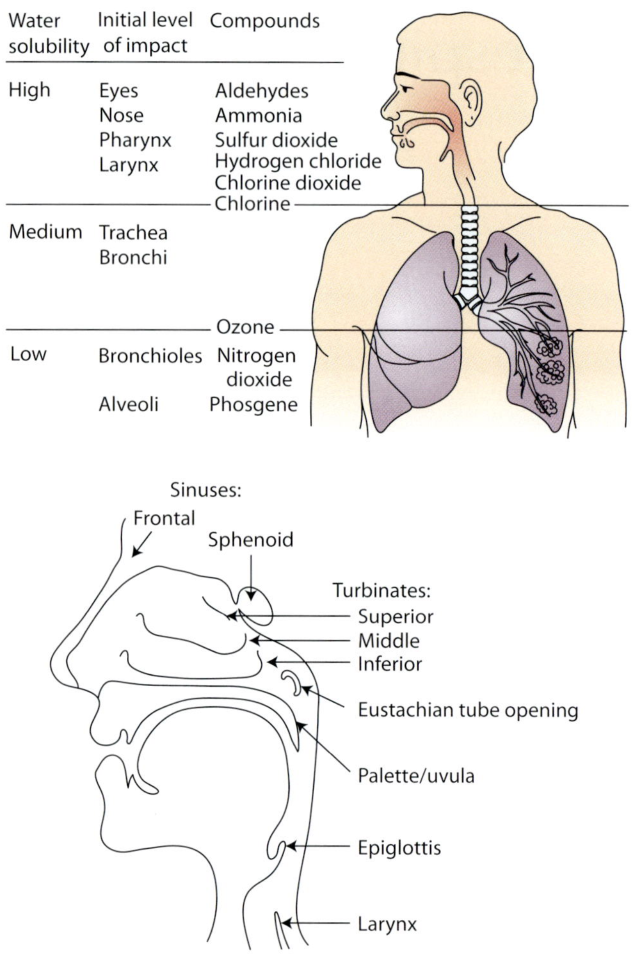

FIGURE 27.1 Anatomical features of the upper respiratory tract and the effects of water solubility of a gas or vapour. (Reproduced from Shusterman, D. 2002. *Environ Health Perspect* 110:649–53.)

dust particles or aerosols (>10 μm diameter) that impact in the upper airway. Highly water-soluble and reactive irritant gases or vapours (such as chlorine, ammonia, sulphur dioxide and formaldehyde) dissolve readily in the upper airways' mucous membrane water and are more likely to have an effect on the upper respiratory tract (Figure 27.1) (Shusterman, 2011).

WORK-RELATED RHINITIS

Occupational rhinitis (OR) has been defined as an 'inflammatory disease of the nose, which is characterized by intermittent or persistent symptoms (i.e. nasal congestion, sneezing, rhinorrhoea, itching), and/or variable nasal airflow limitation and/or hypersecretion due to causes and conditions attributable to a particular work environment and not to stimuli encountered outside the workplace' by the European Academy of Allergology and Clinical Immunology (EAACI) in 2009 (Moscato et al., 2009). The central feature of this definition is the causal relationship between work and the development of rhinitis. Although OR is two- to four-times more common than occupational asthma (OA), this condition receives considerably less recognition, despite its significant negative impact on quality of life (Airaksinen et al., 2009).

OR has been classified into two groups: allergic OR (including IgE-mediated and non-IgE-mediated types) and non-allergic OR. Pre-existing rhinitis may also be aggravated by occupational exposures, and this has been referred to as work-exacerbated rhinitis (WER). Analogous to the classification scheme for work-related asthma, the term 'work-related rhinitis' has been proposed to encompass both OR (rhinitis caused by workplace exposures) and WER (Figure 27.2) (Tarlo et al., 2008; Moscato et al., 2009).

Allergic OR

Allergic OR is caused by an immunologically mediated nasal hypersensitivity response (Moscato et al., 2008). Allergic OR is characterised by a period of latency during which immunological sensitisation develops, but the worker is yet to experience symptoms. The duration of the latent period is variable, but is typically weeks to months from the onset of exposure. Following the onset of symptomatic allergic OR, nasal symptoms will recur with exposure to the causative agent, even at very low doses. Sensitisers that are reported to cause allergic OR are similar to those associated with sensitiser-induced OA. Allergic OR includes IgE-mediated and non-IgE-mediated types:

1. IgE-mediated allergic OR is associated with a wide range of high-molecular-weight (HMW; >5 kDa) occupational agents (including wheat, grain dust, animal-derived allergens, latex and biological enzymes) and some low-molecular-weight (LMW; <5 kDa) agents (such as platinum salts and reactive dyes). IgE-mediated OR is driven by T-helper 2 cells producing cytokines such as IL-4, IL-5 and IL-13, which activate B lymphocytes, causing them to secrete allergen-specific IgE. Further exposure to the allergen results in cross-linking of the allergen with its specific mast cell-bound IgE, causing degranulation with local release of histamine, tryptase and leukotrienes (Hox et al., 2014). This is the same mechanism that is associated with non-occupational allergic rhinitis, such as with dust mite and pollen allergies (Greiner et al., 2011).

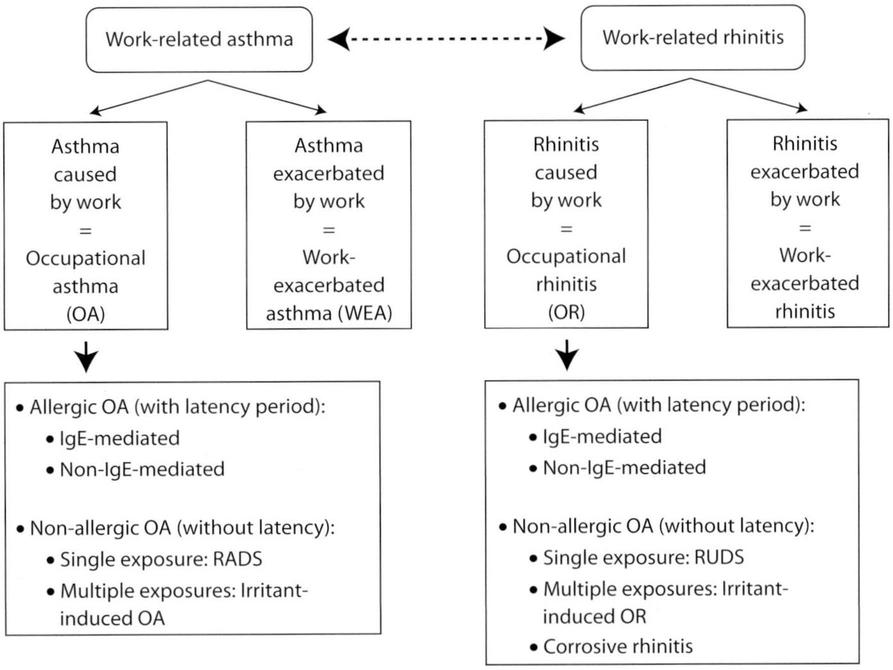

FIGURE 27.2 Parallel classification of occupational asthma and rhinitis. (Reproduced from Moscato, G. et al. 2009. *Respir Res* 10:16. With permission.)

2. Non-IgE-mediated allergic OR has been described in association with some LMW sensitisers, including isocyanates, western red cedar and persulfate salts (Hox et al., 2014). The allergic mechanism has not been fully characterised; however, LMW agents are capable of sensitising the adaptive immune response by acting as haptens in conjugation with proteins, such as albumin (Table 27.1) (Hox et al., 2014).

Non-Allergic OR

Non-allergic (non-immunological) OR includes forms of rhinitis caused by irritant exposures at the workplace. Transient or persistent rhinitis symptoms may develop following single or multiple exposures to upper airway irritants without a period of latency (Moscato et al., 2009). Several forms of non-allergic OR have been described.

Corrosive rhinitis is a severe form of non-allergic OR associated with high-level exposure to corrosive chemicals, which can cause severe trauma to the nasal passages, resulting in ulceration and possibly septum perforation. Chronic exposure to hexavalent chromium from welding fumes or metal plating operations has been described to cause corrosive rhinitis (Lin et al., 1994).

The term 'reactive upper airway dysfunction syndrome' (RUDS) has been proposed to describe the development of chronic rhinitis following a single high-intensity exposure to an irritant, analogous to reactive airways dysfunction syndrome (a form of irritant-induced OA) (Meggs, 1994). Nasal biopsies of patients with RUDS after chlorine exposure showed an increased number of nerve fibres, which may explain persistent sensitivity and symptoms following a single irritant exposure (Meggs, 1997). A positive feedback loop may be developed, with epithelial damage leading to a lower threshold at which chemicals produce inflammation. Inflammation in turn leads to ongoing loss of epithelial integrity (Meggs, 1997).

Irritant-induced OR may develop with repeated exposure to irritants at work (such as dust, fumes and vapours) without a specific episode of 'high'-level exposure, leading to transient or persistent symptoms of rhinitis (Moscato et al., 2008). Irritant occupational exposures associated with rhinitis include ozone, grain dust, volatile organic compounds (VOCs), formaldehyde, wood dust and chlorine gas (Hellgren et al., 2003; Moscato et al., 2009).

'Non-specific building-related illness' is a contentious entity that comprises a constellation of symptoms, including nasal irritation and congestion, as well as ocular irritation, headache and difficulty concentrating. This condition has been associated with exposure to low levels of airway irritants such as VOCs, formaldehyde and bio-aerosols, but also personal factors such as stress (Laumbach and Kipen, 2005; Menzies and Kreiss, 2006; Shusterman and Murphy, 2007).

TABLE 27.1
Agents and Occupations Associated with Occupational Rhinitis

Agent	Occupation	Prevalence (%)
High Molecular Weight		
Laboratory animals	Laboratory workers	6–33
Other animal-derived allergens	Swine confinement workers	8–23
Insects and mites	Laboratory workers, farms workers	2–60
Grain dust	Grain elevators	28–64
Flour	Bakers	18–29
Latex	Hospital workers, textile factory workers	9–20
Other plant allergens	Tobacco, carpet, hot pepper, tea, coffee, cocoa, dried fruit and saffron workers	5–36
Biological enzymes	Pharmaceutical and detergent industries	3–87
Fish and seafood proteins	Trout, prawn, shrimp, crab and clam workers, fish-food factory workers	5–24
Low Molecular Weight		
Diisocyanates	Painters, urethane mould workers	36–42
Anhydrides	Epoxy resin production, chemical workers, electrical condenser workers	10–48
Wood dust	Carpentry and furniture making	10–36
Platinum	Platinum refinery workers	43
Chemicals	Manufacturing of reactive dyes, persulphate, shoes, synthetic fibres, pulp and paper, hairdressing	3–30
Drugs (psyllium, spiramycin, piperacillin)	Healthcare and pharmaceutical workers	9–41

Source: Reproduced from Moscato, G. et al. 2009. *Respir Res* 10:16; Siracusa, A., Desrosiers, M. and Marabini, A. 2000. *Clin Exp Allergy* 30:1519–34. With permission.

Occupational vasomotor rhinitis has been used to describe a form of non-allergic rhinitis associated with nasal reactivity to non-specific physical stimuli at work, such as low humidity, rapid changes in temperature and excessive air motion (Balkissoon, 2002). Rhinorrhoea is the predominant symptom rather than nasal itch or sneezing.

WER is pre-existing or concurrent (non-allergic or allergic) rhinitis that is worsened by workplace exposures (Moscato et al., 2008). Many workplace conditions and exposures may exacerbate rhinitis, such as irritant agents (dusts, chemicals and fumes), physical factors (temperature and humidity level), strong smells (such as perfumes) and common environmental allergens (such as grass pollens and dust mites) (Moscato et al., 2008). Symptoms of WER are similar to OR; therefore, thorough assessment for the presence of a potential workplace sensitiser should be undertaken prior to making a diagnosis of WER.

Irritant exposure may also interact with non-occupational allergic rhinitis (Shusterman, 2011). Pre-existing nasal allergies can intensify responses to nasal irritants. Exposure to some pollutants such as diesel exhaust can reinforce sensitisation or intensify allergy responses (Diaz-Sanchez et al., 2000). Conversely, exposure to air pollutants can intensify responses in the setting of allergic rhinitis and reinforce sensitisation (Shusterman, 2011).

Epidemiology

Allergic rhinitis is very common in the general population, affecting 10%–40% of people in the United States and other industrialised countries (Uzzaman and Story, 2012; Canuel and Lebel, 2014). Non-allergic rhinitis has been noted to affect approximately 7% of the US population (Settipane and Kaliner, 2013). There has, however, been very little study of the prevalence of OR in the general population.

Occupations that pose a risk for workers developing OR are similar to those that pose a risk for workers developing OA. Data from Finland note that at-risk occupations include furriers, bakers, livestock breeders, food processing workers, veterinarians, farmers, electronic/electrical product assemblers and boat builders (Hytonen et al., 1997).

The prevalence of OR in some high-risk industries has been well studied, including animal-exposed laboratory workers (6%–33%), bakers (18%–29%) and grain elevator workers (28%–64%) (Siracusa et al., 2000; Moscato et al., 2009). Studies of diisocyanate-exposed workers noted a prevalence of work-related nasal symptoms ranging from 36% to 42%, but specific IgE antibodies were found in only 1% (Siracusa et al., 2000). Similarly, specific IgE has low predictive sensitivity for the diagnosis of diisocyanate OA (Kimber et al., 2014).

The dose of exposure to the sensitiser and a background of atopy are the main established risk factors for the development of HMW-associated OR (Siracusa et al., 2000).

Relationship between OR and OA

In the non-occupational setting, asthma and rhinitis often coexist, and rhinitis typically precedes the development of asthma (Shaaban et al., 2008). The association between rhinitis and asthma has led to the description of 'united airways disease', in which an inflammatory response of the upper airway affects the lower respiratory tract and vice versa (Compalati et al., 2010).

OA is the most frequently reported occupational lung disease in developed countries; however, studies suggest that OR is two- to four-times more prevalent than OA (Siracusa et al., 2000; Ruoppi et al., 2004). In workers with OA, coexistent rhinitis symptoms are very common, occurring in 76%–92% of such workers (Malo et al., 1997). A French national study observed a high frequency of OR in association with OA caused by HMW flour (78.6%) and some LMW agents (quaternary ammoniums, 66.2% and persulphate salts, 60.5%) (Ameille et al., 2013).

OR caused by HMW agents usually develops prior to the onset of asthmatic symptoms (Malo et al., 1997). Data from Finland demonstrated a 4.8-fold increased risk of developing asthma in patients with OR in comparison to subjects with other occupational diseases (Karjalainen et al., 2003). The greatest risk of asthma was in the year after reported rhinitis, but increased risk persisted for several years. In a study of laboratory animal allergy, OR occurred before OA in 45% of subjects and at the same time in 55%, but never afterwards (Gross, 1980; Siracusa et al., 2000). The interval between onset of nasal and respiratory symptoms was 4.6 months. In a study of rat-exposed laboratory workers, nasal symptoms were noted to develop after a median interval of 12 months, and asthma symptoms after 18 months (Cullinan et al., 1999). The prevalence of OR in subjects with OA caused by LMW agents has been reported to be similar, but with less intense symptoms and fewer cases developing before the onset of asthma (Malo et al., 1997).

Clinical Features

Diagnostically, it can be very difficult to differentiate forms of work-related rhinitis and to differentiate these from non-work related rhinitis. The clinical history should attempt to identify whether there is a temporal association of nasal symptoms with reference to work activities (Moscato et al., 2009). Improvement in symptoms whilst away from the workplace, such as on holidays, would be expected for a workplace cause of rhinitis. A thorough occupational history should be undertaken, including the worker's current job duties, duration of employment, workplace hygiene standards, personal protective equipment used, agents or tasks associated with symptoms, processes in adjacent work areas and changes in work processes or materials (Moscato et al., 2009). Safety datasheets of products that are used at the workplace may assist in the identification of potential sensitisers or respiratory irritants.

Nasal examination should be undertaken using anterior rhinoscopy and nasal endoscopy (Moscato et al., 2009). Visualisation of the nasal mucosa provides the ability to identify other nasal pathologies that may mimic rhinitis or contribute to nasal obstruction (septal deviation and nasal polyps) in patients with rhinitis. Clinical features of asthma should always be assessed, as these conditions often coexist.

Investigations

Objective tests are required in order to confirm that rhinitis is caused by a particular work environment. Assessment should include evaluation of other causes of rhinitis, such as allergy to common non-occupational aeroallergens (house dust mites, pollens and pet dander). An EAACI position paper on OR has developed a diagnostic algorithm for this purpose (Moscato et al., 2009). Initially, a thorough medical and occupational assessment with nasal examination should be undertaken. When available, immunological tests in order to demonstrate IgE-mediated sensitisation (skin-prick tests and/or specific serum IgE antibodies) should be performed towards the suspected occupational allergen based on the history obtained and the review of safety datasheets. Well-standardised extracts for only a limited number of occupational allergens (mostly HMW agents) are available. The results of such an approach are sensitive but not specific for the diagnosis of OR, as many exposed but asymptomatic workers may be sensitised (demonstrating specific IgE) towards the allergen. The diagnosis of OR may be considered 'probable' in the setting of a consistent clinical history and the demonstration of a positive marker of sensitisation (Moscato et al., 2009).

Despite exposure to a well-described HWM cause of OR, in one study of workers who were exposed to laboratory animals, 24% of subjects reported incident occupational rhinoconjunctivitis symptoms, yet only 9.6% had symptoms combined with skin sensitisation to an animal-derived allergen (Rodier et al., 2003). This suggests that nasal symptoms in such a cohort may also be due to irritant exposures, such as to dust and ammonia. High rates of non-allergic rhinitis symptoms have also been described in pastry-making apprentices, in whom the incidence of allergic OR was only a tenth of the rate of rhinitis without specific sensitisation (Gautrin et al., 2002).

Specific nasal provocation challenge testing (NPT) under controlled conditions in a laboratory is recommended (Moscato et al., 2008). Workplace challenges may be considered when a laboratory challenge is not feasible. HWM agents may be administered directly to the nasal mucosa via a spray or dropper. Challenge rooms can be used for water-insoluble agents or for mimicking exposure conditions at the workplace, similarly to the 'realistic method' used in the assessment of sensitiser-induced OA (Vandenplas and Malo, 1997). Few studies have been performed regarding the use of NPT with LMW agents, apart from with persulphates, wood dust and isocyanates (Airaksinen et al., 2007; Diab et al., 2009). Nasal responses to the agents may be assessed by symptom scoring, visual analogue scales, nasal patency measures and assessment of the volume and inflammatory composition of secretions (Scadding et al., 2011). Specific levels of response that define a positive challenge have, however, not been well defined.

All patients with symptoms of OR should be thoroughly evaluated for the presence of OA in accordance with best practice guidelines, as these conditions frequently coexist (Figure 27.3) (Moscato et al., 2009).

Management

The management of OR aims to control nasal symptoms for the worker and prevent the development of OA (Moscato et al., 2009). Avoidance of exposure to the causative agent is the optimal management approach. Complete avoidance, however, may require a change in job or role, which could lead to considerable socioeconomic consequences for the worker, as has been demonstrated in the management of sensitiser-induced OA (Vandenplas et al., 2003). Reduction of exposure could be considered if close, ongoing medical surveillance is provided; however, this approach has not been specifically investigated.

Pharmacotherapy of OR is similar to non-OR and should follow best practice guidelines (Brozek et al., 2010). In the management of allergic OR, medication

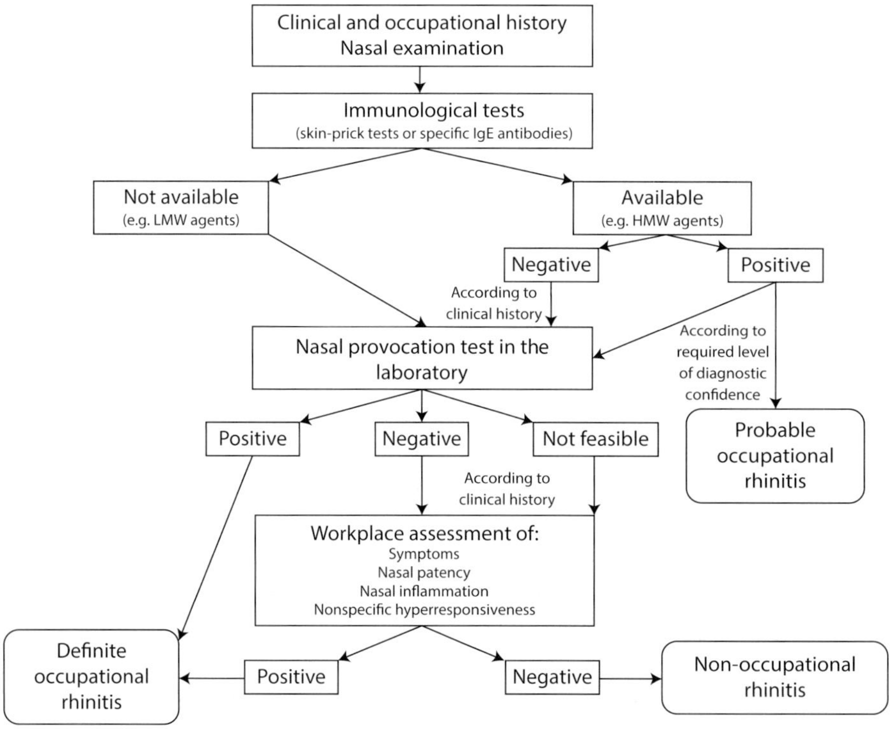

FIGURE 27.3 Algorithm for diagnosing occupational rhinitis. LMW: low-molecular-weight; HMW: high-molecular-weight. (Reproduced from Moscato, G. et al. 2009. *Respir Res* 10:16. With permission.)

should not be used as an alternative to exposure control. Specific immunotherapy with occupational agents has received little study, and there is a lack of standardised allergen extracts for most occupational agents. Some improvement in respiratory symptoms has been demonstrated with purified rodent proteins, wheat flour and natural rubber latex (Hansen et al., 2004; Sastre and Quirce, 2006; Moscato et al., 2009). Currently, allergen immunotherapy should be used with caution and under close supervision (Moscato et al., 2009).

Primary prevention of allergic OR requires accurate identification of a sensitiser at the workplace and the implementation of measures in order to minimise exposure as far as is possible. This has been demonstrated to be effective in detergent enzyme production, platinum refining workers and research laboratory workers (Hughes, 1980; Gordon and Preece, 2003; Sarlo, 2003). Engineering controls that are utilised in order to minimise exposure to animal allergens in research facilities include one-way airflow systems in animal holding rooms, task-specific local exhaust ventilation, automation of the emptying of soiled cages and individually ventilated cage systems (Thulin et al., 2002; Gordon and Preece, 2003). Cage design has been demonstrated to be important, with the replacement of open-top cages with filter-top cages resulting in reductions of allergen concentrations by >75% (Gordon et al., 1992).

Atopy, despite being a risk factor for the development of allergic OR associated with HMW agents, is very common in the general population and should not be used in order to determine the suitability of employment in a particular role. Atopic individuals should be educated regarding the risk of OR and OA in certain industries and be aware of potential symptoms in order to enable early identification. Education should be provided for students regarding the risk of occupational respiratory allergies in certain industries prior to commencing vocational training so that they can make informed career choices (Cullinan et al., 2003; Tarlo and Liss, 2003).

Surveillance programmes in high-risk occupations should be implemented as early as possible following employment. OR frequently develops following a short latency period from the onset of exposure to the occupational agent, especially over the first year of exposure. Surveillance programmes include periodic administration of a work-related symptoms questionnaire, detection of markers of sensitisation by skin-prick testing or serum-specific IgE when available, early specialist referral of symptomatic or sensitised workers and evaluation of possible OA in workers who are confirmed to have OR (Moscato et al., 2008, 2009).

SINUSITIS

Inflammation of the nasal mucosa (rhinitis) through allergy or chemical irritation can cause obstruction of osteomeatal complexes, resulting in impaired mucociliary clearance and subsequent sinusitis (Kennedy, 2004). Typical symptoms of chronic rhinosinusitis (CRS) are mucopurulent nasal drainage (anterior or posterior), nasal congestion/obstruction, facial pain/pressure and reduction/loss of sense of smell. The association between sinusitis and occupational exposures has received little study and has mostly been based on self-reported symptoms of sinusitis, rather than objective investigations.

A Korean population-based study of CRS symptoms noted increased prevalence in plant and machinery operators and assemblers, elementary occupations, crafts and related trade workers (Koh et al., 2009). Several occupations with exposure to organic dusts, including spice workers, furriers, hemp workers and workers in pharmaceuticals, paper recycling, textiles, farming and vegetable pickling have been reported in association with sinusitis symptoms (Shusterman, 2011). Non-organic exposures associated with sinusitis symptoms include ozone, car exhaust and water-based machining fluids (Shusterman, 2011). A cross-sectional survey of 3099 Danes noted self-reported symptoms of CRS to be associated with occupational exposure to gases, fumes, dust or smoke, and in women was more frequent in 'blue collar' than 'white collar' workers (Thilsing et al., 2012).

SINONASAL CANCER

Cancers arising in the paranasal sinuses are rare, constituting approximately 3% of head and neck malignancies (Ansa et al., 2013). The majority of these tumours arise in the maxillary sinuses and most of the remainder start in the ethmoid sinuses. Sinonasal cancer has, however, been identified as one of the most likely cancer sites to be associated with occupational exposures (Rushton et al., 2012). In Great Britain, it has been estimated that 43.5% (95% confidence interval [CI]: 27.3%–74.0%) of sinonasal cancers were attributable to occupational exposures (Rushton et al., 2012). Exposures identified in association with sinonasal cancer include wood dust, leather dust, formaldehyde, hexavalent chromium, mineral oils, mustard gas, selected nickel compounds and tobacco smoke (Battista et al., 1995; 't Mannetje et al., 1999; Luce et al., 2002; IARC, 2012; Rushton et al., 2012). The International Agency for Research on Cancer (IARC) Monograph Working Group notes that the most important occupational exposures associated with the development of sinonasal cancers are in furniture and woodworking industries, leather and shoe manufacturing and in nickel workers (IARC, 2012). Survival may also be influenced by occupational factors, as a study of 98 patients with sinonasal adenocarcinoma noted that the length of occupational exposure to metals was associated with 5-year survival ($p = 0.31$) (Tripodi et al., 2011).

OLFACTORY DYSFUNCTION

Up to 20% of the population have impaired sense of smell; however, only a small proportion of people complain of the problem (Croy et al., 2012). Loss of sense of smell can lead to significant impairment of quality of life and health risks, such as through loss of olfactory warning of leaking natural gas or spoiled food (Santos et al., 2004). Slight increases in the risks for social insecurity, depressive symptoms and household accidents have been identified (Croy et al., 2012). Olfaction may be very important in some occupations, such as for chefs and firefighters, and thus dysfunction could lead to work disability. Olfaction is also required for accurate fit testing of respiratory protection devices.

The most common causes of olfactory dysfunction are post-infectious and post-traumatic, followed by idiopathic, congenital, toxic and neurological causes (Fonteyn et al., 2014). Occupational exposure to airborne substances can lead to anosmia (loss of the sense of smell) or to hyposmia (diminished sense of smell) through direct toxicity to the olfactory epithelium, injury to the central nervous system and impaired delivery of odorants to the olfactory epithelium (due to nasal obstruction or congestion) (Shusterman, 2002). Olfactory fatigue will develop after a short period of time with repeated inhalation of any chemical, resulting in a transiently decreased ability to accurately detect and identify an odour (Greenberg et al., 2013).

Exposures noted in association with persistently impaired smell include acetone, acrylates, ammonia (chemical plant workers), metals (welders), cadmium (battery workers and braziers), sulphuric acid (chemical plant workers), methacrylate (dental technicians), hydrocarbons (paint formulators and tank cleaners), butyl acetate, wood dust, alkaline dusts, irritant gases, solvents, hydrogen sulphide and carbon disulphide (Gobba, 2006; Antunes et al., 2007; Smith et al., 2009; Shusterman, 2011).

Objective assessment of smell may be performed with qualitative screening tests, such as the 40-odour University of Pennsylvania Smell Identification Test (UPSIT), administered in a clinic or workplace (Doty et al., 1984). For each item, the subject scratches a microencapsulated odorant label that is present on the bottom of each page with a pencil tip and then chooses the best descriptor of the odour quality from a set of four alternatives (Doty, 2006). The level of absolute smell function (normosmia, mild hyposmia, moderate hyposmia, severe hyposmia and total anosmia) and a percentile rank for each age and gender group is determined by the test. Following the identification of impaired smell, otolaryngological and neurological examination is required, including nasal endoscopy and imaging.

Clinical history may note immediate-onset hyposmia following a discrete toxin exposure at work. Olfactory dysfunction associated with chronic exposure is likely to be more difficult to diagnose (Gobba, 2006). Little is known about the natural history of occupational toxin-associated olfactory dysfunction, but recovery of smell is likely to be associated with the specific chemical, duration of exposure and potential future exposures (Smith et al., 2009). Avoidance of further exposure to the occupational cause is therefore recommended.

UPPER AIRWAY TRAUMA

Acute upper airway inhalational injuries caused by thermal or chemical irritant exposure can cause life-threatening airway obstruction. Upper airway injury from smoke inhalation is primarily due to the rapid dissipation of heat in the upper airway, which may result in massive swelling of the tongue, epiglottis and aryepiglottic folds (Dries and Endorf, 2013). Swelling can develop over hours; therefore, continuous monitoring is required in order to assess the need for airway support. Acute external trauma to the upper airway, such as that which is caused by a motor vehicle accident or physical assault, is uncommon, but may also cause life-threatening airway obstruction (Schaefer, 2014).

Sinus barotrauma (tissue damage resulting from the direct effects of pressure) may occur in occupations such as divers or aviators, in which workers are exposed to significant changes in barometric pressure (Becker and Parell, 2001; Weitzel et al., 2008). If sinus outflow is compromised, equalisation of pressure through the nose is prevented. During descent, a relative vacuum in the sinus cavity develops, causing pain, mucosal oedema and mucosal haemorrhage (Weitzel et al., 2008). More severely but less commonly, as ambient pressure decreases during ascent, trapped expanding air can fracture the sinus walls, with resultant subcutaneous or orbital emphysema. Neurologic complications have been reported, including blindness, pneumocephalus, meningitis and trigeminal nerve dysfunction (Becker and Parell, 2001). Management requires the treatment of any underlying predisposing condition, such as polyps or ostial insufficiency. Functional endoscopic sinus surgery has been shown to assist aviators with recurrent sinus barotrauma to return to flying duties and reduce the risk of further sinus barotrauma (Parsons et al., 1997).

WORK-RELATED VOCAL CORD DYSFUNCTION

There is growing recognition of the importance of vocal cord dysfunction (VCD) as a cause of episodic respiratory symptoms and as a condition that is difficult to differentiate from asthma (Barnes and Woolcock, 1998; Ayres and Mansur, 2011; Balkissoon and Kenn, 2012). The primary feature of VCD is variable upper airway obstruction caused by inappropriate intermittent paradoxical adduction of the vocal folds, mainly during inspiration, causing dyspnoea of varying intensity (Morris and Christopher, 2010). There is a lack of consensus regarding the appropriate terminology to describe this condition. VCD has been widely used by pulmonologists; however, as laryngeal structures apart from the vocal 'cords' also adduct, 'paradoxical vocal fold motion disorder' and 'periodic occurrence of laryngeal obstruction' have been proposed as alternative terms for the syndrome (Morris and Christopher, 2010). Historically, many other terms, such as 'Munchausen's stridor' or 'hysterical croup', have been used, contributing to the confusion regarding this disorder (Andrianopoulos et al., 2000). 'Irritable larynx syndrome' (ILS) has been coined in order to describe more generalised laryngeal hype-reactivity presenting with VCD and other symptoms of laryngeal dysfunction, including chronic cough, globus pharyngeus (sense of a lump in the throat) and muscular tension dysphonia (Table 27.2) (Morrison et al., 1999; Andrianopoulos et al., 2000).

TABLE 27.2
Alternative Terminology Used to Describe Vocal Cord Dysfunction

Atypical asthma	Laryngeal dysfunction
Benign paradoxical vocal cord motion	Laryngeal dyskinesia
Episodic laryngeal dyskinesia	Munchausen stridor
Episodic laryngeal wheeze	Non-organic upper airway obstruction
Emotional paradoxical laryngospasm	Paradoxical vocal fold dysfunction
Exercise-induced laryngospasm	Paradoxical vocal fold motion
Expiratory laryngeal stridor	Periodic occurrence of laryngeal obstruction
Factitious asthma	Pseudoasthma
Factitious upper airway obstruction	Pseudo-steroid-resistant asthma
Functional laryngeal dyskinesia	Psychogenic laryngeal dysfunction
Functional stridor	Psychogenic stridor
Glottic dysfunction	Psychogenic upper airway obstruction
Hysterical croup	Spasmodic croup
Irritable larynx syndrome	Vocal cord dyskinesia
Irritant-induced vocal cord dysfunction	Work-associated irritable larynx syndrome

Source: Reproduced from Morris, M. J. and Christopher, K. L. 2010. *Chest* 138:1213–23. With permission.

VCD may masquerade with symptoms that are suggestive of asthma and may coexist with asthma (Christopher et al., 1983; Barnes and Woolcock, 1998). It has been estimated that 3%–5% of people with a diagnosis of asthma actually have VCD (Kenn and Hess, 2008). In patients who are thought to have difficult-to-treat asthma, this proportion is likely to be much greater. A retrospective study of 292 patients attending an outpatient asthma and allergy clinic demonstrated that 42% of subjects with the primary diagnosis of VCD were misdiagnosed with asthma for an average of 9.0 years (Traister et al., 2013). Large series of subjects with VCD noted coexistent asthma in 35%–56% of cases (Newman et al., 1995; O'Connell et al., 1995). Failure to diagnose VCD may lead to iatrogenic complications from inappropriate asthma treatments, such as high-dose steroid therapy. Medical utilisation and oral steroid therapy have been demonstrated to be very high in patients with VCD (Newman et al., 1995; Traister et al., 2013).

Work-related asthma guidelines refer to the need to consider other causes of asthma-like symptoms, including VCD, especially when objective investigations fail to confirm the diagnosis of asthma (Tarlo et al., 2008; Tarlo et al., 2009). Workplace exposures, particularly to respiratory irritants, have been reported to precipitate laryngeal dysfunction and also to trigger recurrent symptoms (Perkner et al., 1998; Balkissoon, 2002; Hoy et al., 2010). A retrospective study of 340 subjects with work-related respiratory symptoms identified 90 subjects with work-related asthma and 30 with work-associated ILS (WILS) (Hoy et al., 2010). Five patients had concurrent diagnoses of WILS and work-related asthma. VCD has been well described in association with several occupational groups, including elite athletes, military recruits and individuals who have had high-level irritant exposures (Balkissoon and Kenn, 2012).

Pathogenesis

Current concepts of VCD have progressed from this being considered exclusively as a psychological or somatisation disorder (Kenn and Balkissoon, 2011).

Some hypotheses have focused on alteration of the larynx's normal role in the protection of the lower respiratory tract, particularly lowering the threshold for reflex response to stimuli (Ayres and Gabbott, 2002). It is suggested that both intrinsic and environmental (including occupational) factors are involved in altering neurological responses (Morrison et al., 1999). Morrison et al. hypothesised that nociceptive stimuli (such as airborne irritants or gastroesophageal reflux) may lead to 'plastic' changes in central neurons, lowering their threshold for initiating the glottic closure reflex (Morrison et al., 1999). As the larynx is in a 'spasm-ready' state, symptoms of cough, dysphonia, globus and laryngospasm may then occur at relatively low levels of stimuli. Similarly, Ayres and Gabbott suggested that following an initial inflammatory insult to the upper airway, a state of altered autonomic balance develops, causing 'laryngeal hyper-responsiveness' (Ayres and Gabbott, 2002). The state of 'hyper-responsiveness' may be transient or persistent. Further stimuli, including irritant exposures, olfactory triggers or stress, then result in triggering local parasympathetic reflexes, causing airway narrowing at the glottis (Shusterman, 1992; Ayres and Gabbott, 2002). At the workplace, exposure to 'low-level' stimuli, such as perfumes, cleaning products, odours and irritants, may then result in triggering the laryngeal reflex inappropriately (Hoy et al., 2010).

Occupational Exposures

Irritant Exposures

'Irritant-associated VCD' was described in a study comparing 11 cases of laryngoscopically confirmed irritant-associated VCD, with 33 VCD controls (Perkner et al., 1998). Ten cases of irritant-associated VCD developed following workplace exposures, including to ammonia vapour, fumes from the inappropriate mixing of flux and solder, an aerosolised cleaning solution, a noxious odour while cooking 'Cajun salmon', ceiling tile dust and smoke (Perkner et al., 1998). In a retrospective review of patients with WILS, 14 out of 30 patients identified a specific precipitating event at the workplace at the time of the onset of their symptoms, and five of these patients presented to an emergency department following the event (Hoy et al., 2010).

World Trade Center Responders

Rescue and recovery workers at the World Trade Center (WTC) site following the terrorist attacks of 11 September 2001, were exposed to high levels of alkaline dust capable of causing irritation and inflammation of the upper respiratory tract (de la Hoz et al., 2010).

Analysis of spirometry performed on former WTC rescue and clean-up workers and volunteers attending the WTC Health Effects Treatment Program identified inspiratory flow–volume loop limitation that was consistent with variable extra-thoracic airflow obstruction in 18.6% (32/172) of subjects (de la Hoz et al., 2008). VCD was diagnosed in ten workers by flexible laryngoscopic examination. All subjects had coexistent findings of laryngopharyngitis suggestive of acid reflux-related disease. It has been proposed that upper airway dysfunction in this group is likely to have been precipitated by upper airway inflammation due to acute irritant dust exposure and perpetuated by gastroesophageal reflux, rhinitis and coexistent psychopathology, stemming from the psychological stressors of the WTC disaster (de la Hoz et al., 2008, 2010).

Professional Athletes

VCD has frequently been reported in elite and professional athletes (McFadden and Zawadski, 1996; Rundell and Spiering, 2003; Al-Alwan and Kaminsky, 2012). VCD may be difficult to clinically differentiate from exercise-induced bronchospasm, and the two conditions may coexist. Exercise-associated VCD may present with exertional dyspnoea with associated inspiratory stridor. Throat rather than chest tightness may be described, with symptoms beginning soon after exercise starts and resolution occurring within 5 minutes of stopping exercise (Rundell and Spiering, 2003).

The prevalence of inspiratory stridor was investigated in 370 athletes from a wide range of predominately winter sports (169 competed in outdoor sports, such as biathlon, kayaking and cross-country skiing, and 201 competed in indoor sports, such as skating and ice hockey) at the US Olympic training centre in Lake Placid (Rundell and Spiering, 2003). Participants provided a medical history and underwent spirometry and exercise challenge in cold, dry ambient conditions. Exercise-induced bronchospasm was present in 30% of subjects and inspiratory stridor in 5.1% (18 female and 1 male). Ten of the subjects (52%) with inspiratory stridor also had exercise-induced bronchospasm. Inspiratory stridor was also more common in outdoor athletes than indoor athletes (8.3% vs. 2.5%; $p < 0.05$), suggesting exercising in cold, dry ambient air may increase the sensitivity of the extra-thoracic airway, resulting in VCD (Rundell and Spiering, 2003). Others have speculated that VCD is a conversion reaction that is associated with personality traits that may be common to some elite athletes, such as success orientation and vulnerability to pressure not to fail (McFadden and Zawadski, 1996; Chiang et al., 2013).

Military Personnel

In a study of 40 active-duty military patients undergoing evaluation for exertional dyspnoea, Morris et al. performed flexible laryngoscopy with direct visualisation of the vocal cords before and after exercise in order to evaluate the presence of inspiratory vocal cord adduction (Morris et al., 1999). VCD was present in 15% of prospectively studied subjects. Sixty percent of patients with VCD had a positive methacholine challenge. The cause of VCD in military personnel has not been determined; however, extreme psychological stress during wartime and training may contribute, as may the high level of regular strenuous exercise that is required (Craig et al., 1992; Morris et al., 1999).

Clinical Features

Symptoms of intermittent dyspnoea, wheeze and cough are common to both asthma and VCD (Bahrainwala and Simon, 2001). This may result in a delayed diagnosis and the potentially adverse effects of unnecessary corticosteroid therapy (Newman et al., 1995).

Features that suggest VCD include a sensation of inspiratory limitation, rather than expiratory limitation as is usual in asthma, and tightness in the throat rather than the chest. Typically, episodes are of sudden onset and are self-limiting (Morris and Christopher, 2010; Balkissoon and Kenn, 2012). During an acute episode, the wheeze can be loudest over the neck and upper thorax, but is transmitted throughout the chest. (Morris and Christopher, 2010). Hyperventilation during an episode may lead to symptoms such as tingling of the perioral area and digits, dizziness and lightheadedness. Other symptoms of laryngeal dysfunction, apart from those caused by variable upper airway obstruction, have been described as ILS and include acute dysphonia (muscular tension dysphonia), sensation of tension in the throat (globus pharyngeus), recurrent cough and, sometimes, dysphagia (Morrison et al., 1999; Hoy et al., 2010).

Occupational exposures may both induced VCD and be associated with recurrent symptoms (Perkner et al., 1998; Tonini et al., 2009; Huggins et al., 2004; Hoy et al., 2010). Exposure of the upper respiratory tract to an irritant, such as an accidental spill of a water-soluble agent, may be associated with the onset of symptoms (Perkner et al., 1998; Hoy et al., 2010). The event may have been psychologically traumatic and have required emergency medical treatment. Perkner et al. described a short latency following occupational irritant exposure and the onset of VCD symptoms, ranging from 1 hour or less to 24 hours (Perkner et al., 1998).

Recurrent symptoms of laryngeal dysfunction may be primarily related to occupational factors, including irritant exposures, physical exertion and psychogenic factors (Craig et al., 1992; McFadden and Zawadski, 1996; Huggins et al., 2004; Hoy et al., 2010; Morris and Christopher, 2010). Andrianopoulos et al. noted ten out of 27 patients with VCD having sensory triggers for symptoms, including exposures to environmental stimuli that may be present in a work environment, such as perfumes, air pollutants and chemical agents (Andrianopoulos et al., 2000). Members of the military involved in combat and elite athletes in sports competitions may experience periods of acute and extreme stress, which may act as triggers for episodes of VCD (Craig et al., 1992; McFadden and Zawadski, 1996).

Patients with VCD should also be clinically evaluated for the adverse effects of steroid therapies, gastroesophageal reflux, post-nasal secretions and psychological comorbidities, such as anxiety and depression (Kenn and Balkissoon, 2011; Balkissoon and Kenn, 2012).

Diagnosis

Exposure to irritants at the workplace may result in the development of respiratory symptoms due to range of conditions, including irritant-induced OA, OR and VCD. Objective evaluation of pulmonary function is necessary for the diagnosis of work-related asthma (Tarlo et al., 2008). Normal lung function tests in the setting of a clinical suspicion of asthma should raise the possibility of VCD as the cause of the symptoms (Morris and Christopher, 2010).

Between symptomatic episodes, spirometry is usually normal in patients with VCD. When symptoms are present, spirometry may identify truncation of the inspiratory limb of the flow–volume curve, with a mid-inspiratory flow:mid-expiratory flow ratio of less than 1, a feature that is suggestive of variable extra-thoracic airway obstruction (Balkissoon and Kenn, 2012). Bronchial provocation testing with methacholine has been reported to induce VCD; however, truncation of the inspiratory flow–volume loop during non-specific challenge testing has not been validated as diagnostic for VCD (Perkner et al., 1998). Specific provocation tests in order to induce symptoms of VCD have been performed based on the patient's history of provoking exposures, including specific irritants, cold air and exercise (Balkissoon and Kenn, 2012). Nonetheless, standardised methods have not been developed. Normal spirometry does not exclude the diagnosis of VCD and should not influence the decision to perform further investigation (Figure 27.4) (Watson et al., 2009).

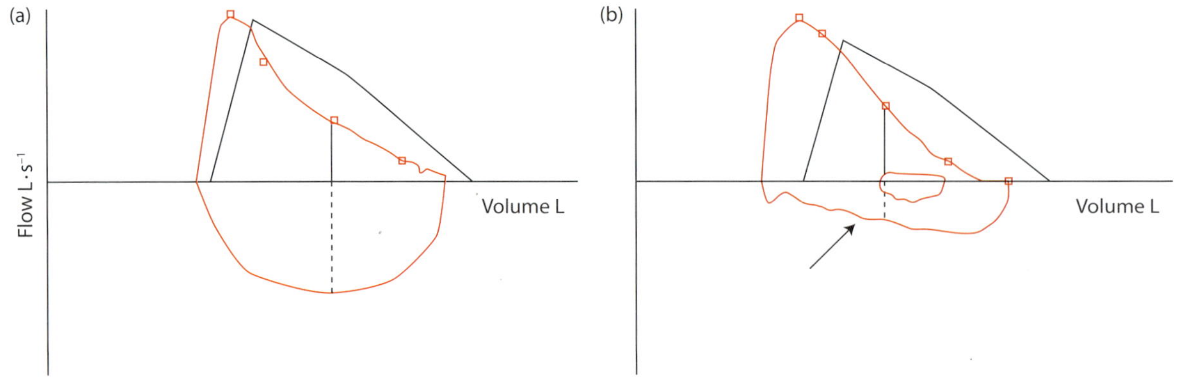

FIGURE 27.4 (a) Pre- and (b) post-methacholine changes in flow–volume loop. Inspiratory curve flattened (black arrow) following methacholine challenge leads to reversal in maximal inspiratory flow at 50% of forced vital capacity (MIF50)/maximal expiratory flow at 50% of forced vital capacity (MEF50) ratio from (a) .1 to (b) ,1 (i.e. MIF50 smaller MEF50). ——: MEF50; - - - -: MIF50. Red line: patient result; black line: predicted result. (Reproduced from Kenn, K. and Balkissoon, R. 2011. *Eur Respir J* 37:194–200. With permission of the European Respiratory Society.)

The current gold standard investigation for confirming VCD is through examination of the larynx by flexible fibre optic laryngoscopy (Morris and Christopher, 2010; Kenn and Balkissoon, 2011). In a symptomatic patient, paradoxical adduction of the cords during inspiration may be observed. Laryngoscopy also enables assessment of the upper airway for aggravating factors such as post-nasal secretion or laryngopharyngeal reflux. Laryngoscopy is required in order to examine the upper airway for anatomical and neurological causes of symptoms, particularly tumours, laryngomalacia, subglottic stenosis from thyroid compression and vocal cord paralysis. Limitations of laryngoscopy include the lack of access to appropriately skilled physicians, the subjective nature of some diagnostic features and the procedure possibly being poorly tolerated in some patients with acute symptoms (Figure 27.5) (Jain et al., 2006).

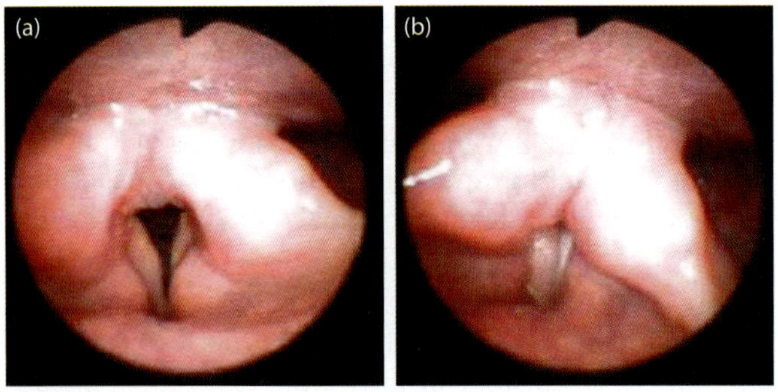

FIGURE 27.5 Laryngoscopic view of classic vocal cord dysfunction with (a) early paradoxical adduction of the vocal folds with formation of a 'posterior chink' and (b) complete closure of the vocal folds. (From Kenn, K. and Balkissoon, R. 2011. *Eur Respir J* 37:194–200. Reproduced with permission of the European Respiratory Society.)

VCD should not be ruled out until the vocal cords have been directed visualised whilst a patient is symptomatic (Kenn and Balkissoon, 2011), Provocation tests, with the challenge agent determined based on the patient's history, have been noted to be of value for inducing symptoms when performing laryngoscopy. Reported specific challenges to occupational agents include alkaline persulphate, eucalyptus, glutaraldehyde and iroko and western red cedar wood dust (Huggins et al., 2004; Galdi et al., 2005; Munoz et al., 2007; Herin et al., 2012). The investigation of exercise-associated VCD has been achieved with continuous fibre optic laryngoscopy performed during an exercise test and was noted to be easy to perform, well tolerated and useful in the diagnosis of exercise-associated VCD (Heimdal et al., 2006; Tervonen et al., 2009).

Morris and Christopher have proposed diagnostic criteria for VCD including: (1) clinical symptoms of noisy breathing and dyspnoea; (2) laryngoscopic evidence of vocal cord adduction; and (3) confirmatory pulmonary function test findings of an abnormal flow–volume loop (most commonly the inspiratory limb) or a lack of airway hyper-reactivity (Morris and Christopher, 2010).

Recent modalities for investigating VCD include high-resolution, 320-slice dynamic volume computed tomography scans and endospirometry, a technique that combines endoscopy timed with spirometric reading (Kenn and Hess, 2008; Holmes et al., 2009).

Management

The management of VCD requires careful explanation of the condition and feedback regarding the cause of dyspnoea (Balkissoon and Kenn, 2012). This should be done without the implication that the disorder is purely psychological. The management of acute VCD episodes may include relaxation techniques such as pursing lips and active reassurance despite the sensation of severe dyspnoea (Pitchenik, 1991; Andrianopoulos et al., 2000). Continuous positive airway pressure and Heliox (a gas mixture of 80% helium and 20% oxygen) inhalation has been shown to be effective in a proportion of patients during acute episodes (Reisner and Borish, 1995).

Chronic therapy is usually necessary and requires a multidisciplinary approach (Andrianopoulos et al., 2000; Kenn and Balkissoon, 2011). Patients with work-associated symptoms should be questioned regarding specific triggers, and measures should be put in place in order to minimise exposure to triggers. Factors contributing to laryngeal irritation such as post-nasal secretions and laryngopharyngeal reflux should be addressed. Speech therapy and relaxation techniques may be useful in order to manage ongoing symptoms (Murry and Sapienza, 2010; Kenn and Balkissoon, 2011). In a study of 20 adolescent female athletes, 95% were able to control their symptoms after speech therapy (Sullivan et al., 2001). Biofeedback has been found to be beneficial in some athletes with VCD (Chiang et al., 2013; Marcinow et al., 2014). Psychological evaluation and therapy may be required in order to address anxiety or post-traumatic stress disorder (Morrison et al., 1999; Andrianopoulos et al., 2000; Kenn and Balkissoon, 2011). Unilateral vocal cord injection with botulinum toxin has recently been investigated as a treatment for VCD in association with treatment-resistant asthma, but has not been evaluated in the setting of occupational triggers (Baxter et al., 2014).

REFERENCES

Airaksinen, L. K., Luukkonen, R. A., Lindstrom, I., Lauerma, A. I. and Toskala, E. M. 2009. Long-term exposure and health-related quality of life among patients with occupational rhinitis. *J Occup Environ Med* 51(11):1288–97.

Airaksinen, L., Tuomi, T., Vanhanen, M., Voutilainen, R. and Toskala, E. 2007. Use of nasal provocation test in the diagnostics of occupational rhinitis. *Rhinology* 45(1):40–6.

Al-Alwan, A. and Kaminsky, D. 2012. Vocal cord dysfunction in athletes: Clinical presentation and review of the literature. *Phys Sports Med* 40(2):22–7.

Ameille, J., Hamelin, K., Andujar, P., Bensefa-Colas, L., Bonneterre, V., Dupas, D., Garnier, R. et al. 2013. Occupational asthma and occupational rhinitis: The united airways disease model revisited. *Occup Environ Med* 70(7):471–5.

Andrianopoulos, M. V., Gallivan, G. J. and Gallivan, K. H. 2000. PVCM, PVCD, EPL, and irritable larynx syndrome: What are we talking about and how do we treat it? *J Voice* 14(4):607–18.

Ansa, B., Goodman, M., Ward, K., Kono, S. A., Owonikoko, T. K., Higgins, K., Beitler, J. J. et al. 2013. Paranasal sinus squamous cell carcinoma incidence and survival based on surveillance, epidemiology, and end results data, 1973 to 2009. *Cancer* 119(14):2602–10.

Antunes, M. B., Bowler, R. and Doty, R. L. 2007. San Francisco/Oakland Bay Bridge Welder Study: Olfactory function. *Neurology* 69(12):1278–84.

Ayres, J. G. and Gabbott, P. L. 2002. Vocal cord dysfunction and laryngeal hyperresponsiveness: A function of altered autonomic balance? *Thorax* 57(4):284–5.

Ayres, J. G. and Mansur, A. H. 2011. Vocal cord dysfunction and severe asthma: Considering the total airway. *Am J Respir Crit Care Med* 184(1):2–3.

Bahrainwala, A. H. and Simon, M. R. 2001. Wheezing and vocal cord dysfunction mimicking asthma. *Curr Opin Pulm Med* 7(1):8–13.

Balkissoon, R. 2002. Occupational upper airway disease. *Clin Chest Med* 23(4):717–25.

Balkissoon, R. and Kenn, K. 2012. Asthma: Vocal cord dysfunction (VCD) and other dysfunctional breathing disorders. *Semin Respir Crit Care Med* 33(6):595–605.

Barnes, P. J. and Woolcock, A. J. 1998. Difficult asthma. *Eur Respir J* 12(5):1209–18.

Battista, G., Comba, P., Orsi, D., Norpoth, K. and Maier, A. 1995. Nasal cancer in leather workers: An occupational disease. *J Cancer Res Clin Oncol* 121(1):1–6.

Baxter, M., Uddin, N., Raghav, S., Leong, P., Low, K., Hamza, K., Holmes, P. W. et al. 2014. Abnormal vocal cord movement treated with botulinum toxin in patients with asthma resistant to optimised management. *Respirology* 19(4):531–7.

Becker, G. D. and Parell, G. J. 2001. Barotrauma of the ears and sinuses after scuba diving. *Eur Arch Otorhinolaryngol* 258(4):159–63.

Brozek, J. L., Bousquet, J., Baena-Cagnani, C. E., Bonini, S., Canonica, G. W., Casale, T. B., van Wijk, R. G. et al. 2010. Allergic Rhinitis and its Impact on Asthma (ARIA) guidelines: 2010 revision. *J Allergy Clin Immunol* 126(3):466–76.

Canuel, M. and Lebel, G. 2014. Epidemiology of allergic rhinitis in Quebec: From a 2008 population-based survey. *Chronic Dis Inj Can* 34(2–3):163–8.

Chiang, T., Marcinow, A. M., deSilva, B. W., Ence, B. N., Lindsey, S. E. and Forrest, L. A. 2013. Exercise-induced paradoxical vocal fold motion disorder: Diagnosis and management. *Laryngoscope* 123(3):727–31.

Christopher, K. L., Wood, R. P. 2nd, Eckert, R. C., Blager, F. B., Raney, R. A. and Souhrada, J. F. 1983. Vocal-cord dysfunction presenting as asthma. *N Engl J Med* 308(26):1566–70.

Chung, K. F. and Pavord, I. D. 2008. Prevalence, pathogenesis, and causes of chronic cough. *Lancet* 371(9621):1364–74.

Compalati, E., Ridolo, E., Passalacqua, G., Braido, F., Villa, E. and Canonica, G. W. 2010. The link between allergic rhinitis and asthma: The united airways disease. *Expert Rev Clin Immunol* 6(3):413–23.

Craig, T., Sitz, K., Squire, E., Smith, L. and Carpenter, G. 1992. Vocal cord dysfunction during wartime. *Mil Med* 157(11):614–6.

Croy, I., Negoias, S., Novakova, L., Landis, B. N. and Hummel, T. 2012. Learning about the functions of the olfactory system from people without a sense of smell. *PLoS One* 7(3):e33365.

Cullinan, P., Cook, A., Gordon, S., Nieuwenhuijsen, M. J., Tee, R. D., Venables, K. M., McDonald, J. C. et al. 1999. Allergen exposure, atopy and smoking as determinants of allergy to rats in a cohort of laboratory employees. *Eur Respir J* 13(5):1139–43.

Cullinan, P., Tarlo, S. and Nemery, B. 2003. The prevention of occupational asthma. *Eur Respir J* 22(5):853–60.

de la Hoz, R. E., Shohet, M. R., Bienenfeld, L. A., Afilaka, A. A., Levin, S. M. and Herbert, R. 2008. Vocal cord dysfunction in former World Trade Center (WTC) rescue and recovery workers and volunteers. *Am J Ind Med* 51(3):161–5.

de la Hoz, R. E., Shohet, M. R. and Cohen, J. M. 2010. Occupational rhinosinusitis and upper airway disease: The World Trade Center experience. *Curr Allergy Asthma Rep* 10(2):77–83.

Diab, K. K., Truedsson, L., Albin, M. and Nielsen, J. 2009. Persulphate challenge in female hairdressers with nasal hyperreactivity suggests immune cell, but no IgE reaction. *Int Arch Occup Environ Health* 82(6):771–7.

Diaz-Sanchez, D., Penichet-Garcia, M. and Saxon, A. 2000. Diesel exhaust particles directly induce activated mast cells to degranulate and increase histamine levels and symptom severity. *J Allergy Clin Immunol* 106(6):1140–6.

Doty, R. L. 2006. Olfactory dysfunction and its measurement in the clinic and workplace. *Int Arch Occup Environ Health* 79(4):268–82.

Doty, R. L., Shaman, P., Kimmelman, C. P. and Dann, M. S. 1984. University of Pennsylvania Smell Identification Test: A rapid quantitative olfactory function test for the clinic. *Laryngoscope* 94(2 Pt 1):176–8.

Dries, D. J. and Endorf, F. W. 2013. Inhalation injury: Epidemiology, pathology, treatment strategies. *Scand J Trauma Resusc Emerg Med* 21:31.

Fonteyn, S., Huart, C., Deggouj, N., Collet, S., Eloy, P. and Rombaux, P. 2014. Non-sinonasal-related olfactory dysfunction: A cohort of 496 patients. *Eur Ann Otorhinolaryngol Head Neck Dis* 131(2):87–91.

Galdi, E., Perfetti, L., Pagella, F., Bertino, G., Ferrari, M. and Moscato, G. 2005. Irritant vocal cord dysfunction at first misdiagnosed as reactive airway dysfunction syndrome. *Scand J Work Environ Health* 31(3):224–6.

Gautrin, D., Ghezzo, H., Infante-Rivard, C. and Malo, J. L. 2002. Incidence and host determinants of work-related rhinoconjunctivitis in apprentice pastry-makers. *Allergy* 57(10):913–8.

Gobba, F. 2006. Olfactory toxicity: Long-term effects of occupational exposures. *Int Arch Occup Environ Health* 79 (4):322–31.

Gordon, S. and Preece, R. 2003. Prevention of laboratory animal allergy. *Occup Med (Lond)* 53(6):371–7.

Gordon, S., Tee, R. D., Lowson, D., Wallace, J. and Newman Taylor, A. J. 1992. Reduction of airborne allergenic urinary proteins from laboratory rats. *Br J Ind Med* 49(6):416–22.

Greenberg, M. I., Curtis, J. A. and Vearrier, D. 2013. The perception of odor is not a surrogate marker for chemical exposure: A review of factors influencing human odor perception. *Clin Toxicol (Phila)* 51(2):70–6.

Greiner, A. N., Hellings, P. W., Rotiroti, G. and Scadding, G. K. 2011. Allergic rhinitis. *Lancet* 378(9809):2112–22.

Gross, N. J. 1980. Allergy to laboratory animals: Epidemiologic, clinical, and physiologic aspects, and a trial of cromolyn in its management. *J Allergy Clin Immunol* 66(2):158–65.

Hansen, I., Hormann, K. and Klimek, L. 2004. [Specific immunotherapy in inhalative allergy to rat epithelium]. *Laryngorhinootologie* 83(8):512–5.

Heimdal, J. H., Roksund, O. D., Halvorsen, T., Skadberg, B. T. and Olofsson, J. 2006. Continuous laryngoscopy exercise test: A method for visualizing laryngeal dysfunction during exercise. *Laryngoscope* 116(1):52–7.

Hellgren, J., Karlsson, G. and Toren, K. 2003. The dilemma of occupational rhinitis: Management options. *Am J Respir Med* 2(4):333–41.

Herin, F., Poussel, M., Renaudin, J. M., Leininger, A., Moreau-Colson, C., Menard, O. and Paris, C. 2012. A 38-year-old hairdresser with irritant-associated vocal cord dysfunction. *Int J Tuberc Lung Dis* 16(1):138–9.

Holmes, P. W., Lau, K. K., Crossett, M., Low, C., Buchanan, D., Hamilton, G. S. and Bardin, P. G. 2009. Diagnosis of vocal cord dysfunction in asthma with high resolution dynamic volume computerized tomography of the larynx. *Respirology* 14(8):1106–13.

Hox, V., Steelant, B., Fokkens, W., Nemery, B. and Hellings, P. W. 2014. Occupational upper airway disease: How work affects the nose. *Allergy* 69:282–91.

Hoy, R. F., Ribeiro, M., Anderson, J. and Tarlo, S. M. 2010. Work-associated irritable larynx syndrome. *Occup Med (Lond)* 60(7):546–51.

Huggins, J. T., Kaplan, A., Martin-Harris, B. and Sahn, S. A. 2004. Eucalyptus as a specific irritant causing vocal cord dysfunction. *Ann Allergy Asthma Immunol* 93(3):299–303.

Hughes, E. G. 1980. Medical surveillance of platinum refinery workers. *J Soc Occup Med* 30(1):27–30.

Hytonen, M., Kanerva, L., Malmberg, H., Martikainen, R., Mutanen, P. and Toikkanen, J. 1997. The risk of occupational rhinitis. *Int Arch Occup Environ Health* 69(6):487–90.

IARC. 2012. Arsenic, metals, fibres, and dusts. *IARC Monogr Eval Carcinog Risks Hum* 100(Pt C):11–465.

Jain, S., Bandi, V., Officer, T., Wolley, M. and Guntupalli, K. K. 2006. Role of vocal cord function and dysfunction in patients presenting with symptoms of acute asthma exacerbation. *J Asthma* 43(3):207–12.

Karjalainen, A., Martikainen, R., Klaukka, T., Saarinen, K. and Uitti, J. 2003. Risk of asthma among Finnish patients with occupational rhinitis. *Chest* 123(1):283–8.

Kenn, K. and Balkissoon, R. 2011. Vocal cord dysfunction: What do we know? *Eur Respir J* 37(1):194–200.

Kenn, K. and Hess, M. M. 2008. Vocal cord dysfunction: An important differential diagnosis of bronchial asthma. *Dtsch Arztebl Int* 105(41):699–704.

Kennedy, D. W. 2004. Pathogenesis of chronic rhinosinusitis. *Ann Otol Rhinol Laryngol Suppl* 193:6–9.

Kimber, I., Dearman, R. J. and Basketter, D. A. 2014. Diisocyanates, occupational asthma and IgE antibody: Implications for hazard characterization. *J Appl Toxicol* 34(10):1073–7.

Koh, D. H., Kim, H. R. and Han, S. S. 2009. The relationship between chronic rhinosinusitis and occupation: The 1998, 2001 and 2005 Korea National health and nutrition examination survey (KNHANES). *Am J Ind Med* 52(3):179–84.

Laumbach, R. J. and Kipen, H. M. 2005. Bioaerosols and sick building syndrome: Particles, inflammation, and allergy. *Curr Opin Allergy Clin Immunol* 5(2):135–9.

Lin, S. C., Tai, C. C., Chan, C. C. and Wang, J. D. 1994. Nasal septum lesions caused by chromium exposure among chromium electroplating workers. *Am J Ind Med* 26(2):221–8.

Luce, D., Leclerc, A., Begin, D., Demers, P. A., Gerin, M., Orlowski, E., Kogevinas, M. et al. 2002. Sinonasal cancer and occupational exposures: A pooled analysis of 12 case–control studies. *Cancer Causes Control* 13(2):147–57.

Malo, J. L., Lemiere, C., Desjardins, A. and Cartier, A. 1997. Prevalence and intensity of rhinoconjunctivitis in subjects with occupational asthma. *Eur Respir J* 10(7):1513–5.

Marcinow, A. M., Thompson, J., Chiang, T., Forrest, L. A. and deSilva, B. W. 2014. Paradoxical vocal fold motion disorder in the elite athlete: Experience at a large division I university. *Laryngoscope* 124(6):1425–30.

McFadden, E. R. Jr. and Zawadski, D. K. 1996. Vocal cord dysfunction masquerading as exercise-induced asthma. A physiologic cause for 'choking' during athletic activities. *Am J Respir Crit Care Med* 153(3):942–7.

Meggs, W. J. 1994. RADS and RUDS—The toxic induction of asthma and rhinitis. *J Toxicol Clin Toxicol* 32(5):487–501.

Meggs, W. J. 1997. Hypothesis for induction and propagation of chemical sensitivity based on biopsy studies. *Environ Health Perspect* 105(Suppl. 2):473–8.

Menzies, D. and Kreiss, K. 2006. Building-related illness. In I.L. Bernstein, M. Chan-Yeung, J. L. Malo, D. I. Bernstein (eds), *Asthma in the Workplace*. New York, NY: Taylor & Francis Group. pp. 737–83.

Morris, M. J. and Christopher, K. L. 2010. Diagnostic criteria for the classification of vocal cord dysfunction. *Chest* 138(5):1213–23.

Morris, M. J., Deal, L. E., Bean, D. R., Grbach, V. X. and Morgan, J. A. 1999. Vocal cord dysfunction in patients with exertional dyspnea. *Chest* 116(6):1676–82.

Morrison, M., Rammage, L. and Emami, A. J. 1999. The irritable larynx syndrome. *J Voice* 13(3):447–55.

Moscato, G., Vandenplas, O., Gerth Van Wijk, R., Malo, J. L., Quirce, S., Walusiak, J., Castano, R. et al. 2008. Occupational rhinitis. *Allergy* 63 (8):969–80.

Moscato, G., Vandenplas, O., Van Wijk, R. G., Malo, J. L., Perfetti, L., Quirce, S., Walusiak, J. et al. 2009. EAACI position paper on occupational rhinitis. *Respir Res* 10:16.

Munoz, X., Roger, A., De la Rosa, D., Morell, F. and Cruz, M. J. 2007. Occupational vocal cord dysfunction due to exposure to wood dust and xerographic toner. *Scand J Work Environ Health* 33(2):153–8.

Murry, T. and Sapienza, C. 2010. The role of voice therapy in the management of paradoxical vocal fold motion, chronic cough, and laryngospasm. *Otolaryngol Clin North Am* 43(1):73–83, viii–ix.

Newman, K. B., Mason, U. G. 3rd and Schmaling, K. B. 1995. Clinical features of vocal cord dysfunction. *Am J Respir Crit Care Med* 152(4 Pt 1):1382–6.

O'Connell, M. A., Sklarew, P. R. and Goodman, D. L. 1995. Spectrum of presentation of paradoxical vocal cord motion in ambulatory patients. *Ann Allergy Asthma Immunol* 74(4):341–4.

Parsons, D. S., Chambers, D. W. and Boyd, E. M. 1997. Long-term follow-up of aviators after functional endoscopic sinus surgery for sinus barotrauma. *Aviat Space Environ Med* 68(11):1029–34.

Perkner, J. J., Fennelly, K. P., Balkissoon, R., Bartelson, B. B., Ruttenber, A. J., Wood, R. P., Newman, L. S. et al. 1998. Irritant-associated vocal cord dysfunction. *J Occup Environ Med* 40(2):136–43.

Pitchenik, A. E. 1991. Functional laryngeal obstruction relieved by panting. *Chest* 100(5):1465–7.

Reisner, C. and Borish, L. 1995. Heliox therapy for acute vocal cord dysfunction. *Chest* 108(5):1477.

Rodier, F., Gautrin, D., Ghezzo, H. and Malo, J. L. 2003. Incidence of occupational rhinoconjunctivitis and risk factors in animal-health apprentices. *J Allergy Clin Immunol* 112(6):1105–11.

Rundell, K. W. and Spiering, B. A. 2003. Inspiratory stridor in elite athletes. *Chest* 123(2):468–74.

Ruoppi, P., Koistinen, T., Susitaival, P., Honkanen, J. and Soininen, H. 2004. Frequency of allergic rhinitis to laboratory animals in university employees as confirmed by chamber challenges. *Allergy* 59(3):295–301.

Rushton, L., Hutchings, S. J., Fortunato, L., Young, C., Evans, G. S., Brown, T., Bevan, R. et al. 2012. Occupational cancer burden in Great Britain. *Br J Cancer* 107(Suppl. 1): S3–7.

Santos, D. V., Reiter, E. R., DiNardo, L. J. and Costanzo, R. M. 2004. Hazardous events associated with impaired olfactory function. *Arch Otolaryngol Head Neck Surg* 130(3):317–9.

Sarlo, K. 2003. Control of occupational asthma and allergy in the detergent industry. *Ann Allergy Asthma Immunol* 90(5 Suppl. 2):32–4.

Sastre, J. and Quirce, S. 2006. Immunotherapy: An option in the management of occupational asthma? *Curr Opin Allergy Clin Immunol* 6(2):96–100.

Scadding, G., Hellings, P., Alobid, I., Bachert, C., Fokkens, W., van Wijk, R. G., Gevaert, P. et al. 2011. Diagnostic tools in Rhinology EAACI position paper. *Clin Transl Allergy* 1(1):2.

Schaefer, S. D. 2014. Management of acute blunt and penetrating external laryngeal trauma. *Laryngoscope* 124(1):233–44.

Settipane, R. A. and Kaliner, M. A. 2013. Chapter 14: Nonallergic rhinitis. *Am J Rhinol Allergy* 27(Suppl. 1):S48–51.

Shaaban, R., Zureik, M., Soussan, D., Neukirch, C., Heinrich, J., Sunyer, J., Wjst, M. et al. 2008. Rhinitis and onset of asthma: A longitudinal population-based study. *Lancet* 372(9643):1049–57.

Shusterman, D. 1992. Critical review: The health significance of environmental odor pollution. *Arch Environ Health* 47(1):76–87.

Shusterman, D. 2002. Review of the upper airway, including olfaction, as mediator of symptoms. *Environ Health Perspect* 110(Suppl. 4):649–53.

Shusterman, D. 2011. The effects of air pollutants and irritants on the upper airway. *Proc Am Thorac Soc* 8(1):101–5.

Shusterman, D. and Murphy, M. A. 2007. Nasal hyperreactivity in allergic and non-allergic rhinitis: A potential risk factor for non-specific building-related illness. *Indoor Air* 17(4):328–33.

Siracusa, A., Desrosiers, M. and Marabini, A. 2000. Epidemiology of occupational rhinitis: Prevalence, aetiology and determinants. *Clin Exp Allergy* 30(11): 1519–34.

Smith, W. M., Davidson, T. M. and Murphy, C. 2009. Toxin-induced chemosensory dysfunction: A case series and review. *Am J Rhinol Allergy* 23(6):578–81.

Sullivan, M. D., Heywood, B. M. and Beukelman, D. R. 2001. A treatment for vocal cord dysfunction in female athletes: An outcome study. *Laryngoscope* 111(10): 1751–5.

't Mannetje, A., Kogevinas, M., Luce, D., Demers, P. A., Begin, D., Bolm-Audorff, U., Comba, P. et al. 1999. Sinonasal cancer, occupation, and tobacco smoking in European women and men. *Am J Ind Med* 36(1):101–7.

Tarlo, S. M., Balmes, J., Balkissoon, R., Beach, J., Beckett, W., Bernstein, D., Blanc, P. D. et al. 2008. Diagnosis and management of work-related asthma: American College of Chest Physicians Consensus Statement. *Chest* 134(3 Suppl.):1S–41S.

Tarlo, S. M. and Liss, G. M. 2003. Practical implications of studies in occupational rhinoconjunctivitis. *J Allergy Clin Immunol* 112(6):1047–9.

Tarlo, S. M., Malo, J. L. and Participants Third Jack Pepys Workshop on Asthma in the Workplace. 2009. An official ATS proceedings: Asthma in the workplace: The Third Jack Pepys Workshop on Asthma in the Workplace: Answered and unanswered questions. *Proc Am Thorac Soc* 6(4):339–49.

Tervonen, H., Niskanen, M. M., Sovijarvi, A. R., Hakulinen, A. S., Vilkman, E. A. and Aaltonen, L. M. 2009. Fiberoptic videolaryngoscopy during bicycle ergometry: A diagnostic tool for exercise-induced vocal cord dysfunction. *Laryngoscope* 119(9):1776–80.

Thilsing, T., Rasmussen, J., Lange, B., Kjeldsen, A. D., Al-Kalemji, A. and Baelum, J. 2012. Chronic rhinosinusitis and occupational risk factors among 20- to 75-year-old Danes-A GA(2) LEN-based study. *Am J Ind Med* 55(11):1037–43.

Thulin, H., Bjorkdahl, M., Karlsson, A. S. and Renstrom, A. 2002. Reduction of exposure to laboratory animal allergens in a research laboratory. *Ann Occup Hyg* 46(1):61–8.

Tonini, S., Dellabianca, A., Costa, C., Lanfranco, A., Scafa, F. and Candura, S. M. 2009. Irritant vocal cord dysfunction and occupational bronchial asthma: Differential diagnosis in a health care worker. *Int J Occup Med Environ Health* 22(4):401–6.

Traister, R. S., Fajt, M. L., Whitman-Purves, E., Anderson, W. C. and Petrov, A. A. 2013. A retrospective analysis comparing subjects with isolated and coexistent vocal cord dysfunction and asthma. *Allergy Asthma Proc* 34(4):349–55.

Tripodi, D., Ferron, C., Malard, O., de Montreuil, C. B., Planche, L., Sebille-Rivain, V., Roedlich, C. et al. 2011. Relevance of both individual risk factors and occupational exposure in cancer survival studies: The example of intestinal type sinonasal adenocarcinoma. *Laryngoscope* 121(9):2011–8.

Uzzaman, A. and Story, R. 2012. Chapter 5: Allergic rhinitis. *Allergy Asthma Proc* 33(Suppl. 1):S15–8.

Vandenplas, O. and Malo, J. L. 1997. Inhalation challenges with agents causing occupational asthma. *Eur Respir J* 10(11):2612–29.

Vandenplas, O., Toren, K. and Blanc, P. D. 2003. Health and socioeconomic impact of work-related asthma. *Eur Respir J* 22(4):689–697.

Watson, M. A., King, C. S., Holley, A. B., Greenburg, D. L. and Mikita, J. A. 2009. Clinical and lung-function variables associated with vocal cord dysfunction. *Respir Care* 54(4):467–73.

Weitzel, E. K., McMains, K. C., Rajapaksa, S. and Wormald, P. J. 2008. Aerosinusitis: Pathophysiology, prophylaxis, and management in passengers and aircrew. *Aviat Space Environ Med* 79(1):50–3.

28 Acute Inhalation Injuries

Johanna Feary, Sherwood Burge and Paul Cullinan

CONTENTS

INTRODUCTION

Acute inhalation injuries are fortunately rare and occur sporadically, and both the nature of exposures and the affected populations are highly heterogeneous. Together, these factors make such injuries a difficult subject of study, and much of the literature is in the form of uncontrolled case reports or series, a selection of which are presented below. There is an almost complete absence of evidence relating to issues of clinical management, and much practice is based on precedent and analogy.

Definitions

There is no universally accepted definition of an acute inhalation injury; the focus of this chapter is on the sequelae of acute—usually single—high-intensity exposure to an agent that may be toxic, an irritant or an asphyxiant. Generally, the relevant exposure is far in excess of permissible workplace limits or recommended limits for population-wide environmental levels. Exposures may occur inside or outside of a workplace or, importantly, during the transport of products between sites. Frequently, more than one individual is exposed; in some cases, the numbers are very large, most catastrophically in the explosion at the Union Carbide India pesticide plant in Bhopal in 1984, when approximately a quarter of the city's 1 million inhabitants were exposed to toxic gas following an explosion in the plant's storage facility (Cullinan et al., 1997). Exposures resulting in inhalation injury may be categorised in a variety of ways: as single or recurrent; by their intensity or nature (either a specific chemical or a mixture, such as fire-smoke); and as accidental (as is normally the case) or deliberate.

TABLE 28.1
Relationship between Water Solubility and Site of Injury of Inhaled Irritants

Water Solubility	Agent	Typical Sites of Response
High	Ammonia Hydrogen chloride Sulphur dioxide	Eyes and upper airway inflammation (rhinitis and laryngeal oedema)
Intermediate	Chlorine	Upper and lower airways
Low	Oxides of nitrogen Phosgene Ozone	Delayed onset of lower airway inflammation at 24–48 hours with pneumonitis and pulmonary oedema and small airways obstruction

Epidemiology

The epidemiology of acute inhalation injury is poorly documented. Inhalation accidents are the fifth most common cause of illness reported to the UK surveillance of work-related and occupational respiratory disease (SWORD) surveillance scheme, with an estimated 1180 cases in the period from 1989 to 1994, with the highest annual incident rate (164 cases/million employees) in chemical processors (Sallie and McDonald, 1996).

Chemistry

Respiratory injury may occur from the inhalation of substances encountered in various physical states, including gases, vapours (gaseous forms of substances that are in liquid or solid form at normal temperatures and pressures) or fumes (solid materials, often metals, of small particle sizes [most <1.0 μm and many <0.1 μm] suspended in a gaseous medium that has condensed from a vaporised state). 'Aerosols' comprise a mix of potential states (liquid droplets or fine particulates dispersed in a gaseous medium), with smoke being a subset of the group resulting from incomplete combustion (Blanc, 2015).

Effects of Exposure

The anatomical distribution of injury and speed of onset of symptoms depend largely on the solubility of the gas, vapour or fume concerned; other important factors include the quantity inhaled, the duration of exposure and other characteristics of the agent, such as its pH and temperature, and, in the case of a fume, the physical characteristics of the particles. Host factors such as age, use of respiratory-protective equipment and pre-existing respiratory disease may also be important.

Highly water-soluble agents such as ammonia, hydrogen chloride and sulphur dioxide cause immediate irritation to the eyes and upper airways. In contrast, materials that are insoluble or have low solubility—such as oxides of nitrogen, phosgene and ozone—cause no acute injury, but delayed effects are seen, mainly involving the small airways. Chlorine has intermediate solubility and can cause upper and lower airway inflammation (Table 28.1).

If the inhaled material is hot, and particularly if it contains particles, thermal injury to the airways may result. Overwhelming exposure may result in asphyxia or catastrophic pulmonary oedema. Gases that are heavier than air can cause asphyxiation in poorly ventilated, enclosed or low-lying areas; a striking example was chlorine used as an agent of warfare in the trenches of the First World War. Similarly, gases that are lighter than air may displace oxygen in situations in which individuals are situated at a higher elevation.

SPECIFIC AGENTS

Asphyxia

Hypoxia due to lack of inspired oxygen is mostly an out-of-hospital issue for workers in areas where oxygen has been depleted (such as by combustion in an underground mine) or who have entered confined spaces where oxygen has been displaced by lighter or heavier gases as described above. Some workplaces, such as computer suites, have deliberately reduced oxygen environments in order to reduce the risk of fire or to preserve materials such as rare manuscripts. Common gases that are heavier than air include carbon dioxide, North Sea gas, ethane, argon, propane and phosgene. Gases that are lighter than air include methane (in mines), ethylene and acetylene. Hypoxia can occur in domestic dwellings due to seepage of foul air from disused underground mines, which inspire air when atmospheric pressure is high and expire air with a low FiO_2 when atmospheric pressure is low (Hendrick and Sizer, 1992). Cases of occupational fatalities due to asphyxia have also been reported with the use of epoxy resin paint in confined spaces (Centers for Disease Control [CDC], 1990).

Acetic Acid

Acetic acid is used in the production of plastics and a variety of chemicals and in the dye, rubber, pharmaceutics, food and textiles industries. Vapour may produce immediate irritation to the eyes and upper respiratory tract, and if exposure is high, pulmonary oedema may occur. A report from 1989 describes reversible airflow obstruction in a maintenance fitter who was exposed to hot glacial (anhydrous) acetic acid when disconnecting a pressurised pump for overhaul. He had first-degree burns and developed exertional dyspnoea over 7 days with inspiratory basal crackles, scattered wheeze and bilateral reticulonodular infiltration, particularly at the lung bases, on chest radiograph. Trans-bronchial biopsy showed a diffuse, mainly mononuclear interstitial pneumonitis, and bronchial lavage contained excess macrophages and lymphocytes; his symptoms resolved with oral corticosteroids (Rajan and Davies, 1989). Acute exposure to glacial acetic acid in a hospital resulted in three of the 14 workers with high exposure fulfilling the criteria for acute irritant asthma (Kern, 1991).

Acetaldehyde (CH_3CHO)

Acetaldehyde is a volatile, colourless liquid with a pungent smell produced by the oxidation of ethylene gas. It is used in the manufacture of chemicals, synthetic resins and rubbers, plastics and disinfectants. Low concentrations cause ocular irritation and hyper-secretion of mucus in the upper and lower respiratory tracts, with the development of acute pulmonary oedema at up to 48 hours after exposure. At higher concentrations, it has narcotic properties, and headache and stupor may occur.

Acrolein (Acrylic Aldehyde, CH_2CHCO)

Acrolein is an oily liquid that is produced by catalytic oxidation of propylene. In liquid state it is relatively harmless, but it has a high vapour pressure and may quickly form a colourless, pungent gas. It is used in the manufacture of plastics, acrylates and synthetic pharmaceuticals and can be formed when oils and fats are heated to high temperatures, such as in the production of soap and linseed oils and in cooking. It is also present in tobacco smoke and is released when biomass is burned (Bein and Leikauf, 2011). Intensely irritant at concentrations exceeding 5 ppm, exposure results in a range of predominantly lower airway symptoms with productive cough and dyspnoea. Fatalities have been reported (Committee on Aldehydes, 1981).

Ammonia (NH_3)

Ammonia is a colourless, highly soluble, pungent, irritant alkaline gas that is widely used in soil fertiliser production, refrigeration and in the pharmaceutical and chemical industries (Figure 28.1). Anhydrous ammonia is used in the illicit manufacture of methamphetamine, and inhalation injuries have become common in small, makeshift ‘meth labs’ in areas such as Illinois, USA, where there is ready access to agricultural fertilisers (Bloom et al., 2008). When ammonia combines with water, it forms ammonium hydroxide, a strong alkali that causes chemical burns to the eyes and upper respiratory tract. Victims describe severe oropharyngeal pain followed quickly by a feeling of suffocation with cough, copious watery sputum and breathlessness. Asphyxia due to obstructive laryngeal oedema can occur. A range of sequelae may develop in both the upper and lower airways, including pneumonitis and pulmonary oedema. Those surviving the acute phase may develop chronic pulmonary disease including bronchiectasis, obstruction of the small and large airways and interstitial lung disease (Ortiz-Pujols et al., 2014). Clinical signs at

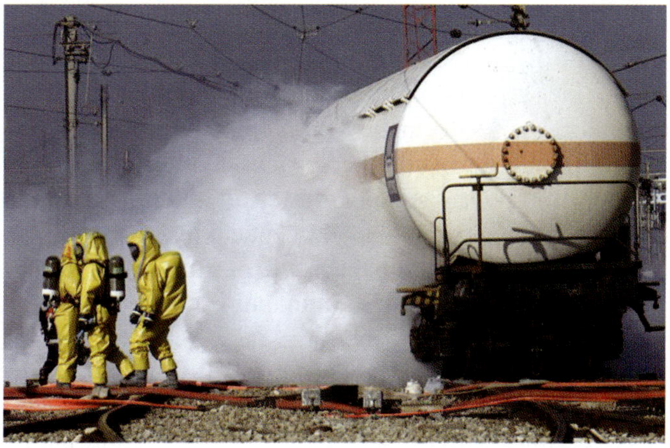

FIGURE 28.1 Leak from a truck carrying ammonia; France, 2001. (From http://www.ibtimes.com/ammonia-gas-leak-northern-indian-city-kills-least-5-100-hospitalized-1965562. With permission.)

24 hours are a good guide to prognosis (Montague and Macneil, 1980).

Blast and Blunt Injury

Blast injuries may occur from explosions in factories, ships and mines, in warfare and in water where divers and armed forces personnel may be affected. Blunt trauma may occur with falls from height into water or from a blow to the chest wall. Alveolar rupture can occur due to shearing injury of the lungs with fatalities in the absence of other signs of external trauma. Clinical features include cough with frothy blood-stained sputum and crackles. Subcutaneous and mediastinal emphysema and pneumothoraces may develop, and delayed pulmonary oedema is common. Management includes conventional ventilator support using lung-protective strategies (Mackenzie and Tunnicliffe, 2011).

Cadmium

Cadmium, a heavy metal, is a component of certain metal solders, including 'gold carat' used in jewellery. Acute inhalation occurs when it is liberated during the welding or flame cutting or brazing of cadmium-containing materials and can cause acute pneumonitis and diffuse alveolar damage. Chronic exposure may result in emphysema (Scott, 1980; Fuortes et al., 1991; Moitra et al., 2013).

Carbon Monoxide (CO)

Carbon monoxide is used in the synthesis of many chemicals, including isocyanates, ethylene, methanol and aldehydes, as well as in nickel refining in the Mond process; it results from incomplete combustion of carbon. Petrol engines are particular sources of carbon monoxide, especially in confined spaces such as underground carparks. It can be a problem in mines and a danger to firefighters in confined spaces. Domestic exposure occurs from poorly ventilated fires and boilers.

Carbon monoxide poisoning needs exclusion in all patients with acute inhalation exposures, particularly following significant smoke inhalation. In patients with subacute exposures, symptoms are often non-specific and include headache (often described as being in the centre of the skull), fatigue, confusion and breathlessness. Oximetry may be normal, as most transcutaneous oximeters cannot differentiate between oxy- and carboxy-haemoglobin. The PaO_2 is usually normal, as carbon monoxide does not interfere with the dissolved oxygen measured during blood gas measurement. In all suspected cases, carboxyhaemoglobin should be measured in arterial or venous blood. Carbon monoxide in exhaled breath can be measured with devices that are used to monitor cigarette smoking. It binds to haemoglobin 240-times more avidly than oxygen and also shifts the oxygen dissociation curve to the left, inhibiting the offloading of oxygen in the tissues. It enters cells and there inactivates cytochrome oxidase, further inhibiting the availability of oxygen to mitochondria and producing greater effects of tissue hypoxia than would be anticipated from the blood gases. Treatment is with 100% oxygen via a rebreathing bag, with a somewhat controversial role for hyperbaric oxygen for patients who have been unconscious. For survivors, there are no known long-term respiratory consequences, but neuropsychiatric effects including memory loss, personality changes and Parkinsonism can occur, particularly when peak carboxyhaemoglobin exceeds 25% (Weaver et al., 2007).

Chlorine

Chlorine is a greenish–yellow gas that is 2.5-times heavier than air. It is used in the chemical industry in the production of polymers (such as polyvinyl chloride [PVC]) and other chemicals, and as a bleaching agent in the paper industry. It can result from the accidental mixture of bleach with an acid in domestic or industrial cleaning. Chlorine is used as a sterilising agent and biocide in industrial and domestic settings, including the treatment of fruit and vegetables. Historically, it was used in gaseous form as a water treatment for swimming pools, resulting in gassings of workers in basement water treatment rooms following leaks from cylinders. Chlorine reacts with nitrogen-forming chloramines, which are thought to be responsible for causing asthma in elite swimmers (the prevalence of which is nearly 50%). Exposures are also significant in cleaners (Das and Blanc, 1993; Helenius et al., 1998; Thickett et al., 2002). Large community exposures have resulted from release from bulk transport tankers (Jones et al., 1986).

Exposure in confined spaces may result in death from hypoxia. On inhalation, chlorine reacts with water to form hydrochloric and hypochlorous acids and free oxygen radicals. Lower levels of exposure cause eye and upper airway inflammation, often with airflow obstruction and vomiting. Larger exposures may result in laryngeal oedema or (delayed-onset) pulmonary oedema; longstanding anosmia has been reported following industrial exposure (Benjamin and Pickles, 1997). Brief concentrations of 3–5 ppm appear to be tolerated without injury; exposure to 5–8 ppm may cause mild acute illness; levels of 14–21 ppm are dangerous; and at over

40 ppm, acute pulmonary oedema occurs. Long-term exposure of chlorine gas workers to concentrations of less than 1 ppm is not associated with significant impairment of ventilatory function (Chester et al., 1969). A study followed up residents in Youngstown, Florida, in 1978 following the derailment of a freight train carrying 50 tons of liquid chlorine, which produced a 1000-feet high chlorine cloud measuring 3 m by 4 m. Eight deaths occurred immediately; longitudinal follow-up of 60 residents for 6 years showed expected differences in decline of forced expiratory volume in 1 second (FEV_1) due to smoking, but no evidence of persistent disease related to the chlorine exposure (Jones et al., 1986).

Cyanide (Hydrogen Cyanide)

Major exposures to hydrogen cyanide can occur in electroplating or in precious metal recovery from scrap (such as silver recovery from old X-ray plates), as well as from the combustion of many materials. It should be suspected in the absence of any obvious cause for severe hypoxia and in all victims of smoke inhalation, particularly those with raised carboxyhaemoglobin. On inhalation, cyanide molecules bind to cytochrome a_3, inhibiting mitochondrial utilisation of oxygen. Since the release of oxygen into tissues is impaired, the venous PvO_2 may be nearer the arterial PaO_2 than usual (so-called arteriolarisation of the venous blood) and serum lactate may be raised. The treatment of choice is high-flow oxygen and parenteral hydroxocobalamin, which should be administered before blood or urine cyanide levels are available. Older treatment was with sodium nitrite and sodium thiosulphate, but these promote methaemoglobin formation, which has a high affinity for hydrogen cyanide (Fortin et al., 2006; Borron et al., 2007).

Environmental Particulates

There are several studies of asthmatics or the previously healthy exposed to high levels of particulates from natural or man-made disasters, with the best documented being those exposed to dust from the collapsed World Trade Center buildings in New York in 2001. A longitudinal study of firefighters who had regular spirometry before the disaster showed that 1 year after exposure to World Trade Center dust, their FEV_1 values fell by a mean 372 mL compared with 31 mL/year in the previous 5 years; this correlated with increased reporting of respiratory symptoms. Surprisingly few wore respiratory protection (Banauch et al., 2006).

Particulate exposures were also high following the eruption from Mount St Helens in 1980. Although there was an increase in emergency room visits after the eruption, a study of children in a residential asthma school that was covered with ash showed little change in FEV_1 (Buist et al., 1983). Conversely, asthma increased in children in Soufrière Hills, Montserrat, following the eruption in 1995 (Forbes et al., 2003). Most of the health-related research of these exposures has focused on the silica content of the respirable particulates. These differences may be explained by the pH of the inspired material: alkaline in the cement dust from the World Trade Center, neutral in the Mount St Helens eruption and acid (due to the sulphur content) in the Montserrat eruption (Horwell and Baxter, 2006).

Fire Smoke and Plastics

Smoke from fires potentially comprises a huge range of toxic gases and pyrolysis products, the chemical components of which may be different from the unheated state and are generally unknown. Respiratory injury may occur in the absence of cutaneous burns. Despite heavy exposures, the outcomes in survivors are variable and it is difficult to generalise or predict outcomes. This is due in part to the heterogeneity at baseline of the affected populations and the lack of pre-exposure clinical assessment. In 1985, the engine of an aircraft exploded on take-off at Manchester Airport; 52 of the 137 passengers died on-board. Fifteen of the survivors were hospitalised for treatment of smoke inhalation and burns, with six requiring invasive ventilation for laryngeal oedema, acute respiratory distress syndrome (ARDS) or exacerbation of pre-existing asthma. Lung function measured 3 months later in 13 of these survivors found that long-term physical sequelae were rare (O'Hickey et al., 1987). In 1987, a fire at an underground station in London caused over 30 deaths; follow-up of 14 survivors with smoke inhalation injuries at 6 months found nine with persistent respiratory symptoms and 11 with evidence of small airways obstruction on lung function testing (Fogarty et al., 1991).

A standard approach should be used (Lee and Mellins, 2006) for anyone with a fire-smoke inhalation injury, with assessment of carbon monoxide levels being particularly important and exposure to hydrogen cyanide managed separately, as described above. Inspection of upper airways may reveal signs of inhaled burnt material and the patient should be observed for the development of laryngeal oedema. Although frequently used, there is no reliable evidence of a beneficial effect of systemic steroids in the acute phase of inhalation injury. Antibiotics should be reserved for patients with clinical evidence of infection, including those with ventilator-associated pneumonia.

Hydrogen Chloride (HCl)

Hydrogen chloride is a colourless or yellowish gas with a pungent odour that, when exposed to atmospheric moisture, condenses to form a dense, white corrosive vapour. It is used in hydrochloric acid manufacture, the refining of mineral ores, petroleum well extraction, leather tanning and the refining of fats, soaps and edible oils. It is also used in the production of polymers and plastics, rubber, fertilisers, dyes and pigments. Serious inhalational exposures are rare because of the vapour's highly irritant nature. Inhalation of substantial amounts causes inflammation, corrosion and subsequent oedema of the upper and lower respiratory tracts.

Hydrogen Fluoride (Hydrofluoric Acid, HF)

Hydrogen fluoride is a strongly acidic colourless gas that can etch glass. It is detectable by smell (the odour is similar to that of chlorine) at concentrations lower than irritating levels and is readily soluble in water, forming a dense white vapour in moist air. It is used in the chemical industry in the synthesis of a variety of fluoropolymers, in the oil industry as a catalyst, in the refining of certain metals, as a constituent of some welding electrodes and as a catalyst for the electro-tinning of steel. Hydrogen fluoride vapour may also be produced in fires as a breakdown product of fluorocarbon fire-extinguishing agents and in the combustion of fluoropolymers (Kelly, 1998). It is highly irritant to skin and mucus membranes; inhalation causes burning of the upper airways and delayed development (24–48 hours) of pulmonary oedema. Prolonged exposure to very low quantities does not appear to have any adverse effects.

Hydrogen Sulphide (H_2S)

Hydrogen sulphide is a colourless gas with a distinctive smell and is heavier than air. It is produced by petrochemical refineries—Alberta, Canada, has particular experience due to its high sulphur-containing oil and gas fields—and is also a problem in farm slurry pits and tankers containing rotting vegetation. At low concentrations, hydrogen sulphide smells of rotten eggs; at high concentrations, it paralyses the sense of smell, removing the warning signs. Inhalation of high concentrations of hydrogen sulphide can stop respiration suddenly through 'knockdown' hypoxia; the rescue of affected individuals is particularly hazardous, often leading to the death of the rescuer (Figure 28.2). Respiration probably ceases due to inhibition of monoamine oxidase in the brainstem, with the intra-mitochondrial detoxification mechanism for sulphide ions being abruptly saturated. There may also be inhibition of cytochrome oxidase, as with hydrogen cyanide. Exposure to lower levels (300–600 ppm) can cause upper and lower airway symptoms, headache and dizziness, followed by pulmonary oedema. Exposure to concentrations above 700 ppm causes rapid death from asphyxia. The presence of thiosulphate in the blood can confirm the diagnosis; nitrite therapy can be useful if administered immediately after exposure; otherwise, treatment is supportive (Guidotti, 1994; Gerasimon et al., 2007).

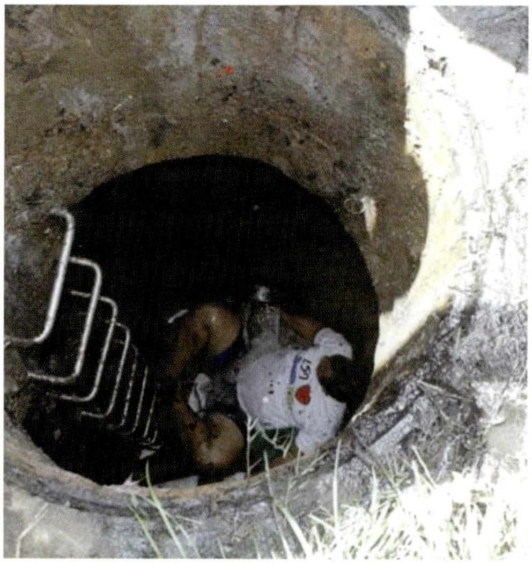

FIGURE 28.2 Man dies from hydrogen sulphide fumes whilst carrying out maintenance work on a sewer. His three colleagues died trying to rescue him one by one; Thailand, 2014. (Reproduced from *Phuket Gazette*. With permission.)

Methyl Bromide (Bromoethane, CH_3Br)

Methyl bromide is a gas that is used as an insecticidal fumigant in food supplies, warehouses, barges, buildings and furniture. It is also used as a refrigerant, herbicide and fire-extinguishing agent and in aniline dye manufacture. It is one of the most toxic halides, dispersing slowly and giving little warning of its presence; exposure prevention therefore includes mixing it with a pungent substance in order to enable early detection. In California, the most frequent cause of death from methyl bromide exposure in recent years has been unauthorised entry into structures that are undergoing fumigation. Acutely, it is highly toxic to the respiratory system (causing acute bronchitis, pulmonary oedema and haemorrhagic pleural effusions) and central nervous system (resulting in pyramidal and extra-pyramidal features); symptoms usually develop at between 2 and 4 hours after exposure. At lower concentrations, neurological symptoms are generally most prominent (Yang et al., 1995).

Nitrogen Mustard (Phosgene, 'Mustard Gas', Carbonyl Chloride, $COCl_2$)

Nitrogen mustards were used as chemical warfare agents in the First World War and have been better understood since their widespread use in the Iran–Iraq war of 1983–1988. Inhalation may occur in the chemical industry, where carbonyl chloride is used as a chlorinating agent in the synthesis of organic compounds such as dyes. It is also released when chlorinated hydrocarbons (e.g. carbon tetrachloride) are heated, such as during the welding of metals that have been cleaned with chlorinated hydrocarbons, in firefighting and in the use of paint removers in heated enclosed spaces. It can be produced in fires where PVC is burned, even where the quantity is small.

An alkylating agent that is far more toxic than chlorine, it is 3.5-times heavier than air and has a sweet, pungent smell resembling freshly mowed hay, which may be undetectable at low concentrations. Exposure initially causes blistering and burning of the skin and eyes and rhinitis; lower respiratory symptoms may start after a few hours, with pulmonary oedema developing at 24–48 hours and being dose dependant. Significant quantities of the gas may therefore be inhaled before symptoms develop. High-level exposure results in constrictive rings of inflammation in the trachea and main airways; lesser exposure can result in bronchiectasis and air trapping. Systemic absorption can lead to bone marrow and organ failure and an ARDS picture (Balali-Mood and Hefazi, 2006).

Oxides of Nitrogen

Acute exposures to nitrogen oxides occur in workers entering silage towers, in welders and in the manufacture of explosives and chemical engraving. Although high exposures can cause airflow obstruction and pulmonary oedema, their importance lies in the lack of acute effects (due to their poor solubility and lack of irritant properties) and their ability to cause delayed bronchiolitis obliterans, often starting 2–6 weeks after exposure. All patients with significant acute exposures should be monitored regularly after exposure in order to identify bronchiolitis, for which there is some evidence of benefit from corticosteroids (Zwemer et al., 1992).

Ozone

Ozone is a highly toxic gas and one of the most powerful oxidising substances known. It is normally present in the atmosphere in minute quantities without any harmful effect, but occurs at increased concentrations at high altitudes and is produced by lightning; significant amounts may enter aircraft cabins at altitudes over 9000 m. In industry, it is used for sterilising water, bleaching paper, flour and oils and deodorising organic factory effluent by masking the odour. Potentially dangerous levels of ozone can be produced by ultraviolet (UV) radiation during gas shielding, welding and arc-air gouging. UV radiation from air-conditioning equipment and office photocopiers may give rise to low levels that are unlikely to be harmful in ordinarily ventilated areas. The effects of ozone in animal models have been widely studied. Heavy exposure (>2 ppm) can cause an acute illness with rapid onset of severe headache, substernal pain and dyspnoea or a more insidious development of ocular and nasal irritation, cough, dyspnoea, haemoptysis and fever. Exposure exceeding 5–20 ppm for 1 hour or more can be fatal. Concentrations of 0.4–0.5 ppm inhaled for 3 hours a day for 5 days caused a short-lived reduction in forced vital capacity and specific airway conductance in healthy volunteers. There is some discrepancy in the reporting of respiratory symptoms by commercial aircrew, where ozone concentrations of up to 1 ppm have been recorded.

Paraquat

Paraquat is a non-selective herbicide that is in widespread use. Considering its toxicity by ingestion, it has proved remarkably safe in agricultural use. For instance, a large study of Sri Lankan rubber plantation workers spraying paraquat showed no changes in spirometry after an average of 12 years of spraying. It is, however, extremely toxic to the lungs, kidneys and liver after ingestion, being concentrated in the lungs, resulting in pulmonary haemorrhage, ARDS and acute pulmonary fibrosis (Senanayake et al., 1993; Dinis-Oliveira et al., 2008).

Sarin

Sarin has recently been used in conflicts in Syria and Iraq, although the best reported descriptions come from terrorist use in Matsumoto, Japan. It is a cholinesterase inhibitor, so most of its effects are on the central nervous system (constricted pupils and bradycardia being clues), but lesser exposures may present with predominantly respiratory symptoms, particularly wheeze and salivation. Respiratory muscle paralysis and pulmonary oedema occur in more severe poisonings. Medical personnel are at risk from skin and clothing contamination. Treatment is with atropine in order to reverse salivation and bronchospasm. Intravenous pralidoxime mesylate reactivates cholinesterase and is given together with atropine for more severe poisoning (Volans, 1996).

Sulphur Dioxide (SO_2)

Sulphur dioxide is a dense, colourless gas with an unpleasant smell of burnt matches and is one of the more commonly encountered toxic gases. Inhaled sulphur dioxide readily reacts with the moisture of mucous membranes to form sulphurous acid (H_2SO_3), which is a severe respiratory irritant. Sulphur dioxide is a major air pollutant that is released primarily from the combustion of fossil fuel; other sources include the smelting of sulphide ores and volcanic emissions. It is used extensively in the chemical manufacturing industries to bleach wood pulp and paper, in food preservation (including the preservation of dried fruit due to its antimicrobial properties), in winemaking and for waste and water treatment. It has been extensively studied: acute exposures of 50–100 ppm may be tolerated for up to 60 minutes, but higher exposures can cause asphyxiation. Chronic low-level exposure from air pollution may cause some respiratory symptoms (mainly bronchospasm) in healthy individuals and can worsen pre-existing asthma.

Tear Gas (Lacrimators)

Although banned as chemical warfare agents under the 1977 Chemical Weapons Convention, these agents are widely used for crowd control. Their use has increased and the methods of delivery escalated; dispersion can be from a hand-held pressured canister with the agent in solution applied in a one-on-one situation, but more commonly the agents are fired from a gun or dispersed in aerosols. The shells shot into crowds often cause serious injuries. The agents used may be unknown. Mace (CN or 2-chloroacetophenone) has largely been replaced by CS (a cyanocarbon structure named after its British discoverers Corson and Stoughton). At room temperature and on the skin, CS is a white crystalline material; although it contains cyanogenic groups, it is unlikely that it causes significant cyanide poisoning.

Pepper spray (capsaicin) or its synthetic equivalent pelargonic acid vanillylamide is a direct stimulator of TRIP receptors, resulting in neurogenic inflammation by reflex action. All are designed to cause acute irritation to the eyes and exposed skin, but irritation to the upper respiratory tract is common. Severe or fatal reactions from the chemicals themselves are rare, but include exacerbations of pre-existing asthma, the development of acute irritant asthma, chemical pneumonitis, pulmonary oedema and death. Medical attendants are also at risk when exposed to contaminated victims (Schep et al., 2015).

Waterproofing Sprays (Fluorocarbon Aerosol)

Acute chemical pneumonitis following the application of fluorocarbon-containing aerosols in confined spaces has emerged as an important syndrome since the early 1990s (Vernez et al., 2006). Examples of this (often in the domestic setting) include the use of waterproofing sprays for footwear, the application of floor stain protectors (Lazor-Blanchet et al., 2004) and the use of grout sealant (Daubert et al., 2009). The underlying mechanism of action is unclear, but cases often occur following changes in the formulation or particle size of a product. A variety of non-specific respiratory symptoms develop within several hours of exposure (including dyspnoea, chest pain, dry cough and sometimes influenza-like symptom) and range from mild and self-limiting to severe, requiring hospitalisation (Figure 28.3). Persistent symptoms and lung function abnormalities have been reported, and in one case, pulmonary fibrosis developed (Schicht et al., 1982).

Zinc Chloride

Most zinc salts are not harmful to the lungs; exceptions are zinc oxide, which can cause metal fume fever and zinc chloride smoke. Zinc chloride is used in galvanising iron, oil refining, dry batteries and taxidermy, and has been used for smoke bombs (formed when zinc oxide and hexachloroethane are burned together) and in firefighting exercises (Schenker et al., 1981). It is not hazardous

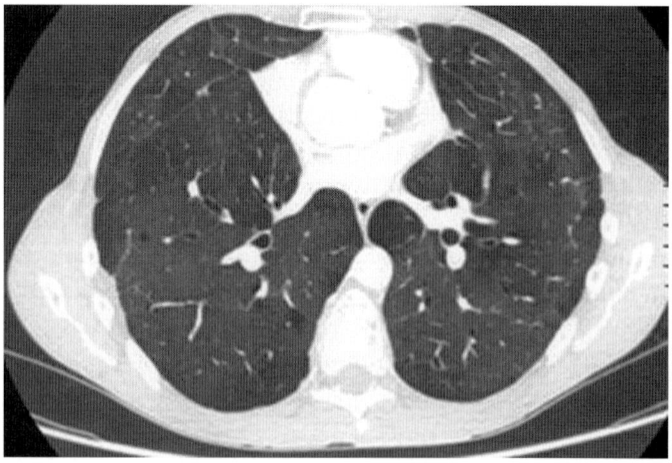

FIGURE 28.3 Computed tomography scan of a 35 year old man demonstrating mosaic attenuation that is suggestive of small airways airflow obstruction.

in well-ventilated spaces, but in confined spaces it may cause lethal acute chemical pneumonitis and delayed pulmonary oedema.

MANAGEMENT

Patients often do not know what agent they have encountered, and in most situations, the best approach is to observe the response, treat any symptoms and recognise the possibility of ongoing evolution of disease over 24 hours or more. Exposures requiring specific therapy are rare and are described above. Those involved in rescue have a difficult task, as the risks of delayed extraction of a victim must be weighed against the delays needed in order to provide rescuers with self-contained breathing apparatus.

Victims who have been unconscious or hypoxic should be observed for at least 24 hours after exposure. Signs of nasal, oral or laryngeal burns, oedema or ulceration can be helpful as indicators of significant exposure. Carbon monoxide poisoning should be excluded by measuring exhaled breath carbon monoxide, or if not available, carboxyhaemoglobin in venous or arterial blood. If there is evidence of breathlessness, wheeze or crackles on auscultation, measurement of spirometry is needed as much as a chest X-ray. Radiological changes are rare and, again, suggest significant exposure. Progressive airway oedema and bronchorrhoea may develop, accompanied by bronchoconstriction and bronchial mucosal sloughing. In the distal airways, injury may vary from mild interstitial oedema to diffuse alveolar damage. These may develop within hours or, depending on the agent, may be delayed by up to 48 hours. Acute complications include pneumothorax and pneumomediastinum. In severe cases, pre-emptive intubation and invasive ventilation may be appropriate in order to protect the airway from progressive airway and pulmonary oedema and for the treatment of hypoxaemia. Diffuse alveolar damage should be managed in the same way as for other causes, including protective ventilator strategies.

If there is evidence of airflow obstruction, treatment reasonably includes inhaled bronchodilators and corticosteroids until all of the respiratory symptoms have resolved and the patient has been reviewed at respiratory follow-up; there are, however, no controlled trials to support this. Asthma symptoms may persist at follow-up, in which case the measurement of non-specific reactivity is indicated (Wang et al., 2005).

Epidemiological data suggest that the majority of those with an acute inhalation injury have no long-term adverse health outcomes (Sallie and McDonald, 1996). A small minority will develop longer-term complications, but these are generally defined through case reports in which there is little information on exposure measurement or pre-existing lung function. The most common of these complications are airflow obstruction and non-specific airway hyper-responsiveness in individuals with acute irritant injuries (acute irritant-induced asthma or RADS). There are some data available from larger studies; for example, follow-up data of 454 survivors of the Union Carbide explosion suggest a dose-dependent relationship between exposure and the development of fixed small airways obstruction (Cullinan et al., 1997). Other potential complications include upper airway symptoms such as chronic rhinitis and vocal cord dysfunction (Blanc, 2015). Where ARDS and diffuse alveolar damage have occurred, patients are susceptible to the same range of complications, including obliterative bronchiolitis and bronchiectasis, which arise when these conditions are due to other causes. Finally, patients with inhalational injuries of either major or minor consequence may have been extracted from frightening and even life-threatening situations; post-traumatic stress may develop and may colour recovery.

REFERENCES

Balali-Mood, M. and Hefazi, M. 2006. Comparison of early and late toxic effects of sulfur mustard in Iranian veterans. *Basic Clin Pharmacol Toxicol* 99:273–82.

Banauch, G. I., Hall, C., Weiden, M., Cohen, H. W., Aldrich, T. K., Christodoulou, V., Arcentales, N. et al. 2006. Pulmonary function after exposure to the World Trade Center collapse in the New York City Fire Department. *Am J Respir Crit Care Med* 174:312–9.

Bein, K. and Leikauf, G. D. 2011. Acrolein—A pulmonary hazard. *Mol Nutr Food Res* 55:1342–60.

Benjamin, E. and Pickles, J. 1997. Chlorine-induced anosmia. A case presentation. *J Laryngol Otol* 111:1075–6.

Blanc, P. D. 2015. Acute pulmonary responses to toxic exposures. In Broaddus, V. C. et al. (eds), *Murray & Nadel's Textbook of Respiratory Medicine.* 6th ed. Philadelphia: Elsevier Saunders, pp. 1343–53.

Bloom, G. R., Suhail, F., Hopkins-Price, P. and Sood, A. 2008. Acute anhydrous ammonia injury from accidents during illicit methamphetamine production. *Burns* 34:713–8.

Borron, S. W., Baud, F. J., Barriot, P., Imbert, M. and Bismuth, C. 2007. Prospective study of hydroxocobalamin for acute cyanide poisoning in smoke inhalation. *Ann Emerg Med* 49:794–801, 801.e1–2.

Buist, A. S., Johnson, L. R., Vollmer, W. M., Sexton, G. J. and Kanarek, P. H. 1983. Acute effects of volcanic ash from Mount Saint Helens on lung function in children. *Am Rev Respir Dis* 127:714–9.

Centers for Disease Control (CDC). 1990. Occupational fatalities associated with exposure to epoxy resin paint in an underground tank—Makati, Republic of the Philippines. *MMWR Morb Mortal Wkly Rep* 39(22):379–80.

Chester, E. H., Gillespie, D. G. and Krause, F. D. 1969. The prevalence of chronic obstructive pulmonary disease in chlorine gas workers. *Am Rev Respir Dis* 99:365–73.

Committee on Aldehydes. 1981. *Formaldehyde and Other Aldehydes.* Washington, DC: National Academy Press.

Cullinan, P., Acquilla, S. and Dhara, V. R. 1997. Respiratory morbidity 10 years after the Union Carbide gas leak at Bhopal: A cross sectional survey. The International Medical Commission on Bhopal. *BMJ* 314:338–42.

Das, R. and Blanc, P. D. 1993. Chlorine gas exposure and the lung: A review. *Toxicol Ind Health* 9:439–55.

Daubert, G. P., Spiller, H., Crouch, B. I., Seifert, S., Simone, K. and Smolinske, S. 2009. Pulmonary toxicity following exposure to waterproofing grout sealer. *J Med Toxicol* 5:125–9.

Dinis-Oliveira, R. J., Duarte, J. A., Sanchez-Navarro, A., Remiao, F., Bastos, M. L. and Carvalho, F. 2008. Paraquat poisonings: Mechanisms of lung toxicity, clinical features and treatment. *Crit Rev Toxicol* 38:13–71.

Fogarty, P. W., George, P. J., Solomon, M., Spiro, S. G. and Armstrong, R. F. 1991. Long term effects of smoke inhalation in survivors of the King's Cross underground station fire. *Thorax* 46:914–8.

Forbes, L., Jarvis, D., Potts, J. and Baxter, P. J. 2003. Volcanic ash and respiratory symptoms in children on the island of Montserrat, British West Indies. *Occup Environ Med* 60:207–11.

Fortin, J. L., Giocanti, J. P., Ruttimann, M. and Kowalski, J. J. 2006. Prehospital administration of hydroxocobalamin for smoke inhalation-associated cyanide poisoning: 8 years of experience in the Paris Fire Brigade. *Clin Toxicol (Phila)* 44(Suppl. 1):37–44.

Fuortes, L., Leo, A., Ellerbeck, P. G. and Friell, L. A. 1991. Acute respiratory fatality associated with exposure to sheet metal and cadmium fumes. *J Toxicol Clin Toxicol* 29:279–83.

Gerasimon, G., Bennett, S., Musser, J. and Rinard, J. 2007. Acute hydrogen sulfide poisoning in a dairy farmer. *Clin Toxicol (Phila)* 45:420–3.

Guidotti, T. L. 1994. Occupational exposure to hydrogen sulfide in the sour gas industry: Some unresolved issues. *Int Arch Occup Environ Health* 66:153–60.

Helenius, I. J., Rytila, P., Metso, T., Haahtela, T., Venge, P. and Tikkanen, H. O. 1998. Respiratory symptoms, bronchial responsiveness and cellular characteristics of induced sputum in elite swimmers. *Allergy* 53:346–52.

Hendrick, D. J. and Sizer, K. E. 1992. 'Breathing' coal mines and surface asphyxiation from stythe (black damp). *BMJ* 305:509–10.

Horwell, C. J. and Baxter P. J. 2006. The respiratory health hazards of volcanic ash: A review for volcanic risk mitigation. *Bull Volcanol* 69:1–24.

Jones, R. N., Hughes, J. M., Glindmeyer, H. and Weill, H. 1986. Lung function after acute chlorine exposure. *Am Rev Respir Dis* 134:1190–5.

Kelly, D. 1998. A review of the inhalation toxicity of hydrogen fluoride. Presented at: *Halon Options Technical Working Conference.* Albuquerque, NM, May 12–14, 1998.

Kern, D. G. 1991. Outbreak of the reactive airways dysfunction syndrome after a spill of glacial acetic acid. *Am Rev Respir Dis* 144:1058–64.

Lazor-Blanchet, C., Rusca, S., Vernez, D., Berry, R., Albrecht, E., Droz, P. O. and Boillat, M. A. 2004. Acute pulmonary toxicity following occupational exposure to a floor stain protector in the building industry in Switzerland. *Int Arch Occup Environ Health* 77:244–8.

Lee, A. S. and Mellins, R. B. 2006. Lung injury from smoke inhalation. *Paediatr Respir Rev* 7:123–8.

Mackenzie, I. M. and Tunnicliffe, B. 2011. Blast injuries to the lung: Epidemiology and management. *Philos Trans R Soc Lond B Biol Sci* 366:295–9.

Moitra, S., Blanc, P. D. and Sahu, S. 2013. Adverse respiratory effects associated with cadmium exposure in small-scale jewellery workshops in India. *Thorax* 68:565–70.

Montague, T. J. and Macneil, A. R. 1980. Mass ammonia inhalation. *Chest* 77:496–8.

O'Hickey, S. P., Pickering, C. A., Jones, P. E. and Evans, J. D. 1987. Manchester air disaster. *Br Med J (Clin Res Ed)* 294:1663–7.

Ortiz-Pujols, S., Jones, S. W., Short, K. A., Morrell, M. R., Bermudez, C. A., Tilley, S. L. and Cairns, B. A. 2014. Management and sequelae of a 41-year-old Jehovah's witness with severe anhydrous ammonia inhalation injury. *J Burn Care Res* 35:e180–3.

Rajan, K. G. and Davies, B. H. 1989. Reversible airways obstruction and interstitial pneumonitis due to acetic acid. *Br J Ind Med* 46:67–8.

Sallie, B. and McDonald, C. 1996. Inhalation accidents reported to the SWORD surveillance project 1990–1993. *Ann Occup Hyg* 40:211–21.

Schenker, M. B., Speizer, F. E. and Taylor, J. O. 1981. Acute upper respiratory symptoms resulting from exposure to zinc chloride aerosol. *Environ Res* 25:317–24.

Schep, L. J., Slaughter, R. J. and McBride, D. I. 2015. Riot control agents: The tear gases CN, CS and OC—A medical review. *J R Army Med Corps* 161:94–9.

Schicht, R., Hartjen, A. and Sill, V. 1982. [Alveolitis after inhalation of leather-impregnation spray (author's transl)]. *Dtsch Med Wochenschr* 107:688–91.

Scott, R. 1980. Fatal cadmium fume inhalation. *Lancet* 2:429–30.

Senanayake, N., Gurunathan, G., Hart, T. B., Amerasinghe, P., Babapulle, M., Ellapola, S. B., Udupihille, M. et al. 1993. An epidemiological study of the health of Sri Lankan tea plantation workers associated with long term exposure to paraquat. *Br J Ind Med* 50:257–63.

Thickett, K. M., McCoach, J. S., Gerber, J. M., Sadhra, S. and Burge, P. S. 2002. Occupational asthma caused by chloramines in indoor swimming-pool air. *Eur Respir J* 19:827–32.

Vernez, D., Bruzzi, R., Kupferschmidt, H., De-Batz, A., Droz, P. and Lazor, R. 2006. Acute respiratory syndrome after inhalation of waterproofing sprays: *A posteriori* exposure–response assessment in 102 cases. *J Occup Environ Hyg* 3:250–61.

Volans, A. P. 1996. Sarin: Guidelines on the management of victims of a nerve gas attack. *J Accid Emerg Med* 13:202–6.

Wang, J., Winskog, C., Edston, E. and Walther, S. M. 2005. Inhaled and intravenous corticosteroids both attenuate chlorine gas-induced lung injury in pigs. *Acta Anaesthesiol Scand* 49:183–90.

Weaver, L. K., Valentine, K. J. and Hopkins, R. O. 2007. Carbon monoxide poisoning: Risk factors for cognitive sequelae and the role of hyperbaric oxygen. *Am J Respir Crit Care Med* 176:491–7.

Yang, R. S., Witt, K. L., Alden, C. J. and Cockerham, L. G. 1995. Toxicology of methyl bromide. *Rev Environ Contam Toxicol* 142:65–85.

Zwemer, F. L. Jr., Pratt, D. S. and May, J. J. 1992. Silo filler's disease in New York State. *Am Rev Respir Dis* 146:650–3.

29 Subacute Inhalation Injuries (Inhalation Fevers)

C. A. C. Pickering

CONTENTS

INTRODUCTION

This group of inhalation injuries is now known collectively as the inhalation fevers and is associated with various types of exposures, including metal fumes, polymer fumes, organic dusts and bio-aerosols. The term 'inhalation fevers' for these diverse types of exposures was first suggested in 1992 (Rask-Anderson and Pratt, 1992). At the time, the construct was criticised since the underlying mechanisms are likely to vary between types of exposure. Nevertheless, this descriptive terminology has persisted and is widely accepted as encompassing a distinct clinical entity.

Inhalation fever is by definition benign, being a self-limited syndrome associated with influenza-like symptoms of fever, chills, malaise, myalgia, joint pains and headache. Respiratory symptoms if present are typically mild. The symptoms develop 3–8 hours after initiation of exposure to the triggering agent or environment and usually resolve spontaneously over 24–36 hours. The syndrome, in most instances, follows a higher-than-normal exposure to fume, dust or aerosol through vocational activities. There is a high attack rate among persons who are similarly exposed, without a pattern of response suggesting sensitisation or an idiosyncratic response. Another hallmark of inhalation fevers as a group is tachyphylaxis; that is, a blunted response with repeated or ongoing exposure. Thus, an attack of inhalation fever may be more likely after a return to work following days off, and so the term 'Monday morning fever' has been applied to more than one exposure scenario associated with inhalation fever.

Unfortunately, grossly similar inhalation exposure scenarios to other agents can cause responses that are not self-limited and should not be confused with inhalation fever. The presence of respiratory compromise or other signs or symptoms of lung injury should not be approached as benign inhalation fever. Similarly, a clinical history that is indicative of an anamnestic response consistent with prior sensitisation is also inconsistent with inhalation fever. This chapter will summarise the major known subtypes of inhalation fever, while at the same time highlighting potential confusion arising from misdiagnosis due to other exposures that are linked to alternative clinical outcomes.

METAL FUME FEVER

Metal fume fever (MFF) is the most common and best appreciated of the inhalation fevers. It has been known under a variety of different names in the past determined by the trade involved, including brass founders' ague, galvanisers' fever, welders' shakes, Monday morning fever, zinc chills and the smothers. As the names suggest, the MFF syndrome is linked to zinc inhalation.

It occurs most commonly through electric arc welding on welding-galvanised mild steel; that is, steel coated with a thin layer of zinc (Blanc et al., 1993). Welding in an oxygen-containing atmosphere efficiently produces high concentrations of highly respirable zinc oxide fume. Galvanising itself is rarely associated with MFF because the temperatures involved do not produce zinc oxide fume. In contrast, zinc smelting operations and arc-air gouging processes (Sanderson, 1968) can generate such fume. Historically, brass foundry work was an endemic source of zinc oxide fume though mixing zinc with copper, the latter melting at a temperature at which the former is easily volatilised. Rarely, finely generated zinc dust, as opposed to freshly formed zinc oxide fume, has been implicated in MFF.

Although a number of reviews of MFF variously invoke a range of other metal fumes as causing MFF, there are no consistent modern data that support this. For example, older experimental data implicated magnesium oxide as a cause, but controlled human experimentation did not observe such an effect. Most importantly, certain metals that are often cited as causing MFF are actually potent causes of severe metal fume-caused acute lung injury, which can be fatal, the most important of which being cadmium and mercury. One modern report implicates copper fume as potentially causing a MFF-like response (Borak et al., 2000), although this has not be observed consistently. Indeed, inhaled copper may cause acute lung injury in a manner that is similar to other toxic metals.

Clinical Features

The symptoms of MFF develop some hours after exposure and can include a sweet metallic taste, dry cough, malaise, headache, rigors, profuse sweating, muscle and joint pains and breathlessness. Repeated exposure over the working week, which is typical in brass foundries but is less characteristic of welding operations, is associated with the resolution of symptoms recurring after periods away from work on days off and after holidays. The body temperature may increase to 39°C or more. Physical examination and chest radiography are usually normal. Recovery occurs in 24–48 hours. Infrequently, reports of transient radiographic changes have appeared in the literature, but this is inconsistent, nor does lung function impairment manifest as a routine component of the MFF syndrome. At the case report level, bronchospasm and allergic-type responses following zinc oxide fume exposure has been observed, but this rare finding is not a part of the classic MFF syndrome (Malo et al., 1990).

Pathogenesis

Early experimental evidence showed that MFF could be produced in human subjects who were intentionally exposure to zinc oxide fume (Anon, 1927). In the modern period, bronchoalveolar lavage in clinical investigation demonstrated that an inflammatory cellular response in the lungs was present in MFF (Vogelmeier, 1987). Later investigations of the mechanisms underlying MFF (Blanc et al., 1991) following zinc oxide fume inhalation exposure in volunteer subjects confirmed that bronchoalveolar lavage showed a marked pulmonary inflammatory response, predominantly made up of polymorphonuclear cells. This cellular response occurred even in the absence of frank symptoms. In further studies (Blanc et al., 1993), it was concluded that MFF was cytokine related. The key mediator appeared to be tumour necrosis factor (TNF), presumed to be secreted by alveolar macrophages and leading in turn to the release of IL-6 and IL-8 by other cells that are present in the lung. A statistically significant, exposure-dependant increase in these other cytokines occurred after the 3-hour TNF peak, with early TNF correlating statistically with IL-8 at 8 hours and with IL-6 at 22 hours.

Prevention, Diagnosis and Treatment

MFF should be prevented by the use of engineering controls, including local exhaust and/or general ventilation. In some circumstances when working in confined spaces or in emergency situations, respirators may be required. The diagnosis of MFF is made on clinical grounds. There is no role for zinc measurement in the blood or urine. It is important not to misdiagnose evolving acute lung injury as MFF. Respiratory impairment or radiographic abnormalities should shift diagnostic consideration to other entities, particularly cadmium pneumonitis, when there has been antecedent welding or flame cutting exposure. There is no specific treatment for MFF given its self-limited nature.

POLYMER FUME FEVER

Polymer fume fever (PFF) is caused by the pyrolysis products of fluoropolymers, most frequently polytetrafluoroethylene (PTFE or Teflon). Other commonly used long-chain fluoropolymers include polyvinyl fluoride and polyvinylidine fluoride.

PTFE resin is produced by controlled polymerisation of tetrafluoroethylene emulsion under pressure. It is then moulded in sintering ovens or by pressure processes. Physiologically, it is inert and causes neither irritation nor allergic sensitisation of body tissues. However, if heated to between 315°C and 375°C, particles—probably consisting of polymer chain fragments—are evolved. Above 380°C, small amounts of the toxic gases hexafluoropropylene and octafluoroisobutylene are produced, and at temperatures in excess of 500°C (when the rate of pyrolysis increases), perfluoroisobutylene and carbonyl fluoride, which is also toxic, are formed. These toxic compounds can cause pulmonary oedema in experimental animals (Harris, 1951) and acute lung injury in exposed humans and their pets.

PTFE resins are used extensively in the plastics industry for most modern plastic products including insulating materials, electrical components, bearings, gaskets, piping, coatings for wires, chemical vessels, 3D printing, non-stick cooking utensils and dirt-repellent starch sprays. Short-chain fluoropolymers are used in architectural and industrial coatings, mould-release sprays, lubricants and paper, leather and textile finishing.

There is no hazard to health from polymer fume unless the polymer is subjected to heat in excess of 300°C. This may occur in a variety of circumstances, with the most common giving rise to PFF being smoking cigarettes contaminated with the polymer either by direct contact or by particles suspended in the workplace atmosphere (the temperature in the burning zone of a cigarette exceeds 800°C). The workplace processes that use polymers include the operation of moulding and extruding machines, high-speed machining of components, welding of metal coated with PTFE or attached to PTFE resin blocks and ironing clothes sprayed with polymer–starch mixture for prolonged periods.

The inhalation of the fluoropolymers contained in products that are delivered by aerosol spray, including waterproofing sprays and sealants, can lead to acute lung injury (Wallace and Brown, 2005). Outbreaks of respiratory failure have been described in Europe, the USA, Canada and Japan, with most of these outbreaks following the marketing of new or reformulated products (Vernez et al., 2006).

Clinical Features

There is always a delay of 3–4 hours between exposure to the ‘fume’ or particulate before symptoms develop. The complaints include tightness of the chest, malaise, shortness of breath, headache, cough, chills and a temperature of 37.8–40°C (Lewis and Kerby, 1965). Physical signs in the lung are usually absent and the chest radiograph is normal. Recovery is complete in 1–2 days.

The illness is frequently regarded as influenza or some other acute infection both by the patient and doctor, unless there are recurrences. Hence, ‘PFF’ should be borne in mind in cases of ‘pyrexia of unknown origin’.

Pathogenesis

The pathogenesis of the symptoms is not known, but may involve similar mechanisms as MFF. Animal experiments (Cavagna et al., 1961) have suggested that particulate-phase PTFE pyrolysis products generated at 400–500°C are implicated in the development of the delayed fever.

Prognosis

Although PFF is, in general, a benign, self-limited syndrome, this is not always the case. Prolonged exposures and exposures to a polymer subjected to high temperatures (e.g. following welding) may result in the development of pulmonary oedema. This is marked by respiratory distress and the physical and radiographic signs of oedema of the lungs. Recovery is usually rapid. However, one fatality has been described (Lee et al., 1997). Repeated episodes of PFF in workers should be avoided. Such exposures have been associated with a rapid decline in lung function, which may occur in susceptible individuals (Kales and Christiani, 1994).

Management and Prevention

The majority of outbreaks of PFF have implicated the smoking of PTFE-contaminated cigarettes as being the source of exposure (Shusterman, 1993). The banning of smoking in the workplace and the introduction of handwashing when leaving the work area will prevent most outbreaks. In instances in which mechanical breakdown leads to the release of high levels of polymer fume, appropriate respiratory protection should be immediately available.

There is no specific therapy for PFF, and in most instances, the symptoms resolve spontaneously.

BIO-AEROSOLS

Organic Dust Toxic Syndrome

Introduction

An acute febrile illness following the inhalation of massive amounts of fungi was first described in 1975 in a group of farmworkers (Emanuel et al., 1975). They named the condition 'pulmonary mycotoxicosis' because they regarded a toxin from the fungus as the likely cause. Febrile episodes in the absence of other evidence of alveolitis have been well described in farmers (Malmberg et al., 1988). These have in the past been referred to as precipitin-negative farmers' lung (Edwards et al., 1974) and atypical farmers' lung (Jones, 1982). In 1986, it was proposed that this group of disorders should be referred to as the organic dust toxic syndrome (ODTS) (doPico, 1986).

Epidemiology

Similar episodes have been described in a number of different environments, including grain elevators (doPico et al., 1982), sewage treatment plants (Rylander et al., 1976), grain silos (Pratt and May, 1984) and sawmills (Rask-Andersen et al., 1994), in swine confinement workers (Vogelzang et al., 1999), in animal feed workers (Kuchuk et al., 2000), in urban landscape workers (Boehmer et al., 2009), in health spas via seaweed (Holm et al., 2009) and in a grass seed plant (Madsen et al., 2012).

Clinical Features

The clinical features of ODTS have been well described in farmers (Rask-Andersen, 1989). The predominating symptom is fever (39.4–41°C) followed by chills, difficulty in breathing, cough, muscle aches and pains and headache. Less common symptoms are nausea and chest tightness. The duration of episodes lasts between 1 and 3 days in the majority of farmers, with a minority experiencing symptoms lasting from 5 to 7 days.

On physical examination, the patient is febrile and tachypnoeic with a tachycardia and inspiratory crackles may be present at the lung bases (May et al., 1986). Pulmonary function tests in the majority of patients are normal, as is the chest radiograph. A leucocytosis is present with a relative increase in neutrophils. Bronchoalveolar lavage shows a neutrophilia in the acute phase at days 1–3 (Lecours et al., 1986), with a rapid transition by 7 days to a lymphocytic profile (Raymenants et al., 1990).

The prevalence of precipitating antibodies to the organic dust does not differ significantly between farmers with or without a history of ODTS.

Pathogenesis

Organic dusts are a mixture of dust particles, including Gram-positive and Gram-negative bacteria, fungi, ammonia and mycotoxins. The respirable fraction of the various dusts varies and may account for some of the conflicting findings of the studies exploring the causative factors that are involved in the inflammatory process of ODTS. The sources of pro-inflammatory cytokines are respiratory epithelial cells and alveolar macrophages. Recent research has suggested that peptidoglycans may play a role in this inflammatory process, in addition to bacterial endotoxin.

Endotoxin or lipopolysaccharide (LPS) derived from the cell wall of Gram-negative bacteria was first identified (Marx et al., 1981) as a possible cause of ODTS.

There is increasing evidence that other factors are involved in the inflammatory process. High exposures to endotoxin may occur in the absence of symptoms (Rask-Andersen, 1989). Bronchial challenge testing in farmers using a workplace exposure and a LPS challenge at a 200-fold higher dose than the dust exposure produced a much stronger pro-inflammatory response in the dust exposure compared to the LPS exposure (Sundblad et al., 2009).

The non-endotoxin agents called peptidoglycans are mainly derived from the cell wall of anaerobic Gram-positive bacteria and have been shown to induce inflammation in alveolar and epithelial cells (Larsson et al., 1999). Muramic acid is a principle component of peptidoglycans and has been associated with inflammation in swine farmers. High levels have been found in swine confinement facilities and dairy barns (Poole et al., 2010). The inhalation of swine dust in healthy subjects may induce fever and pro-inflammatory cytokine release in the upper and lower airways (Wang et al., 1997), with increases in IL-6 and TNF-α in serum, nasal and bronchoalveolar fluid.

The repeated exposure of agricultural workers to organic dusts leads to a reduced inflammatory response (Sundblad et al., 2009), which is consistent with the clinical history of exposed workers.

Occupational Exposure Limit

A health-based exposure limit for endotoxin of 90 endotoxin units (EU)/m^3 over an 8-hour period has been recommended by the Dutch Expert Committee on Occupational Heath (DECOS) following an extensive review of human volunteer and workplace studies (Health Council of The Netherlands; Endotoxin, 2010).

Management and Prevention

Most cases of ODTS are mild and treatment is symptomatic and supportive.

The prevention of episodes of ODTS in which exposures to dusts are likely to be high involves the provision of respirators with high-efficiency particulate arrestance (HEPA) filters, which will prevent significant dust exposure. The prolonged use of respiratory protection is difficult for workers, but if the exposure source cannot be controlled, this may be required. An example of this is in the agricultural seed processing industry (Smit et al., 2006), in which potential exposures to endotoxin in the quality inspection laboratory at levels of 274,000 EU/m^3 were measured. In general, farmers learn to avoid heavy-exposure situations.

Other Organic Dusts: Cotton Dust

Mill fever (factory fever) is characterised by fever, cough, malaise, rigors and rhinitis occurring in some workers upon first exposure to cotton, flax, soft hemp or kapok dust (Greenhow, 1860; Doig, 1949). The symptoms are mild and last for a few hours, but cease with repeated exposure. In some occupational environments, such as the ginning of kapok, symptoms may last for 1–14 days (Uragoda, 1977). The cause is uncertain, but may be due to endotoxins derived from Gram-negative bacteria in the vegetable dusts and in the mill air (Rylander and Lundholm, 1978).

Organic Aerosol Toxic Syndrome (Humidifier Fever)

Introduction

Exposure to microbiological aerosols in the workplace has been associated with episodes of respiratory disease in offices, operating theatres and factories. Usually, these episodes arise from cold water spray humidification within air-conditioning systems, but any mechanical system that aerosolises water into the working environment (e.g. vacuum ring pumps, spinning disc humidifiers and sump bays) and is not properly maintained may result in the development of 'humidifier fever'.

'Humidifier fever' or 'Befeuchterfieber' was first described in 1959 by Pestalozzi (Pestalozzi, 1959) in a group of workers in a carpentry shop who had been exposed to air from a humidifier that was contaminated by bacteria and fungi.

Epidemiology

Investigations of outbreaks of humidifier fever in Britain, including in factories involved in printing and stationary and textile manufacture, an operating theatre and sump bay equipment, have shown that only a minority of workers are usually affected, with prevalence rates varying between 2.5% and 57% (Mamolen et al., 1993). Mists of used metal working fluid have been reported as causing humidifier fever (7 cases), extrinsic alveolitis (19 cases) and occupational asthma (74 cases) in the same work area, comprising 10.4% of the total workforce (Robertson et al., 2007).

Clinical Features

Humidifier fever is an illness that varies between mild influenza-like symptoms with myalgia associated with a low-grade fever and an acute illness consisting of malaise, myalgia, fever, headache and breathlessness. These symptoms usually resolve over 24 hours.

In humidifier fever, the symptoms are most severe on the first day of the working week, improving rapidly over the remainder of the working week. They recur upon re-exposure after an absence from work, such as over a weekend or a holiday. The intermittent use of humidification can give rise to diagnostic difficulties in individual cases (Anderson et al., 1989). The workforce is often unaware of when humidification is running. In areas of a country in which the relative humidity is high, the humidification may only be required for a few days a month. The individual then presents as a pyrexia of unknown origin. In one worker, this led to four hospital admissions and invasive investigations before the correct diagnosis was made (Newman Taylor et al., 1978). At presentation, the physical examination of the worker is usually normal. Bronchial provocation studies demonstrate a febrile response with inspiratory crackles at the lung bases (Friend et al., 1977) at the height of the response. The differentiating features between humidifier fever and all types of extrinsic allergic alveolitis (including humidifier lung) are, in the former, the symptom periodicity, the absence of chest x-ray (CXR) changes and the lack of any evidence of long-term lung damage despite repeated febrile episodes over a number of years.

An investigation of a printing works (Pickering et al., 1976) measured simple spirometry over the working week and demonstrated work-related impairment with maximum and similar falls in forced expiratory volume in 1 second (FEV_1) and forced vital capacity (FVC) across the working shift on the first day of the working week, with progressive improvement over the working week and lung function returning to normal by the weekend.

Pathogenesis

Several causes of humidifier fever have been proposed on the basis of serological testing including bacterial endotoxins (Rylander et al., 1978; Flaherty et al., 1984), *Bacillus subtilis* (Parrott and Blyth, 1980) and amoebae (Medical Research Council Symposium, 1977; Edwards, 1980). However, a study of four outbreaks of humidifier fever (Finnegan et al., 1987) found no correlation between the presence of antibodies to amoebae and the presence of humidifier symptoms.

Airborne endotoxin was also implicated among printers who were exposed to water contaminated with *Pseudomonas* spp. (Rylander and Haglind, 1984). A more recent publication (Koschel et al., 2005) described two cases of humidifier fever associated with the use of ultrasonic domestic humidifiers. Inhalation challenge tests with the water from their own humidifiers resulted in positive systemic responses, but no changes in pulmonary function.

In an estimation of the potential risk to human health of endotoxin inhalation from ultrasonic and impeller (cool mist) humidifiers, which produce large numbers of respirable particles, it was concluded that airway inflammation could occur if humidifier reservoirs were filled with tap water (Anderson et al., 2007). The authors commented that this was unlikely to occur at typical drinking water endotoxin concentrations, but at higher levels (>1000 EU/mL), which are occasionally found in drinking water, symptoms of chills and fever were likely to occur.

Attempts to identify a specific responsible organism by bronchial provocation studies using organisms identified in the workplace and to which the symptomatic workers had precipitating antibodies have been unsuccessful (Pickering et al., 1976).

A provocation study (Figure 29.1) using an extract of contaminated cooling tower water in a symptomatic stationary worker reproduced influenza-like symptoms, with a fever, inspiratory crackles at the lung bases, falls in FEV_1 and FVC and acute impairment of gas transfer (Friend et al., 1977). A control challenge using water from the mains supply was negative.

A consistent finding in outbreaks of humidifier fever is the presence of serum precipitins against crude humidifier extracts in both affected and unaffected but exposed workers. In workers who are exposed to heavily contaminated humidifiers, the presence and amounts of antibodies are determined by the individual's length of service and smoking habits (Finnegan et al., 1985). There is a strong inverse relationship between current smoking and precipitins. This smoking effect is reversed 3 years after stopping smoking. The duration of exposure also

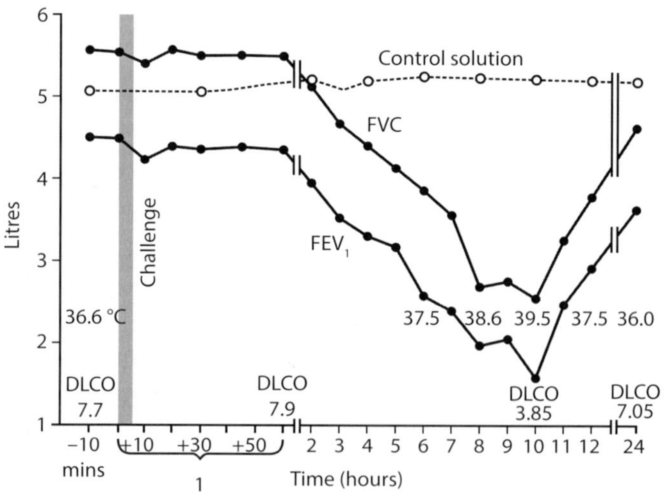

FIGURE 29.1 Lung function after inhalation of water extract (1 mg/mL) and control solution. FVC: forced vital capacity; FEV_1: forced expiratory volume in 1 second. (From Friend, J. A. R. et al. 1977. *Lancet* 1:297–300.)

has a major effect, with a clear dose–response relationship demonstrable between length of employment and the presence and amounts of antibodies. In general, no consistent relationships between precipitins and individual fungi or bacteria have been evident.

Management and Prevention

The symptoms of humidifier fever resolve spontaneously with the removal of the individual from exposure.

Prevention of the growth of organisms in the humidifier system will avoid the development of disease. A rich flora grows readily in recirculated and static water, particularly if the humidifier has a cleaning as well as a humidification function. The design of the humidifier being easily accessible for cleaning is important. In the past, the growth of organisms has been controlled by the introduction of biocides. This should be discouraged, as exemplified by the recent development of progressive pulmonary fibrosis, with a high mortality, following the introduction of a new class of biocide, which was used in the humidifier water while the humidifier was functioning (Pickering, 2014). This effect was seen both in domestic and commercial usage. In the printing works outbreak of humidifier fever (Pickering et al., 1976), the introduction of extensive cleaning and a biocide failed to control microbial growth or symptoms in the workforce. The substitution of cold water humidification with steam humidification led to the disappearance of microbial growth on the eliminator plates and complete resolution of symptoms in the workforce.

SPECIFIC MICROORGANISMS

Pontiac Fever

Introduction

In July 1968, an acute febrile illness occurred in both the staff and visitors to a governmental public building in Pontiac, Michigan, USA The attack rate was high, with 95 out of 100 staff developing the illness. At the time, an unidentified bacterium was isolated from guinea pigs exposed to the air within the building and exposed to water from an evaporative condenser within the air-conditioning system. A defect within this system was implicated as both the source and spread of the causative factor and the organism was later identified as *Legionella pneumophila* (Glick et al., 1978).

Epidemiology

Pontiac fever (PF) is caused by the aerosol generation of contaminated water from man-made structures or processes. Although the causative organism is the same as that leading to active infection in Legionnaires' disease, the latter is an active pneumonia, while PF is a self-limited, non-infective syndrome. They are therefore preventable with appropriate mechanical design, water treatment and maintenance. Vapour drift from wet cooling towers has been frequently implicated in various settings, such as a hospital (O'Mahony et al., 1990), a military base (Ambrose et al., 2014) and an office block (Ward et al., 2010), as well as communal sources such as hot tubs and whirlpool spas (Goldberg et al., 1989; Miller et al., 1993) and an aerosolised potting mixture in a horticultural nursery (Cramp et al., 2010). Outbreaks of travel-related PF (Huhn et al., 2005) may present a particular diagnostic problem, since the individual(s) may have left the exposure source before developing symptoms, presenting as a pyrexia of unknown origin (PUO). A similar problem has been reported from an outbreak of PF associated with a restaurant (Jones et al., 2003). High-pressure cleaning in confined spaces has also been reported to cause PF in a steam turbine condenser (Fraser et al., 1979) and an evaporative vessel in a sugar-beet processing plant (Castor et al., 2005). An aerosol exposure from a decanter in a closed room in a sewage treatment plant led to five cases amongst workers (Gregersen et al., 1999).

Clinical Features

PF is a benign, self-limited disease. It has an incubation period of between 4 and 120 hours (Jones et al., 2003). The attack rate is usually high (70%–95%). However, sporadic cases occurring in the community may easily be overlooked in view of the non-specific presenting symptoms of PF. The cardinal symptoms are malaise, myalgia, fever, chills and headache. Less frequently, cough, dizziness, painful neck, nausea, chest and joint pain may occur (Glick et al., 1978).

Physical examination is normal, apart from the presence of a fever. There are no specific radiological abnormalities.

Patients recover in 2–7 days without treatment.

Microbiological Investigations

The detection of *Legionella* species in water samples may be achieved by culture, fluorescent in situ hybridisation (FISH) or polymerase chain reaction. Culture is the 'gold standard', but the relatively high specificity, sensitivity and speed of the FISH test has advantages over the other tests. The isolation of legionellae on direct culture of environmental samples in an outbreak of PF may prove to be negative (Fallon and Rowbotham, 1990). In this instance, co-cultivation of the whirlpool water and *Acanthamoeba polyphaga* led to the isolation *Legionella micdadei*.

Outbreaks of PF have been caused by *L. pneumophila* serogroups 1, 6 and 7 (Kaufmann et al., 1981), *Legionella feeleii* (Spitalny et al., 1984), *Legionella anisa* (Jones et al., 2003) and *Legionella longbeachae* serogroup 2 (Cramp et al., 2010).

In two outbreaks of PF, the investigators have attempted to define a risk threshold for the development of PF in populations exposed to shower water (Tossa et al., 2006; Hautemaniere et al., 2011). Both studies used similar methodologies of culturable and in-situ hybridisation techniques (Fish Method). The risk threshold, achieving statistical significance, varied between 10^4·L/water (Tossa et al., 2006) and 10^3 colony forming units (cfu) legionella/L water (Hautemaniere et al., 2011).

Pathogenesis

The pathogenesis of PF remains poorly understood. Following the initial outbreak of PF in 1968 (Kaufmann et al., 1981), it was suggested that PF resulted from the toxic effect of inhaling dead *L. pneumophila* bacteria.

In some outbreaks of PF, high levels of endotoxin—varying between 14,400 and 22,200 endotoxin units (Fields et al., 2001; Castor et al., 2005)—have been reported. In view of the similar features of PF and ODTS, with the latter believed to be caused by exposure to bacterial endotoxin, the presence of endotoxin may have an adjuvant role in outbreaks of PF.

The presence of free-living amoebae is a consistent finding in the water biofilm. Bacteria are their main food source. However, some bacteria, including *Legionella* spp., are able to resist intracellular death following phagocytosis and grow in amoebic cells. The amoebic cells themselves are resistant to some disinfectants. The possible role of amoebae in outbreaks of PF is unknown, but studies have suggested a role for amoebae in the development and transmission of Legionnaires' pneumonia (Philippe et al., 2006). This may also be relevant to outbreaks of PF where adequate concentrations of disinfectant are present in the water.

It has been proposed (Edelstein, 2007) that PF is probably due to a toxic mix of live and dead microorganisms and their products, including endotoxin made by non-*Legionella* bacteria, as well as low-dose live or dead *Legionella* bacteria that are unable to cause pneumonia in the affected host.

Diagnosis

In view of the association of cases of PF and cases of Legionnaires' disease occurring from the same exposure source, the rapid establishment of the diagnosis and appropriate intervention is important. The diagnosis is based on the patient's symptoms and the pattern of their symptoms, combined with an exposure to aerosolised water contaminated with *Legionella* species. At the present time, serological testing for antibodies has a low sensitivity, and the need for paired samples has reduced its use. Urine antigen detection—the most frequently used diagnostic test—has led to the early recognition of outbreaks and subsequent intervention. As urinary antigen detection mainly detects *L. pneumophila* serogroup 1, accounting for approximately 70% of outbreaks of Legionnaires' disease and PF, other serogroups and species may be missed.

In most outbreaks of PF, the detection of urinary antigen has been low or absent. However, in a recent outbreak (Burnsed et al, 2007), 36% of those with PF had detectable antigenuria. The sensitivity of the test may be improved by concentrating the urine.

REFERENCES

Ambrose, J., Hampton, L. M., Fleming-Dutra, K. E., Marten, C., McClusky, C., Perry, C., Clemmons, N. A. et al. 2014. Large outbreak of Legionnaires' disease and Pontiac fever at a military base. *Epidemiol Infect* 142:2336–46.

Anderson, K., Watt, A. D., Sinclair, D., Lewis, C., McSharry, C. P. and Boyd, G. 1989. Climate intermittent humidification, and humidifier fever. *BR J Ind Med* 46:671–4.

Anderson, W. B., Dixon, D. D. and Mayfield, C. I. 2007. Estimation of endotoxin inhalation from shower and humidifier exposure reveals potential risk to human health. *J Water Health* 5:553–72.

Anon. 1927. Editorial. Metal fume fever. *Lancet* June:1194–5.

Anonymous. 1978. Inhalation fevers. *Lancet* 1:249.

Blanc, P., Wong, H., Berstein, M. S. and Boushey, H. A. 1991. An experimental model of metal fume fever. *Ann Intern Med* 114:930–6.

Blanc, P. D., Boushey, H. A., Wong, H., Wintermeyer, S. F and Bernstein, M. S. 1993. Cytokines in metal fume fever. *Am Rev Respir Dis* 147:134–8.

Boehmer, T. K., Jones, T. S., Ghosh, T. S., McCammon, C. S. and Vogt, R. L. 2009. Cluster of presumed organic dust toxic syndrome cases among urban landscape workers—Colorado. *Am J Ind Med* 52:534–8.

Borak, J., Cohen, H. and Hethmon, T. A. 2000. Copper exposure and metal fume fever: Lack of evidence for a causal relationship. *Am Ind Hyg Assoc* 61:832–6.

Burnsed, L. J., Hicks, L. A., Smithee, L. M. K., Fields, B. S., Bradley, K. K., Pascoe, N., Richards, S. M. et al. 2007. A large travel-associated outbreak of legionellosis among hotel guests: Utility of the urine antigen assay in confirming Pontiac fever. *Clin Infect Dis* 44:222–8.

Castor, M. L., Wagstrom, E. A., Danila, R. N., Smith, K. E., Naimi, T. S., Besser, J. M., Peacock. K. A. et al. 2005. An outbreak of Pontiac fever with respiratory distress among workers performing high-pressure cleaning at a sugar-beet processing plant. *J Infect Dis* 191:1530–7.

Cavagna, G., Finulli, M. and Vigliani, E. C. 1961. Experimental study on the pathogenesis of fevers caused by the inhalation of Teflon (polytetrafluoroethylene) fumes. *Med Lav* 52:251–61.

Cramp, G. J., Harte, D., Douglas, N. M., Graham, F., Schousboe, M. and Sykes, K. 2010. An outbreak of Pontiac fever due to *Legionella longbeachae* serogroup 2 found in a potting mix in a horticultural nursery in New Zealand. *Epidemiol Infect* 138:15–20.

Doig, A, T. 1949. Other lung diseases due to dust. *Postgrad Med J* 25:639–49.

doPico G. A. 1986. Report on diseases. *Am J Ind Med* 10:261–5.

doPico, G. A., Flaherty, D., Bhansali, P. and Chavaje, N. 1982. Grain fever syndrome induced by inhalation of airborne grain dust. *J Allergy Clin Immunol* 69:435–43.

Edelstein, P. H. 2007. Urine antigen tests positive for Pontiac fever: Implications for diagnosis and pathogenesis. *Clin Infect Dis* 44:229–31.

Edwards, J. H., Baker, J. T. and Davies, B. H. 1974. Precipitin test negative farmer's lung—Activation of the alternate pathway of complement by mouldy hay dust. *Clin Allergy* 4:379–88.

Edwards, J. H. 1980. Microbial and immunological investigations and remedial action after an outbreak of humidifier fever. *Br J Ind Med* 37:55–62.

Emanuel, D. A., Wenzel, F. J. and Lawton, B. R. 1975. Pulmonary mycotoxicosis. *Chest* 67:293–7.

Fallon, R. J. and Rowbotham, T. J. 1990. Microbiological investigations into an outbreak of Pontiac fever due to *Legionella micdadei* associated with use of a whirlpool. *J Clin Pathol* 43:479–83.

Finnegan, M. J., Pickering, C. A. C., Davies, P. S., Austwick, P. K. C. and Warhurst, D. C. 1987. Amoebae and humidifier fever. *Clin Allergy* 17:235–42.

Finnegan, M. J., Pickering, C. A. C., Davies, P. S. and Austwick, P. K. C. 1985. Factors affecting the development of precipitating antibodies in workers exposed to contaminated humidifiers. *Clin Allergy* 15:281–92.

Fields, B. S., Haupt, T., Davis, J. P., Arduino, M. J., Miller, P. H. and Butler, J. C. 2001. Pontiac fever due to *Legionella micdadei* from a whirlpool spa: Possible role of bacterial endotoxin. *J Infect Dis* 184:1289–92.

Flaherty, D. K., Deck, F. H., Cooper, J., Bishop, K., Winzenburger, P. A., Smith, L. R., Bynum, L. et al. 1984. Bacterial endotoxin isolated from a water spray air humidification system as a putative agent of occupation-related lung disease. *Infect Immunol* 43:206–12.

Fraser, D. W., Deubner, D. C., Hill, D. L. and Gilliam, D. K. 1979. Nonpneumonic, short-incubation-period legionellosis (Pontiac fever) in men who cleaned a steam turbine condenser. *Science* 205:690–1.

Friend, J. A. R., Gaddie, J., Palmer, K. N. V., Pickering, C. A. C. and Pepys, J. 1977. Extrinsic allergic alveolitis and contaminated cooling-water in a factory machine. *Lancet* 1:297–300.

Glick, T. H., Gregg, M. B., Berman, B., Mallison, G., Rhodes, W. W. Jr. and Kassanoff, I. 1978. Pontiac fever: An epidemic of unknown etiology in a Health Department: 1. Clinical and epidemiological aspects. *Am J Epidemiol* 107:149–60.

Goldberg, D. J., Collier, P. W., Fallon, R. J., McKay, T. M., Marwick, T. A., Wrench, J. G., Emslie, J. A. et al. 1989. Lochgoilhead fever: Outbreak of non-pneumonic legionellosis due to *Legionella micdadei*. *Lancet* 1:316–8.

Greenhow, H. 1860. *Third Report of the Medical Officer of the Privy Council*. Sir John Simon. p. 152.

Gregersen, P., Grunnet, K., Uldum, S. A., Andersen, B. H. and Madsen, H. 1999. Pontiac fever at a sewage treatment plant in the food industry. *Scand J Work Environ Health* 25:291–5.

Harris, D. K. 1951. Polymer fume fever. *Lancet* 2:1008–11.

Hautemaniere, A., Remen, T., Mathieu, L., Deloge Abarkan, M., Hartemann, P. and Zmirou-Navier, D. 2011. Pontiac fever among retirement home nurses associated with airborne *Legionella*. *J Hosp Infect* 78:269–73.

Health Council of The Netherlands; Endotoxins. 2010. *Health-Based Occupational Exposure Limit*. The Hague: Health Council of The Netherlands.

Holm, M., Johannesson, S., Torén, K. and Dahlman-Höglund, A. 2009. Acute effects after occupational endotoxin exposure at a spa. *Scand J Work Environ Health* 35:153–5.

Huhn, G. D., Adam, B., Ruden, R., Hilliard, L., Kirkpatrick, P., Todd, J., Crafts, W. et al. 2005. Outbreak of travel-related Pontiac fever among hotel guests illustrating the need for better diagnostic tests. *J Travel Med* 12:173–9.

Jones, A. 1982. Farmers' lung: An overview and prospectus. *Ann Am Conf Ind Hyg* 2:171–81.

Jones, T. F., Benson, R. F., Brown, E. W., Rowland, J. R., Crosier, S. C. and Schaffner, W. 2003. Epidemiological investigation of a restaurant-associated outbreak of Pontiac fever. *Clin Infect Dis* 37:1292–7.

Kales, S. N. and Christiani, D. C. 1994. Progression of chronic obstructive pulmonary disease after multiple episodes of an occupational inhalation fever. *J Occup Med* 36:75–8.

Kaufmann, A. F., McDade, J. E., Patton, C. M., Bennett, J. V., Skaliy, P., Feeley, J. C., Andersen, D. C. et al. 1981. Pontiac fever: Isolation of the etiologic agent (*Legionella pneumophila*) and demonstration of its mode of transmission. *Am J Epidemiol* 114:337–47.

Koschel, D., Stark, W., Karmann, F., Sennekamp, J. and Müller-Wening, D. 2005. Extrinsic allergic alveolitis caused by misting fountains. *Respir Med* 99:943–7.

Kuchuk, A. A., Basanets, A. V. and Loehelainen, K. 2000. Bronchopulmonary pathology in workers exposed to organic fodder dust. *Ann Agric Environ Med* 7:17–23.

Kuschner, W. G., D'Alessandro, A., Wong, H. and Blanc, P. D. 1997. Early pulmonary cytokine responses to zinc oxide fume inhalation. *Environ Res* 75:7–11.

Larsson, B. M., Larsson, K., Malmberg, P. and Palmberg, L. 1999. Gram positive bacteria induce IL-6 and IL-8 production in human alveolar macrophages and epithelial cells. *Inflammation* 23:217–30.

Lee, C. H., Guo, Y. L, Tsai, P. J., Chang, H. Y., Chen, C. R., Chen, C. W. and Hsiue, T.-R. 1997. Fatal acute pulmonary oedema after inhalation of fumes from polytetrafluoroethylene (PTFE). *Eur Respir J* 10:1408–11.

Lecours, R., Laviolette, M. and Cormier, Y. 1986. Bronchoalveolar lavage in pulmonary mycotoxicosis (organic dust toxic syndrome). *Thorax* 41:924–6.

Lewis, C. E. and Kerby, G. R. 1965. An epidemic of polymer-fume fever. *JAMA* 191:375–8.

Madsen, A. M., Tendal, K., Schlünssen, V. and Heltberg, I. 2012. Organic dust toxic syndrome at a grass seed plant caused by exposure to high concentrations of bioaerosols. *Ann Occup Hyg* 56:776–88.

Malmberg, P., Rask-Andersen, A., Hoglund, A., Kolmodin-Hedman, B. and Guernsey, J. R. 1988. Incidence of organic toxic dust syndrome and allergic alveolitis in Swedish farmers. *Int Arch Allergy Appl Immunol* 87:47–54.

Malo, J.-L., Malo, J., Cartier, A. and Dolovich, J. 1990. Acute lung reaction to zinc inhalation. *Eur Respir J* 3:111–4.

Mamolen, M., Lewis. D. M., Blanchet, M. A., Satink, S. J. and Vogt, R. L. 1993. Investigation of an outbreak of 'humidifier fever' in a print shop. *Am J Ind Med* 23:483–90.

Marx, J. J., Arden-Jones, M. P., Treuhaft, M. W., Gray, R. L., Motszko, C. S. and Hahn, F. F. 1981. The pathogenic role of inhaled microbial material in pulmonary mycotoxicosis as demonstrated in an animal model. *Chest* 81(Suppl.):76–8.

May, J. J., Stallones, L., Darrow, D. and Pratt, D. S. 1986. Organic dust toxicity (pulmonary mycotoxicosis) associated with silo unloading. *Thorax* 41:919–23.

Medical Research Council Symposium. 1977. Humidifier fever. *Thorax* 32:653–63.

Miller, L. A., Beebe, J. L., Butler, J. C., Martin, W., Benson, R., Hoffman, R. E. and Fields, B. S. 1993. Use of polymerase chain reaction in an epidemiological investigation of Pontiac fever. *J Infect Dis* 168:769–72.

Newman Taylor, A., Pickering, C. A. C., Turner-Warwick, M. and Pepys, J. 1978. Respiratory allergy to a factory humidifier contaminant presenting as pyrexia of undetermined origin. *BMJ* 2:94–5.

O'Mahony, M. C., Stanwell-Smith, R. E., Tillett, H. E., Harper, D., Hutchison, J. G. P., Farrell, I. D., Hutchinson, D. N. et al. 1990. The Stafford outbreak of Legionnaires' disease. *Epidemiol Infect* 104:361–80.

Parrott, W. F. and Blyth, W. 1980. Another causal factor in the production of humidifier fever. *J Soc Occup Med* 30:63–6.

Pestalozzi, C. 1959. Febrile Gruppener Krankungen in einer Modellschreinerei durch Inhalation von mit Schimelpilzen Kontaminiertem Befeuchterwasser ('Befeuchterfieber'). *Schweiz Med Wochenschr* 89:710–3.

Philippe, C., Blech, M. F. and Hartmann, P. 2006. Intra-amoebal development of *Legionella pneumophila* and the potential role of amoeba in the transmission of Legionaire's disease. *Med Maladies Infect* 36:196–200.

Pickering, C. A. C., Moore, W. K. S., Lacey, J., Holford-Strevens, V. C. and Pepys, J. 1976. Investigation of a respiratory disease associated with an air-conditioning system. *Clin Allergy* 6:109–18.

Pickering, C. A. C. 2014. Humidifiers: The use of humidifiers and lung disease. *Thorax* 69:692–3.

Poole, J. A., Dooley, G. P., Saito, R., Burrell, A. M., Bailey, K. L., Romberger, D. J., Mehaffy, J. et al. 2010. Muramic acid, endotoxin, 3-hydroxy fatty acids and ergosterol content explain monocyte and epithelial cell inflammatory responses to agricultural dusts. *J Toxicol Environ Health A* 73:684–700.

Pratt, D. S. and May, J. J. 1984. Feed-associated respiratory illness in farmers. *Arch Environ Health* 39:43–8.

Rask-Andersen, A. 1989. Organic dust toxic syndrome. *Br J Ind Med* 46:233–8.

Rask-Anderson, A. and Pratt, D. S. 1992. Inhalation fever: A proposed unifying term for febrile reactions to inhalation of noxious substances. *Br J Ind Med* 49(1):40.

Rask-Andersen, A., Land, C. J., Enlund, K. and Lundin, A. 1994. Inhalation fever and respiratory symptoms in the trimming department of Swedish sawmills. *Am J Ind Med* 25:65–7.

Raymenants, E., Demendts, M. and Nemery, B. 1990. Bronchoalveolar lavage findings in a patient with organic dust toxic syndrome. *Thorax* 45:713–4.

Robertson, W., Robertson. A. S., Burge, C. B., Moore, V. C., Jaakkola, M. S., Dawkins, P. A., Burd, M. et al. 2007. Clinical investigation of an outbreak of alveolitis and asthma in a car engine manufacturing plant. *Thorax* 62:981–90.

Rylander, R., Anderrson, K., Belin, L., Berglund, G., Bergstrum, R., Hanson, L-A., Lundholm, M. et al. 1976. Sewage workers' syndrome. *Lancet* 2:478–9.

Rylander, R., Haglind, P., Lundholm, M., Mattsby, I. and Stenqvist, K. 1978. Humidifier fever and endotoxin exposure. *Clin Allergy* 8:511–6.

Rylander, R. and Haglind, P. 1984. Airborne endotoxins and humidifier disease. *Clin Allergy* 14:109–12.

Rylander, R. and Lundholm, M. 1978. Bacterial contamination of cotton and cotton dust and effects on the lung. *Br J Ind Med* 35:204–7.

Sanderson, J. T. 1968. Hazards of the arc-air gouging process. *Ann Occup Hyg* 11:123–33.

Shusterman, D. J. 1993. Polymer fume fever. *Occ Med* 8(3):519–31.

Smit, L. A. M., Wouters, I. M., Hobo, M. M., Eduard, W., Doekes, G. and Heederik, D. 2006. Agriculteral seed dust as a potential cause of organic dust toxic syndrome. *Ann Occup Hyg* 63:59–67.

Spitalny, K. C., Vogt, R. L., Orciari, L. A., Witherell, L. E., Etkind, P. and Novick, L. F. 1984. Pontiac fever associated with a whirlpool spa. *Am J Epidemiol* 120:809–17

Sundblad, B-M., Von Scheele, I., Palberg, L., Olsson, M. and Larsson, K. 2009. Repeated exposure to organic material alters inflammatory and physiological airway responses. *Eur Respir J* 34:80–8.

Tossa, P., Deloge-Abarkan, M., Zmirou-Navier, D., Hartemann, P. and Mathieu, L. 2006. Pontiac fever: An operational definition for epidemiological studies. *BMC Public Health* 6:112.

Uragoda, C. G. 1977. An investigation into the health of kapok workers. *Br J Ind Med* 34:181–5.

Vernez, D., Bruzzi, R., Kupferschmidt, H., De-Batz, A., Droz, P. and Lazor, R. 2006. Acute respiratory syndrome after inhalation of waterproofing sprays: *A posteriori* exposure–response assessment in 102 cases. *J Occup Environ Hyg* 3:250–61.

Vogelmeier, C., König. G., Bencze, K. and Fruhmann, G. 1987. Pulmonary involvement in zinc fume fever. *Chest* 92(5):947–8.

Vogelzang, P. F., van der Guilden, J. W., Folgering, H. and van Schayck, C. P. 1999. Organic toxic dust syndrome in swine confinement farming. *Am J Ind Med* 35:332–4.

Wallace, G. M. F. and Brown, P. H. 2005. Horse rug lung: Toxic pneumonitis due to fluorocarbon inhalation. *Occup Environ Med* 62:414–6.

Wang, Z., Larsson, K., Palmberg, L., Malmberg, P., Larsson, P. and Larsson, L. 1997. Inhalation of swine dust induces cytokine release in the upper and lower airways. *Eur Respir J* 10:381–7.

Ward, M., Boland, M., Nicolay, N., Murphy, H., McElhiney, J., Collins, C., Lynch, M. et al. 2010. A cluster of Legionnaires' disease and associated Pontiac fever on office workers, Dublin, June–July 2008. *J Environ Public Health* 2010:463926.

30 Cotton Dust

David Fishwick

CONTENTS

BACKGROUND AND INTRODUCTION

The global textile and clothing industry continues to provide work to large numbers of workers, although the markets for these textile products are constantly changing. Shifts in textile production worldwide have occurred; China, India, Pakistan, Turkey, the United States and Brazil now lead the world in both the production and consumption of cotton.

Various naturally occurring fibres have been historically used, and continue to be used, for producing textiles. Exposure to the dust from these materials has long been linked to the development of respiratory ill health; this chapter summarises the literature in relation primarily to ill health associated with cotton dust exposure, although the health effects of jute, hemp and sisal dust will also be considered.

JUTE

Jute is a commonly used vegetable fibre that can be spun into thread. It has a diverse set of uses, including fishing, construction, art and in the manufacture of certain fabrics. Exposure to dust from its processing has been identified as a cause of respiratory illness.

Workplace-Based Studies

Modern-day descriptions of the health consequences of jute dust exposure are relatively limited. Choudat et al. (1987) studied both cotton and jute workers, comparing exposed to non-exposed workers. The prevalence of respiratory symptoms was not significantly different between the two groups, although lung function changes differed following 5 days of work. For example, mid expiratory flows (at 75% of exhaled forced vital capacity [FVC]) were lower in exposed workers, although there were no differences seen between jute and cotton workers.

Subsequent study of jute exposure in a West African factory (Ankrah, 1989) identified high levels of reported symptoms and dust exposure, with the former related to both dust exposure and tobacco smoking. Interestingly, chest tightness and wheeze on the first working day were rarely reported.

Jute mill workers have also been investigated in China (Zhou et al., 1989). A total of 404 jute mill workers were studied who were exposed to jute dust with less than 5% silica content. Cough and chest tightness were more frequently reported by males in comparison to a control group, and female workers were also reported to have an excess of chronic bronchitis and shortness of breath. Dust-exposed workers had greater levels of abnormal lung function (forced expiratory volume in 1 second [FEV_1] and FVC) in comparison to a control group. The authors identified that dust exposure was the main cause of the reported respiratory symptoms, but both cigarette smoking and dust exposure contributed to abnormal lung function.

Burmese textile workers have also been identified as being exposed to high levels of dust, including jute dust (Noweir et al., 1990). A total of 799 male and female workers in two jute mills and two cotton textile mills and a group of 153 control non-exposed workers were studied by Noweir et al. (1990). Whilst chronic bronchitis, cough and wheezing were reported more commonly among all workers than in the control group, byssinosis was only found in the cotton-exposed workers. The prevalence of byssinosis was related both to the level and duration of textile dust exposure. Smoking of cheroots was found to contribute both to the presence of non-specific respiratory disease and also to the reduction in FEV_1.

The association between jute exposure and respiratory ill health has been confirmed in a study of jute textile workers (Zuskin et al., 1992c). It was identified that dust exposure was associated with respiratory symptoms, but additionally that follow-up over 19 years demonstrated an excess annual FEV_1 decline of 35 mL per year.

Further data from a prospective study of jute workers (Zuskin et al., 1994a) again confirmed the association between dust exposure and chronic respiratory symptoms (significantly so only for shortness of breath), and also identified two workers from the 19 who were subsequently studied at follow-up from an initial population of 70 with symptoms that were consistent with occupational asthma, one of whom had a positive skin-prick test to jute extract.

Evidence to support an acute lung function response following dust exposure is found in Indian jute workers (Chattopadhyay et al., 1995). Thirty-two such workers demonstrated cross-shift falls in FEV_1, and these were noted both on the first and last working days of the week. The falls in lung function were dictated by process type, dust concentration and smoking status.

The more recent paper from the same group reported that a high proportion of workers in Indian jute mills reported typical symptoms of byssinosis (typical symptoms along with acute post-shift FEV_1 changes reported in 31.8% of workers) and reduced lung function in exposed workers (reduced FEV_1 in 43.2% of exposed workers). High levels of airborne endotoxin were also measured in this study: mean endotoxin levels in the hatching, spinning and weaving and beaming areas were 2.319, 0.956 and 0.041 $\mu g/m^3$, respectively (Chattopadhyay et al., 2003).

Further work, again by the same group, confirmed an association between the presence of byssinosis and endotoxin exposure (Mukherjee et al., 2004), with batching, spinning and weaving areas of the jute mill having measured endotoxin levels of 0.22–4.42, 0.04–1.47 and 0.01–0.07 $\mu g/m^3$, respectively. There are also recent limited, uncontrolled data to support decrements in lung function in Nepalese jute mill workers (Das and Jha, 2009).

Experimental Studies

Very few experimental data offer potential mechanisms by which jute exposure causes respiratory ill health. A study of jute and sisal workers assessed the responses to skin-prick testing using jute and sisal allergens. Based on the responses seen in 41 jute and sisal process workers, 5.0% of the jute workers and 9.5% of the sisal workers demonstrated positive skin reactions to at least one allergen (Zuskin et al., 1993). Among the 35 control workers, however, similar reactions were seen: 11.4% reacted with a positive skin-prick reaction to the jute or sisal allergen and 2.9% had increased IgE. It was also evident that there was no relationship between respiratory symptoms and the presence of a positive skin-prick test, leading the authors to conclude that immunological reactions were not likely to be responsible for the development of respiratory impairment in textile workers exposed to jute and sisal dust.

In summary, jute exposure has been associated with the development of respiratory symptoms and excess annual decline in FEV_1, although the evidence base is rather limited.

HEMP

Hemp is a term that is used for varieties of the cannabis plant and its associated products. These include hemp fibre, seed and hemp oil. Subsequent processing produces hemp-based textiles, seed-based foods, hemp oil, wax, resin, rope, hemp pulp, hemp-based paper products and fuels.

Workplace-Based Studies

Early associations between primarily soft hemp exposure and respiratory ill health (Bouhuys et al., 1969) were found in a study of 216 active and retired Spanish hemp workers and a similar number of non-exposed workers. Older hemp workers (50–69 years old) had very high levels of chronic cough and phlegm production, shortness of breath and abnormal lung function.

Approximately two-thirds of these older hemp workers had FEV_1 values recorded to be less than 80% of predicted, and under a fifth (18.5%) were severely disabled by 'ventilatory insufficiency', with FEV_1 values below 1 L. It was also noted that 91% of these older workers had reported shortness of breath on the first working day, consistent with a possible diagnosis of byssinosis. The authors concluded that byssinosis was a preferable diagnosis to chronic bronchitis, and that it had been essential to include retired workers, as otherwise the healthy worker effect may well have influenced their findings.

Further follow-up work by the same group (Bouhuys and Zuskin, 1976) identified that, after 7 years of work, chronic productive cough and shortness of breath were over-represented in hemp workers in comparison to non-exposed workers. Furthermore, there was evidence of accelerated FEV_1 decline over time in the exposed group, and this was not confined only to older workers.

The same group added further to the evidence in relation to hemp exposure by reporting the findings of a study that was designed to assess symptom prevalence and lung function changes in three groups of textile workers; cotton-, hemp- and synthetic fibre-exposed workers (Valic and Zuskin, 1977). The prevalence of shortness of breath (Medical Research Council [MRC] grades 3–4) was lower in workers with a history of exposure to synthetic fibres only. Lung function values were significantly reduced during the work shift on the first and fourth working days. Specifically, the maximum expiratory flow when 50% of the FVC has been exhaled (MEF_{50}) pre-shift values on the first working day were significantly lower than expected in all three groups of workers, suggesting an acute effect of exposure on airway function.

Subsequent work reaffirmed these findings in a workplace-based study of soft hemp workers processing *Cannabis sativa*. A higher prevalence of respiratory symptoms was seen in comparison to control workers (Pokrajac et al., 1990), with interesting additional findings in men of both nasal and sinus-based symptoms. Again, significant cross-shift changes in lung function measures were identified. For example, the FEV_1 fell by a mean of 7.1% over a working shift, whilst mid-expiratory flows (forced expiratory flow when 50% of the FVC has been exhaled [FEF_{50}]) fell by a mean of 15.1% from baseline.

Chronic lung function changes seen over time have been measured in relatively small groups of hemp textile workers over a 3-year period (Zuskin et al., 1992d). In addition to confirming acute shift-related falls in lung function, mean annual declines of FVC (range: 0.014–0.065 L), FEV_1 (range: 0.041–0.068 L), FEF_{50} (range: 0.020–0.220 L/second) and FEF_{25} (range: 0.030–0.140 L/second) were seen. These were identified to be considerably greater than in healthy non-exposed subjects and greater in those with byssinosis.

Longer-term follow-up of this group identified that accelerated annual declines in FEV_1 were again observed in the context of high measured dust levels (Zuskin et al., 1994c).

More recent UK-based work also identified significant reporting of respiratory symptoms in hemp processing workers in a cross-sectional study of hemp fibre processors (Fishwick et al., 2001a,b) and identified that 64% reported respiratory symptoms, with a suggestion that two workers had developed acute responses to hemp. Whilst the numbers that were studied were very small, serial FEV_1 measurements in two workers with work-related symptoms showed a mean fall in FEV_1 on the first working day of 12.9%, contrasting to a 6.25% increase on the last working day. By comparison, the values for the two workers without work-related symptoms were a fall of 1.4% and an increase of 3.2%.

The biologically active nature of this hemp dust was also confirmed. Levels of inhalable dust, endotoxin and fungal and bacterial contamination were all higher than the levels found in similar vegetable fibre processing factories. Measured inhalable dust levels ranged from 10.4 to 79.8 mg/m^3 and inhalable bacterial levels ranged from 4.7 to 190×10^6 CFU/m^3. Additionally, various measured parameters appeared to be correlated: soluble protein and endotoxin ($r = 0.99$, $p < 0.0001$), endotoxin and inhalable dust ($r = 0.94$, $p < 0.005$) and inhalable dust and protein ($r = 0.98$, $p < 0.0001$). This suggested that there was low variation in the composition of the dust between different workplace sites or activities.

Experimental Studies

Various experimental data are available to assist in the understanding of hemp-related respiratory disease. A study of the immunological status of hemp workers using a skin-prick test to hemp and flax dust extracts (Zuskin et al., 1992a) was performed in a relatively small group of female textile workers. Generally, high levels of positive skin-prick tests were found, and were much lower in control non-exposed females. For example, a mixture of hemp and flax extracts elicited a response in 64% of exposed workers. Interestingly, however, the skin-prick test response was found to relate to the reporting of respiratory symptoms, but not to other health endpoints, including abnormalities of lung function.

UK-based work has added to these early experimental observations, with the description of the ability of textile dust extracts to increase lung permeability in a guinea pig model (Bates et al., 1995). Lung permeability was assessed by absorption into blood from the lung of inhaled technetium-99m diethylenetriamine penta-acetate using γ-scintigraphy. Aqueous extracts of various textile dusts were inhaled over a 4-week period, and responses were compared to saline inhalation. Longer-term, repeated inhalations were associated with a reduced half-life of absorption, whereas single inhalations were not. The authors postulated that the increased permeability seen might be due to a loss of the epithelial tight junction.

In summary, hemp dust exposure has been associated with the development of general respiratory symptoms, nasal and sinus symptoms and byssinosis. Cross-sectional, cross-shift and longitudinal declines in lung function have been linked to exposure to this biologically active dust, although its mechanisms of action are relatively unclear.

SISAL

Sisal (*Agave sisalana*) is a species of agave that produces a stiff fibre than can be used to produce rope and twine, although extended uses include paper, carpets and wall fabrics.

Workplace-Based Studies

Relatively little is published about the respiratory health effects seen in sisal workers. Early modern work suggested that there may be an acute effect on lung function of sisal exposure in a group of rope makers (Baker et al., 1979), notably interpreting the absence of a drift up in lung function seen in non-exposed workers. Shortly after its publication, Nicholls et al. postulated that the pulmonary response may be determined in part by changes in blood histamine (Nicholls et al., 1973).

Subsequent study of sisal workers (Zuskin et al., 1992e) reported that the prevalence of respiratory symptoms was higher in sisal-exposed workers in comparison to non-exposed workers (significant only for chest tightness in a relatively small group of workers), and at a 20-year follow-up, significantly higher levels of new symptoms had developed (Zuskin et al., 1994b). The same group studied the role of IgE in various textile dusts including jute and sisal, and concluded that the immunological reactions that were tested for were not likely to be responsible for the development of respiratory impairment in textile workers who were exposed to jute and sisal dust (Zuskin et al., 1993). However, subsequent work, including the measuring of cross-shift lung function changes, raised the possibility that IgE testing might assist with the identification of occupational asthma in this group (Zuskin et al., 1994b).

Tanzanian sisal workers were the subject of a selection of workplace-based studies. The first, published in 2007, identified high levels of respiratory symptoms in sisal brushing and decortication workers (Kayumba et al., 2007). These were predominantly cough and nasal symptoms. When followed up, decortication and brushing workers had higher levels of acute symptoms throughout the week in comparison to non-exposed workers. Chronic sputum (30%) and chest tightness (48%) were identified at high levels in brushing workers (Kayumba et al., 2008a).

The utility of IgE to sisal (dry sisal extract and fresh sap) was again tested in this new group of workers (Kayumba et al., 2008b). On this occasion, it was concluded that sisal exposure was associated with IgE sensitisation (four-times higher than non-exposed workers), but that their ability to distinguish between those with and without symptoms was not clear.

Most recently, further study of this group has reported lung function abnormalities (Kayumba et al., 2011). The presence of a reduced FEV_1:FVC ratio, which is commonly seen in this group, was found to relate to years of work in the brushing department, after adjusting for age and smoking.

In summary, sisal dust exposure has been associated with the presence of various upper and lower respiratory tract symptoms, and abnormalities of lung function (cross-shift and cross-sectional) in certain studies. The role of immunological mechanisms is poorly understood, as the evidence base relating to sisal exposure is relatively limited.

COTTON

Introduction

Over 60 million people worldwide work in the textile or clothing industry (Lai and Christiani, 2013). There is a significant evidence base relating cotton dust exposure to the development of acute respiratory symptoms, abnormalities in lung function and, longer-term, accelerated annual decline in FEV_1 (Christiani and Wang, 2003). There are also many studies specifically describing byssinosis, the classical cotton-related lung disease.

Medical interest in cotton-related ill health is longstanding, and the Trades' Unions, representing the textile workers' plight, were also important historically (Bowden and Tweedale, 2003). Accounts of the representation of workers suggested that a sustained period of Union support was seen from the early 1900s for at least 70 years. Better dust control, compensation for affected workers and support for medical research were the focuses of their activities.

It is of interest that supporting evidence for cotton dust causing lung problems was not sourced only from traditional workplace and laboratory-based studies. Large epidemiological studies have also identified this link. An example is the findings of the Singapore Chinese Health Study (LeVan et al., 2006) that recruited over 52,000 participants. Whilst exposure to dusts from cotton, wood, metal, minerals and/or asbestos was associated with cough and phlegm production, chronic bronchitis and adult-onset asthma, cotton dust exposure was specifically identified as the major contributor to reported respiratory symptoms.

The intent of this section is to summarise the evidence supporting the development of respiratory illness linked to cotton dust exposure.

The Nature of Cotton

Cotton (genus *Gossypium*) is a naturally occurring fibre that is found in many tropical and subtropical regions, consisting almost entirely of cellulose. The fibres grow in a boll configuration around the seed-containing part of the plant. The fibres are either manually or mechanically removed prior to processing. During the subsequent production of cotton yarn, a set of process stages are completed, which include opening, blowing, carding, drawing, spinning and finally weaving in order to produce cloth. Traditionally, the earlier processes in this continuum produce more inhalable dust.

Definitions

Byssinosis is an occupational lung disease that is normally associated with exposure to cotton dust, and less commonly to other textile dusts. Typically, affected workers complain of chest tightness on the first working day after a break from work, with improvement in symptoms over the remaining working week. The cycle repeats, so that following a further cessation of exposure (normally on rest days from work), the chest tightness again appears on the next first working day. Such a description was probably first attributed to Mareska and Hay in 1845.

Schilling et al. proposed an initial classification of byssinosis (Schilling et al., 1963) based on the number of days a worker reported symptoms, and this classification was most recently adapted by the World Health Organization (WHO) in 1983 to include acute and chronic lung function changes (WHO, 1983). This classification is seen in Table 30.1.

Various other rarer or novel diseases have been described in cotton textile workers. These include, for example, mill fever, weavers' cough, mattress makers' fever and, less commonly again, alveolar proteinosis (Thind, 2009) and kaolinosis (Levin et al., 1996). These will not be described further in this chapter.

Workplace-Based Studies

Longitudinal

Various longitudinal studies of cotton workers have been carried out in differing geographies, and the main features of these are summarised in Table 30.2.

Given their design, most have been able to comment on changes in symptoms and lung function over time. Notwithstanding the difficulties associated with the interpretation of a mixed group of studies, variable consideration for smoking and the inevitable reporting of positive studies over negative studies, these findings support, on average, a greater-than-expected FEV_1 loss associated specifically with cotton dust exposure.

Glindmeyer et al. identified that textile work was associated with dose-related declines in lung function (Glindmeyer et al., 1991), and subsequently, large declines in a small group of cotton workers were reported; for example, 68 mL per year for FEV_1 in male workers (Zuskin et al., 1991). Larger declines were recently identified (Wang et al., 2002); for example, 70 mL FEV_1 declines over a single year seen in newly hired female cotton workers.

TABLE 30.1
Classification of Byssinosis

Classification	Definition
Byssinosis Grade	
B0	No complaints of breathing problems
B1/2	Chest tightness and/or shortness of breath sometimes on the first day of the workweek
B1	Chest tightness and/or shortness of breath always on the first day of the workweek
B2	Chest tightness and/or shortness of breath on the first workday and on other days of the workweek
Lung Function Grades	
Acute Changes	
No effect	A consistent[a] decline in FEV_1 of less than 5% or an increase in FEV_1 during the working shift
Mild effect	A consistent[a] decline of between 5% and 10% in FEV_1 during the working shift
Moderate effect	A consistent[a] decline of between 10% and 20% in FEV_1 during the working shift
Severe effect	A decline of 20% or more in FEV_1 during the working shift
Chronic Changes[b,c]	
No effect	FEV_1 80% of the predicted value or greater
Mild to moderate effect	FEV_1 60%–79% of the predicted value
Severe effect	FEV_1 less than 60% of the predicted value

Abbreviation: FEV_1: forced expiratory volume in 1 second.

[a] A decline occurring in at least three consecutive tests made after an absence from dust exposure of 2 days or more.

[b] Predicted values based on data obtained from local populations or similar ethnic and social class groups.

[c] By a pre-shift test after an absence from dust exposure of 2 days or more.

Certain studies have, however, identified more moderate decline values. A study of US-based cotton workers (Glindmeyer et al., 1994) measured a rate of decline of 24.7 mL per year for FEV_1, and the magnitude of this fall was determined not only by tobacco smoking, but also by a combination of cotton dust exposure and the presence of an acute cross-shift change in FEV_1. The latter relationship between longer-term FEV_1 decline and cross-shift change was subsequently confirmed in Shanghai cotton workers (Christiani et al., 2001); it was additionally noted that this acute cross-shift change related to the presence of measured airway hyper-reactivity (Wang et al., 2003b). Further work confirmed the lung function loss that was attributed to additive contributions from dust exposure and smoking (Wang et al., 2005).

The natural history of FEV_1 decline in textile workers is not well understood, although one paper suggested that the fall seen over time in lung function may be 'front ended', with lesser declines seen sequentially over time. Lung function data from the Shanghai cotton workers identified greater declines in comparison to the Glindmeyer et al. (1994) data, and also that these declines were greater in the first 5 years of follow-up: 40 mL per year in the first 5 years of follow-up, then 18 mL per year thereafter in cotton workers. It is of note that within this group, endotoxin exposure was predictive of both the reporting of respiratory symptoms (Shi et al., 2010b) and annual FEV_1 declines (Christiani et al., 2001; Wang et al., 2005).

Not all findings from the literature were necessarily intuitive; Glindmeyer et al., for example, also identified synthetic textile workers as having greater annual FEV_1 declines (36.6 mL per year) in comparison to cotton exposed workers.

A study of Turkish textile workers exposed to cotton dust (Bakirci et al., 2006) was conducted in order to identify early leavers. A total of 198 new workers were followed with questionnaire, lung function and skin prick testing. Fifty-three percent of this group left work in the first 12 months of their employment, and leaving work was found to be associated with increasing age and reporting a work-related lower respiratory tract symptom. Interestingly, atopic status, measured dust and endotoxin levels and lung function changes were not useful predictors of workers who left work.

This relationship was explored further by identifying which early signs of response to inhaled cotton dust were predictive of later health outcomes at 12 months of employment (Bakirci et al., 2007). An acute airway response was defined as either a cross-first-shift or a cross-week fall in FEV_1. In the first week of exposure, smoking tobacco, endotoxin exposure and cotton dust concentrations were all predictive of the presence

TABLE 30.2
Summary of Longitudinal Lung Function Studies of Cotton Workers

Study	Population	Main Findings
Elwood et al. (1986)	Ex-cotton workers	After allowing for age, height and smoking, lung function was approximately 2%–8% lower in the ex-textile workers than in controls who had never been exposed to any dust.
Glindmeyer et al. (1991)	1817 US cotton and synthetic textile workers; 5-year follow-up period	Dose-response FEV_1, FVC and FEF_{25-75} (the average flow from the point at which 25 percent of the FVC has been exhaled to the point at which 75 percent of the FVC has been exhaled) declines were seen and these were with higher in synthetic textile workers in comparison to cotton.
Zuskin et al. (1991)	66 Yugoslavian textile workers; 10-year follow-up period	Mean annual lung function decline was greater than expected; for example, male workers had FEV_1 declines of 68 mL per year and FVC decline of 59 mL per year. High levels of byssinosis were seen in this small group of workers.
Glindmeyer et al. (1994)	611 workers with repeatable spirometry; 5-year follow-up period	A significant association between the acute and chronic effects of cotton dust exposure was identified. Both dust exposure and across-shift change proved to be significant predictors of annual change in FEV_1. Excess annual FEV_1 declines were predicted for exposures of 200 μg/m^3 and across-shift drops in FEV_1 of 200 mL.
Christiani et al. (1994)	447 cotton workers in China; 5-year follow-up period	Accelerated FEV_1 decline was seen in those with symptoms and greater acute lung function responses to cotton dust. Large variability was seen in study responses with time; overall, 'Among cotton workers, consistent responders to either symptom questionnaire or across-shift FEV_1 decrements of less than or equal to 5% appear to be at increased risk for lung function impairment'.
Christiani et al. (1999)	445 and 467 cotton and silk textile workers, respectively, in Shanghai, China; 11-year follow-up period	Cotton workers had a larger loss of FEV_1 during the first 5 years of study (40 mL per year decline) as compared with the second 6 years of follow-up (18 mL per year decline). During the same periods, the average decline among silk workers was slightly higher in the first period, but was more consistent (30 versus 27 mL per year). Declines in lung function were related to dust exposure, not endotoxin.
Christiani et al. (2001)	Same cohort as Christiani et al. (1999) paper, describing 15-year follow-up period findings	The number of years worked in cotton mills, high level of exposure to endotoxin and across-shift drops in FEV_1 were found to be significant determinants for longitudinal change in FEV_1, after controlling for appropriate confounders. No byssinosis found in silk workers.
Wang et al. (2002)	225 newly employed female non-smoking cotton workers; 1-year follow-up period	FEV_1 declined by 70 mL and FVC by 124 mL over the year of follow-up, and workers reporting respiratory symptoms at 3 months showed a significantly greater cross-shift change in FEV_1 (−2.3%) than those without the symptoms (−0.7%).
Wang et al. (2003b)	101 newly employed cotton textile workers; 18-month follow-up period	Increasing airway responsiveness was strongly correlated with cross-shift change in FEV_1.
Wang et al. (2004)	15-year follow-up of cotton and silk workers	Greater FEV_1 declines were seen in cotton workers compared with silk workers. Retirement was identified by regression as a predictor of reduced lung function loss.
Wang et al. (2005)	Same cohort as Wang et al. (2004)	Endotoxin exposure was a stronger predictor of lung function loss than cotton dust exposure. Workers with byssinosis had an accelerated FEV_1 decline in comparison to those without this condition. Excess declines were associated with other symptoms, including chronic bronchitis and cough at an earlier follow-up period.
Shi et al. (2010b)	Same cohort as Wang et al. (2004)	Recent endotoxin exposure was significantly associated with byssinosis, chronic bronchitis and chronic cough.

Abbreviations: FEV_1: forced expiratory volume in 1 second; FVC: forced vital capacity.

of work-related respiratory symptoms. Acute airway responses were seen in the first week, and female gender was the predictive factor for these.

After 1 year of exposure, the mean fall in FEV_1 was 65.5 mL. Increasing age, early respiratory symptoms and early falls in cross-week FEV_1 were found to influence this. It was also interesting to note that cross-first-shift and cross-week falls in FEV_1 were reduced in magnitude during the course of the study. These findings suggested that early responses to cotton dust predicted later health outcomes, but that tolerance to such early responses developed in certain workers.

Elwood et al.'s early study of cotton workers (Elwood et al., 1986), whilst not strictly a longitudinal workplace study, set the scene for subsequent longer-term follow-up of health consequences, and suggested that there may have been other health consequences associated with cotton work, including perhaps nutritional issues, which led to a shorter adult stature.

In summary, the published longitudinal studies of cotton dust-exposed workers are heterogeneous, documenting variable lung function declines measured against differing control or comparator populations. Notwithstanding these issues, certain well-conducted studies identify cotton exposure as an independent predictor of lung function loss when other pertinent factors are corrected for. The presence of accelerated lung function loss was associated across the entire evidence base with self-reported symptoms, cross-shift changes in lung function and both dust and endotoxin exposure.

Whether these changes in lung function represent the development of chronic obstructive pulmonary disease (COPD) per se or are reflections of chronic asthma or indeed another clinical process is not as-yet accurately characterised. In the interim, it seems reasonable to include cotton dust exposure as a contributing factor to the development of COPD in certain cotton-exposed workers who develop the typical features of this condition.

Cross-Shift Studies

In addition to the longitudinal studies discussed above, cross-shift changes in FEV_1 have been identified to relate to the presence of respiratory symptoms (Choudat et al., 1987; Zuskin et al., 1994c; Chattopadhyay et al., 1995, 2003)

Early evidence of an acute effect from exposure on lung function came from a large study of 23 US-based cotton mills (Rylander et al., 1979). Selected more recent examples of studies addressing this issue are shown in Table 30.3. Changes in lung function across shift were also found to relate to dust levels (Zhong et al., 2002) and an interaction between atopy and exposures to dictate lung function fall. Certain studies supported a better relationship with exposure when bacterial counts were used as the exposure parameter (Jones et al., 1980).

There are also data to support a relationship between bronchial hyper-reactivity and cross-shift changes in FEV_1. This was specifically studied in a group of cotton spinners (Fishwick et al., 2010). Available information included the presence of respiratory symptoms, serial peak flow records, FEV_1 cross-shift changes and airway reactivity, and cross-shift changes were best related to both the presence of symptoms and airway hyper-reactivity.

It is important to note that not all studies produce consistent results. Both Costa et al. (2004) and Oldenburg et al. (2007) did not identify significant relationships between exposure levels and cross-shift changes in lung function, and further work is needed in order to better clarify these relationships.

In summary, both longitudinal and cross-sectional studies have identified cross-shift falls in FEV_1 in cotton workers. Their exact cause remains uncharacterised. Given that these falls appear to relate to respiratory symptoms and dust levels but also, importantly, to the presence of airway reactivity, it is perhaps reasonable to conclude that these are a type of asthmatic airway response, the presence of which in longitudinal studies influences accelerated subsequent annual decline. However, there are no longer-term studies that document profile changes in airway reactivity after exposure cessation.

Other Cross-Sectional Studies

Many cross-sectional studies have reported symptoms or abnormalities of lung function in particular groups of textile workers. The differing study population demographics, geographies and study time periods represented by this group make differences and similarities particularly difficult to synthesise.

Prevalence of Byssinosis

Many studies have reported the prevalence of byssinosis, although it is likely that varying definitions will have been adopted between these studies. Table 30.4 highlights certain studies that reported byssinosis as an outcome.

There are examples of both rather unexpectedly low historic levels of byssinosis (2.4%) in New South Wales workers (Barnes and Simpson, 1976) and a recent high prevalence of byssinosis (10.5%) in Karachi cotton workers (Nafees et al., 2013). One paper identified relatively low levels of byssinosis but high levels of mill fever, suggesting either the development of a differential response to the same exposure between groups of workers or a diagnostic labelling issue (Holness et al., 1983).

Workplace Factors Associated with Byssinosis

Many studies supported work in the following cotton process areas as being associated with the development of byssinosis; opening, cleaning, blowing, picking, carding and combing. These are mostly traditionally dusty work areas. One study additionally identified cotton spinning as a risk factor (Nafees et al., 2013).

TABLE 30.3
Selected Examples (not Already Included in Table 30.2) of Cross-Shift Changes in Lung Function and Their Determinants in Cotton-Exposed Workers

Study	Population	Main Findings
Woldeyohannes et al. (1991)	595 Ethiopian cotton textile workers	Prevalence of chronic bronchitis ranged from 17.6% to 47.7% and asthma from 8.5% to 20.5% across all sections. Cross-shift lung function changes were greater in those with respiratory symptoms in comparison to those without symptoms.
Zhong et al. (2002)	110 textile workers initially studied, and comparisons made with those who did or did not remain in employment 3 years later	Atopy and dust exposure both interacted in order to influence cross-shift changes in lung function. Those with cross-shift changes had on average more hyper-reactive airways than those without. Leaving the work environment was predicted by the development of symptoms, but not the presence of atopy.
Costa et al. (2004)	PEF variation and dust levels measured on each day of a working week in a single cotton mill; 47 workers included	Greatest levels of cotton dust and endotoxin seen on a Friday. No differences in across-shift changes in lung function were seen with differing cotton dust and endotoxin exposures. Workers with reported asthma had greater levels of airway reactivity and across-shift lung function changes. The latter were associated with endotoxin exposure, but not with cotton dust levels.
Oldenburg et al. (2007)	150 German cotton textile workers in a cross-sectional study	Relationships between endotoxin exposure and lung function abnormalities (airways obstruction) were seen, with significant effects seen at very high endotoxin levels (above 450 EU/m^3). However, the development of airways obstruction across shift did not relate to endotoxin exposure.
Fishwick et al. (2010)	UK-based cotton and manmade fibre workers	Relationships between lung function, cross-shift lung function, serial peak expiratory flow (PEF) and airway hyper-responsiveness were assessed in 53 textile workers. Work-related respiratory symptoms were best associated with airway hyper-responsiveness and across-shift changes in FEV_1. While a positive peak flow chart suggestive of a work effect was associated with increased airway responsiveness, it was not associated with the presence of work-related symptoms.

Abbreviation: FEV_1: forced expiratory volume in 1 second.

In terms of dust exposure and byssinosis risk, various studies identified current and cumulative cotton dust levels (Liu, 1987; Fishwick et al., 1992; Nafees et al., 2013) as risk factors. Grade of cotton also appeared to be relevant. Coarse cotton appeared to be more potent than fine cotton in a single study (Awad elKarim and Onsa, 1987), and weaving appeared to be associated with low levels of byssinosis, presumably because of the relatively lower dust levels generated from this process.

Intriguingly, byssinosis has also occasionally been identified in non-cotton-exposed workers (Massin et al., 1991) and in blue collar workers (Engelberg et al., 1985). Whether these findings related to other workplace causes for first working day chest tightness or misinterpretation of the questionnaire remains to be elucidated.

Host Factors Associated with Byssinosis

Whilst data supporting each assumption are variable, gender and smoking habit appeared not to influence the development of byssinosis (Zuskin et al., 1989; Fishwick et al., 1994b). Historic data also do not support atopy as a risk factor for the development of byssinosis. The relationship between specific ethnicity and byssinosis was noted in one study (Nafees et al., 2013), although it is not clear whether this related to a true risk or differences in interpretation of a study questionnaire. The latter study also cited lack of education as a risk factor for reporting symptoms of byssinosis, although this must similarly be interpreted with caution.

Byssinosis was found to be associated with cross-shift declines in lung function (Noweir et al., 1984; Liu 1987; Parikh et al., 1990; Altin et al., 2002), although not all studies (Barnes and Simpson, 1976) identified this as a feature. Cross-shift lung function changes related to measured cotton dust levels (Holness et al., 1983) have also been reported.

In terms of the physiological nature of byssinosis, one study identified that workers with byssinosis had significantly greater levels of airway hyper-responsiveness in comparison to those with symptoms that were not consistent with byssinosis (Fishwick et al., 1992), and one study confirmed normal gas transfer estimates in

TABLE 30.4
Details of Studies that Have Commented on Byssinosis Prevalence and its Determinants

Study	Study Type	Main Findings
Barnes and Simpson (1976)	Cotton mills workers from New South Wales	Low levels of byssinosis were identified (12 of 493 workers with byssinosis).
Martin and Higgins (1976)	6631 cotton textile workers	Low numbers of byssinosis seen; its presence was related to the presence of bronchitis. Work opening, picking and carding were specifically associated with byssinosis. The majority of those with byssinosis did not have a cross-shift change in FEV_1. (Byssinosis rates overall were 3% based on history, but only 0.8% when defined using associated 10% fall in the FEV_1 across shift).
Barman (1979)	Cotton compress and warehouse workers	No symptoms were consistent with byssinosis. Respiratory symptoms were related to cross-shift changes in FEV_1.
Morgan and Ong (1981)	Hong Kong textile workers	First description of Hong Kong byssinosis (attributed to 7-day working masking the condition, given no usual break in the working week). No workers were reported to have asthma.
Holness et al. (1983)	Cotton felt workers	5% identified with byssinosis and 31% with mill fever. Dust levels were associated with cross-shift lung function changes.
Noweir et al. (1984)	Egyptian cotton workers	Byssinosis was seen in 21% of workers in opening and cleaning sections and in 13% of workers in carding and combing rooms. Acute cross-shift lung function changes were also seen.
Engelberg et al. (1985)	Cotton waste industry	260 workers studied, 5.9% of whom had byssinosis. Average dust exposures ranged from 0.28 to 7.80 mg/m^3. Cross-shift lung function was increased in cotton workers. Relatively high levels of byssinosis symptoms (4.7%) were also seen in the non-exposed blue collar groups.
Honeybourne and Pickering (1986)	153 cases of grade 2 and 3 byssinosis seen in a hospital clinic	Transfer factor measured and reductions were thought to relate to smoking primarily. The authors consequently suggested that emphysema was not a clinically significant feature of byssinosis.
Li et al. (1987)	Two cotton mills; one dusty (dust levels at 57–159 mg/m^3) and one less so (dust levels at 6.8 mg/m^3)	High levels of byssinosis were seen in the very dusty mill that was studied of 22.2%. 177 mL average significant cross-shift falls in FEV_1 were seen in those with byssinosis (elevation in lung function was seen across shift in non-byssinotics, and controls had a rise in FEV_1 across shift). Byssinosis was related to the total duration of employment.
Liu (1987)	289 cotton workers in Beijing	4.2% with byssinosis. Byssinosis was related to current and cumulative cotton dust exposure. Byssinosis was more common in tobacco smokers.
Kawamoto et al. (1987)	128 cotton workers	10% with symptoms that were consistent with byssinosis (as defined by the presence of Monday chest tightness). Dust levels were measured at a mean of 0.72 mg/m^3.
Awad elKarim et al. (1987)	186 male spinners in two Sudanese textile mills	Prevalence of byssinosis was 37% among Khartoum spinners (coarse cotton) and 1% among Hassaheisa spinners (fine cotton).
Cinkotai et al. (1988)	Lancashire byssinosis trends	Noted significant declines in levels of byssinosis symptoms over time.
Zuskin et al. (1989)	112 cotton workers	High levels of byssinosis that were similar by gender; male: 29.5%, female: 29.4%. Most were byssinosis grade 1/2.
Parikh et al. (1990)	214 cotton-exposed workers in Ahmedabad; control population used	Cross-shift lung function changes were more marked in byssinosis.
Massin et al. (1991)	774 French textile workers and a control population	6.2% had Monday chest tightness consistent with byssinosis, which was also seen in 1.9% of the non-exposed control population. The presence of byssinosis was linked to exposure, and not to smoking.

(*Continued*)

TABLE 30.4 (*Continued*)
Details of Studies that Have Commented on Byssinosis Prevalence and its Determinants

Study	Study Type	Main Findings
Woldeyohannes et al. (1991)	595 Ethiopian cotton textile workers	The prevalence of byssinosis was 43.2% among blowers and 37.5% in carders in comparison with 4%–24% among workers in other sections.
Sigsgaard et al. (1992)	Cross-sectional study of 409 Danish textile workers	Low alpha 1 anti-trypsin (A1A) levels associated with byssinosis. In addition, high mould spore levels were seen in the wool mills. Lung function abnormalities were related to cumulative endotoxin exposures.
Fishwick et al. (1992)	645 UK-based cotton workers	3.6% had byssinosis. The majority of byssinotic workers (18 out of 23) had BHR. Levels of BHR were higher than in those with symptoms that were not consistent with byssinosis (21 out of 56) and asymptomatic workers (14 out of 84). The cumulative cotton dust exposure index was the only dust parameter to be significantly greater in those with BHR (mean mg-year/m^3 [95% CI]: 14.13 [13.1–15.1]) than those with normal airway reactivity (5.35 [3.9–6.8]).
Beckett et al. (1994)	Cross-sectional, 973 cotton workers	9 with grade 1 byssinosis, all production workers.
Fishwick et al. (1994b)	404 man-made fibre-exposed workers and 1048 cotton-exposed workers	The presence of byssinosis (3.7%) was related significantly to cumulative lifetime cotton dust exposure, total years spent carding and currently working in the carding area. Smoking habit did not differ significantly between byssinotic and non-byssinotic workers.
Jiang et al. (1995)	1320 cotton workers, 1306 control workers; cross-sectional study	9% with symptoms that were typical of byssinosis, 1.7% with symptoms of byssinosis and a cross-shift fall in lung function of at least 5%. Median total dust concentrations ranged from 3.04 to 12.32 mg/m^3.
Raza et al. (1999a)	Cross-sectional study of Lancashire weavers	4 out of 1295 weavers had byssinosis, noting a low prevalence of 0.3%. Dust levels were measured between 0.095 and 0.413 mg/m^3.
Altin et al. (2002)	223 cotton mill workers	14.2% with byssinosis, over 50% of whom had evidence of a cross-shift effect.
Su et al. (2003)	Two cross-sectional studies in Taiwanese cotton workers	High levels of byssinosis seen, but lower in a second study (in 1996; 12.6%) than in the first (in 1991; 21.9%).
Wang et al. (2003a)	15-year follow-up of cotton and silk workers	Noted a cumulative incidence of byssinosis of 24% and high levels of chest tightness.
Boubopoulos et al. (2010)	443 Greek cotton mill workers	7.7% with byssinosis, and dust levels were measured; the mean breathing zone cotton dust concentration was 0.16 mg/m^3 and the mean work area cotton dust concentration was 0.14 mg/m^3.
Nafees et al. (2013)	372 male Karachi cotton workers	Byssinosis was found in 10.5% of workers. Work in the spinning section, lack of education, prolonged duration of work and Sindhi ethnicity were identified as important risk factors for respiratory endpoints.

Abbreviations: FEV_1: forced expiratory volume in 1 second; BHR: bronchial hyper-reactivity.

byssinosis (Honeybourne and Pickering, 1986), suggesting that emphysema was not a feature.

Other Symptoms and Diagnoses

There are a large number of studies in the literature that have described other respiratory symptoms and their associations either with cotton dust exposures or measured lung function values. Table 30.5 shows the details of a selection of the main studies.

Bronchitis Various publications supported the relationship between cotton dust exposure and the development of bronchitis. An excess of bronchitis in cotton workers with a low duration of exposure has been reported (Engelberg et al., 1985), although chronic bronchitis was later confirmed in other cotton-exposed populations (Niven et al., 1997), including Lancashire cotton weavers and cotton spinners. The presence of bronchitis in the latter group was related to levels of

TABLE 30.5
Details of Studies that Have Commented on Other Cotton Textile-Related Symptoms, Lung Function Abnormalities and Their Determinants

Study	Study Type	Main Findings
Engelberg et al. (1985)	Cotton waste industry	Excess of bronchitis seen in cotton workers with less than 2 years of employment.
Zuskin et al. (1992b)	Small group of cotton textile workers and non-exposed bottle packers	Poor correlation between immunological findings (cotton skin-prick testing and IgE) and clinical end points.
Beckett et al. (1994)	Cross-sectional; 973 cotton workers	Excess of other respiratory symptoms in comparison to non-exposed workers. Analysis corrected for indoor smoke usage; For example, OR for wheeze: 2.96, shortness of breath: 4.54.
Fishwick et al. (1994a)	1048 cotton and man-made fibre workers	17.5% with work-related eye symptoms and 11% with work-related nasal symptoms. Ethnicity, female gender and younger age were associated with both of these symptoms.
Fishwick et al. (1996)	1057 cotton and man-made fibre workers; cross-sectional study	Although lung function seemed to be affected by high dust exposures when operatives were stratified into high- and low-exposure groups, regression analysis did not identify current dust concentration as an independent factor influencing loss. Smoking habit was found to explain most of the measured change in FEV_1 and FVC. A total of 212 static work area dust samples (range: 0.04–3.23 mg/m^3) and 213 personal breathing zone samples (range: 0.14–24.95 mg/m^3) were collected.
Da Costa et al. (1997)	3529 Portuguese textile workers (natural and man-made fibres)	High levels of both respiratory and nasal symptoms; higher in cotton workers. Adjusted analyses suggested that duration of cotton exposure was a risk factor for symptoms.
Zuskin et al. (1996), Zuskin et al. (1997)	Cross-sectional study of 97 textile dyeing workers and 76 controls	Higher levels of chronic respiratory symptoms and shift-related symptoms in exposed workers. Occupational asthma described in dyers.
Raza et al. (1999b)	Cross-sectional study of Lancashire weavers	6% prevalence of chronic bronchitis and generally low levels of other symptoms associated primarily with smoking habit.
Niven et al. (1997)	2991 cotton and man-made fibre textile workers	High levels of chronic bronchitis. Cumulative exposure to cotton dust was significantly associated with chronic bronchitis after the effects of age, sex, smoking and ethnic group were accounted for ($p < 0.0005$).
Raza et al. (1999a)	Textile weavers with various exposures in a cross-sectional study	Reduced FEV_1 and FVC were predicted by smoking, male sex, age, not working in the weaving shed, ethnicity and personal dust concentrations.
Mberikunashe et al. (2010)	Zimbabwe textile workers	High prevalence of symptoms and measured airways obstruction; for example, 50% of blowers had airways obstruction.
Chaari et al. (2009)	Cotton apprentice study of 600 workers	Allergic-type symptoms common; 120 workers developed these in training. Conjunctivitis and rhinitis the most common symptoms, which were more common in atopic exposed workers.
Nafees et al. (2013)	372 male Karachi cotton workers	High levels of respiratory complaints; chronic cough: 7.5%, chronic phlegm: 12.9%, wheeze with shortness of breath: 22.3%, shortness of breath (grade 2): 21%, chest tightness ever: 33.3%.

Abbreviations: OR: odds ratio; FVC: forced vital capacity; FEV_1: forced expiratory volume in 1 second.

dust exposure after correction for other factors, including smoking. A study of Karachi cotton workers also recently confirmed this association between dust exposure and bronchitis (Nafees et al., 2013).

In a study of bronchitis in Lancashire cotton textile workers using a cross-sectional and nested case-referent study design (Niven et al., 1997), chronic bronchitis was seen at higher levels in workers over the age of 45 years (odds ratio [OR]: 2.51). Its presence was associated with a cumulative cotton dust exposure estimate after the effects of age, sex, smoking and ethnicity were taken into account. Chronic bronchitis was also associated with a small decrement in lung function. For example, the mean percentage predicted FEV_1 in cases of chronic bronchitis was 81.4% (95% confidence interval [CI]: 78.3%–84.6%) compared to a mean of 86.7% (95% CI: 84.9%–88.5%) in the control population.

Cough, Chest Tightness, Wheeze and Shortness of Breath These are commonly reported in many studies, although study design does not often allow for a more precise clinical diagnosis to be made. General comment is made in many study outputs relating to the presence of wheeze (often not distinguished from asthma), chest tightness (as distinct from byssinosis) and ocular and nasal irritation.

High levels of frequent cough, wheeze and shortness of breath have been reported in Chinese cotton workers (Beckett et al., 1994), with respective corrected ORs of 2.23, 2.96 and 4.54. Chronic respiratory symptoms in this group of non-smoking female workers were associated with job category, even after correction for domestic indoor air quality. Similarly, recent work from Karachi (Nafees et al., 2013) has identified current high levels of respiratory symptoms in cotton workers. Non-byssinotic symptoms were generally found to be highly prevalent in this group; for example, chest tightness ever reported by 33.3% of the population, although low levels of asthma were reported. More specifically, work in the spinning section predicted frequent wheeze, wheeze with shortness of breath and airways obstruction. Additionally, prolonged duration of work predicted reductions in both FEV_1 and the FEV_1:FVC ratio. The authors also raised the issue of worker education level (lack of) as a predictor of certain symptoms (Nafees et al., 2013).

Upper airway and ocular symptoms are variably described and documented in the literature. The best documented are those in Lancashire textile workers (Fishwick et al., 1994a), in whom high levels of these complaints have been reported, the presence of which being related to certain ethnicities, female gender and younger age. Similar symptoms have been described in Portuguese workers (Beckett et al., 1994), and conjunctivitis and rhinitis were reported in a large cohort of cotton apprentices (Chaari et al., 2009). In the latter study, the development of rhinitis appeared to relate strongly, although not universally, to the presence of asthma, in addition to dust exposure and atopy.

Asthma The presence or development of asthma is also specifically described in certain studies, although the designs did not generally allow for inference as to whether this should be regarded as occupational asthma.

Early work from the Ethiopian textile mills (Woldeyohannes et al., 1991) described a high prevalence of asthma in textile workers (ranging across sections between 8.5% and 20.5%) that was distinct from additional very high levels of byssinosis and bronchitis. Measured dust levels were relatively high, ranging between 0.86 and 3.52 mg/m^3. Again, no comments were made about the cause of the asthma identified.

Asthma in workers dyeing textiles has been reported (Zuskin et al., 1996), with 7.2% of workers having symptoms that are consistent with occupational asthma, although no further objective assessment of that possible diagnosis was made.

Subsequently, the development of asthma in a small proportion of French cotton textile apprentices has been described (Chaari et al., 2009). Whilst most apprentices who developed allergic consequences did so with new-onset conjunctivitis and rhinitis, 4.6% developed asthma. The development of these conditions was related to atopy. No information was given about measured exposures in this group of clothing apprentices who were presumably working with primarily finished cloth.

Extraordinarily high levels of asthma have been described in a study of Greek cotton workers (Boubopoulos et al., 2010), with 57.7% reporting the onset of asthma after the age of 30 years in the context of relatively modest dust levels (mean breathing zone cotton dust concentration of 0.16 mg/m^3 and mean work area cotton dust concentration of 0.14 mg/m^3). Similarly, in a study that was designed to assess working conditions on each day of a working week, 32% of the study group reported asthma (Costa et al., 2004).

The finding of high levels of asthma in textile workers is by no means universal. Very early byssinosis descriptions from Hong Kong (Morgan and Ong, 1981) particularly mention the absence of asthma in their study population, and much more recent work from Karachi (Nafees et al., 2013) has identified very low levels of asthma (4%) in cotton workers.

In summary, levels of reported asthma vary widely from study to study, and interpretation of this range is compounded by differing populations, exposures and questionnaire types. There currently does not appear to be sufficient evidence to support cotton exposure as a common cause of occupational asthma as distinct from byssinosis.

Lung Function Data from Cross-Sectional Studies

Cross-sectional lung function is recorded in many studies, which are too numerous to detail here. Some identify an effect of measured exposure on cross-sectional lung function estimates, whilst others identify less of an effect following correction for other potential influences.

One example of a lack of effect is seen in Lancashire cotton workers (Fishwick et al., 1996). The FEV_1

measured in 1057 workers was, as anticipated, reduced in smokers (mean of the percentage predicted value: 89.5%; 95% CI: 88%–91%) in comparison with non-smokers (mean of the percentage predicted value: 93.1%; 95% CI: 90.5%–94.1%), and FVC was reduced in those currently working with man-made fibres (mean of the percentage predicted value: 95.3%; 95% CI: 93.8%–96.9%) in comparison with cotton (mean of the percentage predicted value: 97.8%; 95% CI: 96.6%–99.0%). Regression analysis significantly identified smoking, increasing age, increasing time worked in the waste room and male sex as predictive of a lower FEV_1 and FVC. Measured cotton dust level exposures did not appear to predict lower lung function, although years of work in the waste room, which is traditionally dusty, was predictive.

Subsequently, an association between personal breathing zone dust levels and lung function decrements in textile weavers was confirmed (Raza et al., 1999a). When exposed to mean personal dust levels of 1.98 mg/m^3, lung function loss on regression was found to be associated with dust levels in addition, independently, to male sex, age, not working in the weaving shed and not being of white Caucasian ethnicity.

More recently, the presence of airways obstruction in cotton workers has been associated (OR: 3.53; 95% CI: 1.61–7.79) with work in the traditionally dusty cotton blowing department of a Zimbabwe textile mill (Mberikunashe et al., 2010). Work in the weaving department of the same mill was significantly protective (OR: 0.16; 95% CI: 0.04–0.59) of having airways obstruction.

In summary, previous cross-sectional studies, perhaps as anticipated, have varying conclusions, although certain of these support exposure effects on the development of abnormal lung function, including airways obstruction.

Exposure-Only Studies

Various publications have dealt more specifically with cotton-related exposures per se, without associated health information.

Early work from Chinese cotton mills (Christiani et al., 1993) confirmed a positive correlation between measured dust levels and endotoxin levels. Based on data from 11 work areas of two cotton mills, there was a good correlation between dust and endotoxin in both mills. Contemporary work from the UK (Niven et al., 1992) confirmed that an approach using personal rather than work area dust sampling was superior, and less likely to underestimate worker exposure.

Canadian work (Marchand et al., 2007) reaffirmed the association between endotoxin exposure and cotton textile work in a study of four cotton mills measuring levels of endotoxin and identifying which particular processes were responsible for greatest exposures. The highest measured concentrations were found in the weaving and drawing areas, with samples estimating up to 10,000 EU endotoxin/m^3. Opening, cleaning, carding, spinning and drawing processes returned lower and variable estimates of endotoxin exposure, varying between 24 and 8700 EU endotoxin/m^3.

Subsequent work from the Nepalese textile industry (Paudyal et al., 2011), specifically garment making, carpet making, weaving and recycling, identified generally high levels of endotoxin exposure on personal sampling. For example, the highest levels were seen in the recycling sector (mean: 5110 EU/m^3) and weaving (mean: 2440 EU/m^3), with lower levels in the garment area (mean: 157 EU/m^3). It is interesting to note that despite these high levels of endotoxin, total dust levels were generally low: only 18% of workers sampled exceeded the UK-based limit of 2.5 mg/m^3. This study reaffirmed the good correlation seen between the inhalable dust and endotoxin concentrations.

More recent work has identified not only the anticipated Gram-negative bacteria in cotton, but also significant fungal presence, including *Aspergillus*, *Cladosporium* and *Fusarium* species (Lane and Sewell, 2006).

Studies of Mortality

A limited number of publications have dealt with the mortality of textile workers, with varying results. Early data from Rhode Island (Dubrow and Gute, 1988) suggested that male textile workers had a significantly elevated proportional mortality ratio (PMR) for non-malignant respiratory disease (PMR: 110; 95% CI: 102–120). The highest PMR values were seen in workers from traditionally dusty occupations, including carding, lapping and combing.

Data from Finnish cotton mills (Koskela et al., 1990) are also available from a cohort of workers exposed to raw cotton dust who were employed between 1950 and 1971. Whilst there were varying levels of individual worker exposure, each was exposed for at least 5 years. At follow-up in 1985, there did not appear to be an excess mortality for respiratory or cardiovascular diseases when compared to the general Finnish population. There were excessive rates of respiratory diseases ($p < 0.001$), musculoskeletal diseases ($p < 0.01$) and, interestingly, new cases of rheumatoid arthritis ($p < 0.05$).

A meta-analysis of cancer risk in textile workers (Mastrangelo et al., 2002) identified that, in studies published after 1990, there was a general tendency towards unity for all of the cancer risk estimates. Previous more historic estimates (e.g. lung cancer) had shown reduced risks in cotton workers.

Cancer mortality in a group of 444 Shanghai textile workers was more recently reported (Fang et al., 2013). Mortality from gastrointestinal cancers and all cancers combined, excluding lung cancer, were increased in cotton workers when compared to silk workers. Risks were greater with medium exposure, when a lag period of 20 years was used in the analysis. In this group, excesses of lung cancer were not seen, and this led the authors to postulate that endotoxin may have had a protective effect on its development and that this effect persisted following cessation of exposure.

The latter assertion was also supported by further recent evidence (McElvenny et al., 2011) from a study of mortality from lung cancer in a group of 3551 UK-based cotton workers. Here, it was identified that cumulative endotoxin exposure was associated (corrected for smoking) with a reduced risk of lung cancer mortality. For example, the highest cumulative endotoxin exposure of >600,000 endotoxin units was associated with a rate ratio of 0.5 (95% CI: 0.3–0.9).

Finally, a study of mortality from COPD in a group of silk textile workers from 1989 to 2000 has been reported (Cui et al., 2011). Age-adjusted standardised mortality ratios (SMRs) were calculated for each of ten textile work sectors. Most sectors did not have elevated SMR values when compared to the general Nanjing Chinese female population; for example, the age-adjusted SMRs ranged between 0.58 and 1.15. Elevated SMRs were, however, seen for cotton (1.02; 95% CI: 0.81–1.28) and silk workers (2.03; 95% CI: 1.13–3.34). There was greater COPD mortality among all cotton workers (hazard ratio [HR]: 1.40; 95% CI: 1.03–1.89) and silk workers (HR: 2.54, 95% CI: 1.47–4.39).

Studies of the Effectiveness of Interventions

Very few studies have specifically dealt with workplace-based interventions that are designed to reduce ill health associated with cotton dust exposure.

Work from the Karachi cotton mills have supplied limited data supporting the use of respiratory-protective equipment (Farooque et al., 2008). Their experience in a relatively small number of cotton mill workers reported that 19% of the 83 workers had symptoms that were consistent with byssinosis relating to work in the ring and carding areas, those who worked overtime and those who reported using less respiratory-protective equipment. Whilst only small numbers of subjects were included, the authors concluded that hours of work and lack of face mask use were risk factors for developing respiratory ill health.

Interventions that limit workplace cotton dust exposures are only described in relation to workers who subsequently retire and cease exposure. Improvements are described in the annual declines in FEV_1 seen in both cotton and silk workers, with greater gains seen in smoking textile workers (Shi et al., 2010a). In terms of the magnitude of the changes seen, years elapsed since stopping work was positively associated with magnitude of change, with gains of 11.3 mL per year and 5.6 mL per year in 5-year FEV_1 changes for, respectively, cotton and silk workers.

Previous work has also investigated the potential benefits of pre-treating cotton dust prior to processing in order to reduce longer-term health problems. The pre-treatment of cotton dust with the bactericidal benzododecinium bromide prior to workplace processing has been reported (Hend et al., 2003). Treated and non-treated cotton was incubated in order to determine endotoxin development. It was identified that in non-treated cotton samples, the endotoxin content grew to over 5000 ng/mg compared to lower rates in the treated bales. No data, however, were provided regarding subsequent health effects in exposed workers.

Studies of Possible Mechanisms of Cotton-Related Respiratory Ill Health

Various mechanistic studies are reported in the literature that were designed to improve the understanding of the more basic mechanisms involved in the development of cotton-related respiratory disease. Whilst a detailed summary is not possible here, a summary of certain papers is given in Table 30.6.

Despite the broad range of such approaches experimentally, there does not yet appear to be a single accepted mechanism of action for cotton dust on the human airway that causes respiratory ill health, although evidently many approaches are being actively considered.

Diagnoses

The diagnosis of byssinosis remains a clinical one, and would be supported by:

1. A known exposure to a causative agent, with cotton as the most common cause. It would be unusual to develop byssinosis prior to 10 years of cotton dust exposure.

TABLE 30.6
A Summary of Cotton-Related Mechanistic Studies

Study	Study Type	Main Finding
Animal studies		
Muscle		
Mundie et al. (1983)	Bioassay for smooth muscle contracting agents found in cotton bract extract	Various approaches were used to assess contraction of rat stomach smooth muscle and ability to block contractions. It was concluded that increased synthesis and release of arachidonic acid metabolites might be major mechanisms in the bronchoconstriction observed in the acute byssinotic reaction.
Airway		
Gordon and Harkema (1995)	Cotton dust exposure to rat airway	Dose-dependent increased stored intraepithelial mucosubstances in the respiratory tract. The authors postulated a link to the development of chronic bronchitis in humans exposed to cotton dust.
Bates et al. (1995)	Guinea pig lung permeability was assessed by absorption of inhaled technetium-99m diethylenetriamine penta-acetate using γ-scintigraphy	Airway permeability increased after 4 weeks of inhaled exposures. There was a partial return to normal after 7 days. The authors postulated that this increase might relate to loss of epithelial tight junction integrity.
Lai et al. (2012)	Animal model of chronic endotoxin exposure	Airway reactivity increased following endotoxin exposure, followed by an increase in central airway resistance. A balance between dendritic cells (increased) and macrophages (decreased) was seen and postulated as a mechanism for propagating lung inflammation.
Human studies		
Cytokines		
Beshir et al. (2013)	Study of TNF-α, IL-6 and IL-1β in 63 textile workers and 65 non-exposed subjects	IL-1β and IL-6 appeared to show a differential response between those with and without respiratory symptoms. The significance of these findings is as-yet uncertain for exposed textile workers.
Nasal		
Keman et al. (1998)	Nasal lavage carried out in 11 cotton workers following a 2-week break from exposure	Some elevation was seen in IL-8, sTNF-R75 and albumin over the study period, although the changes were not significantly associated with the reduction in measured lung function.
Borm et al. (2000)	Nasal lavage to assess endotoxin binding proteins (same group as Keman et al., 1998)	Increases in bactericidal permeability increasing protein (BPI), albumin and BPI:LBP ratio seen following challenge and lavage. The significance of these findings is uncertain for exposed textile workers
Genes		
Zhang et al. (2013)	SNP assessment in a group of textile workers	Two specific SNPs were identified as potentially relevant to accelerated lung function decline: rs1910047 and rs9469089. The significance of these findings is as-yet uncertain for exposed textile workers.
Blood Markers		
Fishwick et al. (2002)	Cotton workers; study of cross-shift and cross-week blood markers, including monocyte CD14	Cotton workers developed a significant up-regulation in CD14 in comparison to office workers ($p = 0.016$) following 6 hours of work. The significance of these findings is as-yet uncertain for exposed textile workers, although they may suggest a human in vivo-based mechanism for the action of cotton dust and endotoxin exposure.
Venkatakrishna-Bhatt et al. (2001)	Successive weekday study of cotton workers, including blood histamine levels	Histamine levels were significantly higher in the cotton dust-exposed workers in association with decreased FEV_1, peak expiratory flow rate (PEFR) and FEF_{25-75}. The significance of these findings is as-yet uncertain for exposed textile workers, although they may suggest a human in vivo-based mechanism for the action of cotton dust.

Abbreviations: BPI: bactericidal permeability increasing protein; LBP: lipopolysaccharide binding protein; SNP: single-nucleotide polymorphism; FEV_1: forced expiratory volume in 1 second.

2. A typical history of respiratory symptoms (chest tightness and/or shortness of breath) as described in Table 30.1.
3. An acute cross-shift fall in FEV_1, although absence of this finding does not exclude a diagnosis of byssinosis.

No other diagnostic tests (radiological, immunological or physiological) will assist in further confirming a diagnosis of byssinosis, although they may suggest alternative diagnoses such as asthma or COPD. All lung function results must be interpreted, as with all respiratory diseases, in light of other risk factors, including tobacco smoking.

In terms of making a diagnosis of COPD relating to cotton dust exposure, this remains difficult. Whilst there is a substantial body of evidence associating COPD with self-reported occupational exposure to vapours, gases, dusts and fumes, the most likely causes in an individual (cotton dust exposure, smoking, genetics and so on) must be estimated on an individual basis.

Health Surveillance and Periodic Medical Examination

There is no clearly agreed guidance to health surveillance and periodic medical examination in this area, and approaches will vary globally. Previous versions of this text have recommended periodic medical examination and surveillance. Local legislation will most likely dictate a workplace's approach.

In general terms, for those who are at risk of byssinosis, it would be considered good practice to carry out a periodic health assessment with a questionnaire and lung function measurement. This would be carried out in order to identify workers who are developing the typical symptoms of byssinosis so that workplace actions could be taken in order to reduce further risk of progression.

Prevention of Byssinosis

This relates primarily to controlling exposure to cotton dust. This will be achieved by using a combination of approaches. In the UK, for example, a risk-based approach to exposure control is adopted, using a hierarchy of workplace control measures. In general terms, use of respiratory-protective equipment should be regarded as a final control approach when other approaches have failed.

REFERENCES

Altin, R., Ozkurt, S., Fisekçi, F., Cimrin, A. H., Zencir, M. and Sevinc, C. 2002. Prevalence of byssinosis and respiratory symptoms among cotton mill workers. *Respiration* 69(1):52–6.

Ankrah, T. C. 1989. Respiratory symptoms and lung function tests in an African jute factory workers. *West Afr J Med* 8(2):98–105.

Awad elKarim, M. A. and Onsa, S. H. 1987. Prevalence of byssinosis and respiratory symptoms among spinners in Sudanese cotton mills. *Am J Ind Med* 12(3):281–9.

Baker, M. D., Irwig, L. M., Johnston, J. R., Turner, D. M. and Bezuidenhout, B. N. 1979. Lung function in sisal ropemakers. *Br J Ind Med* 36(3):216–9.

Bakirci, N., Kalaca, S., Fletcher, A. M., Pickering, C. A., Tumerdem, N., Cali, S., Oldham, L. et al. 2006. Predictors of early leaving from the cotton spinning mill environment in newly hired workers. *Occup Environ Med* 63(2):126–30.

Bakirci, N., Kalaca, S., Francis, H., Fletcher, A. M., Pickering, C. A., Tumerdem, N., Cali, S. et al. 2007. Natural history and risk factors of early respiratory responses to exposure to cotton dust in newly exposed workers. *J Occup Environ Med* 49(8):853–61.

Barman, M. L. 1979. Prevalence of respiratory disease in a cotton compress and warehouse. A preliminary survey. *J Occup Med* 21(4):273–5.

Barnes, R. and Simpson, G. R. 1976. Variations of pulmonary function amongst workers in cotton mills. *J Occup Med* 18(8):551–5.

Bates, P. J., Farr, S. J. and Nicholls, P. J. 1995. Effect of cotton, hemp and flax dust extracts on lung permeability in the guinea pig. *Exp Lung Res* 21(5):643–65.

Beckett, W. S., Pope, C. A., Xu, X. P. and Christiani, D. C. 1994. Women's respiratory health in the cotton textile industry: An analysis of respiratory symptoms in 973 non-smoking female workers. *Occup Environ Med* 51(1):14–8.

Beshir, S., Mahdy-Abdallah, H. and Saad-Hussein, A. 2013. Ventilatory functions in cotton textile workers and the role of some inflammatory cytokines. *Toxicol Ind Health* 29(2):114–20.

Borm, P. J., Jetten, M., Keman, S. and Schins, R. P. 2000. Endotoxin-binding proteins in nasal lavage: Evaluation as biomarkers to occupational endotoxin exposure. *Biomarkers* 5(2):108–18.

Boubopoulos, N. J., Constandinidis, T. C., Froudarakis, M. E. and Bouros, D. 2010. Reduction in cotton dust concentration does not totally eliminate respiratory health hazards: The Greek study. *Toxicol Ind Health* 26(10):701–7.

Bouhuys, A., Barbero, A., Schilling, R. S. and Van de Woestijne, K. P. 1969. Chronic respiratory disease in hemp workers. *Am J Med* 46(4):526–37.

Bouhuys, A. and Zuskin, E. 1976. Chronic respiratory disease in hemp workers. A follow-up study, 1967–1974. *Ann Intern Med* 84(4):398–405.

Bowden, S. and Tweedale, G. 2003. Mondays without dread: The Trade Union response to byssinosis in the Lancashire cotton industry in the twentieth century. *Soc Hist Med* 16(1):79–95.

Chaari, N., Amri, C., Khalfallah, T., Alaya, A., Abdallah, B., Harzallah, L., Henchi, M. A. et al. 2009. Rhinitis and asthma related to cotton dust exposure in apprentices in the clothing industry. *Rev Mal Respir* 26(1):29–36.

Chattopadhyay, B. P., Alams, J., Gangopadhyay, P. K. and Saiyed, H. N. 1995. Effect of jute dust exposure on ventilatory function and the pertinence of cough and smoking to the response. *J UOEH* 17(2):91–104.

Chattopadhyay, B. P., Saiyed, H. N. and Mukherjee, A. K. 2003. Byssinosis among jute mill workers. *Ind Health* 41(3):265–72.

Choudat, D., Neukirch, F., Brochard, P., Korobaeff, M., Dallet-Grand, A., Perdrizet, S., Marsac, J. et al. 1987. Variation of lung function during the workshift among cotton and jute workers. *Int Arch Occup Environ Health* 59(5):485–92.

Christiani, D. C. and Wang, X. R. 2003. Respiratory effects of long-term exposure to cotton dust. *Curr Opin Pulm Med* 9(2):151–5.

Christiani, D. C., Wang, X. R., Pan, L. D., Zhang, H. X., Sun, B. X., Dai, H., Eisen, E. A. et al. 2001. Longitudinal changes in pulmonary function and respiratory symptoms in cotton textile workers. A 15-yr follow-up study. *Am J Respir Crit Care Med* 163(4):847–53.

Christiani, D. C., Wegman, D. H., Eisen, E. A., Ye, T. T., Lu, P. L. and Olenchock, S. 1993. A. Cotton dust and Gram-negative bacterial endotoxin correlations in two cotton textile mills. *Am J Ind Med* 23(2):333–42.

Christiani, D. C., Ye, T. T., Wegman, D. H., Eisen, E. A., Dai, H. L. and Lu, P. L. 1994. Pulmonary function among cotton textile workers. A study of variability in symptom reporting, across-shift drop in FEV_1 and longitudinal change. *Chest* 105(6):1713–21.

Christiani, D. C., Ye, T. T., Zhang, S., Wegman, D. H., Eisen, E. A., Ryan, L. A., Olenchock, S. A. et al. 1999. Cotton dust and endotoxin exposure and long-term decline in lung function: Results of a longitudinal study. *Am J Ind Med* 35(4):321–31.

Cinkotai, F. F., Rigby, A., Pickering, C. A., Seaborn, D. and Faragher, E. 1988. Recent trends in the prevalence of byssinotic symptoms in the Lancashire textile industry. *Br J Ind Med* 45(11):782–9.

Costa, J. T., Ferreira, J. A., Castro, E., Vaz, M., Barros, H. and Marques, J. A. 2004. One-week variation of cotton dust and endotoxin levels in a cotton mill. Relation with the daily variation of the expiratory flow rates. *Acta Med Port* 17(2):149–56.

Cui, L., Gallagher, L. G., Ray, R. M., Li, W., Gao, D., Zhang, Y., Vedal, S. et al. 2011. Unexpected excessive chronic obstructive pulmonary disease mortality among female silk textile workers in Shanghai, China. *Occup Environ Med* 68(12):883–7.

da Costa, J. T., Barros, H., Macedo, J. A., Ribeiro, H., Mayan, O. and Pinto, A. S. 1997. Respiratory symptoms in the textile industry. Their prevalence in the Vale do Ave. *Acta Med Port* 10(1):7–14.

Das, P. K. and Jha, N. 2009. Occupational exposure and pulmonary function of jute mill workers in Sunsari, Nepal. *Nepal Med Coll J* 11(4):275–7.

Dubrow, R. and Gute, D. M. 1988. Cause-specific mortality among male textile workers in Rhode Island. *Am J Ind Med* 13(4):439–54.

Elwood, P. C., Sweetnam, P. M., Bevan, C. and Saunders, M. J. 1986. Respiratory disability in ex-cotton workers. *Br J Ind Med* 43(9):580–6.

Engelberg, A. L., Piacitelli, G. M., Petersen, M., Zey, J., Piccirillo, R., Morey, P. R., Carlson, M. L. et al. 1985. Medical and industrial hygiene characterization of the cotton waste utilization industry. *Am J Ind Med* 7(2):93–108.

Fang, S. C., Mehta, A. J., Hang, J. Q., Eisen, E. A., Dai, H. L., Zhang, H. X., Su, L. et al. 2013. Cotton dust, endotoxin and cancer mortality among the Shanghai textile workers cohort: A 30-year analysis. *Occup Environ Med* 70(10):722–9.

Farooque, M. I., Khan, B., Aziz, E., Moosa, M., Raheel, M., Kumar, S. and Mansuri, F. A. 2008. Byssinosis: As seen in cotton spinning mill workers of Karachi. *J Pak Med Assoc* 58(2):95–8.

Fishwick, D., Allan, L. J., Wright, A., Barber, C. M. and Curran, A. D. 2001a. Respiratory symptoms, lung function and cell surface markers in a group of hemp fibre processors. *Am J Ind Med* 39(4):419–25.

Fishwick, D., Allan, L. J., Wright, A. and Curran, A. D. 2001b. Assessment of exposure to organic dust in a hemp processing plant. *Ann Occup Hyg* 45(7):577–83.

Fishwick, D., Barraclough, R., Pickering, T., Fletcher, A., Lewis, R., Niven, R. and Warburton, C. J. 2010. Comparison of various airflow measurements in symptomatic textile workers. *Occup Med (Lond)* 60(8):631–4.

Fishwick, D., Fletcher, A. M., Pickering, C. A., McL Niven, R. and Faragher, E. B. 1996. Lung function in Lancashire cotton and man made fibre spinning mill operatives. *Occup Environ Med* 53(1):46–50.

Fishwick, D., Fletcher, A. M., Pickering, C. A., Niven, R. M. and Faragher, E. B. 1992. Lung function, bronchial reactivity, atopic status and dust exposure in Lancashire cotton mill operatives. *Am Rev Respir Dis* 145(5):1103–8.

Fishwick, D., Fletcher, A. M., Pickering, C. A., Niven, R. M. and Faragher, E. B. 1994a. Ocular and nasal irritation in operatives in Lancashire cotton and synthetic fibre mills. *Occup Environ Med* 51(11):744–8.

Fishwick, D., Fletcher, A. M., Pickering, C. A., Niven, R. M. and Faragher, E. B. 1994b. Respiratory symptoms and dust exposure in Lancashire cotton and man-made fibre mill operatives. *Am J Respir Crit Care Med* 150(2):441–7.

Fishwick, D., Raza, S. N., Beckett, P., Swan, J. R., Pickering, C. A., Fletcher, A. M., Niven, R. M. et al. 2002. Monocyte CD14 response following endotoxin exposure in cotton spinners and office workers. *Am J Ind Med* 42(5):437–42.

Glindmeyer, H. W., Lefante, J. J., Jones, R. N., Rando, R. J., Abdel Kader, H. M. and Weill, H. 1991. Exposure-related declines in the lung function of cotton textile workers. Relationship to current workplace standards. *Am Rev Respir Dis* 144(3 Pt 1):675–83.

Glindmeyer, H. W., Lefante, J. J., Jones, R. N., Rando, R. J. and Weill, H. 1994. Cotton dust and across-shift change in FEV_1 as predictors of annual change in FEV_1. *Am J Respir Crit Care Med* 149(3 Pt 1):584–90.

Gordon, T. and Harkema, J. R. 1995. Cotton dust produces an increase in intraepithelial mucosubstances in rat airways. *Am J Respir Crit Care Med* 151(6):1981–8.

Hend, I. M., Milnera, M. and Milnera, S. M. 2003. Bactericidal treatment of raw cotton as the method of byssinosis prevention. *AIHA J (Fairfax, Va)* 64(1):88–94.

Holness, D. L., Taraschuk, I. G. and Pelmear, P. L. 1983. Effect of dust exposure in the cotton felt industry. *J Occup Med* 25(3):191–5.

Honeybourne, D. and Pickering, C. A. 1986. Physiological evidence that emphysema is not a feature of byssinosis. *Thorax* 41(1):6–11.

Jiang, C. Q., Lam, T. H., Kong, C., Cui, C. A., Huang, H. K., Chen, D. C., He, J. M. et al. 1995. Byssinosis in Guangzhou, China. *Occup Environ Med* 52(4):268–72.

Jones, R. N., Butcher, B. T., Hammad, Y. Y., Diem, J. E., Glindmeyer H. W. 3rd, Lehrer, S. B., Hughes, J. M. et al. 1980. Interaction of atopy and exposure to cotton dust in the bronchoconstrictor response. *Br J Ind Med* 37(2):141–6.

Kawamoto, M. M., Garabrant, D. H., Held, J., Balmes, J. R., Patzman, J., Dimick, D. V., Simonowitz, J. A. et al. 1987. Respiratory effects of cotton dust exposure in the cotton garnetting industry. *Am J Ind Med* 11(5):505–15.

Kayumba, A., Moen, B. E., Bratveit, M., Eduard, W. and Mashalla, Y. 2011. Reduced lung function among sisal processors. *Occup Environ Med* 68(9):682–5.

Kayumba, A. V., Bråtveit, M., Mashalla, Y. J., Baste, V. and Moen, B. E. 2008a. Prevalence of respiratory symptoms among sisal processors in Tanzania. *Arch Environ Occup Health* 63(2):76–86.

Kayumba, A. V., Bråtveit, M., Mashalla, Y. and Moen, B. E. 2007. Acute respiratory symptoms among sisal workers in Tanzania. *Occup Med (Lond)* 57(4):290–3.

Kayumba, A. V., Van-Do, T., Florvaag, E., Bråtveit, M., Baste, V., Mashalla, Y., Eduard, W. et al. 2008b. High prevalence of immunoglobulin E (IgE) sensitization among sisal (*Agave sisalana*) processing workers in Tanzania. *Ann Agric Environ Med* 15(2):263–70.

Keman, S., Jetten, M., Douwes, J. and Borm, P. J. 1998. Longitudinal changes in inflammatory markers in nasal lavage of cotton workers. Relation to endotoxin exposure and lung function changes. *Int Arch Occup Environ Health* 71(2):131–7.

Koskela, R. S., Klockars, M. and Järvinen, E. 1990. Mortality and disability among cotton mill workers. *Br J Ind Med* 47(6):384–91.

Lai, P. S. and Christiani, D. C. 2013. Long-term respiratory health effects in textile workers. *Curr Opin Pulm Med* 19(2):152–7.

Lai, P. S., Fresco, J. M., Pinilla MA Pinilla, M. A., Macias, A. A., Brown, R. D., Englert, J. A., Hofmann, O. et al. 2012. Chronic endotoxin exposure produces airflow obstruction and lung dendritic cell expansion. *Am J Respir Cell Mol Biol* 47:209–17.

Lane, S. R. and Sewell, R. D. 2006. The fungal profile of cotton lint from diverse sources and implications for occupational health. *J Occup Environ Hyg* 3(9):508–12.

LeVan, T. D., Koh, W. P., Lee, H. P., Koh, D., Yu, M. C. and London, S. J. 2006. Vapor, dust and smoke exposure in relation to adult-onset asthma and chronic respiratory symptoms: The Singapore Chinese Health Study. *Am J Epidemiol* 163(12):1118–28.

Levin, J. L., Frank, A. L., Williams, M. G., McConnell, W., Suzuki, Y. and Dodson, R. F. 1996. Kaolinosis in a cotton mill worker. *Am J Ind Med* 29(2):215–21.

Li, D. H., Lu, S. X., Ding, M. B. and Zhang, C. J. 1987. Preliminary approach to the diagnosis of byssinosis. *Am J Ind Med* 12(6):731–5.

Liu, M. Z. 1987. The health investigation of cotton textile workers in Beijing. *Am J Ind Med* 12(6):759–64.

Marchand, G., Lalonde, M., Beaudet, Y., Boivin, G., Villeneuve, S. and Pépin, C. 2007. Documentation of the endotoxins present in the ambient air of cotton fibre textile mills in Québec. *Environ Monit* 9(8):869–76.

Mareska, J. and Heyman, J. 1845. Enquête sur le travail et la condition physique et morale des ouvriers employés dans les manufactures de coton, à Gand. *Ann Soc Med Gand* 16. 11:267 p.

Martin, C. F. and Higgins, J. E. 1976. Byssinosis and other respiratory ailments: A survey of 6,631 cotton textile employees. *J Occup Med* 18(7):455–62.

Massin, N., Moulin, J. J., Wild, P., Meyer-Bisch, C. and Mur, J. M. 1991. A study of the prevalence of acute respiratory disorders among workers in the textile industry. *Int Arch Occup Environ Health* 62(8):555–60.

Mastrangelo, G., Fedeli, U., Fadda, E., Milan, G. and Lange, J. H. 2002. Epidemiologic evidence of cancer risk in textile industry workers: A review and update. *Toxicol Ind Health* 18(4):171–81.

Mberikunashe, J., Banda, S., Chadambuka, A., Gombe, N. T., Shambira, G., Tshimanga, M. and Matchaba-Hove, R. 2010. Prevalence and risk factors for obstructive respiratory conditions among textile industry workers in Zimbabwe, 2006. *Pan Afr Med J* 6:1.

McElvenny, D. M., Hurley, M. A., Lenters, V., Heederik, D., Wilkinson, S. and Coggon, D. 2011. Lung cancer mortality in a cohort of UK cotton workers: An extended follow-up. *Br J Cancer* 105(7):1054–60.

Morgan, P. G. and Ong, S. G. 1981. First report of byssinosis in Hong Kong. *Br J Ind Med* 38(3):290–2.

Mukherjee, A. K., Chattopadhyay, B. P., Bhattacharya, S. K. and Saiyed, H. N. 2004. Airborne endotoxin and its relationship to pulmonary function among workers in an Indian jute mill. *Arch Environ Health* 59(4):202–8.

Mundie, T. G., Cordova-Salinas, M., Bray, V. J. and Ainsworth, S. K. 1983. Bioassays of smooth muscle contracting agents in cotton mill dust and bract extracts: Arachidonic acid metabolites as possible mediators of the acute byssinotic reaction. *Environ Res* 32(1):62–71.

Nafees, A. A., Fatmi, Z., Kadir, M. M. and Sathiakumar, N. 2013. Pattern and predictors for respiratory illnesses and symptoms and lung function among textile workers in Karachi, Pakistan. *Occup Environ Med* 70(2):99–107.

Nicholls, P. J., Evans, E., Valić, F. and Zuskin, E. 1973. Histamine-releasing activity and bronchoconstricting effects of sisal. *Br J Ind Med* 30(2):142–5.

Niven, R. M., Fishwick, D., Pickering, C. A., Fletcher, A. M., Warburton, C. J. and Crank, P. 1992. A study of the performance and comparability of the sampling response to cotton dust of work area and personal sampling techniques. *Ann Occup Hyg* 36(4):349–62.

Niven, R. M., Fletcher, A. M., Pickering, C. A., Fishwick, D., Warburton, C. J., Simpson, J. C., Francis, H. et al. 1997. Chronic bronchitis in textile workers. *Thorax* 52(1):22–7.

Noweir, M. H., Noweir, K. H., Myo Tint, U., Win, Z. and Myint, H. 1990. A comparative environmental and medical study of dust exposure in jute and cotton mills in Burma. *J Egypt Public Health Assoc* 65(3–4):349–75.

Noweir, M. H., Noweir, K. H., Osman, H. A. and Moselhi, M. 1984. An environmental and medical study of byssinosis and other respiratory conditions in the cotton textile industry in Egypt. *Am J Ind Med* 6(3):173–83.

Oldenburg, M., Latza, U. and Baur, X. 2007. Exposure–response relationship between endotoxin exposure and lung function impairment in cotton textile workers. *Int Arch Occup Environ Health* 80(5):388–95.

Parikh, J. R., Majumdar, P. K., Shah, A. R., Rao, N. M. and Kashyap, S. K. 1990. Acute and chronic changes in pulmonary functions among Indian textile workers. *J Soc Occup Med* 40(2):71–4.

Paudyal, P., Semple, S., Niven, R., Tavernier, G. and Ayres, J. G. 2011. Exposure to dust and endotoxin in textile processing workers. *Ann Occup Hyg* 55(4):403–9.

Pokrajac, D., Schachter, E. N. and Witek, T. J. Jr. 1990. Respiratory symptoms and lung function in hemp workers. *Br J Ind Med* 47(9):627–32.

Raza, S. N., Fletcher, A. M., Pickering, C. A., Niven, R. M. and Faragher, E. 1999a. Ventilatory function and personal breathing zone dust concentrations in Lancashire textile weavers. *Occup Environ Med* 56(8):520–6.

Raza, S. N., Fletcher, A. M., Pickering, C. A., Niven, R. M. and Faragher, E. B. 1999b. Respiratory symptoms in Lancashire textile weavers. *Occup Environ Med* 56(8):514–9.

Rylander, R., Imbus, H. R. and Suh, M. W. 1979. Bacterial contamination of cotton as an indicator of respiratory effects among card room workers. *Br J Ind Med* 36(4):299–304.

Schilling, R. S. F., Vigliani, E. C., Lammers, B., Valic, F. and Gilson, J. C. 1963. *A report on a Conference on Byssinosis. 14th International Conference on Occupational Health.* Madrid, 137–45. Amsterdam: Execpta Medica.

Shi, J., Hang, J. Q., Mehta, A. J., Zhang, H. X., Dai, H. L., Su, L., Eisen, E. A. et al. 2010a. Long-term effects of work cessation on respiratory health of textile workers: A 25-year follow-up study. *Am J Respir Crit Care Med* 182(2):200–6.

Shi, J., Mehta, A. J., Hang, J. Q., Zhang, H., Dai, H., Su, L., Eisen, E. A. et al. 2010b. Chronic lung function decline in cotton textile workers: Roles of historical and recent exposures to endotoxin. *Environ Health Perspect* 118(11):1620–4.

Sigsgaard, T., Pedersen, O. F., Juul, S. and Gravesen, S. 1992. Respiratory disorders and atopy in cotton, wool and other textile mill workers in Denmark. *Am J Ind Med* 22(2):163–84.

Su, Y. M., Su, J. R., Sheu, J. Y., Loh, C. H. and Liou, S. H. 2003. Additive effect of smoking and cotton dust exposure on respiratory symptoms and pulmonary function of cotton textile workers. *Ind Health* 41(2):109–15.

Thind, G. S. 2009. Acute pulmonary alveolar proteinosis due to exposure to cotton dust. *Lung India* 26(4):152–4.

Valic, F. and Zuskin, E. 1977. Respiratory-function changes in textile workers exposed to synthetic fibres. *Arch Environ Health* 32(6):283–7.

Venkatakrishna-Bhatt, H., Mohan-Rao, N. and Panchal, G. M. 2001. Differential diagnosis of byssinosis by blood histamine and pulmonary function test: A review and an appraisal. *Int J Toxicol* 20(5):321–7.

Wang, X. R., Eisen, E. A., Zhang, H. X., Sun, B. X., Dai, H. L., Pan, L. D., Wegman, D. H. et al. 2003a. Respiratory symptoms and cotton dust exposure; results of a 15 year follow up observation. *Occup Environ Med* 60(12):935–41.

Wang, X. R., Pan, L. D., Zhang, H. X., Sun, B. X., Dai, H. L. and Christiani, D. C. 2002. Follow-up study of respiratory health of newly-hired female cotton textile workers. *Am J Ind Med* 41(2):111–8.

Wang, X. R., Pan, L. D., Zhang, H. X., Sun, B. X., Dai, H. L. and Christiani, D. C. 2003b. A longitudinal observation of early pulmonary responses to cotton dust. *Occup Environ Med* 60(2):115–21.

Wang, X. R., Zhang, H. X., Sun, B. X., Dai, H. L., Hang, J. Q., Eisen, E. A., Wegman, D. H. et al. 2005. A 20-year follow-up study on chronic respiratory effects of exposure to cotton dust. *Eur Respir J* 26(5):881–6.

Wang, X. R., Zhang, H. X., Sun, B. X., Dai, H. L., Pan, L. D., Eisen, E. A., Wegman, D. H. et al. 2004. Is chronic airway obstruction from cotton dust exposure reversible? *Epidemiology* 15(6):695–701.

WHO. 1983. *Recommended Health-based Occupational Exposure Limits for Selected Vegetable Dusts. Report of a WHO Study Group. Technical Report Series 684.* Geneva: World Health Organization.

Woldeyohannes, M., Bergevin, Y., Mgeni, A. Y. and Theriault, G. 1991. Respiratory problems among cotton textile mill workers in Ethiopia. *Br J Ind Med* 48(2):110–5.

Zhang, R., Zhao, Y., Chu, M., Mehta, A., Wei, Y., Liu, Y., Xun, P. et al. 2013. A large scale gene-centric association study of lung function in newly-hired female cotton textile workers with endotoxin exposure. *PLoS One* 8(3):e59035.

Zhong, Y., Li, D., Ma, Q. and Rylander, R. 2002. Lung function and symptoms among cotton workers and dropouts three years after the start of work. *Int J Occup Environ Health* 8(4):297–300.

Zhou, C., Liu, Z. L., Ho, C. S. and Lou, J. Z. 1989. Respiratory symptoms and lung function in jute processing workers: A primary investigation. *Arch Environ Health* 44(6):370–4.

Zuskin, E., Gregurincić, S., Ivanković, D., Kanceljak, B. and Tonković-Lojović, M. 1989. Ventilatory function and allergic skin tests in cotton mill workers. *Arh Hig Rada Toksikol* 40(1):37–46.

Zuskin, E., Ivankovic, D., Schachter, E. N. and Witek, T. J. Jr. 1991. A ten-year follow-up study of cotton textile workers. *Am Rev Respir Dis* 143(2):301–5.

Zuskin, E., Kanceljak, B., Mustajbegović, J. and Kern, J. 1993. Immunologic reactions, respiratory symptoms and ventilatory capacity in jute and sisal textile workers. *Arh Hig Rada Toksikol* 44(1):45–54.

Zuskin, E., Kanceljak, B., Mustajbegovic, J., Schachter, E. N. and Kern, J. 1994a. Respiratory function and immunological reactions in jute workers. *Int Arch Occup Environ Health* 66(1):43–8.

Zuskin, E., Kanceljak, B., Mustajbegovic, J., Schachter, E. N. and Kern, J. 1994b. Respiratory function and immunological reactions in sisal workers. *Int Arch Occup Environ Health* 66(1):37–42.

Zuskin, E., Kanceljak, B., Schachter, E. N., Witek, T. J., Maayani, S., Goswami, S., Marom, Z. et al. 1992a. Immunological findings in hemp workers. *Environ Res* 59;350–61.

Zuskin, E., Kanceljak, B., Schachter, E. N., Witek, T. J., Mustajbegovic, J., Maayani, S., Buck, M. G. et al. 1992b. Immunological findings and respiratory function in cotton textile workers. *Int Arch Occup Environ Health* 64(1):31–7.

Zuskin, E., Mustajbegović, J. and Kanceljak, B. 1992c. Follow-up of respiratory symptoms and pulmonary ventilatory function in jute textile workers. *Lijec Vjesn* 114(9–12):216–20.

Zuskin, E., Mustajbegović, J., Kanceljak, B. and Budak, A. 1992d. Monitoring of respiratory function in hemp-processing workers. *Arh Hig Rada Toksikol* 43(3):237–47.

Zuskin, E., Mustajbegović, J., Kanceljak, B. and Kern, J. 1992e. Monitoring of respiratory symptoms and pulmonary ventilatory function in sisal processing workers. *Arh Hig Rada Toksikol* 43(4):339–47.

Zuskin, E., Mustajbegović, J., Kern, J., Doko-Jelinić, J. and Pavicić, F. 1996. Respiratory findings in textile workers employed in dyeing wool and cotton. *Arh Hig Rada Toksikol* 47(3):295–306.

Zuskin, E., Mustajbegovic, J. and Schachter, E. N. 1994c. Follow-up study of respiratory function in hemp workers. *Am J Ind Med* 26(1):103–15.

Zuskin, E., Mustajbegovic, J., Schachter, E. N. and Doko-Jelinic, J. 1997. Respiratory function of textile workers employed in dyeing cotton and wool fibres. *Am J Ind Med* 31(3):344–52.

31 Chronic Obstructive Pulmonary Disease Including Obstructive Bronchiolitis

Chris Stenton, David J. Hendrick and Cecile Rose

CONTENTS

BACKGROUND

Definitions

Chronic obstructive pulmonary disease (COPD) is characterised by airflow limitation that is not fully reversible, is usually progressive and is associated with an inflammatory response of the lungs to noxious particles or gases (Global Initiative for Chronic Obstructive Lung Disease, 2011). It is the most common form of chronic lung disease in industrially developed countries, and affects some 5%–10% of their populations. It has a substantial adverse effect on work ability (Yelin et al., 2006), quality of life and life expectancy.

The airflow obstruction of COPD can be quantified simply in most individuals as a reduction in the ratio of forced expiratory volume in 1 second (FEV_1) to forced vital capacity (FVC; FEV_1/FVC) on spirometric testing. Recognition is more difficult when there is accompanying fibrotic lung disease caused, for example, by pneumoconiosis. The combination of fibrosis with COPD may lead to normalisation of FEV_1/FVC, albeit with marked impairment of gas transfer and associated disability. FEV_1/FVC is unimodally distributed in the population at large, and so the choice of a threshold with which to define COPD is arbitrary. The Global initiative for Chronic Obstructive Lung Disease (GOLD) criterion of a post-bronchodilator FEV_1/FVC of less than 70% is commonly used, but FEV_1/FVC declines with age, and the GOLD criterion leads to relative under-diagnosis of COPD at younger (working) ages and to relative over-diagnosis in the elderly. The lower limit of normal based on population predicted values is more complex to calculate, but is more appropriate for identifying COPD in working populations (Swanney et al., 2008). Tests of small airway function, such as mid-expiratory flow rates, are sometimes used, but their clinical significance is uncertain when they are not accompanied by reductions in FEV_1 or FEV_1/FVC.

In normal individuals, FEV_1 gradually falls by 20–35 mL/year (Rennard and Vestbo, 2008) from its peak in early adult life. The rate of decline is more rapid in those who are destined to develop COPD: cigarette smokers, for example, have an average annual loss of FEV_1 that is 10–20 mL greater than that of non-smokers (Lange et al., 1989). The adverse effect of cigarette smoking on FVC is less marked than the effect on FEV_1, leading to progressive lowering of the FEV_1/FVC ratio. Serial measurements of FEV_1 that show a more rapid than expected rate of decline serve as a means of detecting COPD at an early stage, provided they are accompanied by a falling FEV_1/FVC ratio. While the average effect of smoking is modest, there is a wide range of individual susceptibility, with most smokers being affected little, but some losing FEV_1 at a rate of 90 mL/year or more. This leads to marked impairment of lung function over two to three decades (Nishimura et al., 2012). The adverse effect of smoking is well understood, and can serve as a useful benchmark against which to assess the effects of occupational and other exposures.

The main site of the airflow obstruction of COPD is in the small airways i.e. those less than 2 mm in diameter). The principal histological components are: the destruction of alveolar walls (emphysema) with loss of support for the small airways; epithelial thickening and peri-bronchiolar fibrosis; and a reduction in the number of small airways (Burgel et al., 2011). COPD associated with chronic asthma is associated with less emphysema than COPD associated with cigarette smoking (Zhang et al., 2014). Both emphysema and small airways disease have been described in association with occupational exposures, but there has been no systematic evaluation of the relative contribution of each or of whether that may vary by cause.

Small airway disease is a feature of hypersensitivity pneumonitis and bronchiolitis. A number of occupational diseases centred on the bronchioles have been recognised to cause fixed airway obstruction in recent decades, although typically with a subacute timescale and often with involvement of the adjacent gas-exchanging tissues and the lung interstitium. These are discussed separately under the heading 'Occupational bronchiolitis'.

Non-Occupational Factors

Cigarette smoking is the most important cause of COPD and, until the 1980s, it was considered to be the only established environmental cause. It is now recognised that COPD occurs in non-smokers and that cigarette smoking is responsible for only 50%–70% of the variation in COPD prevalence found in epidemiological studies (Eisner et al., 2010). There are clearly other important aetiological factors.

Failure to achieve maximum lung growth because of intrauterine or early-life influences can contribute, as can genetic factors; however, with the exception of α1 antitrypsin deficiency, these are poorly understood. Asthma and its functional hallmark, airway hyperresponsiveness, are important determinants of COPD in adults (Harber et al., 2007). Childhood asthma that persists into adult life is associated with a risk of fixed airflow obstruction that is similar to that associated with a 40-pack-year smoking history (Perret et al., 2013). Asthma is an important consideration in studies of COPD, as it causes similar symptoms and lung function abnormalities. A meta-analysis of 116 COPD studies (Forey et al., 2011) found that 18 excluded asthmatics, 69 ignored asthma and the remainder either included asthma in the definition of COPD or dealt with it in some other way. The way asthma was considered markedly influenced the estimated effects of smoking. Similar considerations are likely to be important in studies of occupational exposures.

Aside from smoking and work, exposure to particulates from biomass cooking is probably the most important environmental cause of COPD. Studies have shown adverse effects that are of similar magnitude to those of smoking (Kurmi et al., 2010). There is evidence of an association between outdoor air pollution and impaired lung growth during childhood and adolescence, and a growing body of literature links outdoor particulate matter exposures during adult life to impaired lung function, COPD diagnosis and hospital admissions (Garshick, 2014).

Occupational Bronchitis

The term COPD is a relatively modern one, and much of the earlier literature discusses separately the conditions chronic bronchitis and emphysema. Approximately 30%–40% of individuals with COPD report symptoms of chronic bronchitis, defined as a productive daily cough for at least 3 consecutive months per year for at least 2 consecutive years (Kim and Criner, 2013). Bronchitis can develop without airflow obstruction (Pelkonen et al., 2006), and it is unclear why some individuals develop it and others do not. In those with COPD, it is associated with poorer outcomes, including an increased rate of symptom exacerbations, accelerated decline in lung function, poorer health-related quality of life and possibly increased mortality (Kim and Criner, 2013). These adverse outcomes may be related to the heightened systemic inflammation that is often a feature of COPD.

Bronchitic symptoms are common in those with occupational exposures to dust and fume. Historically, cough and phlegm were reported by approximately two-thirds of coal miners (Rogan et al., 1973) and were more common in those with heavy exposures (Marine et al., 1988). Individuals with occupational bronchitis are more likely than others to have airflow obstruction (Rogan et al., 1973; Attfield and Hodous, 1992; Henneberger and Attfield, 1996), but the airflow obstruction can precede or follow the bronchitis (Beeckman et al., 2001), and the relationship is not causal. Bronchitic symptoms can be identified using questionnaires and so are easier to study than abnormalities of lung function. Symptom reporting is prone to recall bias, but the frequency with which bronchitic symptoms are reported in association with occupational exposures to dust or fume provides persuasive evidence that they can have adverse effects on the airways.

AETIOLOGIES OF OCCUPATIONAL COPD

Cigarette smoke is a complex mixture of particles, vapours and gases, and in that respect can be considered similar to many occupational exposures. No individual constituent of cigarette smoke has been identified as the cause of COPD, and it is biologically plausible that other exposures, such as those encountered in workplaces, might have the same effect.

The evidence that occupational exposures cause COPD has emerged slowly over the last few decades and with much controversy (Nemery, 1990). COPD caused by occupational exposures does not have any clinical or pathophysiological features that allow it to be distinguished from COPD of non-occupational origin. There is evidence from animal studies that occupational gas and dust exposures cause inflammatory changes in the lung, but the characterisation of occupational COPD has primarily been through epidemiological investigation.

Studies of working populations are subject to a number of biases that limit their power to identify associations. Healthy worker and survivor biases are difficult to quantify, but are likely to be substantial. In a study of South African gold miners exposed to silica, younger miners started their working lives with FEV_1 values that were higher than those expected in non-miners by an amount that was approximately equal to the adverse effect of a working lifetime's exposure (Hnizdo, 1992). In some studies of cotton workers, more than 50% of the workforce had left within a year, with those who were most symptomatic being most likely to be among them (Bakirci et al., 2006). Studies of coal miners have found average adverse effects of working lifetime exposures in older miners that were half or less than half of those found in younger miners (Rogan et al., 1973; Lewis et al., 1996). This is probably because miners who developed early adverse health effects stopped mining, leaving a relatively resistant workforce. In general, healthy worker and survivor biases are likely to lead to underestimation of the effects of occupational exposures.

Age and smoking strongly influence COPD prevalence and can be difficult to control for in epidemiological studies. Much of the evidence relating to occupational exposures has emerged from the establishment of exposure–response relationships within working populations. The three main determinants of lung function—cumulative exposure, age and smoking pack-years—can be highly correlated, making their effects difficult to distinguish, particularly when relatively crude measures of cumulative exposure (such as the number of years worked) are used.

The relationship between cumulative exposure and smoking may be complicated further because individuals who can tolerate tobacco smoke may be more likely to choose to work in environments that are contaminated by dust or fume (Beach et al., 1996) and may be more likely to tolerate the adverse effects of exposure without leaving. Occasionally, as with cadmium, there is a good biomarker that allows cumulative exposure to be quantified, but this is usually not the case. Given these epidemiological challenges, it has generally not been possible to demonstrate conclusively from a single study that a particular exposure can cause COPD, even if the magnitude of the effect appears relatively large (i.e. on a par with that of smoking) (Nemery, 1990). The weight of numerous studies, however, points to causal associations.

There are two principal sources of evidence relating occupational exposures to COPD: studies of specific workforces and general population surveys, each with strengths and weaknesses. At their best, workforce studies include a large number of subjects, have detailed measures of exposure, have sufficient variability across the workforce to allow for the effects of age and smoking to be distinguished and include ex-workers as well as those who are currently employed. General population studies allow for a broader range of exposures to be evaluated and can quantify the overall contribution of occupational exposures to COPD.

COAL

Emphysema associated with dust accumulation around terminal bronchioles has long been known to be an early histological feature of coal workers' pneumoconiosis, and clinically significant emphysema a feature of progressive massive fibrosis. Early studies demonstrated the lack of association between the degree of simple coal workers' pneumoconiosis and impairment of lung function, leading to the view that in the absence of progressive massive fibrosis, coal mine dust exposure was relatively benign. However, extensive investigation from the 1950s involving more than 50,000 miners demonstrated clear negative associations between lung function and cumulative coal mine dust exposure that were independent of the presence or severity of simple pneumoconiosis and of smoking. These were attributed to COPD. The estimates of the effects of coal mine dust exposure varied between studies, but overall the effect was on a par with that of cigarette smoking (Table 31.1). Thus, Rogan et al. (1973) showed that every year worked with dust exposures of 3 mg/m^3 (the current UK exposure standard) was associated with a reduction in FEV_1 of approximately 3 mL. This was similar to the average excess loss of FEV_1 associated with smoking 20 cigarettes per day.

There is no clear interaction between smoking and coal mine dust exposure, and the effects appear to be additive (Attfield and Hodous, 1992). More importantly, there appears to be a wide variation in individual susceptibility, with the adverse effects varying markedly in severity amongst exposed individuals. The probability of a miner having an FEV_1 of less than 65% of the predicted value has been shown to be approximately doubled both by 35 years of smoking and by 35 years of work with relatively heavy dust exposures (in the region of 6 mg/m^3) (Marine et al., 1988). Coal miners have a standardised mortality ratio (SMR) for COPD that is increased to 110%–120% and is related to the extent of their lifetime dust exposure (Miller and MacCalman, 2010; Graber et al., 2014).

The adverse effects of coal mine dust have been less consistently demonstrated in longitudinal studies compared with cross-sectional studies. Four large studies demonstrated associations between earlier cumulative exposures and the current rate of decline of FEV_1, but were unable to demonstrate clear associations with exposure during the study period (Love and Miller, 1982; Attfield, 1985; Seixas et al., 1993; Henneberger and Attfield, 1996). This suggests that the adverse effects of coal mine dust can be ongoing after exposures cease and that the maximum effect might only be seen several years later. The first few years of mining have been shown in some studies to have a much more marked adverse effect than later exposures—by as much as 20-fold (Seixas et al., 1993; Wang et al., 2005)—with some subsequent recovery of lung function despite ongoing exposures. There may be differential effects of exposure at different ages, with the developing lungs of young miners being particularly susceptible. It may also be the case that some of the adverse effects seen in miners are related to exposures other than coal dust (e.g. silica, fumes from shot blasting, roof bolting resins or microbially contaminated water sprays) (Wang et al., 1999). The relationship with occupational exposures is likely to be more complex than that assumed by a simple COPD model of gradual decline of lung function that is proportional to cumulative exposure to dust.

There is little evidence directly addressing the structural basis of the impaired lung function of coal miners, but there is no good evidence to suggest that it differs from that associated with cigarette smoking. In general, exposure to coal mine dust appears to cause airflow obstruction more than restriction, with a dust-related effect on FEV_1 that is greater than the effect on FVC (Figure 31.1), although not all studies have demonstrated this (Soutar and Hurley, 1986). Only one study of sufficient size has included gas transfer measurements (Carta et al., 1996). It showed dust-related impairment that was of similar magnitude to that seen with cigarette smoking, suggesting that emphysema contributes to coal miners' airflow obstruction. More direct evidence of emphysema comes from autopsy studies showing relationships between lifetime dust exposure, post-mortem lung dust content and the presence and severity of emphysema. The effects of dust exposure in these autopsy studies were of similar magnitude to those associated with cigarette smoking (Kuempel et al., 2009).

The centrilobular ('focal') emphysema associated with coal workers' pneumoconiosis was previously assumed to be the cause of coal miners' airflow obstruction, but this does not appear to be the case, as there is no relationship between the presence or extent of simple coal workers' pneumoconiosis and airflow obstruction (Rogan et al., 1973). While both are related to the extent of exposure, they appear to be independent processes. A UK study showed no association between regional mortality rates from pneumoconiosis and from COPD, supporting the view that the two diseases are not directly related to each other (Coggon et al., 1995).

Underground coal mining provides the clearest example of occupational COPD with a large body of evidence, consistently demonstrated associations between the extent of exposure and the degree of lung function impairment, a lack of any association with simple pneumoconiosis, obstructive lung function abnormalities, independence from smoking and a close association with the presence of emphysema. Open cast (surface) mining has been less extensively investigated than underground mining in relation to the risk of COPD. One study of surface miners with relatively low average dust exposures (i.e. less than 1 mg/m^3) failed to identify any adverse effects (Love et al., 1997). Some surface miners have heavy dust exposures, and it is likely that they face COPD risks that are similar to those of underground miners. Associations between residential proximity to coal

TABLE 31.1

Comparative Negative Effects on Forced Expiratory Volume in 1 Second (mL) of Dust Exposure, Smoking and Ageing on Lung Function

Study	Year	References	Exposure	n	Effect of Dust Exposure (per mg/m³-year)	Effect of Smoking (per pack-year)	Effect of Ageing (per year)
Coal							
Attfield	1992	Attfield and Hodous (1992)	Coal mine dust	7139	0.7	11.9[a]	31
Rogan	1973	Rogan et al. (1973)	Coal mine dust	3581	1.0	3.0[a]	47
Cowie	2006	Cowie et al. (2006)	Coal mine dust	7115	1.1	8.6[a]	35
Henneberger (1985–1988)	1998	Henneberger and Attfield (1996)	Coal mine dust	1915	1.2	14.9[a]	27
Soutar and Hurley	1986	Soutar and Hurley (1986)	Coal mine dust	4059	1.3	13.0[a]	41
Marine	1988	Marine et al. (1988)	Coal mine dust	3380	1.6		35
Seixas (1985–1988 survey)	1993	Seixas et al. (1993)	Coal mine dust	977	5.9	10.5[a]	42
Carta[b]	1996	Carta et al. (1996)	Coal mine dust	909	7.6	8.0	
Seixas (1972–1975 survey)	1993	Seixas et al. (1993)	Coal mine dust	977	27.5	9.4[a]	42
Silica-Containing Dusts							
Wild	2007	Wild et al. (2008)	Talc mining/milling	378	0.7	6.2	25
Hertzberg[b]	2003	Hertzberg et al. (2002)	Foundry workers	242	1.1		
Johnsen	2010	Johnsen et al. (2010)	Smelting	2620	3.6	6.0[c]	
Humerfelt	1998	Humerfelt et al. (1998)	Quartz containing	2542	4.3[d]	6.9	5
Johnsen	2013	Johnsen et al. (2013)	Silicon carbide	456	7.4[d]	6.1[c]	
Osterman	1989	Osterman et al. (1989)	Silicon carbide	156	12.0	7.3	
Ehrlich	2010	Ehrlich et al. (2011)	Gold mining	520	16.2[e]	NS	
Mohner[b]	2012	Möhner et al. (2013)	Uranium miners	1942	21.0	3.9	27[f]
Cowie	1991	Cowie and Mabena (1991)	Gold mining	1197	21.2[a,g]	6.9	
Hertzberg	2002	Hertzberg et al. (2002)	Foundry workers	523	26.0	7.8	26
Hnizdo	1992	Hnizdo (1992)	Gold mining	1625	28.0[h]	3.9	35
Non-Silica-Containing Dusts							
Harber	2003	Harber et al. (2003)	Carbon black	1753	0.7	6.6[a]	35
Gardiner	2001	Gardiner et al. (2001)	Carbon black	2646	1.2		
Lotz	2006	Lotz et al. (2008)	Potash mining	840	12.7		

Note: Average annual adverse effects of exposure to 1 mg/m^3 dust, cigarette smoking and ageing in studies of occupational chronic obstructive pulmonary disease where the information is available in the paper. NS = not significant.

[a] Assumes starting smoking at 16 years with a constant effect after that.

[b] Longitudinal study.

[c] Figure for average smoking.

[d] Per year of exposure.

[e] Excludes additional contributions from silicosis and duration of work.

[f] At 50 years of age (term for age^2 included).

[g] Includes effect of category 1/1 pneumoconiosis.

[h] Assumes 1740 working hours per year (Rogan et al., 1973).

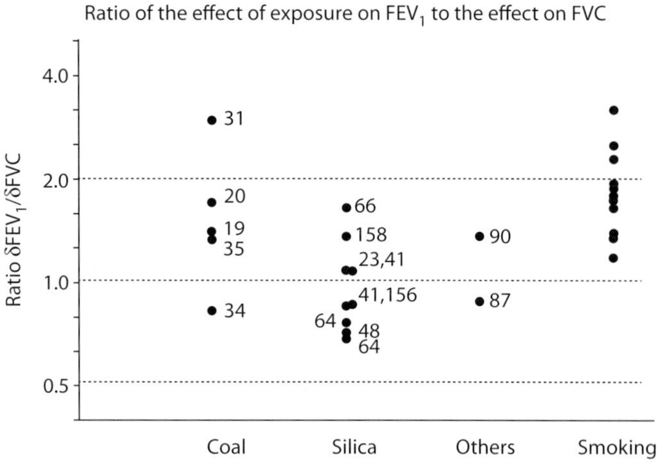

FIGURE 31.1 Ratios of the regression coefficients relating forced expiratory volume in 1 second (FEV_1) to exposure to coefficients relating forced vital capacity (FVC) to exposure in 20 studies of coal mining, silica-containing dusts (gold mining, talc, silicon carbide, cement, ceramics and mixed exposures) and other exposures (potash mining and carbon black). The ratios of the regression equations relating smoking to FEV_1 and FVC are taken from the same studies. The scale is logarithmic. A ratio of 1.0 indicates an equal effect on FEV_1 and FVC, but because FEV_1 is less than FVC, any ratio greater than approximately 0.75 will indicate airflow obstruction. Smoking generally has twice the effect on FEV_1 compared with FVC (ratio of coefficients = 2).

mining and respiratory ill health have been reported, but the mechanism is unclear (Hendryx and Luo, 2015).

Silica and Silica-Containing Dusts

Respirable silica causes pneumoconiosis (silicosis) at much lower levels of exposure than coal dust. It also appears to be a more potent cause of impaired lung function. South African gold miners exposed to dust with 30% silica content were shown in three large cross-sectional surveys to have exposure-related lung function decrements (Cowie and Mabena, 1991; Hnizdo, 1992; Ehrlich et al., 2011). The negative effect on FEV_1 was up to 28 mL for every year worked with respirable silica exposures of 1 mg/m^3 (i.e. more than an order of magnitude greater than the typical effects of coal mine dust) (Table 31.2). German uranium miners who were exposed to dust containing 13% quartz had a 21-mL reduction in FEV_1 for each year of silica exposure at 1 mg/m^3 (Möhner et al., 2013). Similar effects have been reported in hard rock miners and granite quarry workers exposed to dusts containing 6%–11% crystalline silica (Manfreda et al., 1982; Kreiss et al., 1989; Graham et al., 1994; Vacek et al., 2011; Verma et al., 2011).

Several studies (Kreiss et al., 1989; Hnizdo, 1992; Hochgatterer et al., 2013) have shown clearer adverse effects of silica exposure in smokers than in non-smokers, suggesting a multiplicative interaction between the two (Hnizdo et al., 1990). Some studies have shown associations between the presence of silicotic nodules and airflow obstruction (Cowie and Mabena, 1991; Hnizdo et al., 2000; Ehrlich et al., 2011). In others, the exposure-related reductions in FEV_1 and FVC were of similar magnitude (Figure 31.1) (Hnizdo, 1992), suggesting additional fibrotic effects of exposure or effects that are otherwise atypical of COPD.

SMRs for COPD of up to 440% have been reported in silica-exposed workers (Calvert et al., 2003; Scarselli et al., 2011; Cherry et al., 2013; Kreuzer et al., 2013; Tse et al., 2014), with evidence of an exposure–response relationship in some studies (Scarselli et al., 2011; Cherry et al., 2013). Initial reports suggested a strong association between silica exposure and the presence of emphysema at autopsy (Becklake et al., 1987), but this was not confirmed in subsequent larger studies (Hnizdo et al., 1991, 1994, 2000). The absence of a close association between silica exposure and the presence of emphysema has led some to suggest that its dominant effects are in the small airways (Hnizdo et al., 2000). Silica and other mineral dusts are associated with inflammation and fibrosis of the walls of membranous and respiratory bronchioles and alveolar ducts, a condition known as mineral dust airway disease (Churg and Wright, 1983). The histological appearances are considered to be distinguishable from those associated with cigarette smoking. Relatively small studies have shown the lesions of mineral dust airway disease to be associated with abnormalities of lung function, including decreases in FEV_1 and mid expiratory flow (FEF_{25-75}). An autopsy study of 700 gold miners identified little association between antemortem lung function and the presence of bronchitis and bronchiolitis at autopsy after controlling for emphysema severity (Hnizdo et al., 2000). The clinical significance of abnormalities of the small airways for obstructive lung disease associated with respirable silica is therefore uncertain.

Many workers other than metal miners are exposed to dusts with typically lower concentrations of silica. Airflow obstruction has been reported in construction workers (Ulvestad et al., 2000), cement workers (Nordby et al., 2011), tunnellers (Ulvestad et al., 2000), brick makers (Chen et al., 2001), foundry workers (Hertzberg et al., 2002), smelter workers (Johnsen et al., 2010) and in general population surveys (Humerfelt et al., 1998). As the silica content of a dust falls, it becomes increasingly difficult to attribute adverse effects to it, rather than to other

TABLE 31.2
Agents Causing or Suspected of Causing Chronic Obstructive Pulmonary Disease

Agent	Industry	References
Coal/carbon	Coal mining	Rogan et al. (1973), Marine et al. (1988), Attfield and Hodous (1992), Henneberger and Attfield (1996), Beeckman et al. (2001), Lewis et al. (1996), Beach et al. (1996), Miller and MacCalman (2010), Graber et al. (2014), Love and Miller (1982), Attfield (1985), Seixas et al. (1993), Wang et al. (2005), Wang et al. (1999), Soutar and Hurley (1986), Carta et al. (1996), Kuempel et al. (2009), Coggon et al. (1995), Love et al. (1997)
	Carbon black	Gardiner et al. (2001), Harber et al. (2003)
Silica	Mining: gold, uranium, others	Cowie and Mabena (1991), Ehrlich et al. (2011), Möhner et al. (2013), Manfreda et al. (1982), Hnizdo et al. (1990), Hnizdo et al. (2000), Kreuzer et al. (2013), Becklake et al. (1987), Hnizdo et al. (1991), Hnizdo et al. (1994)
	Quarrying	Kreiss et al. (1989), Verma et al. (2011), Graham et al. (1994), Vacek et al. (2011)
	Construction	Ulvestad et al. (2000), Bergdahl et al. (2004)
	Tunnelling	Ulvestad et al. (2000)
	Cement production	Nordby et al. (2011)
	Pottery/ceramic work	Cherry et al. (2013)
	Foundry work	Hertzberg et al. (2002)
	Smelting	Johnsen et al. (2010)
	Silicon carbide production	Johnsen et al. (2013), Osterman et al. (1989)
Metals/inorganic dusts	Iron/steel	Kauffman et al. (1982), Wang et al. (1997)
	Cadmium	Davison et al. (1988), Moitra et al. (2013)
Fibres	Asbestos	Wright and Churg (1985), Wilken et al. (2011), Piirila et al. (2009), Ameille et al. (2010), Miller and Rom (2010), American Thoracic Society (2004)
	Cotton, hemp	Glindmeyer et al. (1994), Christiani et al. (1994), Wang et al. (2008), Bouhuys and Zuskin (1976), Christiani et al. (2001)
	Silk	Cui et al. (2011)
	Wool	Love et al. (1991), Zuskin et al. (1995)
Organic dusts	Grain	Becklake (2007), Huy et al. (1991), Tabona et al. (1984)
	Wood	Jacobsen et al. (2010), Dahlqvist and Ulfvarson (1994), Jacobsen et al. (2013)
	Farming	Szczyrek et al. (2011), Monso et al. (2005), Lamprecht et al. (2007), Eduard et al. (2009)
Gases/fumes	Welding	Szram et al. (2013), Thaon et al. (2012)
	Coke fumes	Hu et al. (2006)
	Bleach (Cl/SO_2), sulphur dioxide	Mehta et al. (2005)
	Ammonia	Kauffman et al. (1982)
	Firefighting	Choi et al. (2014)
	Diesel exhaust	Lotz et al. (2008), Hart et al. (2012)
Chemical agents	Isocyanates	Diem et al. (1982)
	Pesticides	de Jong et al. (2014)
Others	Rubber/plastics/leather, Armed Forces	Hnizdo et al. (2002)

concomitant exposures (Humerfelt et al., 1998; Bergdahl et al., 2004). Coal mine dust in the USA and UK contains on average 4%–5% silica. Mortality studies of coal miners have shown relationships between silica exposure and death from COPD (Miller and MacCalman, 2010; Graber et al., 2014), but these are no closer than the relationships with total dust exposure, suggesting that the silica content is not an important independent determinant of the effect.

While the association between silica exposure and airflow obstruction is often considered to be convincing, the nature of the lung function abnormalities (sometimes obstructive, sometimes restrictive), their pathological basis (the lack of association with emphysema), their association with pneumoconiosis in some studies and their interaction with smoking all imply greater complexity than appears to be the case with coal mine dust exposure.

Asbestos

Asbestos is an important cause of pneumoconiosis (asbestosis). In animal studies, the earliest lesion of asbestosis is thickening and fibrosis of the bronchiolar walls with associated airway narrowing similar to the small airways disease described with silica and other mineral dusts. Small airway abnormalities have been described in the lungs of asbestos miners (Wright and Churg, 1985), and there is reason to suspect from the pathological appearances that asbestos exposures might cause airflow obstruction.

A number of early studies purported to demonstrate airflow obstruction in asbestos-exposed populations, but they generally had poorly matched control populations or relied solely on tests of small airways function. A meta-analysis of ten studies (2192 subjects) of airway function in asbestos-exposed workers showed FEV_1/FVC to be reduced by approximately 5%, but there was potential for confounding by smoking and the effects of other occupational exposures (Wilken et al., 2011). More recent studies (Piirila et al., 2009; Ameille et al., 2010) have failed to provide consistent or conclusive information on the issue (Miller and Rom, 2010). An American Thoracic Society review concluded that asbestos has a relatively small effect on airways function that, by itself, is unlikely to result in functional impairment (American Thoracic Society, 2004). It seems likely that, under most circumstances, any functional effects of asbestos on the airways are overwhelmed by its effects on the pleura and the lung parenchyma.

Metals and Metal Compounds

Cadmium is a constituent of cigarette smoke and is a possible though unlikely contributor to smoking-induced COPD (Mannino et al., 2004). It can cause emphysema along with a variety of other inflammatory responses in animal lungs (Zhang et al., 2010). It is encountered in industry in battery manufacture, alloy, plastic and fertiliser production and soldering/brazing. Human studies have demonstrated associations between exposure, impaired lung function (including gas transfer measurements) and radiological abnormalities suggestive of emphysema (Davison et al., 1988; Moitra et al., 2013). Aluminium refinery workers have been shown to have reductions of FEV_1 of approximately 4 mL per (mg/m^3)-year of dust exposure (Townsend et al., 1985), although this may have been related in part to the known asthmagenic effect of aluminium smelting. Chromium exposure in stainless steel workers has also been reported to be associated with airflow obstruction, but this might also be related to its asthmagenic properties (Huvinen et al., 1996).

One small study from Iran showed lower lung function with obstructive features in manganese miners compared with a control population (Boojar and Goodarzi, 2002). A larger study of 1658 workers from Guangxi in China showed associations between exposure and impaired small airway function, but not with FEV_1 or FVC (Wang et al., 2015). There have been suggestions of airway effects from exposure to cobalt (or hard metal) and titanium dioxide, although abnormalities have not been reported consistently (Nemery, 1990). Beryllium workers have been reported to have an increased SMR for COPD (Schubauer-Berigan et al., 2011), and one study identified very marked exposure-associated decrements of lung function characterised by airflow obstruction (Kriebel et al., 1988). Titanium dioxide nanoparticles have been shown to induce a number of inflammatory effects in the lung and have been implicated in the development of emphysema in rats (Chen et al., 2006). There are as yet no human studies of long-term effects, but it is possible that titanium dioxide and other nanoparticles might have an adverse effect on the airways because of their very small size and hence high surface area to mass ratio.

Other Inorganic Dusts

Many industrial workers are exposed to poorly soluble dusts that are generally considered to be of low toxicity. They are sometimes termed 'nuisance' dusts. A meta-analysis of 27 studies examining the relationship between such 'bio-persistent granular dust' exposures and COPD (Brüske et al., 2013) showed the mean FEV_1 of exposed workers to be 160 mL less than that of reference populations, and the risk of COPD to be increased by 7% for each mg/m^3 of average exposure. Exposures examined included those associated with smelting, steel working and rubber production. The magnitude of the adverse effect varied widely, with average declines in FEV_1 ranging from 1 to 33 mL for every year of exposure to dust concentrations of 1 mg/m^3.

Carbon black has an ultrafine particle size in the range of 10–500 nm, giving it a very high surface area to mass ratio and hence rendering it potentially biologically active. Eleven studies have investigated its effects, mainly in the rubber industry where it is widely used. Two large studies (Gardiner et al., 2001; Harber et al., 2003) showed dust-related respiratory effects that were of similar magnitude to those demonstrated in coal miners, with FEV_1 reduced by 0.7–1.2 mL for every year of exposure to concentrations of 1 mg/m^3. The effect was clearly obstructive in only one of the studies. Carbon black is also the main component of photocopier toner.

Exposures have been reported to cause respiratory symptoms and pneumoconiosis (Gallard et al., 1994), but three studies involving over 2100 subjects failed to identify an exposure-related impairment of lung function (Kitamura et al., 2009).

German potash miners were shown to have very marked adverse effects of exposure on ventilatory function in cross-sectional and longitudinal studies (Lotz et al., 2008), with FEV_1 falling by 12.7 mL for each mg/m^3-year of exposure. There were close correlations between exposure to dust, nitrogen oxides from blasting and diesel exhaust fumes, and it was not possible to separate these effects. No effect of exposure was found in a study of Saskatchewan potash miners (Graham et al., 1984). Polyvinylchloride dust exposure has been associated with a reduction in FEV_1 of 4 mL per year of exposure at 1 mg/m^3 (Soutar et al., 1980). However, this decline was associated with a parallel fall in FVC and with pneumoconiosis, suggesting that the underlying disease process was not typical of COPD.

Although less influential than the studies of coal and silica exposures, these studies of other dusts are important in suggesting that a COPD-inducing effect is not confined to fibrogenic dusts. It may be a generic property of almost any inorganic dust, depending on particle size and exposure level.

Specific Fume and Gas Exposures

Welding fume is a complex mixture of respirable metal oxide particles and reactive gases such as ozone and nitrogen oxides, which are potentially damaging to the airways. Cross-sectional and longitudinal surveys of welders have indicated an effect on lung function of similar magnitude to that caused by smoking (Chinn et al., 1990). Szram et al. carried out a meta-analysis of seven longitudinal studies involving 732 welders (Szram et al., 2013). Overall, welding fume exposure was associated with a 9-mL per annum greater fall in FEV_1 compared with controls, although this did not reach statistical significance in the meta-analysis. There was a suggestion of a synergistic effect with smoking. A recent study of 543 welders reported a similar effect (7-mL reduction of FEV_1 per year of exposure) that was of borderline statistical significance and approximately two-thirds of the magnitude of the effect associated with smoking (Thaon et al., 2012).

Diesel exhaust also contains a complex mixture of particulates, gases and vapours. There are suggestions that exposed workers in mining, construction (Lotz et al., 2008), railways (Hart et al., 2009) and other industries are at increased risk of COPD, but the evidence is limited (Hart et al., 2012). Coke oven emissions comprise a mixture of particulates and volatile organic compounds. A study of 712 coke oven workers (Hu et al., 2006) showed an exposure-related increased risk of COPD that was of similar magnitude to that associated with smoking, with a more than additive interaction between the two. One study of 674 asphalt workers exposed to bitumen fumes showed a higher prevalence of COPD compared with construction workers (Randem et al., 2004), and asphalt workers have been shown to have an increased SMR for non-malignant respiratory disease. Firefighters have been reported to have a higher than expected prevalence of respiratory symptoms and a more rapid rate of decline of ventilatory function (Choi et al., 2014).

There is limited evidence relating the risk of airflow obstruction to the effects of other chemical agents. A recent study of a largely rural population showed a strong association between pesticide exposures and accelerated decline of lung function, with FEV_1 falling by an additional 6.2 mL/year in those with heavy exposures (de Jong et al., 2014). Chlorine and sulphur dioxide exposures in paper pulp mill workers have been associated with airflow obstruction (Mehta et al., 2005). A Polish study identified chemical exposures generally as a significant predictor of FEV_1 decline (Krzyzanowski et al., 1988). Some studies have identified exposure to variable temperature as a predictor of FEV_1 decline, but the mechanism for this is uncertain (Kauffman et al., 1982; Krzyzanowski et al., 1988).

Organic Dusts and Asthmagenic Agents

Workers exposed to organic dusts are at risk of a number of respiratory diseases, at least some of which (such as allergic alveolitis and asthma) are immunologically mediated and caused either by the dust itself or by contaminating microbes (or their products, such as endotoxin). Organic dusts also cause COPD, although whether this too is immunologically mediated or develops through separate mechanisms is unknown.

Farming is associated with a high prevalence of COPD (Szczyrek et al., 2011), at least in animal farmers (Rushton, 2007). Non-smoking European farmers have a reported prevalence of COPD of 17% (Monso et al., 2005), while Austrian farmers (Lamprecht et al., 2007) and Norwegian livestock farmers (Eduard et al., 2009) have an approximately 1.5-fold increased risk of COPD. Grain workers can develop acute grain fever, eye and mucus membrane irritation, cross-shift declines in lung function and asthma. A series of Canadian studies showed that they also had higher prevalences of chronic respiratory symptoms, poorer lung function compared with a reference population and a more rapid rate of longitudinal lung function decline (Becklake, 2007). The effects were exposure related, with 1 mg/m^3 of grain dust having approximately a sixth of the effect of smoking (Huy et al., 1991).

Dust from cotton processing is a prime example of an organic substance that is associated with COPD. Studies have demonstrated higher prevalences of bronchitic symptoms, airflow obstruction and a rapid rate of decline of FEV_1 in exposed workers (Lai and Christiani, 2013). The quantitative relationship with cotton dust exposure is poor, possibly because the main effect is caused by contaminating endotoxin, but overall the effect of cotton dust exposure appears to be similar to that which is associated with smoking (Christiani et al., 1994; Glindmeyer et al., 1994; Wang et al., 2008). There is conflicting evidence regarding whether cotton processing is associated with emphysema or whether the chronic airflow obstruction is associated with airway disease only (Lai and Christiani, 2013). Similar effects are seen in hemp workers (Bouhuys and Zuskin, 1976). Silk workers have been shown to have slightly slower rates of decline of FEV_1 than cotton workers (Christiani et al., 2001), although they also have a higher SMR for COPD (Cui et al., 2011). Studies of wool textile workers have also suggested associations between dust exposures and chronic respiratory symptoms and impairment of lung function. A UK study showed exposure-related effects, but only in female workers (Love et al., 1991). A Croatian study showed lower mid-expiratory flow rates in workers with more than 10 years of exposure (Zuskin et al., 1995).

Most studies of wood dust-exposed workers have shown evidence of a COPD-like effect (Jacobsen et al., 2010), although in some it was difficult to distinguish COPD from airflow obstruction caused by asthma. Several studies of paper pulp workers have shown dust- and fibre-related impairment of lung function, although the effect on FEV_1 has not always been greater than the effect on FVC (Kraus et al., 2004). There are reports of work-related symptoms and lung function impairment in those exposed to coffee, tobacco and other organic dusts. A survey of 1032 UK workers exposed to a variety of organic dusts showed a high prevalence of respiratory symptoms (Simpson et al., 1998). A separate Croatian survey of 3011 workers in the food processing, textile and dairy industries also identified a high prevalence of work-related respiratory symptoms, but no clear exposure-related impairments of lung function (Schachter et al., 2009).

For several organic dust exposures, a relationship has been shown between acute effects measured as cross-shift changes in FEV_1 and the rate of longitudinal decline of lung function. These include the exposures encountered by cotton, grain and swine confinement workers (Tabona et al., 1984; Christiani et al., 1994; Glindmeyer et al., 1994; Kirychuk et al., 1998). The association has been less consistently demonstrated in wood workers (Dahlqvist and Ulfvarson, 1994; Jacobsen et al., 2013). Such effects are not generally seen with mineral dusts (Naidoo et al., 2007; Hankinson and Hodous, 1983). This suggests that at least some organic agents cause COPD through mechanisms related to their acute inflammatory effects on the airways, which are possibly immunologically mediated, and that these differ from the mechanisms leading to COPD from mineral dusts.

Chronic asthma can lead to fixed airflow obstruction, and so the outcome of occupational asthma can be similar to that of COPD. Workers with occupational asthma lose lung function at a rapid rate, mimicking a COPD effect, but this accelerated decline diminishes when exposures cease (Anees et al., 2006). Some studies have suggested that isocyanate-exposed workers without asthma have an accelerated rate of decline of lung function (Diem et al., 1982), but this has not been observed widely. There is no good evidence that other occupational asthmagens cause COPD through mechanisms that are distinct from those associated with chronic non-occupational asthma.

Generic 'Vapour, Gas, Dust and Fume Exposures'

Further evidence of the effects of occupational exposures comes from a series of general population surveys examining associations between respiratory symptoms or lung function and a range of possible explanatory variables. Omland et al. (2014) and Cullinan (2012) have reviewed 30 such studies. Many examined the effect of exposure to any vapour, gas, dust or fume (VGDF) rather than a specific exposure. In general, they have demonstrated associations between impaired lung function, albeit with considerable differences in the ranges and strengths of the associations with VGDF. A 2002 American Thoracic Society review of some of the earlier studies concluded that, on average, occupational VGDF exposures caused 15% of COPD (Balmes et al., 2003). A later systematic review of a further 14 studies supported this estimate (Blanc and Toren, 2007). This 15% estimate is now widely accepted and gives a useful overall summary of the likely public health importance of occupational exposures as contributors to the COPD disease burden. It is based on studies with very disparate findings and cannot be applied uncritically to any specific population. It does, however, provide a starting point when considering legislative and other preventative approaches in the management of occupational COPD.

OCCUPATIONAL BRONCHIOLITIS

Small airways of less than 2 mm in diameter—both membranous and respiratory bronchioles—may be affected by workplace inhalational exposures that cause fixed airflow limitation. Despite being incompletely characterised, the pathogenesis of this occupational form of bronchiolitis is likely to involve exposure-mediated inflammatory injury to the bronchiolar epithelium, followed by excessive proliferation of granulation tissue during the repair process. This leads to concentric narrowing (constrictive bronchiolitis) or obliteration (obliterative bronchiolitis) of the airway lumen (Barker et al., 2014).

Acute, high-dose inhalational exposures to a number of toxic workplace agents—classically the oxides of nitrogen and sulphur—are associated with rare cases of acute or subacute obliterative bronchiolitis, often with organising pneumonia. Industries in which these exposures occur include agricultural settings such as silo filling and unloading (silo fillers' lung) and in the manufacture and use of sulphuric and nitric acid.

A more insidious form of work-related bronchiolitis has been linked recently to chronic exposures to diacetyl and other chemicals that are used in the manufacture of artificial butter flavourings. Workers producing microwave popcorn have been most frequently affected (popcorn workers' lung) (Kreiss, 2002), but cases have also been described in association with the production of flavourings and fragrance generally (Centers for Disease Control and Prevention, 2007) and the upstream manufacture of the flavouring chemicals (van Rooy et al., 2007).

Military personnel deployed to Iraq and Afghanistan have also been reported to develop subacute bronchiolitis, although the causal agent or agents are uncertain. Exposures to sulphur dioxide from a mine fire, incinerated waste, desert dusts and other inhalational hazards in the theatre of war are possible causes (King et al., 2011). Six fibreglass boat builders working with styrene and other chemicals used in glass-reinforced plastics developed rapidly progressive obliterative bronchiolitis without acute exposures; two required lung transplant and one died of the disease (Cullinan et al., 2013).

The diagnosis of occupational bronchiolitis requires a high index of suspicion, as the clinical findings are often non-specific. Moreover, a work-related pattern of respiratory symptoms is generally lacking in its subacute and chronic forms. As with emphysema, accelerated decline in FEV_1 is a hallmark of disabling cases, although the decline is likely to be apparent over weeks or months rather than years. Air trapping is often reflected in an elevated residual lung volume. Pulmonary diffusing capacity (DLCO) is typically normal. Chest radiographs are generally also normal in early disease stages, but may show hyperinflation. High-resolution chest computed tomographic scanning is a useful diagnostic tool. In early disease, characteristic findings include segmental or lobular areas of hypo-attenuation (air trapping) associated with narrowing of pulmonary vessels (mosaic perfusion). The abnormalities may be usefully enhanced in expiratory images, but are then less specific. Peripheral cylindrical bronchiectasis is a frequently associated radiologic finding (Lynch, 1993).

In workers in at-risk industries, early detection of abnormal spirometry or unusual decreases in longitudinal spirometry measurements are important in management. Although long-acting inhaled steroids, oral corticosteroids and immunosuppressive agents have been tried in some cases, there are no published data supporting the efficacy of pharmacological therapy. The lack of effective treatment, the progressive nature of the disease with ongoing exposure and the severity of fixed obstruction often seen in affected workers underscore the need for early recognition and control of causal exposures.

PRACTICAL ISSUES

The contribution of occupational exposures to COPD prevalence and severity, although complex, is not merely a matter of academic interest. It has important practical implications for the determination of occupational exposure standards, the need for workplace engineering controls and surveillance schemes and the management of potentially affected individuals. There are many uncertainties in our current knowledge base, but with the inherent limitations of occupational epidemiology, it may well be that no study will ever fully answer these questions. As with other complex issues, public health policy decisions need to be made in advance of a full understanding of the problem.

Regulatory Exposure Limit

There are few occupational exposures for which there are sufficient data to inform exposure standards aimed at preventing COPD. Coal is the principal exception. It is estimated that 2–6 per 1000 non-smoking miners are likely to experience a reduction of FEV_1 to less than 65% of the predicted value following 45 years of exposure to coal mine dust at 1 mg/m^3 (National Institute for Occupational Safety and Health, 1995). The current exposure standard for coal mine dust is 3 mg/m^3 in the UK and 1.5 mg/m^3 in the USA.

The features of coal dust that give rise to COPD are poorly understood, but it is conceivable that they relate to the total surface area of contact with the airways rather than any chemical or mineralogical property. Other dust exposures would then be expected to have similar effects. The epidemiological evidence that a wide range of other exposures do have similar potency to coal in causing COPD has led some to call for a reduction in occupational exposure standards for so-called 'nuisance' or 'inert' dusts to match those for coal mine dust (Cherrie et al., 2013). To date, no regulatory authority has adopted this approach. The situation is more complex with gas and fume exposures, as there are no good data upon which to base an exposure standard. Organic dusts present additional problems, as they may act through inflammatory or immunological mechanisms that differ from those of mineral dusts and thus may have different potencies.

Surveillance

Occupational COPD is preventable with appropriate reductions in exposure, and its effects overall can be ameliorated by early detection in the minority who are particularly susceptible. A single spirometric survey of a workforce will identify those with advanced COPD, but will be of limited value in detecting early disease. Most individuals start their working lives with normal or supra-normal lung function, and serial measurements to quantify its rate of decline are essential for detecting early disease. There are numerous practical issues to consider. Careful attention to factors such as spirometry technician training, reproducibility of effort and calibration of equipment is important to minimising variability and obtaining optimum results (Redlich et al., 2014). FEV_1 is the most useful measurement as it is less affected by technical factors than FVC or measures of small airway function. The choice of reference values can importantly influence the interpretation of the tests. Post-bronchodilator measurements are preferable in cross-sectional surveys, but they add to the complexity and cost of surveillance and they have little effect on the interpretation of longitudinal changes (Tashkin et al., 2012).

The optimum frequency of serial lung function measurement is uncertain. Obtaining several measurements over the first few years of exposure helps establish a firm baseline. Thereafter, there is little benefit in obtaining measurements more frequently than every 3 years if the sole purpose of surveillance is to detect COPD (Hnizdo et al., 2010). However, if asthma, bronchiolitis or alveolitis are possibilities, then more frequent measurements will be needed. Rates of change of lung function can be calculated simply as the difference between the first and most recent measurement, but when sufficient measurements are available, it is preferable to use a linear regression analysis (Redlich et al., 2014). Spirometry Longitudinal Data Analysis (SPIROLA; http://www.cdc.gov/niosh/topics/spirometry/spirola-software.html) is a publically available software programme that can store and display serial lung function measurements, compare them to population reference values, determine whether an individual's decline in FEV_1 or FVC is excessive and predict when lung function is likely to become moderately or severely impaired.

Given the variability of repeated measurements of FEV_1, an individual must show relatively large decrements before they can be identified as excessive and hence potentially caused by occupational exposures. The smallest rate of decline that can generally be detected as excessive within 5 years is 80 mL/year; this is equivalent to a loss of FEV_1 of 2.8 L over a 35-year working lifetime. If caused by COPD, such a decline is likely to be experienced by only a small minority of workers, even with relatively poorly controlled exposures. Large-magnitude changes over relatively short periods are more likely to be seen with asthma or bronchiolitis. The potential benefits of a COPD surveillance programme to industry need to be balanced against both the costs and the risks of misattributing changes in lung function that are unrelated to occupational exposures (Townsend, 2011). Analysis of pooled lung function data is important, as even a small decline in the average lung function of a workforce might suggest poor control of exposures.

Questionnaires are often used as adjuncts to lung function measurements in surveillance programmes, but their value specifically in relation to COPD is uncertain. Their sensitivity and specificity are both low. A study of 5008 French workers found that only 11% of those who reported breathlessness had COPD (Roche et al., 2008). Changes in lung function often predate symptoms and so lung function measurements should be the primary means of identifying occupational COPD.

Management

If an individual is found via a workplace surveillance scheme to be developing COPD, the possible causes—and particularly the contribution of occupational exposures—will need to be considered. The evidence base for managing patients with suspected occupational COPD is sparse. A 2013 semi-systematic review of health surveillance for occupational respiratory disease identified only three papers relating to COPD and noted that no data were available to inform the interpretation of longitudinal FEV_1 decline (Lewis and Fishwick, 2013).

An accelerated rate of decline of lung function will not necessarily be caused by COPD or be attributable to occupational exposures. Weight gain (Wang et al., 1997) or the development of coincidental asthma (Peters et al., 2010) can contribute importantly to deteriorating lung function. In a recent survey of US coal miners, only a third of the abnormalities of lung function were classified as obstructive (Blackley et al., 2014). More detailed lung function with measures of gas transfer factor along with chest computed tomography scanning may be needed in order to clarify the diagnosis.

While few workers should develop COPD caused solely by occupational exposures, more will be at risk of disease caused by the combination of smoking and work. Attempts to apportion responsibility between the two may be undertaken when determining, for example, whether a worker with COPD should be redeployed. Data on coal miners suggest that relatively heavy dust exposures are approximately equipotent to smoking in causing COPD, but there is no other reliable evidence base upon which to determine the contribution of occupational exposures in those who also smoke. In assessing the impact of occupational COPD, consideration should be given to possible ongoing excess decline in lung function after job reassignment, as there is evidence that an adverse effect can continue after the cessation of exposure. The full effect may not be realised until several years after exposure ceases. Treatment of COPD with inhaled corticosteroids and bronchodilators does not have any clear effect on slowing the rate of decline of lung function or protecting against occupational exposures, although this approach may provide individual symptomatic relief.

Compensation

Most industrialised countries have compensation schemes for those with occupational COPD, although their scope is generally confined to a limited range of exposures. In the UK, the Industrial Injuries Benefit scheme will provide compensation for COPD in coal miners and cotton workers and for emphysema in those exposed to cadmium. In the case of coal miners, disability is apportioned according to the judgement that coal mine dust of a degree that is sufficient to pose a risk of pneumoconiosis is equipotent to average smoking in causing COPD. In the United States, emphysema and industrial bronchitis are included in the spectrum of coal mine dust lung diseases and are potentially compensable under the rubric of 'legal pneumoconiosis' by the federal Department of Labor.

COPD due to other occupational exposures is not recognised for state compensation in the UK Bronchiolitis caused by diacetyl exposures is compensated separately. Welding fumes have been accepted by UK courts to cause COPD and have been the subject of much civil litigation. It is likely that the effects of other exposures will be tested in the courts in the future. In the USA, with increasing recognition of the potential work-relatedness of COPD, individuals may qualify for state-based workers' compensation benefits when there is a reasonable medical probability that workplace exposures were causally important.

REFERENCES

Ameille, J., Letourneux, M., Paris, C., Brochard, P., Stoufflet, A., Schorle, E., Gislard, A. et al. 2010. Does asbestos exposure cause airway obstruction in the absence of confirmed asbestosis? *Am J Respir Crit Care Med* 182:526–530.

American Thoracic Society. 2004. Diagnosis and initial management of nonmalignant diseases related to asbestos. *Am J Respir Crit Care Med* 170:691–715.

Anees, W., Moore, V. C. and Burge, P. S. 2006. FEV_1 decline in occupational asthma. *Thorax* 61:751–5.

Attfield, M. D. 1985. Longitudinal decline in FEV_1 in United States coalminers. *Thorax* 40:132–7.

Attfield, M. D. and Hodous, T. K. 1992. Pulmonary function of U.S. coal miners related to dust exposure estimates. *Am Rev Respir Dis* 145:605–9.

Bakirci, N., Kalaca, S., Fletcher, A. M., Pickering, C. A., Tumerdem, N., Cali, S., Oldham, L., Francis, H. and Niven, R. 2006. Predictors of early leaving from the cotton spinning mill environment in newly hired workers. *Occup Environ Med* 63:126–130.

Balmes, J., Becklake, M., Blanc, P., Henneberger, P., Kreiss, K., Mapp, C., Milton, D. et al. 2003. American Thoracic Society Statement: Occupational contribution to the burden of airway disease. *Am J Respir Crit Care Med* 167:787–97.

Barker, A. F., Bergeron, A., Rom, W. N. and Hertz, M. I. 2014. Obliterative bronchiolitis. *N Engl J Med* 370:1820–8.

Beach, J. R., Dennis, J. H., Avery, A. J., Bromly, C. L., Ward, R. J., Walters, E. H., Stenton, S. C. et al. 1996. An epidemiologic investigation of asthma in welders. *Am J Respir Crit Care Med* 154(5):1394–1400.

Becklake, M. R. 2007. Grain dust and lung health: Not just a nuisance dust. *Can Respir J* 14(7):423–5.

Becklake, M. R., Irwig, L., Kielkowski, D., Webster, I., De Beer, M. and Landau, S. 1987. The predictors of emphysema in South African gold miners. *Am Rev Respir Dis* 135:1234–41.

Beeckman, L. A., Wang, M. L., Petsonk, E. L. and Wagner, G. R. 2001. Rapid declines in FEV_1 and subsequent respiratory symptoms, illnesses, and mortality in coal miners in the United States. *Am J Respir Crit Care Med* 163(3 Pt 1):633–9.

Bergdahl, I. A., Toren, K., Eriksson, K., Hedlund, U., Nilssonz, T., Flodin, R. and Jarvholm, B. 2004. Increased mortality in COPD among construction workers exposed to inorganic dust. *Eur Respir J* 23:402–6.

Blackley, D. J., Halldin, C. N., Wang, M. L. and Laney, A. S. 2014. Small mine size is associated with lung function abnormality and pneumoconiosis among underground coal miners in Kentucky, Virginia and West Virginia. *Occup Environ Med* 71:690–4.

Blanc, P. D. and Toren, K. 2007. Occupation in chronic obstructive pulmonary disease and chronic bronchitis: An update. *Int J Tuberc Lung Dis* 11:251–7.

Boojar, M. M. and Goodarzi, F. 2002. A longitudinal follow-up of pulmonary function and respiratory symptoms in workers exposed to manganese. *J Occup Environ Med* 44(3):282–90.

Bouhuys, A. and Zuskin, E. 1976. Chronic respiratory disease in hemp workers. A follow-up study, 1967–1974. *Ann Intern Med* 84:398–405.

Brüske, I., Thiering, E., Heinrich, J., Huster, K. and Nowak, D. 2013. Biopersistent granular dust and chronic obstructive pulmonary disease: A systematic review and meta-analysis. *PLoS One* 8(11):e80977.

Burgel, P. R., Bourdin, A., Chanez, P., Chabot, F., Chaouat, A., Chinet, T., de Blic, J. et al. 2011. Update on the roles of distal airways in COPD. *Eur Respir Rev* 20(119):7–22.

Calvert, G. M., Rice, F. L., Boiano, J. M., Sheehy, J. W. and Sanderson, W. T. 2003. Occupational silica exposure and risk of various diseases: An analysis using death certificates from 27 states of the United States. *Occup Environ Med* 60:122–9.

Carta, P., Aru, G., Barbieri, M. T., Avataneo, G. and Casula, D. 1996. Dust exposure, respiratory symptoms, and longitudinal decline of lung function in young coal miners. *Occup Environ Med* 53:312–19.

Centers for Disease Control and Prevention. 2007. Fixed obstructive lung disease among workers in the flavor-manufacturing industry—California, 2004–2007. *MMWR Morb Mortal Wkly Rep* 56:389–93.

Chen, H. W., Su, S. F., Chien, C. T., Lin, W. H., Yu, S. L., Chou, C. C., Chen, J. J. and Yang, P. C. 2006. Titanium dioxide nanoparticles induce emphysema-like lung injury in mice. *FASEB J* 20:2393–5.

Chen, Y. H., Wu, T. N. and Liou, S. H. 2001. Obstructive pulmonary function defects among Taiwanese firebrick workers in a 2-year follow-up study. *Occup Environ Med* 43(11):969–75.

Cherrie, J. W., Brosseau, L. M., Hay, A. and Donaldson, K. 2013. A commentary for the *Annals of Occupational Hygiene*: Low-toxicity dusts: Current exposure guidelines are not sufficiently protective. *Ann Occup Hyg* 57(6):685–691.

Cherry, N., Harris, J., McDonald, C., Turner, S., Newman Taylor, A. J. and Cullinan, P. 2013. Mortality in a cohort of Staffordshire pottery workers: Follow-up to December 2008. *Occup Environ Med* 70(3):149–55.

Chinn, D. J., Stevenson, I. C. and Cotes, J. E. 1990. Longitudinal respiratory survey of shipyard workers: Effects of trade and atopic status. *Br J Ind Med* 47:83–90.

Choi, J. H., Shin, J. H., Lee, M. Y. and Chung, I. S. 2014. Pulmonary function decline in firefighters and non-firefighters in South Korea. *Ann Occup Environ Med* 25(26):9.

Christiani, D., Wang, X., Pan, L., Zhang, H. X., Sun, B. X., Dai, H., Eisen, E. A., Wegman, D. H. and Olenchock, S. A. 2001. Longitudinal changes in pulmonary function and respiratory symptoms in cotton textile workers. A 15-yr follow-up study. *Am J Respir Crit Care Med* 163:847–53.

Christiani, D. C., Ve, T.-T., Wegman, D. H., Eisen, E. A., Dai, H.-L. and Lu, P. L. 1994. Cotton dust exposure, across-shift drop in FEV_1 and five-year change in lung function. *Am J Respir Crit Care Med* 150:1250–5.

Churg, A. and Wright, J. L. 1983. Small-airway lesions in patients exposed to nonasbestos mineral dusts. *Hum Pathol* 14:688–93.

Coggon, D., Inskip, H., Winter, P. and Pannett, B. 1995. Contrasting geographical distribution of mortality from pneumoconiosis and chronic bronchitis and emphysema in British coal miners. *Occup Environ Med* 52:554–5.

Cowie, H. A., Miller, B. G., Rawbone, R. G. and Soutar, C. A. 2006. Dust related risks of clinically relevant lung functional deficits. *Occup Environ Med* 63:320–5.

Cowie, R. L. and Mabena, S. K. 1991. Silicosis, chronic airflow limitation, and chronic bronchitis in South African gold miners. *Am Rev Respir Dis* 143:80–4.

Cui, L., Gallagher, L., Ray, R., Li, W., Gao, D., Zhang, Y., Vedal, S., Thomas, D. B. and Checkoway, H. 2011. Unexpected excessive chronic obstructive pulmonary disease mortality among female silk textile workers in Shanghai, China. *Occup Environ Med* 68:883–7.

Cullinan, P. 2012. Occupation and chronic obstructive pulmonary disease (COPD). *Br Med Bull* 104:143–61.

Cullinan, P., McGavin, C. R., Kreiss, K., Nicholson, A. G., Maher, T. M., Howell, T., Banks, J. et al. 2013. Obliterative bronchiolitis in fibreglass workers: A new occupational disease? *Occup Environ Med* 70:357–9.

Dahlqvist, M. and Ulfvarson, U. 1994. Acute effects on forced expiratory volume in one second and longitudinal change in pulmonary function among wood trimmers. *Am J Ind Med* 25:551–8.

Davison, A. G., Newman Taylor, A. J., Darbyshire, J., Chetlle, D. R., Gutherie, C. J. G., O'Malley, D., Mason, H. J. et al. 1988. Cadmium fume inhalation and emphysema. *Lancet* 1:663–7.

de Jong, K., Boezen, H. M., Kromhout, H., Vermeulen, R., Postma, D. S. and Vonk, J. M. 2014. Association of occupational pesticide exposure with accelerated longitudinal decline in lung function. *Am J Epidemiol* 179(11):1323–30.

Diem, J. E., Jones, R. N., Hendrick, D. J., Glindmeyer, H. W., Dharmarajan, V., Butcher, B. T., Salvaggio, J. E. et al. 1982. Five-year longitudinal study of workers employed in a new toluene diisocyanate manufacturing plant. *Am Rev Respir Dis* 126(3):420–8.

Eduard, W., Pearce, N. and Douwes, J. 2009. Chronic Bronchitis, COPD, and lung function in farmers the role of biological agents. *Chest* 136:716–25.

Ehrlich, R. I., Myers, J. E., te Water Naude, J. M., Thompson, M. L. and Churchyard, G. J. 2011. Lung function loss in relation to silica dust exposure in South African gold miners. *Occup Environ Med* 68:96–101.

Eisner, M. D., Anthonisen, N., Coultas, D. et al. 2010. An official American Thoracic Society public policy statement: Novel risk factors and the global burden of chronic obstructive pulmonary disease. *Am J Respir Crit Care Med* 2010;182:693–718.

Forey, B. A., Thornton, A. J. and Lee, P. N. 2011. Systematic review with meta-analysis of the epidemiological evidence relating smoking to COPD, chronic bronchitis and emphysema. *BMC Pulm Med* 11:36.

Gallard, M., Romero, P., Sanchez-Quevedo, M. C. and López-Caballero, J. J. 1994. Siderosilicosis due to photocopier toner dust. *Lancet* 344:412–3.

Gardiner, K., van Tongeren, M. and Harrington, M. 2001. Respiratory health effects from exposure to carbon black: Results of the phase 2 and 3 cross sectional studies in the European carbon black manufacturing industry. *Occup Environ Med* 58:496–503.

Garshick, E. 2014. Effects of short- and long-term exposures to ambient air pollution on COPD. *Eur Respir J* 44(3):558–61.

Glindmeyer, H. W., Lefante, J. J., Jones, R. N., Rando, R. J. and Weill, H. 1994. Cotton dust and across-shift change in FEV, as predictors of annual change in FEV. *Am J Respir Crit Care Med* 149:584–90.

Global Initiative for Chronic Obstructive Lung Disease (GOLD). 2011. Global Strategy for the Diagnosis, Management and Prevention of Chronic Pulmonary Disease. Available at: http://www.goldcopd.org/Guidelines/guidelines-resources.html.

Graber, J. M., Stayner, L. T., Cohen, R. A., Conroy, L. M. and Attfield, M. D. 2014. Respiratory disease mortality among US coal miners; results after 37 years of follow-up. *Occup Environ Med* 71:30–9.

Graham, B. L., Dosman, J. A., Cotton, D. J., Weisstock, S. R., Lappi, V. G. and Froh, F. 1984. Pulmonary function and respiratory symptoms in potash workers. *J Occup Med* 26(3):209–14.

Graham, W. G., Weaver, S., Ashikaga, T. and O'Grady, R. V. 1994. Longitudinal pulmonary function losses in Vermont granite workers. A re-evaluation. *Chest* 106:125–30.

Hankinson, J. L. and Hodous, T. K. 1983. Short-term prospective spirometric study of new coal miners. Morgantown, WV: U.S. Department of Health and Human Services, Public Health Service, Centers for Disease Control, National Institute for Occupational Safety and Health, Clinical Investigations Branch.

Harber, P., Muranko, H., Solis, S., Torossian, A. and Merz, B. 2003. Effect of carbon black exposure on respiratory function and symptoms. *J Occup Environ Med* 45:144–55.

Harber, P., Tashkin, D. P., Simmons, M., Crawford, L., Hnizdo, E., Connett, J; Lung Health Study Group. 2007. Effect of occupational exposures on decline of lung function in early chronic obstructive pulmonary disease. *Am J Respir Crit Care Med* 176(10):994–1000.

Hart, J. E., Eisen, E. A. and Laden, F. 2012. Occupational diesel exhaust exposure as a risk factor for chronic obstructive pulmonary disease. *Curr Opin Pulm Med* 18(2):151–4.

Hart, J. E., Laden, F., Eisen, E. A., Smith, T. J. and Garshick, E. 2009. Chronic obstructive pulmonary disease mortality in railroad workers. *Occup Environ Med* 66(4):221–6.

Hendryx, M. and Luo, J. 2015. An examination of the effects of mountaintop removal coal mining on respiratory symptoms and COPD using propensity scores. *Int J Environ Health Res* 25:265–76.

Henneberger, P. K. and Attfield, M. D. 1996. Coal mine dust exposure and spirometry in experienced miners. *Am J Respir Crit Care Med* 153:1560–6.

Hertzberg, V. S., Rosenman, K. D., Reilly, M. J. and Rice, C. H. 2002. Effect of occupational silica exposure on pulmonary function. *Chest* 122:721–8.

Hnizdo, E. 1992. Loss of lung function associated with exposure to silica dust and with smoking and its relation to disability and mortality in South African gold miners. *Br J Ind Med* 49:472–9.

Hnizdo, E., Baskind, E. and Sluis-Cremer, G. K. 1990. Combined effect of silica dust exposure and tobacco smoking on the prevalence of respiratory impairments among gold miners. *Scand J Work Environ Health* 16:411–22.

Hnizdo, E., Glindmeyer, H. W. and Petsonk, E. L. 2010. Workplace spirometry monitoring for respiratory disease prevention: A methods review. *Int J Tuberc Lung Dis* 14(7):796–805.

Hnizdo, E., Murray, J. and Davison, A. 2000. Correlation between autopsy findings for chronic obstructive airways disease and in-life disability in South African gold miners. *Int Arch Occup Environ Health* 73:235–44.

Hnizdo, E., Sluis-Cremer, G. K. and Abramowitz, J. A. 1991. Emphysema type in relation to silica dust exposure in South African gold miners. *Am Rev Respir Dis* 143:1241–7.

Hnizdo, E., Sluis-Cremer, G. K., Baskind, E. and Murray, J. 1994. Emphysema and airway obstruction in non-smoking South African gold miners with long exposure to silica dust. *Occup Environ Med* 51:557–63.

Hnizdo, E., Sullivan, P. A., Bang, K. M. and Wagner, G. 2002. Association between chronic obstructive pulmonary disease and employment by industry and occupation in the US population: A study of data from the third national health and nutrition examination survey. *Am J Epidemiol* 156(8):738–46.

Hochgatterer, K., Moshammer, H. and Haluza, D. 2013. Dust is in the air: Effects of occupational exposure to mineral dust on lung function in a 9-year study. *Lung* 191:257–63.

Hu, Y., Chen, B., Yin, Z., Jia, L., Zhou, Y. and Jin, T. 2006. Increased risk of chronic obstructive pulmonary diseases in coke oven workers: Interaction between occupational exposure and smoking. *Thorax* 61:290–5.

Humerfelt, S., Eide, G. E. and Gulsvik, A. 1998. Association of years of occupational quartz exposure with spirometric airflow limitation in Norwegian men aged 30–46 years. *Thorax* 53:649–55.

Huvinen, M., Uitti, J., Zitting, A., Roto, P., Virkola, K., Kuikka, P., Laippala, P. et al. 1996. Respiratory health of workers exposed to low levels of chromium in stainless steel production. *Occup Environ Med* 53:741–7.

Huy, T., De Schipper, K., Chan-Yeung, M. and Kennedy, S. M. 1991. Grain dust and lung function. Dose–response relationships. *Am Rev Respir Dis* 144:1314–21.

Jacobsen, G., Schaumburg, I., Sigsgaard, T. and Schlunssen, V. 2010. Non-malignant respiratory diseases and occupational exposure to wood dust. Part I. Fresh wood and mixed wood industry. *Ann Agric Environ Med* 17(1):15–28.

Jacobsen, G. H., Schlünssen, V., Schaumburg, I. and Sigsgaard, T. 2013. Cross-shift and longitudinal changes in FEV_1 among wood dust exposed workers. *Occup Environ Med* 70(1):22–8.

Johnsen, H. L., Bugge, M. D., Føreland, S., Kjuus, H., Kongerud, J. and Søyseth, V. 2013. Dust exposure is associated with increased lung function loss among workers in the Norwegian silicon carbide industry. *Occup Environ Med* 70(11):803–9.

Johnsen, H. L., Hetland, S. M., Benth, J. S., Kongerud, J. and Søyseth, V. 2010. Dust exposure assessed by a job exposure matrix is associated with increased annual decline of FEV_1. *Am J Respir Crit Care Med* 181(11):1234–40.

Kauffman, F., Drouet, D., Lellouch, L. and Brille, D. 1982. Occupational exposure and 12-year spirometric changes among Paris area workers. *Br J Ind Med* 39:221–32.

Kim, V. and Criner, G. J. 2013. Chronic bronchitis and chronic obstructive pulmonary disease. *Am J Respir Crit Care Med* 187(3):228–37.

King, M. S., Eisenberg, R., Newman, J. H., Tolle, J. J., Harrell, F. E. Jr, Nian, H. and Ninan, M. 2011. Constrictive bronchiolitis in soldiers returning from Iraq and Afghanistan. *N Engl J Med* 365:222–30.

Kirychuk, S., Senthilselvan, A., Dosman, J. A., Zhou, C., Barber, E. M., Rhodes, C. S. and Hurst, T. S. 1998. Predictors of longitudinal changes in pulmonary function among swine confinement workers. *Can Respir J* 5:472–8.

Kitamura, H., Terunuma, N., Kurosaki, S., Hata, K., Ide, R., Kuga, H., Kakiuchi, N. et al. 2009. Cross-sectional study on respiratory effect of toner-exposed work in manufacturing plants, Japan: pulmonary function, blood cells, and biochemical markers. *Hum Exp Toxicol* 28:331–8.

Kraus, T.1, Pfahlberg, A., Zöbelein, P., Gefeller, O. and Raithel, H. J. 2004. Lung function among workers in the soft tissue paper-producing industry. *Chest* 25(2):731–6.

Kreiss, K., Gomaa, A., Kullman, G., Fedan, K., Simoes, E. J. and Enright, P. L. 2002. Clinical bronchiolitis obliterans in workers at a microwave-popcorn plant. *N Engl J Med* 347(5):330–8.

Kreiss, K., Greenberg, L. M., Kogut, S. J. H., Lezotte, D. C., Irvin, C. G. and Cherniack, R. M. 1989. Hard-rock mining exposure affects smokers and non-smokers differently. *Am Rev Respir Dis* 139:1487–93.

Kreuzer, M., Sogl, M., Brüske, I., Möhner, M., Nowak, D., Schnelzer, M. and Walsh, L. 2013. Silica dust, radon and death from non-malignant respiratory diseases in German uranium miners. *Occup Environ Med* 70(12):869–75.

Kriebel, D., Sprince, N. L., Eisen, E. A. and Greaves, I. A. 1988. Beryllium exposure and pulmonary function: A cross sectional study of beryllium workers. *Occup Environ Med* 45:167–73.

Krzyzanowski, M.1, Jedrychowski, W. and Wysocki, M. 1988. Occupational exposures and changes in pulmonary function over 13 years among residents of Cracow. *Br J Ind Med* 45(11):747–54.

Kuempel, E. D., Wheeler, M. W., Smith, R. J., Vallyathan, V. and Green, F. H. Y. 2009. Contributions of dust exposure and cigarette smoking to emphysema severity in coal miners in the United States. *Am J Respir Crit Care Med* 180:257–64.

Kurmi, O. P., Semple, S., Simkhada, P., Cairn, S. W., Smith, S. and Ayres, J. G. 2010. COPD and chronic bronchitis risk of indoor air pollution from solid fuel: A systematic review and meta-analysis. *Thorax* 65:221–8.

Lai, P. S. and Christiani, D. C. 2013. Long term respiratory health effects in textile workers. *Curr Opin Pulm Med* 19(2):152–7.

Lamprecht, B., Schirnhofer, L., Kaiser, B., Studnicka, M. and Buist, A. S. 2007. Farming and the prevalence of non-reversible airways obstruction: Results from a population-based study. *Am J Ind Med* 50:421–6.

Lange, P., Groth, S., Nyboe, G. J., Mortensen, J., Appleyard, M., Jensen, G. and Schnohr, P. 1989. Effects of smoking and changes in smoking habits on the decline of FEV_1. *Eur Respir J* 2:811–6.

Lewis, L. and Fishwick, D. 2013. Health surveillance for occupational respiratory disease. *Occup Med (Lond)* 63:322–34.

Lewis, S., Bennett, J., Richards, K. and Britton, J. 1996. A cross sectional study of the independent effect of occupation on lung function in British coal miners. *Occup Environ Med* 1996; 53:125–8.

Lotz, G., Plitzko, S., Gierke, E., Tittelbach, U., Kersten, N. and Schneider, W. D. 2008. Dose response relationships between occupational exposure to potash, diesel exhaust and nitrogen oxides and lung function: Cross-sectional and longitudinal study in two salt mines. *Int Arch Occup Environ Health* 81:1003–19.

Love, R. G. and Miller, B. G. 1982. Longitudinal study of lung function in coal-miners. *Thorax* 37:193–7.

Love, R. G., Miller, B. G., Groat, S. K., Hagen, S., Cowie, H. A., Johnston, P. P., Hutchison, P. A. et al. 1997. Respiratory health effects of opencast coalmining: A cross sectional study of current workers. *Occup Environ Med* 54(6):416–23.

Love, R. G., Muirhead, M., Collins, H. P. R. and Soutar, C. A. 1991. The characteristics of respiratory ill health of wool textile workers. *Br J Ind Med* 48:221–8.

Lynch, D. A. 1993. Imaging of small airways diseases. *Clin Chest Med* 14(4):623–34.

Manfreda, J., Sidwall, G., Maini, K. et al. 1982. Respiratory abnormalities in employees of the hard rock mining industry. *Am Rev Respir Dis* 126:629–34.

Mannino, D. M., Holguin, F., Greves, H. M., Savage-Brown, A., Stock, A. L. and Jones, R. L. 2004. Urinary cadmium levels predict lower lung function in current and former smokers: Data from the Third National Health and Nutrition Examination Survey. *Thorax* 59:194–8.

Marine, W. M., Gurr, D. and Jacobsen, M. 1988. Clinically important respiratory effects of dust exposure and smoking in British coal miners. *Am Rev Respir Dis* 137:106–12.

Mehta, A. J., Henneberger, P. K., Toren, K. and Olin, A.-C. 2005. Airflow limitation and changes in pulmonary function among bleachery workers. *Eur Respir J* 26:133–9.

Miller, A. and Rom, W. M. 2010. Does asbestos exposure (asbestosis) cause (clinical) airway obstruction (small airway disease)? *Am J Respir Crit Care Med* 182(4):444–5.

Miller, B. G. and MacCalman, L. 2010. Cause-specific mortality in British coal workers and exposure to respirable dust and quartz. *Occup Environ Med* 67:270–6.

Möhner, M., Kersten, N. and Gellissen, J. 2013. Chronic obstructive pulmonary disease and longitudinal changes in pulmonary function due to occupational exposure to respirable quartz. *Occup Environ Med* 70:9–14.

Moitra, S., Blanc, P. D. and Sahu, S. 2013. Adverse respiratory effects associated with cadmium exposure in small-scale jewellery workshops in India. *Thorax* 68:565–70.

Monso, E., Riu, E., Radon, K., Magarolas, R., Danuser, B., Iversen, M., Morera, J. and Nowak, D. 2005. Chronic obstructive pulmonary disease in never-smoking animal farmers working inside confinement buildings. *Am J Ind Med* 46:357–62.

Naidoo, R. N., Robins, T. G., Becklake, M., Seixas, N. and Thompson, M. L. 2007. Cross-shift peak expiratory flow changes are unassociated with respirable coal dust exposure among South African coal miners *Am J Ind Med* 50:992–8.

National Institute for Occupational Safety and Health. 1995. *Criteria for a Recommended Standard. Occupational Exposure to Respirable Coal Mine Dust.* U.S. Government Printing Office. Cincinnati, Ohio: US Department of Health and Human Services. Centers for Disease Control and Prevention, National Institute for Occupational Safety and Health, Education and Information Division.

Nemery, B. 1990. Metal toxicity and the respiratory tract. *Eur Respir J* 3:202–19.

Nishimura, N., Makita, H., Nagai, K., Konno, S., Nasuhara, Y., Hasegawa, M., Shimizu, K. et al. 2012. Annual change in pulmonary function and clinical phenotype in chronic obstructive pulmonary disease. *Am J Respir Crit Care Med* 185(1):44–52.

Nordby, K. C., Fell, A. K., Notø, H., Eduard, W., Skogstad, M., Thomassen, Y., Bergamaschi, A. et al. 2011. Exposure to thoracic dust, airway symptoms, and lung function in cement production workers. *Eur Respir J* 38:1278–86.

Omland, Ø., Würtz, E. T., Aasen, T. B., Blanc, P., Brisman, J., Miller, M. R., Pedersen, O. F. et al. 2014. Occupational chronic obstructive pulmonary disease: A systematic literature review. *Scand J Work Environ Health* 40(1): 19–35.

Osterman, J. W., Greaves, I. A., Smith, T. J., Hammond, S. K., Robins, J. M. and Thériault, G. 1989. Respiratory symptoms associated with low level sulphur dioxide exposure in silicon carbide production workers. *Br J Ind Med* 46:629–35.

Pelkonen, M., Notkola, I. L., Nissinen, A., Tukiainen, H. and Koskela, H. 2006. Thirty year cumulative incidence of chronic bronchitis and COPD in relation to 30-year pulmonary function and 40-year mortality: A follow-up in middle-aged rural men. *Chest* 130:1129–37.

Perret, J. L., Dharmage, S. C., Matheson, M. C., Johns, D. P., Gurrin, L. C., Burgess, J. A. and Marrone, J. 2013. The interplay between the effects of lifetime asthma, smoking, and atopy on fixed airflow obstruction in middle age. *Am J Respir Crit Care Med* 187(1): 42–8.

Peters, C. E., Demers, P. A., Sehmer, J., Karlen, B. and Kennedy, S. M. 2010. Early changes in respiratory health in trades' apprentices and physician visits for respiratory illnesses later in life. *Occup Environ Med* 67:237–43.

Piirila, P., Kivisaari, L., Huuskonen, O., Kaleva, S., Sovija, A. and Vehmas, T. 2009. Association of findings in flow-volume spirometry with high-resolution computed tomography signs in asbestos-exposed male workers. *Clin Physiol Funct Imaging* 29:1–9.

Randem, B. G., Ulvestad, B., Burstyn, I. and Kongerud, J. 2004. Respiratory symptoms and airflow limitation in asphalt workers. *Occup Environ Med* 61:367–9.

Redlich, C. A., Tarlo, S. M., Hankinson, J. L., Townsend, M. C., Eschenbacher, W. L., Von Essen, S. G., Sigsgaard, T. et al. 2014. Official American Thoracic Society technical standards: Spirometry in the occupational setting. *Am J Respir Crit Care Med* 189(8):983–93.

Rennard, S. I. and Vestbo, J. 2008. Natural histories of chronic obstructive pulmonary disease. *Proc Am Thorac Soc* 5:878–83.

Roche, N., Dalmay, F., Perez, T., Kuntz, C., Vergnenegre, A., Neukirche, F., Giordanella, J.-P. et al. 2008. Impact of chronic airflow obstruction in a working population. *Eur Respir J* 31:1227–33.

Rogan, J. M., Attfield, M. D., Jacobsen, M., Rae, S., Walker, D. D. and Walton, W. H. 1973. Role of dust in the working environment in development of chronic bronchitis in British coal miners. *Br J Ind Med* 30:217–26.

Rushton, L. 2007. Occupational causes of chronic obstructive pulmonary disease. *Rev Environ Health* 22:195–212.

Scarselli, A., Binazzi, A., Forastiere, F., Cavariani, F. and Marinaccio, A. 2011. Industry and job-specific mortality after occupational exposure to silica dust. *Occup Med* 61:422–9.

Schachter, E. N., Zuskin, E., Moshier, E. L., Godbold, J., Mustajbegovic, J., Pucarin-Cvetkovic, J. and Chiarelli, A. 2009. Gender and respiratory findings in workers occupationally exposed to organic aerosols: A meta analysis of 12 cross-sectional studies. *Environ Health* 8:1.

Schubauer-Berigan, M. K., Couch, J. R., Petersen, M. R., Carreon, T., Jin, Y. and Deddens, J. A. 2011. Cohort mortality study of workers at seven beryllium processing plants: Update and associations with cumulative and maximum exposure. *Occup Environ Med* 68(5):345–53.

Seixas, N. S., Robins, T. G., Attfield, M. D. and Moulton, L. H. 1993. Longitudinal and cross sectional analyses of exposure to coal mine dust and pulmonary function in new miners. *Br J Ind Med* 50:929–37.

Simpson, J. C. G, Niven, R. M., Pickering, C. A., Fletcher, A. M., Oldham, L. A. and Francis, H. M. 1998. Prevalence and predictors of work related respiratory symptoms in workers exposed to organic dusts. *Occup Environ Med* 55(10):668–72.

Soutar, C. A., Copland, L. H., Thornley, P. E., Hurley, J. F., Ottery, J., Adams, W. G. and Bennett, B. 1980. Epidemiological study of respiratory disease in workers exposed to polyvinylchloride dust. *Thorax* 35(9):644–52.

Soutar, C. A. and Hurley, J. F. 1986. Relation between dust exposure and lung function in miners and ex-miners. *Br J Ind Med* 43:307–20.

Swanney, M. P., Ruppel, G., Enright, P. L., Pedersen, O. F., Crapo, R. O., Miller, M. R., Jensen, R. L. et al. 2008. Using the lower limit of normal for the FEV_1/FVC ratio reduces the misclassification of airway obstruction. *Thorax* 63(12):1046–51.

Szczyrek, M., Krawczyk, P., Milanowski, J., Jastrzębska, I., Zwolak, A. and Daniluk, J. 2011. Chronic obstructive pulmonary disease in farmers and agricultural workers—An overview. *Ann Agric Environ Med* 18(2):310–13.

Szram, J., Schofield, S. J., Cosgrove, M. P. and Cullinan, P. 2013. Welding, longitudinal lung function decline and chronic respiratory symptoms: A systematic review of cohort studies. *Eur Respir J* 42:1186–93.

Tabona, M., Chan-Yeung, M., Enarson, D., MacLean, L., Dorken, E., and Schulzer, M. 1984. Host factors affecting longitudinal decline in lung spirometry among grain elevator workers. *Chest* 85:782–6.

Tashkin, D. P., Wang, H., Halpin, D., Kleerup, E. C., Connett, J., Li, N. and Elashoff, R. 2012. Comparison of the variability of the annual rates of change in FEV_1 determined from serial measurements of the pre- versus postbronchodilator FEV_1 over 5 years in mild to moderate COPD: Results of the lung health study. *Respir Res* 13:70.

Thaon, I., Demange, V., Herin, F., Touranchet, A. and Paris, C. 2012. Increased lung function decline in blue-collar workers exposed to welding fumes. *Chest* 142(1):192–9.

Townsend, M. C. 2011. Occupational and environmental lung disorders committee. Spirometry in the occupational health setting—2011 update. *J Occup Environ Med* 53:569–84.

Townsend, M. C., Enterline, P. E., Sussman, N. B., Bonney, T. B. and Rippey, L. L. 1985. Pulmonary function in relation to total dust exposure at a bauxite refinery and alumina-based chemical products plant. *Am Rev Respir Dis* 132(6):1174–80.

Tse, L. A., Yu, I. T. S., Qiu, H. and Leung, C. C. 2014. Joint effects of smoking and silicosis on diseases to the lungs. *PLoS One* 9(8):e104494.

Ulvestad, B., Bakke, B., Melbostad, E., Fuglerud, P., Kongerud, J. and Lund M. B. 2000. Increased risk of obstructive pulmonary disease in tunnel workers. *Thorax* 55:277–82.

Vacek, P. M.1, Verma, D. K., Graham, W. G., Callas, P. W. and Gibbs, G. W. 2011. Mortality in Vermont granite workers and its association with silica exposure. *Occup Environ Med* 68(5):312–8.

van Rooy, F. G., Rooyackers, J. M., Prokop, M., Houba, R., Smit, L. A. and Heederik, D. J. 2007. Bronchiolitis obliterans syndrome in chemical workers producing diacetyl for food flavorings. *Am J Respir Crit Care Med* 176(5):498–504.

Verma, D. K.1, Vacek, P. M., des Tombe, K., Finkelstein, M., Branch, B., Gibbs, G. W. and Graham, W. G. 2011. Silica exposure assessment in a mortality study of Vermont granite workers. *J Occup Environ Hyg* 8(2):71–9.

Wang, F., Zou, Y., Shen, Y., Zhong, Y., Lv, Y., Huang, D., Chen, K. et al. 2015. Synergistic impaired effect between smoking and manganese dust exposure on pulmonary ventilation function in Guangxi Manganese-Exposed Workers Healthy Cohort (GXMEWHC). *PLoS One* 10(2):e0116558.

Wang, M. L., McCabe, L., Petsonk, E. L., Hankinson, J. L. and Banks, D. E. 1997. Weight gain and longitudinal changes in lung function in steel workers. *Chest* 111:1526–32.

Wang, M. L., Petsonk, E. L., Beeckman, L. A. and Wagner, G. R. 1999. Clinically important FEV_1 declines among coal miners: An exploration of previously unrecognized determinants. *Occup Environ Med* 56:837–844.

Wang, M. L., Wu, Z. E., Du, D. Q., Petsonk, E. L., Peng, K. L., Li, Y. D., Li, S. K. et al. 2005. A prospective cohort study among new Chinese coal miners: The early pattern of lung function change. *Occup Environ Med* 62:800–5.

Wang, X., Zhang, H. X., Sun, B. X, Dai H-L., Hang, J-Q., Eisen, E., Su, L. and Christiani, D. C. 2008. Cross-shift airway responses and long-term decline in FEV_1 in cotton textile workers. *Am J Respir Crit Care Med* 177:316–20.

Wild, P., Leodolter, K., Refregier, M., Schmidt, H. and Bourgkard, E. 2008. Effects of talc dust on respiratory health: Results of a longitudinal survey of 378 French and Austrian talc workers. *Occup Environ Med* 65:261–7.

Wilken, D., Velasco Garrido, M., Manuwald, U. and Baur, X. 2011. Lung function in asbestos-exposed workers, a systematic review and meta-analysis. *J Occup Med Toxicol* 6:21.

Wright, J. L. and Churg, A. 1985. Severe diffuse small airways abnormalities in long term chrysotile asbestos miners. *Br J Ind Med* 42:556–9.

Yelin, E., Katz, P., Balmes, J., Trupin, L., Earnest, G., Eisner, M. and Blanc, P. 2006. Work life of persons with asthma, rhinitis, and COPD: A study using a national, population-based sample. *J Occup Med Toxicol* 1:2.

Zhang, J., Lin, X. and Bai, C. 2014. Comparison of clinical features between non-smokers with COPD and smokers with COPD: A retrospective observational study. *Int J COPD* 9:57–63.

Zhang, W., Fievez, L., Zhang, F., Cheu, E., Antoine, N., Delguste, C., Zhang, Y. et al. 2010. Effects of formoterol and ipratropium bromide on repeated cadmium inhalation-induced pulmonary inflammation and emphysema in rats. *Eur J Pharmacol* 647:178–87.

Zuskin, E., Mustajbegovic, J., Schachter, E. N., Kanceljak, B., Godnic-Cvar, J. and Sitar-Srebocan, V. 1995. Respiratory symptoms and lung function in wool textile workers. *Am J Ind Med* 27:845–57.

32 Respiratory Health Effects of Welding Exposures

Shona C. Fang and David C. Christiani

CONTENTS

INTRODUCTION

Welding is a widespread industrial process that joins metals together using high levels of heat, pressure or both. There are numerous welding processes and process variants (Burgess, 1995); common methods include shielded manual metal arc welding (MMAW; also known as stick welding), gas metal arc welding (GMAW; or metal inert gas welding), flux-cored arc welding and gas tungsten arc welding (GTAW; or tungsten inert gas welding). The process used depends on a variety of factors, including the type, form and thickness of the metal being welded. While there are no official global estimates, some have estimated that there are 2–3 million full-time welders worldwide (Solano-Lopez et al., 2006; Szram et al., 2013). The true number is probably much higher, since many trades without the title 'welder' regularly include welding; examples include assemblers, fabricators, boilermakers, pipefitters, steamfitters and sheet metal workers. In addition, many non-welders are exposed to respiratory hazards while working in the vicinity of welders.

Welding occurs in a wide range of industries with diverse physical settings that include indoor and outdoor work, open or confined spaces, underwater and outer space. Moreover, these have varying types and degrees of ventilation. As a result, welders' exposures are complex and depend further on the specific welding process and metals welded. In addition to metal fumes and gases, welders are commonly exposed to dusts and fibres, sometimes including asbestos. Other potential co-exposures include noise, heat, radiation and vibration. In addition to its adverse respiratory health effects, welding is associated with burns, neurological symptoms and potential dermal and reproductive health effects (Antonini, 2003).

Chemical and Physical Properties of Welding Fumes and Gases

In general, there are three main components needed to create a weld: (1) a heat source; (2) a shielding source to protect the weld from air, commonly an inert gas or flux; and (3) filler material used to join the two pieces together, often provided by a consumable electrode. When the metal is heated above its boiling point, the vapours condense into very fine particles (particulate matter [PM]) comprising the welding fume, a complex mixture of metallic oxides, as well as silicates and fluorides from the filler material; much of the fume is derived from the consumable electrode. Because of their small aerodynamic diameter, welding fume particulates are able to penetrate into the alveolar region of the lungs. Processes with high particle mass emission rates (e.g. MMAW, GMAW and laser welding) show mainly agglomerated particles with diameters above 0.10 μm, while processes with low emission rates (e.g. GTAW and resistance spot welding) emit predominantly ultrafine particles (Brand et al., 2013). In a study of real-world welding of mild steel (MS) using predominantly MMAW, metal particles were found to be in the $PM_{0.1-2.5}$ and $PM_{2.5-10}$ range, with most water-soluble metals in the $PM_{2.5-10}$ range (Chang et al., 2013).

It is generally accepted that stainless steel (SS) fume is more hazardous than MS fume due to its higher chromium and nickel content. SS welding generates fumes with up to 20% chromium (hexavalent and trivalent forms) and 10% nickel (Antonini, 2003) and lesser amounts of iron. MS welding generates fumes composed primarily of iron (>80%), with no to small amounts of additive metals (chromium, nickel, manganese, molybdenum, vanadium, titanium, cobalt, copper, etc.). The solubility of a welding fume affects the bioavailability of the metals; SS fumes are generally highly soluble, while MS fumes are less so.

In addition, welders are exposed to gases during welding and cutting processes; these include shielding and fuel gases and gases produced by the decomposition of fluxes or from the interaction of ultraviolet light or high temperatures with gases or vapours in the air. Decomposition of degreasing agents and organic coatings on the welded metal can also be a source. Gases in welding fume include nitrogen oxides, carbon dioxide, carbon monoxide, shielding gas (e.g. argon and helium) and ozone; the latter is formed in particular during gas-shield welding of aluminium and, to a lesser extent, SS. Carbon monoxide may be formed when carbon dioxide is used as a shielding agent, and nitrogen dioxide may form during gas or arc welding when no shielding is used. An overview of typical inhalation exposures in welding fume and gases and their major sources, potential respiratory health effects and recommended threshold limit values is summarised in the Table 32.1.

RESPIRATORY DISORDERS

Metal Fever

Welders commonly report influenza-like symptoms after welding, a condition known previously as metal fume fever but more recently termed metal fever (MF), a type of inhalation fever. It is most common after welding zinc-containing galvanized steel, but is also recognized after inhalation of fumes containing copper, magnesium or cadmium. The condition is non-specific and characterized by a transient fever with elevated white blood cell counts and little or no pulmonary inflammation. Symptoms typically appear a few hours after a single inhalation exposure and are self-limiting, usually resolving 24–48 hours after onset. Symptoms include thirst, dry cough, a sweet or metallic taste in the mouth, chills, dry throat, nausea, headache, sweating, fatigue, muscle aches, dyspnoea and fever. The effects are often worse at the start of the working week, and both new welders and long-time welders can be affected. The exact pathophysiological mechanisms of MF are unclear, but the observation that it occurs in both new and long-term welders suggests an acute poisoning, rather than an immunological response. It is estimated that in the USA, a minimum of 1500–2000 cases of MF occur each year (Gordon and Fine, 1993). In a survey of 145 male shipyard welders, 35% experienced episodes of MF (Kilburn et al., 1989), but in a more recent study using standardized definitions, the prevalence of possible MF was 19.7% (El-Zein et al., 2003). A strong association between MF and respiratory symptoms suggestive of occupational asthma (OA) has been reported (El-Zein et al., 2003), suggesting that MF may be an early marker for the subsequent development of OA, but this remains unproven. Diagnosis is based on clinical suspicion, clinical findings and rapid resolution; MF does not usually have any lasting ill effects. Treatment is symptomatic.

Pulmonary Function and Respiratory Symptoms

Numerous studies have found welders to have increased respiratory symptoms (Bradshaw et al., 1998; Sobaszek et al. 1998; Hammond et al., 2005), while reports of associations with reduced lung function have been more mixed. Small, transient, acute effects of welding fume exposure on lung function have been noted, which appear to occur at the time of exposure and then reverse spontaneously. The duration of welding history may have an impact, with those with longer work histories having greater cross-shift declines in lung function. Differences by metal type and welding processes have also been observed, with evidence of greater declines associated with SS compared to MS welding, and MMAW compared to GMAW (Sobaszek et al., 2000). The implications of acute changes in lung function in relation to the development of long-term respiratory disease, including OA, are unclear.

Any chronic effects of welding fume exposure on lung function are less certain. A recent meta-analysis of five longitudinal studies of lung function found no significant differences in annual decline in welders and non-exposed controls after controlling for smoking, but there

TABLE 32.1
Common Welding Fume Constituents, Gases, Sources, Potential Respiratory Effects and Threshold Limit Values from the American Conference of Industrial Hygienists

Fume Constituent	Sources	Potential Respiratory Hazard(s)	ACGIH TLV
Metal			
Aluminium	Additive in steels and non-ferrous alloys in electrodes; present within coatings; high in GMAW of aluminium alloys.	Respiratory irritant; asthma	5 mg/m^3
Cadmium	Rust-preventive coating on steel and alloying element; fluxes in flux-cored electrodes; SS containing cadmium or plated materials; zinc alloy	Respiratory irritant; MF; pulmonary oedema	0.01 mg/m^3 (total); 0.002 mg/m^3 (respirable)
Chromium	SS and high-alloy steels, welding rods. Also used as a plating material	Lung carcinogen (Cr^{6+}); asthma	0.5 mg/m^3
Copper	Copper coated GMAW electrodes; alloys such as Monel, brass and bronze	Respiratory irritant; MF	0.2 mg/m^3
Iron	Major constituent in all iron or steel welding	Siderosis	5 mg/m^3
Manganese	Flux agent on coating of electrodes and in flux-cored arc electrodes; alloying element in electrodes	Respiratory irritant; MF	0.2 mg/m^3
Nickel	SS and nickel alloys; welding rods and plated steel	Lung carcinogen; asthma	0.2 mg/m^3
Zinc	Galvanized and painted metal	MF	5 mg/m^3
Gas			
Carbon monoxide	Breakdown of carbon dioxide shielding gas in arc welding	Asphyxiation	25 ppm
Carbon dioxide	Decomposition of fluxes	Increased pulmonary ventilation rates; asphyxiation	5000 ppm
Nitrogen oxides	Oxidation of atmospheric nitrogen from heat produced by arc or flame	Respiratory irritant; pulmonary oedema; bronchiolitis obliterans; COPD	NO: 25 ppm NO_2: 0.2 ppm
Ozone	Interaction of UV radiation from electric arc with atmospheric oxygen	Respiratory irritant; pulmonary oedema; bronchiolitis obliterans; lung function decline; COPD	0.08 ppm (moderate work)
Phosgene	Decomposition of chlorinated hydrocarbon solvents by UV radiation	Bronchiolitis obliterans; pulmonary oedema	0.1 ppm

Abbreviations: ACGIH: American Conference of Industrial Hygienists; TLV: threshold limit value; GMAW: gas metal arc welding; SS: stainless steel; MF: metal fever; COPD: chronic obstructive pulmonary disease; UV: ultraviolet.

was a possible effect on forced expiratory volume in 1 second (FEV_1) in welders who smoke, supporting a focus on smoking cessation as well as control of fume exposure (Szram et al., 2013). In a subsequent report of a cohort of welders in Austria, significant declines in FEV_1 were associated with duration of exposure to welding fumes (Haluza et al., 2014).

Asthma

A clear association between welding fumes and OA is currently lacking, although a recent review of causative agents determined the level of evidence linking welding fume to OA to be 'moderate' (Baur, 2013). Work-related asthma, both occupational and work exacerbated, has been described in a number of case reports of welders welding on commonly used metals (Keskinen et al., 1980; Contreras, 1997; Hannu et al., 2005, 2007; Munoz et al., 2009), and population-based studies suggest that welding more than doubles the risk of asthma (Karjalainen et al., 2002; Kogevinas et al., 2007). Studies in welding populations suggest that welding fume exposure is a possible cause of OA (Wang et al., 1994; Beach et al., 1996); it is believed that SS welding is more likely to cause asthma through exposure to chromium and nickel fumes, each of which is considered to be able to cause airway sensitisation.

In a state-based asthma surveillance programme in the USA, welding was the fifth leading cause of work-related asthma (Banga et al., 2011); notably, a large number of cases were in non-welders who worked around welding fumes. National and regional surveillance systems in the UK (Surveillance of work-related and occupational respiratory disease [SWORD], Occupational Physicians Reporting Activity [OPRA] and Surveillance Scheme for Occupational Asthma [SHIELD]) also report welding fume to be a common exposure among reported cases of OA (McDonald et al., 2005; Bakerly et al., 2008).

Those who are suspected of having work-related asthma should have the diagnosis confirmed by pre- and post-shift or mid-shift pulmonary function testing (depending on when the individual becomes symptomatic) or measurement of peak flow four times per day over a substantial period. Sufficient time off work (2 weeks or more) may be necessary in order to allow recovery and documentation by peak flow measurements. Specific inhalation challenge tests to metals may help to confirm the diagnosis of metal-induced OA in welders (Wittczak et al., 2012), but the test is rarely available and requires hospital confinement. Non-specific bronchial challenge testing using agents such as methacholine is a safe outpatient procedure and can be useful in documenting the presence of bronchial hyper-responsiveness.

Chronic Bronchitis

Findings from studies evaluating the risks of bronchitis and chronic obstructive pulmonary disease (COPD) in welders are inconsistent, although recent reviews strongly suggest that welding is associated with an increased risk of each condition (Baur et al., 2012; Cullinan, 2012). Typically, the high rates of smoking in welders have made identifying a link between welding fume and bronchitis difficult. In general, studies suggest that welding increases the risk of bronchitis regardless of smoking, and that among smoking welders, the risk is even greater (Barhad et al., 1975; Oxhoj et al., 1979; Mur et al., 1985; Cotes et al., 1989). In a sample of welders in New Zealand, current workers had a higher prevalence of bronchitis than non-welders, and the risk of bronchitis increased with the duration of welding exposure, but was also markedly higher in smokers (Bradshaw et al. 1998); lung function was lower in welders with bronchitis compared to those without. More recently, the prevalence of COPD as determined by spirometry was 15% in a population of welders (Koh et al. 2015) and was associated with higher cumulative welding exposures after controlling for smoking. Population-based data from the European Community Respiratory Health Survey have also indicated an increased risk of COPD among welders (Lillienberg et al., 2008); chronic bronchitis symptoms were significantly higher in those who frequently welded galvanized steel or iron and in those who frequently manually welded SS.

Respiratory Infection

Increased upper and lower respiratory tract infections among welders have been reported (Zeidler-Erdely et al., 2012). Specifically, mortality studies have noted an increased risk of death from pneumonia among welders (Doig and Challen, 1964; Beaumont et al., 1980; Coggon et al., 1994; Palmer et al., 2009). Much of the evidence has been from national mortality data from England and Wales (Coggon et al., 1994; Palmer et al., 2009), which show that welders have an excess risk of death from pneumococcal and lobar pneumonia in particular. Retired welders do not appear to have the same risk, suggesting that the susceptibility of welders is reversible. Palmer et al. reported that exposure to welding fumes in the previous year, but not in earlier periods, was associated with an increased risk of lobar pneumonia (Palmer et al., 2003). In a large cohort of construction workers, exposure to metal fumes was also found to increase the risk of mortality from lobar and pneumococcal pneumonia (Toren et al., 2011), and an increased risk of invasive pneumococcal disease in welders has been observed in Canada (Wong et al., 2010); welders who smoked were found to be at particular risk.

Based on the accumulating evidence of risk of pneumonia in welders, the Joint Committee on Vaccination and Immunisation in England recommended in 2011 that all welders be offered a single dose of pneumococcal vaccine; in 2102, this was extended to other workers who are exposed to metal fumes (Palmer and Cosgrove, 2012, 2013).

Epidemiological studies show that acute welding fume exposure is associated with lung injury and inflammation (Kim et al. 2005; Wang et al., 2005, 2008; Boyce et al., 2006; Fireman et al., 2008; Jonsson et al., 2011), a finding that is corroborated by toxicological studies (Antonini et al., 1997, 2010, 2013; Solano-Lopez et al., 2006; Zeidler-Erdely et al., 2012). It is suggested that chronic exposure blunts the local immune response of lung tissues against inhaled PM, which may predispose individuals to the development of lung infection. Evidence of immunosuppression in welders may explain, in part, their increased risks of respiratory infection (Boshnakova et al., 1989; Tuschl et al., 1997).

Pneumoconiosis

Welders' siderosis, a pneumoconiosis caused by inhalation of iron oxide particles, is a common chronic repository health effect in welders (Figure 32.1). It is a generally

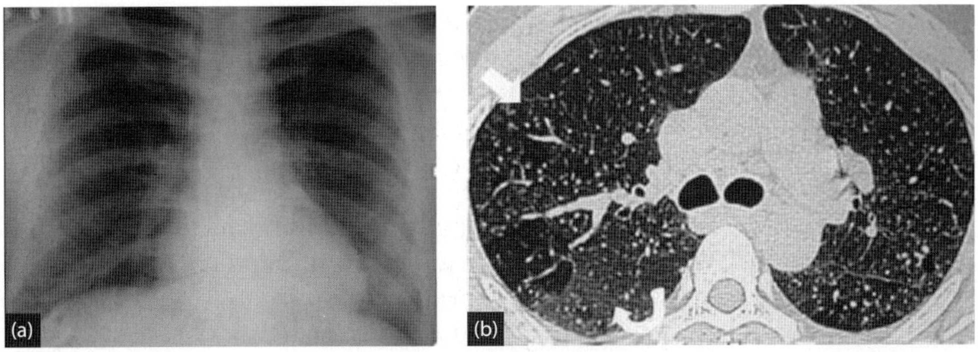

FIGURE 32.1 (a) X-ray and (b) computed tomography scan in a male electric arc welder diagnosed with siderosis. Radiograph is unremarkable, while axial high-resolution computed tomography image shows presence of small, round opacities (straight arrow) in bilateral upper lobes and areas of ground glass opacities (rounded arrow). (Image from Bhawna, S. et al. 2013. *J Clin Imaging Sci* 3:64.)

benign, asymptomatic and non-fibrotic pneumoconiosis. Also referred to as 'welders' lung', the condition was first observed shortly after the introduction of arc welding in the workplace (Doig and McLaughlin, 1936); an abundance of small opacities was observed on the chest radiographs of asymptotic welders with no exposure to coal dust or silica, which on autopsy revealed deposits of significant amounts of iron oxide, mostly present in alveolar macrophages, without the presence of fibrosis. In most cases, regression is observed after cessation of exposure with no impairment of lung function. The iron deposits are usually considered to be confined to the lungs, but systemic iron stores, as evidenced by increased serum ferritin levels, have been reported (Doherty et al., 2004; Patel et al. 2009). A few cases of welders with siderosis and respiratory symptoms or lung function decrements have been reported, although the symptoms were mainly produced by other, non-iron constituents of welding fumes (Billings and Howard, 1993). Rare case reports of fibrosis and symptomatic respiratory disease with siderosis have also been reported, such as in a non-smoker with no known asbestos exposure (McCormick et al., 2008).

Radiographic abnormalities with extensive fibrosis have also been described in welders, mostly in those with exposure to mixed dusts (e.g. silica, asbestos or coalmine dust), but high fume exposure and inadequate ventilation may also lead to interstitial fibrosis (Funahashi et al., 1988; Buerke et al., 2002). In rats, high-dose exposure to welding fume may promote lung fibrosis (Yu et al., 2001). A severe pneumoconiosis, characterized by diffuse pulmonary accumulation of aluminium metal and a corresponding reduction in lung function, is sometimes seen with chronic exposure to high concentrations of fumes during aluminium arc welding (Vallyathan et al., 1982; Hull and Abraham, 2002).

Bronchiolitis Obliterans and Pulmonary Oedema

Exposure to high concentrations of gases and chemical fumes may cause bronchiolitis obliterans, a rare sequela characterized by fibrosis and the narrowing and filling of bronchioles, resulting in irreversible airflow obstruction. Several agents are reported to cause bronchiolitis obliterans, including some found in welding, specifically ozone, nitrogen dioxide and phosgene. Bronchiolitis obliterans must be differentiated from asthma, since both present with wheezing and a clear chest X-ray. High-resolution computed tomography (CT) shows a patchy interstitial pattern in the former.

Exposure to high concentrations of cadmium fume, phosgene, nitrogen dioxide and ozone may also cause pulmonary oedema; in some cases, the effects may be delayed.

Lung Cancer

Occupational exposure to welding fumes is classified as possibly carcinogenic to humans (IARC, 1990). While it is thought that the risk is largely with SS welding due to its high chromium and nickel content, this classification is not limited to SS fume. In vitro toxicity studies indicate that SS welding fumes are mutagenic in mammalian cells while MS fumes are not (Hedenstedt et al., 1977; Maxild et al., 1978; Stern et al., 1988), but epidemiological studies have not been able to make this distinction. Variations in workplaces, in asbestos exposure and a high smoking prevalence among welders have made it difficult to discern a clear association between welding fume and lung cancer, but a recent meta-analysis of 60 studies conducted between 1954 and 2004 found an excess of lung cancer for welders after accounting for smoking, but not for asbestos exposure (Ambroise et al., 2006). Recent epidemiological studies report no increased risk due to welding fumes among moderate to heavy smokers, but a more than twofold excess risk related to both gas and arc welding fumes among light smokers (Vallieres et al., 2012). When controlling for smoking and other occupational exposures, the risk of lung cancer was increased for both MS and SS welders (Sorensen et al., 2007). Siew et al. also observed an increased risk of lung cancer in Finnish male welders after adjusting for smoking and asbestos and silica exposure (Siew et al., 2008). Declines in telomere length associated with cumulative welding PM exposure have been observed, perhaps providing biological plausibility to the association (Wong et al., 2014).

DIAGNOSIS

A history, physical examination, chest X-ray, chest CT imaging and pulmonary function tests are used to diagnose most occupational lung disease. Diagnosis is also helped by finding: (1) a temporal association of work with symptoms; and (2) known aetiological agents in the workplace. An understanding of the specific welding process, base metal and known coatings, type of rod and coating if MMAW is performed and shielding gas is an important part of an occupational history. When assessing risk, it is important to consider how long a welder is actually welding; some welders may spend a significant amount of time setting up before welding. The risk of exposure to non-welders (e.g. helpers or other workers) in the vicinity of welding should also be considered.

TREATMENT

There are no specific treatments for lung disorders caused by welding fumes. Pneumoconiosis management consists of a functional impairment and disability assessment and general health maintenance strategies such as influenza and pneumococcal vaccination. For those with reversible airways obstruction (asthma and some cases of COPD), treatment with bronchodilators and anti-inflammatory agents is warranted. All individuals should be strongly advised to stop smoking. Workers with confirmed OA should be given the option of transferring to areas of non-exposure whenever possible, as sensitized individuals may react at very low levels of exposure.

PREVENTION

Minimizing exposure to welding fumes and gases is an important part of preventing associated occupational lung diseases. Alternative processes that generate lower amounts of fume, reducing the amount of time spent breathing in the fumes directly rising from the torch and minimizing work in enclosed or confined spaces should be considered. Local exhaust ventilation for stationary processes and diluting fumes with general ventilation in mobile tasks can also reduce exposure. Proper personal protective equipment is an important part of exposure minimization; workers should be trained to properly and regularly wear appropriate respirators. Regular annual medical examinations for individuals who are exposed to welding fumes can be an important secondary strategy for preventing respiratory disease caused by the inhalation of welding fumes.

REFERENCES

Ambroise, D., Wild, P. and Moulin, J. J. 2006. Update of a meta-analysis on lung cancer and welding. *Scand J Work Environ Health* 32(1):22–31.

Antonini, J. M. 2003. Health effects of welding. *Crit Rev Toxicol* 33(1):61–103.

Antonini, J. M., Krishna Murthy, G. G. and Brain, J. D. 1997. Responses to welding fumes: lung injury, inflammation, and the release of tumor necrosis factor-alpha and interleukin-1 beta. *Exp Lung Res* 23(3):205–27.

Antonini, J. M., Roberts, J. R., Chapman, R. S., Soukup, J. M., Ghio, A. J. and Sriram, K. 2010. Pulmonary toxicity and extrapulmonary tissue distribution of metals after repeated exposure to different welding fumes. *Inhal Toxicol* 22(10):805–16.

Antonini, J. M., Roberts, J. R., Schwegler-Berry, D. and Mercer, R. R. 2013. Comparative microscopic study of human and rat lungs after overexposure to welding fume. *Ann Occup Hyg* 57(9):1167–79.

Bakerly, N. D., Moore, V. C., Vellore, A. D., Jaakkola, M. S., Robertson, A. S. and Burge, P. S. 2008. Fifteen-year trends in occupational asthma: Data from the Shield surveillance scheme. *Occup Med* 58(3):169–74.

Banga, A., Reilly, M. J. and Rosenman, K. D. 2011. A study of characteristics of Michigan workers with work-related asthma exposed to welding. *J Occup Environ Med* 53(4):415–9.

Barhad, B., Teculescu, D. and Craciun, O. 1975. Respiratory symptoms, chronic bronchitis, and ventilatory function in shipyard welders. *Int Arch Occupational and Environmental Health* 36(2):137–50.

Baur, X. 2013. A compendium of causative agents of occupational asthma. *J Occup Med Toxicol* 8(1):15.

Baur, X., Bakehe, P. and Vellguth, H. 2012. Bronchial asthma and COPD due to irritants in the workplace—An evidence-based approach. *J Occup Med Toxicol* 7(1):19.

Beach, J. R., Dennis, J. H., Avery, A. J., Bromly, C. L., Ward, R. J., Walters, E. H. et al. 1996. An epidemiologic investigation of asthma in welders. *Am J Respir Crit Care Med* 154(5):1394–400.

Beaumont, J. J. and Weiss, N. S. 1980. Mortality of welders, shipfitters, and other metal trades workers in boilermakers Local No. 104, AFL-CIO. *Am J Epidemiol* 112(6):775–86.

Bhawna, S., Ojha, U. C., Kumar, S., Gupta, R., Gothi, D., Pal, R. S. 2013. Spectrum of high resolution computed tomography findings in occupational lung disease: Experience in a tertiary care institute. *J Clin Imaging Sci* 3:64.

Billings, C. G. and Howard, P. 1993. Occupational siderosis and welders' lung: A review. *Monaldi Arch Chest Dis* 48(4):304–14.

Boshnakova, E., Divanyan, H., Zlatarov, I., Marovsky, S., Kisyova, K., Zanev, D. et al. 1989. Immunological screening of welders. *J Hyg Epidemiol Microbiol Immunol* 33(4):379–82.

Boyce, P. D., Kim, J. Y., Weissman, D. N., Hunt, J. and Christiani, D. C. 2006. pH increase observed in exhaled breath condensate from welding fume exposure. *J Occup Environ Med* 48(4):353–6.

Bradshaw, L. M., Fishwick, D., Slater, T. and Pearce, N. 1998. Chronic bronchitis, work related respiratory symptoms, and pulmonary function in welders in New Zealand. *Occup Environ Med* 55(3):150–4.

Brand, P., Lenz, K., Reisgen, U. and Kraus, T. 2013. Number size distribution of fine and ultrafine fume particles from various welding processes. *Ann Occup Hyg* 57(3):305–13.

Buerke, U., Schneider, J., Rosler, J. and Woitowitz, H. J. 2002. Interstitial pulmonary fibrosis after severe exposure to welding fumes. *Am J Ind Med* 41(4):259–68.

Burgess, W. A. 1995. *Recognition of Health Hazards in Industry: A Review of Materials and Processes,* 2nd ed. New York: John Wiley and Sons, Inc.

Chang, C., Demokritou, P., Shafer, M. and Christiani, D. 2013. Physicochemical and toxicological characteristics of welding fume derived particles generated from real time welding processes. *Environ Sci Processes Impacts* 15(1):214–24.

Coggon, D., Inskip, H., Winter, P. and Pannett, B. 1994. Lobar pneumonia: An occupational disease in welders. *Lancet* 344(8914):41–3.

Contreras, G. R. and Chan-Yeung M. 1997. Bronchial reactions to exposure to welding fumes. *Occup Environ Med* 54(11):836–9.

Cotes, J. E., Feinmann, E. L., Male, V. J., Rennie, F. S. and Wickham, C. A. 1989. Respiratory symptoms and impairment in shipyard welders and caulker/burners. *Br J Ind Med* 46(5):292–301.

Cullinan, P. 2012. Occupation and chronic obstructive pulmonary disease (COPD). *Br Med Bull* 104:143–61.

Doherty, M. J., Healy, M., Richardson, S. G. and Fisher, N. C. 2004. Total body iron overload in welder's siderosis. *Occup Environ Med* 61(1):82–5.

Doig, A. T. and Challen, P. J. 1964. Respiratory hazards in welding. *Ann Occup Hyg* 7:223–31.

Doig, A. T. and McLaughlin, A. I. G. 1936. X-ray appearances of the lungs of electric arc welders. *Lancet* 1:771–5.

El-Zein, M., Malo, J. L., Infante-Rivard, C. and Gautrin, D. 2003. Prevalence and association of welding related systemic and respiratory symptoms in welders. *Occup Environ Med* 60(9):655–61.

Fireman, E., Lerman, Y., Stark, M., Schwartz, Y., Ganor, E., Grinberg, N. et al. 2008. Detection of occult lung impairment in welders by induced sputum particles and breath oxidation. *Am J Ind Med* 51(7):503–11.

Funahashi, A., Schlueter, D. P., Pintar, K., Bemis, E. L. and Siegesmund, K. A. 1988. Welders' pneumoconiosis: tissue elemental microanalysis by energy dispersive X ray analysis. *Br J Ind Med* 45(1):14–8.

Gordon, T. and Fine, J. M. 1993. Metal fume fever. *Occup Med* 8(3):504–17.

Haluza, D., Moshammer, H. and Hochgatterer, K. 2014. Dust is in the air. Part II: Effects of occupational exposure to welding fumes on lung function in a 9-year study. *Lung* 192(1):111–7.

Hammond, S. K., Gold, E., Baker, R., Quinlan, P., Smith, W., Pandya, R. et al. 2005. Respiratory health effects related to occupational spray painting and welding. *J Occup Environ Med* 47(7):728–39.

Hannu, T., Piipari, R., Kasurinen, H., Keskinen, H., Tuppurainen, M. and Tuomi T. 2005. Occupational asthma due to manual metal-arc welding of special stainless steels. *Eur Respir J* 26(4):736–9.

Hannu, T., Piipari, R., Tuppurainen, M., Nordman, H. and Tuomi T. 2007. Occupational asthma caused by stainless steel welding fumes: a clinical study. *Eur Respir J* 29(1):85–90.

Hedenstedt, A., Jenssen, D., Lidestein, B. M., Ramel, C., Rannug, U. and Stern, R. M. 1977. Mutagenicity of fume particles from stainless steel welding. *Scand J Work Environ Health* 3(4):203–11.

Hull, M. J. and Abraham, J. L. 2002. Aluminum welding fume-induced pneumoconiosis. *Hum Pathol* 33(8):819–25.

IARC. 1990. *IARC Monographs on the Evaluation of Carcinogenic Risks to Humans, Chromium, Nickel, and Welding.* Geneva: WHO IARC.

Jonsson, L. S., Nielsen, J. and Broberg, K. 2011. Gene expression analysis in induced sputum from welders with and without airway-related symptoms. *Int Arch Occup Environ Health* 84(1):105–13.

Karjalainen, A., Martikainen, R., Oksa, P., Saarinen, K. and Uitti J. 2002. Incidence of asthma among Finnish construction workers. *J Occup Environ Med* 44(8):752–7.

Keskinen, H., Kalliomaki, P. L. and Alanko, K. 1980. Occupational asthma due to stainless steel welding fumes. *Clin Allergy* 10(2):151–9.

Kilburn, K. H., Warshaw, R. H., Boylen, C. T. and Thornton, J. C. 1989. Respiratory symptoms and functional impairment from acute (cross-shift) exposure to welding gases and fumes. *Am J Med Sci* 298(5):314–9.

Kim, J. Y., Chen, J. C., Boyce, P. D. and Christiani, D. C. 2005. Exposure to welding fumes is associated with acute systemic inflammatory responses. *Occup Environ Med* 62(3):157–63.

Kogevinas, M., Zock, J. P., Jarvis, D., Kromhout, H., Lillienberg, L., Plana, E. et al. 2007. Exposure to substances in the workplace and new-onset asthma: An international prospective population-based study (ECRHS-II). *Lancet* 370(9584):336–41.

Koh, D. H., Kim, J. I., Kim, K. H., Yoo, S. W.; on behalf of the Korea Welders Cohort Group. 2015. Welding fume exposure and chronic obstructive pulmonary disease in welders. *Occup Med* 65(1):72–7.

Lillienberg, L., Zock, J. P., Kromhout, H., Plana, E., Jarvis, D., Toren, K. et al. 2008. A population-based study on welding exposures at work and respiratory symptoms. *Ann Occup Hyg* 52(2):107–15.

Maxild, J., Andersen, M. and Kiel, P. 1978. Mutagenicity of fume particles from metal arc welding on stainless steel in the *Salmonella*/microsome test. *Mutat Res* 56(3):235–43.

McCormick, L. M., Goddard, M. and Mahadeva, R. 2008. Pulmonary fibrosis secondary to siderosis causing symptomatic respiratory disease: A case report. *J Med Case Rep* 2:257.

McDonald, J. C., Chen, Y., Zekveld, C. and Cherry, N. M. 2005. Incidence by occupation and industry of acute work related respiratory diseases in the UK, 1992–2001. *Occup Environ Med* 62(12):836–42.

Munoz, X., Cruz, M. J., Freixa, A., Guardino, X. and Morell F. 2009. Occupational asthma caused by metal arc welding of iron. *Respiration* 78(4):455–9.

Mur, J. M., Teculescu, D., Pham, Q. T., Gaertner, M., Massin, N., Meyer-Bisch, C. et al. 1985. Lung function and clinical findings in a cross-sectional study of arc welders. An epidemiological study. *Int Arch Occup Environ Health* 57(1):1–17.

Oxhoj, H., Bake, B., Wedel, H. and Wilhelmsen, L. 1979. Effects of electric arc welding on ventilatory lung function. *Arch Environ Health* 34(4):211–7.

Palmer, K. and Cosgrove, M. 2013. Community-acquired pneumonia and welding. *Clin Med* 13(2):214–5.

Palmer, K. T. and Cosgrove, M. P. 2012. Vaccinating welders against pneumonia. *Occup Med* 62(5):325–30.

Palmer, K. T., Cullinan, P., Rice, S., Brown, T. and Coggon, D. 2009. Mortality from infectious pneumonia in metal workers: A comparison with deaths from asthma in occupations exposed to respiratory sensitisers. *Thorax* 64(11):983–6.

Palmer, K. T., Poole, J., Ayres, J. G., Mann, J., Burge, P. S. and Coggon, D. 2003. Exposure to metal fume and infectious pneumonia. *Am J Epidemiol* 157(3):227–33.

Patel, R. R., Yi, E. S. and Ryu, J. H. 2009. Systemic iron overload associated with welder's siderosis. *Am J Med Sci* 337(1):57–9.

Siew, S. S., Kauppinen, T., Kyyronen, P., Heikkila, P. and Pukkala, E. 2008. Exposure to iron and welding fumes and the risk of lung cancer. *Scand J Work Environ Health*. 34(6):444–50.

Sobaszek, A., Boulenguez, C., Frimat, P., Robin, H., Haguenoer, J. M. and Edme, J. L. 2000. Acute respiratory effects of exposure to stainless steel and mild steel welding fumes. *J Occup Environ Med* 42(9):923–31.

Sobaszek, A., Edme, J. L., Boulenguez, C., Shirali, P., Mereau, M., Robin, H. et al. 1998. Respiratory symptoms and pulmonary function among stainless steel welders. *J Occup Environ Med* 40(3):223–9.

Solano-Lopez, C., Zeidler-Erdely, P. C., Hubbs, A. F., Reynolds, S. H., Roberts, J. R., Taylor, M. D. et al. 2006. Welding fume exposure and associated inflammatory and hyperplastic changes in the lungs of tumor susceptible a/j mice. *Toxicol Pathol* 34(4):364–72.

Sorensen, A. R., Thulstrup, A. M., Hansen, J., Ramlau-Hansen, C. H., Meersohn, A., Skytthe, A. et al. 2007. Risk of lung cancer according to mild steel and stainless steel welding. *Scand J Work Environ Health* 33(5):379–86.

Stern, R. M., Hansen, K., Madsen, A. F. and Olsen, K. M. 1988. *In vitro* toxicity of welding fumes and their constituents. *Environ Res* 46(2):168–80.

Szram, J., Schofield, S. J., Cosgrove, M. P. and Cullinan, P. 2013. Welding, longitudinal lung function decline and chronic respiratory symptoms: A systematic review of cohort studies. *Eur Respir J* 42(5):1186–93.

Toren, K., Qvarfordt, I., Bergdahl, I. A. and Jarvholm, B. 2011. Increased mortality from infectious pneumonia after occupational exposure to inorganic dust, metal fumes and chemicals. *Thorax* 66(11):992–6.

Tuschl, H., Weber, E. and Kovac, R. 1997. Investigations on immune parameters in welders. *J Applied Toxicol* 17(6):377–83.

Vallieres, E., Pintos, J., Lavoue, J., Parent, M. E., Rachet, B. and Siemiatycki, J. 2012. Exposure to welding fumes increases lung cancer risk among light smokers but not among heavy smokers: Evidence from two case–control studies in Montreal. *Cancer Med* 1(1):47–58.

Vallyathan, V., Bergeron, W. N., Robichaux, P. A. and Craighead, J. E. 1982. Pulmonary fibrosis in an aluminum arc welder. *Chest* 81(3):372–4.

Wang, Z., Neuburg, D., Li, C., Su, L., Kim, J. Y., Chen, J. C. et al. 2005. Global gene expression profiling in whole-blood samples from individuals exposed to metal fumes. *Environ Health Perspect* 113(2):233–41.

Wang, Z., Neuberg, D., Su, L., Kim, J. Y., Chen, J. C., Christiani, D. C. 2008. Prospective study of metal fume-induced responses of global gene expression profiling in whole blood. *Inhal Toxicol* 20(14):1233–44.

Wang, Z. P., Larsson, K., Malmberg, P., Sjogren, B., Hallberg, B. O. and Wrangskog K. 1994. Asthma, lung function, and bronchial responsiveness in welders. *Am J Ind Med* 26(6):741–54.

Wittczak, T., Dudek, W., Walusiak-Skorupa, J., Swierczynska-Machura, D., Cader, W., Kowalczyk, M. et al. 2012. Metal-induced asthma and chest X-ray changes in welders. *Int J Occup Med Environ Health* 25(3):242–50.

Wong, A., Marrie, T. J., Garg, S., Kellner, J. D., Tyrrell, G. J. and SPAT Group. 2010. Welders are at increased risk for invasive pneumococcal disease. *Int J Infect Dis* 14(9):e796–9.

Wong, J. Y., De Vivo, I., Lin, X. and Christiani, D. C. 2014. Cumulative $PM_{2.5}$ exposure and telomere length in workers exposed to welding fumes. *J Toxicol Environ Health A* 77(8):441–55.

Yu, I. J., Song, K. S., Chang, H. K., Han, J. H., Kim, K. J., Chung, Y. H. et al. 2001. Lung fibrosis in Sprague–Dawley rats, induced by exposure to manual metal arc-stainless steel welding fumes. *Toxicol Sci* 63(1):99–106.

Zeidler-Erdely, P. C., Erdely, A. and Antonini, J. M. 2012. Immunotoxicology of arc welding fume: Worker and experimental animal studies. *J Immunotoxicol* 9(4):411–25.

33 Pulmonary Infections Including Zoonoses

Julia Heptonstall and Anne Cockcroft

CONTENTS

INTRODUCTION

A wide range of infections may have at least some lung involvement and occur more frequently in some occupational groups. In this chapter, we cover those infections that have important and serious lung consequences, with or without the involvement of other systems, and that present a clear occupational risk. The occupational groups that are most commonly at risk of lung infections include those exposed to animals or animal products, as well as healthcare workers and laboratory workers. We do not cover infections that present a clear occupational risk but rarely involve the lungs (such as brucellosis) or lung infections without a clear occupational risk. These are covered in general texts on occupational diseases (Baxter et al., 2010) and on infection. We describe conditions in three groups: those with a zoonotic source (the largest group); those with an environmental source; and those with a human source.

Many of the infections covered here, particularly those with a zoonotic or environmental source, occur mainly in resource-poor countries, with poor health infrastructure and little, if any, provision of occupational health services for most workers. Therefore, it is likely that the frequency of these infections, and their occupational impact, are underestimated.

INFECTIONS WITH A ZOONOTIC SOURCE

Anthrax

Epidemiology

Anthrax was one of the first diseases to be recognised as work related, and much of the early history of occupational pulmonary medicine is concerned with attempts to control the disease in the textile industry in the United Kingdom, where it was first described in 1847 (LaForce, 1978; Turnbull, 2002). The history of anthrax is covered in detail elsewhere (Stark, 2013).

Anthrax is primarily a disease of herbivores (cattle, sheep, goats, horses, camels, buffalo, etc.). Pulmonary (or inhalational) anthrax is rare in humans, but there is an occupational risk for people who may deal with infected animals (vets, farmers, shepherds and herders, and zookeepers), their carcasses (slaughterhouse and abattoir workers, and butchers) or animal products (textile workers, carpet factory workers, leather importers and tanners, and workers who process or render gelatine, glue, bone or tallow), as well as for workers involved in the storage or transport of infected raw materials, such as dockers and warehousemen.

In developed countries, with risk assessment (Health and Safety Executive, 1997), engineering controls and pre-exposure vaccination (Public Health England, 2014), the disease is very rare. A few sporadic cases of pulmonary anthrax continue to be reported in people making drums from imported untreated goatskin or doing craftwork with imported yarns (Marston et al., 2011), in two cases of people who had separately visited state parks in the USA but had no obvious history of exposure (Griffith et al., 2014; Sprenkle et al., 2014) and in a soldier who had been vaccinated against anthrax before service in Iraq 4 years previously but who had no previous or recent identifiable exposure (Sykes et al., 2013). Pulmonary anthrax with apparently minimal exposure is well recognised (Brachman et al., 1961). Some infections may be asymptomatic: in a wool processing factory in Belgium, where live anthrax spores were identified but no clinical cases occurred, eight out of 66 employees had relevant antibodies, and workers who sorted or processed raw goat hair were more likely to be seropositive (Kissling et al., 2012).

Anthrax as a Bioweapon

The bioweapon potential of *Bacillus anthracis* was first explored early in the twentieth century. The organism is easily grown, has an inhalable and dispersible form that can persist in the environment for long periods, causes a fatal disease in humans and animals and is not directly transmissible from person to person. In the United Kingdom during World War II, cattle cakes laced with anthrax spores were produced, although never used (Hammond and Carter, 2001), and in Sverdlovsk, Ukraine, in 1979, 74 cases of pulmonary anthrax occurred in the local community after the inadvertent dispersal of *B. anthracis* spores from a military research establishment (Meselson et al., 1994).

In 2001, 11 cases of pulmonary anthrax occurred (with seven confirmed and four suspected cutaneous cases) after anthrax spores were sent through the US Postal Service in envelopes addressed to prominent government or media figures (Jernigan et al., 2001, 2002; Guarner et al., 2003). Most cases occurred in people handling or processing the contaminated mail in transit (four mail workers, two of whom died, and two mail processors) or receiving the contaminated mail (a media company mailroom worker, a government office mail processor and a media company employee, who died), but a hospital supply worker and a retired elderly woman, both thought to have become infected after exposure to cross-contaminated mail, also died. Post-exposure antibiotic prophylaxis (a 60-day course of oral ciprofloxacin or doxycycline) was recommended for approximately 10,000 people assessed as being at risk of spore exposure; most of these individuals probably did not complete the course, but no cases of anthrax occurred. A laboratory worker dealing with outbreak-related samples acquired cutaneous anthrax (Jernigan et al, 2002). These were the first cases of pulmonary anthrax in the USA since 1976, and equalled the number of naturally acquired cases of pulmonary anthrax reported throughout the USA from 1955 to 2000. In consequence, there has been an explosion of work on anthrax in research and diagnostic laboratories; several incidents have occurred in which live anthrax has been transferred between laboratories as a result of lapses in laboratory procedure (Centers for Disease Control and Prevention, 2014; Weiss et al., 2015). Some national health authorities recommend pre-exposure vaccination of laboratory workers who are at high risk of exposure to anthrax spores (Public Health England, 2014). Guidance on the management of suspected anthrax (and other infections) in the context of an 'incident' is available from the UK Health Protection Agency (Heptonstall and Gent, 2006).

Pathology, Clinical Features and Management

Inhaled spores of less than 5-μm diameters are carried by macrophages from the terminal bronchioles to the regional lymph nodes, germinating either locally or in the lymph nodes into toxin-producing, rapidly replicating bacilli; haemorrhagic mediastinitis, bacteraemia and anthrax toxinaemia follow. *B. anthracis* has a plasmid-encoded polyglutamate capsule that inhibits phagocytosis; a second plasmid codes for three main toxin components (protective antigen, lethal factor and oedema factor), which act in combination to produce lethal toxin and oedema toxin. These cause cell death and disruption of cell signalling systems, and also hypotension via direct effects on the myocardium and peripheral vasculature. Pathologically, infection is characterised by oedema and haemorrhagic necrosis; typical autopsy findings report haemorrhagic mediastinitis with oedema, large serosanguinous pleural effusions, pericardial effusion, ascites, splenic involvement, cerebral oedema and haemorrhagic meningitis (Albrink et al., 1960).

Pulmonary anthrax may present as a non-specific febrile illness; diagnosis may be delayed unless other cases have recently been reported. In severe cases, a short prodromal phase is followed by a fulminant phase with rapid progression to hypotension, refractory shock and death. The diagnosis is established by culture of *B. anthracis* from blood or other appropriate specimens (cerebrospinal fluid [CSF], pleural fluid or biopsy); immunohistochemistry and serology may also be helpful, especially if antibiotics have already been given. The chest radiograph (Figure 33.1) may show a widened mediastinum, but hilar and para-tracheal node enlargement and pleural and pericardial effusions may be best shown with computed tomography (Plotkin et al., 2002). In the 2001 outbreak, cases treated with antibiotics in the prodromal phase survived; those treated later did not. Combination intravenous antibiotic therapy using a fluoroquinolone (e.g. ciprofloxacin), a carbapenem (e.g. imipenem/cilastin or meropenem) and a protein inhibitor (e.g. clindamycin or linezolid) is recommended, and corticosteroids and antitoxin should be considered

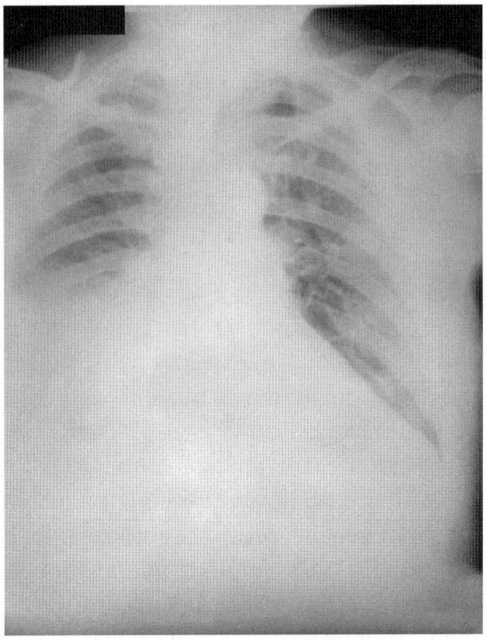

FIGURE 33.1 Chest radiograph of anthrax pneumonia on the fourth day of illness. (From Public domain, accessed via Centers for Disease Control and Prevention [CDC] Public Health Images Library.)

(Hendricks et al., 2014). *B. anthracis* is not sensitive to cephalosporins. Modern intensive care, with haemodynamic monitoring, treatment of coagulopathy or thrombocytopenia and early and aggressive drainage of effusions (which may reduce toxin load as well as improve ventilation), may increase survival.

Bacillus cereus, an organism that is very closely related to *B. anthracis* and normally causes pneumonia only in the immunosuppressed, has been reported as the cause of fulminant bacteraemia, severe pneumonia and an anthrax-like illness in metal workers in Texas and Louisiana (Miller et al., 1997; Avashia et al., 2007). These strains have been shown to be capsulated and to carry anthrax toxin genes. *B. cereus* is often regarded as a contaminant, but when found in pure culture in samples from a patient with severe illness, it should not be automatically discounted as the cause.

Hantavirus Pulmonary Syndrome

Hantavirus pulmonary syndrome (HPS) was first described in an outbreak of severe pulmonary illness in the United States in 1993 (Centers for Disease Control and Prevention, 1993); Sin Nombre virus was isolated from patients and deer mice.

Nearly 30 different hantaviruses (including Bayou, Monongahela, New York, Andes, Oran, Choclo, Bermejo and Lechiguana) have been associated with HPS, reported from the United States, Argentina, Brazil, Chile, Colombia, Uruguay, Panama, Paraguay, Venezuela and Canada. (Pan American Health Organisation, 1999). Each hantavirus has a specific rodent host; humans are infected by inhaling the virus in dust contaminated with rodent excreta or by direct contact with rodents. Occupational groups that are at risk include forestry workers and farmers (Schmaljohn and Hjelle, 1997; Riquelme et al., 2015), field biologists, and construction workers and others exposed to rodent infestations in buildings. Human-to-human transmission has been reported only for Andes virus, which often occurs in household clusters (Wells et al., 1997).

The incubation period is 1–5 weeks. A febrile prodrome of 3–5 days, with myalgia and sometimes headache, nausea and vomiting, is followed by cough and breathlessness, with rapid progression to pulmonary oedema and respiratory failure; 35%–50% of human infections are fatal. There may be thrombocytopenia and atypical lymphocytes and immunoblasts. Diagnosis is usually made by serology (IgM capture enzyme linked immunosorbent assay [ELISA], IgG ELISA on paired acute and convalescent sera), although direct detection of virus by polymerase chain reaction (PCR) in blood and tissue is possible. There is no specific treatment, but early diagnosis and intensive care support may reduce mortality.

Henipavirus Infections

These highly pathogenic paramyxoviruses have a natural reservoir in fruit bats (flying foxes, *Pteropus* spp.). Hendra virus (HeV) is endemic in fruit bats only in Australia (Field et al., 2011). There is evidence of Nipah virus (NiV) infection in fruit bats in South and South East Asia. Infected bats are asymptomatic, but shed virus in urine, faeces, saliva and other body fluids. Human infections are rare.

HeV (formerly equine morbillivirus) was discovered after an outbreak of fatal respiratory and neurological disease in horses in a training stable near Brisbane in 1994 (Murray et al., 1995; Selvey et al., 1995). The trainer died of a fulminant pneumonia; the stable foreman survived an influenza-like illness. Some 50 equine outbreaks have since been reported. Horse-to-horse transmission occurs, but bat-to-human and human-to-human transmission has not been reported. Only seven human cases (two trainers, a stable worker, two vets and two workers in a veterinary hospital) have been reported (O'Sullivan et al., 1997; Hannah et al., 2006; Playford et al., 2008). Three of the four fatal cases died from encephalitis. All cases had exposure to the body fluids of infected horses 5–21 days before disease onset. A commercial vaccine for horses is available in Australia. Other preventative measures include preventing access of horses to bat habitats, segregation of sick horses and use of personal protective equipment (Biosecurity Queensland, 2011). There is published guidance on exposure assessment and the management of cases and their contacts (Australian Government Department of Health, 2012).

NiV was first isolated from a patient in Malaysia in 1999 during an outbreak of severe neurological illness, initially thought to be Japanese encephalitis, among pig farmers and others in contact with pigs in intensive farming units in Malaysia, and abattoir workers in Singapore in contact with imported pigs (Centers for Disease Control and Prevention, 1999; Chua et al., 1999; Paton et al., 1999). Cases in Malaysia presented with encephalitis preceded by 3–14 days of febrile illness, sometimes with a non-productive cough; few had abnormal chest radiographs. Almost half of the affected individuals died; some survivors had long-term neurological sequelae or late relapses. Person-to-person transmission did not occur. The pigs were probably infected via exposure to bat secretions. The dense pig farm populations and transport of infected pigs between farms amplified the porcine epidemic. The epidemic was controlled with the provision of personal protective equipment for workers, a transport ban on pigs and widespread pig culling. Although NiV has been found since 1999 in fruit bats in Malaysia, no further human cases have been reported.

Outbreaks and sporadic cases of human NiV encephalitis have been reported in Bangladesh since 2001, especially in rural areas in winter, with case–fatality rates of approximately 75% (Luby et al., 2009). Outbreaks have also occurred in neighbouring areas in India (Chadha et al., 2006). Two-thirds of NiV cases in Bangladesh have had cough and breathlessness, with diffuse bilateral pulmonary opacities on the chest radiograph. Infection may be through drinking fresh date palm sap contaminated with infected bat secretions (Rahman et al., 2012) or exposure to sick goats, pigs and cows. Person-to-person transmission has occurred frequently (to family caregivers, healthcare workers and a rickshaw driver who transported a case) and NiV has been isolated from human saliva.

In an outbreak of 24 cases of henipavirus infection associated with the slaughter and consumption of meat from sick horses in the Philippines (Ching et al., 2015), 14 out of 17 cases with acute encephalitis died, and five with an influenza-like illness and one with meningitis all survived. Two healthcare workers who had cared for the patients using gloves and masks but without eye protection were infected.

When henipavirus infection is suspected, public health authorities should be alerted. The diagnosis is confirmed by specialist laboratories under containment level 4 conditions using a combination of virus isolation and reverse transcription polymerase chain reaction (RT-PCR) on acute samples (throat swab, blood, urine and CSF), serology and immunohistochemistry. There is no specific treatment, although both ribavirin and virus-specific monoclonal antibody have been used.

Human Avian Influenza Infection

Avian influenza A viruses cause infection in poultry and many wild birds. Most are not serious avian pathogens, but some (highly pathogenic avian influenza A virus) are highly transmissible and cause lethal disease in poultry flocks. In 1997, the first cases of human infection occurred during a poultry outbreak of influenza A (H5N1) in Hong Kong. Influenza A (H5N1) remerged in 2003, and has since become endemic in birds in China and much of South East Asia, and is found widely elsewhere. Avian influenza virus A (H7N9) first infected humans in China in 2013 (Cowling et al., 2013); by February 2015, 571 laboratory-confirmed cases, with 212 deaths (37%), had been reported (World Health Organization, 2015).

Most human influenza A (H5N1) and avian influenza A (H7N9) cases have reported exposure either to birds or to markets in which live birds are sold. Sustained human-to-human transmission has not occurred, but both viruses may have pandemic potential, and both have caused more aggressive human disease than seasonal influenza virus. There is evidence that healthcare workers exposed to patients with influenza A (H5N1) are at risk of contracting the infection (Bridges et al., 2000), as well as a case report of a doctor dying from influenza A (H7N9), possibly contracted from a patient (Pan et al., 2015). Cases present with fever, cough and a rapidly progressive pneumonia that does not respond to antibiotic therapy. There may be lymphopenia, thrombocytopenia, impaired liver and renal function and rapid progression to acute respiratory distress syndrome. Older patients with comorbidity have a greater risk of severe disease and death. Diagnosis is by detection of the virus by real time RT-PCR or isolation from nasopharyngeal aspirate or other respiratory specimens (bronchoalveolar lavage and endotracheal aspirate). If the diagnosis is suspected, empiric antiviral treatment with a neuraminidase inhibitor (oseltamivir, zanamivir or peramivir) is recommended, as it is for close contacts of either birds or humans with known infection who develop fever or respiratory symptoms in the 7 days after exposure. Steroids are not effective; the viruses are resistant to adamantine drugs.

Leptospirosis

This zoonosis is caused by pathogenic spirochetes of the genus *Leptospira*. It occurs worldwide, but especially in the tropics; over half a million cases occur each year. Infected animal hosts (rodents, dogs and many wild and domestic mammals) shed leptospirae in their urine. Humans become infected by direct exposure to an infected animal (vets, dairy and pig farmers, abattoir workers, rodent trappers and field biologists) or more commonly by exposure of broken skin or the eyes, nose or oropharynx to water or damp soil contaminated with animal urine (miners, sewer and canal workers, plantation workers, fish, taro and paddy rice farmers [Figure 33.2], orienteers, canoeists, triathletes and military personnel) (Queensland Government: Department of Industrial Relations Workplace Health and Safety, 2002; Gill et al., 1985; Levett, 2001; Thornley et al., 2002; Hartskeerl et al., 2011; Katz et al., 2011). Large outbreaks have occurred after flooding in urban slums. Person-to-person transmission is unusual.

Many infections are asymptomatic or produce an acute, non-specific febrile illness. Leptospirosis may be mistaken for influenza A, dengue, malaria, viral

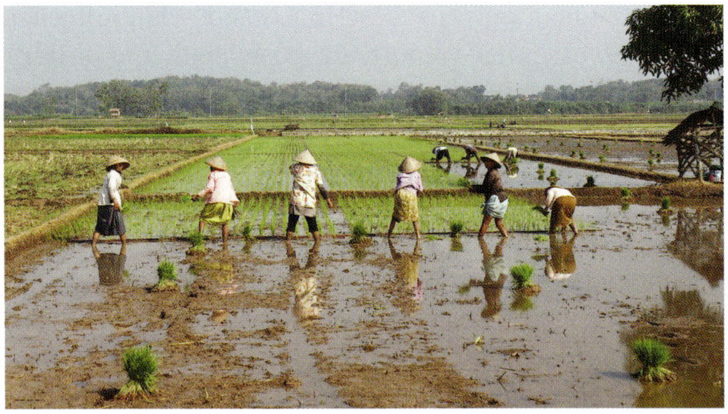

FIGURE 33.2 Workers in a rice paddy field, Indonesia, 2014, during an investigation of an outbreak of leptospirosis in the community. These farmers work all day with their feet in water without any footwear, and this puts them at risk of contracting leptospirosis. (Photo by Evi Susanti Sinaga, Indonesia. Image in public domain, accessed via CDC Public Health Images Library.)

haemorrhagic fever, plague, yellow fever, hantavirus infection or typhoid. The median incubation period is 10 days (2–26 days). Severe leptospirosis is classically biphasic. An initial 'septicaemic' phase lasts for approximately 1 week, with fever, intense myalgia, retro-orbital headache and abdominal pain, and sometimes reddened sclerae and muscle tenderness. Leptospirae are detectable in blood, CSF and tissues. At the end of this phase, leptospirae disappear from the blood and CSF and IgM antibody develops. After several days, the second 'immune' phase begins, with recurrence of fever and the development of severe disease, including aseptic meningitis, jaundice, acute renal failure or myocarditis; leptospirae become detectable in the urine.

Mild respiratory symptoms, including a dry cough, are common in the leptospiraemic phase. Cigarette smoking may be a risk factor (García et al., 2000). In nine large case series, 5%–51% of cases reported haemoptysis at hospital admission (Levett, 2001). Intra-alveolar haemorrhage can occur without obvious respiratory symptoms. Severe pulmonary haemorrhagic syndrome (SPHS) may progress rapidly to acute respiratory distress syndrome (ARDS) and has a mortality of 30%–60% even with optimal treatment. SPHS is more likely with a high leptospiral load and can sometimes occur without jaundice and renal failure. Radiography shows diffuse small opacities ('snowflake' patterning) in the peripheral lung fields, which may later coalesce (Segura et al., 2005; Marchiori et al., 2011).

Laboratory confirmation of leptospirosis is difficult outside of specialist centres. Most diagnoses are made serologically, either by IgM ELISA or, ideally, the microscopic agglutination test (performed in a reference laboratory). PCR-based tests are not widely available. Culture of the organism (from blood and CSF early in infection and later from urine) requires prolonged incubation, so is not helpful for immediate management. There is debate regarding the role of antibiotics given after the initial phase, doubt regarding whether mild disease should be treated and few trials to guide recommendations. High-dose intravenous benzyl penicillin is usually recommended for severe disease, although ceftriaxone has become widely used, with doxycycline, azithromycin or amoxicillin for mild disease (Phimda et al., 2007).

Plague

Yersinia pestis remains endemic in parts of Africa (Madagascar and Democratic Republic of Congo [DRC]), South America, Asia and the western USA (Butler, 2009, 2013; Bertherat et al., 2011; Andrianaivoarimanana et al., 2013; Kugeler et al., 2015). Approximately 750–2000 cases of plague are reported to the World Health Organization (WHO) annually; the true number is probably much higher. Endemic foci are maintained by the cycling of *Y. pestis* between the natural reservoir in small burrowing mammals (rats, gerbils, marmosets, prairie dogs, flying squirrels and others) and their fleas; wild carnivores and domestic pets may become infected if they are bitten by an infected flea or eat infected mammals.

Approximately 90% of human infections are bubonic, with an incubation period of 2–10 days, abrupt onset of high fever and very painful, tender regional lymphadenopathy, caused by the bite of an infected flea or direct contact with an infected mammal. Rarely, secondary pneumonic plague develops through bacteraemic spread. Septicaemic spread can also lead to peripheral gangrene and necrosis (Figure 33.3). The mortality from untreated bubonic plague is 50%–90%, but less than 20% with prompt diagnosis and antibiotic treatment.

Primary pneumonic plague follows inhalation of *Y. pestis* from an infected mammal or in the laboratory (Burmeister et al., 1962). Human-to-human transmission occurs through exposure to large respiratory droplets. The huge epidemics of the pre-antibiotic era, including those in Manchuria in 1910–1911 (~60,000 cases) and 1920–1921 (~9500 cases)—both beginning in groups of marmoset hunters living in overcrowded inns—will probably never be seen again (Kool, 2005). However, outbreaks and sporadic cases still occur. In an outbreak of 16 cases in India in 2002, the index case was a hunter who had killed and skinned a wild cat (Gupta and Sharma, 2007). In DRC in 2004–2005, and in 2006,

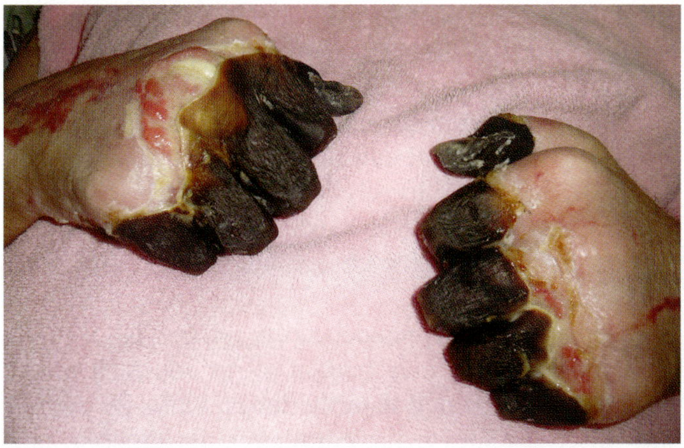

FIGURE 33.3 Gangrene and necrosis of the fingers as a complication of septicaemic plague. This 59 year old man contracted plague after exposure to an infected cat and a dead mouse. Two days after the exposure, he developed fever and myalgia, and by the following day, he had developed a left axillary bubo. Seven days after the initial exposure, he became critically ill with multiple organ failure. Blood cultures were positive for *Yersina pestis*. He was treated with gentamicin and survived, but necrosis of the hands and feet developed and he required amputation of the hands and feet. (Photo by Christina Nelson, MD, MPH, 2012. Image in public domain, accessed via CDC Public Health Images Library.)

outbreaks occurred in communities of miners (Bertherat et al., 2011). In Madagascar, cases continue to occur in highland villages (Andrianaivoarimanana et al., 2013). A recent cluster of four cases in the USA, including two veterinary clinic workers, had been exposed to a sick dog; human-to-human transmission to one case may have occurred (Centers for Disease Control and Prevention, 2015). In Yunnan, China, cases (including a truck driver) were exposed in a truck taking the index case to hospital (Luo et al., 2013). A wildlife biologist in Arizona, who had performed an autopsy on a mountain lion, died of pneumonic plague in 2007; his occupational exposure was missed when he presented with fever and haemoptysis (Wong et al., 2009).

Pneumonic plague has an incubation period of 2–4 days (range: 1–9 days). Initial symptoms of high fever, headache, chills, malaise and dry cough progress very rapidly to an increasingly bloody productive cough, with breathlessness and chest pain. Untreated, the disease is usually fatal within 48–72 hours. In the early stages, pneumonic plague is similar to any other severe pneumonia. The chest radiograph typically shows multi-lobar consolidation, with or without hilar lymphadenopathy and pleural effusion (Figure 33.4). The diagnosis is confirmed by isolation (in containment level 3 conditions) of *Y. pestis* from blood, sputum or other body fluids,

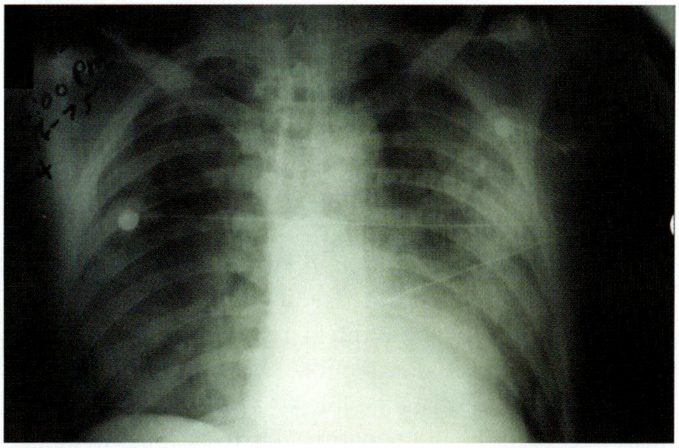

FIGURE 33.4 Chest radiograph showing widespread bilateral infiltrates in pneumonic plague. (Photo by Dr. Jack Poland, 1975. Image in public domain, accessed via CDC Public Health Images Library.)

serology or the detection of *Y. pestis* F1 antigen, for which a rapid dipstick test is in use in Africa (Chanteau et al., 2003; Bertherat et al., 2011). Effective antibiotics include aminoglycosides (gentamicin and streptomycin), doxycycline, chloramphenicol and fluoroquinolones (Inglesby et al., 2000; Mwengee et al., 2006). Molecular techniques may allow isolates from human cases to be linked to their zoonotic source (Lowell et al., 2005). Any suspected case should be discussed urgently with public health authorities. Contacts who have been within 6 feet of a coughing patient with suspected or confirmed pneumonic plague in the preceding 7 days should be given post-exposure prophylaxis, usually doxycycline. Standard and respiratory/droplet (disposable face mask) precautions should be used for suspected cases during the first 48 hours of antibiotic treatment.

Psittacosis (Ornithosis)

Chlamydia psittaci, an obligate intracellular organism, is found worldwide. It infects a wide range of birds; occupationally acquired infection is usually through exposure to psittacine birds (parrots, parakeets, macaws and budgerigars), to poultry or to the organism in the laboratory. Infected birds may be asymptomatic but shed the organism in nasal discharge and faeces, where it can survive in the environment for months. Human infection follows inhalation of the organism during activities such as handling of carcasses, cage cleaning or pet handling (Smith et al., 2005). Outbreaks have been described in poultry processors, duck farm workers, vets and veterinary medical students, bird fanciers, zoo workers, customs officials, workers in breeding aviaries and pet shop workers (Irons et al., 1951; Palmer et al., 1981; Newman et al., 1992; De Schrijver, 1995; Heddema et al., 2006; Vanrompay et al., 2007; Gaede et al., 2008; Matsui et al., 2008; Harkinezhad et al., 2009; Laroucau et al., 2009). Human infection is probably underdiagnosed.

After an incubation period of 1–4 weeks, infection typically presents as an influenza-like illness with features of pneumonia, although milder and asymptomatic infections may occur. Radiographic signs may be more marked than the clinical findings would suggest. Systemic generalised infection, which may be fulminant, has been described, as have myocarditis, endocarditis, encephalitis and hepatitis. There is some evidence from animal models that the severity of infection may be dose related (Knittler et al., 2014). Transmission from a severely ill patient to ten people, including seven hospital caregivers, has been described, highlighting the need for respiratory infection control precautions in all cases of febrile respiratory disease (Wallensten et al., 2014). Diagnosis is made by serology on paired sera (although early antibiotic treatment may blunt the antibody response). *C. psittaci*-specific PCR-based assays can be used for direct detection in respiratory samples, including pharyngeal swabs, sputum and bronchoalveolar lavage, as well as to determine the infecting genovar, which may give a guide to the source. Recommended management of severe community-acquired pneumonia includes treatment with a macrolide (erythromycin, clarithromycin and azithromycin), which will usually treat *C. psittaci* infection. If a definitive diagnosis is made early, doxycycline is a preferred treatment for adult men and for women in whom pregnancy has been excluded. Treatment for 12–14 days is recommended.

Pulmonary Echinococcosis

This parasitic infection is caused by the larval stages of the tapeworm *Echinococcus granulosus*. Adult tapeworms live in the intestine of dogs and wild carnivores; these animals excrete gravid tapeworm segments and eggs in their faeces. Sheep, cattle, goats and other herbivore intermediate hosts eat these; the oncospheres released in the gastrointestinal tract then migrate, usually to the liver or lungs, where they mature into a hydatid (metacestode) cyst. The cycle is perpetuated when dogs eat infected meat or viscera. *E. granulosus* is found worldwide and remains a serious public health problem in Africa, Asia and Central and South America and throughout the Mediterranean and Eastern Europe.

Humans are infected by hand-to-mouth transfer of eggs after handling an infected dog or its faeces or, less often, by eating contaminated food. Children are most often infected, but adults who are at occupational risk include shepherds and farmers who keep sheep (or camels, yaks or other intermediate hosts) and dogs. Dog deworming programmes, improved abattoir and carcass disposal practices and education decrease transmission to humans, and have largely prevented it in high-income countries. However, WHO estimates that there are 1 million people living with echinococcosis worldwide (Eckert et al., 2001).

Human cystic echinococcosis (CE) is initially asymptomatic, and may remain so. In adults, the liver is affected more often than the lungs, although pulmonary disease tends to present earlier; in children, pulmonary disease is more common than hepatic disease (Santivanez and Garcia, 2010). CE may be an incidental finding of a calcified cyst wall on the chest radiograph. It may present with pressure symptoms from an enlarging cyst, including cough, chest pain and breathlessness, or a cyst may rupture into the bronchial tree or pleural space. Secondary bacterial infection of a cyst may mimic a lung abscess. Diagnosis and management require specialist advice and assessment (Tamarozzi et al., 2015).

Q Fever

This highly infectious zoonosis caused by *Coxiella burnetii* was first described after an outbreak of febrile respiratory illness in abattoir workers in Queensland, Australia, in 1935 (Derrick, 1937) and is now known to occur worldwide. Infection in the main animal reservoirs (domesticated mammals, especially cattle, sheep and goats) is usually asymptomatic, although abortion, stillbirth and infertility may occur, and 'abortion storms' in affected flocks or herds may precede a human outbreak. Infected animals shed the organism in blood, amniotic fluid and other birth products (concentrations may reach 10^9 organisms/g), as well as in milk, urine and faeces; it may survive for years in the environment in a spore-like form. *C. burnetii* is also found in ticks and other arthropods, which may maintain the infection in animal reservoirs. Humans are usually infected by inhalation of the organism, in aerosols created at animal birthing or in the laboratory or in dusts contaminated with dried blood and excreta. Windborne spread has caused outbreaks miles from the originating site (Tissot-Dupont et al., 1999; Wallensten et al., 2010). Rarely, infection is acquired by eating or drinking unpasteurised milk or milk products, or by tick bite. Person-to-person transmission is rare; cases have been reported in pathologists conducting autopsies, obstetricians caring for infected pregnant women and in recipients of blood or bone marrow from infected donors (Porter, 2011).

Agricultural workers, meat processing workers, veterinarians and laboratory workers are at occupational risk. Infection may also occur through exposures such as 'hobby' farming, visiting a petting zoo or contact with a family pet. However, infection without recognised direct contact with animals is common. The infective dose is low: fewer than ten organisms may produce clinical disease. Infections are often seasonal, occurring at times of lambing, kidding or manure spreading. In The Netherlands, from 2007 to 2010, over 4000 people became infected in an outbreak linked to large-scale dairy goat farming (Delsing et al., 2010). Nearly 300 visitors and vendors at a farmers' market in Soest, Germany, were infected on a single day when an infected ewe lambed (Porten et al., 2006). Other reported outbreaks have involved: people living on a road along which sheep descended from their mountain pastures (Dupuis et al., 1987; Lovey et al., 1999); workers in a cosmetics supply factory that handled ovine products (Wade et al., 2006); visitors and workers at a ranch that introduced a herd of goats (Bamberg et al., 2007); workers in a machine tool factory next door to a herd of goats (Naranjo et al., 2011); and workers in a cardboard manufacturing plant exposed to straw-board dust (van Woerden et al., 2004). Exposure to aerosols generated by helicopter has been implicated in some outbreaks, including in a community near a sheep slaughterhouse in France (Carrieri et al., 2002) and in military personnel deployed in Bosnia (Splino et al., 2003) and Iraq (Faix et al., 2008; Royal et al., 2013). Three-toed sloths were the source of an outbreak in a military camp in French Guiana (Davoust et al., 2014).

The incubation period is usually 2–3 weeks (range: 4–40 days), but may be shorter after exposure to a large inoculum. Approximately half of human infections are asymptomatic. Symptomatic cases present with fever and influenza-like symptoms and often a non-productive cough, and may progress to pneumonia or hepatitis. A maculopapular or purpuric rash may occur. The pattern (hepatitis or pneumonia) and severity of clinical illness may relate to the genotype of the infecting organism. In the Dutch outbreak, 96% of cases had radiological evidence (although not necessarily physical signs) of pneumonia. Acute infection has a mortality rate of less than 2%. Without treatment, fever and other symptoms usually resolve in approximately 10 days; older patients may have more prolonged fever and more severe symptoms. Response to antibiotics is usually rapid. Uncommon complications include pericarditis, myocarditis, cholecystitis and meningoencephalitis. Infection in pregnancy may be associated with adverse pregnancy outcomes. Recent guidelines on management include detailed advice on the diagnosis and management of the infection in children (Anderson et al., 2013).

Sporadic infections are indistinguishable clinically and radiologically from other causes of community-acquired pneumonia or viral hepatitis, and if the diagnosis is not considered and specific testing requested, it will not be made. Some national guidelines now counsel against routine microbiological testing of community-acquired pneumonia of low severity (British Thoracic Society, 2015), which may mean that more Q fever infections pass undetected. Routine blood cultures are negative and the white blood cell count is typically normal, although there may be a thrombocytopenia and raised transaminases. Serology is the mainstay of diagnosis, using immunofluorescence or complement fixation, ideally on paired acute and convalescent sera, to detect *C. burnetii* phase 1 and phase 2 antigens. Antibodies to phase 2 antigens suggest acute infection (especially if there is an IgM response), whereas high-titre antibodies to phase 1 antigens suggest chronic infection. Interpretation of test results may be complex, and specialist advice should be sought. Acute Q fever in adults is usually treated with doxycycline, to which most isolates remain sensitive (Rouli et al., 2012).

Persistent fatigue post-*C. burnetii* infection is well recognised. In a few infections (<5%), what is currently still called 'chronic' Q fever develops weeks or years after the primary infection. The most common forms are endocarditis and infections of arterial aneurysms or vascular grafts, but osteomyelitis, chronic hepatitis and chronic pulmonary infection have been reported. Affected individuals may not recall an acute infection (Kampschreur et al., 2014).

Some authorities now suggest that all cases of acute infection should be assessed for risk of progression to chronic infection at initial diagnosis, and those with an identified risk (prosthetic cardiac valve, bicuspid aortic valve, mitral valve prolapse, moderate mitral insufficiency, congenital cardiac defects, vascular prosthesis, pregnancy and immunosuppression) should be followed up clinically and serologically long-term; those without risk factors should be reviewed at 6 months post-diagnosis for signs of potential progression to chronic disease (Anderson et al., 2013; Million and Raoult, 2015).

In Australia, Q fever is a notifiable disease, and a vaccine has been licensed and is recommended for at-risk occupational groups (Australian Government Department of Health, 2015). A national vaccination programme targeted abattoirs and farms from 2001 to 2006; the number of notified cases fell by 50% between

2002 and 2005 (Gidding et al., 2009). Vaccine is contraindicated in those previously exposed to *C. burnetii*, in whom severe local reactions may occur at the vaccination site, so pre-vaccination serology and skin testing are required. The vaccine is not available outside Australia. Guidelines on safety in laboratories and sheep research facilities cover risk reduction for workers and visitors (World Health Organization, 2004); there is also guidance for farmers (Health Protection Agency, 2010).

Rhodococcus equi (Previously *Corynebacterium equi*) Infections

Rhodococcus equi is primarily an equine pathogen, causing pneumonia in foals, but is also found in other grazing animals (Prescott, 1991). The first human infection was described in 1967 in an immunosuppressed stockyard hand who cleaned animal pens (Golub et al., 1967). Most human infections occur in the immunosuppressed, but can occur rarely in the immunocompetent (Weinstock and Brown, 2002). Approximately half of cases have a history of exposure to herbivores or their manure. Person-to-person transmission has been reported in immunosuppressed patients.

The infection presents as pulmonary disease much more commonly in immunosuppressed patients (Kedlaya et al., 2001). It presents subacutely with fever, cough, breathlessness, pleuritic chest pain and weight loss. There may be abscess formation at distant sites. The chest radiograph shows dense nodular infiltrates, usually with cavitation. Pleural effusion, empyema, mediastinal lymphadenopathy and spontaneous pneumothorax have also been reported (Donisi et al., 1996; Muntaner et al., 1997).

Diagnosis is by culture of the organism from blood, sputum, bronchial washings, pleural fluid or biopsy. *R. equi* is variably acid-fast and may be mistaken for *Mycobacterium* spp. or *Nocardia* spp.; differential diagnosis can be difficult, as these pathogens also cause cavitating lung disease (Le et al., 2015). *R. equi* is resistant to many antibiotics. There may be rifampicin resistance if patients have previously received anti-mycobacterial therapy; rifampicin- and erythromycin-resistant *R. equi* has been reported on horse-breeding farms that use the drugs to treat disease in foals (Burton et al., 2013). Combination antibiotic therapy should be guided by sensitivity testing (Hseuh et al., 1998) and may need to continue for months in immunosuppressed patients. Recommended combinations include rifampicin plus erythromycin, with or without a fluoroquinolone, or vancomycin plus imipenem.

Severe Acute Respiratory Syndrome and Middle East Respiratory Syndrome

Coronaviruses (CoVs) cause respiratory infections ranging from the common cold to severe acute respiratory syndrome (SARS) and Middle East respiratory syndrome (MERS).

SARS CoV, which probably has its natural reservoir in Chinese horseshoe bats (Ge et al., 2013), emerged in Guandong, China, in 2002. Rapid person-to-person spread caused outbreaks in Hong Kong, Vietnam, Singapore and Canada in 2003, with more than 8000 cases in 30 countries. Further clusters, some originating from laboratory-acquired infection, occurred in Singapore, Taiwan and China in 2004. Overall, 15% of hospitalised cases died. Person-to-person spread by respiratory droplet infection occurred in hospitals when early cases were cared for without effective respiratory infection control precautions (NHS England, 2014); 22% of SARS cases in Hong Kong and over 40% in Singapore and in Toronto, Canada, occurred in healthcare workers. After an incubation period of 3–5 days (range: 2–10 days), an initial influenza-like illness is followed 2–4 days later by a non-productive cough, breathlessness and pneumonia, with rapid progression to respiratory failure in severe cases (Peiris et al., 2003). Asymptomatic contacts are not infectious.

MERS-CoV (Figure 33.5) was first identified in Saudi Arabia in 2012 (de Groot et al., 2013). As of July 2015, 1437 (507 fatal) laboratory-confirmed cases had been reported to WHO (World Health Organization, 2015). Most cases have been reported from Saudi Arabia and the Arabian Peninsula, but imported cases have caused outbreaks in the Republic of South Korea and elsewhere. MERS-CoV has been isolated from dromedary camels in Saudi Arabia, Qatar and Egypt. These may be the main animal reservoir; seroprevalence studies suggest that workers on camel farms, markets and slaughterhouses are at increased risk. Transmission to healthcare workers and others has occurred in healthcare facilities. The incubation period is 5–6 days (range: 2–14 days). Some infections are asymptomatic or produce a mild upper respiratory illness. Initial symptoms include fever, cough and breathlessness, sometimes with diarrhoea. In severe cases, this is followed by rapidly progressive pneumonitis, with a high risk of respiratory and renal failure and death. The chest radiograph may show unilateral or bilateral consolidation and pleural effusion. Management of MERS and SARS includes isolation of cases, contact tracing, standard and respiratory droplet precautions and supportive and intensive care.

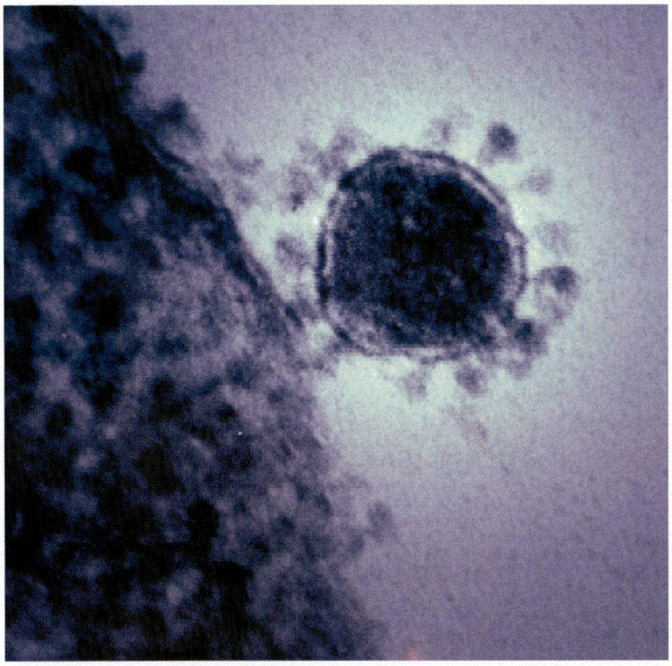

FIGURE 33.5 Transmission electron micrograph showing a single, spherical-shaped Middle Eastern respiratory syndrome coronavirus virion. (Photo by National Institute of Allergy and Infectious Diseases [NIAID], USA, 2014. Image in public domain, accessed via CDC Public Health Images Library.)

Tularaemia

Francisella tularensis primarily infects small mammals (rodents, hares, rabbits, muskrats, lemmings, squirrels and hamsters). Most infections are caused by two subspecies: *F. tularensis* subsp. *holoarctica* ('type B'), the most common isolate in Scandinavia, Russia, eastern and central Europe and Japan, but not found in the United Kingdom; and *F. tularensis* subsp. *tularensis* ('type A'), which is most common in North America and may (genotype A1b) be more virulent (Staples et al., 2006).

Localised human tularaemia infection has signs at the site of entry of the organism, accompanied by an influenza-like illness. The incubation period is 3–5 days (range: 1–21 days). Percutaneous exposure via a bite from an infected tick or biting insect or direct contact with an infected animal (e.g. during skinning, butchering or trapping) results in ulceroglandular infection, with a cutaneous ulcer and regional lymphadenopathy (Figure 33.6). Exposure of the conjunctivae results in oculoglandular disease; ingestion of contaminated food or water results in oropharyngeal disease. Localised infection may progress to systemic, septicaemic disease, and secondary pneumonia may occur. Human-to-human transmission has not been reported (Dennis et al., 2001; Tarnvic, 2007).

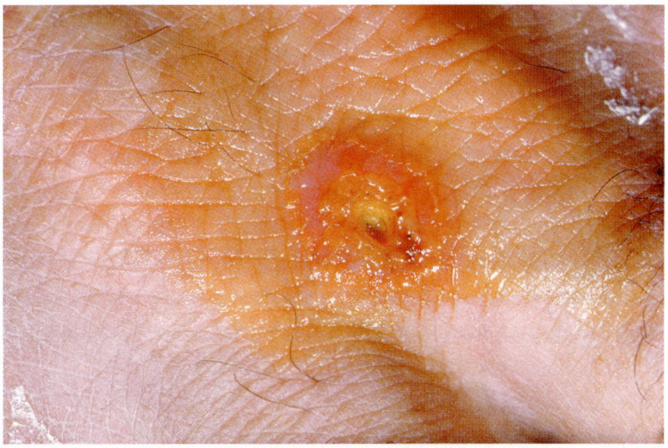

FIGURE 33.6 A tularaemia ulcer at the site of inoculation on the right hand. (Photo by Dr. Brachman. Image in public domain, accessed via CDC Public Health Images Library.)

Pneumonic tularaemia follows inhalation of the organism in contaminated aerosols or dusts. *F. tularensis* is highly infectious (<10 organisms may infect). Most infections are sporadic, although outbreaks have been reported (Teutsch et al., 1979; Hauri et al., 2010). Aerosol exposure may occur when agricultural workers move rodent-contaminated hay (Dahlstrand et al., 1971; Syrjälä et al., 1985) or landscapers and gardeners use lawnmowers, power blowers or drive a machine over a dead animal (Feldman et al., 2001; Feldman et al., 2003). Laboratory-acquired infection was once common, and cases still occur (Rusnak et al., 2004). Primary pneumonic tularaemia is rare (perhaps 5% of all tularaemia infections), but given a virulent infecting strain, untreated infection has a mortality of 30%. In severe infections, there is abrupt onset of fever, chills, malaise, relative bradycardia, cough, pleuritic chest pain, breathlessness and weight loss; the illness can rapidly become life threatening. Mild cases are indistinguishable from any other community-acquired pneumonia. The chest radiograph may show lung nodules or masses, usually within one lobe, sometimes with pleural effusions or hilar lymphadenopathy. The radiographic features and general symptoms may lead to suspicion of lung cancer (Fachinger et al., 2015).

Sporadic cases are difficult to diagnose, and the sentinel case in an outbreak may be recognised only in retrospect (Dembek et al., 2003). *F. tularensis* is fastidious and relatively slow growing, so is rarely isolated from routine blood cultures or sputum, and when it is, may take some time to identify, unless the laboratory has been informed of the possible diagnosis in advance (Shapiro and Schwartz, 2002). If the diagnosis is suspected, a presumptive diagnosis can be made by direct detection (by direct fluorescent antibody, immunohistochemistry or PCR-based tests) of *F. tularensis* in sputum or other respiratory samples. Laboratory work with known or suspected isolates that is likely to generate aerosols requires containment level 3 conditions. The diagnosis is usually confirmed serologically, ideally on paired sera taken at presentation and after 4 weeks. Aminoglycosides (streptomycin or gentamicin), doxycycline or a fluoroquinolone are recommended antibiotics for 10–21 days. Relapse may occur on cessation of therapy. Post-exposure prophylaxis may be appropriate for laboratory exposure (Centers for Disease Control and Prevention, 2011).

INFECTIONS WITH AN ENVIRONMENTAL SOURCE

Fungal Infections

Histoplasmosis

Histoplasmosis is caused by *Histoplasma capsulatum*, a dimorphic fungus found in soil enriched by faeces of birds or bats. *H. capsulatum* is found worldwide, but illness is reported mainly from the Ohio and Mississippi River valleys of the United States, St Lawrence River valley in Canada and Central America (Cano and Hajjeh, 2001). High concentrations of spores are found in bird roosts, old buildings, poultry houses, caves or schoolyards. People who clean bird roosts, visit bat caves, demolish older contaminated buildings or perform excavations for road or building construction are at occupational risk (Taylor et al., 1997; Huhn et al., 2005).

In endemic areas, rural dwellers have a high prevalence of positive skin tests to *H. capsulatum* antigens. Many infections are asymptomatic. Mild cases have an influenza-like illness with dry cough and chest pain. The chest radiograph shows non-specific, patchy, segmental infiltrates, often with hilar or mediastinal lymphadenopathy. Progressive pneumonic histoplasmosis is characterised by prostration, cough productive of purulent sputum and haemoptysis. The chest radiograph shows multiple nodules, lobar consolidation and dense, multilobar interstitial infiltrates. Acute respiratory distress syndrome may develop. Some cases (often patients with emphysema or other pre-existing lung disease) progress to chronic pulmonary histoplasmosis, with cavitating apical lung lesions. Approximately 20% of cases have other features, including arthritis, erythema nodosum and pericarditis (Wheat et al., 1981, 1984). Immunosuppressed patients may develop disseminated histoplasmosis (Wheat et al., 1982), and this was often the AIDS-defining illness in HIV-infected patients living in endemic areas, especially before the advent of highly active antiretroviral therapy.

There is an assay for histoplasma antigen in the urine, serology is useful in some cases and culture of the organism is possible. Treatment is now mainly with imidazoles, usually itraconazole, either alone for primary treatment of mild to moderate disease or following a few weeks of amphotericin B for severe infections. Most cases respond to treatment, but relapses are common (Kauffman, 2007).

There is no effective vaccine. Suggested methods of reducing exposure include pre-wetting soil in order to reduce aerosolisation or decontamination with formaldehyde and the use of personal respiratory protection.

Other Fungal Infections

Other fungal lung infections posing a potential risk for construction workers, agricultural workers and other outdoor workers include blastomycosis, coccidioidomycosis, paracoccidioidomycosis and cryptococcosis, caused by *Blastomyces dermatitidis*, *Coccidioides immitis*, *Paracoccidioides brasiliensis* and *Cryptococcus neoformans*, respectively. *Penicillium marneffei* can also cause human infection in agricultural workers. Infections with these fungi are rare and more likely in those who are immunosuppressed. Although the fungi are widespread, some have a recognised endemic area. Blastomycosis occurs mainly in the eastern and central United States and parts of Canada, coccidioidomycosis in areas of the south-western United States, paracoccidioidomycosis in South and Central America and *P. marneffei* infection in South East Asia.

The clinical presentation of blastomycosis, coccidioidomycosis or paracoccidioidomycosis is similar to histoplasmosis. Blastomycosis may present as pulmonary, cutaneous or systemic disease. The most common presentation is a chronic cough with pneumonia similar to tuberculosis. Most patients with blastomycosis also have extra-pulmonary lesions involving the skin, bones or genito-urinary system (Saccente and Woods, 2010). In coccidioidomycosis, most infections are asymptomatic; progressive disease with extra-pulmonary dissemination to multiple organs occurs mainly in the immunosuppressed (Saubolle et al., 2007). As well as lung involvement, lymphadenopathy and mucocutaneous lesions are characteristic of paracoccidioidomycosis (Ameen et al., 2010). In cryptococcal disease, extra-pulmonary dissemination is a particular concern, and cryptococcal meningo-encephalitis is a recognised risk for patients with HIV. Patients with disseminated *P. marneffei* infection present with fever, weight loss, skin lesions, lymphadenopathy and hepatomegaly, and sometimes with respiratory symptoms (Vanittanakom et al., 2006).

Diagnosis of these fungal infections is confirmed by direct demonstration of the organism in biopsies and aspirates. Immunofluorescence can be useful in some cases. The organisms can also be cultured from suspicious lesions. A positive cryptococcal antigen assay in CSF is consistent with cryptococcal meningoencephalitis.

Legionnaires' Disease

In 1976, an outbreak of severe pneumonia affected members of the American Legion attending a conference in Philadelphia (Fraser et al., 1977). A previously unrecognised pathogen, *Legionella pneumophila,* was isolated from post-mortem lung tissue (McDade et al., 1977). There are now 50 recognised species of legionellae; approximately half have been associated with human disease. In their natural freshwater habitat, they are found in low numbers and do not cause human disease. However, in warm (25–42°C) artificial water systems, they may multiply rapidly in the right conditions, and if the water is aerosolised and inhaled or aspirated, human infection can occur.

Most (80%–90%) human infections are caused by *L. pneumophila* serogroups 1, 4 and 6. Cases are usually sporadic, but community- and travel-associated outbreaks have been associated with water from cooling towers, hotel and campsite showers, whirlpool spas, hot-tubs and fountains, and nosocomial cases or outbreaks have been associated with hospital cooling towers, showers, birthing pools, respiratory therapy equipment and dental unit waterlines (Atlas et al., 1995; Fields et al., 2002; Ricci et al., 2012). Groups at higher risk include men, older people, smokers and those who are immunosuppressed, are heavy drinkers or have diabetes mellitus or chronic renal disease. Person-to-person transmission does not occur. In Australia, Japan and New Zealand, infection with *Legionella longbeachae* after exposure to potting mixes, soil or compost is reported as often as infection with *L. pneumophila*. In Australia, commercial potting mixes carry a health warning (Whiley and Bentham, 2011).

Occupational infections of *Legionella* pneumonia are rare. Small clusters have been reported in maintenance workers at a water cooling plant (Isozumi et al., 2005), in construction workers (Abbas et al., 2003) and in workers in car engine manufacturing plants, sewage treatment plants and factories (Fry et al., 2003). Exhibitors at a floral trade show where a whirlpool spa was linked to an outbreak had higher *Legionella* antibody levels than the general population, related to proximity to the whirlpool (Boshuizen et al., 2001). An analysis of cases in New York City suggested an increased risk for transport and construction workers and janitorial and cleaning staff (Farnham et al., 2014), and there is some evidence that dentists and hospital staff with a known exposure to legionellae may have a higher prevalence of *Legionella* antibodies (Reinthaler et al., 1988; Pankhurst et al., 2003; Rudbeck et al., 2009). Prevention of potential occupational risk is mainly by good management of water systems (European Agency for Safety and Health at Work, 2016).

Legionella pneumonia has an incubation period of 2–14 days. There is abrupt onset of high fever, myalgia, cough and breathlessness, sometimes with headache, confusion, abdominal pain and diarrhoea, with clinical signs of pneumonia (Figure 33.7). Acute respiratory and renal failure may follow. Routine blood and sputum cultures are negative. Diagnosis is confirmed by detection of antigen in urine, direct immunofluorescence testing of sputum, serology on paired sera and ideally by isolation of the organism from sputum or other respiratory specimens. Urinary antigen tests often detect only *L. pneumophila* serogroup 1. Culture is slow, but allows for rarer species of *Legionella* to be isolated, and can allow cases to be linked to an environmental source.

Treatment is with a macrolide (erythromycin, clarithromycin or azithromycin) or a respiratory fluoroquinolone. The infection is notifiable in the UK, USA and other countries.

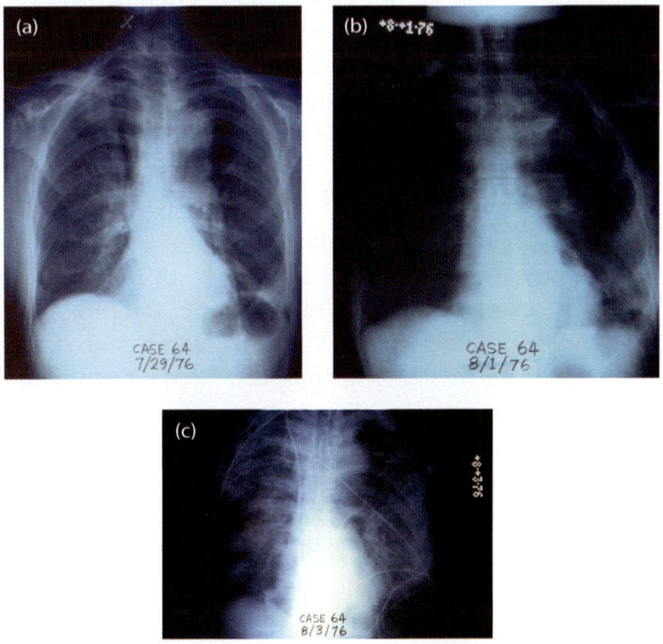

FIGURE 33.7 Chest radiographs from a patient with legionnaires' disease in 1976. (a) Initial appearances. (b) Three days later, showing bilateral infiltrates. (c) After a further 2 days, progression of the infiltrates is shown. (From Betty Partin. Image in public domain, accessed via CDC Public Health Images Library.)

Melioidosis

Melioidosis, caused by *Burkholderia pseudomallei* (found in moist soil and surface water), is endemic in South East Asia and northern Australia, and has been reported from Central and South America and Africa (Currie et al., 2008). In north-east Thailand, melioidosis occurs in paddy rice farmers and their families and is a leading cause of fatal community-acquired pneumonia (Cheng and Currie, 2005). In a large series from Darwin, Australia, 18% (96/540) of cases were directly exposed through occupational activities such as gardening and outdoor maintenance, plumbing and military exercises (Currie et al., 2010). Short-stay visitors to endemic areas may also be at risk (Amadasi et al., 2015). Infection usually follows inoculation or inhalation; many infections are asymptomatic.

Most (85%) cases of melioidosis present acutely, after an incubation of 1–21 days (Currie et al., 2010). Reactivation of latent infection is rare, but may occur many years after exposure (Ngauy et al., 2005), and has been reported in military personnel (Dance, 1991). Approximately half of melioidosis cases present with pneumonia; some 20% of these are septicaemic at presentation. Approximately 20% of cases with an extrapulmonary presentation (prostatic, splenic or hepatic abscess, osteomyelitis, septic arthritis, pyomyositis and meningo-encephalitis) develop secondary pneumonia, especially if blood cultures are positive (Meumann et al., 2012). The risk of severe infection and death is higher among older patients, heavy drinkers and those with diabetes mellitus and chronic lung, renal or cardiac disease.

Acute pulmonary melioidosis may present with fever, chills, cough, chest pain and breathlessness, or as fever and prostration with few focal signs, despite radiographic evidence of pneumonia. The illness may progress rapidly to septic shock and death. In the Darwin study, the overall mortality rate was 7%, ranging from 49% (43/88) among cases with pneumonia and septic shock to 3% (3/101) among non-bacteraemic pneumonia cases (Meumann et al., 2012).

Chronic pulmonary melioidosis may mimic tuberculosis, with fever, night sweats, weight loss and haemoptysis, with cavities, nodules and alveolar infiltrates on radiography, and with involvement of the upper lobes in approximately two-thirds of cases. Pleural effusion and lung abscesses occur in both acute and chronic pulmonary melioidosis (Dhiensiri et al., 1988; Meumann et al., 2012). Diagnosis is made by culture of *B. pseudomallei* (in level 3 containment) from blood, throat swab, sputum, other respiratory specimens, urine or pus. Other foci of deep-seated infection (spleen, liver and prostate) should be sought. Serology using an indirect haemagglutination assay may help to confirm the diagnosis if cultures are negative, but results require expert interpretation.

Initial parenteral treatment (ceftazidime or a carbapenem, with amoxicillin/calvulanate as an alternative) for at least 10 days should be followed by oral treatment aimed at preventing relapse, with trimethoprim-sulphamethoxazole (with amoxicillin/clavulanate as an alternative) for a total of at least 20 weeks of antibiotic therapy (Cheng et al., 2008). Fluoroquinolone-based regimens have poorer outcomes and should not be used (Dance, 2014). Pleural effusions and collections of pus should be drained. Early diagnosis and antibiotic therapy and high-quality intensive care management reduce mortality.

INFECTIONS WITH A HUMAN SOURCE

Invasive Pneumococcal Disease

In the 1980s, authors in the USA and UK reported excess mortality among shipyard welders exposed to metal fumes (Beaumont and Weiss, 1980; Newhouse et al., 1985). Further analysis of mortality data suggested that the excess was due mainly to lobar pneumonia (Coggon et al., 1994), and that exposure to ferrous metal fumes was particularly hazardous (Palmer and Coggon, 1997). Invasive pneumococcal disease (IPD) is a serious condition in which *Streptococcus pneumoniae* is found in blood or other normally sterile body fluids, and is associated with lobar pneumonia, empyema and meningitis; analysis of cases of IPD found an excess risk, especially of pneumonia, among welders, with a higher risk among those who smoked (Wong et al., 2010). Since 2011, the UK government has advised that giving welders and others who are exposed to metal fumes a single dose of pneumococcal vaccine (PPV23) should be considered, as well as minimising exposure through engineering controls and personal protective equipment and encouraging welders not to smoke (Public Health England, 2013). A review of the evidence for the increased risk of pneumococcal disease in welders concluded that vaccination was justified (Palmer and Cosgrove, 2012), and there is evidence that increased mortality from pneumococcal disease persists in welders in the UK despite improved engineering controls (Coggon et al., 2015). A recent outbreak of four cases of IPD in welders in a Belfast shipyard highlights the continuing risk (Patterson et al., 2015).

Tuberculosis

There has been a recrudescence of pulmonary tuberculosis worldwide, largely related to the HIV epidemic. This includes multidrug-resistant tuberculosis (MDR-TB) and extensively drug-resistant tuberculosis (XDR-TB). In the 1950s, healthcare workers were recognised as being at increased risk of contracting tuberculosis, including those with direct patient contact, pathologists and mortuary workers and laboratory workers (Sepkowitz, 1994). More recent studies have shown continuing increased risk for healthcare workers (Meredith et al., 1996; Baussano et al., 2011), including increased risk of MDR-TB and XDR-TB in areas where these are prevalent (O'Donnell et al., 2010). Prison officers are also at increased risk (Steenland et al., 1997). Workers with HIV or with immunosuppression for some other reason are at greater risk of contracting MDR-TB or XDR-TB (Jarand et al., 2010). Silica exposure (with or without silicosis) increases the risk of developing pulmonary tuberculosis, and silicotuberculosis remains a problem in countries such as South Africa with high rates of silicosis, tuberculosis and HIV (teWaterNaude et al., 2006).

The clinical features of pulmonary tuberculosis include fever, weight loss, cough, malaise, sweats and haemoptysis. The diagnosis should be considered in any healthcare worker (or other exposed worker) who presents with such symptoms and no other apparent cause. Radiographs may be normal in early infection or show a diffuse bronchopneumonia; in more advanced cases there is typically upper-lobe pneumonia with cavitation.

Guidelines in the UK cover the health clearance of new and transferring National Health Service workers, protection of workers against infection (including the use of Bacille Calmette-Guérin vaccine [BCG]) and safe working practices (National Institute for Health and Care Excellence, 2011; Public Health England, 2013). In the UK, BCG is recommended for healthcare workers, whatever their age, who will have contact with patients or clinical material and who are not tuberculin skin test positive as a result of previous BCG immunisation. BCG should not be used in HIV-infected workers. Healthcare workers found to be HIV positive during employment should be assessed for tuberculosis risk, and may need to be redeployed in order to reduce exposure. The guidance also covers the management of healthcare workers who have a significant occupational exposure to tuberculosis, and of those who are infected with tuberculosis. There are also UK infection control guidelines for preventing the spread of tuberculosis in relation to HIV and MDR-TB (National Institute for Health and Care Excellence, 2011). Tuberculosis in an occupation involving contact with sources of tuberculous material is a prescribed disease in the UK In the USA, detailed guidelines for preventing the transmission of *Mycobacterium tuberculosis* in healthcare facilities cover: administrative controls to prevent exposure cases of infectious tuberculosis; engineering controls to reduce spread of infectious droplet nuclei; and the use of personal respiratory-protective equipment where there is still a risk of exposure to infection (Centers for Disease Control and Prevention, 2005).

Mycobacterium bovis is found in cattle, bison, deer and elks. Human infection by ingesting unpasteurised milk or milk products is rare in industrialised countries, but more frequent in countries where the infection is still prevalent in cattle. Meat industry and slaughterhouse workers are at risk through inhalation of droplets in these countries. Hunters and trappers may also be at risk. Evidence of person-to-person transmission is rare. Lung infections with *M. bovis* are clinically similar to those with *M. tuberculosis*, and the combination chemotherapy used for *M. tuberculosis* is usually effective against *M. bovis* infections (Thoen et al., 2006).

Other Infections in Healthcare Workers

In addition to the infections covered in this chapter, healthcare workers may be at risk of measles, chickenpox, seasonal influenza and pertussis. They may develop lung complications from these infections acquired as adults, and those with direct patient contact may pass the infection to immunosuppressed patients. For healthcare workers who have direct patient contact, UK guidelines recommend vaccinating those who are non-immune against measles (using the measles, mumps and rubella [MMR] vaccine) and chickenpox, and offering them annual vaccination against seasonal influenza (Public Health England, 2013). Guidelines in the USA also recommend MMR and varicella vaccine for non-immune healthcare workers (Advisory Committee on Immunization Practices, 2011).

REFERENCES

Introduction

Baxter, P. J., Aw, T. C., Cockcroft, A., Durrington, A. and Harrington, J. M. (eds). 2010. *Hunter's Diseases of Occupations,* tenth edition. London: Hodder Arnold.

Anthrax

Albrink, W. S., Brooks, S. M., Biron, R. E. and Kopel, M. 1960. Human inhalation anthrax: A report of three fatal cases. *Am J Pathol* 36(4):457–71.

Avashia, S. B., Riggins, W. S., Lindley, C., Hoffmaster, A., Drumgoole, R., Nekomoto, T., Jackson, P. J. et al. 2007. Fatal pneumonia among metalworkers due to inhalation exposure to *Bacillus cereus* containing *Bacillus anthracis* toxin gene. *Clin Infect Dis* 44(3):414–6.

Brachman, P. S., Pagano, J. S. and Albrink, W. S. 1961. Two cases of fatal inhalation anthrax, one associated with sarcoidosis. *N Engl J Med* 265:203–8.

Centers for Disease Control and Prevention. 2014. CDC Lab Incident: Anthrax, June 2014. Available at: http://www.cdc.gov/anthrax/news-multimedia/lab-incident/index.html (accessed 13 March 2016).

Griffith, J., Blaney, D., Shadomy, S., Lehman, M., Pesik, N., Tostenson, S., Delaney, L. et al.; and the Anthrax Investigation Team. 2014. Investigation of inhalation anthrax case, United States. *Emerg Infect Dis.* 20(2):280–3.

Guarner, J., Jernigan, J. A., Shieh, W.-J., Tatti, K., Flannagan, L. M., Stephens, D. S., Popovic, T. et al.; and the Inhalational Anthrax Pathology Working Group. 2003. Pathology and pathogenesis of bioterrorism-related inhalational anthrax. *Am J Pathol* 163(2):701–9.

Hammond, P. M. and Carter, G. B. 2001. *From Biological Warfare to Healthcare. Porton Down, 1940–2000.* Basingstoke: Palgrave.

Health and Safety Executive. 1997. *Anthrax: Safe Working and the Prevention of Infection (HSG 174).* London: HSE. Available at: http://www.hse.gov.uk/pUbns/priced/hsg174.pdf (accessed 13 March 2016).

Hendricks, K. A., Wright, M., Shadomy, S., Bradley, J., Morrow, M. G., Pavia, A. T., Rubinstein, E. et al. 2014. Centers for Disease Control and Prevention expert panel meetings on prevention and treatment of anthrax in adults. *Emerg Infect Dis* 20(2):e130687.

Heptonstall, J. and Gent, N. 2006. *CRBN Incidents: Clinical Management and Health Protection.* London: Health Protection Agency. Available at: https://www.gov.uk/government/publications/chemical-biological-radiological-and-nuclear-incidents-recognise-and-respond (accessed 13 March 2016).

Jernigan, D. B., Raghunathan, P. L., Bell, B. P., Brechner, R., Bresnitz, E. A., Butler, J. C., Cetron, M. et al.; and the National Anthrax Epidemiologic Investigation Team. 2002. Investigation of bioterrorism-related anthrax, United States, 2001: Epidemiologic findings. *Emerg Infect Dis* 8(10):1019–28.

Jernigan, J. A., Stephens, D. S., Ashford, D. A., Omenaca, C., Topiel, M. S., Galbraith, M., Tapper, M. et al.; and Anthrax Bioterrorism Investigation Team. 2001. Bioterrorism-related inhalational anthrax: The first 10 cases reported in the United States. *Emerg Infect Dis* 7(6):933–44.

Kissling, E., Wattiau, P., China, B., Poncin, M., Fretin, D., Pirenne, Y. and Hanquet, G. 2012. *B. anthracis* in a wool-processing factory: Seroprevalence and occupational risk. *Epidemiol Infect* 140(5):879–86.

LaForce, F. M. 1978. Woolsorters' disease in England. *Bull NY Acad Sci* 54(10):956–63.

Marston, C. K., Allen, C. A., Beaudry, J., Price, E. P., Wolken, S. R., Pearson, T., Keim, P. et al. 2011. Molecular epidemiology of anthrax cases associated with recreational use of animal hides and yarn in the United States. *PLoS One* 6(12):e28274.

Meselson, M., Guillemin, J., Hugh-Jones, M., Langmuir, A., Popova, I., Shelokov, A. and Yampolskaya, O. 1994. The Sverdlovsk anthrax outbreak of 1979. *Science* 266(5188):1202–8.

Miller, J. M., Hair, J. G., Hebert, M., Hebert, L., and Roberts F. J. Jr. 1997. Fulminating bacteremia and pneumonia due to *Bacillus cereus. J Clin Microbiol* 35(2):504–7.

Plotkin, S. A., Brachman, P. S., Utell, M., Bumford, F. H. and Atchison, M. M. 2002. An epidemic of inhalation anthrax, the first in the twentieth century: I. Clinical features. 1960. *Am J Med* 112(1):4–12.

Public Health England. 2014. 13. Anthrax; guidance, data and analysis. In *Immunisation Against Infectious Disease.* London: Public Health England, 91–7.

Sprenkle, M. D., Griffith, J., Marinelli, W., Boyer, A. E., Quinn, C. P., Pesik, N. T., Hoffmaster, A. et al. 2014. Lethal factor and anti-protective antigen IgG levels associated with inhalation anthrax, Minnesota, USA. *Emerg Infect Dis* 20(2):310–4.

Stark, J. F. 2013. *The Making of Modern Anthrax, 1875–1920: Uniting Local, National and Global Histories of Disease.* London/Vermont: Pickering and Chatto.

Sykes, A., Brooks, T., Dusmet, M., Nicholson, A. G., Hansell, D. M. and Wilson, R. 2013. Survival of inhalational anthrax in a previously vaccinated soldier. *Eur Respir J* 42:285–7.

Turnbull, P. C. B. 2002. Introduction: Anthrax history, disease and ecology. *Curr Top Microbiol Immunol* 271:1–19.

Weiss, S., Yitzhaki, S. and Shapira, S. C. 2015. Lessons to be learned from recent biosafety incidents in the United States. *IMAJ* 17:269–73.

Hantavirus Pulmonary Syndromes

Centers for Disease Control and Prevention. 1993. Outbreak of acute illness—Southwestern United States, 1993. *MMWR Morb Mortal Wkly Rep* 42:421–4.

Pan American Health Organisation. 1999. Hantavirus in the Americas: Guidelines for diagnosis, treatment, prevention and control. Available at: http://www1.paho.org/english/ad/dpc/cd/hantavirus-americas.htm (accessed 13 March 2016).

Riquelme, R., Rioseco, M. L., Bastidas, L., Trincado, D., Riquelme, M., Loyola, H. and Valdivieso, F. 2015. Hantavirus pulmonary syndrome, Southern Chile, 1995–2012. *Emerg Infect Dis* 21(4):562–8.

Schmaljohn, C. S. and Hjelle, B. 1997. Hantaviruses: A global disease problem. *Emerg Infect Dis* 3:95–104.

Wells, R. M., Estani, S. S., Yadon, Z. E., Enria, D., Padula, P., Pini, N., Mills, J. N. et al.; and the Hantavirus Pulmonary Syndrome Study Group for Patagonia. 1997. An unusual Hantavirus outbreak in southern Argentina: Person-to-person transmission? *Emerg Infect Dis* 3:171–4.

Henipa Virus Infections

Australian Government Department of Health. 2012. Hendra Virus: National Guidelines for Public Health Units. Available for: http://www.health.gov.au/internet/main/publishing.nsf/Content/cdna-song-hendra.htm (accessed 13 March 2016).

Biosecurity Queensland. 2013. Guidelines for Veterinarians Handling Potential Hendra Virus Infection in Horses. Brisbane, 2013. Available at: https://www.daf.qld.gov.au/_data/assets/pdf_file/0009/97713/2355-guidelines-for-veterinarians-sept-2013.pdf (accessed 13 March 2016).

Centers for Disease Control and Prevention. 1999. Outbreak of Hendra-like virus—Malaysia and Singapore, 1998–1999. *MMWR Morb Mortal Wkly Rep* 48(3):265–9.

Chadha, M. S., Comer, J. A., Lowe, L., Rota, P. A., Rollin, P. E., Bellini, W. J., Ksiazek, T. G. et al. 2006. Nipah virus-associated encephalitis outbreak, Siliguri, India. *Emerg Infect Dis* 12(2):235–40.

Ching, P. K. G., de los Reyes, V. C., Sucaldito, M. N., Tayag, E., Columna-Vingno, A. B., Malbas F. F. Jr., Bolo, G. C. Jr. et al. 2015. Outbreak of henipavirus infection, Philippines, 2014. *Emerg Infect Dis* 21(2):328–31.

Chua, K. B., Goh, K. J., Wong, K. T., Kamarulzaman, A., Tan, P. S. K., Ksiazek, T. G., Zaki, S. R. et al. 1999. Fatal encephalitis due to Nipah virus among pig-farmers in Malaysia. *Lancet* 354(9186):1257–9.

Field, H., de Jong, C., Melville, D., Smith, C., Smith, I., Broos, A., Kung, Y. H. et al. 2011. Hendra virus infection dynamics in Australian fruit bats. *PLoS One* 6(12):e28678.

Hanna, J. N., McBride, W. J., Brookes, D. L., Shield, J., Taylor, C. T., Smith, I. L., Craig, S. B. et al. 2006. Hendra virus infection in a veterinarian. *Med J Aust* 185(10):562–4.

Luby, S. P., Gurley, E. S. and Hossain, M. J. 2009. Transmission of human infection with Nipah virus. *Clin Infect Dis* 49(11):1743–8.

Murray, K., Selleck, P., Hooper, P., Hyatt, A., Gould, A., Gleeson, L., Westbury, H. et al. 1995. A morbillivirus that caused fatal disease in horses and humans. *Science* 268:94–7.

O'Sullivan, J. D., Allworth, A. M., Paterson, D. L., Snow, T. M., Boots, R., Gleeson, L. J., Gould, A. R. et al. 1997. Fatal encephalitis due to novel paramyxovirus transmitted from horses. *Lancet* 349(9045):93–5.

Paton, N. I., Leo, Y. S., Zaki, S. R., Auchus, A. P., Lee, K. E., Ling, A. E., Chew, S. K. et al. 1999. Outbreak of Nipah-virus infection among abattoir workers in Singapore. *Lancet* 354(9186):1253–6.

Playford, E. G., McCall, B., Smith, G., Slinko, V., Allen, G., Smith, I., Moore, F. et al. 2008. Human Hendra virus encephalitis associated with equine outbreak, Australia, 2008. *Emerg Infect Dis* 16(2):219–23.

Rahman, M. A., Hossain, M. J., Sultana, S., Homaira, N., Khan, S. U., Rahman, M., Gurley, E. S. et al. 2012. Date palm sap linked to Nipah virus outbreak in Bangladesh, 2008. *Vector Borne Zoonotic Dis* 12(1):65–73.

Selvey, L. A., Wells, R. M., McCormack, J. G., Ansford, A. J., Murray, K., Rogers, R. J., Lavercombe, P. S. et al. 1995. Infection of humans and horses by a newly described morbillivirus. *Med J Aust* 162:642–5.

Human Avian Influenza Infection

Bridges, C. B., Katz, J. M., Seto, W. H., Chan, P. K. S., Tsang, D., Ho, W., Mak, K. H. et al. 2000. Risk of influenza A (H5N1) infection among health care workers exposed to patients with influenza A (H5N1), Hong Kong. *J Infect Dis* 181(1):344–8.

Cowling, B. J., Jin, L., Lau, E. H. Y., Liao, Q., Wu, P., Jiang, H., Tsang, T. K. et al. 2013. Comparative epidemiology of human infections with avian influenza A(H7N9) and A(H5N1) viruses in China. *Lancet* 382(9887):129–37.

Pan, H., Zhang, X., Hu, J., Chen, J., Pan, Q., Teng, Z., Zheng, Y. et al. 2015. A case report of avian influenza H7N9 killing a young doctor in Shanghai, China. *BMC Infect Dis* 15:237.

World Health Organization. 2015. Avian influenza A (H7N9) virus. Available at: http://www.who.int/influenza/human_animal_interface/influenza_h7n9/en/ (accessed 13 March 2016).

Leptospirosis

García, M. M. A., de Diego Damiá, A., Villanueva, R. M. and López Hontagas, J. L. 2000. Pulmonary involvement in leptospirosis. *Eur J Clin Microbiol Infect Dis* 19:471–4.

Gill, O. N., Coghlan, J. D. and Calder, I. M. 1985. The risk of leptospirosis in United Kingdom fish farm workers. Results from a 1981 serological survey. *J Hyg* 94:81–6.

Hartskeerl, R. A., Collares-Pereira, M. and Ellis, W. A. 2011. Emergence, control and re-emerging leptospirosis: Dynamics of infection in the changing world. *Clin Microbiol Infect* 17(4):494–501.

Katz, A. R., Buchholz, A. E., Hinson, K., Park, S. Y. and Effler, P. V. 2011. Leptospirosis in Hawaii, USA, 1999–2008. *Emerg Infect Dis* 17(2):221–6.

Levett, P. N. 2001. Leptospirosis. *Clin Microbiol Rev* 14:296–326.

Marchiori, E., Lourenço, S., Setúbal, S., Zanetti, G., Gasparetto, T. D. and Hochhegger, B. 2011. Clinical and imaging manifestations of hemorrhagic pulmonary leptospirosis: A state-of-the-art review. *Lung* 189(1):1–9.

Phimda, K., Hoontrakul, S., Suttinont, C., Chareonwat, S., Losuwanaluk, K., Chueasuwanchai, S., Chierakul, W. et al. 2007. Doxycycline versus azithromycin for treatment of leptospirosis and scrub typhus. *Antimicrob Agents Chemother* 51(9):3259–63.

Queensland Government: Department of Industrial Relations Workplace Health and Safety. Leptospirosis and the Banana Industry: Information and Risk Minimisation Guidelines. 2002. Available at: https://www.health.qld.gov.au/ph/documents/tphn/29073.pdf (accessed 13 March 2016).

Segura, E. R., Ganoza, C. A., Campos, K., Ricaldi, J. N., Torres, S., Silva, H., Céspedes, M. J. et al.; and Peru–United States Leptospirosis Consortium. 2005. Clinical spectrum of pulmonary involvement in leptospirosis in a region of endemicity, with quantification of leptospiral burden. *Clin Infect Dis* 40(3):343–51.

Thornley, C. N., Baker, M. G., Weinstein, P. and Maas, E. W. 2002. Changing epidemiology of human leptospirosis in New Zealand. *Epidemiol Infect* 128:29–36.

Plague

Andrianaivoarimanana, V., Kreppel, K., Elissa, N., Duplantier, J.-M., Carniel, E., Rajerison, M. and Jambou, R. 2013. Understanding the persistence of plague foci in Madagascar. *PLoS Negl Trop Dis* 7:e2382.

Bertherat, E., Thullier, P., Shako, J. C., England, K., Koné, M. L., Arntzen, L., Tomaso, H. et al. 2011. Lessons learned about pneumonic plague diagnosis from 2 outbreaks, Democratic Republic of the Congo. *Emerg Infect Dis* 17(5):778–84.

Burmeister, R. W., Tigertt, W. D. and Overholt, E. L. 1962. Laboratory-acquired pneumonic plague: Report of a case and review of previous cases. *Ann Intern Med* 56:789–800.

Butler, T. 2009. Plague into the 21st century. *Clin Infect Dis* 49:736–42.

Butler, T. 2013. Plague gives surprises in the first decade of the 21st century in the United States and worldwide. *Am J Trop Med Hyg* 89(4):788–93.

Centers for Disease Control and Prevention. 2015. Outbreak of human pneumonic plague with dog-to-human and possible human-to-human transmission—Colorado, June–July 2014. *MMWR Morb Mortal Wkly Rep* 64(16):429–34.

Chanteau, S., Rahalison, L., Ralafiarisoa, L., Foulon, J., Ratsitorahina, M., Ratsifasoamanana, L., Carniel, E. et al. 2003. Development and testing of a rapid diagnostic test for bubonic and pneumonic plague. *Lancet* 361:211–6.

Gupta, M. L. and Sharma, A. 2007. Pneumonic plague, northern India, 2002. *Emerg Infect Dis* 13(4):664–6.

Inglesby, T. V., Dennis, D. T., Henderson, D. A., Bartlett, J. G., Ascher, M. S., Eitzen, E., Fine, A. D. et al.; for the Working Group on Civilian Biodefense. 2000. Plague as a biological weapon: medical and public health management. *JAMA* 284:2281–90.

Kool, J. L. 2005. Risk of person-to-person transmission of pneumonic plague. *Clin Infect Dis* 40:1166–72.

Kugeler, K. J., Staples, E., Hinckley, A. F., Gage, K. L. and Mead, P. S. 2015. Epidemiology of human plague in the United States, 1900–2012. *Emerg Infect Dis* 21(1):16–22.

Lowell, J. L., Wagner, D. M., Atshabar, B., Antolin, M. F., Vogler, A. J., Keim, P., Chu, M. C. et al. 2005. Identifying sources of human exposure to plague. *J Clin Microbiol* 43(2):650–6.

Luo, H., Dong, X., Li, F., Xie, X., Song, Z., Shao, Z., Li, Z. et al. 2013. A cluster of primary pneumonic plague transmitted in a truck cab in a new enzootic focus in China. *Am J Trop Med Hyg* 88 (5):923–8.

Mwengee, W., Butler, T., Mgema, S., Mhina, G., Almasi, Y., Bradley, C., Formanik, J. B. et al. 2006. Treatment of plague with gentamicin or doxycycline in a randomized clinical trial in Tanzania. *Clin Infect Dis* 42:614–21.

Wong, D., Wild, M. A., Walburger, M. A., Higgins, C. L., Callahan, M., Czarnecki, L. A., Lawaczeck, E. W. et al. 2009. Primary pneumonic plague contracted from a mountain lion carcass. *Clin Infect Dis* 49:e33–8.

Psittacosis (Ornithosis)

De Schrijver, K. 1995. A psittacosis outbreak in Belgian customs officers. *Euro Surveill* 1995;0(0):pii=173.

Gaede, W., Reckling, K. F., Dresenkamp, B., Kenklies, S., Schubert, E., Noack, U., Irmscher, H. M. et al. 2008. *Chlamydophila psittaci* infections in humans during an outbreak of psittacosis from poultry in Germany. *Zoonoses Public Health* 55:184–8.

Harkinezhad, T., Verminnen, K., De Buyzere, M., Rietzschel, E., Bekaert, S. and Vanrompay, D. 2009. Prevalence of *Chlamydophila psittaci* infections in a human population in contact with domestic and companion birds. *J Med Microbiol* 58:1207–12.

Heddema, E. R., van Hannen, E. J., Duim, B., de Jongh, B. M., Kaan, J. A., van Kessel, R., Lumeij, J. T. et al. 2006. An outbreak of psittacosis due to *Chlamydophila psittaci* genotype A in a veterinary teaching hospital. *J Med Microbiol* 55:1571–5.

Irons, J. V., Sullivan, T. D. and Rowen, J. 1951. Outbreak of psittacosis (ornithosis) from working with turkeys or chickens. *Am J Pub Health* 41:931–7.

Knittler, M. R., Berndt, A., Böcker, S., Dutow, P., Hänel, F., Heuer, D., Kägebein, D. et al. 2014. *Chlamydia psittaci*: New insights into genomic diversity, clinical pathology, host–pathogen interaction and anti-bacterial immunity. *Int J Med Microbiol* 304(7):877–93.

Laroucau, K., de Barbeyrac, B., Vorimore, F., Clerc, M., Bertin, C., Harkinezhad, T., Verminnen, K. et al. 2009. Chlamydial infections in duck farms associated with human cases of psittacosis in France. *Vet Microbiol* 135:82–9.

Matsui, T., Nakashima, K., Ohyama, T., Kobayashi, J., Arima, Y., Kishimoto, T., Ogawa, M. et al. 2008. An outbreak of psittacosis in a bird park in Japan. *Epidemiol Infect* 136:492–5.

Newman, C. P., Palmer, S. R., Kirby, F. D. and Caul, E. O. 1992. A prolonged outbreak of ornithosis in duck processors. *Epidemiol Infect* 108:203–10.

Palmer, S. J., Andrews, B. E. and Major, R. 1981. A common-source outbreak of ornithosis in veterinary surgeons. *Lancet* 8250:798–9.

Smith, K. A., Bradley, K. K., Stobierski, M. G. and Tengelsen, L. A. 2005. Compendium of measures to control *Chlamydophila psittaci* (formerly *Chlamydia psittaci*) infection among humans (psittacosis) and pet birds. *J Am Vet Med Assoc* 226:532–9.

Vanrompay, D,, Harkinezhad, T., van de Walle, M., Beeckman, D., van Droogenbroeck, C., Verminnen, K., Leten, R.

et al. 2007. *Chlamydophila psittaci* transmission from pet birds to humans. *Emerg Infect Dis* 13(7):1108–10.

Wallensten A., Fredlund, H. and Runehagen, A. 2014. Multiple human-to-human transmission from a severe case of psittacosis, Sweden, January–February 2013. *Euro Surveill* 19(42):20937.

Pulmonary Echinococcosis

Eckert J., Gemmell, M. A., Meslin, F.-X. and Pawlowski, Z. S. 2001. *WHO/OIE Manual on Echinococcosis in Humans and Animals: A Public Health Problem of Global Concern*. Paris/Geneva: World Organization for Animal Health/World Health Organization. Available at: http://whqlibdoc.who.int/publications/2001/929044522X.pdf (accessed 13 March 2016).

Santivanez, S. and Garcia, H. H. 2010. Pulmonary cystic echinococcosis. *Curr Opin Pulm Med* 16(3):257–61.

Tamarozzi, F., Rossi, P., Galati, F., Mariconti, M., Nicoletti, G. J., Rinaldi, F., Casulli, A. et al. 2015. The Italian registry of cystic echinococcosis (RIEC): The first prospective registry with a European future. *Euro Surveill* 20(18):21115.

Q Fever

Anderson, A., Bijlmer, H., Fournier, P.-E., Graves, S., Hartzell, J., Kersh, G. J., Limonard, G. et al. 2013. Diagnosis and management of Q fever—United States, 2013: Recommendations from CDC and the Q fever working group. *MMWR Morb Mortal Wkly Rep* 62(RR03):1–23.

Australian Government Department of Health. 2015. Q fever. In *Australian Immunisation Handbook*. Available at: http://www.health.gov.au/internet/immunise/publishing.nsf/Content/Handbook10-home ~ handbook-10part4 ~ handbook10-4-15 (accessed 13 March 2016).

Bamberg, W. M., Pape, W. J., Beebe, J. L., Nevin-Woods, C., Ray, W., Maguire, H., Massung, R. F. et al. 2007. Outbreak of Q fever associated with a horse-boarding ranch, Colorado, 2005. *Vector Borne Zoonotic Dis* 7(3):394–402.

British Thoracic Society. 2015. Annotated BTS Guideline for the management of CAP in adults 2015. Available at: https://www.brit-thoracic.org.uk/guidelines-and-quality-standards/community-acquired-pneumonia-in-adults-guideline/annotated-bts-guideline-for-the-management-of-cap-in-adults-2015/ (accessed 13 March 2016).

Carrieri, M. P., Tissot-Dupont, H., Rey, D., Brousse, P., Renard, H., Obadia, Y. and Raoult, D. 2002. Investigation of a slaughterhouse-related outbreak of Q fever in the French Alps. *Eur J Clin Microbiol Infect Dis* 21(1):17–21.

Davoust, B., Marié, J.-L., de Santi, V. P., Berenger, J.-M., Edouard, S. and Raoult, R. 2014. Three-toed sloth as putative reservoir of *Coxiella burnetii*, Cayenne, French Guiana. *Emerg Infect Dis* 20(10):1760–1.

Delsing, C. E., Kullberg B. J. and Bleeker-Rovers, C. P. 2010. Q fever in The Netherlands from 2007 to 2010. *Neth J Med* 68(12):382–7.

Derrick, E. H. 1937. "Q" fever, a new fever entity: Clinical features, diagnosis and laboratory investigation. *Med J Aust* 2:281–99.

Dupuis, G., Petite, J., Péter, O. and Vouilloz, M. 1987. An important outbreak of human Q fever in a Swiss Alpine valley. *Int J Epidemiol* 16(2):282–7.

Faix, D. J., Harrison, D. J., Riddle, M. S., Vaughn, A. F., Yingst, S. L., Earhart, K. and Thibault, G. 2008. Outbreak of Q fever among US military in western Iraq, June–July 2005. *Clin Infect Dis* 46(7):e65–8.

Gidding, H. F., Wallace, C., Lawrence, G. L. and McIntyre, P. B. 2009. Australia's national Q fever vaccination program. *Vaccine* 27:2037–41.

Health Protection Agency. 2010. Q fever: Information for farmers. Available at: https://www.gov.uk/government/uploads/system/uploads/attachment_data/file/322815/Q_fever_information_for_farmers.pdf (accessed 13 March 2016).

Kampschreur, L. M., Delsing, C. E., Groenwold, R. H. H., Wegdam-Blans, M. C. A., Bleeker-Rovers, C. P., de Jager-Leclercq, M. G., Hoepelman, A. I. et al. 2014. Chronic Q fever in The Netherlands 5 years after the start of the Q fever epidemic: Results from the Dutch chronic Q fever database. *J Clin Microbiol* 52(5):1637–43.

Lovey, P.-Y., Morabia, A., Bleed, D., Péter, O., Dupuis, G., and Petite, J. 1999. Long term vascular complications of *Coxiella burnetii* infection in Switzerland: Cohort study. *BMJ* 319(7205):284–6.

Million, M. and Raoult, D. 2015. Recent advances in the study of Q fever epidemiology, diagnosis and management. *J Infect* 71(Suppl. 1):S2–9.

Naranjo, J. D., Fustel, E. A., Gamarra, I. A., Lobato, G. E. and Agirre, N. M. 2011. Study and management of a Q fever outbreak among machine tool workers in the Basque Country (Spain). *Epidemiol Res Int* 2011:136946.

Porten, K., Rissland, J., Tigges, A., Broll, S., Hopp, M., Lunemann, M., van Treeck, U. et al. 2006. A superspreading ewe infects hundreds with Q fever at a farmers' market in Germany. *BMC Infect Dis.* 6:147.

Porter, S. R., Czaplicki, G., Mainil, J., Guattéo, R. and Saegerman, C. 2011. Q fever: Current state of knowledge and perspectives of research of a neglected zoonosis. *Int J Microbiol* 2011:248418.

Rouli, L., Rolain, J. M., El Filali, A., Robert, C. and Raoult, D. 2012. Genome sequence of *Coxiella burnetii* 109, a doxycycline-resistant clinical isolate. *J Bacteriol* 194(24):6939.

Royal, J., Riddle, M. S., Mohareb, E., Monteville, M. R., Porter, C. K. and Faix, D. J. 2013. Seroepidemiologic survey for *Coxiella burnetii* among US military personnel deployed to Southwest and Central Asia in 2005. *Am J Trop Med Hyg* 89(5):991–5.

Splino, M., Beran, J. and Chlíbek, R. 2003. Q fever outbreak during the Czech Army deployment in Bosnia. *Mil Med* 168(10):840–2.

Tissot-Dupont, H., Torres, S., Nezri, M. and Raoult, D. 1999. Hyperendemic focus of Q fever related to sheep and wind. *Am J Epidemiol* 150(1):67–74.

van Woerden, H. C., Mason, B. W., Nehaul, L. K., Smith, R., Salmon, R. L., Healy, B., Valappil, M. et al. 2004. Q fever outbreak in industrial setting. *Emerg Infect Dis* 10(7):1282–9.

Wade, A. J., Cheng, A. C., Athan, E., Molloy, J. L., Harris, O. C., Stenos, J. and Hughes, A. J. 2006. Q fever outbreak at a cosmetics supply factory. *Clin Infect Dis* 42(7):e50–2.

Wallensten, A., Moore, P., Webster, H., Johnson, C., van der Burgt, G., Pritchard, G., Ellis-Iversen, J. et al. 2010. Q fever outbreak in Cheltenham, United Kingdom, in 2007 and the use of dispersion modelling to investigate the possibility of airborne spread. *Euro Surveill* 15(12):9521.

World Health Organization. 2004. *Laboratory Biosafety Manual,* third edition. Available at: http://www.who.int/csr/resources/publications/biosafety/en/Biosafety7.pdf (accessed 13 March 2016).

Rhodococcus equi (Previously *Corynebacterium equi*) Infections

Burton, A. J., Giguère, S., Sturgill, T. L., Berghaus, L. J., Slovis, N. M., Whitman, J. L., Levering, C. et al. 2013. Macrolide- and rifampin-resistant *Rhodococcus equi* on a horse breeding farm, Kentucky, USA. *Emerg Infect Dis* 19(2):282–5.

Donisi, A., Suardi, M. G., Casari, S., Longo, M., Cadeo, G. P. and Carosi, G. 1996. *Rhodococcus equi* infection in HIV-infected patients. *AIDS* 10:359–62.

Golub, B., Falk, G. and Spink, W. W. 1967. Lung abscess due to *Corynebacterium equi*: Report of first human infection. *Ann Intern Med* 66:1174–7.

Hsueh, P.-R., Hung, C.-C., Teng, L.-J., Yu, M.-C., Chen, Y.-C., Wang, H.-K. and Luh, K.-T. 1998. Report of invasive *Rhodococcus equi* infections in Taiwan, with an emphasis on the emergence of multidrug-resistant strains. *Clin Infect Dis* 27:370–5.

Kedlaya, I., Ing, M. B. and Wong, S. S. 2001. *Rhodococcus equi* infections in immunocompetent hosts: Case report and review. *Clin Infect Dis* 32:E39–46.

Le, T., Cash-Goldwasser, S., Tho, P. V., Lan, N. P. H., Campbell, J. I., van Doorn, H. R., Lam, N. T. et al. 2015. Diagnosing *Rhodococcus equi* infections in a setting where tuberculosis is highly endemic: A double challenge. *J Clin Microbiol* 53(4):1431–3.

Muntaner, L., Leyes, M., Payeras, A., Herrera, M. and Gutierrez, A. 1997. Radiologic features of *Rhodococcus equi* pneumonia in AIDS. *Eur J Radiol* 24:66–70.

Prescott, J. F. 1991. *Rhodococcus equi*: An animal and human pathogen. *Clin Microbiol Rev* 4:20–34.

Weinstock, D. M. and Brown, A. E. 2002. *Rhodococcus equi*: An emerging pathogen. *Clin Infect Dis* 34:1379–85.

Severe Acute Respiratory Syndrome and Middle East Respiratory Syndrome

de Groot, R. J., Baker, S. C., Baric, R. S., Brown, C. S., Drosten, C., Enjuanes, L., Fouchier, R. A. M. et al. 2013. Middle East respiratory syndrome coronavirus (MERS-CoV): Announcement of the coronavirus study group. *J Virol* 87(14):7790–2.

Ge, X.-Y., Li, J.-L., Yang, X.-L., Chmura, A. A., Zhu, G., Epstein, J. H., Mazet, J. K. et al. 2013. Isolation and characterization of a bat SARS-like coronavirus that uses the ACE2 receptor. *Nature* 503:535–8.

NHS England. 2014. Infectious respiratory viruses—The use of face masks and respirators. Available at: http://www.england.nhs.uk/ourwork/eprr/id/ (accessed 13 March 2016).

Peiris, J. S. M., Yuen, K. Y., Osterhaus, A. D. M. E. and Stöhr, K. 2003. The severe acute respiratory syndrome. *N Engl J Med* 349:2431–41.

World Health Organization. Middle East respiratory syndrome coronavirus (MERS-CoV). Available at: http://www.who.int/emergencies/mers-cov/en/ (accessed 13 March 2016).

Tularaemia

Centers for Disease Control and Prevention. 2011. Managing potential laboratory exposures to *Francisella tularensis*. Available at: http://www.cdc.gov/tularemia/laboratory-exposure/index.html (accessed 13 March 2016).

Dahlstrand, S., Ringertz, O. and Zetterberg, B. 1971. Airborne tularemia in Sweden. *Scand J Infect Dis* 3(1):7–16.

Dembek, Z. F., Buckman, R. L., Fowler, S. K. and Hadler, J. L. 2003. Missed sentinel case of naturally occurring pneumonic tularemia outbreak: Lessons for detection of bioterrorism *J Am Board Fam Pract* 16:339–42.

Dennis, D. T., Inglesby, T. V., Henderson, D. A., Bartlett, J. G., Ascher, M. S., Eitzen, E., Fine, A. D. et al. for the Working Group on Civilian Biodefense. 2001. Tularemia as a biological weapon: Medical and public health management. *JAMA* 285(21):2763–73.

Fachinger, P., Tini, G. M., Grobholz, R., Gambazzi, F., Fankhauser, F. and Irani, S. 2015. Pulmonary tularaemia: All that looks like cancer is not necessarily cancer—Case report of four consecutive cases. *BMC Pulm Med* 15:27.

Feldman, K. A., Enscore, R. E., Lathrop, S. L., Matyas, B. T., McGuill, M., Schriefer, M. E., Stiles-Enos, D. et al. 2001. An outbreak of primary pneumonic tularemia on Martha's Vineyard. *N Engl J Med* 345:1601–6.

Feldman, K. A., Stiles-Enos, D., Julian, K., Matyas, B. T., Telford S. R. III, Chu, M. C., Petersen, L. R. et al. 2003. Tularemia on Martha's Vineyard: Seroprevalence and occupational risk. *Emerg Infect Dis* 9(3):350–4.

Hauri, A. M., Hofstetter, I., Seibold, E., Kaysser, P., Eckert, J., Neubauer, H. and Splettstoesser, W. D. 2010. Investigating an airborne tularemia outbreak, Germany. *Emerg Infect Dis* 16(2):238–43.

Rusnak, J. M., Kortepeter, M. G., Hawley, R. J., Anderson, A. O., Boudreau, E. and Eitzen, E. 2004. Risk of occupationally acquired illnesses from biological threat agents in unvaccinated laboratory workers. *Biosecur Bioterror* 2(4):281–93.

Shapiro, D. S. and Schwartz, D. R. 2002. Exposure of laboratory workers to *Francisella tularensis* despite a bioterrorism procedure. *J Clin Micobiol* 40(6):2278–81.

Staples, J. E., Kubota, K. A., Chalcraft, L. G., Mead, P. and Petersen, J. M. 2006. Epidemiologic and molecular analysis of human tularemia, United States, 1964–2004. *Emerg Infect Dis* 12(7):1113–8.

Syrjälä, H., Kujala, P., Myllylä, V. and Salminen, A. 1985. Airborne transmission of tularemia in farmers. *Scand J Infect Dis* 17(4):371–5.

Tarnvik, A. 2007. *WHO Guidelines on Tularaemia. WHO/CDS/EPR/2007.7.* Geneva: World Health Organization.

Teutsch, S. M., Martone, W. J., Brink, E. W., Potter, M. E., Eliot, G., Hoxsie, R., Craven, R. B. et al. 1979. Pneumonic tularemia on Martha's Vineyard. *N Engl J Med* 301:826–8.

Histoplasmosis and Other Fungal Infections

Ameen, M., Talhari, C. and Talhari, S. 2010. Advances in paracoccidioidomycosis. *Clin Exp Dermatol* 35:576–80.

Cano, M. V., and Hajjeh, R. A. 2001. The epidemiology of histoplasmosis: A review. *Sem Resp Infect* 16(2):109–18.

Huhn, G. D., Austin, C., Carr, M., Heyer, D., Boudreau, P., Gilbert, G., Eimen, T. et al. 2005. Two outbreaks of occupationally acquired histoplasmosis: More than workers at risk. *Environ Health Perspect* 113:585–9.

Kauffman, C. A. 2007. Histoplasmosis: A clinical and laboratory update. *Clin Microbiol Rev* 20:115–32.

Saccente, M. and Woods, G. L. 2010. Clinical and laboratory update on blastomycosis. *Clin Microbiol Rev* 23:367–81.

Saubolle, M. A., McKellar, P. P. and Sussland, D. 2007. Epidemiologic, clinical, and diagnostic aspects of coccidioidomycosis. *J Clin Microbiol* 45:26–30.

Taylor, M. L., Pérez-Mejía, A., Yamamoto-Furusho, J. K. and Granados, J. 1997. Immunologic, genetic and social human risk factors associated to histoplasmosis: Studies in the State of Guerrero, Mexico. *Mycopathologia* 138:137–41.

Vanittanakom, N., Cooper C. R. Jr., Fisher, M. C. and Sirisanthana, T. 2006. *Penicillium marneffei* infection and recent advances in the epidemiology and molecular biology aspects. *Clin Microbiol Rev* 19:95–110.

Wheat, L. J., Slama, T. G., Eitzen, H. E., Kohler, R. B., French, M. L. V. and Biesecker, J. L. 1981. A large urban outbreak of histoplasmosis: Clinical features. *Ann Intern Med* 94(3):331–7.

Wheat, L. J., Slama, T. G., Norton, J. A., Kohler, R. B., Eitzen, H. E., French, M. L. V. and Sathapatayavongs, B. 1982. Risk factors for disseminated or fatal histoplasmosis: Analysis of a large urban outbreak. *Ann Intern Med* 96(2):159–63.

Wheat, L. J., Wass, J., Norton, J., Kohler, R. B. and French, M. L. V. 1984. Cavitary histoplasmosis occurring during two large urban outbreaks: Analysis of clinical, epidemiologic, roentgenographic, and laboratory features. *Medicine (Baltimore)* 63:201–9.

Legionnaires' Disease

Abbas Z., Nolan, L., Landry, L., Galanis, E. and Egan, C. 2003. Investigation of an outbreak of Legionnaires' disease in a hospital under construction: Ontario, September–October 2002. *Can Commun Dis Rep* 29(17):145–52.

Atlas, R. M., Williams, J. F. and Huntington, M. K. 1995. Legionella contamination of dental unit waters. *Appl Environ Microbiol* 61:1208–13.

Boshuizen, H. C., Neppelenbroek, S. E., van Vliet, H., Schellekens, J. F. P., den Boer, J. W., Peeters, M. F. and Conyn-van Spaendonck, M. A. E. 2001. Subclinical *Legionella* infection in workers near the source of a large outbreak of Legionnaires disease. *J Infect Dis* 184 (4):515–8.

European Agency for Safety and Health at Work. 2016. *Legionella* in the workplace. OSH-Wiki. Available at: http://oshwiki.eu/wiki/Legionella_in_the_workplace (accessed 13 March 2016).

Farnham A., Alleyne, L., Cimini, D. and Balter, S. 2014. Legionnaires' disease incidence and risk factors, New York, New York, USA, 2002–2011. *Emerg Infect Dis* 20(11):1795–802.

Fields, B. S., Benson, R. F. and Besser, R. E. 2002. *Legionella* and Legionnaires' disease: 25 years of investigation. *Clin Microbiol Rev* 15(3):506–26.

Fraser, D. W., Tsai, T. R., Orenstein, W., Parkin, W. E., Beecham, H. J., Sharrar, R. G., Harris, J. et al. 1977. Legionnaires' disease: Description of an epidemic of pneumonia. *N Engl J Med* 297:1189–97.

Fry, A. M., Rutman, M., Allan, T., Scaife, H., Salehi, E., Benson, R., Fields, B. et al. 2003. Legionnaires' disease outbreak in an automobile engine manufacturing plant. *J Infect Dis* 187(6):1015–8.

Isozumi R., Ito, Y., Ito, I., Osawa, M., Hirai, T., Takakura, S., Iinuma, Y. et al. 2005. An outbreak of *Legionella pneumonia* originating from a cooling tower. *Scand J Infect Dis* 37(10):709–11.

McDade, J. E., Shepard, C. C., Fraser, D. W., Tsai, T. R., Redus, M. A. and Dowdle, W. R.. 1977. Legionnaires' disease: Isolation of a bacterium and demonstration of its role in other respiratory disease. *N Engl J Med* 297:1197–203.

Pankhurst, C. L., Coulter, W., Philpott-Howard, J. J., Harrison, T., Warburton, F., Platt, S., Surman, S. et al. 2003. Prevalence of *Legionella* waterline contamination and *Legionella pneumophila* antibodies in general dental practitioners in London and rural Northern Ireland. *Br Dent J* 195(10):591–4.

Reinthaler F. F., Mascher, F. and Stünzner, D. 1988. Serological examinations for antibodies against *Legionella* species in dental personnel. *J Dent Res* 67(6):942–3.

Ricci, M. L., Fontana, S., Pinci, F., Fiumana, E., Pedna, M. F., Farolfi, P., Sabattini, M. A. et al. 2012. Pneumonia associated with a dental unit waterline. *Lancet* 379(9816):684.

Rudbeck, M., Viskum, S., Mølbak, K. and Uldum, S. A. 2009. *Legionella* antibodies in a Danish hospital staff with known occupational exposure. *J Environ Public Health* 2009:812829.

Whiley, H. and Bentham, R. 2011. *Legionella longbeachae* and legionellosis. *Emerg Infect Dis* 17(4):579–83.

Melioidosis

Amadasi, S., Zoppo, S. D., Bonomini, A., Bussi, A. Pedroni, P., Balestrieri, G., Signorini, L. et al. 2015. A case of melioidosis probably acquired by inhalation of dusts during a helicopter flight in a healthy traveler returning from Singapore. *J Travel Med* 22:57–60.

Cheng, A. C. and Currie, B. J. 2005. Melioidosis: Epidemiology, pathophysiology, and management. *Clin Microbiol Rev* 18:383–416.

Cheng, A. C., Chierakul, W., Chaowagul, W., Chetchotisakd, P., Limmathurotsakul, D., Dance, D. A. B., Peacock, S. J. et al. 2008. Consensus guidelines for dosing of amoxicillin–clavulanate in melioidosis. *Am J Trop Med Hyg* 78:208–9.

Currie, B. J., Dance, D. A. B. and Cheng, A. C. 2008. The global distribution of *Burkholderia pseudomallei* and melioidosis: An update. *Trans R Soc Trop Med Hyg* 102(Suppl. 1):S1–4.

Currie, B. J., Ward, L. and Cheng, A. C. 2010. The epidemiology and clinical spectrum of melioidosis: 540 cases from the 20 year Darwin prospective study. *PLoS Negl Trop Dis* 4(11):e900.

Dance, D. 2014. Treatment and prophylaxis of melioidosis. *Int J Antimicrob Agents* 43(4):310–8.

Dance, D. A. B. 1991. Melioidosis: The tip of the iceberg? *Clin Microbiol Rev* 4(1):52–60.

Dhiensiri, T., Puapairoj, S. and Susaengrat, W. 1988. Pulmonary melioidosis: Clinical–radiologic correlation in 183 cases in northeastern Thailand. *Radiology* 166:711–5.

Meumann, E. M., Cheng, A. C., Ward, L. and Currie, B. J. 2012. Clinical features and epidemiology of melioidosis pneumonia: Results from a 21-year study and review of the literature. *Clin Infect Dis* 54(3):362–9.

Ngauy, V., Lemeshev, Y., Sadkowski, L. and Crawford, G. 2005. Cutaneous melioidosis in a man who was taken as a prisoner of war by the Japanese during World War II. *J Clin Microbiol* 43:970–2.

Invasive Pneumococcal Disease

Beaumont, J. J. and Weiss, N. S. 1980. Mortality of welders, shipfitters, and other metal trades workers in boilermakers Local No. 104, AFL-CIO. *Am J Epidemiol* 112:775–86.

Coggon, D., Harris, E. C., Cox, V. and Palmer, K. T. 2015. Pneumococcal vaccination for welders. *Thorax* 70:198–9.

Coggon, D., Inskip, H., Winter, P. and Pannett, B. 1994. Lobar pneumonia: An occupational disease in welders. *Lancet* 344(8914):41–3.

Newhouse, M. L., Oakes, D. and Woolley, A. J. 1985. Mortality of welders and other craftsmen at a shipyard in NE England. *Br J Ind Med* 42:406–10.

Palmer, K. and Coggon, D. 1997. Does exposure to iron promote infection? *Occup Environ Med* 54:529–34.

Palmer, K. T. and Cosgrove, M. P. 2012. Vaccinating welders against pneumonia. *Occup Med* 62:325–30.

Patterson, L., Irvine, N., Wilson, A., Doherty, L., Loughrey, A. and Jessop, L. 2015. Outbreak of invasive pneumococcal disease at a Belfast shipyard in men exposed to welding fumes, Northern Ireland, April–May 2015: Preliminary report. *Euro Surveill* 20(21):21138.

Public Health England. 2013. Pneumococcal: The green book, Chapter 25. Available at: http://www.gov.uk/government/publications/pneumococcal-the-green-book-chapter-25 (accessed 13 March 2016).

Wong, A., Marrie, T. J., Garg, S. and Tyrrell, G. J. 2010. Welders are at increased risk for invasive pneumococcal disease. *Int J Infect Dis* 14(9):e796–9.

Tuberculosis

Baussano, I., Nunn, P., Williams, B., Pivetta, E., Bugiani, M. and Scano, F. 2011. Tuberculosis among health care workers. *Emerg Infect Dis* 17(3):488–94.

Centers for Disease Control and Prevention. 2005. Guidelines for preventing the transmission of *Mycobacterium tuberculosis* in health-care settings, 2005. *MMWR Morb Mortal Wkly Rep* 54(17):1–141.

Jarand, J., Shean, K., O'Donnell, M., Loveday, M., Kvasnovsky, C., Van der Walt, M., Adams, S. et al. 2010. Extensively drug-resistant tuberculosis (XDR-TB) among health care workers in South Africa. *Trop Med Int Health* 15(10):1179–84.

Meredith, S., Watson, J. M., Citron, K. M., Cockcroft, A. and Darbyshire, J. H. 1996. Are healthcare workers in England and Wales at increased risk of tuberculosis? *Br Med J* 313:522–5.

National Institute for Health and Care Excellence. 2011. Clinical diagnosis and management of tuberculosis, and measures for its prevention and control (CG117). Available at: www.nice.org.uk/guidance/cg117 (accessed 13 March 2016).

O'Donnell, M. R., Jarand, J., Loveday, M., Padayatchi, N., Zelnick, J., Werner, L., Naidoo, K. et al. 2010. High incidence of hospital admissions with multidrug-resistant and extensively drug-resistant tuberculosis among South African health care workers. *Ann Intern Med* 153(8):516–22.

Public Health England. 2013. Tuberculosis: The green book, Chapter 32. Available at: https://www.gov.uk/government/uploads/system/uploads/attachment_data/file/148511/Green-Book-Chapter-32-dh_128356.pdf (accessed 13 March 2016).

Sepkowitz, K. A. 1994. Tuberculosis and the health care worker: A historical perspective. *Ann Intern Med* 120(1): 71–9.

Steenland, K., Levine, A. J., Sieber, K., Schulte, P. and Aziz, D. 1997. Incidence of tuberculosis infection among New York State prison employees. *Am J Public Health* 87(12):2012–4.

teWaterNaude, J. M., Ehrlich, R. I., Churchyard, G. J., Pemba, L., Dekker, K., Vermeis, M., White, N. W. et al. 2006. Tuberculosis and silica exposure in South African gold miners. *Occup Environ Med* 63:187–92.

Thoen, C., LoBue, P. and de Kantor, I. 2006. The importance of *Mycobacterium bovis* as a zoonosis. *Vet Microbiol* 112:339–45.

Other Infections in Healthcare Workers

Advisory Committee on Immunization Practices. 2011. Immunization of health-care personnel. *MMWR Morb Mortal Wkly Rep* 60(RR07):1–45.

Public Health England. 2013. Immunisation against infectious disease. Available at: https://www.gov.uk/government/publications/immunisation-against-infectious-disease-the-green-book-front-cover-and-contents-page (accessed 13 March 2016).

34 Diving

Mark Glover

CONTENTS

DIVING PRACTICE AND EQUIPMENT

INTRODUCTION

Humans have dived in water for work and for pleasure over many thousands of years. The principal limit on the duration of a dive is a human's inability to breathe underwater. The advent of equipment that allows a diver to carry extra gas to breathe revolutionised human exploitation of the underwater world, but also introduced new hazards. The lungs have an important role in the majority of diving-related disorders but, depending on the specific disorder, they can act as victim, guardian, accomplice or perpetrator.

Diving is normally associated with immersion in fluid (water in the vast majority of cases), but many of the same environmental effects act on an individual who enters a dry pressurised environment. Diving will almost always be associated with a raised environmental pressure and usually with immersion. It is important to distinguish between the effects of these two components of diving when assessing individual cases.

'Dry diving' can take place in the following circumstances:

- Underground work, such as in a tunnel, a section of which is pressurised to prevent the ingress of water
- A caisson, an open-bottomed vessel that is placed on a seabed or riverbed, is pressurised to prevent the ingress of water and allows construction workers direct access to the enclosed space without the need for diving apparatus
- A hyperbaric chamber used for the treatment of decompression illness and other medical conditions

SURFACE-ORIENTATED DIVING AND SATURATION DIVING

The majority of diving while immersed is 'surface orientated', meaning that the diver returns to surface pressure after each immersion.

In saturation diving, the diver returns to a diving bell that is suspended just above the diver's worksite, is open to the water and remains at approximately the same pressure as the worksite. The diver completes the planned work, returns to the bell, which contains respirable gas, and then a hatch is closed in order to prevent the internal pressure from changing as the bell is hoisted to the surface. At the surface, the bell occupants transfer to a living chamber and remain at elevated pressure until the next working shift, when the pressurised bell will deliver the diver back to the worksite. The diver is able to complete several long-duration dives but decompresses to surface pressure only once at the end of the dive series. Saturation diving requires more sophisticated technical support and is used almost exclusively for deep commercial diving projects.

SELF-CONTAINED UNDERWATER BREATHING APPARATUS

Divers carry their own breathing gas in compressed form or have it delivered to them via a hose. Self-contained underwater breathing apparatus (SCUBA) has the advantage that it is possible to be completely independent of the surface. The disadvantages are the practical limitation on gas supply and difficulty locating the diver if lost. Gas is stored at high pressure in vessels that are typically cylindrical or spherical in shape. Reducing valves allow the gas to be delivered to the diver at ambient pressure. The main distinguishing characteristic of different forms of self-contained equipment is whether the exhaled gas is exhausted into the water (open circuit), partially recycled (semi-closed circuit) or reused to the maximum extent possible (closed circuit). Equipment that recycles breathing gas will include a counter-lung into which exhaled gas is collected and can be returned to the diver with carbon dioxide scrubbed out and oxygen levels replenished.

HOSE SUPPLY

Hose supply (also known as surface supply in surface-orientated diving) can provide plentiful quantities of gas and permits other services to be delivered to the diver alongside the breathing gas, such as hot water for heating, hard-wired communications, camera surveillance, electricity for lighting and reclaim of exhaled gas for recycling. Hose-supplied divers usually carry a supplementary self-contained source of gas that gives a short-term 'bail-out' supply that will allow them to retreat to safety if the hose fails.

In modern equipment, delivery of breathing gas is actuated by the negative pressure that is created as the diver inhales. Older diving equipment, such as the classic standard diving helmet, provided a free flow of gas.

THE WORKING ENVIRONMENT

For a working diver, the dive is a means of reaching work that could involve heavy manual labour in an area akin to a construction site, skilled tasks or inspection for commercial, scientific, archaeological, entertainment, instructional, police or defence purposes. A wide range of tools and other equipment have been adapted for underwater use, introducing hazards that are familiar to those working at the surface (such as vibration and trauma from an angle grinder or cognitive decrement due to respirable heavy metal particles from grinding and welding in an enclosed space) and new ones (such as uncontrolled depressurisation due to entanglement with a buoyant lifting bag that breaks free).

PHYSICS AND PHYSIOLOGY RELEVANT TO DIVING

Physical Principles

Ambient pressure increases by approximately 100 kPa for every 10 m of descent underwater. Since the pressure at sea level is approximately 100 kPa, this means that pressure will be doubled at 10 m depth below sea level. This contrasts dramatically with the changes in pressure experienced in air where, in order to halve the ambient pressure, an ascent to an altitude of approximately 5500 m (18,000 feet) would be required. Boyle's Law describes how the volume of a fixed mass of gas is inversely proportional to the absolute pressure and, as the gas is compressed, the partial pressure of each component in a mixture of gases will increase in the same proportion as the change in total pressure. Although air contains other gases in very small amounts, it is made up almost completely from a mixture of approximately 79% nitrogen and 21% oxygen. Table 34.1 shows how volume and partial pressures in a fixed mass of air would vary with depth.

As the lungs contain free gas, the partial pressures are affected in a similar way. Alveolar gas does not, however, have exactly the same composition as inspired gas due to inward diffusion of carbon dioxide, outward diffusion of oxygen and saturation of the gas in the alveolar space with water vapour at body temperature. Oxygen is essential for aerobic metabolism and, therefore, for survival. Nitrogen is considered to be chemically and physiologically inert at normal atmospheric pressure. As the partial pressures rise, however, the properties of these gases change. Oxygen at high partial pressures, for instance, becomes toxic to many tissues by overwhelming antioxidant defences and then causing oxidative damage.

Immersion

The magnitude of change in pressure with increasing depth in water means that the pressure exerted on the feet of a human immersed in a vertical position with the head out of the water will be significantly greater than that acting on the head and thorax. This contrasts with the situation in air where the pressure applied to all parts of the body is almost equal. The pressure differential in the water acts on blood, which typically occupies the more distensible blood vessels in the lower limbs and redistributes it more evenly. Intrathoracic vessels become engorged with the displaced blood and reduce pulmonary capacity. The redistribution of blood also depends on the degree of vasoconstriction caused by ambient water temperature.

The pressure exerted on the abdominal wall will exceed that applied to the chest. In a similar way, the pressure exerted on the chest wall will exceed that applied to the mouth and nose. These two effects add extra force against which the diaphragm and inspiratory muscles must act in order to inhale. It is not surprising, therefore, that human maximal inspiratory volume is reduced when immersed compared with when on land (Table 34.2).

TABLE 34.1
Changes in Volumes and Partial Pressures in Air as Pressure Changes with Increasing Depth

Depth (m)	Approximate Pressure (kPa)	Volume (L)	Partial Pressure of Oxygen (kPa)	Partial Pressure of Nitrogen (kPa)
Surface (0)	100	1	21	79
1	110	10/11	23	87
5	150	2/3	31.5	118.5
10	200	1/2	42	158
20	300	1/3	63	237
30	400	1/4	84	316
40	500	1/5	105	395
50	600	1/6	126	474
90	1000	1/10	210	790

TABLE 34.2
Changes in Vital Capacity Associated with Immersion in Water of Different Temperatures

Water Temperature	40°C	35°C	20°C
Reduction in vital capacity in immersed human with 'head out'	2%	5%	10%

Source: Data from Camporesi, E. M. and Bosco, G. 2003. Ventilation, gas exchange and exercise under pressure. In A. O. Brubakk and T. S Neuman (eds), *Bennett and Elliott's Physiology and Medicine of Diving*, fifth edition. London: Saunders, 77–114.

Submersion

If head-out immersion progresses to complete submersion, the redistribution of blood remains unchanged irrespective of posture in the water due to the similarity in density of blood and water. The relationship between pressure exerted on the abdominal wall, chest wall and at the level of the mouth and nose will depend on the diver's attitude within the water. When in water, the usual functional residual capacity of the lung on land can be restored by delivering gas to the mouth at the same pressure as a notional point within the chest known as the lung centroid. This is approximately 19 cm below and 7 cm behind the sternal notch in an average human male (Francis and Denison, 1999). Any deviations from lung centroid pressure will either increase or decrease functional residual capacity and encourage the diver to breathe around a state of expansion associated with decreased lung compliance.

The diver's attitude in the water will influence ventilation with standard SCUBA equipment, which delivers gas at the same pressure as that acting on the demand valve attached directly to diver's mouthpiece. If the diver's head is down, then the pressure of the gas delivered to the mouth exceeds the pressure exerted on the thorax, so it assists inspiration and resists expiration. The situation is reversed if the diver's head is uppermost. Another consequence of total immersion is that the diver can breathe from nothing other than the compressed gas supply and, in the event of a problem, aspiration or, worse still, asphyxia and drowning can occur.

The diver can vary breathing mixtures in order to optimise them for different phases of the dive.

Descent

The pressure increases rapidly as the diver descends in water. At 10 m depth in seawater, ambient pressure will be approximately doubled compared with the surface, at 20 m it will be tripled, and so on. The partial pressures of the component gases in the breathing mixture will also increase by the same proportion, and this can change a gas mixture from one that is safe into one that is not.

There is some evidence that cartilaginous reinforcement of the small airways in some marine mammals permits more complete alveolar emptying during a dive, isolating the compressed gas from pulmonary capillary blood (Denison et al., 1971). Humans do not have the same reinforcing structures so, even on a breath-hold dive, the partial pressures of gases in the arterial circulation closely follow those in the alveoli. Breathing from a compressed gas supply will, of course, resist the compression of the lungs altogether and the alveolar gas will remain accessible to the pulmonary capillaries throughout the dive. The raised tensions of gases dissolved in the blood establish a gradient that encourages gas to diffuse from capillaries into the tissues. This does not cause a problem at this stage but, depending on the amount of additional gas that accumulates, might do so later in the dive. The density of the gas will also increase in proportion with the ambient pressure. The work of breathing increases as the mass per unit volume of the gas and the tendency for turbulent flow in the airways rise. As a result, maximum voluntary ventilation rates fall. The thermal capacity of the gas mixture increases and significant heat can be lost via the breathing gas, unless it is warmed for very deep dives (greater than 90 m); this cooling effect can cause chest discomfort, excessive upper respiratory tract secretions and bronchoconstriction (Flynn, 1999), and if these are tolerated, continued heat loss can induce hypothermia (Flynn, 1999).

Ascent

Eventually, the diver must return to surface pressure. During the ascent, ambient pressure falls, the partial pressures of the component gases in the breathing mixture decline and gas within the lungs will expand.

DIVING-RELATED PROBLEMS THAT INVOLVE THE LUNGS

Immersion Pulmonary Oedema

This is characterised by the onset of pulmonary oedema while immersed and in the absence of obvious aspiration or pulmonary or cardiac abnormality; the prevalence was 1.1% among recreational divers in one survey (Pons et al., 1995). Complete submersion is not required and cases have been reported after strenuous swimming at the surface (Weiler-Ravell et al., 1995). Presenting features include cough, which is sometimes productive of blood and/or frothy sputum, and syncope. There is no history of cardiac chest pain. It typically occurs in cold water or with strenuous exercise and excessive rehydration. Inspiratory resistance from airway narrowing or faulty equipment might also play a part. The diversion of blood to the pulmonary vasculature due to the hydrostatic effect of immersion is presumed to be the common contributory factor. A series of cases induced by cold had abnormally high resting vascular resistance and the resistance increased much more than in controls when presented with a cold challenge (Wilmshurst et al., 1989). The condition usually resolves within hours if the diver rests and receives supplemental oxygen therapy, although diuretics or vasodilators might be required in more severe cases. It can, however, lead to fatality, and as yet there is no a way to determine with accuracy the risk of recurrence after an episode. Although recurrences have been reported in up to 30% of cases (Edmonds et al., 2012), many swimmers and divers have not suffered any recurrences on returning to the water. It is not unusual, however, for such individuals to adopt more conservative diving habits (Slade et al., 2001).

Salt Water Aspiration Syndrome

The diver presents with a cough soon after diving. After a delay of between 1 and 15 hours, the diver develops a productive element to the cough (occasionally with a frothy haemoptysis), dyspnoea (sometimes with wheeze) plus extra-pulmonary symptoms such as shivering, anorexia, nausea, vomiting, headaches, more generalised aches, malaise, fever and even impaired consciousness. Retrosternal pain is experienced by the majority of cases. Crackles are often audible on examining the lungs and 50% of cases have patchy consolidation on chest X-ray. Pulmonary symptoms require treatment with no more than supplemental oxygen. Warmth appears to help the other symptoms (Edmonds, 2002b). Various mechanisms have been suggested, including a very mild variant of near drowning, a direct inflammatory or osmotic effect of hypertonic saline or inflammation provoked by irritants, particles or organisms in the seawater. It might be that several different provoking agents present with the same symptoms and signs. Whatever the cause, the natural history is one of spontaneous recovery within 6–24 hours of onset (Mitchell, 2002).

Pulmonary Barotrauma of Descent

In breath-hold diving or in circumstances in which the compressed gas supply fails, the gas remaining in the diver's lungs can be compressed. A large part of the reduction in gas volume is compensated for by the redistribution of peripheral venous blood and the distensible vessels within the lungs becoming increasingly engorged. As a result, the lungs can compress well beyond residual volume and sustain little or no damage. For instance, the official world record for a 'no-limits' breath-hold dive at the time of writing is 214 m (AIDA, 2015), at which depth the gas would occupy less than a twentieth of its original volume. Excursions to extreme depths with no gas supply would, however, result in lung damage with bleeding into the airways.

Inert Gas Narcosis

Air is suitable for breathing at the surface and for diving in the normal recreational range. At high partial pressures, however, nitrogen has narcotic properties that first become apparent when breathing air at 30–50 m. Mild impairment of performance is the first manifestation, then overconfidence, a sense of well-being (anxiety and distress in some), sleepiness, confusion, dizziness, loss of memory, hallucinations, stupefaction and unconsciousness as the partial pressure rises further. Some inert gases are more narcotic than nitrogen, and others less so. Helium, for instance, does not cause narcosis and is much less dense than nitrogen, making it a very suitable diluent for deep diving gas mixtures.

Pulmonary Oxygen Toxicity

The tissues most often affected by oxygen toxicity in diving are the nervous system and the lungs, although eyesight changes have been reported in some cases. Atelectasis is observed in patients and healthy volunteers who breathe high fractions of oxygen at normal atmospheric pressure for any prolonged period of time. This can be avoided by including a substantial fraction of inert diluent gas in the breathing mixture. Even after taking this precaution, problems can occur if oxygen is breathed at an inspired partial pressure greater than 50 kPa. This is known as pulmonary oxygen toxicity, and is characterised by inflammation spreading from the carina. If unchecked, it can proceed to respiratory failure due to impaired gas exchange across inflamed and fibrosed respiratory epithelium. Deterioration in lung volumes, flows, compliance and gas transfer all usually precede symptoms. Onset is not immediate, but is more rapid with higher inspired partial pressures of oxygen. Symptoms usually improve substantially within hours of reducing inspired partial pressures to normal values, and improved flows and volumes soon follow, but total resolution of symptoms and normalisation of gas transfer values can take several days (Clark and Thom, 2003).

Central Nervous System Oxygen Toxicity

A mixture containing a 40% fraction of oxygen could be breathed at the surface for many hours with no ill effect. At 50 m depth, the inspired partial pressure of the same mixture exceeds 240 kPa and would increase the risk of a range of central nervous system (CNS) symptoms, including generalised seizure. In the tonic phase of the seizure, which is usually short lived, the vocal cords can appose in spasm. Sometimes there are premonitory symptoms; those that are usually taught to divers are visual disturbances, tinnitus, nausea, twitching, irritability and dizziness. It is worth noting that respiratory problems have also been attributed to CNS oxygen toxicity. The relevant features include episodic spasm of the diaphragm (mimicking problems with gas supply) and unexpectedly rapid and early reductions in forced expiratory volume in 1 second (FEV_1) and mid-expiratory flows that are thought to be vagally mediated (Clark and Thom, 2003). In order to minimise the risk of CNS oxygen toxicity, the inspired partial pressure of oxygen is typically not allowed to exceed an upper limit of 140–150 kPa when the diver is active and 160 kPa when resting. Immersion reduces the seizure threshold, and it is unusual for seizures to be provoked at an inspired partial pressure of less than 200 kPa when at rest in a dry hyperbaric chamber.

Contaminated Gas Mixture

A mixture that contains a contaminant (such as carbon monoxide, carbon dioxide or volatile hydrocarbons) in non-toxic concentrations at the surface can become toxic as the partial pressure of the contaminant rises when the diver descends and breathes the gas at increased pressure.

Hypercapnia

Even with equipment that is optimised to minimise dead space, divers develop a moderate hypercapnia when breathing a gas mixture of increased density. Introducing an external resistance to breathing in normal atmospheric conditions will cause hypercapnia in a non-diver, and this is exaggerated further as workload rises. Denser gas increases the work of breathing, and the additional internal resistance created within the diver's chest is thought to have a similar effect. In fact, elimination of carbon dioxide, rather than oxygen delivery, is the most important factor limiting workload in a diver. Hypercapnia is unwelcome as the resulting vasodilatation potentiates heat loss from the skin and increases the delivery of inert gas to tissues. It also lowers the threshold for inert gas narcosis and cerebral oxygen toxicity.

A minority population of divers are classed as carbon dioxide retainers. They develop high alveolar carbon dioxide levels by hypoventilating even in moderately raised pressures and the magnitude of this effect is often more pronounced during exercise. These divers benefit from economical gas consumption, but they remain vulnerable to hypercapnic narcosis and the other effects of hypercapnia mentioned above. In addition, a lack of dyspnoeic symptoms will deprive them of an early warning of rising inspired carbon dioxide levels in equipment that is starting to malfunction. It is difficult to identify retainers reliably with standard tests such as end breath-hold carbon dioxide levels and response at surface to different fractions of carbon dioxide. Exercise at depth appears to be the best form of screening.

Fortunately, the use of a less dense breathing mixture, such as oxygen in helium, reduces the tendency to hypercapnia in normal divers and in retainers (Lanphier and Bookspan, 1999).

Decompression Illness

During the dive, inert gases accumulate in the tissues. The reduction in partial pressure of inert gas in the lungs is reflected in the arterial blood, and if this is lower than the tension of the same gas dissolved in any of the tissues, the gas will begin to diffuse out of the tissue. Oxygen does not accumulate, as it is metabolised constantly. Carbon dioxide production is limited by metabolic rate, but tissue levels are likely to be slightly higher due to equilibration with blood, which has itself equilibrated with alveolar levels of carbon dioxide elevated by the effects of diving on ventilation. Carbon dioxide is very soluble, however, and contributes little to the overall gas burden within a tissue. As a result, inert gas is likely to contribute a large proportion of any free gas that is released into the tissues, including the blood. If the total pressure of the free gas exceeds ambient to the extent that it can also overcome surface tension and the mechanical resistance offered by surrounding tissue, the bubble will grow. Many bubbles arise in the venous circulation as it is low pressure and offers little mechanical resistance to expansion. The bubble-laden blood is transported to the lungs where, in normal circumstances, the bubbles are trapped in the alveolar capillaries until they have equilibrated with the intra-alveolar gas, at which point the bubble will no longer be able to sustain itself and will collapse. As a result, in normal circumstances, the left heart receives fully oxygenated blood from which the bubbles and excess inert gas have been filtered. Problems arise when:

1. Bubbles develop in solid tissue
2. Venous gas emboli accumulate in such numbers that they impair perfusion of the tissues in which they originate or they overwhelm the pulmonary filter
3. Venous gas emboli circumvent the pulmonary filter via a right–left circulatory shunt and are delivered to the systemic circulation

In these circumstances, divers develop a medical condition known as decompression illness, decompression sickness or, more colloquially, 'the bends'. The most frequent manifestations are either an ill-defined pain in one or more large limb joints or neurological problems, some of which can be very subtle, but more serious deficits such as quadriplegia can also occur. Less commonly reported manifestations include: cardiopulmonary compromise, which can range from cough or mild dyspnoea through shortness of breath, chest pain, haemoptysis, cyanosis and oedema to frank cardiopulmonary arrest; cutaneous symptoms, ranging from pruritus through erythema and papular rash to tender, marbled ischaemic skin; enlarged, tender lymph nodes; and a selection of non-specific symptoms such as headache and inappropriate fatigue. Manifestations can be trivial and self-limiting, disabling or life-threatening. First aid for decompression illness involves basic life support and high-fraction inspired oxygen; the accepted definitive treatment is recompression.

Divers minimise the risk of this disorder by breathing mixtures of gases that minimise the accumulation of inert gas and by ascending according to a schedule, sometimes stopping for a set duration at one or more depths, which is designed to release the inert gas from the tissues at a safe rate.

Saturation divers often remain at pressure for many days. UK health and safety regulations limit exposure to 28 days, but this limit is arbitrary in terms of decompression obligation. After a day or so, all of the tissues in the divers' bodies are 'saturated' with as much inert gas that can accumulate at the pressure at which they are being stored and, therefore, the decompression schedule will not change, however long they remain thereafter. The decompression may take several days, but the risk of decompression illness is minimised by adopting a single very slow decompression as opposed to the multiple shorter schedules that would have been required if the same task was undertaken using surface-orientated techniques.

Divers with a large right–left circulatory shunt are at increased risk of decompression illness (Bove, 1998) and are more likely to suffer from decompression illness after a dive that observes safe limits. A large shunt has been shown to be a statistically significant risk factor for neurological (Wilmshurst and Bryson, 2000) and cutaneous (Wilmshurst et al., 2001) decompression illness. Many of the large shunts are due to a patent foramen ovale, but some cases have features that are consistent with the presence of pulmonary arteriovenous fistulae, such as delayed arrival of bubbles in the left heart on bubble contrast echocardiography and orthodeoxia on pulse oximetry (Wilmshurst and Bryson, 2000). The time from surfacing to first symptoms of decompression illness associated with a large right–left shunt had a mode range of 11–20 minutes and a median of 20 minutes (Wilmshurst and Bryson, 2000).

Pulmonary Barotrauma of Ascent

Intact fresh cadaveric lungs cannot tolerate a sustained overpressure of much more than 9 kPa (equivalent to an ascent from less than 1 m to the surface) and will rupture (Francis and Denison, 1999). Therefore, a diver who makes an ascent and does not exhale is at risk of pulmonary barotrauma as gas expands in the lungs. For this reason, a casualty suffering from an oxygen toxicity seizure should not be surfaced during the tonic phase of the episode due to the possibility that the glottis has closed. Rupture is not always associated with over-inflation of the whole lung, and localised abnormalities within the lung can also trap expanding gas during ascent, despite the best efforts of the diver to exhale completely. Rapid, uncontrolled and unexpected ascents can predispose an individual to this pulmonary barotrauma of ascent. The consequences can include one or more of interstitial emphysema, pneumothorax, pneumomediastinum and pneumoperitoneum. In addition, arterial gas embolism (AGE) can occur when the expanding gas ruptures into a pulmonary vessel and is delivered to the left heart, which pumps it into the systemic circulation. The bubbles are delivered preferentially to tissues with a high blood flow, and gravity might also play a part. The two outcomes with the greatest impact are cerebral AGE and coronary AGE. There is a short latency between reaching the surface and first symptoms; this is usually no longer than 10 minutes and, due to the mechanism, symptoms can sometimes occur before the diver reaches the surface. A typical presentation is a sudden onset of diminished consciousness, hemiplegia or hemiparesis. It is not unusual for the symptoms to improve quickly as the gas emboli traverse and are expelled from the capillaries, and then for the casualty to deteriorate later due to the mechanical damage to the vascular endothelium caused by the original bubbles.

AGE occurs more often in divers than other victims of pulmonary rupture. The reason for this is not known, but it might be that splinting of the chest by immersion and/or tight-fitting equipment resists overexpansion. After anything other than the most shallow and short dive, excess inert gas will be loaded in the tissues, and this might magnify the effects of emboli that would otherwise have had no clinical effect as they passed through the capillary bed. It is often not possible to find any evidence of pulmonary damage, but if a casualty has symptoms that are consistent with AGE, clinical features of pulmonary barotrauma must be excluded. Conversely, anyone who sustains pulmonary barotrauma of ascent must undergo neurological examination in order to exclude AGE.

First aid for AGE involves basic life support and high-fraction inspired oxygen; the accepted definitive treatment is recompression. It is often not possible to determine whether the gas that is causing the symptoms is escaped from a ruptured lung, evolved from that accumulated in tissues or a combination of both, but their treatment does not differ. As a result, the term 'decompression illness' also includes AGE (Francis and Smith, 1991). Decompression sickness, however, is reserved for describing the symptoms caused by evolved gas.

A pneumomediastinum is often asymptomatic and only some 50% of spontaneous cases are visible on posteroanterior (PA) chest X-ray. The most common presenting symptom is retrosternal pain. It can present solely with voice change and the gas can track upwards and manifest as subcutaneous emphysema (Francis and Denison, 1999).

Hypoxia of Ascent

Sometimes, in order to avoid oxygen toxicity, a diver will use a breathing gas mixture that contains a much lower fraction of oxygen than is found in air. Although the mixture will give an adequate partial pressure of oxygen at depth due to the raised ambient pressure, these 'lean' mixtures will not maintain consciousness near the surface, and if the diver does not change to a more suitable mixture, there is a risk of blackout as the partial pressure of oxygen declines during the ascent. A similar phenomenon is seen in breath-hold divers. This is sometimes described as 'shallow-water blackout', although this term was originally used to describe severe hypercapnia caused by rudimentary rebreather equipment that was unable to scrub all of the carbon dioxide from the gas exhaled at high levels of exertion.

Dilution Hypoxia

Semi-closed rebreather diving equipment based on a constant mass flow principle will inject the same mass of gas mixture into the counter-lung, irrespective of the diver's depth and level of exertion. It would be wasteful to set the flow to accommodate maximum oxygen consumption for the diver, so a compromise is made based on the assumption that the diver will not exercise maximally for long periods and, therefore, will not exhaust the supply of oxygen in the counter-lung. It is sometimes possible for oxygen consumption during prolonged, unusually strenuous exertion to deplete the mixture in the counter-lung to the extent that it becomes hypoxic. The presence of a diluent inert gas means that the diver is unaware that the oxygen is being exhausted until the symptoms of hypoxia arise. Sometimes, the mixture has adequate oxygen to sustain consciousness at depth, but will cause hypoxia of ascent if the diver begins to surface immediately. In order to avoid this, the well-trained diver will empty the counter-lung and fill it with fresh gas prior to ascent (Figure 34.1).

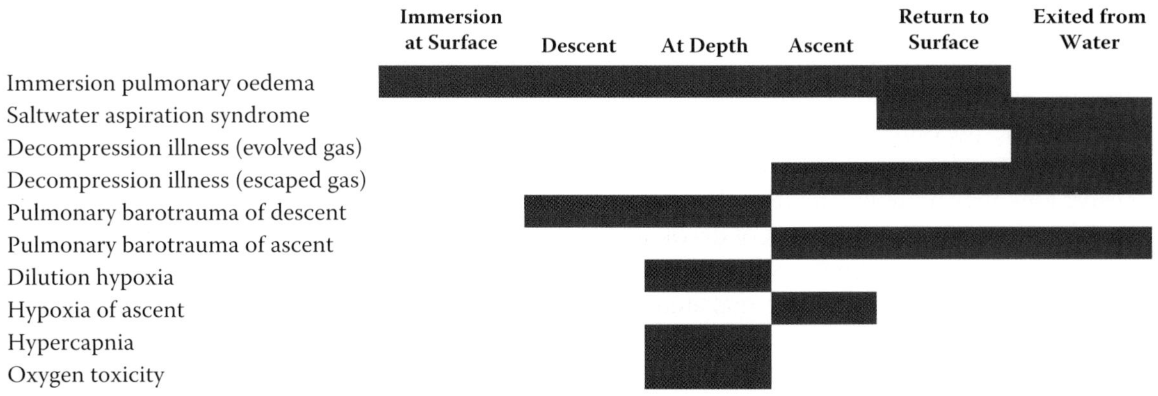

FIGURE 34.1 Phase of dive in which a particular problem is more likely to manifest.

PULMONARY ASPECTS OF FITNESS TO DIVE

Background

There are many hazards in diving, although these are generally well controlled for those who work in areas with good health and safety oversight. There were 23 cases of decompression illness in the UK offshore sector in the 10 years up to 2014, with three cases in 2013/2014. There were no diving fatalities in the UK offshore sector in 2013/2014, the last being in 2011/2012 (UK Health and Safety Executive, 2014).

General Considerations

When considering respiratory fitness for a dive, the following should also be taken into account:

- Capacity to support physical activity while breathing dense gas
- Risk of incapacitation
- Risk factors for barotrauma
- Impact of any medication (or sudden withdrawal of it) in a challenging environment (e.g. systemic steroids and immunosuppressants)

Other sources of advice on fitness for occupational diving can be found from UK Health and Safety Executive (HSE) (2015), the European Diving Technology Committee (EDTC) (2003) and the National Oceanic and Atmospheric Administration (NOAA) (2010).

Some specific issues that might arise in a consultation with a diver are considered in the following sections.

Long-Term Pulmonary Effects of Diving

Divers tend to have larger lung volumes than expected. This might be because divers are, in general, a self-selecting fit population who have, in addition, received respiratory muscle training from breathing against resistance for long periods. Forced vital capacity (FVC) is enlarged proportionately more than FEV_1, which gives many divers a lower FEV_1:FVC expiratory ratio than might otherwise be expected. Mid- and late-expiratory flows are lower and there is some evidence of a relationship between these flows and length of diving career. Some consider that this might be an indication of small airway changes. Lung volumes appear to decline at a faster rate than expected in some longitudinal studies of divers, but other studies show that this might be more closely related to smoking history (Tetzlaff et al., 2006). Diffusing capacity is impaired after a saturation dive, and this has been attributed to low-grade oxygen toxicity or bubble damage. It appears, however, to recover gradually following the exposure, no structural changes have been demonstrated on imaging and, most importantly, no clinically relevant consequences of the changes have been found.

Pulmonary Barotrauma: Primary Screening

In a study of submarine escape trainees, victims of pulmonary barotrauma were more likely to have a low FVC. This might be due to reduced lung compliance and/or a lack of support to the lungs from the chest wall. The analysis of this population did not show that a low expiratory ratio (FEV_1:FVC) was a risk factor, but it must be borne in mind that candidates with significant obstructive defects are likely to have been disqualified from submarine escape training. Nevertheless, a low FEV_1, FVC or peak expiratory flow (PEF) (<80% of predicted) or low expiratory ratio (<70%) deserves investigation in order to exclude airway narrowing or gas trapping in all diving candidates.

Some case reports have raised the question of whether a large FVC is a risk factor for pulmonary barotrauma during a free ascent, but to date, the relationship has not been established with certainty (van Hulst et al., 2011). In the meantime, it is prudent to consider carefully any candidate whose spirometry is clearly outside upper or lower boundaries of the normal range.

Pulmonary Barotrauma: Post-Incident

Divers who sustain pulmonary barotrauma of ascent will need to be assessed prior to returning to dive. The main goal is to exclude gas trapping, fixed or reversible airway narrowing or any other predisposition to pulmonary rupture or over-inflation. Meticulous history taking, careful respiratory examination and spirometry are important components of this assessment. Some authorities advise routine use of high-resolution computed tomography (HRCT), while others advocate this only if there is any uncertainty. It is unusual to find any residual pulmonary damage, but even if no abnormality is found, time should be allowed for the respiratory tract to heal. Recommended periods typically vary between 1 and 3 months. Traumatic pneumothorax should be assessed in a similar way.

Spontaneous Pneumothorax

Assessment for return to diving after spontaneous pneumothorax is similar to the above. The British Thoracic Society recommends that a candidate would normally be considered fit to dive only after bilateral surgical pleurectomy and if they have normal pulmonary function tests and thoracic computed tomography (CT) imaging (British Thoracic Society Fitness to Dive Group, 2003). The UK Diving Medical Committee accepts that, in a candidate who has not had a pleurectomy but has had no pneumothorax for 5 years, the risk of pulmonary barotrauma is small and not significantly greater than for many in the general population. These individuals are allowed to dive provided that a CT scan of the chest and lung function tests, including flow–volume loops, show no reason to suggest that there is significant residual lung disease.

Bullae

Bullae are often found retrospectively in many cases of barotrauma, and it is frequently not possible to ascertain whether they are the cause or consequence of the incident. HRCT is more sensitive than plain chest X-ray and many more bullae are being found, but we are not yet sure of the risk represented by these findings. There are a few case reports of pre-existing bullae enlarging over time and eventually causing AGE symptoms (Germonpré et al., 2008). More prospective studies are required, but in the meantime, large bullae contraindicate diving, especially those that are visible on plain chest X-ray.

Decompression Illness

It is helpful to decide whether a case of decompression illness was more likely to have been due to evolved gas or escaped gas. In cases of the former, presence of a right–left shunt should be considered when the decompression profile was within accepted limits, especially if symptoms present within or near the interval of 11–20 minutes after surfacing. A history of migraine with aura increases the likelihood of the presence of a right–left shunt. If a shunt is considered likely, the diver should be counselled regarding how to dive safely with a shunt (UK Diving Medical Committee) and referred for testing if they wish. Some shunts are amenable to closure using percutaneous techniques.

It is important to consider whether it is necessary to screen for predisposition to barotrauma prior to return to diving, especially if the history was consistent with AGE. This would normally require pulmonary function tests and at least plain chest X-ray imaging. Many authorities would now advise HRCT, although, as mentioned earlier, interpretation is not straightforward.

Recompression might be necessary in order to treat AGE after pulmonary barotrauma, in which case the treatment should proceed with caution and any significant pneumothorax should be relieved before the chamber is decompressed.

Asthma

Asthma was implicated in 8% of recreational diving deaths in one study. Only 1% of divers in that population were asthmatic, leading the authors to conclude that the condition was a genuine risk factor for diving fatality (Edmonds, 2002a). Diving is associated with several potential provocative stimuli for asthma, such as exertion, resistance to breathing and inhalation of cold, dry air and hypertonic saline.

Assessment would require history, examination, inspection of a peak expiratory flow diary and spirometry with exercise challenge and/or reversibility studies. The acceptability of asthma in a diver, and whether diving while on treatment is permissible, will depend on the body that is responsible for advising on fitness standards. The British Thoracic Society (2003) guidelines permit diving if the diver has acceptable control at the time of assessment, self-monitors (with regular twice-daily peak flow) and remains stable on medication up to British Thoracic Society (BTS) Step 2 (regular inhaled anti-inflammatory agents). The criteria suggested are

- Free of asthma symptoms
- Normal spirometry (FEV_1 >80% predicted and FEV_1:FVC ratio >70% predicted)
- Negative exercise test (<15% fall in FEV_1 after exercise)

The guidelines recommend no diving if the diver has:

- Asthma symptoms requiring relief medication in the 48 hours preceding the dive
- Reduced Peak Expiratory Flow (more than 10% fall from best values)
- Increased peak flow variability (more than 20% diurnal variation)

Causes of Shortness of Breath

The list of differential diagnoses for shortness of breath in a diver is long and includes pulmonary barotrauma, oxygen toxicity, immersion pulmonary oedema, saltwater aspiration syndrome, underwater blast, cardiopulmonary decompression illness and hypercapnia. Always consider the circumstances (depth, breathing mixture, ascent rate, etc.) in which the problem arose in order to focus on only the most plausible causes.

CONCLUSION

Diving can be very hard work, especially in an emergency, and there is no doubt that significant cardiovascular and respiratory capacity is required for the more demanding roles. Many pulmonary problems will have a direct significant effect on a diver.

When assessing fitness to dive from a pulmonary perspective, the principal considerations are whether there is adequate gas flow and exchange to support the necessary level of activity and whether there is any predisposition to lung rupture.

Obstruction or restriction is likely to compromise activity, limit gas movement and predispose to barotrauma. Pulmonary barotrauma itself will compromise ventilation, the discomfort could distract the diver and any gas-filled spaces that arise at depth would expand further on ascent to the surface, potentially converting a simple pneumothorax into tension. A tension pneumothorax or an AGE could incapacitate the diver, who might then drown. Bullae can be large enough to compromise ventilation or to be at significant risk of rupture during ascent, although their fate cannot be predicted with any certainty. An acute respiratory infection would disqualify from diving on the grounds of general impairment, respiratory compromise and the possibility of barotrauma.

Connective tissue and inflammatory disorders can weaken or stiffen the lung tissue and cause obstruction and restriction that will, in turn, compromise ventilation and predispose to barotrauma.

A careful history is important in the acute situation, when reviewing a diver after an incident and also during a routine assessment of fitness to dive. It will help to identify episodes of saltwater aspiration syndrome or immersion pulmonary oedema. As mentioned earlier, a large pulmonary arteriovenous shunt will increase the risk of decompression illness, so an episode following a decompression that was within normal limits should prompt further investigation.

REFERENCES

AIDA. 2015. Association Internationale pour le Développement de l'Apnée. World records. Available at: https://www.aidainternational.org/worldrecords (accessed 25 April 2016).

Bove, A. A. 1998. Risk of decompression sickness with patent foramen ovale. *Undersea Hyper Med* 25(3):175–8.

British Thoracic Society Fitness to Dive Group. 2003. British Thoracic Society guidelines on respiratory aspects of fitness for diving. *Thorax* 58:3–13.

Clark, J. M. and Thom, S. R. 2003. Oxygen under pressure. In A. O. Brubakk and T. S. Neuman (eds), *Bennett and Elliott's Physiology and Medicine of Diving*, fifth edition. London: Saunders, 358–418.

Denison, D. M., Warrell, D. A. and West, J. B. 1971. Airway structure and alveolar emptying in the lungs of sea lions and dogs. *Respir Physiol* 13(3):253–60.

Edmonds, C., Lippmann, J., Lockley, S. and Wolfers, D. 2012. Scuba divers' pulmonary oedema: Recurrences and fatalities. *Diving Hyperb Med* 42(1):40–4.

Edmonds, C. 2002a. Asthma. In C. Edmonds C. Lowry, J. Pennefather and R. Walker (eds), *Diving and Subaquatic Medicine*, fourth edition. London: Arnold, 559–74.

Edmonds, C. 2002b. Drowning syndromes: Saltwater aspiration syndrome. In C. Edmonds, C. Lowry, J. Pennefather and R. Walker (eds), *Diving and Subaquatic Medicine*, fourth edition. London: Arnold, 273–6.

European Diving Technology Committee (EDTC). 2003. Fitness to Dive Standards. Guidelines for Medical Assessment of Working Divers. Available at: http://www.edtc.org/EDTC-Fitnesstodivestandard-2003.pdf (accessed 25 April 2016).

Flynn, E. T. 1999. Temperature effects. In C. E. G. Lundgren and J. N. Miller (eds), *The Lung at Depth*. New York, NY: Marcel Dekker, Inc., 129–64.

Francis, T. J. R. and Denison, D. M. 1999. Pulmonary barotrauma. In C. E. G. Lundgren and J. N. Miller (eds), *The Lung at Depth*. New York, NY: Marcel Dekker, Inc., 259–374.

Francis, T. J. R. and Smith, D. J. (eds). 1991. *Describing Decompression Illness. 42nd Undersea and Hyperbaric Medical Society Workshop*. Bethesda, MD: Undersea and Hyperbaric Medical Society.

Germonpré, P., Balestra, C. and Pieters, T. 2008. Influence of scuba diving on asymptomatic isolated pulmonary bullae. *Diving Hyperb Med* 38(4):206–11.

Lanphier, E. H. and Bookspan, J. 1999. Carbon dioxide retention. In C. E. G. Lundgren and J. N. Miller (eds), *The Lung at Depth*. New York, NY: Marcel Dekker, Inc., 211–36.

Mitchell, S. J. 2002. Salt water aspiration syndrome. *J SPUMS* 32(4):205–6.

National Oceanic and Atmospheric Administration (NOAA). 2010. Diving Medical Standards and Procedures Manual. Available at: http://www.ndc.noaa.gov/pdfs/NOAA_Medical_Standards_Procedures_Manual.pdf (accessed 25 April 2016).

Pons, M., Blinkenstorfer, D., Oechslin, E., Hold, G., Greminger, P., Franzeck, U. K. and Russi, E. W. 1995. Pulmonary oedema in healthy persons during SCUBA-diving and swimming. *Eur Respir J* 8(5):762–7.

Slade, J. B., Hattori, T., Ray, C. S., Bove, A. A. and Cianci, P. 2001. Pulmonary edema associated with SCUBA diving. Case reports and review. *Chest* 120:1686–94.

Tetzlaff, K., Theysohn, J., Stahl, C., Schlegel, S., Koch, A. and Muth, C. M. 2006. Decline of FEV_1 in SCUBA divers. *Chest* 130(1):238–43.

U.K. Health and Safety Executive. 2011. The medical examination and assessment of divers (MA1). Available at: http://www.hse.gov.uk/pubns/ma1.pdf (accessed 25 April 2016).

U.K. Health and Safety Executive. 2014. Annual Offshore Statistics and Regulatory Activity Report 2013/2014. Available at: http://www.hse.gov.uk/offshore/statistics/hsr1314.pdf (accessed 25 April 2016).

U.K. Diving Medical Committee. Intracardiac Shunts. Available at: http://ukdmc.org/2015/09/29/intracardiac-shunts/ (accessed 25 April 2016).

U.K. Diving Medical Committee. Pneumothorax and Diving. Available at: http://ukdmc.org/2015/09/29/pneumothorax (accessed 25 April 2016).

Weiler-Ravell, D., Shupak, A., Goldenberg, I., Halpern, P., Shoshani, O., Hirschhorn, G. and Margulis, A. 1995. Pulmonary oedema and hemoptysis induced by strenuous swimming. *BMJ* 311:361–2.

van Hulst, R., van Ooij, P. J., Houtkooper, A. and Schlosser, N. J. 2011. Large lungs in divers, risk for pulmonary barotrauma? Undersea and Hyperbaric Medicine meeting abstract. Available at: http://archive.rubicon-foundation.org/9889 (accessed 30 July 2015).

Wilmshurst, P. and Bryson, P. 2000. Relationship between the clinical features of neurological decompression illness and its causes. *Clin Sci* 99:65–75.

Wilmshurst, P. T., Nuri, M., Crowther, A. and Webb-Peploe, M. M. 1989. Cold-induced pulmonary oedema in SCUBA divers and swimmers and subsequent development of hypertension. *Lancet* 1(8629):62–5.

Wilmshurst P. T., Pearson, M. J., Walsh, K. P., Morrison, W. L. and Bryson, P. 2001. Relationship between right-to-left shunts and cutaneous decompression illness. *Clin Sci* 100:539–42.

35 Work at High Altitudes

Matthew C. Frise, Nayia Petousi and Peter A. Robbins

CONTENTS

INTRODUCTION

The Physical Environment at High Altitude Poses a Number of Physiological Challenges

Work in many regions of the Earth involves exposure to high altitude. Workers may be native highlanders—those who were born and have lived their whole lives in an elevated region—or lowlanders, ordinarily resident at or close to sea level. It is increasingly necessary for work at altitude to be performed by lowlanders, who may either commute or remain there for extended periods. This is due to a combination of increasing manpower requirements as industries expand and the limited availability of requisite skills within the indigenous population. Mining activities in particular are moving higher and higher as economically important deposits are exhausted at lower altitudes. High altitude poses a variety of occupational challenges, although those faced by lowlanders have historically been somewhat neglected (West, 2014).

The geological processes that are responsible for the creation of mountainous regions (Figure 35.1) led also to the concentration in many of these areas of valuable mineral and fossil fuel deposits. Industries concerned with extracting and processing these materials therefore cluster at high altitudes, as do the towns and villages that have grown up in order to accommodate those who work

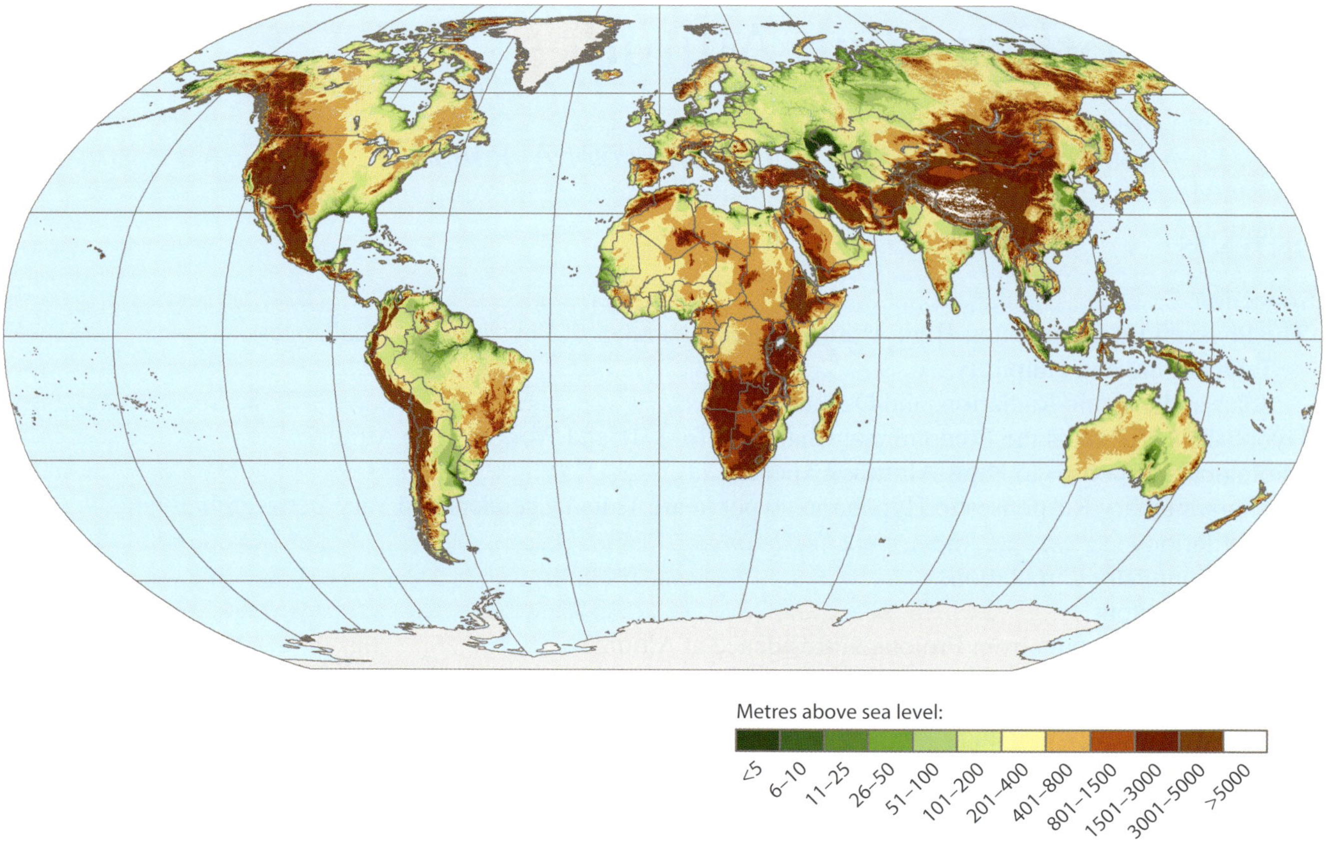

FIGURE 35.1 Global land elevation. (Reproduced under Creative Commons 3.0 Attribution License, Centre for International Earth Science Information Network/Columbia University. 2012. National Aggregates of Geospatial Data Collection: Population, Landscape, and Climate Estimates, Version 3. Palisades, NY: NASA SEDAC. Available at: http://sedac.ciesin.columbia.edu/data/set/nagdc-population-landscape-climate-estimates-v3.)

within them. The beauty of these areas, snow cover and challenges posed by the terrain make these environments very popular for outdoor pursuits. Leisure and tourism industries are therefore another reason workers find themselves at altitude, perhaps with seasonal exposures year after year. The difficulties confronting the very large numbers of people who travel to altitude for recreational purposes, and the huge industries that have grown up to support such activities, are a considerable stimulus for research. Many principles are equally applicable to high-altitude occupational medicine more generally.

Of the challenges that come with high altitude, hypobaric hypoxia rightly receives the most attention because of the potential severity of high-altitude illness (HAI) that may result. Additional problems are encountered in the form of extremes of temperature, humidity, cosmic and solar radiation, traumatic injury and certain infections that are restricted to particular geographic areas. A comprehensive discussion of these aspects can be found in works on wilderness medicine (Auerbach, 2012). For the worker at high altitude, many of these difficulties may be mitigated relatively simply, but hypobaric hypoxia is not easily avoided. The most extreme altitudes are encountered with air and space travel, which are made possible only by pressurised craft. Since this text is concerned with the pulmonary pathologies associated with work at high altitude, hypobaric hypoxia and its consequences will be the focus of this chapter.

Temperature and Humidity

For every 150-m increase in altitude, the ambient air temperature falls by approximately 1°C (West et al., 2013) and wind chill factor is an added complication (Huey and Eguskitza, 2001). Working outdoors at even relatively modest elevations therefore mandates special attention to clothing, particularly if strenuous physical work is being carried out, in order to ensure proper thermoregulation is not compromised (Ainslie and Reilly, 2003). The fact that even native highlanders who have lived and worked at altitude for many years are not immune to the dangers of thermal injury underscores the threats posed (Subedi et al., 2010). From a pulmonary perspective, temperature is particularly important when considering high-altitude pulmonary oedema (HAPE), since cold is a predisposing factor. The very low absolute humidity at altitude is also a challenge; insensible water losses are much greater when breathing dry air, and this is compounded by the increased minute ventilation in response to alveolar hypoxia. Although it is clear that this effect is important (Ferrus et al., 1984), actual measurements of its magnitude at different altitudes are lacking.

Solar and Cosmic Radiation, and Ozone

At high altitude anywhere in the world, the thinner, drier air permits a greater amount of solar radiation to reach the Earth's surface. An additional factor is the propensity of the ground to reflect ultraviolet (UV) radiation, termed albedo, which is particularly marked in desert locations or those with snow cover. Some of the highest levels of UV radiation in the world have been recorded at high altitude, including in Hawaii (Bodhaine et al., 1997), Tibet (Dahlback et al., 2007) and Chile (Cordero et al., 2014). For those working long term in the open at high altitude, such as mountain guides, very high levels of UV exposure have been documented (Moehrle et al., 2003). Whilst this has obvious implications for skin damage and cutaneous malignancies, UV radiation promotes the generation of ozone from atmospheric oxygen, and this, coupled with other climatic factors, can lead to high concentrations of ozone at high altitude. In urban areas, elevated atmospheric ozone levels are associated with a significant increase in the risk of death from respiratory causes independent of airborne particular matter (Jerrett et al., 2009). A number of studies have implicated ozone in exacerbating existing respiratory conditions (Dey et al., 2010), although the extent to which this effect is important at altitude is unknown. Exposure to cosmic radiation is also greater at altitude, although even in those with the greatest exposure (i.e. pilots and cabin crew), it is uncertain whether an apparent increase in breast and skin malignancies is real and, if so, whether it is accounted for by this or other factors (Sigurdson and Ron, 2004). An increase in primary pulmonary malignancies has not been reported.

Hypobaric Hypoxia is the Predominant Challenge for Life and Work at High Altitude

The partial pressure of oxygen falls on ascent as a consequence of the decline in barometric pressure (Table 35.1 and Figure 35.2). This relationship is not straightforward, as the dependence of barometric pressure upon altitude varies with latitude, whilst seasonal changes may cause barometric pressure to vary in a given location depending on the time of year (West et al., 1983b), which can become important for workers at extreme altitudes. The early literature relating to studies of hypobaric hypoxia provides numerous examples of the hazards posed (Bert, 1878). What these accounts have in common is the recognition that, with rapid ascent to extreme altitude, the scarcity of oxygen leads to profound mental and physical impairment, followed swiftly by loss of consciousness and death if descent is not begun. While most workers will be exposed to more modest altitudes, there still exist very real risks, even for previously completely healthy individuals.

It is useful to draw a distinction between those processes that allow any healthy human to function at high altitude in the short term (acclimatisation) and those that have operated over many thousands of years to permit

TABLE 35.1
Falling Barometric Pressure and Inspired Partial Pressure of Oxygen with Increasing Altitude

Location	Elevation (m)	Atmospheric Pressure (mmHg)	P_IO_2 (mmHg)	Sea-Level Equivalent F_IO_2
Sea level	0	760	149	0.209
Mount Hutt, New Zealand	2086	598	115	0.161
Commercial aircraft cabin	2438	574	110	0.154
Telluride, Colorado	2600	563	108	0.151
Cusco, Peru	3300	518	99	0.139
Lhasa, Tibet	3600	499	95	0.133
Pike's Peak, Colorado	4300	458	86	0.121
Beijing–Lhasa railway peak	5074	416	79	0.111
Mount Everest summit, Nepal	8848	253	43	0.060

Source: Data from Seccombe, L. M. and Peters, M. J., *J Appl Physiol (1985)*, 116(5), 478–85, 2014.
Abbreviations: P_IO_2: inspired partial pressure of oxygen; F_IO_2: fraction of inspired oxygen.

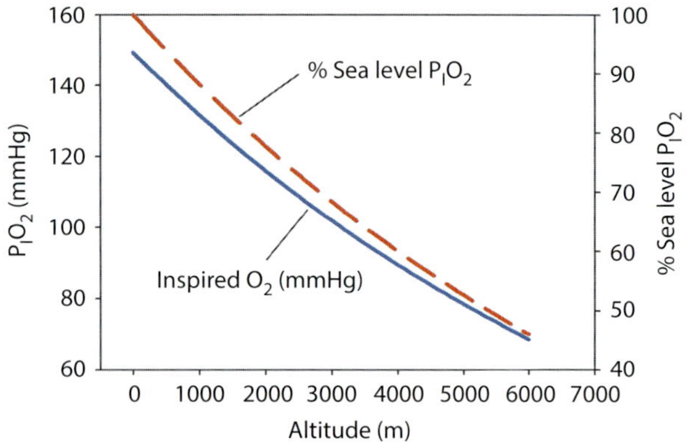

FIGURE 35.2 The relationship between altitude and inspired partial pressure of oxygen (P_IO_2). (Redrawn from Beall, C. M. 2007. *Proc Natl Acad Sci USA* 104 (Suppl. 1):8655–60. With permission. Copyright 2007, National Academy of Sciences, USA)

certain peoples to thrive in environments at high or very high altitudes (evolutionary adaptation) (West, 2006). The inhabitants of the Tibetan plateau, at approximately 4000 m above sea level, are an excellent example of the latter. This group has lived at very high altitude for in excess of 25,000 years (Aldenderfer, 2011). In that time, selection pressure has been such that this population shows alterations in the physiological responses to hypoxia that may serve to protect against chronic HAI, mediated at least partly by alterations in the hypoxia-inducible factor (HIF) transcription factor system (Beall et al., 2010; Petousi and Robbins, 2014). Individuals from certain ethnic groups are thus particularly well suited to work at high altitudes; Sherpas are an obvious example, although it is important to stress that even these populations are not immune to HAI (Droma et al., 2006).

Whilst lowlanders all acclimatise to an extent on ascent to high altitude, there are limits to the level of hypobaric hypoxia that can be tolerated, even with the considerable physiological responses that occur. At extreme altitude, it becomes impossible for humans to survive for extended periods. A brief increase in altitude in an already acclimatised individual, such as a climber attempting to summit Mount Everest, will be met with physiological responses that sustain life until descent, but these are associated with considerable physiological impairment if they are allowed to continue for any significant length of time. Thus, one does not encounter sizeable permanent human settlements at altitudes very much greater than 5000 m (West, 2002b). Occupations that demand such extreme ascent on the surface of the Earth are rare, although some do involve long-term exposure to altitudes that are close to that which can be tolerated.

PHYSIOLOGICAL RESPONSES TO HIGH-ALTITUDE EXPOSURE

Cardiopulmonary Responses to Hypobaric Hypoxia are Time Dependent and Vary Between Individuals

The human race as a whole has not been subjected to significant selection pressure on physiological responses to profound sustained alveolar hypoxia. It should therefore not come as a surprise that the physiological responses that occur on ascent to altitude are not universally helpful. The successful ascent of Everest without the use of supplemental oxygen demonstrates that humans can survive for short periods despite profound hypobaric hypoxia. Acute exposure to that degree of alveolar hypoxia, however, such as might occur during aircraft cabin depressurisation, quickly incapacitates non-acclimatised individuals. Thus, acclimatisation must occur, and rate of ascent is an important determinant.

Ventilation

Ventilatory responses to hypoxia vary greatly between individuals and also vary with repeated measurement in the same individual (Zhang and Robbins, 2000). The acute hypoxic ventilatory response is brought about by direct hypoxic stimulation of the peripheral chemoreceptors in the carotid bodies and occurs within seconds to minutes, before a brief hypoxic ventilatory decline (HVD) supervenes after approximately 10 minutes (Figure 35.3). The mechanisms behind HVD are a subject of debate and may involve both the peripheral chemoreceptors and the central respiratory centres (Robbins, 1995). Ventilatory acclimatisation refers to the subsequent progressive rise in ventilation that occurs over hours to days following ascent to high altitude. Increased minute ventilation results in a fall in alveolar carbon dioxide tension and respiratory alkalosis. Historically, the resulting 'braking effect' on ventilation was emphasised, and early ventilatory acclimatisation to hypoxia (VAH) was attributed to increased renal bicarbonate excretion countering this phenomenon (Berger et al., 1977; Crawford and Severinghaus, 1978). A body of evidence from human and animal studies conclusively demonstrates that VAH over the first 2 days at altitude is not dependent on respiratory alkalosis, and in fact, changes in peripheral chemoreceptor function are driven directly by hypoxia, with renal acid–base changes becoming important later (Robbins, 2007). Work contrasting the fall in alveolar carbon dioxide with increasing hypoxia in acclimatised versus non-acclimatised individuals illustrates the magnitude of the effect (Figure 35.4) (Rahn and Otis, 1949). At very high altitude, minute ventilation rises exponentially, such that alveolar oxygen

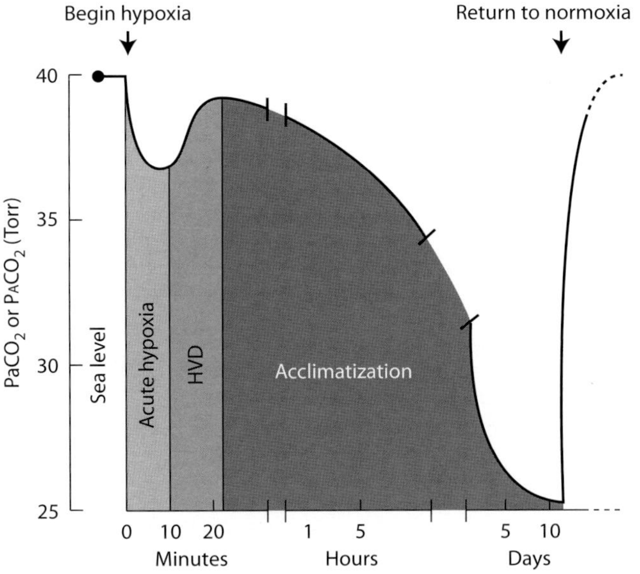

FIGURE 35.3 The time course of ventilatory acclimatisation to hypoxia, with alveolar ($PaCO_2$) or arterial (P_ACO_2) partial pressure of oxygen as an index of ventilation. HVD: hypoxic ventilatory decline. (Redrawn from Smith, C. A., Dempsey, J. A. and Hornbein, T. F. 2001. Control of breathing at high altitude. In T. F. Hornbein and R. B. Schoene (eds), *High Altitude: An Exploration of Human Adaptation*, New York, NY: Marcel Dekker, 139–73. With permission.)

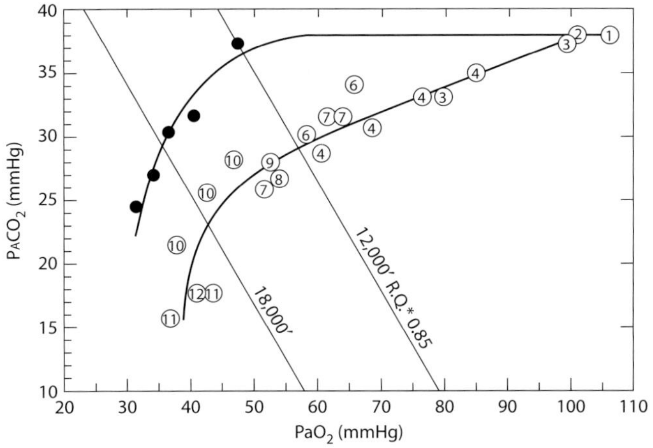

FIGURE 35.4 Fall in alveolar carbon dioxide tension ($PaCO_2$), reflecting increased alveolar minute ventilation, with increasing severity of alveolar hypoxia. Filled circles (upper line) are non-acclimatised individuals; open circles (lower line) are acclimatised individuals. The two diagonal lines indicate a respiratory quotient (R.Q.) of 0.85 at altitudes of 12,000 and 18,000 feet. The circled numbers indicate data from primary studies (see original reference). (Redrawn from Rahn, H. and Otis, A. B. 1949. *Am J Physiol* 157(3):445–62. With permission.)

tension does not fall below approximately 35 mmHg, leading to the concept of a physiological 'defence zone' (West et al., 1983a).

The Pulmonary Circulation

Hypoxic pulmonary vasoconstriction (HPV) describes the propensity of the pulmonary vascular bed to vasoconstrict in response to a fall in oxygen tension, in contrast to the systemic circulation, which vasodilates in response to the same stimulus. HPV occurs rapidly; an initial rise in pulmonary arterial pressure begins within seconds and plateaus within a few minutes, and a second phase is detectable from approximately 40 minutes onwards (Talbot et al., 2005), with pressures continuing to rise for at least another 2 hours (Dorrington et al., 1997; Talbot et al., 2005). The magnitude of HPV appears to vary by nearly fivefold between individuals (Grünig et al., 2000). Pulmonary vascular 'acclimatisation' is characterised by the resultant elevation in pulmonary arterial pressure and by an accompanying increase in the sensitivity of the pulmonary vascular response to any additional acute hypoxic stimulus (Dorrington et al., 1997). Once a week or more has been spent at high altitude, prolonged alveolar hypoxia will initiate pulmonary vascular remodelling, and HPV will no longer be reasonably quickly reversed by inhalation of supplemental oxygen (Groves et al., 1987). It is clear that the pulmonary hypertensive response to alveolar hypoxia is, in contrast to VAH, unhelpful; this maladaptive process contributes to several forms of HAI, which are discussed later (Hackett and Roach, 2001; Penaloza and Arias-Stella, 2007). That HPV occurs rapidly and with even modest degrees of hypobaric hypoxia is demonstrated by the finding that commercial air travel is sufficient to raise pulmonary artery pressure in healthy passengers (Smith et al., 2012).

Cardiac Output

Acute hypoxia triggers a reflex increase in heart rate and cardiac output as part of a sympathetic chemoreflex response. At high altitude, an increase in cardiac output is observed over the course of several days, which is associated with an elevation in heart rate rather than stroke volume. This returns to normal as individuals acclimatise, but heart rate often remains elevated with a concomitant reduction in stroke volume (Vogel and Harris, 1967).

Polycythaemia Results from Prolonged Residence at Altitude

Polycythaemia has been recognised for well over a century as a consequence of residence at altitude (Viault, 1891), with careful measurements by Mabel Fitzgerald during the Pike's Peak expedition of 1911 confirming a relationship between elevation of altitude and elevation of haematocrit (FitzGerald, 1913). An acute increase in haemoglobin concentration on ascent may arise from a reduced plasma volume in response to increased renal sodium excretion, driven in turn by hypoxic stimulation of atrial natriuretic peptide release, although the hormonal responses involved are complex and appear to vary between individuals (Bartsch et al., 1988). Serum erythropoietin levels rise within 90 minutes of the onset of hypoxia (Eckardt et al., 1989), peak within 2 days and thereafter decline towards sea-level values over a period of 2 weeks (Milledge and Cotes, 1985; Richalet et al., 1994). Again, there is huge interindividual variation in the magnitude of the erythropoietin response. Haemoglobin concentration and haematocrit are elevated within days of exposure to high-altitude hypoxia (Richalet et al., 1994) and continue to rise for up to 8 months, causing a total increase in red cell mass of up to 50% at 4500 m (Reynafarje et al., 1959). Haemoglobin concentrations greater than 21 g/dL have been reported in humans acclimatising to extreme high altitude (Winslow et al., 1984).

PATHOLOGIES ASSOCIATED WITH WORK AT HIGH ALTITUDE

The most common pathologies encountered in workers at high altitude are those that are directly related to hypobaric hypoxia and thus may afflict anyone from workers in leisure and tourism industries to miners. Most of these predominantly affect lowlanders who have gone up high, but others can complicate long-term residence in these areas, even in native high-altitude dwellers. Of course, there are also many existing medical conditions, not confined to respiratory pathologies, which may deteriorate with the hypobaric hypoxia of high altitude. Finally, pathologies that are specific to certain occupations, particularly mining, are associated with high altitude as a geographical coincidence, although the possibility that hypobaric hypoxia may in some way modify the exposure–risk profile is an important consideration.

For the purposes of considering the challenges of life and work at higher climes, altitude may be classified arbitrarily as high (1500–3500 m), very high (3500–5500 m) or extreme (>5500 m) (Hackett and Roach, 2012). A variety of related conditions exist that may afflict workers. These HAIs share the aetiological factor of hypobaric hypoxia, but the absence of a detailed understanding of the pathophysiology in each case is unfortunately another common characteristic, despite considerable research efforts. Most attention is usually given to those conditions that occur in the hours and days following ascent. These afflict usually healthy individuals who ascend rapidly to altitudes above 2500 m, and appear to share common pathophysiological mechanisms, leading many to view them as a spectrum rather than separate entities. The acute conditions are of great relevance to any worker who is usually resident at sea level but needs to travel to elevated areas for work, who may do so rapidly by road or air. They are especially problematic for those who repeatedly travel to attitude for short periods but do not reside long enough for acclimatisation to occur; for example, telescope operators on Mauna Kea, Hawaii (West, 2012). For individuals who need to spend prolonged periods working at altitude, such as workers in high-altitude mines, there are additional problems that may occur later even if acute HAI has been avoided.

Acute Mountain Sickness and High-Altitude Cerebral Oedema

In 1991, the criteria for acute mountain sickness (AMS) were defined by consensus and embodied in the Lake Louise scoring system (Hackett, 1992). The hallmark of AMS is headache, occurring in conjunction with at least one of a selection of other symptoms, including constitutional, gastrointestinal and those of the central nervous system. This high-altitude headache (HAH) must be in the setting of ascent of a non-acclimatised individual to above 2500 m and, importantly, occurs in the absence of any clear physical signs (Table 35.2).

TABLE 35.2
Lake Louise Consensus Definition for the Diagnosis of Acute Mountain Sickness

Altitude ≥ 2500 m above sea level
Headache present
Any one of the following:

- Gastrointestinal symptoms (nausea, vomiting, anorexia)
- Sleep symptoms (insomnia, disturbed sleeping)
- Fatigue or weakness
- Dizziness or light-headedness

Source: Hackett, P. H. and Oelz, O. 1992. The Lake Louise consensus on the definition and quantification of altitude illness. In J. R. Sutton, G. Coates and C. S. Houston (eds), *Advances in the Biosciences Vol. 84: Hypoxia and Mountain Medicine: Proceedings of the 7th International Hypoxia Symposium Held at Lake Louise, Canada, February 1991*, Oxford: Pergamon Press, 327–30.

Note: All three features are required; the severity can be further graded by scoring the degree of symptoms in each domain.

Typically, symptoms are first noticed 6 or more hours after arrival at altitude, and are particularly troublesome during the first night, although they may develop as early as 1 hour after ascent. Sleep disturbance is also prominent and is multifactorial, with apnoeas, headache and dyspnoea all contributing. The incidence of AMS increases with elevation and rate of ascent. With rapid ascent by air, as many as 40% of individuals might experience symptoms at 3000 m, with that figure doubled at 3750 m; however, the incidence varies very widely between studies (Figure 35.5).

AMS may evolve to the much rarer entity of high-altitude cerebral oedema (HACE), with the development of clinical signs including altered consciousness and ataxia. Thus, whereas AMS is a subjective syndrome, HACE is a clinical diagnosis (Hackett and Roach, 2001). The condition can progress rapidly, with unconsciousness supervening within 24 hours of the first appearance of clinical signs. It is important to exclude other causes, such as hypothermia, which can similarly cause confusion and ataxia at altitude, as well as alcohol or drug intoxication. However, it is essential that these features are considered indicative of possible HACE and not misattributed, since HACE is generally fatal if appropriate therapy is not instituted quickly. Fortunately, HACE is much rarer than AMS. The incidence has been reported at approximately 1% of trekkers at very high altitude, although considerably more may be affected at extreme altitude and with rapid ascent (Hackett and Roach, 2004). Many deaths in mountaineers are likely to reflect continued ascent in the face of symptoms that are indicative of HACE.

The fundamental mechanisms underlying AMS and HACE are not well understood. Experimental models using normobaric hypoxia seem to differ slightly from those using hypobaric hypoxia (Millet et al., 2012). Further discussion of this point, which is the subject of much debate, is beyond the scope of this text, but is mentioned in order to highlight the difficulties encountered when investigating the pathophysiology of altitude illnesses in general. The pathogenesis of AMS almost certainly involves hypoxia-driven vasodilatation of cerebral vessels with a degree of mild cerebral oedema. Individual anatomical variation may therefore underlie the apparently random nature of AMS, with the capacity for the cranial vault to accommodate mild cerebral swelling determining the presence or absence of symptoms. Cross-sectional imaging of the brain in those with more severe AMS and that which progresses to frank HACE demonstrates vasogenic oedema, likely due to a combination of increased hydrostatic pressure and altered vascular permeability (Hackett et al., 1998). Sometimes, these features

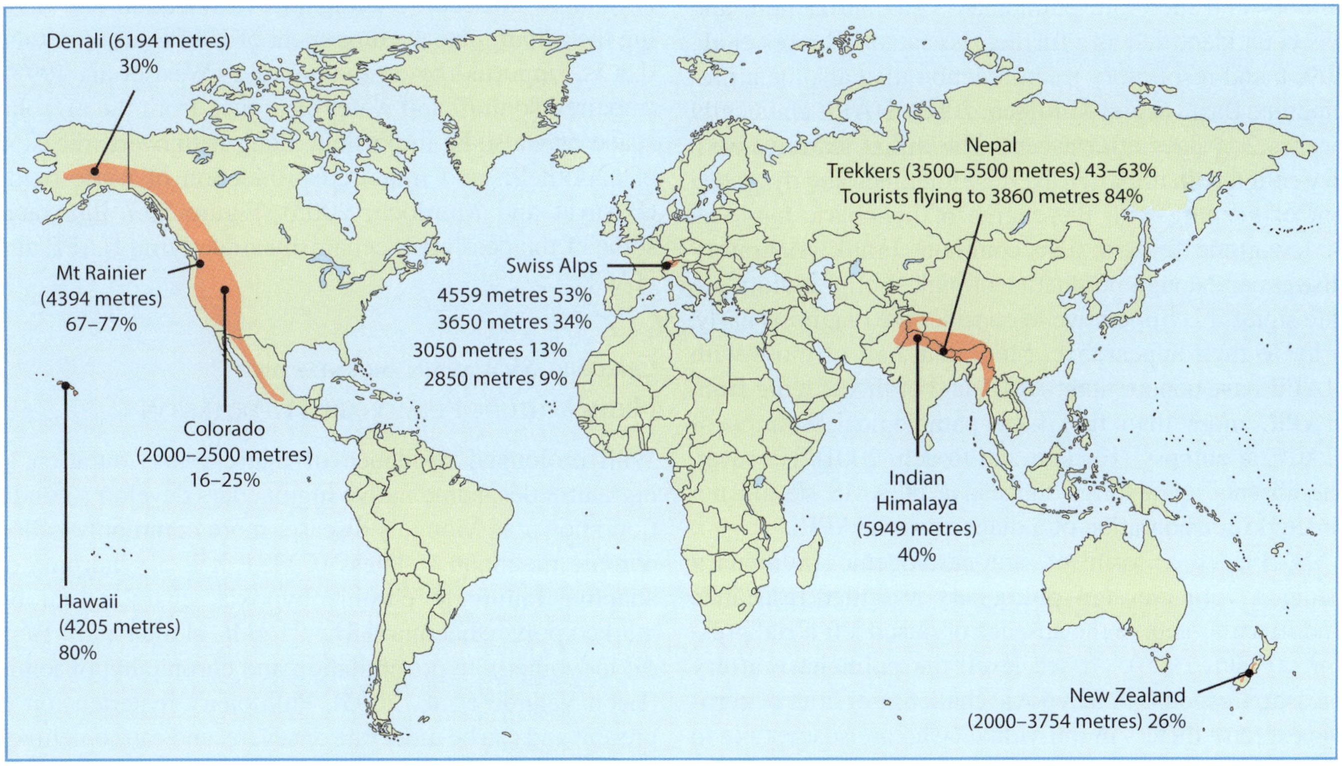

FIGURE 35.5 Reported incidence rates of acute mountain sickness at various high-altitude locations. (Reproduced from Barry, P. W. and Pollard, A. J. 2003. *BMJ* 326(7395),915–9. With permission.)

manifest as retinal haemorrhages on fundoscopy, with or without papilledema as a result of raised intracranial pressure. There may be associated cranial nerve palsies, but seizures are rare. HACE should be viewed as a generalised encephalopathy that, without treatment, leads to coning and death.

Given that hypoxia drives the processes leading to AMS and HACE, it might be anticipated that variation between individuals in the ventilatory response to hypoxia may in part explain an individual's predisposition to developing these conditions. Whilst this appears to be true at the extremes, which is to say that those with a very low ventilatory response to hypoxia are at increased risk of AMS and that those with a vigorous response are to an extent protected, the ventilatory response to hypoxia at sea level is not in isolation a useful predictor of an individual's AMS risk. Similarly, whilst fluid retention may play a role in AMS and diuresis seems to be protective, there is very considerable interindividual variation.

High-Altitude Pulmonary Oedema

HAPE is the HAI accounting for most fatalities. As with AMS and HACE, rate of ascent and final altitude influence the likelihood of its occurrence. A low ambient temperature may increase sympathetic nervous system activity and therefore pulmonary vasoconstriction, and has been identified as a further risk factor (Reeves et al., 1993), and respiratory tract infection may also be a precipitant (Basnyat and Murdoch, 2003). HAPE classically occurs 2–4 days after ascent. The initial features are a dry cough with impaired exercise tolerance and dyspnoea out of keeping with the degree of hypobaric hypoxia. A low-grade fever is also common. Frank respiratory distress and cough productive of pink, frothy sputum are late signs; it is imperative to consider the diagnosis early, prior to their appearance. More than half of those with HAPE have concomitant AMS, and of those dying from HAPE, more than half have pathological features of HACE at autopsy (Hackett and Roach, 2001). However, the absence of features suggestive of AMS should not preclude consideration of a diagnosis of HAPE.

HAPE is a form of non-cardiogenic pulmonary oedema with elevated pulmonary vascular resistance and vascular leak in the absence of raised left atrial pressure (Figure 35.6). At sea level, the pulmonary artery pressure response to a hypoxic challenge or bout of aerobic exercise differs in individuals who are susceptible to HAPE as a group (Grünig et al., 2000), suggesting interindividual variation in the potency of HPV as a factor. Heterogeneity in HPV may also be important, supported by observations that those with an anomalous pulmonary circulation are at higher risk (Hackett et al., 1980). Ultimately, stress failure of the pulmonary capillaries is thought to occur, leading to extravasation and driving the inflammatory component of HAPE, a suggestion that is supported by animal studies (West et al., 1995). Impaired sodium and water clearance from the alveolar space may also be important, along with overexpression of endothelin and impaired production of nitric oxide (Basnyat and Murdoch, 2003). Figure 35.7 illustrates some of the possible mechanisms underlying HAPE and HACE.

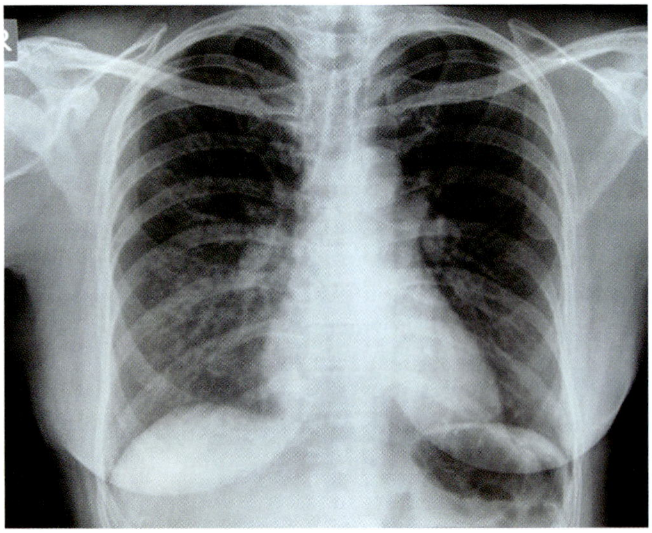

FIGURE 35.6 Chest radiograph showing high-altitude pulmonary oedema in a 55 year old female evacuated by air from an altitude of 4410 m in the Nepalese Himalayas. (Reproduced from Shrestha, P., Pun, M. and Basnyat, B. 2014. *Extrem Physiol Med* 3(1):6. Reproduced under Creative Commons 2.0 Attribution License.)

Chronic Mountain Sickness and High-Altitude Pulmonary Hypertension

With prolonged residence of many years' duration at high altitudes, some native highlanders develop a condition known as Monge's disease, more commonly called chronic mountain sickness (CMS). It is a syndrome of adaptive failure to chronic hypoxia, characterised by marked polycythaemia (Hb > 21 g/dL in men and >19 g/dL in women), hypoventilation and chronic hypoxaemia (Leon-Velarde et al., 2005). Pulmonary hypertension is present and can be moderate or severe, and can sometimes lead to right ventricular failure. The symptoms of CMS include headache, dizziness, breathlessness, palpitations, sleep disturbance, progressive fatigue and impairment of

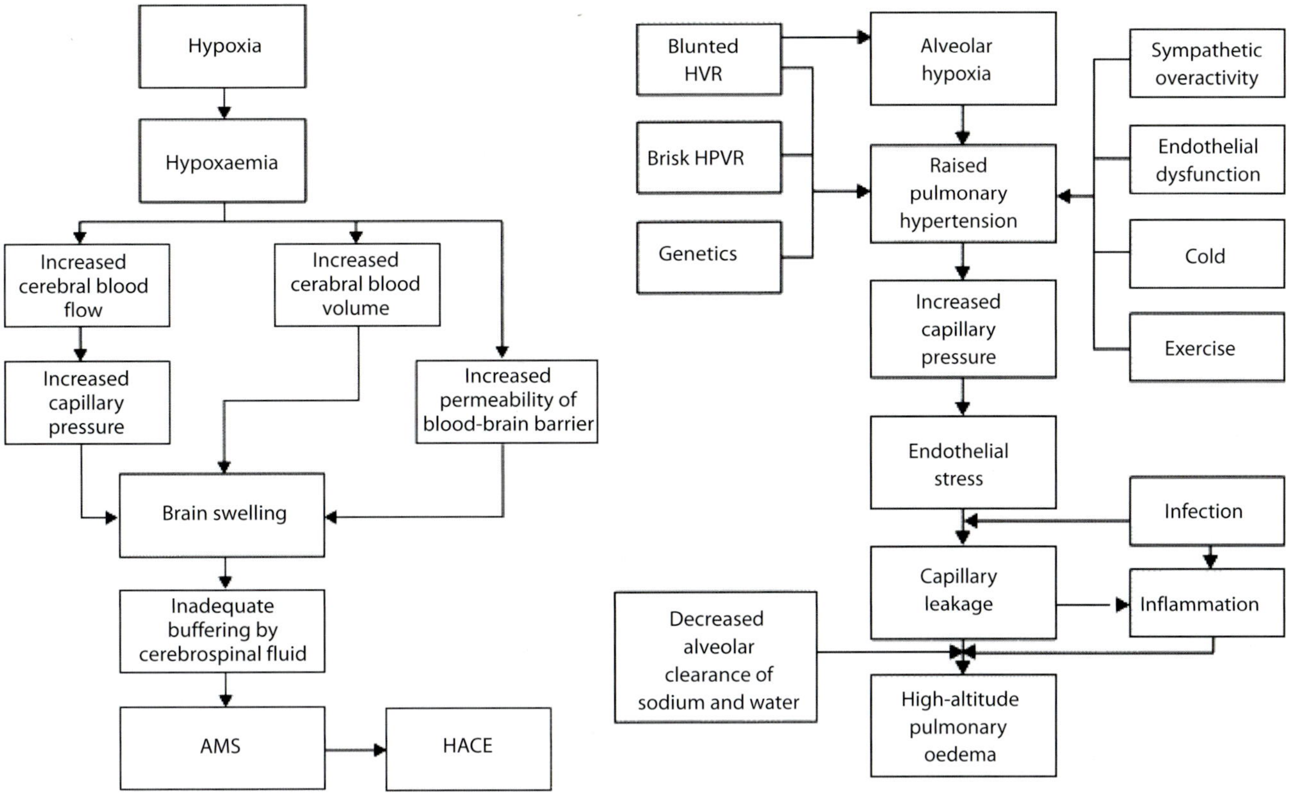

FIGURE 35.7 Schematic representation of the putative mechanisms underlying high-altitude cerebral oedema and high-altitude pulmonary oedema. (Reproduced from Basnyat, B. and Murdoch, D. R. 2003. *Lancet* 361(9373):1967–74. With permission.)

performance. Moreover, CMS patients have an elevated risk of stroke and myocardial infarction, likely related to increased blood viscosity and tissue hypoxia.

The prevalence of CMS varies according to race and region. As many as 15% of Andeans above 3200 m are afflicted (Monge et al., 1992). In contrast, Tibetan highlanders are relatively protected from CMS; the overall prevalence of CMS in Tibetans living on the Qinghai–Tibetan plateau was 1.2% compared with 5.6% in Han Chinese living at the same plateau (Wu et al., 1998). Figure 35.8 shows the prevalence of CMS in various different groups over a range of altitudes. Acclimatised lowlanders are similarly at risk of pulmonary hypertension with continued residence at high altitude, although there are clearly pathophysiological differences between classical CMS and the decompensated right heart failure that has been described with residence of a few months at very high and extreme altitudes, notably in Indian soldiers (Anand et al., 1990).

Genetic differences have been implicated in the different patterns of adaptation seen from one high-altitude population to another, which may also account for differences in the prevalence of CMS. Tibetan highlanders

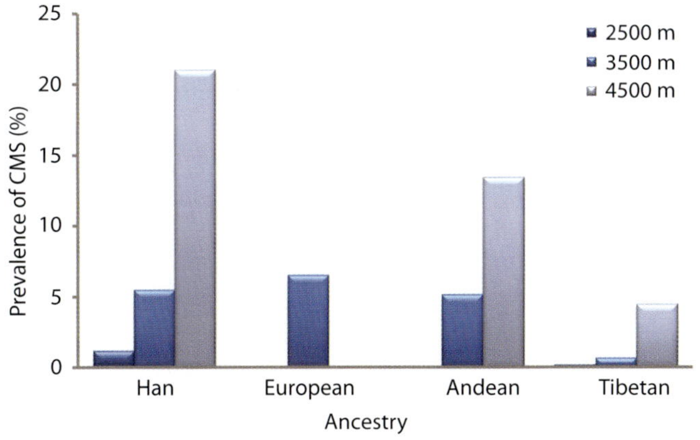

FIGURE 35.8 Differing prevalence of chronic mountain sickness (CMS) in Han Chinese, individuals of European extraction living in Colorado, Andeans and Han Tibetans over a range of altitudes. Europeans at 2500 m and 4500 m and Andeans at 2500 m have no consistent data available, whilst the prevalence of CMS in Tibetans at 2500 m is effectively zero. (Drawn using data taken from Moore, L. G. 2001. *High Alt Med Biol* 2(2):257–79.)

have lower haemoglobin levels and are resistant to the development of pulmonary hypertension compared to their Andean counterparts. Genome-wide analyses in Tibetans have identified positive selection on genes that belong to the HIF pathway, namely *EPAS1* (Figure 35.9) and *EGLN1*, thus providing evidence of genetic adaptation in Tibetans to the hypoxia of high altitude (Beall et al., 2010; Simonson et al., 2010; Yi et al., 2010). A laboratory study of Tibetan individuals who were resident at sea level (Petousi et al., 2014) has confirmed that they exhibit attenuated HPV compared to Han Chinese individuals (Figure 35.10). This difference in behaviour, which is likely related to genetic differences, no doubt contributes to the lower prevalence of conditions such as CMS in this ethnic group. These genes appear to play less of a role in the high-altitude adaptation of Andeans. A whole-genome study of Andean highlanders investigating the genetic basis of CMS reported two genes—*SENP1* (an erythropoiesis regulator) and *ANP32D* (an oncogene)—as showing significant genetic differences between the CMS and non-CMS individuals, consistent with natural selection (Zhou et al., 2013).

Intermittent Exposure to Hypoxia

There is a great deal of interest in the ways in which the pathophysiological consequences of repeated short hypoxic exposures, usually termed chronic intermittent hypoxia, differ from those of a sustained hypoxic exposure. From an occupational perspective, the consequences of prolonged work at altitude might differ between workers who are intermittently exposed (commuters) and those who reside at altitude for long periods of time. Hypoxic exposures may last 8–12 hours' duration for the daily commuter, such as a telescope operator, or 1–2 weeks for a miner, depending on shift pattern. One clear implication is for acclimatisation, since it does not appear that these workers ever fully acclimatise in the same way that they would with chronic residence at high altitude (West, 2012). Unfortunately, the risk of acute HAI appears to persist at the beginning of each block of work following ascent (Richalet et al., 2002). Interestingly, high rates of obesity, systemic hypertension, dyslipidaemia and impaired glucose tolerance have been reported in mining industry workers exposed to intermittent high-altitude hypoxia (Esenamanova et al., 2014), although the extent to which this association is causal is unclear.

Sleep Disturbance

Impaired sleep is frequently reported by visitors to high altitude (Windsor and Rodway, 2012). Periodic breathing is common, following an oscillating pattern with central hypopnoeas or apnoeas followed by arousals and hyperventilation. The prevalence of sleep-disordered breathing increases with the degree of elevation, but considerable differences in magnitude and time course are reported in different studies. While sleep quality appears to improve

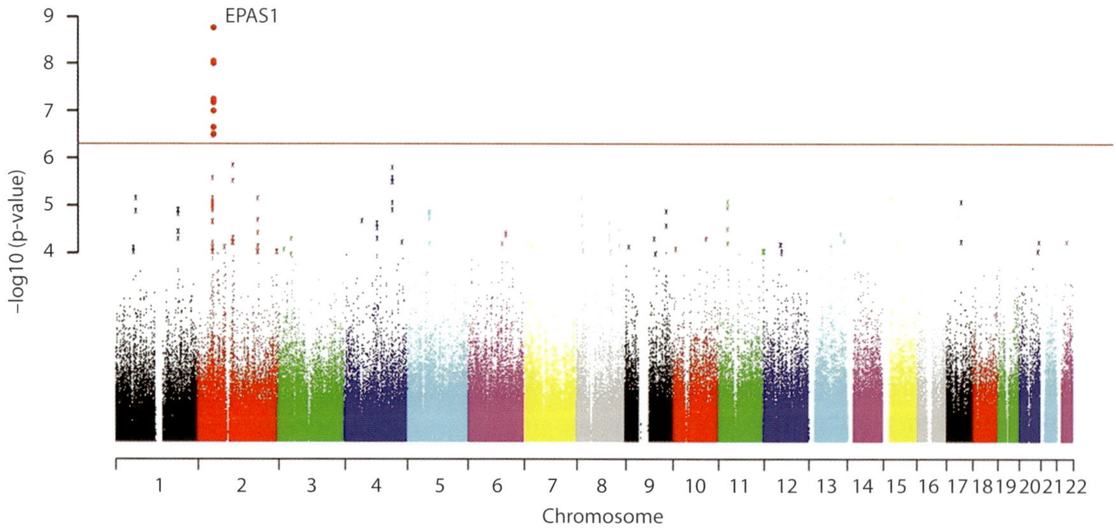

FIGURE 35.9 Genome-wide allelic differentiation scan comparing Tibetans with Han Chinese. Genomic position is shown on the horizontal axis; individual chromosomes are represented by different colours. The vertical axis indicates the negative logarithm of single-nucleotide polymorphism (SNP)-by-SNP p-values generated from a Tibetan versus HapMap Han Chinese comparison. Eight SNPs that are near one another and *EPAS1* have genome-wide significance (below threshold of $p = 5 \times 10^{-7}$, illustrated by the red line). (Reproduced from Beall, C. M. et al. 2010. *Proc Natl Acad Sci U S A* 107(25):11459–64. With permission. Copyright 2007 National Academy of Sciences, USA)

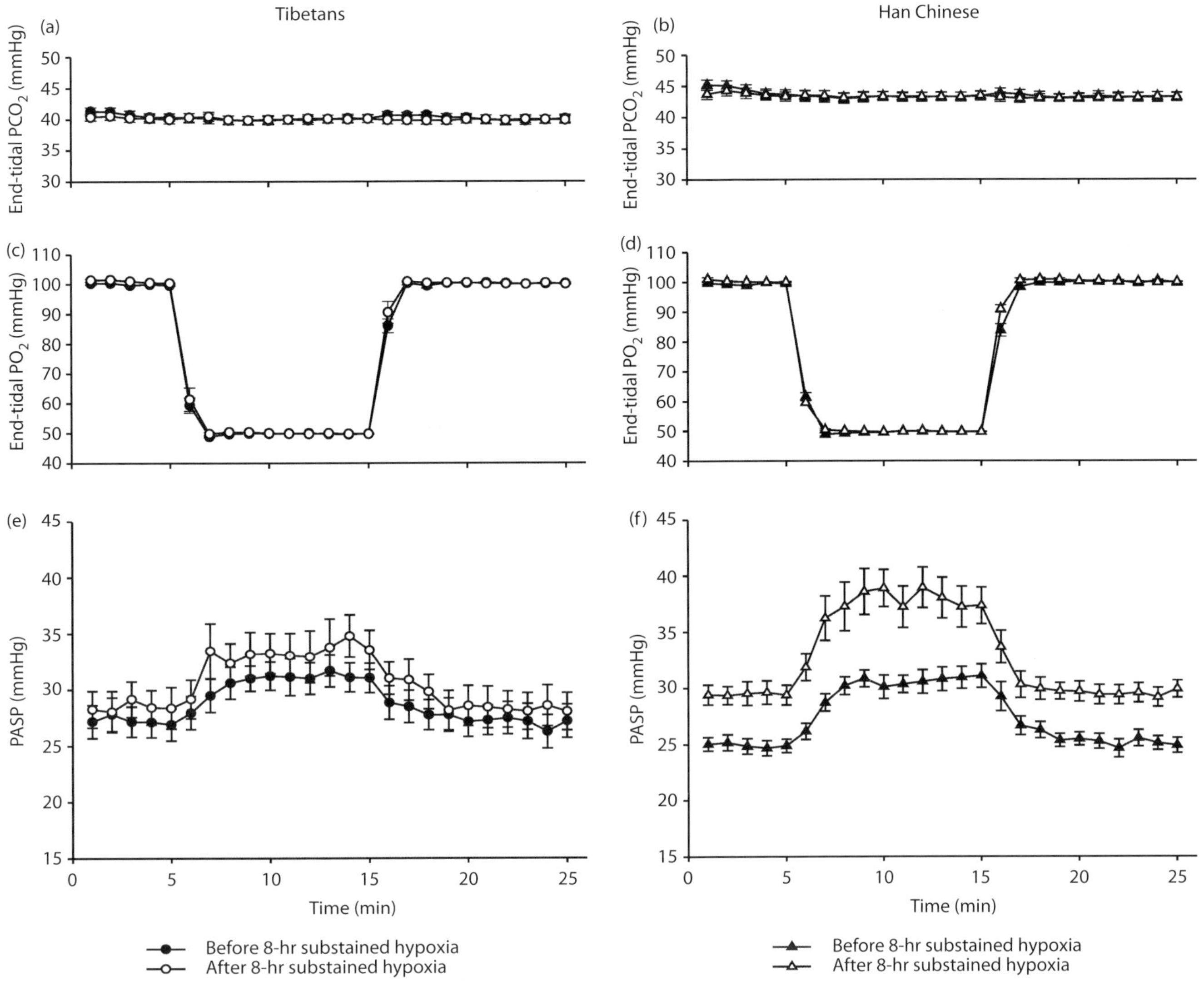

FIGURE 35.10 Pulmonary arterial systolic pressure (PASP) elevation during acute isocapnic hypoxia before and after an 8-hour exposure to sustained isocapnic hypoxia. The rise in PASP is an index of the potency of hypoxic pulmonary vasoconstriction. (a and b) End-tidal partial pressures of carbon dioxide over time. (c and d) End-tidal partial pressures of oxygen over time. (e and f) PASP values over time. All data are for ten Tibetan and ten Han Chinese volunteers, respectively. Values are means; error bars represent standard error of the mean. (Reproduced from Petousi, N. et al. 2014. *J Appl Physiol (1985)* 116(7):893–904. With permission.)

over days (Nussbaumer-Ochsner et al., 2012), periodic breathing itself persists despite prolonged exposure to hypobaric hypoxia (Tellez et al., 2014). From an occupational perspective, poor sleep quality at high altitude may lead to daytime somnolence, compromising productivity and perhaps even safety in certain professions, such as those requiring the operation of heavy machinery.

Pre-Existing Medical Conditions

Many passengers on commercial aircraft and those enjoying recreational activities in mountainous regions have existing medical conditions that may be exacerbated by hypobaric hypoxia, and so too may those whose occupations take them to high altitude. For those wishing to fly with existing medical conditions, strict guidance exists (Seccombe and Peters, 2014), because of the difficulty in managing medical emergencies in the air and the cost of diverting an aircraft for what is a foreseeable problem. Whilst conditions such as hypertension, coronary disease, diabetes and chronic obstructive pulmonary disease do not, perhaps surprisingly, appear manifestly to increase the risk of HAI (Hackett and Roach, 2001; Barry and Pollard, 2003), these conditions may deteriorate at altitude; Table 35.3 gives a summary. Data on the manner in which drug metabolism is affected at altitude are very

TABLE 35.3
Considerations for Work at High Altitude in Those with Existing Medical Conditions

Condition	Considerations
Ischaemic heart disease	• Risk of coronary events not apparently increased in previously well individuals • Sympathetically mediated increases in circulatory demand mean exertional angina is likely to worsen and may be precipitated in patients with previously stable coronary disease
Cardiac failure and valvular heart disease	• Potential inability adequately to increase cardiac output • Increased work of breathing
Hypertension	• Well-controlled hypertension is not a contraindication
Asthma	• Generally unaffected by altitude • Very high levels of ozone may increase risk of exacerbation • Peak flow meters may be inaccurate at altitude
Chronic obstructive pulmonary disease	• Inability adequately to increase alveolar ventilation and increased work of breathing mean symptoms and performance deteriorate • Infectious exacerbations are a greater risk • Risk of barotrauma and pneumothorax with rapid ascent • Chronic obstructive pulmonary disease mortality increased with increasing altitude of residence
Pulmonary hypertension	• Increased demand on right ventricle due to further elevated pulmonary vascular resistance may lead to decompensation
Diabetes mellitus	• Exposure to altitude in itself probably does not worsen diabetes; changes in diet and activity may contribute to deteriorating control • Symptoms of hypoglycaemia may be confused with high-altitude cerebral oedema • Blood glucose monitors may be inaccurate at altitude • Extremes of temperature may shorten storage life of insulin
Epilepsy	• No clear increased risk of seizures in patients with well-controlled epilepsy • Consequences of a seizure may be more severe in remote areas

Source: Cote, T. R. et al. 1993. *Chest* 103(4):1194–7; Barry, P. W. and Pollard, A. J. 2003. *BMJ* 326(7395):915–9; Richards, P. and Hillebrandt, D. 2013. *High Alt Med Biol* 14(3):197–204; Seccombe, L. M. and Peters, M. J. 2014. *J Appl Physiol (1985)* 116(5):478–85.

limited; a reduction in the rate of clearance of certain metabolites by cytochrome P450 (Jurgens et al., 2002; Fradette et al., 2007), for example, has not been demonstrated to translate into a clinically meaningful effect.

Pulmonary Complications of Particular High-Altitude Occupations

The occupation that takes an individual to altitude may have implications for respiratory health in its own right, and these are addressed comprehensively elsewhere in this text. Industrial lung disease related to dust exposure in miners is a particular consideration. The question arises as to whether involvement in such occupations carries a risk that is in any way different to that at sea level: does hypobaric hypoxia modify the exposure–risk profile in any way? There is no good evidence in this area; it has been suggested that mining at altitude might accelerate the development of silicosis (Voznesenskii, 1996). Altitude has consequences for the efficiency of the internal combustion engine (Vearrier and Greenberg, 2011), but it is unknown whether as a result exhaust emissions cause more harm to respiratory health at high altitude than at sea level.

STRATEGIES FOR PREDICTING, PREVENTING AND TREATING HIGH-ALTITUDE ILLNESS (HAI)

The Strongest Risk Factor for Future HAI is a History of the Condition during Previous Exposure

Not unexpectedly, individuals who have encountered difficulties during previous sojourns at altitude are at the highest risk of HAI. For example, the risk of recurrent HAPE may be as high as 60% (Bartsch et al., 1991). However, this is clearly not a particularly useful observation for those needing to work for the first time at altitude, who would wish to avoid the development of

HAI altogether. The ability to predict risk would inform decisions regarding rate of ascent and pharmacological prophylaxis, and permit better education and planning regarding the management of HAI. It is not ideal for workers to arrive at altitude and then be incapacitated for a period of days, or worse, require evacuation.

Unfortunately, there is no simple or reliable way to identify who will develop HAI, but several approaches exist that can give an indication of the likelihood of problems. At sea level, various stressors can be applied in order to elicit a physiological response that is similar to that which is brought about at altitude. In the case of measuring an individual's hypoxic ventilatory drive, the unfortunate lack of predictive value for AMS has already been discussed. Echocardiography can be performed during exercise or hypoxic gas inhalation in order to give a measure of the potency of HPV, and therefore the risk of HAPE. Again, whilst, as already discussed, those with previous episodes of HAPE show, as a group, exaggerated HPV (Figure 35.11), the test is not useful for prospectively identifying healthy individuals who will encounter significant difficulty on ascent. Of course, it is possible to expose those who are planning to work at altitude to either normobaric or hypobaric hypoxia in a chamber at sea level, but this approach simply induces HAI, so cannot really be considered any more 'predictive' than a previous ascent that ended in difficulty, although it does permit relatively rapid termination of the exposure. More recently, attempts have been made to develop assessment systems incorporating a number of variables including physiological responses to hypoxia (Canoui-Poitrine et al., 2014). These show promise, but require further validation before they can be recommended as part of occupational health pre-deployment assessment. At present, the best strategy remains to estimate an individual worker's risk based on the planned rate of ascent and history (Table 35.4). This allows modification of the initial journey to altitude and appropriate pharmacological prophylaxis to be offered.

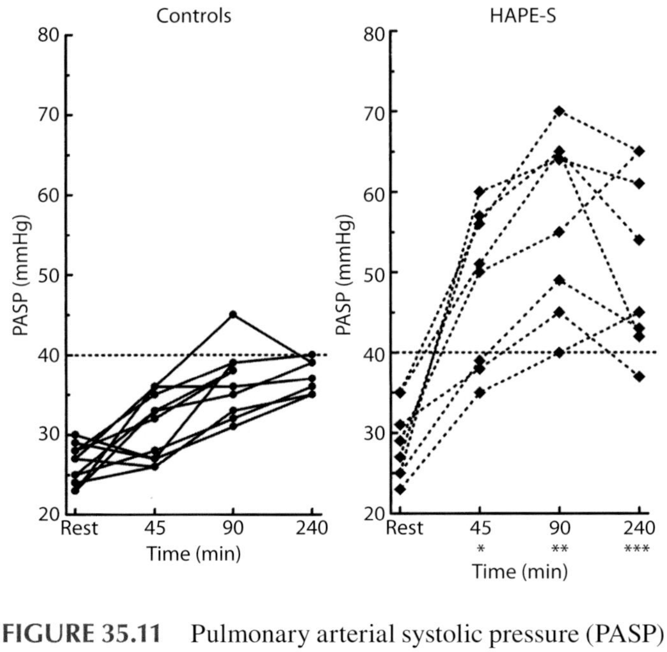

FIGURE 35.11 Pulmonary arterial systolic pressure (PASP) response to sustained hypoxia (fraction of inspired oxygen: 12%) measured using Doppler echocardiography. Note the differences between controls and subjects who are susceptible to high-altitude pulmonary oedema (HAPE-S). Despite no significant difference at rest between groups, PASP in HAPE-S subjects was higher at all subsequent time points. (Reproduced from Grünig, E. et al. 2000. *J Am Coll Cardiol* 35(4):980–7. With permission.)

TABLE 35.4
Estimating Risk of High-Altitude Illness Based on Ascent Profile and Personal History

Risk Level	Characteristics of Individual and Ascent
Low	Ascending to ≤2800 m; no history of HAI
	Ascending to 2500–3000 m over ≥2 days; subsequent increases in sleeping elevation <500 m/day
Moderate	Ascending to 2500–2800 m in 1 day; history of AMS
	Ascending to >2800 m in 1 day; no history of AMS
	Increase in sleeping elevation >500 m/day at altitudes above 3000 m
High	Ascending to >2800 m in 1 day; history of AMS
	History of HAPE or HACE
	Ascending to >3500 m in 1 day
	Increase in sleeping elevation >500 m/day at altitudes above 3500 m
	Very rapid ascents, such as at Mount Kilimanjaro

Source: Modified from Luks, A. M. et al. 2010. *Wilderness Environ Med* 21(2):146–55.
Abbreviations: HAI: high-altitude illness; AMS: acute mountain sickness; HAPE: high-altitude pulmonary oedema; HACE: high-altitude cerebral oedema.

Gradual Ascent Reduces the Likelihood of Altitude-Related Illness

It is perhaps surprising that athletic fitness at sea level does not confer protection against altitude illness. Even more disappointingly for the very physically fit, the converse may be true, although it is unclear if this simply reflects a tendency for the very fit to be more active despite high altitude, thus exacerbating symptoms, or a direct physical effect, perhaps mediated by greater pulmonary vascular reactivity. On the other hand, gradual ascent, which allows time for successful acclimatisation, works exceptionally well—it is the most effective prophylactic measure against HAI. Compared to an ascent to high altitude over 1 hour, this strategy can reduce the incidence of AMS by over 40% (Purkayastha et al., 1995). Various recommendations exist, such as that once above 2500 m, sleeping altitude should increase by no more than 600 m per day and a rest day should be introduced for every increase of 600–1200 m above this. Some individuals may find that they are able to tolerate much less than this—only 100–200 m per day—if they are to remain symptom free. Avoiding strenuous exercise in the initial days at altitude is also protective. Another approach that may prove helpful is pre-exposure, whereby short trips to or one stint of several days at a site above 1500 m for some weeks prior to a spell at higher elevation offers a pre-acclimatisation effect that may subsequently allow for more rapid ascent to the desired altitude. Strategies for the initial journey to high altitude, which may reduce the chance of HAI on or shortly after arrival, may or may not be feasible depending on the nature of work. They may not be appropriate for those only making a brief trip, nor feasible for those who commute to altitude by road for shift work.

Periods at a Lower Altitude with Supplemental Oxygen or at Higher Barometric Pressure Can Facilitate Work at High Altitude

Populations living at high altitudes recognise that there are some activities that are so demanding as to make a spell at lower altitude, and thus higher partial pressure of oxygen, desirable. The best example of this is perhaps pregnancy. For lowlanders needing to work at altitude for a prolonged period, the option of spending the night, and perhaps some of the working day, breathing a higher partial pressure of oxygen is one that can prove very helpful. There are several ways in which this can be achieved. The simplest is for workers to sleep at a lower altitude than that at which they work. This option is not associated with any great expense other than the travel to and from accommodation, usually by road. In very remote, mountainous areas, this may not be practical. The next option is to increase artificially the oxygen content of ambient air, be it by enriching the atmosphere with oxygen from a concentrator, increasing atmospheric pressure or a combination of both approaches. Increasing atmospheric pressure is of course the strategy that is employed in order to make commercial air travel possible. Oxygen enrichment of room air is a very powerful approach for lowering the effective altitude and does not depend on having a gas-tight enclosure, unlike air travel. Very approximately, each absolute increase of 1% in the ambient oxygen concentration lowers the effective altitude by about 300 m (West, 2002a). Thus, it is possible for Chilean radio-telescope operators at a true altitude of over 5000 m to live effectively at 3200 m simply with an increase in oxygen concentration from 21% to 27%. This approach is also taken on the Chinese train to Lhasa, Tibet, which has oxygen concentrators in each passenger car delivering a fraction of inspired oxygen (F_IO_2) of up to 25% in order to mitigate the effects of a railway at altitudes in excess of 4000 m for most of the route. It would also in theory be possible to combine an increase in barometric pressure with oxygen enrichment (West, 2012). The use of oxygen enrichment solely during sleep has been shown to be useful for improving sleep quality and reducing periodic breathing in miners who have already been at altitude for several years (Moraga et al., 2014).

There are now some occupations that involve exposure to normobaric hypoxia by virtue of deliberate nitrogen enrichment of the ambient air as an anti-fire strategy (Angerer and Nowak, 2003). Here, the F_IO_2 levels involved are approximately 13%–15%. This is precisely the opposite effect to that which is achieved at altitude by use of an oxygen concentrator; there would be expected to be similar pulmonary implications for workers being intermittently exposed to this normobaric hypoxia as daily commuters to high altitude.

The Cornerstone of Therapy for HAI is Descent with Supplemental Oxygen if Available

Since hypoxia is central to the pathobiology of this group of conditions, correction of a low oxygen tension is foremost in their treatment. The simplest manner in which alveolar oxygen tension can be increased is descent. If symptoms are recognised early and treated with appropriate seriousness, descent, or in some cases simply arresting ascent temporarily, may be enough to lead to their resolution. If there is any doubt, it is safest simply to descend. Difficulty arises when the geographical location is such that it is not possible to descend quickly, or an individual has become incapacitated by their illness to the point of becoming wholly dependent on others. If supplemental oxygen is available, this can be given. Pressure bags can be used to surround the casualty and increase the effective atmospheric pressure, increasing the partial pressure of oxygen without a need for a concentrated supply of the gas.

Pharmacological Strategies Exist for the Prophylaxis and Treatment of HAI

Proven Therapies

Table 35.5 provides an overview of agents that are effective in the prevention and treatment of HAI. The

TABLE 35.5
Recommended Pharmacological Therapies for the Prevention and Treatment of High-Altitude Illness

Agent	Prophylaxis	Treatment
Acetazolamide	AMS, HACE: 125 mg 12-hourly	AMS, HACE: 250 mg 12-hourly CMS: 250 mg daily
Dexamethasone	AMS, HACE: 4 mg 12-hourly or 2 mg 6-hourly	AMS: 4 mg 6-hourly HACE: 8 mg immediately then 4 mg 6-hourly (can be given IM or IV)
Nifedipine	HAPE: 30 mg 12-hourly or 20 mg 8-hourly (slow-release preparation)	HAPE: 30 mg 12-hourly or 20 mg 8-hourly (slow-release preparation)
Sildenafil	HAPE: 50 mg 8-hourly	Not studied

Source: Modified from Luks, A. M. et al. 2010. *Wilderness Environ Med* 21(2):146–55.
Abbreviations: AMS: acute mountain sickness; HACE: high-altitude cerebral oedema; CMS: chronic mountain sickness; IM: intramuscularly; IV: intravenously; HAPE: high-altitude pulmonary oedema.

carbonic anhydrase inhibitor acetazolamide is effective at reducing the incidence of AMS and HACE (Imray et al., 2010), and is a useful therapy for CMS (Richalet et al., 2008). Its efficacy is traditionally attributed to the generation of a mild metabolic acidosis that counteracts the braking effect of hypocapnia on alveolar ventilation. As already noted however (see ‘Cardiopulmonary Responses to Hypobaric Hypoxia are Time Dependent and Vary Between Individuals’ section), the view that compensation for the respiratory alkalosis occurring with acute altitude exposure is important for early ventilatory acclimatisation is not supported by contemporary physiological studies (Robbins, 2007). Acetazolamide may instead have direct effects on the pulmonary vasculature (Shimoda et al., 2007). Whatever its mechanism of action, if acetazolamide is used for treatment of HACE, this should not be as a monotherapy, but instead in conjunction with dexamethasone.

Dexamethasone is effective in preventing and treating AMS and HACE, but is not useful in HAPE. Dexamethasone may reduce hypoxia-driven increases in vascular permeability; additionally, it appears to enhance VAH (Liu et al., 2013). The calcium channel blocker nifedipine reduces pulmonary vasoconstriction and is advocated in the prophylaxis and treatment of HAPE (Oelz et al., 1989; Bartsch et al., 1991), but the evidence is conflicting (Deshwal et al., 2012). It has not been shown to be useful for AMS or HACE. Phosphodiesterase inhibitors may be effective at reducing the incidence of HAPE (Maggiorini et al., 2006), but evidence to guide their use in the treatment of established HAPE is awaited. Non-steroidal anti-inflammatory drugs are useful for the prevention (aspirin) and treatment (ibuprofen) of HAH; anti-emetics may be used for the gastrointestinal symptoms of AMS.

Uncertainties

Intravenous iron, which may act to down-regulate the HIF system, is being explored as a therapy for preventing and treating HAI. It reduces HPV in those who are already at altitude (Smith et al., 2009) and may reduce the severity of AMS (Talbot et al., 2011). It is not known if iron deficiency predisposes an individual to HAI (Frise and Robbins, 2015), although it is interesting that iron depletion induced by venesection as a treatment for CMS worsens pulmonary hypertension in that setting (Smith et al., 2009). Diuretics are not helpful in HAPE and may be harmful. The evidence for *Ginkgo biloba* in AMS prophylaxis is mixed; given the undoubted efficacy of acetazolamide and the safety profile of this agent, it is preferred.

REFERENCES

Ainslie, P. N. and Reilly, T. 2003. Physiology of accidental hypothermia in the mountains: A forgotten story. *Br J Sports Med* 37(6):548–50.

Aldenderfer, M. 2011. Peopling the Tibetan plateau: Insights from archaeology. *High Alt Med Biol* 12(2):141–7.

Anand, I. S., Malhotra, R. M., Chandrashekhar, Y., Bali, H. K., Chauhan, S. S., Jindal, S. K., Bhandari, R. K. et al. 1990. Adult subacute mountain sickness—A syndrome of congestive heart failure in man at very high altitude. *Lancet* 335(8689):561–5.

Angerer, P. and Nowak, D. 2003. Working in permanent hypoxia for fire protection—Impact on health. *Int Arch Occup Environ Health* 76(2):87–102.

Auerbach, P. S. E. 2012. *Wilderness Medicine*, sixth edition. Philadelphia, PA: Elsevier.

Barry, P. W. and Pollard, A. J. 2003. Altitude illness. *BMJ* 326(7395):915–9.

Bärtsch, P., Maggiorini, M., Ritter, M., Noti, C., Vock, P. and Oelz, O. 1991. Prevention of high-altitude pulmonary edema by nifedipine. *N Engl J Med* 325(18):1284–9.

Bärtsch, P., Shaw, S., Franciolli, M., Gnadinger, M. P. and Weidmann, P. 1988. Atrial natriuretic peptide in acute mountain sickness. *J Appl Physiol (1985)* 65(5):1929–37.

Basnyat, B. and Murdoch, D. R. 2003. High-altitude illness. *Lancet* 361(9373):1967–74.

Beall, C. M. 2007. Two routes to functional adaptation: Tibetan and Andean high-altitude natives. *Proc Natl Acad Sci U S A* 104(Suppl. 1):8655–60.

Beall, C. M., Cavalleri, G. L., Deng, L., Elston, R. C., Gao, Y., Knight, J., Li, C. et al. 2010. Natural selection on *EPAS1 (HIF2alpha)* associated with low hemoglobin concentration in Tibetan highlanders. *Proc Natl Acad Sci U S A* 107(25):11459–64.

Berger, A. J., Mitchell, R. A. and Severinghaus, J. W. 1977. Regulation of respiration. *N Engl J Med* 297(4): 194–201.

Bert, P. 1878. *La Pression Barometrique*. English translation (1943) by M. A. Hitchcock and F. A. Hitchcock. Columbus, OH: College Book Co.

Bodhaine, B. A., Dutton, E. G., Hofmann, D. J., McKenzie, R. L. and Johnston, P. V. 1997. UV measurements at Mauna Loa: July 1995 to July 1996. *J Geophys Res* 102(D15):19265–73.

Canoui-Poitrine, F., Veerabudun, K., Larmignat, P., Letournel, M., Bastuji-Garin, S. and Richalet, J. P. 2014. Risk prediction score for severe high altitude illness: A cohort study. *PLoS One* 9(7):e100642.

Cordero, R. R., Seckmeyer, G., Damiani, A., Riechelmann, S., Rayas, J., Labbe, F. and Laroze, D. 2014. The world's highest levels of surface UV. *Photochem Photobiol Sci* 13(1):70–81.

Cote, T. R., Stroup, D. F., Dwyer, D. M., Horan, J. M. and Peterson, D. E. 1993. Chronic obstructive pulmonary disease mortality. A role for altitude. *Chest* 103(4):1194–7.

Crawford, R. D. and Severinghaus, J. W. 1978. CSF pH and ventilatory acclimatization to altitude. *J Appl Physiol Respir Environ Exerc Physiol* 45(2):275–83.

Dahlback, A., Gelsor, N., Stamnes, J. J. and Gjessing, Y. 2007. UV measurements in the 3000–5000 m altitude region in Tibet. *J Geophys Res* 112:D09308.

Deshwal, R., Iqbal, M. and Basnet, S. 2012. Nifedipine for the treatment of high altitude pulmonary edema. *Wilderness Environ Med* 23(1):7–10.

Dey, R., Van Winkle, L., Ewart, G., Balmes, J., Pinkerton, K.; and ATS Environmental Health Policy Committee. 2010. A second chance. Setting a protective ozone standard. *Am J Respir Crit Care Med* 181(4):297–9.

Dorrington, K. L., Clar, C., Young, J. D., Jonas, M., Tansley, J. G. and Robbins, P. A. 1997. Time course of the human pulmonary vascular response to 8 hours of isocapnic hypoxia. *Am J Physiol* 273(3 Pt 2):H1126–34.

Droma, Y., Hanaoka, M., Basnyat, B., Arjyal, A., Neupane, P., Pandit, A., Sharma, D. et al. 2006. Symptoms of acute mountain sickness in Sherpas exposed to extremely high altitude. *High Alt Med Biol* 7(4):312–4.

Eckardt, K. U., Boutellier, U., Kurtz, A., Schopen, M., Koller, E. A. and Bauer, C. 1989. Rate of erythropoietin formation in humans in response to acute hypobaric hypoxia. *J Appl Physiol (1985)* 66(4):1785–8.

Esenamanova, M. K., Kochkorova, F. A., Tsivinskaya, T. A., Vinnikov, D. and Aikimbaev, K. 2014. Chronic intermittent high altitude exposure, occupation, and body mass index in workers of mining industry. *High Alt Med Biol* 15(3):412–17.

Ferrus, L., Commenges, D., Gire, J. and Varene, P. 1984. Respiratory water loss as a function of ventilatory or environmental factors. *Respir Physiol* 56(1):11–20.

Fitzgerald, M. P. 1913. The changes in the breathing and the blood at various high altitudes. *Philos Trans R Soc B Biol Sci* 203(294–302):351–71.

Fradette, C., Batonga, J., Teng, S., Piquette-Miller, M. and Du Souich, P. 2007. Animal models of acute moderate hypoxia are associated with a down-regulation of CYP1A1, 1A2, 2B4, 2C5 and 2C16 and up-regulation of CYP3A6 and P-glycoprotein in liver. *Drug Metab Dispos* 35(5):765–71.

Frise, M. C. and Robbins, P. A. 2015. Iron, oxygen and the pulmonary circulation. *J Appl Physiol (1985)* 119(12):1421–31.

Groves, B. M., Reeves, J. T., Sutton, J. R., Wagner, P. D., Cymerman, A., Malconian, M. K., Rock, P. B. et al. 1987. Operation Everest II: Elevated high-altitude pulmonary resistance unresponsive to oxygen. *J Appl Physiol (1985)* 63(2):521–30.

Grünig, E., Mereles, D., Hildebrandt, W., Swenson, E. R., Kübler, W., Kuecherer, H. and Bärtsch, P. 2000. Stress Doppler echocardiography for identification of susceptibility to high altitude pulmonary edema. *J Am Coll Cardiol* 35(4):980–7.

Hackett, P. H. and Oelz, O. 1992. The Lake Louise consensus on the definition and quantification of altitude illness. In J. R. Sutton, G. Coates and C. S. Houston (eds), *Advances in the Biosciences Vol. 84: Hypoxia and Mountain Medicine: Proceedings of the 7th International Hypoxia Symposium Held at Lake Louise, Canada, February 1991*, Oxford: Pergamon Press, 327–30.

Hackett, P. H., Creagh, C. E., Grover, R. F., Honigman, B., Houston, C. S., Reeves, J. T., Sophocles, A. M. et al. 1980. High-altitude pulmonary edema in persons without the right pulmonary artery. *N Engl J Med* 302(19):1070–3.

Hackett, P. H. and Roach, R. C. 2001. High-altitude illness. *N Engl J Med* 345(2):107–14.

Hackett, P. H. and Roach, R. C. 2004. High altitude cerebral edema. *High Alt Med Biol* 5(2):136–46.

Hackett, P. H. and Roach, R. C. 2012. High-altitude medicine and physiology. In *Wilderness Medicine*, sixth edition. Philadelphia, PA: Elsevier, 2–33.

Hackett, P. H., Yarnell, P. R., Hill, R., Reynard, K., Heit, J. and McCormick, J. 1998. High-altitude cerebral edema evaluated with magnetic resonance imaging: Clinical correlation and pathophysiology. *JAMA* 280(22):1920–5.

Huey, R. B. and Eguskitza, X. 2001. Limits to human performance: Elevated risks on high mountains. *J Exp Biol* 204(Pt 18):3115–9.

Imray, C., Wright, A., Subudhi, A. and Roach, R. 2010. Acute mountain sickness: Pathophysiology, prevention, and treatment. *Prog Cardiovasc Dis* 52(6):467–84.

Jerrett, M., Burnett, R. T., Pope, C. A. 3rd, Ito, K., Thurston, G., Krewski, D., Shi, Y. et al. 2009. Long-term ozone exposure and mortality. *N Engl J Med* 360(11):1085–95.

Jurgens, G., Christensen, H. R., Brosen, K., Sonne, J., Loft, S. and Olsen, N. V. 2002. Acute hypoxia and cytochrome P450-mediated hepatic drug metabolism in humans. *Clin Pharmacol Ther* 71(4):214–20.

Leon-Velarde, F., Maggiorini, M., Reeves, J. T., Aldashev, A., Asmus, I., Bernardi, L., Ge, R. L. et al. 2005. Consensus statement on chronic and subacute high altitude diseases. *High Alt Med Biol* 6(2):147–57.

Liu, C., Croft, Q. P., Kalidhar, S., Brooks, J. T., Herigstad, M., Smith, T. G., Dorrington, K. L. et al. 2013. Dexamethasone mimics aspects of physiological acclimatization to 8 hours of hypoxia but suppresses plasma erythropoietin. *J Appl Physiol (1985)* 114(7):948–56.

Luks, A. M., McIntosh, S. E., Grissom, C. K., Auerbach, P. S., Rodway, G. W., Schoene, R. B., Zafren, K. et al.; and Wilderness Medical Society. 2010. Wilderness Medical Society consensus guidelines for the prevention and treatment of acute altitude illness. *Wilderness Environ Med* 21(2):146–55.

Maggiorini, M., Brunner-La Rocca, H. P., Peth, S., Fischler, M., Bohm, T., Bernheim, A., Kiencke, S. et al. 2006. Both tadalafil and dexamethasone may reduce the incidence of high-altitude pulmonary edema: A randomized trial. *Ann Intern Med* 145(7):497–506.

Milledge, J. S. and Cotes, P. M. 1985. Serum erythropoietin in humans at high altitude and its relation to plasma renin. *J Appl Physiol (1985)* 59(2):360–4.

Millet, G. P., Faiss, R. and Pialoux, V. 2012. Point: Hypobaric hypoxia induces different physiological responses from normobaric hypoxia. *J Appl Physiol (1985)* 112(10):1783–4.

Moehrle, M., Dennenmoser, B. and Garbe, C. 2003. Continuous long-term monitoring of UV radiation in professional mountain guides reveals extremely high exposure. *Int J Cancer* 103(6):775–8.

Monge, C. C., Arregui, A. and Leon-Velarde, F. 1992. Pathophysiology and epidemiology of chronic mountain sickness. *Int J Sports Med* 13(Suppl. 1):S79–81.

Moore, L. G. 2001. Human genetic adaptation to high altitude. *High Alt Med Biol* 2(2):257–79.

Moraga, F. A., Jimenez, D., Richalet, J. P., Vargas, M. and Osorio, J. 2014. Periodic breathing and oxygen supplementation in Chilean miners at high altitude (4200 m). *Respir Physiol Neurobiol* 203:109–15.

Nussbaumer-Ochsner, Y., Ursprung, J., Siebenmann, C., Maggiorini, M. and Bloch, K. E. 2012. Effect of short-term acclimatization to high altitude on sleep and nocturnal breathing. *Sleep* 35(3):419–23.

Oelz, O., Maggiorini, M., Ritter, M., Waber, U., Jenni, R., Vock, P. and Bärtsch, P. 1989. Nifedipine for high altitude pulmonary oedema. *Lancet* 2(8674):1241–4.

Penaloza, D. and Arias-Stella, J. 2007. The heart and pulmonary circulation at high altitudes: Healthy highlanders and chronic mountain sickness. *Circulation* 115(9):1132–46.

Petousi, N., Croft, Q. P., Cavalleri, G. L., Cheng, H. Y., Formenti, F., Ishida, K., Lunn, D. et al. 2014. Tibetans living at sea level have a hyporesponsive hypoxia-inducible factor system and blunted physiological responses to hypoxia. *J Appl Physiol (1985)* 116(7): 893–904.

Petousi, N. and Robbins, P. A. 2014. Human adaptation to the hypoxia of high altitude: The Tibetan paradigm from the pregenomic to the postgenomic era. *J Appl Physiol (1985)* 116(7):875–84.

Purkayastha, S. S., Ray, U. S., Arora, B. S., Chhabra, P. C., Thakur, L., Bandopadhyay, P. and Selvamurthy, W. 1995. Acclimatization at high altitude in gradual and acute induction. *J Appl Physiol (1985)* 79(2):487–92.

Rahn, H. and Otis, A. B. 1949. Man's respiratory response during and after acclimatization to high altitude. *Am J Physiol* 157(3):445–62.

Reeves, J. T., Wagner, J., Zafren, K., Honigman, B. and Schoene, R. B. 1993. Seasonal variation in barometric pressure and temperature in Summit County: Effect on altitude illness. In *Hypoxia and Molecular Medicine: Proceedings of the 8th International Hypoxia Symposium Held at Lake Louise, Canada.* Burlington, VT: Queen City Printers, 275–81.

Reynafarje, C., Lozano, R. and Valdivieso, J. 1959. The polycythemia of high altitudes: Iron metabolism and related aspects. *Blood* 14(4):433–55.

Richalet, J. P., Donoso, M. V., Jimenez, D., Antezana, A. M., Hudson, C., Cortes, G., Osorio, J. et al. 2002. Chilean miners commuting from sea level to 4500 m: A prospective study. *High Alt Med Biol* 3(2):159–66.

Richalet, J. P., Rivera-Ch, M., Maignan, M., Privat, C., Pham, I., Macarlupu, J. L., Petitjean, O. and Leon-Velarde, F. 2008. Acetazolamide for Monge's disease: Efficiency and tolerance of 6-month treatment. *Am J Respir Crit Care Med* 177(12):1370–6.

Richalet, J. P., Souberbielle, J. C., Antezana, A. M., Dechaux, M., Le Trong, J. L., Bienvenu, A., Daniel, F. et al. 1994. Control of erythropoiesis in humans during prolonged exposure to the altitude of 6,542 m. *Am J Physiol* 266(3 Pt 2):R756–64.

Richards, P. and Hillebrandt, D. 2013. The practical aspects of insulin at high altitude. *High Alt Med Biol* 14(3):197–204.

Robbins, P. A. 1995. Hypoxic ventilatory decline: Site of action. *J Appl Physiol (1985)* 79(2):373–4.

Robbins, P. A. 2007. Role of the peripheral chemoreflex in the early stages of ventilatory acclimatization to altitude. *Respir Physiol Neurobiol* 158(2–3):237–42.

Seccombe, L. M. and Peters, M. J. 2014. Physiology in medicine: Acute altitude exposure in patients with pulmonary and cardiovascular disease. *J Appl Physiol (1985)* 116(5):478–85.

Shimoda, L. A., Luke, T., Sylvester, J. T., Shih, H. W., Jain, A. and Swenson, E. R. 2007. Inhibition of hypoxia-induced calcium responses in pulmonary arterial smooth muscle by acetazolamide is independent of carbonic anhydrase inhibition. *Am J Physiol Lung Cell Mol Physiol* 292(4):L1002–12.

Shrestha, P., Pun, M. and Basnyat, B. 2014. High altitude pulmonary edema (HAPE) in a Himalayan trekker: A case report. *Extrem Physiol Med* 3(1):6.

Sigurdson, A. J. and Ron, E. 2004. Cosmic radiation exposure and cancer risk among flight crew. *Cancer Invest* 22(5):743–61.

Simonson, T. S., Yang, Y., Huff, C. D., Yun, H., Qin, G., Witherspoon, D. J., Bai, Z. et al. 2010. Genetic evidence for high-altitude adaptation in Tibet. *Science* 329(5987): 72–5.

Smith, C. A., Dempsey, J. A. and Hornbein, T. F. 2001. Control of breathing at high altitude. In T. F. Hornbein and R. B. Schoene (eds), *High Altitude: An Exploration of Human Adaptation*. New York, NY: Marcel Dekker, 139–73.

Smith, T. G., Talbot, N. P., Chang, R. W., Wilkinson, E., Nickol, A. H., Newman, D. G., Robbins, P. A. et al. 2012. Pulmonary artery pressure increases during commercial air travel in healthy passengers. *Aviat Space Environ Med* 83(7):673–6.

Smith, T. G., Talbot, N. P., Privat, C., Rivera-Ch, M., Nickol, A. H., Ratcliffe, P. J., Dorrington, K. L. et al. 2009. Effects of iron supplementation and depletion on hypoxic pulmonary hypertension: Two randomized controlled trials. *JAMA* 302(13):1444–50.

Subedi, B. H., Pokharel, J., Thapa, R., Banskota, N. and Basnyat, B. 2010. Frostbite in a Sherpa. *Wilderness Environ Med* 21(2):127–9.

Talbot, N. P., Balanos, G. M., Dorrington, K. L. and Robbins, P. A. 2005. Two temporal components within the human pulmonary vascular response to approximately 2 h of isocapnic hypoxia. *J Appl Physiol (1985)* 98(3):1125–39.

Talbot, N. P., Smith, T. G., Privat, C., Nickol, A. H., Rivera-Ch, M., Leon-Velarde, F., Dorrington, K. L. et al. 2011. Intravenous iron supplementation may protect against acute mountain sickness: A randomized, double-blinded, placebo-controlled trial. *High Alt Med Biol* 12(3):265–9.

Tellez, H. F., Mairesse, O., Macdonald-Nethercott, E., Neyt, X., Meeusen, R. and Pattyn, N. 2014. Sleep-related periodic breathing does not acclimatize to chronic hypobaric hypoxia: A 1-year study at high altitude in Antarctica. *Am J Respir Crit Care Med* 190(1):114–16.

Vearrier, D. and Greenberg, M. I. 2011. Occupational health of miners at altitude: Adverse health effects, toxic exposures, pre-placement screening, acclimatization, and worker surveillance. *Clin Toxicol (Phila)* 49(7):629–40.

Viault, F. 1891. Sur la quantité d'oxygène contenue dans le sang des animaux des hauts plateaux de l'amerique du sud. *CR Acad Sci (Paris)* 112:295–98.

Vogel, J. A. and Harris, C. W. 1967. Cardiopulmonary responses of resting man during early exposure to high altitude. *J Appl Physiol* 22(6):1124–8.

Voznesenskii, N. K. 1996. Characteristics of the progression of silicosis under alpine conditions. *Gig Sanit* (1):16–8.

West, J. B. 2002a. Commuting to high altitude: Value of oxygen enrichment of room air. *High Alt Med Biol* 3(2):223–35.

West, J. B. 2002b. Highest permanent human habitation. *High Alt Med Biol* 3(4):401–7.

West, J. B. 2006. Human responses to extreme altitudes. *Integr Comp Biol* 46(1):25–34.

West, J. B. 2012. High-altitude medicine. *Am J Respir Crit Care Med* 186(12):1229–37.

West, J. B. 2014. Working at high altitude. *High Alt Med Biol* 15(3):307–08.

West, J. B., Colice, G. L., Lee, Y. J., Namba, Y., Kurdak, S. S., Fu, Z., Ou, L. C. et al. 1995. Pathogenesis of high-altitude pulmonary oedema: Direct evidence of stress failure of pulmonary capillaries. *Eur Respir J* 8(4):523–9.

West, J. B., Hackett, P. H., Maret, K. H., Milledge, J. S., Peters, R. M. Jr., Pizzo, C. J. and Winslow, R. M. 1983a. Pulmonary gas exchange on the summit of Mount Everest. *J Appl Physiol Respir Environ Exerc Physiol* 55(3):678–87.

West, J. B., Lahiri, S., Maret, K. H., Peters, R. M. Jr. and Pizzo, C. J. 1983b. Barometric pressures at extreme altitudes on Mt. Everest: Physiological significance. *J Appl Physiol Respir Environ Exerc Physiol* 54(5):1188–94.

West, J. B., Milledge, J. S., Luks, A. M. and Schoene, R. B. 2013. *High Altitude Medicine and Physiology*, fifth edition. Boca Raton, FL: Taylor & Francis.

Windsor, J. S. and Rodway, G. W. 2012. Sleep disturbance at altitude. *Curr Opin Pulm Med* 18(6):554–60.

Winslow, R. M., Samaja, M. and West, J. B. 1984. Red cell function at extreme altitude on Mount Everest. *J Appl Physiol Respir Environ Exerc Physiol* 56(1):109–16.

Wu, T., Li, W., Li, Y., Ge, R.-L., Cheng, Q., Wang, S., Zhao, G. et al. 1998. Epidemiology of chronic mountain sickness: Ten year's study in Qinghai–Tibet. In *Progress in Mountain Medicine and High Altitude Physiology*. Matsumoto, Japan: Dogura & Co, Ltd., 120–5.

Yi, X., Liang, Y., Huerta-Sanchez, E., Jin, X., Cuo, Z. X., Pool, J. E., Xu, X. et al. 2010. Sequencing of 50 human exomes reveals adaptation to high altitude. *Science* 329(5987):75–8.

Zhang, S. and Robbins, P. A. 2000. Methodological and physiological variability within the ventilatory response to hypoxia in humans. *J Appl Physiol (1985)* 88(5):1924–32.

Zhou, D., Udpa, N., Ronen, R., Stobdan, T., Liang, J., Appenzeller, O., Zhao, H. W. et al. 2013. Whole-genome sequencing uncovers the genetic basis of chronic mountain sickness in Andean highlanders. *Am J Hum Genet* 93(3):452–62.

36 Abnormal Sleep Conditions and Work

Anita K. Simonds

CONTENTS

INTRODUCTION

The sleep–wake cycle is governed by neuronal processes that control alertness and the tendency to sleep. This cycle in humans is a balance between endogenous circadian and ultradian (more than one cycle per 24 hours) processes, but is influenced by external factors such as light, temperature and social mores (zeitgebers) that entrain the individual to the environment. Broadly, the abnormalities of sleep that affect daytime function are sleep deprivation and sleep disruption. Clients will present as 'too sleepy' or having insufficient sleep. Both can result from a variety of social pressures or disorders that are either intrinsic to sleep or caused by other medical conditions. This chapter will consider the medical conditions that affect sleep and impact on daytime function, secular changes in sleep habits, primary problems with sleep that affect sickness absence and occupational aspects related to circadian issues—shift work and extended working hours.

MEDICAL CONDITIONS

Obstructive Sleep Apnoea

Obstructive sleep apnoea (OSA) affects 4% of middle-aged males. In women, the prevalence is approximately half that of men, but rises to a similar level after the menopause. Patients usually present with a triad of snoring, apnoeas during sleep witnessed by bed partners and daytime somnolence, which can be quantitated by the Epworth Sleepiness Score or STOP-BANG questionnaire (Table 36.1). The obstructive apnoeas are caused by loss of tone in the pharyngeal airway during sleep, causing partial or total airway obstruction. These apnoeas provoke hypoxaemia, autonomic stimulation and are terminated by brief arousals from sleep, which underlie the sleep fragmentation. The severity of OSA is classified by the Apnoea/Hypopnoea Index (AHI), with an AHI of 5–14 considered to be mild OSA, 15–29 moderate OSA and >30 severe OSA, although the correlation between sleepiness

TABLE 36.1
Screening Questionnaires for Obstructive Sleep Apnoea: Epworth Sleepiness Scale and STOP-BANG Questionnaire

Epworth Sleepiness Scale

How likely are you to doze off or fall asleep during the following situations, in contrast to just feeling tired?

For each of the situations listed below, give yourself a score of 0–3, where:

0 = Would never doze
1 = Slight chance
2 = Moderate chance
3 = High chance

Work out your total score by adding up your individual scores for situations 1–8. (If you have not been in the following situations recently, think about how you would have been affected.)

Situation	Score
Sitting and reading	/3
Watching television	/3
Sitting inactive in a public place (e.g. a theatre/meeting)	/3
As a passenger in a car for an hour with no break	/3
Lying down in the afternoon (when possible)	/3
Sitting and talking to someone	/3
Sitting quietly after lunch without alcohol	/3
In a car, while stopped for a few minutes in traffic	/3
Total	/24

- If your score is below 10, you have a healthy level of daytime sleepiness in comparison to the general population.
- If your score is between 10 and 18, you have an excessive level of daytime sleepiness compared to the general population, which may require further attention. You should consider whether you are obtaining adequate sleep, need to improve your sleep hygiene and consult your doctor for further medical help.
- If your score is 18 or above, you have a very high level of excessive daytime sleepiness and it is vital that you consult your doctor for further medical help.

STOP-BANG questionnaire

1. *Snoring*
   Do you snore loudly (louder than talking or loud enough to be heard through closed doors)?
   Yes/No
2. *Tired*
   Do you often feel tried, fatigued or sleepy during the daytime?
   Yes/No
3. *Observed*
   Has anyone observed you stop breathing during your sleep?
   Yes/No
4. *Blood pressure*
   Do you have or are you being treated for high blood pressure?
   Yes/No
5. *Body mass index*
   Is your body mass index more than 35 kg/m^2?
   Yes/No
6. *Age*
   Age over 50 years?
   Yes/No
7. *Neck circumference*
   Neck circumference greater than 40 cm?
   Yes/No

High risk of obstructive sleep apnoea: answering yes to three or more items.

Low risk of obstructive sleep apnoea: answering yes to fewer than three items.

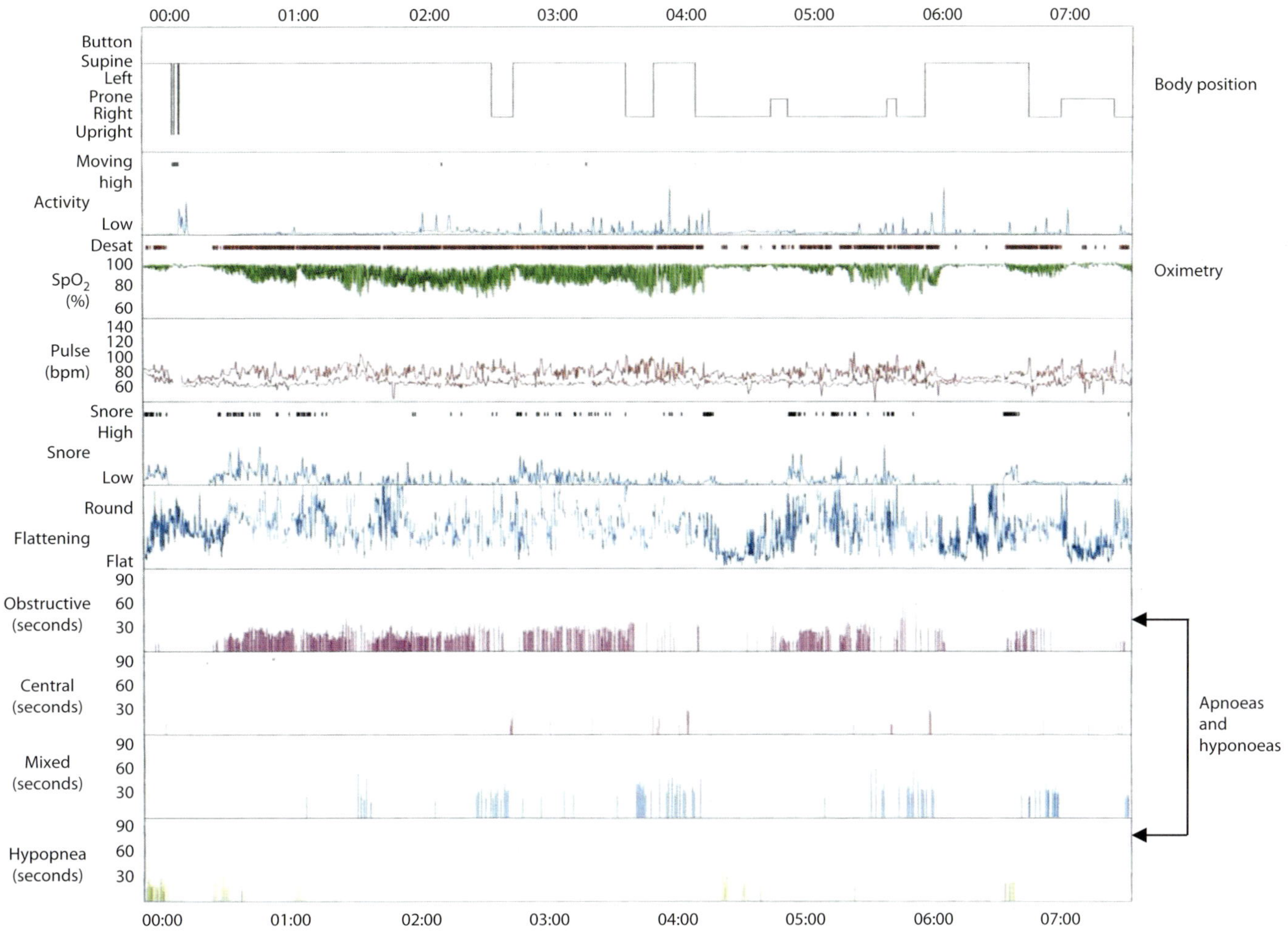

FIGURE 36.1 Respiratory polygraphy sleep study trace of a patient with obstructive sleep apnoea.

and severity is not marked. Figure 36.1 is an example of a respiratory sleep study showing OSA. Predisposing factors to OSA are obesity, as adipose tissue in the neck and surrounding the pharynx will increase the tendency to airway collapse, and upper airway pathology, such as large tonsils and adenoids. Individuals with acromegaly, hypothyroidism, Marfan syndrome and ankylosing spondylitis have an increased risk of OSA. Opiates and nocturnal sedation can exacerbate OSA by reducing pharyngeal muscles tone and ventilatory responses. As well as producing sleepiness, sleep fragmentation and deprivation may adversely affect vigilance, concentration, memory and mood.

Restless Leg Syndrome

Restless leg syndrome (RLS) describes a jumping, uncomfortable sensation in the legs (but it can also occur in the arms). It often occurs before sleep and can delay sleep onset, but if movements occur throughout the night, sleep is fragmented, resulting in daytime tiredness and somnolence. Most cases are idiopathic, but there is an increased incidence in those with renal, hepatic and cardiac failure and neuropathies. The prevalence of RLS increases with age and it is more common in multiparous females than males, in part related to the fact that iron deficiency is a further precipitating factor. The history is virtually diagnostic, but findings can be confirmed by demonstrating characteristic periodic limb movements occurring every 20–40 seconds on sleep monitoring (polysomnography; see Figure 36.2). An isolated finding of periodic limb movements in sleep without symptoms or sleep disturbance does not constitute a diagnosis of restless legs syndrome. After screening for iron deficiency and secondary causes, first-line therapy is usually an anti-Parkinsonian drug such as ropinirole.

Sleep Duration in Adults

The assumption that sleep duration has declined markedly over the last few decades associated with a '24/7'

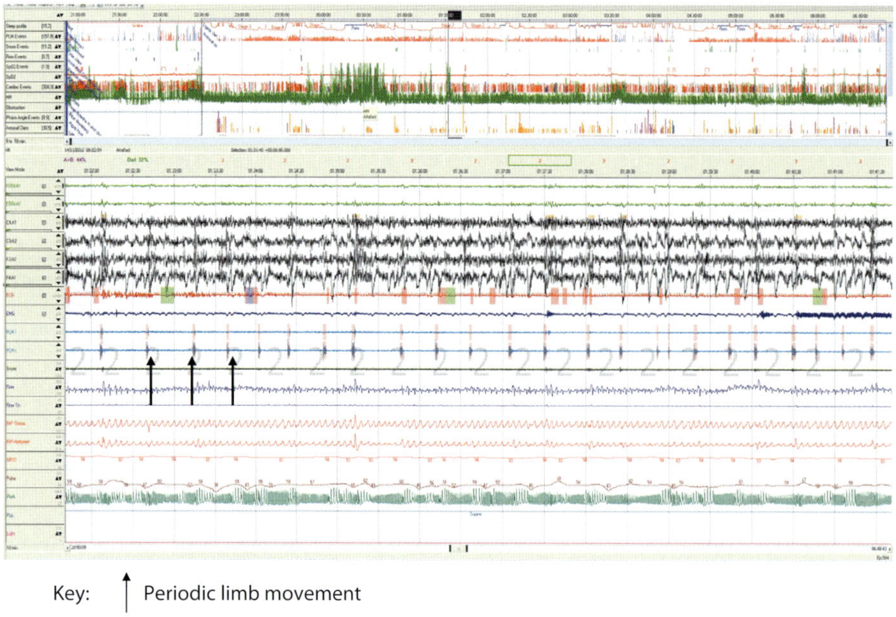

FIGURE 36.2 Polysomnographic trace of periodic leg movements in patients with restless leg syndrome.

society is supported by public polls that suggest that 27% of US citizens now sleep fewer than 6 hours/night (National Sleep Foundation, 2011), while an online survey in Australia (Australian Broadcasting Corporation, 2000) showed that average sleep in 2010 was 7 hours, compared to 8 hours a decade earlier. These reductions have been attributed to the rise in communication technology, television viewing, commute times and longer working hours (Chatzitheochari and Arber, 2009). The objective evidence base to such assertions is less secure, and a systematic review (Bin et al., 2012) of secular trends in adult sleep duration in 15 developed countries from the 1960s to 2000s showed no consistent decrease in self-reported sleep duration, with average sleep duration decreasing in some countries and increasing in others. This discrepancy may be explained by selection and response biases in public polls and the fact that while average sleep duration may be largely unchanged, the proportions of very short and very long sleepers may have increased over that period.

It is also evident that commuting time, work hours and employment status are strong correlates of sleep time (Chatzitheochari and Arber, 2009) and that short sleep time is more common in certain occupations and industries and more pronounced in working-age men and younger women. Socioeconomic status within populations does not appear to have a consistent effect. These findings are important as a public health issue since short sleep duration (defined by less than 6 hours of sleep) is associated with increased rates of hypertension, cardiovascular disease, obesity and diabetes.

Poor Sleep and Work Life

While the average duration of sleep may not have changed greatly, significant numbers complain of poor sleep, with almost 10% of the general population complaining of chronic insomnia. In a large register-based follow-up study in Finland, Lallukka et al. (2014) linked the prevalence of a variety of sleep measures with sickness absence data from the Finnish Social Insurance Institution. A previous register-based Finnish study (Aromaa and Koskinen, 2004) had shown that, compared to controls, cases with sleep apnoea had an increased risk of both sickness absence and disability retirement, with the effect being more marked in females than males.

In the study of Lallukka et al. (2014), participants comprised 1875 working-age women and 1885 working-age men, selected to be representative of the demographics of the Finnish population. Symptoms related to insomnia, early-morning awakenings, tiredness in the day, use of sleeping tablets, excessive daytime sleepiness (EDS) and reported sleep duration were examined as determinants of sickness absence. Additional covariates included nature of employment, educational level, health behaviours (smoking and exercise), obesity and working conditions. In men, after adjusting for age, all sleep disturbances apart from EDS were associated with sickness absence (relative risks: 1.3–2.5). In women, following age adjustment, insomnia-related symptoms, early-morning awakenings, tiredness and use of sleeping pills were associated with sickness absence (relative risks: 1.4–1.8). As an example, men who reported being more tired than others had 9 days of sickness absence per year compared to 4.8 days in those who reported that they were not more tired than others. Men using sleeping tablets often or almost every night had 8.1 days more sickness leave per annum than those who did not use sleeping pills. In women, those reporting insomnia-related symptoms had 5.7 more days of sickness absence per annum. The figures for early-morning awakening, being more tired than others and use of sleeping pills were 2.3, 5.5 and 3.2 days of leave, respectively, in excess of those without these features.

Interestingly, the authors examined optimal sleep duration. Not surprisingly, the relationship between sleep duration and work absence was U-shaped, with a sleep duration of 7.8 hours for men and 7.6 hours for women being associated with the lowest sickness absence rates. The authors suggested that while health problems such as sleep apnoea need to be addressed, the simple move of promoting optimum sleep duration could decrease sickness absence by almost 30% (Lallukka et al., 2014).

EDS and Accidents in Non-Shift Workers

While sleep-related symptoms may be associated with work absence, there can be other serious consequences. It is helpful to examine these first by excluding complicating and confounding circadian factors, such as shift work. The risk of occupational injuries in non-shift daytime workers with EDS injuries was investigated by Melamed and Oksenberg (2002). A sleep disorders assessment was carried out in a group of 740 daytime workers from eight industrial plants, and data on injuries registered by participating factories were recorded. The average Epworth score was just over 9, but 22% of workers had a score of above 10 and were therefore considered to have EDS. EDS was associated with an increased risk of injury (odds ratio [OR]: 2.2; 95% confidence interval: 1.3–3.8) after controlling for factory category, job and environmental conditions. The link between EDS and sleep apnoea was explored with a further questionnaire, in which approximately 37.1% of respondents with EDS had features of OSA. The study had a prospective component in that after completing the sleep questionnaire, subjects received a 90–minute lecture and discussion session in small groups on sleep disorders, sleepiness, the effects of EDS on quality of life and performance, sleep hygiene and treatments for EDS (Figure 36.3). Workers were provided with their sleep assessment results and those with moderate or severe EDS were given a letter of recommendation to attend a sleep disorders clinic. There is no record of the number that availed themselves of this opportunity or who were started on treatment. However, in the year after this intervention, the injury rate in workers who had previously reported EDS fell to the level of those who had not had EDS the year before. Additionally, the injury rate in

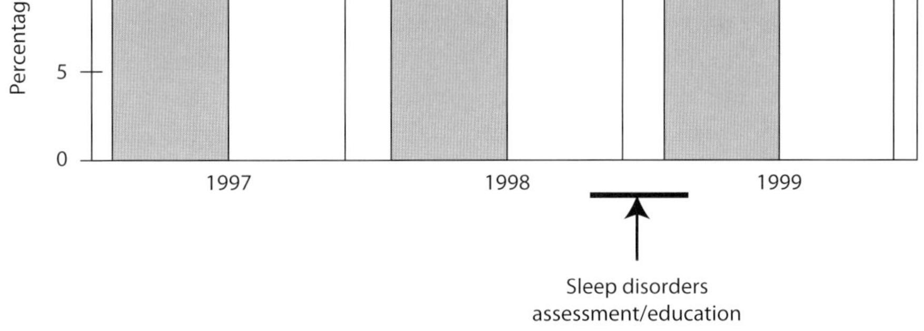

FIGURE 36.3 Percentages of non-shift daytime workers with excessive daytime somnolence (EDS; n = 120) sustaining occupational injuries in 1997, 1998 and 1999, and the corresponding percentages among workers without EDS (n = 412) and the time of the sleep disorders assessment/education procedure and in the year afterwards. (From Melamed, S. and Okenberg, A. 2002. *Sleep* 25:315–22. With permission.)

workers without EDS remained constant in the 3 years surveyed, whereas the rate in those with EDS was a third of the rate recorded before the intervention. It was also seen that workers who regularly slept for less than 6 hours/night had a higher rate of EDS than those who slept for 6–8 hours, but importantly, the minority who reported sleeping for 9 hours or more each night had not only the highest level of EDS, but also experienced more than 2.5-times the number of occupational injuries of those with a normal sleep duration.

Insomnia and Work-Based Accidents

From another sleep disorder perspective, the American Insomnia Survey (Shahly et al., 2012) investigated the association between chronic insomnia and workplace accidents and errors, using a detailed, psychiatrically validated, cross-sectional telephone survey. Accidents and errors were defined as workplace accidents that caused either damage or work disruption with a value of \$500 (US) or more or mistakes that cost the company \$500 (US) or more. The survey was administered to a stratified sample of just over 10,000 adults who were fully insured health plan members. In addition to insomnia-related questions, a total of nine treated and untreated clusters of chronic disorders were identified in the questionnaire, including chronic cardiac and respiratory disease, chronic pain, major depression and other sleep disorders. The results showed an estimated prevalence of insomnia, present for at least 12 months, of 20%. The estimated prevalence (standard errors) of workplace accidents was 1.1% (0.2%), and for errors was 3.4% (0.2%). Accident and error rates were lower in the >65 year olds than in those aged 18–64 years. Reported accidents and errors were also more prevalent in men than women (ORs: 2.8 for accidents and 5.6 for errors). Insomnia was positively associated with all chronic conditions. Those with insomnia had an increased rate of both accidents and errors (ORs: 1.9 for accidents and 1.4 for errors), but only three chronic conditions had significant associations with accidents and or errors: neuropathic pain, sleep apnoea and emotional disorders other than depression. Population-attributable risk proportions (PARPs) were calculated: these represent the proportion of incidents that would not have occurred, according to logistic regression models, if insomnia was absent or effectively treated. The actual survey PARP showed that 14.5% of all costly workplace accidents were attributable to insomnia, a figure reducing to 10.3% when controlled for comorbid conditions. The PARPs for insomnia were higher than those for sleep apnoea, neuropathic pain and emotional disorders. The authors finally estimated that 274,000 workplace accidents and errors per year are attributable to insomnia, representing a combined cost of \$31.1 million (US). It is unclear whether interventions to screen and treat insomnia would be effective in reducing this toll, although the Melamed and Oksenberg (2002) study described above suggests that such a proactive strategy should at least be evaluated.

Circadian Disorders

These describe a misalignment of the sleep–wake cycle with the normal 24-hour body clock and may be intrinsic (e.g. delayed sleep phase syndrome [late bedtime, extreme 'owl'] or advanced sleep phase syndrome [early awakening, extreme 'lark']) or related to extrinsic factors (e.g. jet lag, a new baby or shift work).

Shift work embraces a variety of work practices, including regular night work, rotating day and night work, early-morning starts or evening work. Many workers experience sleep symptoms related to these, meaning that the threshold between a normal reaction and abnormality is difficult to establish, and the matter is complicated by the fact that regardless of sleep quality, on average, shift workers have a shorter sleep duration than non-shift workers. Shift work has been shown to be associated with raised levels of gastrin and pepsinogen; a chronic sleep debt that is more common in shift workers is associated not only with EDS, but also with an elevation of C-reactive protein, which is an inflammatory marker of cardiovascular morbidity. Hormonal changes may well be another factor, since the release of many hormones and precursors is related to sleep stage.

The minimum criteria for the diagnosis of shift work sleep disorder (SWSD) are a primary symptom of either insomnia or EDS that is temporally associated with work period and occurs during habitual sleep phases. Drake et al. (2004) have investigated the prevalence and consequences of SWSD in a population from Detroit, USA. Of the 2570 participants, 360 worked rotating shifts, 174 worked nights and the remainder were day workers. A total of 14.1% of night workers and 8.1% of rotating shift workers met the criteria for SWSD, creating a true prevalence of 10.1% of SWSD in shift workers aged 18–65 years; by extrapolation, this would represent 1% of the US working population. Occupational, behavioural and health-related outcomes were compared between night, rotating shift and day workers. Those individuals who met the criteria for SWSD had higher rates of gastric/duodenal ulcers (OR: 4.18), sleepiness-related accidents, absenteeism and depression. They also failed to attend family and social activities more frequently than those who did not reach the diagnostic criteria. Heart disease was more prevalent in permanent night and rotating workers, but did not differ between those with SWSD and those without.

Shift Work and Occupational Injury

Up to 20% of the working population work at night or on shifts. In reviews dating back several decades, there has been the strong suggestion that occupational injury rates vary according to shifts. For example, Folkard et al. (2005) showed that the risk of occupational injury was 15% higher in afternoon shifts and 28% higher in night shifts compared to morning shifts. They also found that on successive nights, the risk of injury increased from the first to the fourth night shift. Furthermore, in a Scandinavian study (Dembe et al. 2006), rotating shifts increased injury risk by 36% and working irregular shifts increased this by 15%. Construction workers seem prone to the greatest risk of injury from night shifts.

Other factors can come into play. In a glass and steel plant in Canada, injuries occurred maximally just before lunchtime and between 2 and 4 a.m. of the night shift (Woijczak-Jaroszwa and Jarosz, 1987). On drilling rigs, operators had more injuries during day shifts, but there were more staff working in the daytime. For drilling crews on the same rigs, there was no difference in injury rates between day and night shifts. In Australia, female adolescents had almost five-times more injuries when working night shifts than adult co-workers, and male adolescents experienced three-times more injuries than adult men (Loudoun and Allan, 2008).

Rotating shifts are more likely to reduce the chance of successful phase shifts in the body clocks of workers. Those in a German electronic factory had 34% more injuries than day shift workers (Loudoun and Allan, 2008), and in Taiwan, a fixed shift system proved less harmful that rotating shifts (Liou and Wang, 1991).

A recent review by Salminen (2010) shows more complex findings. Cumulating data from the USA alone show the expected trend of increases in occupational injury rates by 31% in afternoon shifts and 30% in night shifts (Dembe et al., 2005). However, this does not tally with findings from Singapore and India, where injury risks fell in the afternoon and evening. Salminen (2010) speculates that there may be fewer supervisors present during night and afternoon shifts and that injuries during these periods may be under-reported; in addition, it is not always clear in published reports whether workers regularly worked night shifts or were on rotating shifts, for example.

Extended Working Hours

The situation is further complicated by the fact that shift workers may work extended hours, which, in its own right, whether associated with shift work or not, is a risk factor for occupational injury. The usual definition of extended working hours is a working week of more than 48 hours. Based on a systematic review, Salminen (2010) concluded that extended hours increased the risk of occupational injury, with working a >12-hour day doubling the risk. Rest breaks can help, and it is important to note that risk was highest in the last hour of the working day. In car assembly workers in the UK (Tucker et al., 2003), accidents rose in the fourth half-hour after a break, but fell immediately after a break; in general, studies support the introduction of a rest break every 2 hours. Having said that, with the pressure to increase 12-hour shifts for financial reasons, a change from an 8- to a 12-hour day in a US police station produced improved efficiency and decreased fatigue and stress in officers (Pierce and Dunham, 1992); as such, work circumstances, nature of work, cycle of days off and worker preference are clearly of importance.

Genotypes and Chronotypes

It is common knowledge that some individuals function better in the morning than at night and vice versa; morning 'lark' and evening 'owl' propensities (chronotypes) can be assessed by standardised questionnaires. There is some evidence to suggest that morning types are sleepier than evening types on night shifts and are better adapted to day shifts, as might be predicted. Furthermore, over the last decade, it has become evident that the circadian clock is determined by a large number of 'clock' genes and proteins. Indeed, it seems that as many as 10,000 mammalian genes are regulated by clock genes. A range of these have been shown to affect sleep duration and sleep phases. For example, a mutation in *PER2* results in advanced sleep phase syndrome, and *PER3* gene polymorphisms are associated with delayed sleep phase syndrome and diurnal sleep preference. These genes may also affect adaption to shift work strategies. In a study of shift working nurses, Gamble et al. (2011) found that chronotype affected the efficiency of adaptation to shift routine. In addition, polymorphisms in the clock *NPA2*, *PER2* and *PER3* genes were associated with use of alcohol and caffeine to manage symptoms and the levels of sleepiness and inertia. Night shift nurses who used sleep deprivation in order to aid adaption to and from diurnal shifts were found to be most poorly adapted to their work schedule; that is, most symptomatic. There are clear practical implications to this, as surveys have shown that one in four nurses report being excessively sleepy, and night shift work is associated with drug administration error. Management decisions that flow from these findings are that the use of sleep deprivation when moving from a day to a night schedule is detrimental, and longer cycles of night and day shifts (e.g. reducing the frequency of switching from day to night shifts) are advantageous.

Impact on Medical Staff

Overwork and long working hours are harmful to medical workers themselves—they experience twice the risk of a road traffic accident when driving home after a 24-hour work period (Berger et al., 2005) and suffer over 60% more needle-stick injuries after the 20th consecutive hour of work (Ayas et al., 2006). This performance decrement seems to be imposed on a 'normal' chronic level of sleep deprivation, as Howard et al. (2002) showed that median sleep latency time (MSLT) was reduced after on-call periods; even at baseline, MSLT was reduced, indicating that short sleep times are a routine lifestyle choice for young interns. Self-assessment and perception of alertness are also impaired, similarly to the effect of alcohol on performance, in that the individual becomes progressively less able to rate alertness accurately and gauge his/her limitations. In fact, a range of studies in physicians has shown that sleep deprivation at a personal level impairs language and mathematics skills, can produce less empathy and poor communication and is associated with significant family and marital stress (Eddy, 2005).

Impact on Working Practice and Patients

In an overview, Lockley et al. (2008) summarised that doctors in training carrying out 24-hour shifts had twice as many attentional errors when on night duty and made five-times as many diagnostic errors and 36% more serious medical errors than those who worked just 16 consecutive hours. A meta-analysis of the impact of sleep deprivation on physician and non-physician performance showed that continuous 24–30-hour shifts reduced overall performance by 1 standard deviation and clinical performance by over 1.5 standard deviations (Philibert, 2005). Similarly, critical care nurses working more than 12.5 hours had twice the risk of medical error (OR: 1.94) compared to those working shorter hours (Scott et al., 2006).

Effect of Change in Working Hours on Patient Outcomes

Interventional studies assessing the benefits of reducing long working hours have shown some benefit. Landrigan et al. (2004) compared the rate of serious medical errors made by interns in intensive care units working a traditional schedule of 24 hours of work every other shift with those working a schedule that reduced the number of working hours per week and abolished extended work shifts. The findings were that the error rates in critical care units with traditional rotas were 22% higher than those with the new rota. The rate of serious diagnostic error was also higher during traditional schedules (18.3 vs. 3.3 per 1000 patient-days, $p < 0.001$).

Examining the implications more widely for patient care is more difficult. Landrigan et al. (2010) further examined temporal trends in rates of patient harm related to medical care across a large stratified sample of hospitals in North Carolina. These adverse events were carefully scrutinised by external reviewers. Despite the fact that changes in work hours had been introduced several years before this study, there was no evidence of a fall in episodes of patient harm, resulting in a debunking headline in the *New York Times* of 5 August 2011 of 'The phantom menace of sleep-deprived doctors'.

Greater reflection is required, however—firstly, absence of evidence of a benefit does not show that some interventions are not worthwhile. A trend in preventable harms was seen, for example. In addition, adverse events occur due to a multiplicity of causes—not all related to staff work times. In mitigation, there are significant data to suggest that evidence-based practice is not practised in many areas—handwashing to prevent cross-infection is a clear example. Furthermore, in some hospitals, the advocated control of long shifts and extended hours had not been introduced and teams still worked long hours. Few hospitals had electronic patient records, and prescribing and recording of events was voluntary. The authors recommended a trigger tool in order to identify events more comprehensively. A respiratory example of a trigger tool is administration of naloxone—this would trigger a review of notes in order to assess whether an opiate overdose had occurred unintentionally.

One should add that there are other consequences of reducing shift hours. This process inevitably results in more frequent handovers of care to incoming teams, which in itself may result in communication errors and omissions of care as a result of poor continuity; awareness of the problem and structured handovers can reduce these limitations. There is an additional impact over the whole training duration of medical staff of fewer hours on duty, resulting in less experience. The consequences of this have been debated but remain an area of concern, and have necessitated important changes in medical education, including increased use of simulation.

Investigation and Management of Sleep Disorders

Following history taking, clients with key symptoms of OSA (snoring, witnessed apnoeas and somnolence) should be referred for a sleep study. Screening tools for somnolence are shown in Table 36.1. Depending on the pre-test probability, respiratory polygraphy (several-channel monitoring without detailed monitoring of sleep stage; see Figure 36.1) in hospital or at home will identify sleep apnoea. If at a moderate or severe level or at a mild level with marked symptoms, continuous positive airway pressure (CPAP) is the treatment of choice (Figure 36.4a). Effective CPAP rapidly reduces sleepiness and vascular morbidity. A mandibular advancement splint can be used in snoring and mild to moderate OSA (Figure 36.4b). Sensible health measure such as weight loss and stopping smoking should be advised, and upper airway problems such as large tonsils, nasal polyps and rhinitis should be evaluated.

(a) (b)

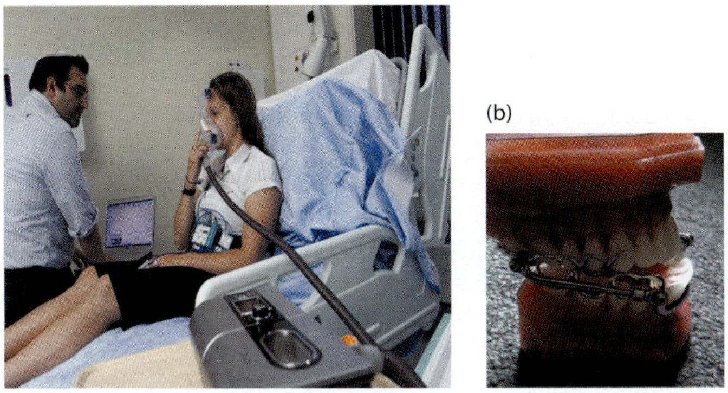

FIGURE 36.4 Treatments for obstructive sleep apnoea. (a) Continuous positive airway pressure therapy set-up. (b) Mandibular advancement split.

Insomnia may be precipitated by a number of issues, but if present for more than 1 month, referral and consideration of cognitive behavioural therapy can be tried. For circadian disorders, use of an Actiwatch that monitors body movement is useful for demonstrating day/night activity over several weeks, as shown by an actogram (Figure 36.5). The application of bright light in order to entrain to the new sleep–wake phase may be helpful, as may be the avoidance of maladaptive strategies such as

(a) (b)

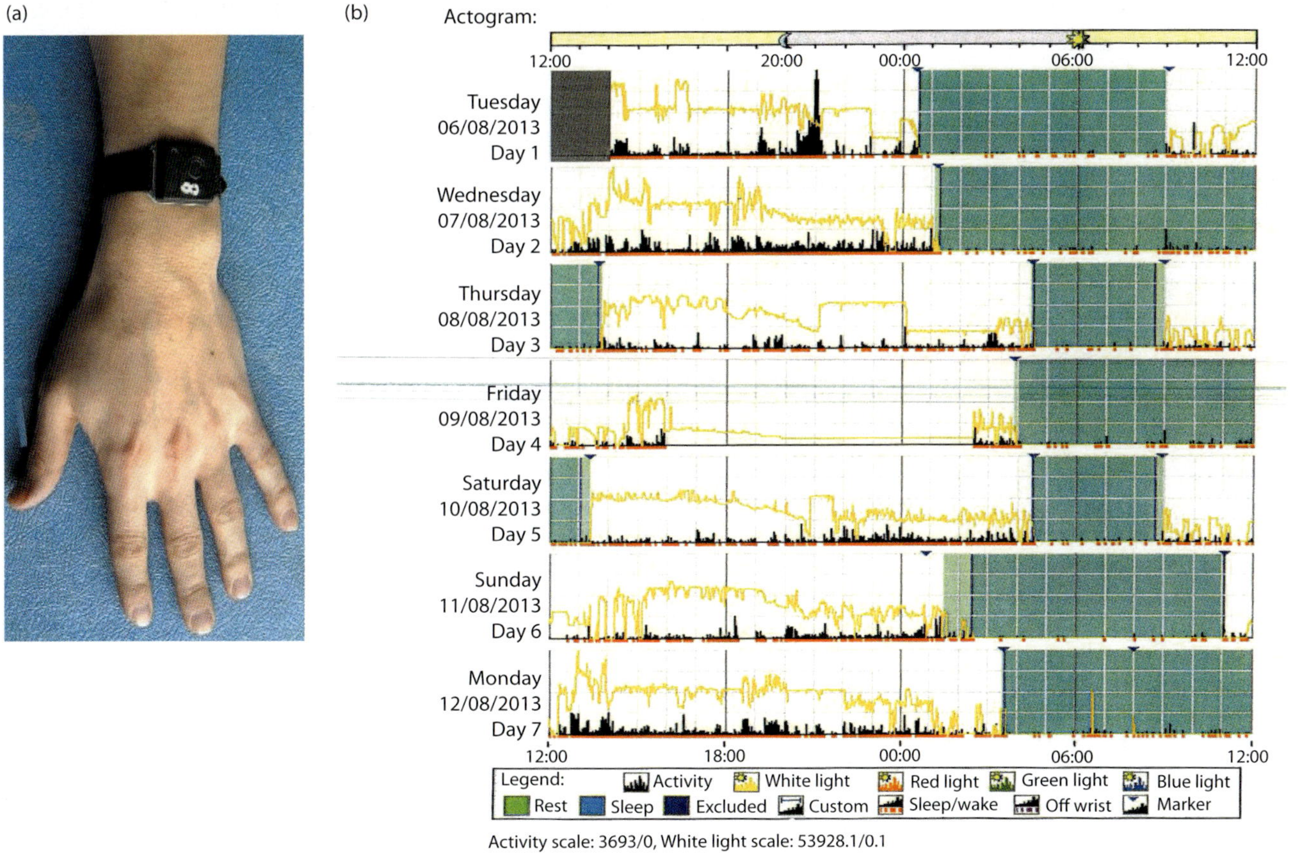

FIGURE 36.5 (a) Actiwatch and (b) actogram trace showing a sleep–wake cycle for the assessment of circadian disorders.

sleep deprivation when shifting from day to night work and vice versa.

CONCLUSION

The evidence is clear that sleep deprivation and disruption have significant adverse effects on daytime function and work performance. Social pressures, financial imperatives and the need for greater productivity mean that shift work and extended hours will always be with us. The burden of sleep disorders is likely to mushroom, as OSA will increase with the growing world prevalence of obesity, and RLS and other sleep disturbances related to age will increase as society ages.

On a positive note, simple interventions such as identifying and advising somnolent workers in the study by Melamed and Oksenberg (2002) can significantly reduce accident rates in those with EDS, and it is possible that a similar strategy could work in those with insomnia. Furthermore, education of employers and manufacturers regarding the increased risks posed by rotating shifts, extended hours and a lack of regular breaks is likely not only to produce a safer work environment, but may also be cost effective. Finally, a less 'bullish' attitude to surviving on little sleep would be beneficial from a societal perspective. It has been shown that performance after a heavy on-call rota is equivalent or worse than after alcohol ingestion, producing a blood level of 0.04–0.05g% (Arnedt et al., 2005). The situation may not improve until the effect of sleep disruption on performance is recognised by society to be as harmful as that of alcohol.

REFERENCES

Arnedt, J. T. et al. 2005. Neurobehavioural performance of residents after heavy night call vs after alcohol ingestion. *JAMA* 294:1025–33.

Aromaa, A., Koskinen, S. (eds). 2004. Health and functional capacity in Finland. Baseline results of the Health 2000 Health Examination. Available at: http://www.terveys2000.fi/julkaisut/baseline.pdf

Australian Broadcasting Corporation. 2000. The National Sleep Research Project. http://www.abc.net.au/science/sleep/

Ayas, N. T. et al. 2006. Extended work duration and the risk of self-reported percutaneous injuries in interns. *JAMA* 296:1055–62.

Berger, L. K. et al. 2005. Extended work shifts and the risk of motor vehicle crashes among interns. *N Engl J Med* 352:125–34.

Bin, Y. S., Marshall, N. M. and Glozier, N. 2012. Secular trends in adult sleep duration: A systematic review. *Sleep Med Rev* 16:223–30.

Chatzitheochari, S. and Arber, S. 2009. Lack of sleep, work and the long hours culture: Evidence from the UK time use survey. *Work Emply Soc* 23:30–48.

Dembe, A. E., Erickson, A. D., Delbos, R. G. and Banks, S. M. 2005. The impact of overtime and long work hours on occupational injuries and illnesses: new evidence from the United States. *Occup Environ Med* 62:588–97.

Dembe, A. E., Erickson, J. B., Delbos, R. G. and Banks, S. M. 2006. Nonstandard shift schedules and the risk of job-related injuries. *Scand J Work Environ Health* 32:232–40.

Drake, C. L., Roehrs, T., Richardson, G., Walsh, J. K. and Roth, T. 2004. Shift work sleep disorder: Prevalence and consequences beyond that of symptomatic day workers. *Sleep* 27:1453–62.

Eddy, R. 2005. Sleep deprivation among physicians. *BMC Med J* 47:176–80.

Folkard, S., Lombardi, D. A. and Tucker, P. T. 2005. Shiftwork: Safety, sleepiness and sleep. *Ind Health* 43:20–3.

Gamble, K. L., Motsinger-Reif, A. A., Hida, A., Borsetti, H. M., Servick, S. V., Ciarleglio, C. M., Robbins, S. et al. 2011. Shift work in nurses: Contribution of phenotypes and genotypes to adaptation. *PLoS One* 6:e18395.

Howard, S. K., Gaba, D. M. and Zarcone, V. P. 2002. The risks and implications of excessive daytime sleepiness in resident physicians. *Acad Med* 77:1019–25.

Lallukka, T., Kaikkonen, R., Harkanen, T., Kronholm, E., Parlonen, T., Rahkonen, O. and Koskinen, S. 2014. Sleep and sickness absence: A nationally representative register-based follow-up study. *Sleep* 37:1413–1425.

Landrigan, C. P., Rothschild, J. M., Cronin, J. W., Kaushai, R., Burdick, E., Katz, J.T., Lilly, C.M. et al. 2004. Effect of reducing interns' work hours on serious medical errors in intensive care units. *N Engl J Med* 351:838–48.

Landrigan, C. P., Parry, G. J., Bones, C. B., Hackbarth, A. D., Goldmann, D. A. and Sharek, P. J. 2010. Temporal trends in rates of patient harm resulting from medical care. *N Engl J Med* 363:2124–34.

Liou, T.-S. and Wang, M.-J. 1991. Rotating-shift system vs fixed-shift system. *Int J Ind Ergon* 7:63–70.

Lockley, S. W., Barger, L. K., Ayas, N. T., Rothschild, J. M., Czeisler, C. A. and Landrigan, C. P. 2008. Effects of health care provider work hours and sleep deprivation on safety and performance. *Jt Comm J Qual Patient Saf* 33:7–18.

Loudoun, R. and Allan, C. 2008. The effect of time of day on injury patterns amongst adolescents in Australia. *Appl Ergon* 39:663–70.

Melamed, S. and Oksenberg, A. 2002. Excessive daytime sleepiness and risk of occupational injuries in non-shift daytime workers. *Sleep* 25:315–22.

National Sleep Foundation. 2011. *Sleep in America Poll: Communications Technology in the Bedroom.*

Philibert, I. 2005. Sleep loss and performance in residents and nonphysicians. A meta-analytic examination. *Sleep* 28:1392–402.

Pierce, J. L. and Dunham, R. B. 1992. The 12-hour work day: A 48-hour, eight day week. *Acad Manag J* 35:1086–98.

Salminen, S. 2010. Shift work and extended working hours as risk factors for occupational injury. *Ergonom Open J* 3:14–8.

Scott, L. D. et al. 2006. Effects of critical are nurses' work hours on vigilance and patients' safety. *Am J Crit Care* 15:30–7.

Shahly, V., Berglund, P. A., Coulouvrat, C., Fitzgerald, T., Hajak, G., Roth, T., Shillington, A. C. et al. 2012. The associations of insomnia with costly workplace accidents and errors. *Arch Gen Psychiatry* 69:1054–63.

Tucker, P., Folkard, S. and Macdonald, I. 2003. Rest breaks and accident risk. *Lancet* 361:680.

Woijczak-Jaroszwa, J. and Jarosz, D. 1987. Time-related distribution of occupational accidents. *J Saf Res* 18:33–41.

Appendix 1: Elements of Geology and Mineralogy

Peter Baxter and Grant Heiken

INTRODUCTION

A basic knowledge of geology and mineralogy is useful, if not essential, to an informed understanding and recognition of the nature and composition of particular rocks and minerals that are encountered in widely differing circumstances in mining operations and in their use or incidental occurrence in industrial processes. Although not a comprehensive account, it is hoped that this chapter may offer some guidance in this respect.

The Earth consists of a superficial crust that is a few miles thick, which rests on a denser mass—the mantle—which is nearly 2000 miles thick, and a central core that is probably solid, but behaves in some respects as if in a molten state. Molten rock material, or magma, which contains gases and steam, also exists as pockets within the crust and mantle. As a consequence of abnormally high temperatures, often with earth movements, magma is forced up into the crust. If it cools and solidifies before reaching the surface, the resulting rocks are termed 'igneous rocks'; because they invade the surrounding rocks—referred to as 'country rocks'—they are called 'intrusive'. However, some of the magma may, periodically, reach and pour out—or explode—onto the surface. Rocks formed in this way are termed 'extrusive' or 'volcanic'. Thus, igneous rocks are divided into two broad groups: intrusive and extrusive.

'Rock' means 'any mass or aggregate of one or more kinds of mineral or of organic matter, whether hard and consolidated or soft and incoherent, which owes its origin to the operation of natural causes. Thus, granite, basalt, limestone, clay, sand, silt and peat are all equally termed rocks' (Geikie, 1908).

Chemically, the average composition of the crust consists of approximately 27.7% silicon, 46.6% oxygen, 8% aluminium and 16.2% in aggregate of calcium, iron, magnesium, potassium and sodium. This gives a total of 98.5%, with the remainder consisting of all of the other elements that are present.

The ingredients that are available for the formation of rocks are known as minerals. A mineral is a naturally occurring, inorganic, homogeneous substance of distinct chemical composition, atomic structure and physical properties. Minerals fall into two broad categories:

1. Primary minerals; that is, rock constituents that crystallized out of the magma. These are of two kinds: essential minerals, which determine the species of rocks; and accessory minerals, which are accidental ingredients (usually in small quantity) in igneous, sedimentary and metamorphic rocks and whose presence or absence does not affect the general character of the rock.
2. Secondary minerals; these are formed by chemical alterations of essential and accessory minerals.

Minerals crystallize into different habits, or forms, under different physical conditions. The term 'habit' denotes the characteristic shapes of crystals caused by variations in the number, size and shape of their faces; for example, prismatic, acicular and platy for single crystals, and columnar, radiating, granular, asbestiform (or fibrous), massive and foliated for crystalline aggregates (Zoltai and Wylie, 1979).

Silicon (Si) and oxygen are the two most predominant elements in the crust. However, silicon does not exist in a free state in nature, although its compounds, which are ubiquitous as oxides and as a large group of silicates, constitute the most important rock-forming minerals.

SILICA

Silicon and oxygen form a fundamental silicon tetraoxide (SiO_4) tetrahedral unit consisting of a central silicon ion with oxygen ions attached three-dimensionally at the four 'corners' of a tetrahedron. All forms of silica—that is, silicon dioxide (SiO_2)—are composed of a 3D network of tetrahedra joined by common oxygen atoms, so that each crystal consists of a giant molecule with an average stoichiometric formula of SiO_2. As they are uncombined, they are referred to as 'free silica'. The tetrahedra are linked in various ways by –Si–O–Si– chains, and the manner in which metallic cations are included in this linkage controls their form and characteristics.

The distinction between free and combined silica is important. Free (uncombined) silica (SiO_2) is by far the major component of the Earth's crust; combined silica is SiO_2 in combination with various cations as silicates. Free silica occurs in three main forms: crystalline, cryptocrystalline (microcrystalline) and amorphous (non-crystalline). Most of the following section owes much to the classic work of Sosman (1965).

The Principal Phases (Polymorphs) of Silica

Crystalline Silica

In nature, crystalline silica occurs in six different polymorphic phases: quartz, tridymite and cristobalite, and keatite, coesite and stishovite; the last three are formed only under conditions of high temperature and pressure—usually in the craters of meteorites.

Quartz

This is the most common polymorph found in nature and is the main constituent of igneous rocks and sandstones formed from the breakdown of igneous rocks; it is a common constituent of many metamorphic rocks. It also occurs in varying amounts, by detrital deposition, at different stages in the development of sedimentary rocks, including carbonaceous rocks.

Tridymite

This is only found in nature in acid volcanic rocks.

Cristobalite

This occurs as minute crystals in some lavas and as small globules (spherulites) in acid lavas and glasses. However, it is frequently present in bentonite clays in the western USA.

Under certain industrial and laboratory conditions, reversible transformation—or inversion—of these phases occurs at different temperatures at atmospheric pressure (Figure A.1). Thus:

$$\text{Quartz} \underset{}{\overset{867^\circ C}{\rightleftharpoons}} \text{Tridymite} \underset{}{\overset{1470^\circ C}{\rightleftharpoons}}$$

$$\text{Cristobalite} \underset{}{\overset{1723^\circ C}{\rightleftharpoons}} \text{Vitreous silica}$$

They are interconvertible at the points of inversion. Inversions, by which one polymorph of silica changes into another, are of two kinds: (1) a slow change that requires a moderate amount of energy, but less than that needed for melting; and (2) a rapid and reversible change requiring much less energy.

Quartz exists in two reversible temperature modifications at constant pressure: α-quartz, which is stable from absolute zero up to 573°C; and β-quartz, which is stable at temperatures between 573°C and 867°C. Below 867°C, therefore, under atmospheric pressure and if the temperature is constant and uniform, quartz remains stable no matter how long heating continues, and it does not change into any other phase (Figure A.1). Between 867°C and 1470°C, over a brief period, pure quartz almost invariably converts to cristobalite, not to tridymite, but if heating is continued below 1470°C, the stable form of tridymite is ultimately formed. However, in the presence of fluxing oxides (such as CaO and Al_2O_3), conversion is accelerated, and crystalline tridymite may then form at temperatures as low as 950°C. Thus, excellent samples of stable tridymite are found in silica brick from open-hearth furnace roofs where temperatures may be held at 867–1470°C for several weeks or longer. Similarly, silica bricks from by-product coke ovens maintained at high temperatures, often for years, are an equally rich source.

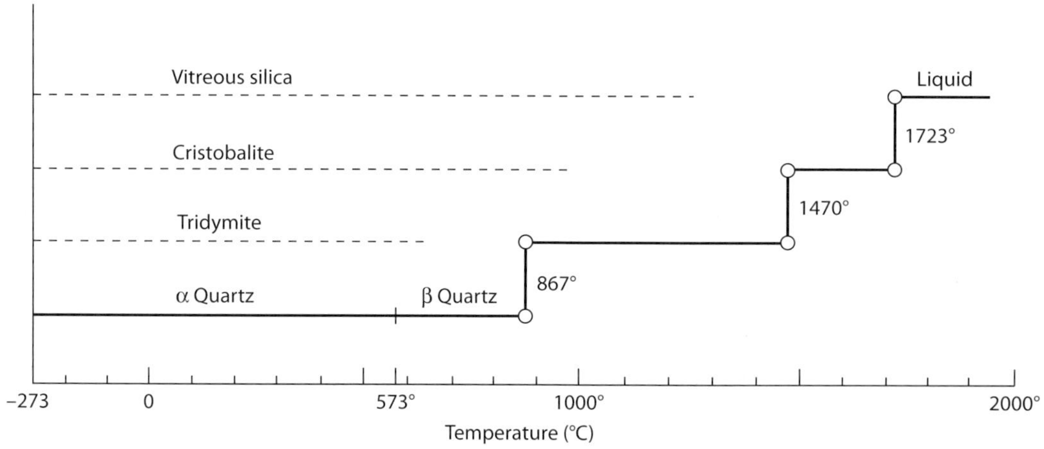

FIGURE A.1 Graphic classification of the better-known phases (polymorphs) of silica in stable states at 1 atmospheric pressure, as controlled by temperature. (Reproduced from Sosman, R. B. 1965. *The Phases of Silica*. New Brunswick, NJ: Rutgers University Press. With permission. Copyright 1965, Rutgers University Press, New Brunswick, NJ.)

Cristobalite is the stable polymorph of silica at atmospheric pressure between approximately 1470°C and 1723°C, its melting point. If the temperature remains uniform and constant, it does not convert permanently to any other crystalline phase. However, cristobalite may also form at temperatures below 1470°C, in which case it is in a metastable state; between 867°C and 1470°C, whether alone or in contact with a melt, it inverts first to the metastable, and then to the stable form of tridymite. Thus, with repeated firings of silica brick below 1470°C, quartz gradually disappears and cristobalite forms and then decreases steadily as the formation of tridymite increases and replaces it; however, for a time, both cristobalite and tridymite may be present.

The rate of conversion of quartz to cristobalite is important and strongly influenced by two factors:

1. The degree of subdivision of quartz: At the same temperature, large homogeneous crystals convert extremely slowly, whereas similar crystals reduced to a fine powder are transformed much more rapidly.
2. Temperature: The rate of conversion is not appreciable at temperatures of less than 1000°C and does not become rapid until they exceed 1470°C. At 1160°C, complete conversion takes 6 days, whereas at 1570°C, it takes 1 hour. These rates of change are in line with the usual exponential increase in speed of a chemical reaction with temperature, but the presence of foreign substances may have accelerating or delaying effects on conversion.

Thus, whether heated alone or with added substances, quartz may be expected to transform into cristobalite at any temperature over 1000°C, but the change is only stable and permanent above 1470°C (Figure A.1).

In summary, if given appropriate conditions of temperature and time, conversion of quartz to cristobalite or tridymite may occur in a variety of industrial processes. Examples of possible sources are fired silica (refractory) bricks and other highly siliceous ceramic products, fired insulation bricks, used refractory bricks and foundry sands and straight and flux calcined diatomite.

The occurrence of these polymorphs of silica under such industrial conditions is important insofar as cristobalite and tridymite are at least as fibrogenic as quartz, if not more so. Indeed, King et al. (1953) showed that, in rats exposed to fused (amorphous) silica, quartz, cristobalite and tridymite of high purity and equal particle size, the rate of development and the severity of fibrosis were least with fused silica, greater in ascending order with quartz and cristobalite and greatest with tridymite, the effect of which was described as 'spectacular'.

Cristobalite is specifically manufactured for a variety of refractory purposes, including investment castings, to increase dimensional accuracy and to compensate for shrinkage of the metal being cast.

At this juncture, it should be noted that stable phases of well-crystallized cristobalite, together with mullite, may be produced, in the absence of quartz, from aluminium silicates such as kaolinite, andalusite, kyanite and sillimanite at high temperatures.

Crypto (Micro) Crystalline Silica

This polymorph of silica, also referred to as 'chalcedonic silica', originates from silica derived from the skeletons of a variety of marine animals, including sponges—so-called biogenic silica. Densely packed, interlocking microscopic crystals are cemented together by amorphous silica. Its three main varieties are flint, chalcedony and jasper. Flint and chert, which is closely similar to flint but normally exhibits less microcrystalline quartz, occur in calcareous rocks in the form of nodules, layers and irregular concretions. Chalcedony occurs in a large number of sub-varieties distinguished chiefly by colour, specifically agate, cornelian, bloodstone and onyx. Jasper is a mixture of microcrystalline silica with clay and iron oxides. Similarly to quartz, all of these varieties undergo inversion to cristobalite with heat, but between 1200°C and 1400°C, the rate of change of flint and chert is, in general, greater than that of pure, crystalline quartz.

Amorphous (Non-Crystalline) Silica

Diatomaceous silica or kieselguhr is the form of amorphous silica that is most relevant to pulmonary disease. It, too, is of biogenic origin, being formed mainly of the siliceous skeletons of diatoms, but various stages of transformation to micro-crystallisation are found in some older deposits (see 'Siliceous deposits' section). It converts to cristobalite at all temperatures between 1000°C and 1723°C. In a pure, dry state, its conversion to tridymite does not seem to occur between 867°C and 1470°C, but it does so in the presence of a flux or water. A flux also facilitates the formation of stable cristobalite at significantly lower temperatures than in its absence (see Chapter 12, p. 326).

Vitreous (fused) silica is formed when any of the other polymorphs are melted (i.e. at temperatures over 1723°C) and quickly cooled. It then remains stable, but if heated for a prolonged period at temperatures over 1150°C (common in many refractories), it devitrifies (re-crystallises) to cristobalite.

TYPES OF ROCK DEFINED

Because free silica is the principal rock-forming constituent, the proportions in which it is present determine the nature of many rocks. There are three great classes of rocks:

1. Igneous
2. Sedimentary
3. Metamorphic

Igneous Rocks

Igneous rocks are the primary rocks of the crust that were formed from magma either by rapid extrusion of magma onto the Earth's surface or by intrusion of magma within the crust; in the first case, cooling occurred quickly and, in the second, slowly. The rate of cooling determines the size of the rock crystals: the quicker the cooling, the smaller the crystals; the slower the process, the larger the crystals. Granite is an important example that varies in texture from micro-crystalline to very coarsely crystalline.

Sedimentary Rocks

Sedimentary rocks are formed in one of two ways:

1. By the gradual breakdown of pre-existing igneous or older sedimentary and metamorphic rocks (see next section) by the action of wind, sun, water, frost and ice in weathering and corrosion processes to form deposits of debris such as sand and mud. The resulting material, in most cases, is transported as solid particles or in solution and deposited at a distance from its origin. Hard and persistent minerals, such as quartz and cristobalite, remain unchanged, whereas less stable feldspars and ferromagnesian minerals decompose to produce clay minerals (hydrous aluminosilicates), iron and manganese hydroxides and solutions containing calcium, magnesium, sodium and potassium ions, which are essential in the formation of non-silicate, rock-forming minerals.
2. By the deposition in former seas or swamps of the shells of marine organisms, rotting vegetation and chemical substances.

As a rule, sedimentary rocks are laid down in layers, or strata, which differ significantly in composition and grain size. Slow or cataclysmic earth movements alter the levels of these accumulations and new sediments are deposited on top of them, squeezing out their water and compressing them into rocks such as sandstone, limestone and coal.

Metamorphic Rocks

Metamorphism implies change of form, structure and constitution in already-existing igneous and sedimentary rocks. This change is brought about in one of four ways:

1. By a local and substantial rise in temperature caused by the intrusion of magma, which bakes the neighbouring rocks (thermal metamorphism)
2. By movement of the crust, which applies shearing or thrusting forces to the rocks and so distorts them such that the formation of new minerals results (dynamic metamorphism)
3. By percolation of hot water through rocks and steam and gases through the magma, which causes important chemical changes (hydrothermal metamorphism)
4. By a combination of thermal and dynamic metamorphism (regional metamorphism)

Composition

For the most part, all such rocks are composed of silicate minerals; that is, silicon dioxide in various combinations with the oxides of other elements such as aluminium, calcium, iron, magnesium and potassium. The proportion of silica that was available in the original magma determined the form that igneous rocks were to take, and this proportion varied from approximately 30% to 75%.

Where the percentage of silicon dioxide was very low, iron and magnesium, which have a strong affinity for it, combined with all that was available, especially if they were predominant among the cations. This gave rise to the 'ferromagnesian' group of minerals (such as the olivine group). When a large quantity of uncombined iron remained, this was deposited as iron ore; when the percentage of silica was of intermediate order, iron and magnesium again combined with it, but if their concentration was low, aluminium, potassium, sodium and calcium combined with the available remaining silica to produce the feldspar group of minerals. Where the percentage of silicon was high, all available cations were absorbed and an excess of silica was left, which crystallised as quartz.

Acid and Basic Rocks

Silica-rich magmas are termed 'acid' and those that contain little silica but large quantities of bases, such as aluminium, iron and magnesium, are termed 'basic'. Four magma types are distinguished according to their content—or percentage—of combined silica. Thus:

- Acid: More than approximately 66% silica
- Intermediate: From approximately 52% to 66% silica
- Basic: From approximately 45% to 52% silica
- Ultrabasic: Less than approximately 45% silica

The more acid the rock, therefore, the more free silica it contains. The proportions of free silica in any rock can only be expressed in general terms. Among the igneous rocks, the quartz content of the acid group (chiefly the granite family) may be as much as 30%. In rocks of the intermediate group, it may be negligible in some, but as much as 5% in others, and in basic and ultrabasic rocks, it is usually very low or absent (see Table A.1).

CLASSIFICATION OF IGNEOUS ROCK-FORMING MINERALS

According to the ways in which magma penetrated or invaded all kinds of rocks, igneous rocks fall into two main divisions—intrusive and extrusive—which can be classified according to the minerals they contain. All, apart from quartz and small amounts of iron oxides, are silicates formed in magma during its gradual cooling. The most important and characteristic are described in the following sections (Table A.1).

Intrusive Rocks

Quartz Group

As has been pointed out already, when silica is present in abundance and all other substances have entered into combination with it, a variable amount remains and crystallises as quartz. This almost pure free silica is found in such important igneous rocks as quartz porphyry, rhyolite and granite. Hence, the sedimentary and metamorphic rocks that were subsequently formed from them also have a high content of silica.

Feldspar Group

Members of this group are the most common of all the rock-forming minerals and are the most important constituents of igneous rocks. They are anhydrous potassium, sodium and calcium aluminium silicates or various combinations of all three; they may comprise as much as 75% of granite. There are two main varieties:

1. Orthoclase feldspars, which are rich in potassium and usually occur in acid rocks with a high percentage of quartz.
2. Plagioclase feldspars, which contain variable proportions of sodium and calcium. Sodium plagioclases occur in more acid rocks and are, therefore, frequently associated with orthoclase, whereas calcium plagioclases are found in basic rocks.

TABLE A.1
A Classification of the Igneous Rocks

Mode of Occurrence	Proportion of Combined Silica (SiO_2)				
	>60% (Acid)	52%–66% (Intermediate)		45%–52% (Basic)	<45% (Ultrabasic)
Volcanic lavas	Rhyolite Obsidian Pitchstone	Trachyte	Andesite	Basalt	
Minor intrusions	Microgranite Quartz–porphyry	Microsyenite	Microdiorite	Dolerite	
Major intrusions	Granite	Syenite	Diorite	Gabbro	Periodolite Dunite Serpentinite
Essential minerals	Quartz Hornblende and/or mica Feldspar (orthoclase or sodium-rich plagioclase)	Hornblende or augite Feldspar (orthoclase or sodium-rich plagioclase)	Augite or hornblende Feldspar (calcium-rich plagioclase)	Olivine Augite Feldspar (plagioclase)	Olivine Augite Hornblende

Source: Reproduced from Bradshaw, M. J. 1968. *A New Geology*. London: The English Universities Press, with permission of Hodder & Stoughton Ltd.

Thus, at the acid end of the series, feldspars contain significant amounts of quartz and, at the basic end, they contain little or none.

As the feldspar minerals that are employed in the ceramic industries are silica rich, they have been an important cause of silicosis. However, feldspars that contain no quartz have not been found to be fibrogenic in the lungs of experimental animals (Mohanty et al., 1953; Goldstein and Rendall, 1970).

Feldspathoid Group

Members of this group are composed of the same elements as feldspars, but in different proportions, and they play a similar, although subordinate, role in rock formation. Primary quartz and feldspathoid do not occur together in the same rock. If free silica had been present during formation, it would have combined with feldspathoid to form feldspar.

Micas and Clay Group

This group is generally associated with acid rocks such as granite. The structure of micas is of the sheet lattice type, which gives them their well-known characteristic of cleavage into layers. Important members of the group are biotite, a complex silicate of magnesium, aluminium, potassium and iron found in many igneous and metamorphic rocks, and muscovite (potassium aluminium silicate), the common white mica. Sericite, once thought to be important in the pathogenesis of coal pneumoconiosis, is a secondary muscovite that may be produced by the alteration of orthoclase feldspar. Vermiculite, which possesses important industrial properties, is a natural alteration product of biotite and phlogopite (magnesium) micas.

The clay minerals are related to the micas and are hydrous aluminium silicates of a sheet lattice type formed by the breakdown of feldspars and ferromagnesian minerals. Kaolinite, the chief constituent of china clay, is one of the most important of these.

Pyroxene Group

The pyroxenes are a large group of rock-forming minerals found in intermediate basic and ultrabasic rocks. Augite, a silicate of calcium, magnesium, iron and aluminium, is the most common member.

Amphibole Group

This group, similarly to the pyroxenes, includes a number of important rock-forming minerals, the physical and chemical character of which link them together as one family. All possess the double chain-type silicate structure (Si_4O_{11}). Hornblende, a complex aluminium, calcium, magnesium, iron and sodium silicate, is the most common member of the group. It occurs as a primary mineral in acid and intermediate igneous rocks such as granites and syenites, as well as in many metamorphic rocks derived from igneous rocks; for example, hornblende–schists and hornblende–gneisses. The asbestos minerals actinolite, tremolite, amosite and crocidolite are members of this group.

Olivine Group

Olivines are magnesium iron silicates in which magnesium is in excess of iron in most varieties. Of all the groups, they have the lowest proportion of combined silica, and quartz is either absent or present in very small amounts. Thus, they are generally confined to basic and ultrabasic rocks.

Extrusive Rocks

These are formed from lava flows or from magmatic and rocky material forcibly blown from volcanoes to considerable distances in order to produce beds of pyroclastic rock. They include basalts, dolerites, pumice, pumicite and perlite.

Basalts are the most common, constituting approximately 80% of lava rocks. They consist, in essence, of calcium-rich plagioclase feldspar and augite with or without olivine, and they are divided into two major groups according to the proportion of olivine that they contain: up to 20% in the one that contains no quartz; and little or none in the other, which may contain small quantities of quartz. Basalts are also abundant as intrusive rocks.

Dolerites are similar to basalts but more coarse grained, and occur more in the form of minor intrusions as olivine–dolerite without quartz and as quartz–dolerites.

Both basalt and quartz–dolerites are quarried extensively in central Scotland for dimension stone, asphalt roofing material, road setts, roadstone chips, as concrete aggregate and for tiles and flooring.

Pumice and pumicite consist of frothy, silicic glass that may contain varying amounts of crystalline silica; perlite is a volcanic glass of rhyolitic composition. They are discussed in more detail later.

Crystalline Structure

The order of crystallization of rocks depended primarily on the composition of the magma. For example, in a magma that was rich in silicon dioxide, quartz tended to crystallize first; hence, quartz–porphyries. Similarly, in basic rocks, feldspar often crystallised before pyroxene.

Within the ferromagnesian and feldspar groups, therefore, fairly well-defined sequences are observed. For example:

Ferromagnesian minerals		Feldspars
Olivine	Plagioclase	Calcium feldspar
↓		↓
Pyroxene		Sodium calcium feldspar
↓		↓
Amphibole		Sodium potassium feldspar
↓		
Biotite		

As a general principle, it is worth noting that some minerals cannot occur together in rocks. In particular, quartz is not present either in rocks of the olivine group (other than those that are almost pure iron–olivine) or in the feldspathoid group. Rocks that contain quartz are often classified as 'oversaturated', and those with little or no quartz, but which contain olivine and feldspathoids, as 'undersaturated'.

Non-Silicate Rock-Forming Minerals

Non-silicate minerals are important constituents of certain sedimentary and metamorphic rock types. They fall into the groups that are outlined in the following sections.

Carbonates

These are the predominant non-silicates and they consist of calcite ($CaCO_3$—the chief constituent of limestone), dolomite ($MgCO_3 \cdot CaCO_3$—which constitutes dolomite limestone) and siderite ($FeCO_3$). Marbles are metamorphosed calcite or dolomite. Siderite occurs in some coal measures.

Halides and Sulphates

Rock salt (NaCl), anhydrite ($CaSO_4$) and gypsum ($CaSO_4 \cdot 2H_2O$), which were deposited by evaporation of lakes and land-locked seas, and fluorspar (CaF_2) contain no free silica unless by detrital deposition.

Oxides and Sulphides

These are chiefly iron minerals. The most important of the oxides are magnetite (Fe_3O_4), haematite (Fe_2O_3) and goethite ($Fe_2O_3 \cdot H_2O$). Magnetite, one of the most valuable iron ores, is an accessory mineral in most igneous rocks and in metamorphic deposits in limestones. Haematite occurs in igneous, hydrothermal metamorphic and volcanic rocks. It is found in limestone beds owing to replacement of the limestone by haematite from overlying ferruginous sandstones in various locations; for example, north Lancashire. The largest deposits in the world—in the Lake Superior district of Minnesota—were formed by alteration and concentration of iron silicates of sedimentary origin.

TYPES OF ROCK DESCRIBED

Igneous Rocks

The rate at which the original magma cooled determined the degree and form of its crystallisation and, therefore, the 'texture' or fundamental structure of the igneous rock.

Intrusive rocks are subdivided into minor intrusions, which are fairly near the surface of the crust, and major intrusions, which lie deep below the surface. More than 600 varieties of igneous rocks have been described, but they can all be placed in a few large groups, as shown in Table A.1.

Intrusive rocks reach the surface of the crust through the action of earth movements and the erosion and disruption of overlying rocks.

Sedimentary Rocks

Sedimentary rocks fall broadly into three categories, according to their origin: fragmental (mechanical) origin; non-fragmental organic origin; and non-fragmental chemical origin (Figure A.2).

Fragmental Rocks

As the chief ingredients of fragmental rocks were produced mechanically by attrition and erosion, they are classed according to the nature and size of the fragments.

Rudaceous (Rubbly) Rocks

These are composed of granules, pebbles or boulders that, when rounded by wear, produce conglomerates, but if angular, they are called breccias. The fragments are cemented together by a mineral such as secondary silica, leached out from elsewhere, or by mud.

Arenaceous (Sandy) Rocks

The raw materials of these are sands and silts cemented by siliceous and clay substances. The chief members of this group are the sandstones and they are composed predominantly of quartz grains.

Origin	Group character	Type	Main features of composition
Fragmental (mechanical) origin	Rudaceous	Conglomerate	Quartz content similar to parent rock; iron oxides (e.g. limonite and haematite); sometimes calcite or dolomite.
		Breccia	Mixed rock fragments; calcite and limonite with fine silt or mud in matrix.
	Arenaceous	Sandstone	Quartz, muscovite and feldspar rock particles cemented by siliceous, ferruginous, calcareous, argillaceous and carbonaceous matter.
		Grilstone	Similar to sandstone; particle slightly different in shape.
		Arkose	Sandstone or gritstone subjected to contact metamorphism and approximately 25% feldspars of various sorts. Siliceous and ferruginous content.
		Quartzite	Sandstone or gritstone subjected to contact metamorphism, and detrital quartz cemented by secondary silica.
		Ganister	Highly siliceous. Quartz, cherts, orthoclase, feldspar, clay minerals such as kaolinite ($Al_2Si_2O_5[OH]_4$). Haematite and limonite are accessory minerals.
		Sillstone	Fine-grained, compact detritus from rivers, lakes and glacial action. Quartz, muscovite, feldspars and iron ores with siliceous, ferruginous and calcareous cementing material.
	Argillaceous	Clay	Fine-grained, earthy material, plastic when wet; hard when dry. Consists of orthoclase and plagioclase feldspars, muscovite and occasionally a little quartz[a].
		Fuller's earth	Mainly montmorillonite ($[Mg \cdot Ca]O \cdot Al_2O_3 \cdot 5SiO_2[5–8]H_2O$)—calcium smectite—but also small amounts of feldspar, mica, glauconite and apatite may be present. Quartz is rare except in intercalated sand layers.
		Volcanic clay	Bentonite: Sodium montmorillonite (sodium smectite) with quartz, cristobalite, feldspar, mica, apatite and ferromagnesian minerals.
		Residual clay	Formed in situ from rock decomposition. Very finely divided; for example, bauxite (hydrous aluminium oxides) and china clay (kaolin)[b].
		Mudstone Fireclay	Consolidated, non-fissile clay with similar constituents. Usually from beneath coal seams ('seatearths'). Content of quartz variable, often secondary.
			Contains quartz, feldspars, mica, secondary silica and iron compounds. Quartz content high.
		Shale	Indurated, laminated, fine-grained clay mineral matter; contains quartz, mica, iron ores, secondary silica, calcite and iron oxides. Quartz content up to 30%.
	Calcareo-argillaceous	Marl	Unconsolidated, non-laminated calcareous clay. Composition as clays, but more calcareous materials as matrix. Quartz content small and variable.
		Calcareous shale	Consolidated, laminated clay with such calcareous material (i.e. consolidated marl with similar composition).
Organic origin	Calcareous	Limestone	$CaCO_3$ mainly of organic origin (e.g. corals, crustaceans, molluscs, algae and foraminifera), occasionally iron ores. Very small quantities of free silica may be present.
		Dolomite	Limestone with a large quantity of $Ca \cdot Mg(CO_3)_2$, much of organic origin; also variable haematite.
		Oolitic and pisolitic limestone	Limestone, more chemical than sedimentary in origin, with large characteristic grains of $CaCO_3$ found in successive layers around a nucleus of shell fragments or quartz grains. ('Grains' resemble fishroe or peas.) Small and variable amounts of free silica.
		Chalk	Almost pure $CaCO_3$. No free silica, but nodules of flint in some chalk deposits.
	Siliceous	Chert and flint	Crystalline and cryptocrystalline silica (microcrystalline quartz) often aggregated into 'nodules' in chalk. Very high free silica content with traces of limonite.
		Siliceous deposits	Mainly organic in origin. Diatomite: Amorphous silica content 60%–90%; cristobalite and quartz integrated from volcanic ash in some deposits. Sinter: Chemical precipitation of amorphous and cryptocrystalline silica from solution.
	Carbonaccous	Carbonaceous rocks	Peat, lignite, bituminous and anthracite coals. Variable amounts of quartz, iron mineral ores (pyrite, siderite and limonite) and clays (e.g. kaolinite) and illite. Oil shale: Combination of essentially sedimentary shale and varying amounts of carbonaceous matter. Contains abundant quartz and mica; 'kerogen' and, sometimes, feldspar and rutile.
			Asphalt, asphaltic bitumen and bituminous impregnations. Mixtures of different hydrocarbons usually as black or brown, pitchy materials; impregnations mainly in limestones in certain locations, as well as in sandstones and shales. Thus, quartz is either absent or abundant according to origin.

FIGURE A.2 Classification of some common sedimentary rocks. [a]The majority of true clays contain very little free silica, and what there is depends upon the nature of the parent rock. Clays with particle size greater than 2 μm may contain a small quantity (occasionally up to 10%), but those of smaller particle size contain an insignificant quantity. [b]'Free silica' refers to crystalline or cryptocrystalline forms unless otherwise stated. (Adapted from Milner, H. B. 1962. *Sedimentary Petrography. Vol. 2*. London: Allen and Unwin. With permission.)

(Continued)

	Group character	Type	Main features of composition
Chemical origin	Calcareous	Calcium carbonate (calcitc)	$CaCO_3$, but some impurity such as limonite. Traces of free silica, detrital and rare.
		Dolomite (partly)	Occurring as mineral, not limestone replacement. $Ca \cdot Mg(CO_3)_2$ with some iron impurities.
	Ferrugineous	Bedded iron ores	From aqueous solutions in mudstones, limestones, primary haematite, magnesite. Variable quartz content.
		Bog iron ores	Small amounts of detrital quartz.
	Saline	Chlorides	Mainly rock salt (NaCl) with various impurities but no quartz. Carnellite ($KMgCl_3 \cdot 6H_2O$)—used as fertiliser and source of potash; quartz absent.
		Sulphates	Barytes ($BaSO_4$), celestite ($SrSO_4$), anhydrite ($CaSO_4$), alunite ($KAl_3[SO_4]_2[OH]_6$), apatite ($Ca_5[FCl][PO_4]_3$) and gypsum ($CaSO_4 \cdot 2H_2O$). Rarely free of some mineral impurity from sands, marls, clays, shales and limestones; thus, small quantities of quartz may be present, but are more substantial in some gypsum formations.

FIGURE A.2 (*Continued*) Classification of some common sedimentary rocks. [a]The majority of true clays contain very little free silica, and what there is depends upon the nature of the parent rock. Clays with particle size greater than 2 μm may contain a small quantity (occasionally up to 10%), but those of smaller particle size contain an insignificant quantity. [b]'Free silica' refers to crystalline or cryptocrystalline forms unless otherwise stated. (Adapted from Milner, H. B. 1962. *Sedimentary Petrography. Vol. 2*. London: Allen and Unwin. With permission.)

Argillaceous (Clayey) Rocks

These consist essentially of naturally plastic clay minerals, but they may also contain significant quantities of free silica derived from older quartz-bearing rocks (detrital quartz). They are laid down as clays and, when consolidated, become rocks known as mudstones and shales. Clays or a mixture of clay and non-clay minerals have considerable commercial importance. They can be considered under two broad headings: clays and mudstones.

Clays These are composed of single clay minerals, the most important of which, industrially, are china clay (known internationally as kaolin), fuller's earth and bentonite. The significant amount of quartz often present in raw china clay and kaolin is an undesirable impurity in most industrial processes (e.g. the manufacture of paper) and is therefore removed, principally by washing with water. The quantity of quartz present in fuller's earth and bentonite varies, but for the most part is small.

Although most deposits of china clay worldwide are sedimentary in origin, the deeper deposits in Cornwall and Devon are of hydrothermal metamorphic origin from granite and thus have different physical characteristics and composition.

Mudstones These are indurated, massive argillaceous sediments that have the texture and composition of shales, but lack their fine lamination and fissility. Both mudstones and shales may contain substantial amounts of quartz.

Unbedded mudstones associated with coal-bearing (carbonaceous) strata are sometimes called 'fireclays', which have been widely exploited in the past for their refractory properties. In British geological terminology, these mudstones, in general, are referred to as seatearths, the composition of which varies widely from almost pure clay rocks (i.e. seatclays), through silty and sandy sediments, to quartz-rich sandstones that, until recently, were also valued as refractory materials (the so-called 'ganisters'). In North America, the term 'underclay' is used to describe clay-rich seatearths. Today, the term 'fireclay', in general, describes seatclays that are of economic interest. They consist of kaolinite, mica and quartz, in varying proportions, with some impurities such as ironstone nodules and carbonaceous matter. Because of their physicochemical properties, fireclays have commercial value for both refractory and non-refractory applications. An essential constituent of fireclays is kaolinite. It is predominant in refractory fireclays, but present in approximately equal proportions with mica and quartz in non-refractory fireclays. Thus, it is kaolinite that confers the valuable refractory properties, whereas clays that contain higher proportions of quartz and mica have important non-refractory applications; for example, in the manufacture of vitrified clay pipes, facing bricks, stoneware, sanitary ware and floor and wall tiles (Highley, 1982).

It is convenient, at this point, to consider the effects of heating fireclays and the resultant mineralogical changes that occur. These are also a paradigm for some other aluminium silicates. The overall chemical equation for the stable phases when kaolinite is heated at temperatures of approximately 1550°C is:

$$\underset{\text{Kaolinite}}{3[Al_2(SiO_5)(OH)_4]} \rightarrow \underset{\text{Mullite}}{3Al_2O_3 \cdot 2SiO_2} + \underset{\text{Cristobalite}}{4SiO_2} + 6H_2O$$

The refractoriness of fireclays is mainly determined by the Al_2O_3:SiO_2 ratio. The effects of differences or changes in this ratio and the temperatures applied are shown in Figure A.3, which is also relevant to other aluminium silicate minerals. The lowest temperatures—1595°C—at which complete melting occurs (i.e. the eutectic) corresponds to a composition of 92.5% by weight SiO_2 and 7.5% by weight Al_2O_3. With increasing alumina and silica, refractoriness increases. Calcined kaolinite containing a maximum of approximately 45% Al_2O_3 is the chief source of alumina in fireclay. For aluminium silicates in general, containing between 7.5% and 72% Al_2O_3, pure mullite is formed between 1595°C and 1850°C (the melting point of mullite), and its needle-shaped crystals occur in a viscous liquid. As the content of alumina falls and temperature increases, more of the liquid phase is formed. Because the crystals of mullite are hard and elongated, their presence in a refractory product denotes a well-fired body: the more it contains, the greater the density and strength of the body, and the better its refractory properties. However, this simple relationship between alumina content and refractoriness is complicated by the presence of alkalis (K_2O, Na_2O), alkaline earths (CaO, MgO) and iron oxide (FeO), which can significantly lower the temperature of the initial formation of the liquid phase and thus greatly reduce the refractoriness of the fireclay. Formation of the liquid phase, for example, begins at 985°C in a mix of K_2O–Al_2O_3–SiO_2. Therefore, a simple model based solely on the content of alumina is not valid when fluxes are present (Highley, 1982).

Cristobalite is seldom present in structural clay products and does not form from the kaolinite of Cornish clay when heated to high temperatures because of its high alkali content, which produces a glass phase instead.

The term 'fuller's earth' refers to clay that has been extracted in Britain since Roman times and is used primarily for cleaning and adsorbing natural oils from woollen cloth (i.e. 'fulling') until the latter part of the nineteenth century. Many clays, and sometimes silts, were used for this purpose and thus became known as 'fuller's earths'. However, modern analytical methods for the identification of clay minerals have shown that the most effective fuller's earths are those that contain a high proportion of clay minerals of the smectite group (i.e. layered silicate clay minerals that are distinct from the mica group), the most commonly occurring member of which is montmorillonite, the essential constituent of fuller's earth in Britain.

There are additional reasons for terminological confusion. The most effective fulling clays are those that

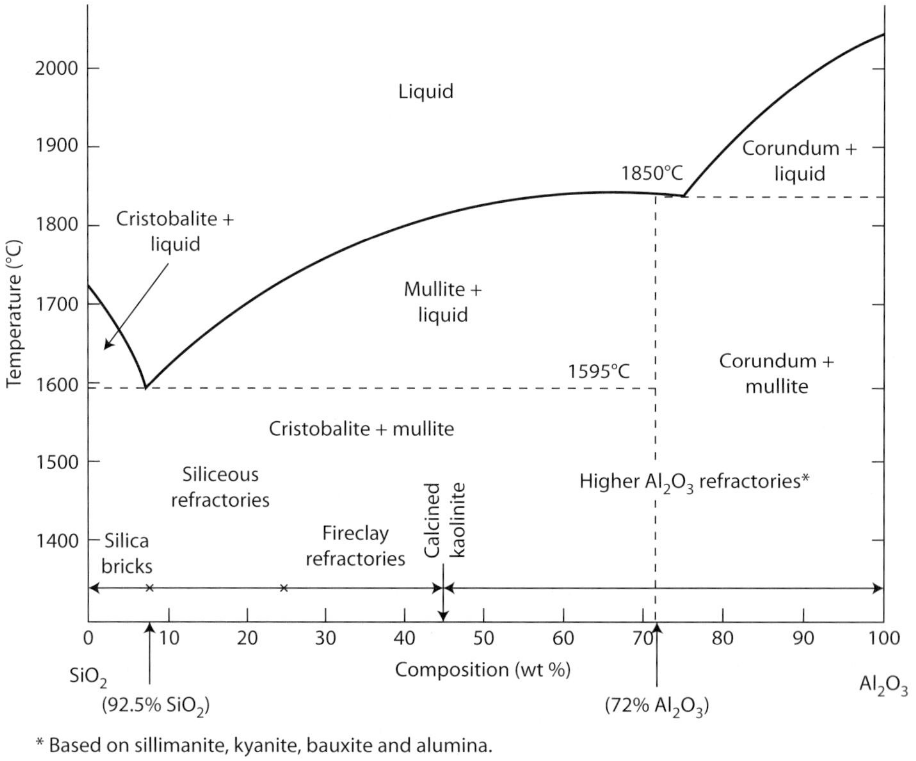

FIGURE A.3 Phase diagram for the Al_2O_3:SiO_2 binary system, broadly illustrating the behaviour of refractory aluminium silicates according to temperature and relative content of Al_2O_3 and SiO_2. (Reproduced from Highley, D. E. 1982. *Fireclay. Mineral Dossier No. 24*. London: HMSO. And after Aramaki, S. and Roy, R. 1959. *J Am Ceram Soc* 42:644–45. With permission.)

are rich in montmorillonite, which contains loosely bonded exchangeable cations, usually calcium, magnesium and sodium. Depending upon the dominant cation present, the clay, either as calcium smectite or sodium smectite, has markedly different properties and thus different industrial applications. In Britain, clay consisting mainly of calcium montmorillonite is known as fuller's earth, while clay containing mainly sodium montmorillonite is known as bentonite. There are two geological formations in Britain in which clays consist essentially of calcium smectite (more than 60%) and are referred to as fuller's earth: the Jurassic Fuller's Earth Formation and the Lower Greensand. The former, which is generally of lower quality, was worked by underground mining near Bath (Somerset) until 1979, and the latter in Surrey (Redhill), Bedfordshire and Oxfordshire by open pit methods. Outside Britain, the term 'bentonite' is used to describe montmorillonite-rich clays irrespective of the dominant cation present. Sodium montmorillonite is comparatively rare worldwide, although large deposits occur in the western USA. Fortunately, however, calcium montmorillonite can easily be converted to sodium montmorillonite by a simple sodium-exchange process. Montmorillonite-rich clays are the alteration products of volcanic ash. In countries other than Britain, particularly the USA, the term 'fuller's earth' applies to any clay that has the capacity to decolourise oil, and may consist of either montmorillonite or attapulgite (palygorskite)—another clay mineral so named because it was found at Attapulgus, in Georgia, USA. Originally, these clays were developed as substitutes for fuller's earth imported from England. Both attapulgite and its magnesium analogue, sepiolite, are imported into Britain for use as granular adsorbents (Moorlock and Highley, 1991).

Differences and misunderstandings regarding the nomenclature undoubtedly help to explain the disparity in reports as to whether or not fuller's earth can cause pulmonary fibrosis. It is important, therefore, to recognise that fuller's earths of comparable grade, but from different localities, may exhibit appreciably different properties. The applied properties of an individual clay are dependent on the crystal structure of the clay mineral, itself a function of the geological history of the deposit, as well as on the nature and amount of impurities present (Moorlock and Highley, 1991). The presence of such impurities, which include quartz, varies widely in different deposits. They are, as a rule, removed by beneficiation from the final products.

Ball clays also consist of kaolinite, mica and quartz and have similar mixed mineral assemblages to fireclays. They are more plastic than fireclays and are white, or near-white, on firing due to their low iron content, which makes them suitable for the manufacture of whiteware ceramics—their major application.

Shales are indurated clay rocks that are characterised by a poorly laminated structure that is parallel to the beading planes along which they split. They represent a further stage in the consolidation of clay, mud and organic remains, and include black, carbonaceous shales, associated with coal measures, and oil shales that contain bitumen and a rubbery hydrocarbon called 'kerogen' derived from deposits of aquatic organisms and small plants. When heated to approximately 500°C, kerogen decomposes to produce shale oil, light hydrocarbon gases and a coke-like carbon residue.

All shales contain varying—and sometimes large—quantities of detrital quartz. For example, in some coal measure shales, it may exceed 20%; in the Green River Formation oil shales in Colorado, Utah and Wyoming, it is reported to range from 10% to 20%, and in the shales used for the manufacture of bricks, pipes and similar materials, it may be as much as 60%.

Non-Fragmental Rocks of Organic Origin

Limestones

These are chiefly of organic origin and consist mostly of calcium carbonate. Small amounts of magnesium carbonate are often present, but when this reaches significant proportions, the rock is referred to as dolomitic limestone or dolomite. Many different types of organism have contributed to their formation, including, among others, corals, crustaceans, foraminifera, molluscs and algae. The calcium carbonate of some limestones, however, is entirely of chemical origin. In general, they do not contain any free silica, but small amounts are sometimes present as an impurity. However, flint also occurs as nodules in some chalk deposits, as well as chert in some limestone deposits.

Tripoli, rottenstone and wollastonite are found in association with limestones and have a wide variety of applications in industry.

Tripoli is a microcrystalline, very finely grained, particulate form of silica (more than 89% silica) that results from the leaching and weathering of siliceous limestone or calcareous chert. Particles commonly range from 1 to 10 μm in diameter. It should be noted that, commercially, it has sometimes been wrongly referred to as 'amorphous silica', although none has been detected by X-ray or scanning electron microscope analysis (Bradbury and Ehrlinger, 1975). Either underground or open-cast methods of mining are used for its extraction, according to the type and location of the deposit.

Tripoli has many uses: As an abrasive in soaps and cleaning powders; in polishing compounds; as a filler and extender in paints, plastics and rubber; for refractories, ceramic glazes and foundry facings; and as a filler in wallboards and plastic wood.

Rottenstone is a siliceous–argillaceous limestone from which calcium carbonate has been removed in solution. It contains up to 15% quartz and 85% alumina, and has been used in industry as a refractory material and filler.

Wollastonite is a naturally occurring calcium melasilicate ($CaSiO_3$) formed mainly by contact metamorphism of quartz-bearing limestone and by silica-bearing emanations from igneous intrusions (often granite) reacting with pure or impure limestone. It is used in some countries as a substitute for flint, quartz, sand, feldspar and china clay in ceramic-bonded abrasives, as well as in other industries.

Carbonaceous Rocks

Coal Coal is an extremely heterogeneous substance, consisting largely of carbon, hydrogen, oxygen and nitrogen, which is difficult to characterise. In essence, it is composed of a number of distinct organic entities, known as 'macerals', and smaller, but important, amounts of minerals. These occur in distinct associations known as lithotypes. The basic units—coal seams—in which coal is found consist of layers of coal lithotypes; individual seams often have a unique set of physical and chemical properties. Even if two coal seams have a similar composition of macerals and minerals, the seams may have significantly different properties if the lithotypes in the two seams differ (Crelling, 1989). Coal seams comprise a small proportion (1%–2%) of the Upper Carboniferous rocks and are known as coal measures.

Coals are the products of progressive change ('coalification') in accumulations of rotting vegetation (trees, ferns and giant club mosses) in swampy conditions. These are subsequently overlaid by deposits of sediment from inundation from rivers, lakes or seas, resulting in layers of sandstones, clays, shales and limestones. Accumulated sediment consolidates the vegetable debris and squeezes out water to form coal of progressively increasing maturity as depth increases. The organic-rich, petrographic components produced by progressive rotting of macerated vegetation—the macerals just referred to—can be regarded as the organic counterparts of the mineral matter in coal. A large number of macerals have been defined. They are derived from different parts of plants and trees degraded under critical conditions, and are optically homogeneous aggregates with distinctive physical and chemical properties. There are, however, three main groups: vitrinites, liptinites and inertines. Most of these contain between 73% and 85% carbon, with more widely differing quantities of hydrogen and oxygen.

The degree of maturity of coal is referred to, and classified, as rank. All coal begins as peat, which is then changed into progressively higher ranks—lignite, sub-bituminous, bituminous and anthracite coals. This transformation occurs in two phases: the first at the peat stage, when most of the plant material in the peat is biochemically altered (diagenesis), although spores and pollens survive without much change; and the second, during which altered peat is buried and subjected to the geological forces of temperature, pressure and time. Temperature, which rises with increasing depth and pressure, is the chief factor in coalification, which takes place between 50°C and 150°C and results in devolatisation and the formation of bituminous and higher-rank coals.

As rank of coal increases, most of its properties change: moisture, volatile matter and ultimate oxygen decrease; fixed and ultimate carbon, calorific value and reflectance increase. Reflectance of coal is a characteristic based upon the amount of light that is reflected from vitrinite macerals in the coal under examination compared with a glass standard of known refractive index and reflectance. All of these properties have been used as measures of rank, but reflectance is the most reliable because, unlike the others, it changes uniformly across most of the coal rank range (Crelling, 1989). However, in medical research, the definition of rank that is normally used is the ratio of carbon to volatile matter in the coal—the so-called fuel ratio. In high-rank anthracite, the content of carbon is high (approximately 92%–95%), and that of volatile substances very low; at the other end of the scale, low-rank lignite contains much less carbon (65%–75%), but a greater quantity of volatile substances (Table A.2).

Although spore cases—either empty or filled with mineral matter—may have survived intact in some coals, organic matter with immunogenic potential does not appear to exist in bituminous or anthracite coals.

Coal contains considerable quantities of important minerals that decrease as rank increases, due to leaching, but are never absent even in coal of the highest rank. They are deposited both during its formation in peat swamps by influx of mineral-containing waters and, in some regions, by fall-out of volcanic ash, and, after it has been formed, also as a result of seepage of mineral-containing waters from a distance. The amounts present vary widely, but commercial coal, in general, must contain less than 10% mineral matter as ash. The most common accessory minerals are clays, quartz, pyrite and

TABLE A.2
Carbon Content of Coals

Coal Type	Rank	Composition (% Dry Mineral, Matter-Free Basis)		
		Carbon	Hydrogen	Oxygen
Peat		50–65	5–7	30–40
Lignite	(Low)	65–75	5–6	20–30
Sub-bituminous	↓	75–80	5–6	13–20
Bituminous	(Intermediate)	80–90	4.9–5.7	5–15
Semi-bituminous	↓	90–92	4.5–4.9	4–5
Anthracite	(High)	92–95	2–4	2–4

calcite; trace metals are also usually present, but with great variability in their nature and amount in different coal seams and in the same seam. The clay minerals and quartz account for between 60% and 90% of the total non-coal mineral matter in coals; the most common species of clay minerals are muscovite – illites (potassium aluminium silicates), kaolinites (aluminium silicates) and mixed-layer illite – montmorillonites of variable composition (Raask, 1985).

There appears to be no clear correlation between the inorganic content of coals and their maceral composition, which indicates that most minerals were introduced by detrition rather than accumulating as a result of peat degradation. Where a transport mechanism for detritus existed, detrital material occurs in the peat in considerable amounts and thus in varying quantity in the subsequent ranks of coal (Davis et al., 1984). Silica usually occurs in coal seams in the form of discrete, fine grains of quartz and, sometimes, cristobalite from ash fall-out in volcanic regions or chalcedony formed by the weathering of feldspar and mica (Mackowsky, 1968). The clay minerals originated from deposited detritus, transformation of other clay minerals and precipitation of a gel or solution (Davis et al., 1984).

The great variability in the distribution of mineral species in different coal strata was exemplified in coal fields in the east Midlands of the UK Examination of more than 50 seams showed that: quartz, kaolin and mica were the principal non-coal minerals in all seam profiles; quartz was more abundant in roof and floor strata and least abundant in the coal layers and inter-seam strata; the highest concentrations of kaolin occurred in the coal and some inter-seam dirt bands; and 20%–90% of mineral matter in the coal seam consisted of non-silicate minerals (Raask, 1985). The majority of US coals have a quartz content of between 1% and 20% of the total mineral matter, and some coal ashes have over 30% quartz (Raask, 1985).

Accessory minerals in coal, including quartz, are disseminated as discrete particles ranging from submicrometre to more than 1 mm in size, but their mean grain size is approximately 5 μm, so that most of them are near, or below, the resolution of the optical microscope, and they are intimately intermixed with maceral material (Finkelman, 1988). In their identification, it is difficult to recognise fine-grained minerals that are intimately mixed with the coal matter by the petrological microscope. Therefore, carefully controlled low-temperature ashing, which has the advantage of providing a relatively unchanged sample for the identification of its constituent minerals, is employed in order to prepare samples that are substantially free of organic matter. However, the yield of ash is slightly lower than the mineral matter in the coal, chiefly because of losses of water and the gaseous products of the decomposition of some minerals, depending on the temperature of the ashing (Swaine, 1990). A variety of methods for identification is employed. These include scanning electron microscopy (SEM), energy-dispersive X-ray analysis (EDXA), combined SEM–EDXA and infrared spectrophotometry. The SEM–EDXA system appears to be the best for studying accessory minerals and their relationships with macerals in situ (Finkelman, 1988). However, it is important to stress that, although the minerals in coal are readily identified by these techniques, accurate determination of their quantities has not yet been achieved (Crelling, 1989).

Beneficiation of Coal In order to improve the quality of coal for commercial purposes, the removal or lessening of unwanted run-of-mine, non-coal constituents is required; that is, beneficiation. The processes involved are often referred to as 'coal cleaning' or 'coal washing'. It is important to understand exactly what this means because, in the medical literature, it is commonly supposed that washing with water frees coal of all non-coal minerals, producing, in effect, 'pure coal'. The facts are otherwise.

Extraneous run-of-mine dirt and relatively large mineral particles or clusters of minerals are readily removed by washing, but finely divided particles, especially when embedded in coaly matter, are impossible to remove by the methods that are normally used for large-scale beneficiation based on density separations in water (Swaine, 1990). This is due to the fact that the vast majority of mineral matter in coal is insoluble in water, as well as being so intimately mixed with macerals and other coal material that, unless the coal is finely ground (which is generally impractical in industry), most of the mineral matter is inaccessible to water (J. W. Patrick, 1992, personal communication). However, such grinding fails to remove fine-grained particles that are encapsulated in organic coaly matter. For the same reasons, methods of beneficiation that depend on separation by differences in specific gravity are unpredictable (Finkelman and Gluskoter, 1983).

Thus, industrial beneficiation has little, if any, effect on removing small particles of quartz (or other polymorphs of silica) and clay silicates from within coals (J. W. Patrick, 1992, personal communication); trace elements, many of which are associated with the clay minerals, are only partially freed (Swaine, 1990). The definitive separation of coal into coal and non-coal minerals that is often implied in the medical literature is, therefore, an oversimplification that overlooks this intimate relationship.

In laboratory conditions, coal can be very finely milled and treated with hydrochloric and hydrofluoric acids. This 'demineralised' coal has been widely used in coal laboratories for experiments in which mineral matter would interfere significantly (J. W. Patrick, 1992, personal communication). However, such techniques for the production of samples of coal dust for animal experiments do not seem to have been described in the medical literature, although finely ground anthracite ('pulverised coal') has been used in some reported inhalation experiments.

The close association of some coal measures with mudstones (fireclays and ganisters) and shales has been discussed earlier (see 'Argillaceous [Clayey] Rocks' section).

Bitumens These, in essence, are hydrocarbons of the paraffin and naphthalene series, different proportions of which occur in different bitumens. They include members ranging from a very liquid, light yellow oil through gradations to solid bitumens.

Natural Petroleum and Crude Oil These are usually found in sandstones and dolomites and seldom in relation to coal measures. They were probably formed from the remains of minute marine organisms in deep muddy seas. Oil shales have been referred to earlier.

Asphalt or Mineral Pitch This is a mixture of different hydrocarbons that occurs as a black semisolid or solid substance at or near the surface of the earth. It may occur as lakes (notably in Trinidad) or impregnations of sandstones or dolomites (rock asphalt), in which as much as 15% of asphalt may be present. Asphaltic rocks have, until recently, been worked for the extraction of asphalt or for natural paving, flooring and roofing material, especially in the USA, France, Germany and Italy. It is possible that the working of impregnated sandstones (blasting, crushing and grading) may have presented a silica hazard.

Siliceous Deposits

Diatomite

Also referred to as diatomaceous earth and kieselguhr, diatomite is the most important member of the group. It consists principally of the fossilised skeletal remains of diatoms, unicellular aquatic plants of the class Bacillariophyceae, related to the algae, It is, in fact, a rock formed by induration of diatomaceous silica, a biogenic amorphous silica closely resembling opal or hydrous silica ($SiO_2 \cdot nH_2O$), secreted by the walls of the cells of living diatoms. Diatomaceous silica is, however, not entirely pure hydrous silica. Particles of rock-forming minerals may be integrated as part of diatomite rock, with sand, feldspar, clay and volcanic ash being some of the typical contaminants. Indeed, diatomites that are richest in silica are associated with volcanism. Analysis of quarry samples (source not stated) by Vorwald et al. (1949) revealed 75% diatomite, 2%–3% crystalline free silica (of which 2% was quartz and 0.3% cristobalite) and 14% feldspar and clay silicates. Thus, these polymorphs of silica may be present in some natural diatomite deposits. In addition, commercial diatomite may contain fossilised fragments and particles of organisms such as Radiolaria and siliceous sponges (Kadey, 1975).

Diatomite forms in freshwater and marine conditions and is deposited in beds in large, shallow ponds and lakes and in proximity to collections of volcanic ash. It is usually extracted by quarrying or open pit mining, although underground methods are used in some small operations.

Cryptocrystalline Silica

Layers of cryptocrystalline silica formed by chemical precipitation are exemplified by some forms of chalcedonic silica, flint and chert, in which remnants of tests of Radiolaria or sponge spicules are sometimes found, as well as by sinter; that is, formed around the mouths of volcanic geysers and some hot springs.

Non-Fragmental Rocks of Chemical Origin

Saline Deposits

These were formed by precipitation in dried-up, enclosed bodies of salt water from seas and lakes, and they include calcite, rock salt, apatite ($Ca_5F[PO_4]_3$ and $Ca_5Cl[PO_4]_3$), anhydrite ($CaSO_4$), gypsum, carnallite ($KMgCl_3 \cdot 6H_2O$) and a form of calcium carbonate known as aragonite.

Gypsum needs further comment. It was formed in one of three ways:

1. As pure saline residues caused by the evaporation of enclosed basins of sea water, notably in Germany and the USA
2. In association with alterations of limestones to dolomite.
3. As a result of the action of sulphuric acid generated by the decomposition of pyrite on $CaCO_3$ in clays such as mudstones and shales, which, as stated earlier, contain variable amounts of fine-grained quartz—30% being fairly common. Deposits of this type occur in the UK in Sussex and Nottingham, but the associated silica is higher in the former than the latter.

Gypsum occurs mainly in tabular, prismatic or acicular habits, but a variety called satin spar has a silky, fibrous form.

Ferruginous Deposits

Iron from aqueous solutions or iron-storing bacteria is found in two forms, as details below.

Bedded Ironstones These are deposits in which iron was deposited in mudstones and limestones as glauconite (hydrous silicate of iron and potassium), haematite (Fe_2O_3) and limonite ($Fe_2O_3 \cdot H_2O$).

Haematite from overlying ferruginous sandstones replaces the limestone in limestone beds in various geological locations (e.g. in Cumbria and north Lancashire) and thus contains quartz, which may become airborne during underground mining operations. The largest of the world's deposits in Lake Superior District of Minnesota was formed by the alteration and concentration of iron silicates of sedimentary origin. The term 'taconite' was used originally to refer to a hard, fine-grained, banded, iron-bearing rock (not a mineral) in this region, which contains magnetite and haematite or both, either banded or disseminated with cherty rocks. However, in recent years, it has been applied more generally to low-grade, iron–quartz iron ores that can be beneficiated and agglomerated to produce high-grade, iron-containing pellets. Hence, mining and beneficiation of haematite and taconite rock may be associated with exposure to dust containing quartz or chert.

Bog Iron Ore This consists of an impure ferruginous deposit formed in swampy ground and associated with clay, which often underlies it. The mineral composition includes limonite, siderite ($FeCO_3$), iron sulphate and iron silicate. Quartz is usually absent. Limonite and siderite are found in many bituminous coals throughout the world. Siderite forms the clay ironstones that are associated with some coal measures in Britain, notably south Wales, Staffordshire and Durham.

Metamorphic Rocks

Only examples of these rocks that are important in industry are considered. They differ widely in type and origin.

The Asbestos Group

'Asbestos' is a collective term that refers to two large, but different, groups of rock-forming minerals and not to one family, nor to a particular type of rock. It is, rather, a commercial term applied to two groups of silicate minerals—serpentines and amphiboles—that are capable of separating readily into long, thin, strong fibres that have many invaluable properties and industrial applications (Figures A.4 and A.5). The non-fibrous variants of these minerals are not equated with asbestos.

Serpentines

Chrysotile, the sole fibrous variety of the group, has a growth form that is readily distinguishable from the non-asbestos serpentines such as anligorite and lizardite (Table A.3). It is the most abundant type of asbestos. Most chrysotiles formed in ultrabasic rocks in which olivines and pyroxenes were altered to serpentine by hydrothermal action—a process completed by intrusion of acid magma and subsequent further hydrothermal action. Talc and magnetite are common impurities and, in some geological regions (e.g. Quebec, Canada and the Xeros–Troodos area in Cyprus), inter-growths of the amphiboles tremolite and actinolite occur in the ore body. Although tremolite occurs in commercial chrysotile in only small quantities (less than 1%), unlike chrysotile, it is apt to resist leaching and decomposition in biological systems for very long periods of time (Hodgson, 1986).

Amphiboles

The paragenesis of amphibole asbestos (crocidolite, amosite, anthophyllite, tremolite and actinolite) occurred at a higher metamorphic grade than that of chrysotile, thus forming minerals with a lower content of water of crystallisation. Bulk formations of tremolite and

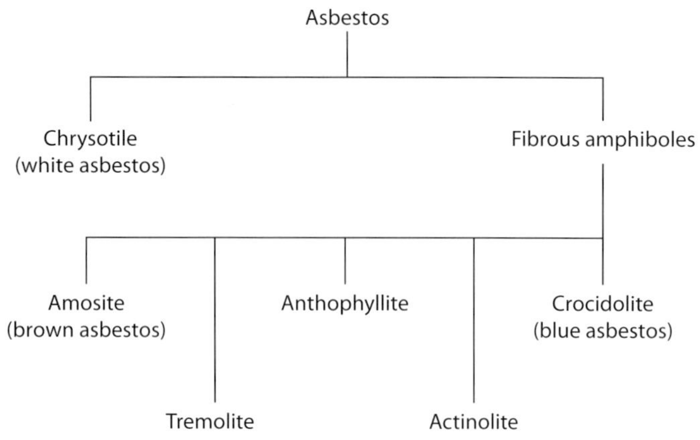

FIGURE A.4 Classification chart of the asbestos minerals.

anthophyllite, and some actinolite, are derived from direct metamorphism of pyroxenites with associated silica by igneous activity, but at the same time, there are localised transitions, particularly to tremolite, in chrysotile-bearing serpentine rocks. Amosite and crocidolite formed in banded ironstones by chemical reaction and crystallisation from original iron hydroxides and colloidal silica under conditions of very high hydrostatic compression and shear. Some actinolite fibre formed in similar conditions.

To mineralogists, the term 'asbestos' implies a pattern of fibrous crystal growth described as the 'asbestiform' or fibrous habit, although these minerals also occur in nature in non-asbestiform (non-fibrous) habit. Whereas chrysotile has a growth and internal crystal structure that is readily distinguishable from non-asbestos, rock-forming serpentines (Zussman, 1957), both the asbestiform and non-asbestiform rock-forming analogues of the amphiboles have the same composition and internal crystal structure; in the cases of tremolite, anthophyllite and actinolite, they have the same names (Table A.3). This, undoubtedly, has sometimes been—and may still be—a source of misinterpretation and error in mineralogical analyses of samples of dust both in the workplace and in the lungs. The basic differences between the two patterns of crystal growth are summarised graphically in Figure A.6, and two examples of microscopic differences are seen in Figure A.7.

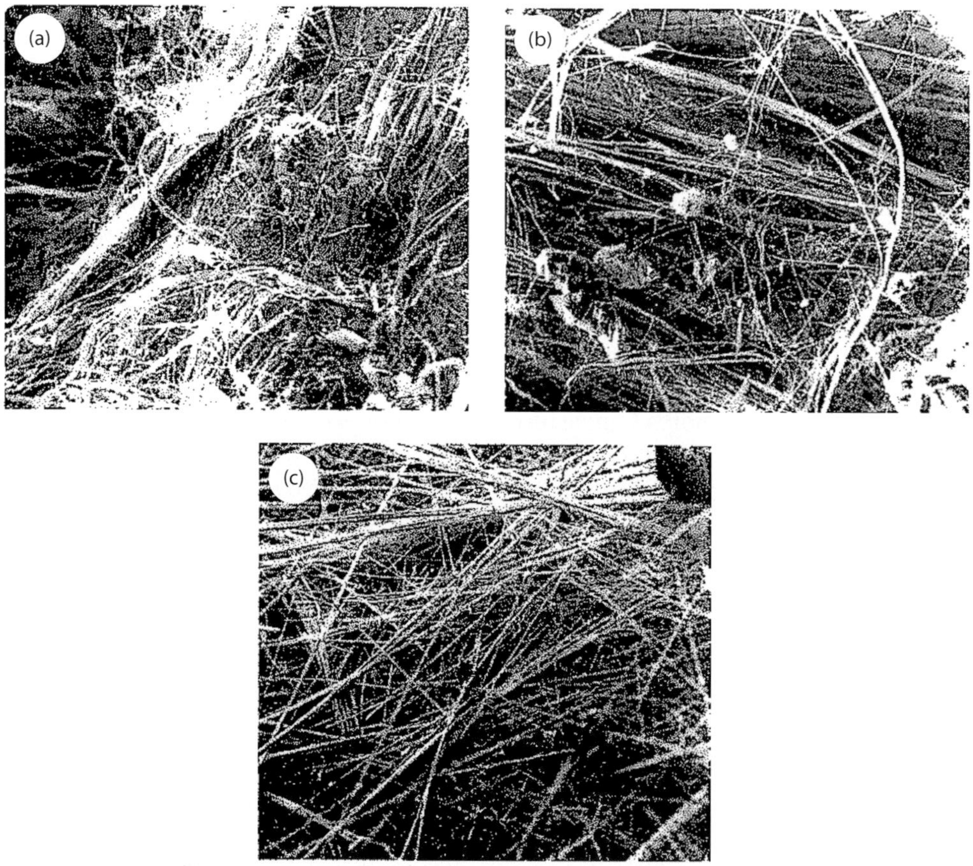

FIGURE A.5 Stereoscan electron micrographs of (a) chrysotile, (b) crocidolite and (c) amosite. Magnification × 550. Compare with electron micrographs in Figure 14.1a–c. (Courtesy of Cape Asbestos Fibers Ltd.)

TABLE A.3
Asbestiform and Non-Asbestiform Varieties of Asbestos

Asbestiform Variety	Chemical Composition	Non-Asbestiform Variety
Serpentine Group		
Chrysotile	$3MgO, 2SiO_3, 2H_2O$	Antigorite, lizardite
Amphibole Group		
Crocidolite	$Na_2O, Fe_2O_3, 3FeO, 8SiO_2, H_2O$	Riebeckite
Grunerite (amosite asbestos)	$5.5FeO, 1.5MgO, 8SiO_2, H_2O$	Cummingtonite–grunerite
Anthophyllite asbestos	$7MgO, 8SiO_2, H_2O$	Anthophyllite
Tremolite asbestos	$2CaO, 5MgO, 8SiO_2, H_2O$	Tremolite
Actinolite asbestos	$2CaO, 4MgO, FeO, 8SiO_2, H_2O$	Actinolite

Source: Reproduced from Kelse, J. W. and Thompson, C. S. 1989. *Am Ind Hyg Assoc J* 50:613–22, by permission of the American Hygiene Association.

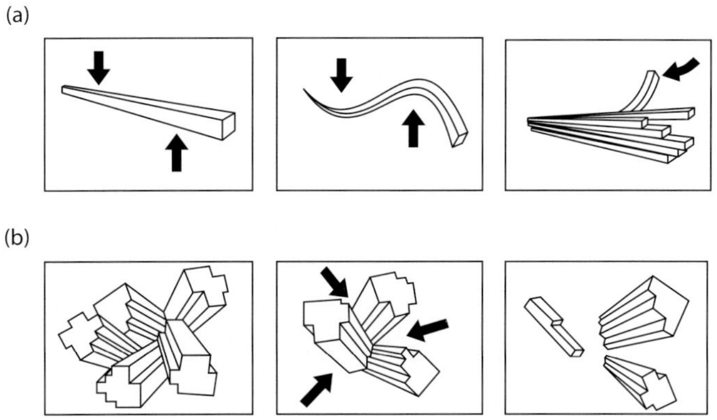

FIGURE A.6 Graphic representation of the distinction between the (a) asbestiform and (b) non-asbestiform habits. (a) In the asbestiform habit, mineral crystals grow in a single dimension, in a straight line, until they form long, thread-like fibres with aspect ratios of 20:1 to 1000:1 and higher. When pressure is applied, the fibres do not shatter, but simply bend much like a wire. Fibrils of a smaller diameter are produced as bundles of fibres and are pulled apart. This bundling effect is referred to as being polyfilamentous. Milling breaks longer into shorter fibres and reduces their diameter. (b) In the non-asbestiform variety, crystal growth is random, forming multi-dimensional prismatic patterns. When pressure is applied, the crystal fractures easily, fragmenting into prismatic particles. Some of the particles or cleavage fragments are acicular or needle shaped as a result of the tendency of amphibole minerals to cleave along the two dimensions, but not along the third. Stair-step cleavage along the edges of some particles is common, and oblique extinction is exhibited under the microscope. Cleavage fragments never show curvature. (Reproduced from Kelse, J. W. and Thompson, C. S. 1989. *Am Ind Hyg Assoc J* 50:613–22, by permission of the American Hygiene Association.)

Rock-forming, non-asbestiform tremolite, anthophyllite and actinolite are of more common occurrence than their asbestiform counterparts.

Asbestos fibres are characterised by high length-to-breadth ratios (aspect ratios), by flexibility (often being curved with splayed ends), by a higher tensile strength than the non-asbestiform habits of the same material and by aggregation in parallel or radiating bundles from which the fibres can easily be separated (Zoltai and Wylie, 1979). A variety of habits occurs in the non-asbestos amphiboles, with the growth forms ranging from blocked, straight-edged laths to acicular (needle-like) particles. As for other rock-forming silicates, they all exhibit prismatic cleavage, the microscopic fragments of which have parallel edges after comminution by grinding. At times, it may be difficult to distinguish these particles from small, short fibres (less than 1 μm in diameter or 5 μm in length)—which also have parallel edges—by optical microscopy, although they are readily differentiated by SEM and transmission electron microscopy (TEM), which render the fibrils making up each fibre visible.

The morphological definition of a fibre given by mineralogists rests on the aspect ratio of the particle being 10:1 or more. The American Society for Testing and Materials, in fact, proposed that mineral particles 'are not demonstrated to be asbestos, in the absence of farther analysis, if their length-to-width ratio is less than 20:1' (Ross et al., 1984); indeed, populations of fibres of asbestiform minerals generally have aspect ratios ranging from 20:1 to 100:1 or higher, and lengths in excess of 5 μm (Kelse and Thompson, 1989), However, differentiation between asbestiform and non-asbestiform amphiboles (cleavage fragments) tends to be blurred when, due to comminution, most of the particles in a sample are less than 1 μm in diameter and 5 μm in length. Even so, cleavage fragments of these minerals are entirely distinct from a similarly sized group of asbestos particles (Pooley, 1987; Langer et al., 1990; Schenk et al., 1990). They can, for example, be differentiated by a systematic approach to the analysis of particles using electron microscopy with selected area electron diffraction (Lee and Fisher, 1979) or high-resolution TEM. If, using such methods, a specimen contains elongated cleavage fragments, some of which have the same widths and lengths as asbestos fibres, 'elongated cleavage fragments will

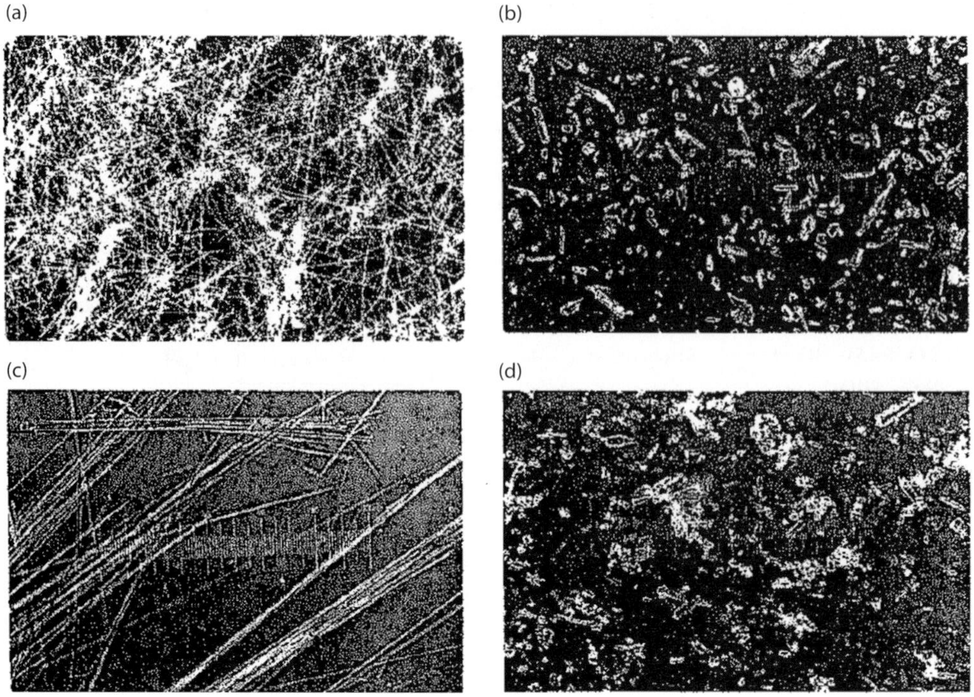

FIGURE A.7 Examples of (a and c) asbestiform and (b and d) non-asbestiform habits in amphiboles with (a and b) different names and (c and d) the same name. (a) Amosite, (b) cummingtonite–grunerite, (c) tremolite and (d) tremolite. Magnification × 265; 2.75 μm per division. (Reproduced from Kelse, J. W. and Thompson, C. S. 1989. *Am Ind Hyg Assoc J* 50:613–22, by permission of the American Hygiene Association.)

have a greater variation in diameter as a function of length than asbestos, tending to have lower aspect ratios' (Langer et al., 1991) (Table A.4).

The morphological difference between asbestiform and non-asbestiform particles is of capital importance in the pathogenesis of disease. However, unfortunately, it has been confused and obscured by a redefinition of 'asbestos' for regulatory health purposes (chiefly airborne particles) by the US Occupational Safety and Health Administration (OSHA) (1986) and the National Institute for Occupational Safety and Health (NIOSH), and supported, particularly in relation to tremolite, by the American Thoracic Society (1990). It defines asbestos as mineral fibres of crystalline hydrated silicates that are 5 μm or more in length and with an aspect ratio of greater than 3:1; although the OSHA statement recognises the difference between asbestiform and non-asbestiform habits, it does not specify methods for their differentiation. Thus, elongated cleavage fragments with these dimensions become 'asbestos fibres'; indeed, the new rule states that the non-asbestiform variants of tremolite, anthophyllite and actinolite are to be treated as if they were asbestos. Apart from this redefinition being a frank departure from established mineralogical taxonomy, it implies that both variants have similar biological effects, although there is no evidence that non-asbestiform amphiboles have the same pathogenic properties as asbestos (McDonald et al., 1978; Cooper et al., 1988). In this respect, it is pertinent to note that most elongated (acicular) amphibole cleavage fragments have aspect ratios of less than 10:1 and are small enough to be completely ingested by alveolar macrophages.

Detailed size distributions of the particles obtained by counting from SEM observations can distinguish one type of asbestos from another (Campbell et al., 1980). Table A.4 shows that, as the aspect ratio increases, the length of particles increases up to 6 μm. It will also be observed that the aspect ratio for non-fibrous tremolite (cleavage fragments) is substantially less than 3:1. In general, this investigation 'gives considerable weight to the extension of aspect ratios well above the currently acceptable 3:1 ratio for purposes of counting by optical microscopy' (Hodgson, 1986). In fact, it has been categorically asserted that a particle with an aspect ratio of 3:1 cannot be considered to be a fibre (Kelse and Thompson, 1989; Langer et al., 1991). Figure A.8 shows, in a graphic form, a clear distinction between the aspect ratios of asbestiform particles and cleavage fragments. Unfortunately, the criterion of a 3:1 aspect ratio has been widely employed for some years by pathologists for interpreting the significance of mineral particles in human lungs, often with erroneous conclusions.

TABLE A.4
Particle Size Distributions by Scanning Electron Microscopy

	Percentage Particles by Aspect Ratio				
Length Range (μm)	**1:1 to 3:1**	**3:1 to 5:1**	**5:1 to 10:1**	**10:1 to 20:1**	**20:1 to 50:1**
Chrysotile					
0–1	25	18	50	7	
1–2	2	4	24	52	16
2–3		1	5	34	50
3–4			2	22	60
4–5				5	71
5–6				6	47
Representing 55% of all particles					
Amosite					
0–2	12	34	43	11	
2–4		10	52	34	4
4–6		6	23	52	18
Representing 26% of all particles					
Crocidolite					
0–1	12	64	24		
1–2	2	15	60	23	
2–3		2	25	57	15
3–4			21	64	15
4–5			2	51	46
5–6			3	36	58
Representing 60% of all particles					
Tremolite (non-fibrous)					
0–1	100				
1–2	92	8			
2–3	75	22	3		
3–4	67	29	4		
4–5	76	18	6		
5–6	67	30	3		
>10	35	37	18	4	
Representing 85% of all particles, below 6 μm					

Source: Reproduced from Hodgson, A. A. 1986. *Scientific Advances in Asbestos, 1967–1985.* Croydon: Anjalena Publications, Jupiter Press. After Campbell, W. J., Huggins, C. W. and Wylie, A G. 1980. *Chemical and Physical Characterization of Amosite, Chrysotile, Crocidolite and Non-Fibrous Tremolite for Oral Ingestion Studies by the National Institute of Environmental Health Sciences.* In Bureau of Mines Report of Investigations, R I 8452. US Department of the Interior, with permission.

Commercial asbestos, in general, is subjected to some form or other of processing in order to increase its degree of 'fiberisation' before it is applied in industry. This results in some reduction in the proportion of long fibres, an increase in that of short fibres and a decrease in the upper limit of the diameter of fibres (Hodgson, 1986). Nonetheless, a significant number of fibres longer than 10 μm, with aspect ratios greater than 10:1, are present in all commercial grades of asbestos, and it is these that are of biological importance. For this reason, and because the presence of a substantial number of short particles or of a few large particles in a sample has a disproportionate distorting effect, in opposite directions, on particle distribution data, the necessity for careful

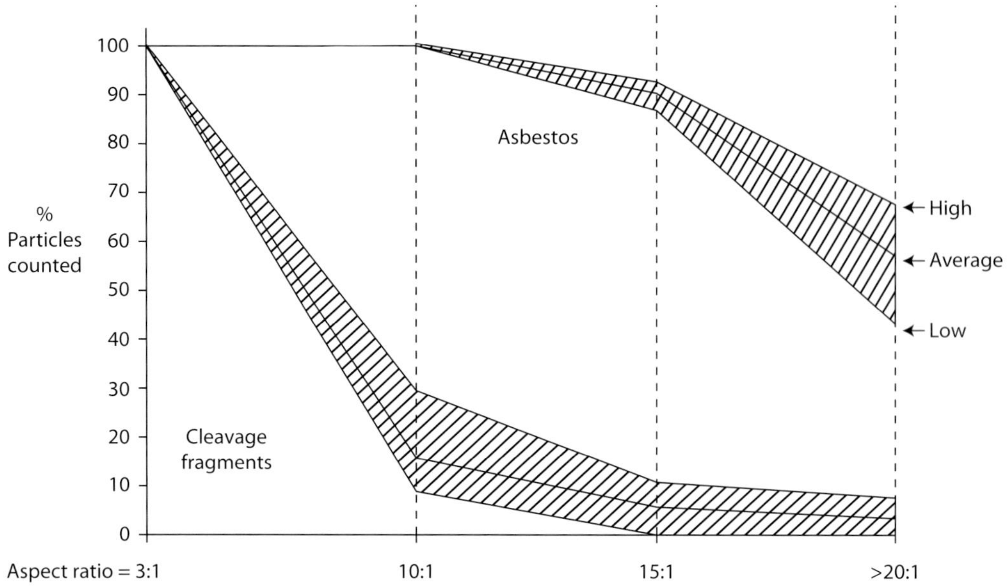

FIGURE A.8 Airborne asbestos versus cleavage fragment aspect ratio comparison (particles with an aspect ratio of 3:1 or greater, >5 μm length and >0.25 μm width). Note that the majority of cleavage fragments do not fall into this range (most reflect lengths of <5 μm). The 100% value therefore represents the starting point for 3:1 aspect ratio particle counting and not the total percentage of airborne cleavage fragments. (Reproduced from Kelse, J. W. and Thompson, C. S. 1989. *Am Ind Hyg Assoc J* 50:613–22, by permission of the American Hygiene Association.)

measurement of size distribution in samples used for biological research has been emphasised. It is necessary to correlate the number of particles in any size range to the weight of the sample; any method used for analysing fibre size must be capable of measuring both long and short fibres (Campbell et al., 1980). This has to be borne in mind when evaluating reports in the medical literature.

Thus, strict mineralogical definitions and criteria of asbestiform and non-asbestiform habits and of fibres (aspect ratios in excess of 10:1) must always be observed when studying (or interpreting) the biological effects of minerals and their presence in the lungs, both animal and human.

Hydrous Magnesium Silicates

Talc (French Chalk)

This is a hydrated magnesium silicate that was formed by regional metamorphic processes applied to dolomitic limestones and ultrabasic igneous rocks. It may take the form of flat, polygonal, flaky plates, granules or short 'fibres'. These are not true fibres, however, but rolled up, flat talc plates—an example of pseudomorphism. The formation of talc was closely akin to that of the production of asbestos minerals and, in fact, the amphiboles actinolite, anthophyllite and tremolite may be present as accessory minerals with talc, which is then often referred to as asbestine; in addition, chlorites, calcite, dolomite, magnesite, magnetite, pyrite, pyrophyllite (see next section) and quartz may be present. The amount of quartz varies from negligible to approximately 20% in some deposits (Weiss and Boettner, 1967). Talc and serpentine share a common origin from metamorphosed ultrabasic rocks, but in the majority of talc deposits, talc has replaced serpentine; hence, chrysotile is rarely found as an accessory mineral.

Analysis of bulk talc samples imported into the UK has shown that quartz is a fairly common contaminant in minor amounts (1%–2% by weight), although it exceeded 5% in one sample; an asbestiform tremolite was an uncommon finding, but chrysotile was absent. No other varieties of asbestos minerals were detected (Pooley and Rowlands, 1977).

Hence, most commercial talc is not a pure mineral. Some examples of 'talc' may contain substantial quantities of quartz and others may consist to a large extent of tremolite (in both asbestiform and non-asbestiform habits) or talcose anthophyllite. This wide variation in the identity and quantity of accessory minerals that depends upon the source of the talc deposits is undoubtedly an important determinant of the pathogenesis and variable characteristics of 'talc' pneumoconiosis. The term 'asbestiform talc' is sometimes found in the medical literature. It is misleading and inaccurate, and should not be used.

Talc has a low refractive index and is strongly birefringent. Its plate-like habit is not destroyed by grinding.

For industrial use, talcs that are virtually free of all impurities are known as 'high grade' and those in which impurities may be as much as 50% are known as 'low grade'. The term 'steatite' (soapstone) has long been applied to an impure, massive form of talc, which can be quarried in large blocks, but it is now often used to designate especially pure forms of talc for industry.

Palygorskite (Attapulgite) and Sepiolite

These are clay materials derived by metamorphism, often hydrothermal, from montmorillonites, amphiboles and pyroxenes. Large deposits exist in the USA. They occur as lath-like particles and fine, very short, intertwined fibres. The compact variety of sepiolite is known as meerschaum.

Vermiculite

Despite being a hydrous magnesium silicate, vermiculite contains varying amounts of iron and aluminium. It is derived from biotite and phlogopite mica by hydrothermal metamorphism, but probably more often from chlorite, an altered product of biotite, itself altered by surface waters and weathering. It occurs as thin plates, similar to talc, and granules, and is often classed with clay minerals when, in very fine particulate form, it has some of the appearance of the montmorillonite group.

Hydrous Aluminium Silicates

China Clay (Kaolin)

This finely divided aluminium silicate (kaolinite) is formed by hydrothermal and pneumatolytic attack on the feldspars of granites in some regions, notably Cornwall and Devon in the UK, but otherwise results from ordinary weathering and sedimentation of feldspar. Thus, most of the commercial china clay in the USA is not metamorphic in origin. In advanced stages of the hydrothermal metamorphism, only quartz may remain unaltered in powdery feldspar, so that it is present in significant, although variable, quantities. This is the form of china clay that is most suitable to the ceramic industry. The content of quartz in Cornish china clay is under 1% and that of ball clays is up to 25%.

It is relevant to point out here that china stone is a largely kaolinised granite composed principally of feldspar and quartz in which the relative absence of iron-bearing minerals makes it suitable for use as a flux in ceramic manufacture. It occurs in general association with metamorphic china clay, but is worked separately. Its content of quartz is that of granite: approximately 25%.

Smectite Group

The term 'smectite' is used, for convenience, as a group name for montmorillonite (by far the most common) and other hydrous aluminium silicates—beidellite, saponite, hectorite and sauconite—because of confusion concerning the meaning of montmorillonite and the difficulty in distinguishing mineralogically between the other species.

All montmorillonites are essentially volcanic in origin and are altered either by weathering of airborne deposits of ash at considerable distances from their origin (e.g. bentonites in England and Wyoming, USA) or by decomposition in situ, often under marine conditions. Thus, cristobalite and some poorly ordered forms of silica, as well as other minerals, are present in many deposits, such as in western USA.

Pyrophyllite ('Fire-Stone')

This is closely similar in origin, structure and properties and is commercially included with, and defined as, 'talc'. However, aluminium replaces the magnesium of talc in its composition and, unlike talc, it does not fuse when fired and thus is valuable for refractory purposes; it is also used as a ceramic raw material and paint extender. It undergoes dehydroxylation at approximately 800°C in order to give a metastable phase that, upon heating in excess of 1100°C, forms a felted mass of cristobalite and mullite needles.

Pyrophyllite is found in metamorphosed volcanic rocks of acid composition. Quartz and sericite are the chief impurities. It occurs as fine-grained, foliated lamellae with platy cleavage, as compact masses of small crystals and, less often, as aggregates of radiating needle-like crystals. All have a low refractive index and are strongly birefringent. It is mined by open-cast and underground methods.

Anhydrous Aluminium Silicates

These comprise a trio of metamorphic minerals—kyanite, sillimanite and andalusite—all of which have the same composition ($Al_2O_3 \cdot SiO_2$), and mullite. Industrially, kyanite is the most important of the trio because it is available in large, easily accessible deposits.

Kyanite, which was formed by regional and hydrothermal metamorphism in granite and pegmatite intrusions, occurs as long, thin, bladed crystals. Large deposits are exploited in India, where it is found in schists associated with quartz and pegmanites. In the USA, it is disseminated in quartzite.

Sillimanite, also known as fibrolite, occurs in argillaceous rocks, schists and slates as long, acicular crystals that shatter readily, as slender prismatic crystals and as wispy, fibrous aggregates.

Andalusite occurs as nearly square prismatic crystals in metamorphosed clayey rocks, in some slates and as an accessory mineral in granite.

All are used, either raw or calcined, in heavy-duty, refractory materials. The low electrical conductivity of sillimanite is exploited in porcelain for electrical equipment. When any of these minerals is heated to temperatures of approximately 1300–1600°C, they are converted to mullite and cristobalite (see Figure A.3). The presence of stable cristobalite probably explains the pulmonary fibrosis that has been attributed to sillimanite in some reports in the past (e.g. Jotten and Eickoff, 1944).

Mullite ($3Al_2O_3 \cdot 2SiO_2$)

This is of exceptionally rare occurrence in nature, being found originally in shales fused by immersion in basic magma in the Isle of Mull, Scotland. However, in synthetic form (the basis of a large industry), it is greatly valued as a 'super-duty' refractory with irreversible expansion characteristics that compensate for the shrinkage of other mineral components after firing, and for electrical and chemical porcelain. It is stable at temperatures of up to 1800°C. It occurs as weakly birefringent crystals of long prismatic habit, laths or needles, but not in fibrous form.

Most calcined kaolins (china clay) such as those used in paper, paints and plastics, however, do not contain mullite because the temperatures to which they are subjected are too low.

Quartzites

These are formed either by thermal, contact metamorphism of sandstones, which re-crystallises their quartz grains into an interlocking mosaic of quartz crystals or by regional metamorphism of detrital sandy rocks, which consist of small grains of quartz cemented by a scanty bond of silica and other minerals such as calcium carbonate and iron oxide. The content of quartz in both is very high, especially in the sedimentary type. Sands formed from these rocks are often called 'quartzite sands'.

Slates

Shales and mudstones containing quartz grains and clay minerals were compressed and flattened by considerable lateral forces (low-grade regional metamorphism) resulting in a reorientation of their crystalline structure to form a rock with well-developed and fine cleavage. The quartz content of all slates is usually high, being approximately 30%–45% by weight. The production of commercial slate powders results in a slight loss; thus, for example, powdered Cornish slate contains approximately 25% quartz, and powdered slate from north Wales, eastern Pennsylvania and eastern New York State contains approximately 30%.

Schists

These rocks are composed largely of flaky minerals such as mica, chlorite and talc or prismatic minerals such as hornblende, characterised by parallel lamellation, which were subjected to medium-grade regional metamorphism. This process greatly altered the structure of sedimentary and igneous rocks, rendering them more plastic. Some sedimentary rocks formed mica–schists and igneous rocks re-crystallised to form hornblende–schists or amphiboles.

Gneisses

The most intense metamorphism—high-grade metamorphism—completely transformed various existing rocks into these coarse-grained, roughly banded rocks that are composed essentially of pyroxenes, feldspar, quartz, biotite mica and hornblende in varying proportions. Quartzo-feld-spathic layers alternate with mica-rich layers.

Marbles

These are the results of thorough re-crystallisation of limestone by thermal and regional metamorphism which obliterated their sedimentary and fossiliferous features. Pure limestone (more than 99% calcium carbonate) yielded white marble, such as Italian Carrara marble. However, if the parent rock was impure limestone or a dolomitic limestone (a mixture of calcium carbonate and calcium magnesium carbonate), prominent, streaky colouring resulted. Most marbles contain small proportions of other minerals in the range of a few percent. Chief among the non-silicate impurities are quartz, graphite, limonite, haematite and pyrite, and among the silicates are mica chlorite, non-asbestiform tremolite, hornblende, diopside and wollastonite. Thus, most marbles, other than those that contain quartz, are unlikely to present a hazard.

It is important, however, to note that, commercially, 'marble' is usually any stone other than granite, and mostly sedimentary, which is of attractive appearance and takes a polish. Geologically, it is not marble.

Mineral Ores

These originated in a number of ways: by early crystallisation from magma and then separation (e.g. chromite [$FeCr_2O_4$]); by percolation and subsequent solidification of magmatic gas or liquid in pockets within native rock that was often of igneous type (e.g. beryl, copper, gold, lead, silver, tin and zinc); and by subterranean, volcanic waters dissolving scattered minerals and depositing them elsewhere in increased concentration. Decay and weathering of aluminium-bearing rocks—igneous rocks high in aluminium silicates and clayey limestones—resulted in the formation of bauxite. Hence, it contains a variety of mineral impurities. Silica, iron oxides and titanium minerals are always present, with the silica usually as quartz, but in some deposits, it is as cristobalite. Others include clay minerals such as kaolinite and chlorite.

Thus, mineral ores are apt to be found deposited in 'pockets' and 'veins' in rocks of widely differing type and composition.

Graphite

This is a soft black form of carbon that is disseminated mostly in mica–schists, micaceous quartzites and, occasionally, in some igneous rocks. Accordingly, it may contain a variety of impurities, especially in the mined material. These include feldspars, pyrites, iron oxides, muscovite and quartz.

EARTH MOVEMENTS

The various rock types have not remained in the order in which they were formed. The effects of weathering and enormous pressures due to earth movements caused by earthquakes and volcanic activity folded, dislocated and fractured the crust. The effects of movements are exemplified by simple folds, over-folds, faults and thrusts of sedimentary rocks, the original strata of which were thereby extensively displaced and intermingled.

This means that in tunnelling and mining or quarrying for a mineral in a particular stratum, a variety of different and unrelated materials will be encountered. Thus, the composition of dusts produced by these processes will vary from locality to locality.

PRODUCTS OF ACTIVE VOLCANIC ERUPTIONS

Particular interest in the possibility of a hazard to the lungs of human beings in the vicinity of active volcanoes was aroused by the dramatic eruption of Mount St Helens in Washington State, USA, in March, 1980. This offered an unprecedented opportunity to evaluate the products of volcanic eruptions from this standpoint.

Violent eruptions are characterised by the forceful ejection of a variety of pyroclastic fragments, hot toxic gases, superheated steam, radiation and lava flows. Thus, apart from physical injury (as may be caused by high-velocity blast waves), the potential hazards to be considered are respirable dust, toxic gases and radiation.

Pyroclastic fragments consist of the following:

1. Ash: Pulverised lava composed of crystals, glass or rock fragments, or a mixture of all three, of less than 4 mm in diameter. The finest particles are dusts.
2. Lapilli: Small stones.
3. Blocks and bombs: Larger rocks up to boulder sized.

These fragments are formed from erupting fluid magma and the fracture and ejection of old rocks and lava in the walls of the volcano's conduit by the force of the eruption. However, it is the composition of ash and dust that is relevant here.

As noted earlier, magmas consist of various gradations of molten basalts, andesites and rhyolites. Free silica may be present in volcanic ash as cristobalite as well as quartz, even though the temperature within the conduits and at the vents of volcanoes is believed to be no more than approximately 1200°C; that is, below the temperature range (1470–1723°C) at which cristobalite is normally stable at atmospheric pressure. This is probably explained by a high ambient water vapour pressure in the conduit, facilitating inversion of quartz to cristobalite at lower temperatures. The surface temperatures of some lavas may be higher due to the burning of hydrogen and other volcanic gases escaping from the lava. Thus, cristobalite is typically a mineral of volcanic rocks and not of igneous (plutonic) rocks formed at depth. However, much of the silica is converted to glass, usually as minute spheroids, during the rapid cooling of magma as it is ejected from the vent.

Ash

The average size of ash-fall deposit fragments at any point decreases exponentially with the distance from the vent, with the largest and heaviest thus being nearest. The distances at which ash-falls occur depend upon the severity of the eruption. When very violent, the ash cloud is projected miles into the air and fall-out occurs over enormously large areas (often hundreds of miles) and is most concentrated downwind. The finest and furthest-travelled ash derived from siliceous magmas (rhyolites and andesites) commonly consists largely of glass shards; some rock minerals such as feldspar may be present, as well as substantial amounts of cristobalite. Long, flexible fibrous particles or threads are a feature of the ash-fall dust and ash of some eruptions, often at very great distances. These are formed of basalitic glass and are known as Pelee's hair—after the legendary goddess of Hawaiian volcanoes.

Analysis of Mount St Helens' ash—in which 90% of particles were less than 10 μm in diameter—showed that crystalline silica ranged from 2.8% to 6.6% by weight of ash and consisted of quartz and approximately two-thirds cristobalite, but there was considerable inter-laboratory variability in the values of cristobalite (Green et al., 1983). Although these concentrations are fairly low, the theoretical possibility exists that exposure to high concentrations of ash particles for a short period could cause 'acute silicosis' or silico-lipoproteinosis, but this does not seem to have been observed. A radiographic study of survivors of a Japanese eruption in 1977 did not reveal any pulmonary disease related to ash exposure. No fibrous particles were identified in the Mount St Helens' ash (Green et al., 1983).

Thus, exposure to ash-fall—which is usually short-lived and only for a matter of days—is unlikely to be a pneumoconiosis hazard, although, as mentioned later, near the source of an eruption, it may cause acute respiratory distress or asphyxia in unprotected individuals. However, when the eruption has ceased, personnel in various occupations (particularly bulldozer and truck drivers; forestry, agricultural and vinicultural workers; and geologists and volcanologists) may be subjected to more prolonged exposure from ash that is re-suspended by their activities and by the wind. However, subsequent rainfall transforms the ash into a cement-like texture. It is worth noting that, experimentally, Mount St Helens' ash appears to be less toxic than quartz, and some studies have suggested that it behaves more like an inert dust; however, this requires confirmation (Martin et al., 1983).

Pumice and pumicite are lavas that are full of gas bubbles, produced by rapid frothing of viscous lava due to a sudden fall in pressure. They consist of silicic glasses, the composition of which varies according to the conditions of their formation. They may be simply a frothy glass, sometimes with streaks of non-cellular glass, or they may contain quartz, cristobalite and feldspars. Thus, crystalline silica is either absent or present in varying and sometimes substantial amounts in different deposits; consequently, prolonged occupational exposure may result in nodular silicosis or 'mixed dust fibrosis'. Pumice usually forms near the vent of a volcano, but pumicite (being composed of small particles) is carried great distances by winds before settling as accumulations of fine-grained 'ash'.

Perlite, a volcanic glass of rhyolitic composition, has a concentric structure consisting of minute spheroids that are a few millimetres in diameter. It often contains inclusions of quartz, feldspar and biotite and sometimes of cristobalite. Because of its content of combined water, it possesses the valuable commercial property of sudden expansion on rapid heating.

Toxic Gases

Another danger of volcanic activity that is not confined to the immediate vicinity of an eruption is the presence of toxic gases. These include sulphur dioxide, sulphur trioxide, hydrogen sulphide, chlorine and hydrogen chloride in varying proportions, as well as carbon dioxide. They are present in ash clouds, and unexpected jets of gas may be expelled from innocent-looking cooling lava flows that are distant from the centre of the eruption. The predominant gas in the early stages of an eruption is sulphur dioxide, but hydrogen sulphide is more common later. Not all eruptions are short and violent; some grumble on for years with episodic emissions of these and other gases. Steam vents (fumaroles) that may be found in the vicinity of both active and dormant volcanoes often produce high concentrations of carbon dioxide and sulphur dioxide.

Sulphur dioxide, hydrogen sulphide and carbon dioxide are potentially the most hazardous of volcanic gases because, being heavier than air, they hug the ground and accumulate in hollows and can thus cause acute respiratory disease or asphyxia in human beings and animals. Carbon dioxide is especially dangerous, as it is odourless and non-irritant and its presence is likely to be unsuspected.

Ionising Radiation

The plume from Mount St Helens was estimated to contain approximately 3 million curies of radon gas, which, in view of the rapid decay of radon, is unlikely to have presented a hazard. The radioactivity of longer-lived radioactive isotopes—^{232}Th, ^{226}Ra and ^{40}K—was similar to that which was present in the Earth's crust. From all the available data, it was computed that, over the period of a lifetime, the radiation effect of exposure to the ash would be a negligible threat to human populations (Soldat et al., 1981; Green et al., 1983).

Clinicopathological Effects

Most acute respiratory complaints associated with the Mount St Helens eruption were cough, wheeze and shortness of breath—symptoms that are similar to those recorded in other eruptions at different geographical locations: the Usu volcano in Japan in 1977, Irazu volcano in Costa Rica in 1963 and Mount Katmai, Alaska, in 1912 (Green et al., 1983). Among individuals who had been fairly close to the eruption and were overtaken by ash clouds projected at high speed near ground level, the most common cause of death was asphyxia from inhalation of ash, which, with mucus, formed occlusive plugs in the upper thoracic airways, particularly the larynx and trachea. In those who were further afield (chiefly loggers) and who survived longer, the ash extended to the peripheral bronchi, but not as far as the bronchioles (Eisele et al., 1981). The findings in two individuals who did not die of asphyxia and survived for 10 and 16 days, respectively, revealed a combination of thermal burns of the large airways, acute alveolar injury and respiratory failure. In the first case, there was alveolar oedema, interstitial infiltration of inflammatory cells with accumulations of ash-containing macrophages in the alveoli and desquamation of type 1 cells; in the second, bronchiolitis obliterans and organising intra-alveolar exudates with occasional granulomas were observed. There was little or no evidence that toxic gases played any part in the pathology (Green et al., 1981; Parshley et al., 1982).

Conclusion

The products of volcanic activity can cause potentially lethal, acute pulmonary disease due to the inhalation of large amounts of ash or toxic gases, and it is possible that survivors of heavy exposure to ash may develop chronic bronchiolitis obliterans. Transient bronchoconstriction (possibly severe in some cases) may be provoked in asthmatic subjects and others with hyperactive bronchial airways exposed to lower levels of ash or toxic gas.

Although the size distribution of airborne ash particles is well within 'respirable' range, and crystalline silica is usually present, a silicosis risk is highly improbable because the duration and intensity of exposure, even if repeated as a result of episodic resuspension of ash, are too short lived (days or weeks rather than years) and the percentage of silica is low. Apart from prolonged occupational exposure to pumice (which is a different matter), pneumoconiosis has not been observed. Ionising radiation from volcanic eruptions does not appear to present any hazard to the lungs.

IONISING RADIATION FROM ROCKS

Uranium-238 and thorium-232 are present in most igneous rocks and in minute amounts in all rocks and soils. Uranium gives rise to decay chain products—of which uranium-238 is the first member—through a series of solid elements to radium-226, which decays to the gas radon-222 that, in turn, when in air, rapidly gives rise to other isotopes—radon 'daughters'. The important members of the series in the present context are those that emit α-particles, namely radon-222 (half-life: 3.8 days) and the three radon daughters, polonium-218 (half-life: 3.05 minutes), polonium-214 (half-life: 26.8 minutes) and polonium-210 (half-life: 19.4 years). Radon-222 leaks from rocks, fallen ore and soil and escapes into the air, although concentrations at ground level are very low (Morgan, 1970). However, in enclosed areas, such as mines, shafts, underground chambers and tunnels—especially if poorly ventilated—concentrations may be high because the gas has less chance to diffuse away. It may also be carried into mine-workings by waters from a distant source.

Thorium, which is also fairly abundant in the Earth's crust, is usually found in association with uranium. It decays into thoron gas (radon-220), thorium A (polonium-216), thorium B (lead-212) and thorium C (bismulh-212). Of these, thoron, thorium B and thorium C are α-emitters.

The amount of radiation that escapes into the atmosphere varies greatly in different areas for three reasons: differing concentrations or uranium and thorium in the bedrock; the nature of their mineralisation; and the permeability of the bedrock. Thus, only a proportion of either gas becomes airborne, and although high levels of radon are associated with granites, this is not always the case. Because of differences in the style of mineralisation of uranium, some granites in which its levels are comparable may have low radon levels. In addition, many basic igneous rocks have low contents of uranium with no production of radon. However, in some regions, other rocks—such as limestones and black shales—may yield high radon levels. Hence, there is considerable global and local variation in the doses of radiation received from this source.

When first formed, the decay products are single ionised atoms, but they readily attach themselves to molecules of water vapour or to dust particles as 'cluster ions'. It has been calculated that their mean radioactivity diameter is approximately 0.25 μm in non-operational mines and approximately 0.4 μm diameter in operational mines (Davies, 1967). In this aerosol state, therefore, they can, on inhalation, penetrate to the trachea, bronchi and peripheral airways, and be retained in the lungs.

α-particles are positively charged helium nuclei with two protons and neutrons that have a greater mass than other radiation particles and great kinetic energy, but, owing to their large mass and positive charge, have only feeble penetrating power. β-particles, being electrons, have greater penetrating capacity, but less ionising power. It is believed that ionisation is the cause of malignant change in living cells.

For this reason, inhaled α-particles are more important than β-particles—although high doses of the latter may induce lung tumours in experimental animals—and there is strong evidence that exposure of human beings to radon-222 and α-emitting radon daughters is responsible for a significantly increased risk of developing carcinoma of the lung. The radiation dose to the lungs of radon and thoron appears to be approximately similar (Albert, 1966).

REFERENCES

Albert, R. E. 1966. *Thorium and its Industrial Hygiene Aspects.* New York and London: Academic Press.

American Thoracic Society. 1990. Official Statement. Health effects of Tremolite. *Am Rev Respir Dis* 142:1453–8.

Andrews, R. W. 1970. *Wollaslonite.* London: Institute of Geological Science, HMSO.

Aramaki, S. and Roy, R. 1959. The mullite-corundum boundary in the systems MgO—Alzoa-SiOz and CaO—Alea—SiOZ, *J Am Ceram Soc* 42:644–45.

Bradbury, J. C. and Ehrlinger H. P. III. 1975. Tripoli. In S. J. Lefond (editor-in-chief), *Industrial Minerals and Rocks.* New York, NY: American Institute of Mining, Metallurgical and Petroleum Engineers, Inc., 1209–18.

Bradshaw, M. J. 1968. *A New Geology.* London: The English Universities Press.

Campbell, W. J., Huggins, C. W. and Wylie, A. G. 1980. *Chemical and Physical Characterization of Amosite, Chrysotile, Crocidolite and Non-Fibrous Tremolite for Oral Ingestion Studies by the National Institute of Environmental Health Sciences.* Bureau of Mines Report of Investigations, R I 8452, U.S. Department of the Interior.

Cooper, W. C., Wong, O. and Graebner, R. 1988. Mortality of workers in two Minnesota taconite mining and milling operations. *J Occup Med* 30:506–11.

Crelling, J. C. 1989. Coal as a material. In H. Marsh (ed.), *Introduction to Carbon Science.* London, Boston, Sydney: Butterworths, 260–84.

Davies, C. N. 1967. *Assessment of Airborne Radioactivity.* Vienna: International Atomic Energy Agency, 3–20.

Davis, A., Russell, S. J., Rimmer, S. M. and Yeakel, D. 1984. Some genetic implications of silica and aluminosilicates in peat and coal. *Int J Coal Geol* 3:293–314.

Dorling, M. and Zussman, J. 1980. Comparative studies of asbestiform and non-asbestiform calcium-rich amphiboles. Presented at: *4th International Asbestos Conference*, Torino, Italy.

Eisele, J. W., O'Halloran, R. L., Reay, D. T., Lindholm, G. R., Lewman, L. V. and Brady, W. J. 1981. Deaths during the 18 May 1980. Eruption of Mount St Helens. *N Engl J Med* 305:931–6.

Finkelman, R. B. 1988. The inorganic chemistry of coal: A scanning electron microscopy view. *Scan Microsc* 2:97–105.

Finkelman, R. B. and Gluskoter, H. J. 1983. Characterization of minerals in coal: Problems and promises. In R.W. Bryers (ed.), *Fouling and Slagging Resulting from Impurities in Combustion Gases. Proceedings of the 1981 Engineers Foundation Conference.* New York, NY, 299–318.

Geikie, J. 1908. *Structural and Field Geology,* second edition. London: Oliver and Boyd.

Goldstein, B. and Rendall, R. E. G. 1970. The relative toxicities of the main classes of minerals. In H. A. Shapiro (ed.), *Pneumoconiosis, Proceedings of International Conference, Johannesburg, 1969.* Cape Town: Oxford University Press, 429–34.

Green, F. H. Y., Dollberg, D., Tucker, J. H. and Keissling, P. 1983. Toxicity of Mount St Helens' volcanic ash and relevance to mining populations. In W. L. Wagner, W. N. Rom and J. A. Merchant (eds), *Health Issues Related to Metal and Nonmctallic Mining.* Boston, London: Butterworths: 105–20.

Green, F. H. Y., Vallyathan, V., Menlnech, M. S., Tucker, J. H., Merchant, J. A., Keissling, P. J., Antonius, J. A. and Parshley, P. 1981. Is volcanic ash a pneumoconiosis risk? *Nature* 293:216–7.

Highley, D. E. 1972. *Fuller's Earth. Mineral Dossier No. 3.* London: Mineral Resources Consultative Committee, HMSO.

Highley, D. E. 1982. *Fireclay. Mineral Dossier No, 24.* London: HMSO.

Hodgson. A. A. 1977. Nature and paragenesis of asbestos minerals. *Phil Trans R Soc London* A286:611–24.

Hodgson, A. A. 1986. *Scientific Advances in Asbestos, 1967–1985.* Croydon: Anjalena Publications, Jupiter Press.

Jotten, K. W. and Eickoff, W. 1944. Lungenveränderungen durch Sillimanislaub. *Arch Gewerbepath Gewerbchyg* 12:223–32.

Kadey, F. L. Jr. 1975. Diatomite. In S. J. Lefond (editor-in-chief), *Industrial Minerals and Rocks.* New York, NY: American Institute of Mining Engineers, 605–35.

Kelse, J. W. and Thompson, C. S. 1989. The regulatory and mineralogical definitions of asbestos and their impact on amphibole dust analysis. *Am Ind Hyg Assoc J* 50:613–22.

King, E. J., Mohanty, G. P., Harrison, C. V. and Nagelschmidt, G. 1953. The action of different forms of pure silica on the lungs of rats. *Br J Ind Med* 10:9–17.

Langer, A. M., Nolan, R. P. and Addison, J. 1991. On talc, tremolite and tergiversation. *Br J Ind Med* 48:359–60.

Langer, A. M., Nolan, R. P. and Pooley, F. D. 1990. Phyllosilicates: associated fibrous minerals. In J. Bignon (ed.), *Health-Related Effects of Phyllosillicates.* Berlin, Paris: Springer Verlag, 59–61.

Lee, R. J. and Fisher, R. M. 1979. Identification of fibrous minerals. *Ann NY Acad Sci* 330:645–60.

Mackowsky, M-Th. 1968. Mineral matter in coal. In D. G. Murchison and T. S. Westoll (eds), *Coal and Coal-Bearing Strata.* London: Oliver and Boyd, 309–21.

Martin, T. R., Wehner, A. P. and Butler, J. 1983. Pulmonary toxicity of Mt St Helens' volcanic ash. *Am Rev Respir Dis* 128:158–62.

McDonald, J. C., Gibbs, G. W., Liddell, F. K. W. and McDonald, A. D. 1978. Mortality after exposure to cummingtonite–grunerite. *Am Rev Respir Dis* 118: 271–7.

Mohanty, G. P., Roberts, D. C., King, E. J. and Harrison, C. V. 1953. The effect of feldspar, slate and quartz on the lungs of rats. *J Pathol Bacteriol* 65:501–12.

Moorlock, B. S. P. and Highley, D. E. 1991. An appraisal of fuller's earth resources in England and Wales. In *British Geological Survey. Technical Report, WA/91/75.*

Morgan, A. 1970. Physical behaviour of radon and its daughters with particular reference to monitoring methods. In H. A. Shapiro (ed.), *Pneumoconiosis: Proceedings of the International Conference, Johannesburg, 1969.* Cape Town: Oxford University Press, 540–3.

Parshley, P. F., Kiessling, P. J., Antonius, J. A., Connell, R. S., Miller, S. H. and Green, F. H. Y. 1982. Pyroclastic flow injury. Mount St Helens, 18 May 1980. *Am J Surg* 143:565–8.

Pooley, F. D. 1987. Asbestos mineralogy. In K. Antman and J. E. Aisner (eds), *Asbestos-Related Malignancy.* Orlando, FL: Grune and Stratton, 21.

Pooley, F. D. and Rowlands, N. 1977. Chemical and physical properties of British talc powders. In W. H. Walton and B. McGovern (eds), *Inhaled Particles IV.* Oxford and New York: Pergamon Press, 639–46.

Raask, E. 1985. *Mineral Impurities in Coal Combustion—Behaviour, Problems and Remedial Measures.* Washington, DC: Hemisphere.

Ross, M., Kuntze, R. A. and Clifton, R. A. 1984. A definition of asbestos. In *A.S.T.M. Special Technical Publication 834.* Philadelphia, PA: American Society for Testing and Materials, 139–47.

Schenk, W. M., Gobb, P. and Kolmer, H. A. 1990. A morphological study of mesomorphs. In J. Bignon (ed.), *Health-Related Effects of Phyllosilicates.* Berlin and Paris: Springer Verlag, 85–6.

Soldat, J. K., Kathren, R. L., Corley, J. P. and Strange, D. L. 1981. Radiation doses from Mount St Helens, May 1980 eruption. *Science* 213:585.

Sosman, R. B. 1965. *The Phases of Silica.* New Brunswick, NJ: Rutgers University Press.

Swaine, D. J. 1990. *Trace Elements in Coal.* London, Boston, Singapore and Sydney: Butterworths.

United States Department of Labor, Occupational Safety and Health Administration. 1986. Occupational exposure to asbestos, tremolite, anthophyllite and actinolite: Final rules. *Federal Register* 51(119):22612–790.

Vorwald, A. J., Durkan, T. M., Pratt, P. C. and Delahant, A. B. 1949. Diatomaceous earth pneumoconiosis. In *Proceedings of the IXth International Congress on Industrial Medicine*. Wright and Bristol, 726–41.

Weiss, B. and Boettner, E. A. 1967. Commercial talc and talcosis. *Arch Environ Health* 14:304–8.

Zoltai, T. and Wylie, A. G. 1979. Definitions of asbestos-related mineralogical terminology. *Ann NY Acad Sci* 330:707–9.

Zussman, J. 1957. Electron diffraction studies of the serpentine minerals. *Am Mineralogist* 42:133–53.

Index

F

G

P

Q

R

T

U

V

W

X

Y

Z